PRECLINICAL SPEECH SCIENCE

PRECLINICAL SPEECH SCIENCE

Anatomy, Physiology, Acoustics, Perception

SECOND EDITION

Thomas J. Hixon
Gary Weismer
Jeannette D. Hoit

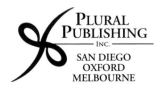

PLURAL
PUBLISHING
INC.

SAN DIEGO
OXFORD
MELBOURNE

PLURAL PUBLISHING
INC.

5521 Ruffin Road
San Diego, CA 92123

e-mail: info@pluralpublishing.com
Web site: http://www.pluralpublishing.com

Typeset in 10/12 Palatino by Flanagan's Publishing Services, Inc.
Printed in Malaysia by Four Colour Print Group

Library of Congress Cataloging-in-Publication Data is available.

Hixon, Thomas J., 1940-2009.
  Preclinical speech science : anatomy, physiology, acoustics, and perception / Thomas J. Hixon, Gary Weismer, Jeannette D. Hoit. -- 2nd ed.
      p. ; cm.
  Includes bibliographical references and index.
  ISBN-13: 978-1-59756-520-2 (alk. paper)
  ISBN-10: 1-59756-520-2 (alk. paper)
  I. Weismer, Gary. II. Hoit, Jeannette D. (Jeannette Dee), 1954- III. Title.
  [DNLM: 1. Speech--physiology. 2. Respiratory System--anatomy & histology. 3. Speech Disorders. 4. Speech Perception. WV 501]

  612.7'8--dc23
                    2012049151

Contents

4 VELOPHARYNGEAL-NASAL FUNCTION AND SPEECH PRODUCTION   155

6 BRAIN STRUCTURES AND MECHANISMS FOR SPEECH, LANGUAGE, AND HEARING   281

8 ACOUSTIC THEORY OF VOWEL PRODUCTION   **415**

Acknowledgments

There are many people to thank for the book you see before you. Maury Aaseng created the artwork for the book; he is in many ways the silent partner/coauthor of this text. His images reflect his enormous talent and add a special dimension to the book. Sandy Doyle oversaw the production of the first edition from beginning to end, and Caitlin Mahon and Scott Barbour guided us through the preparation of this second edition. Many colleagues and students made important contributions through their advice on content and their critiques on different sections. These include Julie Barkmeier-Kraemer, Sam Brown, Kate Bunton, Yun-Ching Chung, Susan Ellis Weismer, Harry Hollien, Kristen Kalend, Joel Kahane, Yunjung Kim, Dave Kuehn, Amy Lederle, Rosemary Lester, Julie Liss, Robin Samlan, Sara Finch Schubert, and Brad Story; a special thanks to Susan Ellis Weismer, who spent countless hours in the final stages of readying this second edition, hours that could have been spent in her own laboratory. Finally, the considerable guidance and encouragement of Angie Singh and Sadanand Singh during the long course of this project, both then and now, deserve special recognition.

For Sadanand Singh, Tom Hixon, and S Gabriel Weismer

1

Introduction

Welcome to *Preclinical Speech Science: Anatomy, Physiology, Acoustics, Perception, Second Edition*. Two preliminaries are offered here. One is a discussion of the focus of the book, the other a discussion of the domain of preclinical speech science.

FOCUS OF THE BOOK

Preclinical Speech Science: Anatomy, Physiology, Acoustics, Perception is designed as an introduction to the fundamentals of speech science (inclusive of voice science) that are important to aspiring clinicians and practicing clinicians. The text is suitable for courses that cover the anatomy and physiology of speech production and swallowing, and the acoustics and perception of speech. The material is user friendly to beginning students, yet integrative and translational for graduate students and practicing speech-language pathologists. Certain topics in the text are novel to the speech science and speech-language pathology literatures and suggest important new conceptualizations.

This book is an outgrowth of the three authors' many years of teaching experience with several thousand undergraduate and graduate students. The development of the book is the result of a sifting and winnowing of the broad range of facts, principles, and methods associated with its topics. The outcome is an integrated fabric that is a logical precursor for clinical study and practice. Chapters in the book are infused with clinical scenarios, sidetracks of clinical and historical interest, considerations of the scientific bases of clinical protocols and methodologies, and discussions of clinical personnel involved in the evaluation and management of disorders of speech production, speech, and swallowing.

The illustrations, done by an extremely talented artist, are a key feature of this book. These original illustrations, largely in full color, are supplemented by a small number of illustrations from other sources. The original illustrations were carefully chosen and drafted to convey only salient features, an approach in line with the written text. Occasional cartoons lighten the material, but carry educational messages.

DOMAIN OF PRECLINICAL SPEECH SCIENCE

The domain of preclinical speech science is portrayed in Figure 1–1. This domain encompasses speech production, speech acoustics, speech perception, and swallowing. Within this domain, consideration is given to levels of observation, subsystems of speech production and swallowing, and applications of data.

Levels of Observation

Speech production and swallowing are processes. They result in acoustic products (more so for speech than swallowing) and perceptual experiences. These processes, products, and experiences involve different levels of observation. Six such levels are represented in Figure 1–1: (a) neural, (b) muscular, (c) structural, (d) aeromechanical, (e), acoustic, and (f) perceptual.

The neural level of observation encompasses nervous system events during speech production and swallowing. These include all events that qualify as motor planning and execution and all forms of afferent and sensory information that influence the ongoing control of speech production and swallowing. The neural level of observation pertains to the parts of

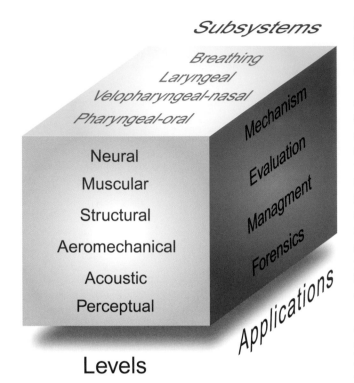

Figure 1-1. Domain of preclinical speech science.

the brain, spinal cord, and cranial and spinal nerves important to speech production and swallowing and to all underlying neural mechanisms, some voluntary and some automatic, some that involve awareness, and some that do not. Neural data are often derived from physical or metabolic imaging methods that reflect patterns of activation of different regions of the brain. Activation at the neural level can also be inferred from events associated with other (downstream) levels of observation.

The muscular level of observation is concerned with the influence of muscle forces on speech production and swallowing. Muscle forces are responsible for powering these two processes. Muscles are effectors that respond to control signals from the nervous system. The muscular events of speech production and swallowing are manifested in mechanical pulls and are often indexed at the periphery through the electrical activities associated with muscle contractions. Inferences about muscle activities are also made from measurements of the forces or movements generated by different parts of the speech production apparatus and swallowing apparatus. Nevertheless, there are ambiguities introduced when attempting to infer individual muscle activities from forces or movements because

forces and movements are usually accomplished by groups of muscles working together. Such inferences, if they can be made at all, require a detailed knowledge of anatomy and physiology.

The structural level of observation deals with movements of the speech production apparatus and swallowing apparatus. This level of observation is concerned with the displacements, velocities, and accelerations/decelerations of structures and how they are timed in relation to the movements of other structures. Certain structural observations can be made with the naked eye, whereas others are hidden from view or are too rapid to be followed with the naked eye and require the use of instrumental monitoring. To the person on the street, the structural level of observation is public evidence of speech production and swallowing. Speech reading (lip reading) has its roots at this level of observation.

The structural movements of speech production and swallowing give rise to an aeromechanical level of observation. It is at this level that air comes into play. Movements of structures impart energy to the air by compressing and decompressing it and causing it to flow from one region to another. The raw airstream generated in association with the aeromechanical level is modified by structures of the speech production apparatus and swallowing apparatus that lie along various passageways. The products of the aeromechanical level are complex, rapid, and nearly continuous changes in air pressures, airflows, and air volumes. These products are usually "invisible," especially for swallowing. However, those who speak and smoke at the same time or who speak in subfreezing temperatures often provide the observer with the opportunity to visualize certain aeromechanical events.

The acoustic level of observation is fully within the public domain. Although certain aspects of swallowing may be accompanied by sounds, primacy at this level pertains to the generation of speech sounds. The raw material of the acoustic level is the buzzlike, hisslike, and poplike sounds that result from the speaker's valving of the airstream in different ways and at different locations within the speech production apparatus. This raw material is filtered and conditioned by its passage through the apparatus and radiates from the mouth or nose, or both, in the form of nearly continuous changes in atmospheric pressure. The sound waves that are formed propagate spherically from the speaker and can be coded in terms of frequency, sound pressure level, and time. These sound waves are what constitute speech, an acoustic representation of language. The acoustic level is important in face-to-face communication and in the use of telephones, radios, televisions, and various forms of recording. It is this level that makes it possible for many listeners to be engaged simultaneously and makes it possible to communicate effectively around corners, through obstacles, in the dark, and over long distances.

The perceptual level of observation has somewhat different manifestations for speech production and swallowing. For speech production, it pertains primarily to auditory events. Kinesthesia (movement sensation), proprioception (position-in-space sensation), and touch-pressure sensation are important as bases for staying informed about ongoing speech production events, but the principal factor is audition (hearing sensation). Visual information is sometimes important as well, and experience and knowledge of the language is critical for extracting meaning from speech. In contrast, swallowing is highly dependent on kinesthesia, touch-pressure sensation, and even taste, with relatively little reliance on auditory or visual information. Cognitive processes contribute to various degrees at the perceptual level of observation for both speech production and swallowing.

The levels of observation portrayed in Figure 1–1 are not completely separate entities, but have important interactions. These interactions are not shown in the figure, but are discussed in subsequent chapters.

Subsystems of Speech Production and Swallowing

The speech production apparatus and the swallowing apparatus perform different activities. However, they share many structural and functional components and, although different in their control and movement, can be viewed along similar lines. It is convenient, for discussion purposes, to partition the speech production apparatus and swallowing apparatus into subsystems. Speech production subsystems may differ when chosen by a linguist versus a speech scientist versus a speech-language pathologist. And swallowing subsystems may differ when chosen by a swallowing scientist versus a gastroenterologist versus a speech-language pathologist. For the purposes of this book, four subsystems are used for speech production and swallowing. As illustrated in Figure 1–1, these include the: (a) breathing apparatus, (b) laryngeal apparatus, (c) velopharyngeal-nasal apparatus, and (d) pharyngeal-oral apparatus. The role of each of these subsystems is considered in detail in subsequent chapters. The functional significance of each of the four subsystems dif-

fers between speech production and swallowing, but each subsystem is critically important to its respective behaviors and each manifests in clinical signs that can reveal abnormality.

The breathing apparatus is defined in the present context to include structures below the larynx within the neck and torso. These are, most importantly, the pulmonary apparatus (pulmonary airways and lungs) and chest wall apparatus (rib cage wall, diaphragm, abdominal wall, and abdominal content). During speech production, the breathing apparatus provides the necessary driving forces, while simultaneously serving the functions of ventilation and gas exchange. During swallowing, the breathing apparatus engages in a period of apnea (breath holding) to protect the pulmonary airways and lungs from the intrusion of unwanted substances (food and liquid). The breathing apparatus is the largest of the subsystems and its role in speech production and swallowing is fundamentally important.

The laryngeal apparatus lies between the trachea (windpipe) and the pharynx (throat) and adjusts the coupling between the two. At times, the laryngeal airway is open to allow air to move in and out of the breathing apparatus, whereas at times it is adjusted to obstruct or constrict the airway. During speech production, obstructions and constrictions enable the generation of transient and sustained noises, respectively. Very rapid to and fro movements of the vocal folds within the larynx create voiced sounds and give the laryngeal apparatus its colloquial label "voice box." During swallowing, the laryngeal apparatus is active in closing the laryngeal airway to protect the pulmonary airways. Food and liquid are then able to pass over and around the larynx and into the esophagus on their way to the stomach.

The velopharyngeal-nasal apparatus consists of the upper pharynx, velum, nasal cavities, and outer nose. When breathing through the nose, the velopharyngeal-nasal airway is open. When speaking, the size of the velopharyngeal port varies, depending on the nature of the speech produced. For example, consonant sounds that require high oral air pressure are typically associated with airtight closure of the velopharyngeal port, whereas nasal consonants are produced with an open velopharyngeal port. Function of the velopharyngeal-nasal apparatus during swallowing is concerned mainly with keeping the velopharynx sealed airtight. This prevents the passage of food and liquid into the nasal cavities, while substances are moved backward and downward through the oropharynx.

The pharyngeal-oral apparatus comprises the middle and lower pharynx, oral cavity, and oral vestibule. During running speech production, the apparatus is typically open during inspiration and makes different adjustments for consonant and vowel productions during expiration, including the generation of transient, voiceless, and voiced sounds and the filtering of those sounds. During swallowing, the pharyngeal-oral apparatus prepares food and liquid and propels it to the esophagus.

Applications of Data

There are many applications of data obtained about speech production and swallowing. These applications depend on who selects and defines the data and what the goals are for collecting and analyzing them. For the purposes of this book, applications of data are categorized into four areas: (a) mechanism, (b) evaluation, (c) management, and (d) forensics. These are shown in Figure 1–1.

One application of data is the understanding of mechanism. This use provides the foundational bases for knowing how speech is produced and how swallowing is performed. Such foundational bases are important for their heuristic value in elucidating fundamental processes and working principles and for differentiating normal from abnormal.

Another application of data is its use in evaluation. This use is usually practical in nature and involves quantitative determinations of the status and functional capabilities of an individual's speech production, speech, and swallowing. Evaluation first enables a determination as to whether or not abnormality exists. If abnormality does exist, then appropriate evaluation may contribute to: (a) making a diagnosis, (b) developing a rational, effective, and efficient management plan, (c) monitoring progress during the course of management, and (d) providing a reasonable prognosis as to the extent and speed of improvement to be expected. For example, a specific use of subsystems analysis in the evaluation of speech production is the determination of how individual subsystems contribute to deficits in speech intelligibility. Two individuals may have equivalent intelligibility problems as determined by formal tests, but have different subsystems "explanations" for their deficits. The careful evaluation of subsystems performance can point to which parts of the speech production apparatus may be particularly responsible for speech intelligibility deficits, and how those parts should be addressed in management. Evaluation relies on an understanding of what constitutes normal function.

A third application of data is management. Different interventions may be based on any of the six levels of observation and include any of the four subsystems of speech production and swallowing. Different management strategies may include adjusting individual variables or combinations of variables, staging the order of different interventions, and providing feedback about speech production and swallowing processes, products, and experiences. Management data provide information about outcome and whether or not interventions are effective, efficient, and long lasting. Management data can also be used to compare and contrast different interventions to arrive at optimal choices.

The remaining application of data is their use in forensics. This application is concerned with scientific facts and expert opinion as they relate to legal issues. The speech scientist and speech-language pathologist are sometimes called on to give legal depositions or to testify in courts of law in a variety of forensic contexts. Forensic uses of data may include issues pertaining to speaker identification, speaker status under the influence of drugs or alcohol, and speaker intent at deceit, among others. Forensic uses of data may also relate to personal injury claims or malpractice claims. These may involve speech production, speech, or swallowing alone, or in different combinations, and may include adversarial depositions and testimonies of other experts. Under such circumstances, the status and capabilities of the individuals claiming personal injury or malpractice may be considered from the perspective of underlying mechanism, evaluation, and management.

REVIEW

Preclinical Speech Science: Anatomy, Physiology, Acoustics, Perception is intended as an introduction to the fundamentals of speech science (inclusive of voice science) that are important to aspiring clinicians and practicing clinicians.

The text is suitable for different courses that cover anatomy and physiology of speech production and swallowing, and the acoustics and perception of speech.

The material in the text is strongly integrative and translational, applicable to both undergraduate and graduate students, and a source of continuing education and reference for practicing speech-language pathologists.

The domain of preclinical speech science encompasses different levels of observation, different subsystems of speech production and swallowing, and different applications of data.

Levels of observation include the neural, muscular, structural, aeromechanical, acoustic, and perceptual levels.

Subsystems of speech production and swallowing include the breathing apparatus, laryngeal apparatus, velopharyngeal-nasal apparatus, and pharyngeal-oral apparatus.

Applications of data include the understanding of mechanism, evaluation, management, and forensics.

Sidetracks

Throughout the book you'll find a series of sidetracks. These are short asides that relate to topics being discussed in the main text. Many of the sidetracks in the book are a bit less formal and a bit more lighthearted than the main text they complement. This is intended to enhance your reading enjoyment and to put some fun in your study of the material. We hope you enjoy reading these sidetracks as much as we enjoyed writing them.

Breathing and Speech Production

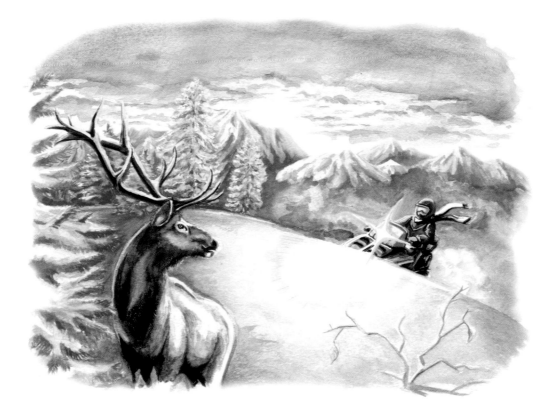

Scenario

The continental divide was in sight. It was near dusk and the peaks of the San Juan Mountains were pink with the last sun of December. This was a time of day she loved. She had just turned 20. He was 4 years old. He weighed 500 lbs, was massive through the shoulders, and respected. She weighed less than 100 lbs, was petite, and a college sophomore favorite of her classmates. His winter life was about survival and moving slowly. Hers was about thrills and a craving for speed.

When she crested the hill they met. The headlight of her snow machine momentarily shined on his eyes and his massive antlers. The impact was full on and it was over in a few seconds. She never managed to scream. His life was snapped and hers changed forever. She awoke to a new vibration and the sound of a voice on a radio. She was strapped down, her head, neck, and body braced. She heard talk of Durango and the activation of landing pad lights. She tried to move but could not. Her arms and legs had taken leave from her control. Her worst fears were confirmed in the emergency room. It was an unmercifully long night full of tears.

The morning's choice was Denver or Albuquerque, where a new mountain would have to be climbed, one higher than any she had ever seen or imagined. By midday a decision was made, with her family, and she again would hear the sound of a voice on a radio. This time it was in a fixed-wing air ambulance that was given clearance for takeoff on runway 9 with a straight-out departure. From then on she slept, with a flight nurse and her mother at her side. Denver came into sight below the front range of the Rocky Mountains. She was now on a leave of absence of indeterminate duration from her studies in veterinary science.

Six months passed and her abilities and disabilities were now known and part of her new life. Her spirit was returning and she had some optimism, some of it realistic and some of it not. She had a cervical spinal cord lesion (C6) and was quadriplegic, except for some movement in her arms and hands. She was thinking about getting a service dog to assist her with daily activities. A counselor from an agency visited with her and expressed some concern about whether or not she could control a dog because her voice was so soft. Her neurologist made a referral to a speech-language pathologist with a request to determine her potential to increase the power of her voice.

Auditory-perceptual examination revealed problems with reading aloud, extemporaneous speaking, and conversational speaking. Her speech was low in loudness, characterized by short breath groups (typically about 4 syllables each), and interspersed with relatively slow inspirations. Her speech phrasing was abnormal and her voice trailed off and became inaudible toward the ends of her expirations. She could not increase her loudness much, could not generate heavily stressed syllables, and could not increase the lengths of her speech expirations. She tired when speaking for more than a couple of minutes and needed to take frequent breaks while conversing to "catch her breath." Her conversational style was low keyed and gave the impression that she lacked energy. She reported that her breathing was uncomfortable when she spoke for too long and that it took a lot of effort to speak.

Physical examination revealed paralysis of the abdominal wall and severe paresis of the rib cage wall for both inspiration and expiration. Neck muscle function and diaphragm function were intact. During forced inspiration, the intercostal spaces were sucked inward and the upper rib cage wall moved inward (paradoxically). She required trunk support to maintain an upright body position. The abdominal wall was distended and the rib cage wall was positioned low. Forced expiration was weak, as was cough.

Her inspiratory capacity was 0.90 L and her expiratory reserve volume was 0.04 L. These values were 35% and 3% of their predicted values, respectively. Maximum inspiratory pressure was -28 cmH$_2$O and maximum expiratory pressure was 3 cmH$_2$O, as measured at the resting tidal end-expiratory level, 31% and 2% of their predicted values, respectively. She failed a screening of alveolar pressure for speech production (criterion 5 cmH$_2$O for 5 seconds). Impairment of inspiratory function was rated as moderate to severe and impairment of expiratory function was rated as severe to profound. Measurements on a breathing discomfort scale revealed moderate dyspnea in association with reading and mild dyspnea in association with conversational speaking.

Diagnostic interventions were tested and results were positive. With intervention, she could be made to inspire deeper and more forcefully and increase her loudness and phrase length. Certain intervention probes also reduced her dyspnea. A report was prepared for the neurologist with recommendations that included mechanical intervention and subsequent behavioral management.

Meanwhile, life continued as usual in the San Juan Mountains. It was now summer. The creeks were swollen, the meadows in color, and Lobo Lookout revealed the splendor of Wolf Creek Pass and the Weminuche Wilderness. She wondered about her chances of returning there.

INTRODUCTION

Speech breathing disorders are often encountered in clinical practice. It has been estimated that among individuals who present with speech disorders, 15% will have problems that are caused, at least in part, by one or more abnormalities of speech breathing. A speech breathing disorder may be the result of functional and/or organic causes and may present as a problem of breathing movement, gas exchange, breathing comfort, or any combination of these (Hixon & Hoit, 2005).

This chapter begins by considering the fundamentals of breathing, then turns to the consideration of breathing for normal speech production. This is followed by description of selected methods for the measurement of breathing. Next, general information about speech breathing disorders and the clinical professionals who work with them is considered as a bridge between the areas of basic science discussed in the chapter and their clinical application. The chapter ends with a review and the completion of its opening scenario.

FUNDAMENTALS OF BREATHING

The breathing apparatus is a mechanical air pump. This pump includes an energy source and passive components that couple this source to the air it moves. The present section considers the nature of this pump and how it functions. Topics discussed include the anatomical bases of breathing, forces and movements of breathing, adjustments of the breathing apparatus, output variables of breathing, neural control of breathing, and ventilation and gas exchange during tidal breathing. For the purposes of this chapter, the breathing apparatus is considered to include the pulmonary apparatus and chest wall (both defined below). Structures of the laryngeal apparatus, velopharyngeal-nasal apparatus, and pharyngeal-oral apparatus are covered in other chapters.

Coming to Terms

Terms can enlighten you or get you into verbal quagmires. Respiratory physiologists have gone out of their way to be precise in their use of terms. They've even held conventions to iron out their differences in language. It's a good idea to take a little extra time and care when reading the early sections of this chapter. Let the lexicon of the respiratory physiologist take firm root. Don't be tempted to skip over parts just because the words in the headings look familiar to you. You may be surprised to find that a term you thought you understood actually has an entirely different meaning to a respiratory physiologist.

Anatomical Bases of Breathing

The breathing apparatus is located within the torso (body trunk). A skeleton of bone and cartilage forms a superstructure for the torso. This superstructure is depicted in Figure 2–1.

Skeletal Superstructure

At the back of the torso, 34 irregularly shaped vertebrae (bones) form the vertebral column or backbone. The uppermost 7 of these vertebrae are termed cervical (neck), the next lower 12 are called thoracic (chest), and the next three lower groups of 5 each are referred to as lumbar, sacral, and coccygeal (collectively, abdominal). The vertebral column constitutes a back centerpost for the torso.

The ribs comprise most of the upper skeletal superstructure. They are 12 flat, arch-shaped bones on each side of the body. The ribs slope downward from back to front along the sides of the torso, forming the rib cage and giving roundness to the superstructure.

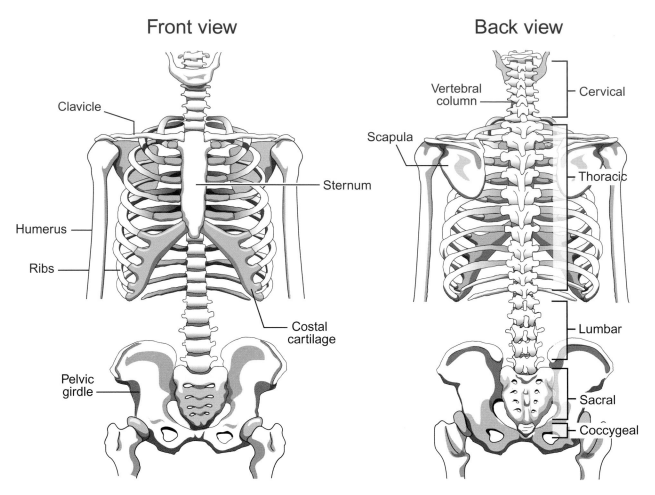

Figure 2–1. Skeletal superstructure of the torso.

At the front, most of the ribs attach to bars of costal (rib) cartilage, which, in turn, attach to the sternum or breastbone. The sternum serves as a front centerpost for the rib cage. The typical rib cage includes upper pairs of ribs attached to the sternum by their own costal cartilages, lower pairs that share cartilages, and the lowest two pairs that float without front attachments.

The remainder of the upper skeletal superstructure is formed by the pectoral girdle (shoulder girdle). This structure is near the top of the rib cage. The front of the pectoral girdle is formed by the two clavicles (collar bones), each of which is a strut extending from the sternum over the first rib toward the side and back of the rib cage. At the back, the clavicles attach to two triangularly shaped plates, the scapulae (shoulder blades). The scapulae cover most of the upper back portion of the rib cage.

Two large, irregularly shaped coxal (hip) bones are located in the lower skeletal superstructure. These two bones, together with the sacral and coccygeal vertebrae, form the pelvic girdle (bony pelvis). The pelvic girdle comprises the base, lower back, and sides of the lower skeletal superstructure.

Breathing Apparatus and Its Subdivisions

The breathing apparatus (breathing pump) and its subdivisions are depicted in Figure 2–2. The torso, which houses the apparatus, consists of upper and lower cavities that are partitioned by the diaphragm. The upper cavity, the thorax or chest, is almost totally filled with the heart and lungs, whereas the lower cavity, the abdomen or belly, contains much of the digestive system and other organs and glands. The structures of the breathing apparatus form two major subdivisions, the pulmonary apparatus and chest wall. These subdivisions are concentrically arranged, with the pulmonary apparatus being surrounded by the chest wall.

Pulmonary Apparatus. The pulmonary apparatus is the air containing, air conducting, and gas exchanging

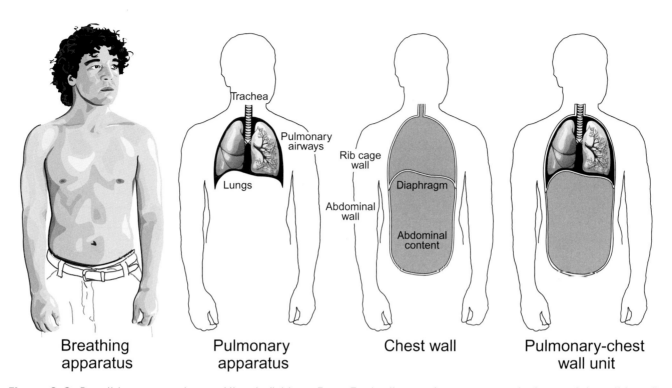

Breathing
apparatus

Pulmonary
apparatus

Chest wall

Pulmonary-chest
wall unit

Figure 2–2. Breathing apparatus and its subdivisions. From *Evaluation and management of speech breathing disorders: Principles and methods* (p. 13), by T. Hixon and J. Hoit, 2005, Tucson, AZ: Redington Brown. Copyright 2005 by Thomas J. Hixon and Jeannette D. Hoit. Modified and reproduced with permission.

part of the breathing apparatus. Figure 2–3 portrays some of its salient features. The pulmonary apparatus provides oxygen to the cells of the body and removes carbon dioxide from them. The apparatus can itself be subdivided into two components, the pulmonary airways and lungs.

Pulmonary Airways. The pulmonary airways constitute a complex network of flexible tubes through which air can be moved to and from the lungs and between different parts of the lungs. These tubes are patterned like the branches of an inverted deciduous tree. The network, in fact, is commonly referred to as the pulmonary tree.

The trunk of the pulmonary tree (the top part) is the trachea or windpipe. The trachea is a tube attached to the bottom of the larynx (voice box). It runs down through the neck into the torso. The trachea is composed of a series of C-shaped cartilages whose open ends face toward the back where the structure is completed by a flexible wall shared with the esophagus (a muscular tube leading to the stomach). At its lower end, the trachea divides into two smaller tubes, one running to the left lung and one running to the right lung. These two tubes, called the main-stem bronchi, branch

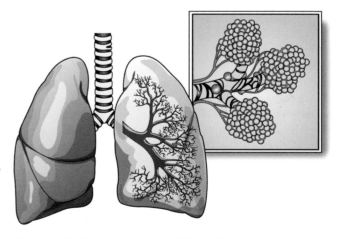

Figure 2–3. Salient features of the pulmonary apparatus.

into what are called lobar bronchi, tubes that run to the five lobes of the lungs (two on the left and three on the right). The five lobar bronchi each branch and their offspring also each branch, and so on, through more than 20 generations. Each successive branching leads to smaller and less rigid structures within the pulmonary apparatus. These include, in succession, segmental bronchi, subsegmental bronchi, small bronchi, terminal bronchi, bronchioles, terminal bronchioles, respiratory bronchioles, alveolar ducts, alveolar sacs, and alveoli. The last, the alveoli, are extremely small cul de sacs filled with air. They number more than 300 million and are the sites where oxygen and carbon dioxide are exchanged.

Lungs. The lungs are the organs of breathing. They are a pair of cone-shaped structures that are porous and spongy. Each lung contains an abundance of resilient elastic fibers and behaves like a stretchable bag. The outer surfaces of the lungs are covered with a thin air-tight membrane, the visceral pleura. A similar membrane, the parietal pleura, covers the inner surface of the chest wall where it contacts the lungs. Together these two membranes form a double-walled sac that encases the lungs. Both walls of this sac are covered with a thin layer of liquid, which lubricates them and enables them to move easily upon one another. The same layer of liquid links the visceral and parietal membranes together, in the manner that a film of water holds two glass plates together. Thus, the lungs and chest wall tend to move as a unit—where one goes the other follows.

Chest Wall. The chest wall encases the pulmonary apparatus. There are four parts to the chest wall: the rib cage wall, diaphragm, abdominal wall, and abdominal content.

Rib Cage Wall. The rib cage wall surrounds the lungs and is shaped like a barrel. Recall that the rib cage superstructure includes the thoracic segments of the vertebral column, the ribs, the costal cartilages, the sternum, and the pectoral girdle. The remainder of the rib cage wall is formed by muscular and nonmuscular tissues that fill the spaces between the ribs and cover their inner and outer surfaces.

Diaphragm. The diaphragm forms the convex floor of the thorax and the concave roof of the abdomen. The diaphragm separates the thorax and abdomen, and thus, gets its name — diaphragm meaning "the fence between." The diaphragm is dome-shaped and has the appearance of an inverted bowl. The left side of the structure is positioned slightly lower than the right. At its center, the diaphragm consists of a tough sheet of inelastic tissue, the central tendon. The remainder of the structure is formed by a sheet of muscle that rises as a broad rim from all around the lower portion of the inside of the rib cage and extends upward to the edges of the central tendon.

Abdominal Wall. The abdominal wall provides a casing for the lower half of the torso. This casing is shaped like an oblong tube and runs all the way around the torso. The lower portion of the skeletal superstructure of the torso forms the framework around which the abdominal wall is built. This includes a back centerpost of 15 vertebrae (lumbar, sacral, and coccygeal) that extends from near the bottom of the rib cage to the tailbone and pelvic girdle. Much of the abdominal wall consists of two broad sheets of connective tissue and several large muscles. The two sheets of connective tissue cover the front and back of the abdominal wall and are called the abdominal aponeurosis and lumbodorsal fascia, respectively. Muscles are located all around the abdominal wall—front, back, and flanks—and combine with the abdominal aponeurosis, lumbodorsal fascia, vertebral column, and pelvic girdle to form its encircling casing.

Abdominal Content. The abdominal content is everything in the abdominal cavity. This includes a wide array of structures, such as the stomach, intestines, and various other internal structures. This content is close to unit density (the density of water) and constitutes a relatively homogeneous mass. This mass is suspended from above by a suction force at the undersurface of the diaphragm and is held in place circumferentially and at its base by the casing of the abdominal wall. Together, the abdominal cavity and the abdominal content are the mechanical equivalent of an elastic bag filled with water.

Pulmonary Apparatus-Chest Wall Unit. The pulmonary apparatus and chest wall form a single functional unit that derives from the linkage effected by the pleural membranes. As shown in Figure 2–4, the resting positions of the pulmonary apparatus and chest wall in this intact unit are different from their individual resting positions when the two are separated. When the pulmonary apparatus is removed from the chest wall, its resting position is a collapsed state in which it contains very little air. In contrast, the resting position of the chest wall, with the pulmonary apparatus removed, is a more expanded state. With the pulmonary apparatus and chest wall held together by pleural linkage, the breathing apparatus assumes a resting position between these two separate positions such that the pulmonary apparatus is somewhat expanded and the chest wall is somewhat compressed. This resting position of the linked pulmonary apparatus-chest wall unit involves a mechanically neutral or balanced state in which the force of the pulmonary apparatus to

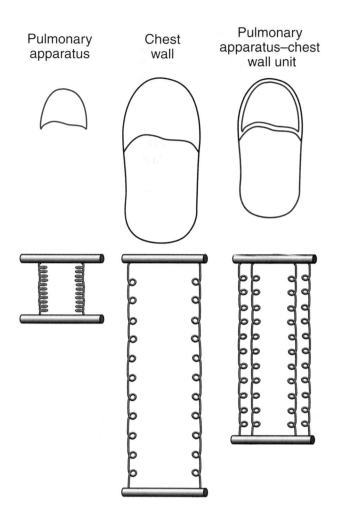

Pulmonary apparatus   Chest wall   Pulmonary apparatus–chest wall unit

Figure 2–4. Resting positions of the pulmonary apparatus, chest wall, and pulmonary apparatus-chest wall unit (breathing apparatus).

collapse is opposed by an equal and opposite force of the chest wall to expand.

Forces and Movements of Breathing

Forces applied to and by different parts of the breathing apparatus result in movements. Such forces and movements constitute breathing at the mechanical level.

Forces of Breathing

Passive and active forces operate on the breathing apparatus. Passive force is inherent and always present. Active force, in contrast, is applied willfully and in accordance with ability.

Passive Force. The passive force of breathing comes from: (a) the natural recoil of muscles, cartilages, ligaments, and lung tissue, (b) the surface tension of alveoli, and (c) the pull of gravity. These factors cause the breathing apparatus to behave like a coil spring, which, when stretched or compressed, tends to recoil toward its resting length.

The sign (inspiratory or expiratory) and magnitude of passive force depends on the amount of air in the breathing apparatus. When the apparatus contains more air than it does at its resting level, it recoils toward a smaller size (expires), like a stretched spring. The more air in the apparatus, the greater the recoil force. In contrast, when the apparatus contains less air than it does at its resting level, it recoils toward a larger size (inspires), like a compressed spring. The less air in the apparatus, the greater the recoil force. Thus, like a coil spring, the more the breathing apparatus is deformed from its resting level, whether in the inspiratory or expiratory direction, the greater the passive recoil force it generates.

Active Force. The active force of breathing comes from the actions of muscles of the chest wall. The sign (inspiratory or expiratory) and magnitude of this force depends on which muscles are active and in what patterns. Active force also depends on the amount of air in the breathing apparatus. The more air in the apparatus, the greater the active force that can be generated to expire, and the less air in the apparatus, the greater the active force that can be generated to inspire.

The roles of individual muscles in generating active force are described below for the rib cage wall, diaphragm, and abdominal wall. These descriptions assume that only the muscle under consideration is active and that it is shortening during contraction. It should be noted, however, that several factors might influence the contribution of an individual muscle, including the actions of other muscles, the mechanical status of different parts of the chest wall, and the breathing activity being performed.

Muscles of the Rib Cage Wall. The muscles of the rib cage wall are defined to include muscles of the neck and rib cage. These muscles are depicted in different views in Figure 2–5.

The *sternocleidomastoid* muscle is a broad, thick structure positioned on the front and side of the neck. It originates in two subdivisions, one at the top and front of the sternum and the other at the top of the sternal end of the clavicle. Fibers from these subdivisions pass upward and backward and insert into the bony skull

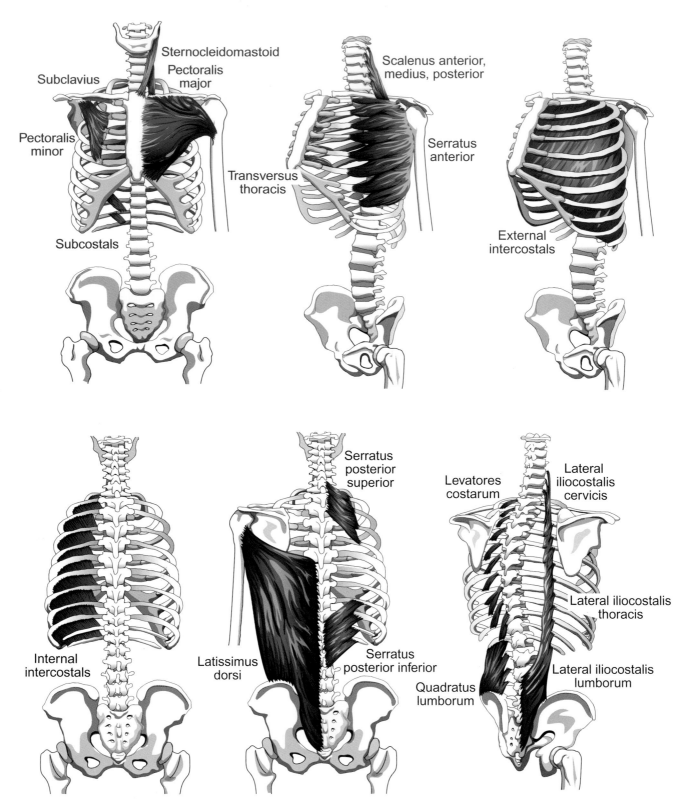

Figure 2–5. Muscles of the rib cage wall. From *Evaluation and management of speech breathing disorders: Principles and methods* (pp. 19–20), by T. Hixon and J. Hoit, 2005, Tucson, AZ: Redington Brown. Copyright 2005 by Thomas J. Hixon and Jeannette D. Hoit. Modified and reproduced with permission.

behind the ear. When the head is fixed in position, contraction of the *sternocleidomastoid* muscle results in elevation of the sternum and clavicle. The force generated is transmitted to the ribs through their connections to the sternum and clavicle. Consequently, the ribs are also elevated.

The *scalenus anterior, scalenus medius,* and *scalenus posterior* muscles are three separate muscles that form a functional group. These are positioned on the side of the neck. The *scalenus anterior* muscle originates from the third through sixth cervical vertebrae and runs downward and toward the side to insert along the inner border of the top of the first rib. The *scalenus medius* muscle arises from the lower six cervical vertebrae and descends along the side of the vertebral column to insert into the first rib behind the point of insertion of the *scalenus anterior* muscle. And the *scalenus posterior* muscle originates from the lower two or three cervical vertebrae and passes downward and toward the side to attach to the outer surface of the second rib. When the head is fixed in position, contraction of the *scalenus anterior* and/or *scalenus medius* muscles results in elevation of the first rib, whereas contraction of the *scalenus posterior* muscle results in elevation of the second rib.

The *pectoralis major* muscle is a broad, fan-shaped muscle positioned on the upper front wall of the rib cage. This muscle has a complex origin that includes the front surface of the upper costal cartilages, sternum, and inner half of the clavicle. Fibers run across the front of the rib cage wall and converge to insert into the humerus (the major bone of the upper arm). When the humerus is held in position, contraction of the *pectoralis major* muscle pulls the sternum and ribs upward.

The *pectoralis minor* muscle is a relatively large, thin muscle that lies underneath the *pectoralis major* muscle. Its fibers originate from the second through fifth ribs near their cartilages. From there, they extend upward and toward the side, where they insert into the front surface of the scapula. When the scapula is fixed in position, contraction of the *pectoralis minor* muscle elevates the second through fifth ribs.

The *subclavius* muscle is a small muscle that originates from the undersurface of the clavicle. It runs slightly downward and toward the midline, where it attaches at the junction of the first rib and its cartilage. When the clavicle is braced, contraction of the *subclavius* muscle elevates the first rib.

The *serratus anterior* muscle is a large muscle positioned on the side of the rib cage wall. It originates from the outer surfaces of the upper eight or nine ribs. Fibers pass backward around the side of the rib cage, where they converge and insert into the front of the scapula. When the scapula is fixed in position, contraction of the *serratus anterior* muscle results in elevation of the upper ribs.

The *external intercostal* muscles are 11 muscles that fill the outer portions of the rib interspaces. Each is a thin layer of muscle that runs between adjacent ribs. The fibers of the muscles are oriented forward and downward. Together, the 11 muscles form a large sheet of muscle that links the ribs to one another. This sheet of muscle is anchored from above to the first rib, the cervical vertebrae, and the base of the skull. When the muscle in any rib interspace contracts, it

---

Rib Torque

Sounds like leftovers. Actually, it refers to rotational stress produced when one end of a rib is twisted out of line with the other. Some have suggested that when the ribs are elevated during resting tidal inspiration they're twisted outward (placed under positive torque) and store energy, which is then supposedly released during expiration. Not so. The ribs are actually twisted inward (are under negative torque) at the resting tidal end-expiratory level. The lungs are pulling inward on the rib cage wall at that level. The ribs untwist during resting tidal inspiration, but do not reach neutral (zero torque) in the upright body position until the 60 %VC (percent vital capacity) level is attained. Resting tidal inspiration involves only about a 10 %VC increase, from say, 40 to 50 %VC. Thus, rib torque actually opposes resting tidal expiration rather than assists it. The only thing left over about rib torque in this context is the folklore.

elevates the rib immediately below and, perhaps, other ribs below through their linkage to the sheet of muscle. The *external intercostal* muscles may activate individually in different rib interspaces or they may activate collectively. En masse activation causes the ribs to move upward as a unit. Muscle activation also stiffens the tissue-filled rib interspaces. This prevents them from being sucked inward and pushed outward as internal pressure is lowered and raised, respectively.

The *internal intercostal* muscles are 11 muscles that lie in the inner portions of the rib interspaces. They are located underneath the *external intercostal* muscles and extend from around the sides of the rib cage to the sternum. The *internal intercostal* muscles do not fill the rib interspaces at the back of the rib age. Fibers of the *internal intercostal* muscles run downward and backward and at a right angle to those of the *external intercostal* muscles. The *internal intercostal* muscles form a large sheet of muscle that links the ribs to one another and to the pelvic girdle through other muscles, especially those of the abdominal wall. When muscle in a rib interspace contracts, it pulls downward on the rib immediately above and, perhaps, on other ribs above through the linkage created by the muscle sheet. The *internal intercostal* muscles may activate individually in any rib interspace or they may activate collectively. For the latter, the ribs tend to move downward as a unit. Muscle contraction stiffens the tissue-filled rib interspaces and prevents them from being sucked inward and bulged outward during the lowering and raising of internal pressure, respectively.

The portion of the *internal intercostal* muscles that lies between the costal cartilages (the *intercartilaginous internal intercostal* muscles) is arranged such that the muscle tissue exerts an upward pull on the rib cage wall rather than the downward pull exerted by the portion of the muscle that lies between the bony ribs (the *interosseous internal intercostal* muscles). Thus, the *internal intercostal* muscles play a functional role in the intercartilaginous region that is similar to that played by their companion *external intercostal* muscles throughout the rib cage wall. Stated otherwise, the two layers of intercostal muscles (external and internal) function similarly toward the front of the rib cage, but dissimilarly at other locations.

The *transversus thoracis* muscle is a fan-shaped structure located on the inside, front wall of the rib cage. It originates at the midline on the inner surface of the lower sternum and fourth or fifth through seventh costal cartilages. From there, it fans out across the rib cage and inserts into the inner surface of the costal cartilages and bony ends of the second through sixth ribs. The upper fibers of the muscle run nearly vertically, whereas the intermediate and lower fibers course at other angles. When the *transversus thoracis* muscle contracts, it exerts a downward pull on the second through sixth ribs.

The *latissimus dorsi* muscle is a large muscle positioned on the back of the body. It has a complex origin from the lower six thoracic, lumbar, and sacral vertebrae, along with the back surfaces of the lower three or four ribs. Fibers run upward across the back of the lower torso at different angles to insert into the humerus. When the humerus is fixed in position, contraction of the fibers of the *latissimus dorsi* muscle that insert into the lower ribs will elevate them. Contraction of the muscle as a whole, in contrast, compresses the lower portion of the rib cage wall. Thus, the *latissimus dorsi* muscle is capable of generating active force of different signs (inspiratory and expiratory).

The *serratus posterior superior* muscle is located on the upper back portion of the rib cage wall. It is a thin muscle that originates from the back of the vertebral column. Points of origin include the seventh cervical and first three or four thoracic vertebrae. Fibers course downward across the back of the rib cage and insert into the second through fifth ribs. When the *serratus posterior superior* muscle contracts, it pulls upward on the second through fifth ribs.

The *serratus posterior inferior* muscle is a thin muscle positioned on the lower back portion of the rib cage wall. It arises from the lower two thoracic and upper two or three lumbar vertebrae and slants upward across the back of the rib cage where it inserts into the lower borders of the lower four ribs. Contraction of the *serratus posterior inferior* muscle results in a downward pull on the lower four ribs.

The *lateral iliocostalis* muscle group includes three muscles located on the back of the torso. These are positioned to the side of the vertebral column and extend between the cervical and lumbar regions. The *lateral iliocostalis cervicis* muscle originates from the outer surfaces of the third through sixth ribs and courses upward and toward the midline to insert into the fourth through sixth cervical vertebrae. The *lateral iliocostalis thoracis* muscle arises from the upper edges of the lower six ribs and courses upward to insert into the lower edges of the upper six ribs. And the *lateral iliocostalis lumborum* muscle originates from the lumbodorsal fascia, lumbar vertebrae, and back surface of the coxal bone. It courses upward and toward the side to insert into the lower edges of the lower six ribs. Contraction of the *lateral iliocostalis cervicis* muscle causes elevation of the third through sixth ribs, whereas contraction of the *lateral iliocostalis lumborum* muscle results in depression of the lower six ribs. Contraction of the *lateral iliocostalis thoracis* muscle stabilizes large segments of the back of the rib cage wall and makes them move in concert with either the rib elevation or depression caused by the cervical and lumbar elements of the muscle group, respectively.

The *levatores costarum* muscles are 12 small muscles positioned on the back of the rib cage wall. Their origin is from the seventh cervical and upper eleven thoracic vertebrae and they extend downward and slightly outward to insert into the back surface of the rib immediately below the vertebra of origin. When an individual muscle of the *levatores costarum* muscle group contracts, it elevates the ribs into which it inserts. When the muscle group contracts collectively, its action is similar to that effected by collective contraction of the *external intercostal* muscles (the ribs elevate as a unit).

The *quadratus lumborum* muscle is a flat, quadrilateral sheet of muscle located on the back of the torso. It arises from the top of the coxal bone and runs upward and toward the midline where it inserts into the first four lumbar vertebrae and lower border of the inner half of the lowest rib. When the *quadratus lumborum* muscle contracts, it pulls downward on the lowest rib.

The *subcostal* muscles comprise a group of thin muscles located on the inside back wall of the rib cage. They differ in number from person to person and are most often located and best developed in the lower portion of the rib cage wall. The *subcostal* muscles originate near the vertebral column on the inner surfaces of ribs and course upward and toward the side where they insert into the inner surfaces of ribs immediately above, or skip a rib or two and insert into higher ribs. When the *subcostal* muscles contract, they pull downward on the ribs into which they are inserted.

Muscle of the Diaphragm. The muscular features of the diaphragm are portrayed in Figure 2–6. The *diaphragm* muscle is a large, complex muscle that subdivides the torso into two compartments. Its origin is around the internal circumference of the lower rib cage. This includes the bottom of the sternum, the lower six ribs and their cartilages, and the first three or four lumbar vertebrae. From this internal rim, muscle fibers radiate upward to insert into the circumference of the central tendon, a broad sheet of inelastic tissue that forms the centermost portion of the diaphragm. When the *diaphragm* muscle contracts, it can effect two actions. As portrayed in Figure 2–7, one of these is to pull the central tendon downward and forward, thus enlarging the thorax vertically, whereas the other is to enlarge the thorax circumferentially through elevation of the lower six ribs. The actions of lowering the base of the thorax and expanding its circumference occur in patterns that depend on the relative stiffness of the rib cage wall and abdominal wall.

Muscles of the Abdominal Wall. The muscles of the abdominal wall are depicted in Figure 2–8. They are located on the front and sides of the abdominal wall.

The *rectus abdominis* muscle is a ribbonlike structure located on the front of the lower rib cage wall and abdominal wall just off the midline. It arises from the upper, front edge of the coxal bone and runs upward vertically to insert into the outer surfaces of the fifth, sixth, and seventh costal cartilages and lower sternum. The *rectus abdominis* muscle is compartmentalized into four or five short segments by tendinous breaks. The entire muscle is encased in a fibrous sheath formed by the abdominal aponeurosis. The muscle and sheath form a centerpost along the front of the abdominal wall that is a continuation of the front centerpost formed by the sternum on the rib cage wall. When the *rectus abdominis* muscle contracts, it pulls the lower ribs and sternum downward and forces the front of the abdominal wall inward. The compartmentalized segments of the muscle are also capable of independent contraction.

The *external oblique* muscle is a broad structure located on the side and front of the lower rib cage wall and abdominal wall. It originates from the upper surface of the coxal bone and abdominal aponeurosis near the midline. Fibers course upward across the abdominal wall at various angles. The most prominent course is upward and toward the side, with insertions being on the outer surfaces and lower borders of the lower eight ribs. When the *external oblique* muscle contracts, it pulls the lower ribs downward and forces the front and side of the abdominal wall inward.

The *internal oblique* muscle is a large muscle positioned on the side and front of the lower rib cage wall and abdominal wall. It lies underneath the *external oblique* muscle. The *internal oblique* muscle originates from the upper surface of the coxal bone and lumbodorsal fascia. Its fibers fan out across the abdominal wall to insert into the abdominal aponeurosis and the lower borders of the costal cartilages of the lower three or four ribs. The fibers of the *internal oblique* muscle run at a right angle to those of the *external oblique* muscle. When the *internal oblique* muscle contracts, it pulls the lower ribs downward and forces the front and side of the abdominal wall inward. Thus, its functional potential is similar to that of the *external oblique* muscle.

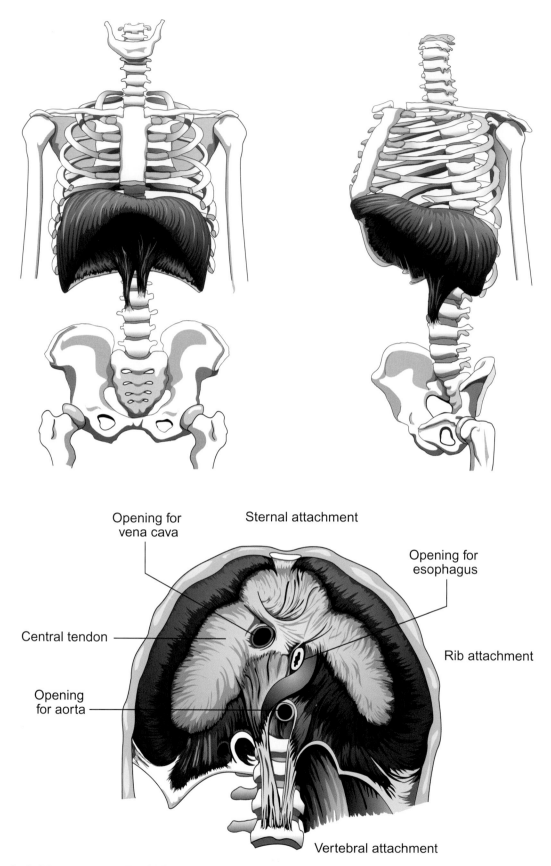

Opening for
vena cava

Sternal attachment

Opening for
esophagus

Central tendon

Rib attachment

Opening
for aorta

Vertebral attachment

Figure 2–6. Muscle of the ***diaphragm***. Upper panels from *Evaluation and management of speech breathing disorders: Principles and methods* (p. 25), by T. Hixon and J. Hoit, 2005, Tucson, AZ: Redington Brown. Copyright 2005 by Thomas J. Hixon and Jeannette D. Hoit. Modified and reproduced with permission.

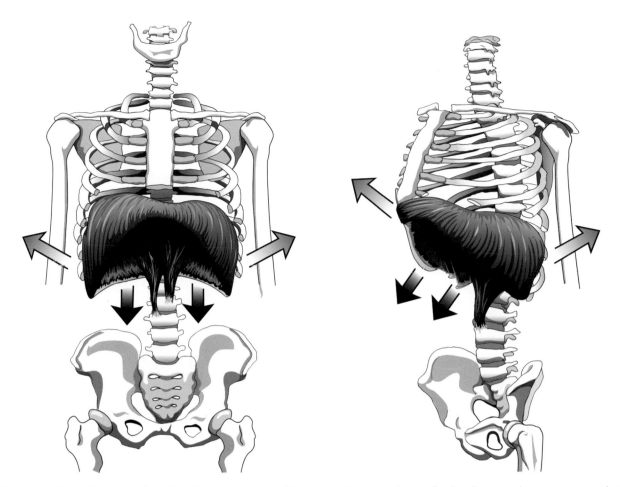

Figure 2–7. Actions of the ***diaphragm*** muscle. Structural features from *Evaluation and management of speech breathing disorders: Principles and methods* (p. 25), by T. Hixon and J. Hoit, 2005, Tucson, AZ: Redington Brown. Copyright 2005 by Thomas J. Hixon and Jeannette D. Hoit. Modified and reproduced with permission.

The ***transversus abdominis*** muscle is a broad structure located on the front and side of the abdominal wall. It lies underneath the ***internal oblique*** muscle. The ***transversus abdominis*** muscle has a complex origin that includes the upper surface of the coxal bone, lumbodorsal fascia, and inner surfaces of the costal cartilages of ribs seven through twelve. Fibers of the muscle run horizontally around the abdominal wall and insert at the front into the abdominal aponeurosis. The paired left and right ***transversus abdominis*** muscles encircle the abdominal wall. When the ***transversus abdominis*** muscle contracts, it forces the front and side of the abdominal wall inward.

The four muscles just described are routinely referred to as "the" abdominal muscles. However, the abdominal wall runs all the way around the torso and includes more than just its front and sides. Three other muscles traverse the abdominal wall at the back and

are as much a part of the abdominal wall as the muscles just discussed. These three muscles are described above in the context of the rib cage wall. They include the ***latissimus dorsi***, ***lateral iliocostalis lumborum***, and ***quadratus lumborum*** muscles. These muscles do not effect major displacements of the abdominal wall. Nevertheless, they can brace the abdominal wall at the back and alter its stiffness. Accordingly, they are important functional partners with the other four abdominal muscles.

Summary of the Chest Wall Muscles. The muscles of the rib cage wall, diaphragm, and abdominal wall comprise the muscles of the chest wall. These muscles, through their activations, can change the volume of the pulmonary apparatus (pulmonary airways and lungs) by increasing or decreasing the circumference of the thorax, increasing or decreasing the vertical length of

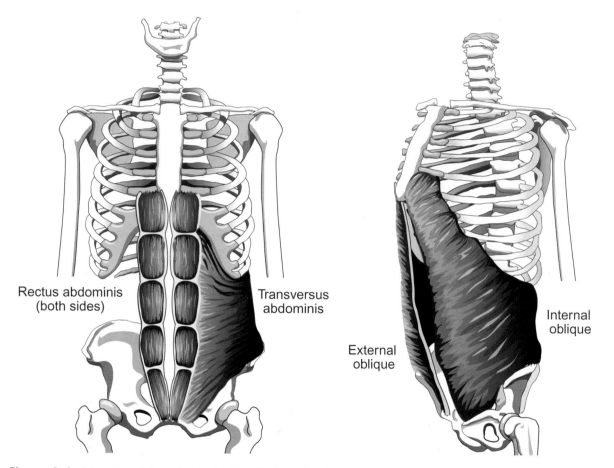

Rectus abdominis
(both sides)

Transversus
abdominis

Internal
oblique

External
oblique

Figure 2–8. Muscles of the abdominal wall. From *Evaluation and management of speech breathing disorders: Principles and methods* (p. 26), by T. Hixon and J. Hoit, 2005, Tucson, AZ: Redington Brown. Copyright 2005 by Thomas J. Hixon and Jeannette D. Hoit. Modified and reproduced with permission.

the thorax (by lowering or raising its floor), or both. Table 2–1 lists the chest wall muscles and their potential actions on the thorax. Increasing thoracic size (and, thus, increasing the volume of the pulmonary apparatus) is an "inspiratory" action, and decreasing thoracic size is an "expiratory" action.

Realization of Passive and Active Forces

Forces of breathing are realized in two ways. One is through pulls on structures and the other is through pressures developed at various locations. Pulling forces are distributed in a complex fashion. Fortunately, they are uniformly distributed at certain points where they manifest as pressures. The locations of the most important of these pressures are indicated in Figure 2–9.

Included among these pressures are alveolar pressure, pleural pressure, abdominal pressure, and transdiaphragmatic pressure. Alveolar pressure is the pressure inside the lungs. Pleural pressure is the pressure inside the thorax but outside the lungs (between the pleural membranes). Abdominal pressure is the pressure inside the abdominal cavity. And transdiaphragmatic pressure is the difference in pressure across the diaphragm (the difference between pleural pressure and abdominal pressure). Although all of these pressures are critical to the function of the breathing apparatus, the pressure of greatest primacy to the understanding of speech production is alveolar pressure.

Movements of Breathing

The movements of breathing occur in the rib cage wall, diaphragm, and abdominal wall. Movement potential is considered here apart from the forces responsible for it.

Movements of Rib Cage Wall. The rib cage wall is able to move because of two sets of joints, those between the ribs and sternum (costosternal joints) and those between the ribs and the vertebral column (costovertebral joints). Actual movement differs somewhat from

Table 2–1. Muscles of the Chest Wall and Their Potential Actions on the Thorax

CIRCUMFERENCE INCREASERS	CIRCUMFERENCE DECREASERS
Sternocleidomastoid	Internal Intercostal (Interosseus)
Scalenes (Anterior, Medius, Posterior)	Transverse Thoracis
Pectoralis Major	Latissimus Dorsi
Pectoralis Minor	Serratus Posterior Inferior
Subclavius	Lateral Iliocostalis Lumborum
Serratus Anterior	Lateral Iliocostalis Thoracis
External Intercostal	Quadratus Lumborum
Internal Intercostal (Intercartilaginous)	Subcostal
Latissimus Dorsi	Rectus Abdominis
Serratus Posterior Superior	External Oblique Abdominis
Lateral Iliocostalis Cervicis	Internal Oblique Abdominis
Lateral Iliocostalis Thoracis	
Levatores Costarum	
Diaphragm	
VERTICAL LENGTH INCREASER	**VERTICAL LENGTH DECREASERS**
Diaphragm	Rectus Abdominis
	External Oblique Abdominis
	Internal Oblique Abdominis
	Transverse Abdominis

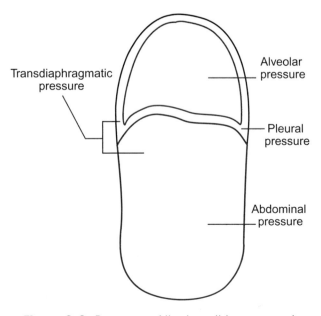

Transdiaphragmatic pressure

Alveolar pressure

Pleural pressure

Abdominal pressure

Figure 2–9. Pressures of the breathing apparatus.

rib to rib, owing the differences in the lengths and shapes of individual ribs. Nevertheless, two forms of rib movements are typical and are illustrated in Figure 2–10.

One form of rib movement involves a vertical excursion of its front end. The excursion is either upward and forward or downward and backward and results in an increase or decrease, respectively, in the front-to-back diameter of the rib cage. Each rib rotates through the axis of its neck (at the back near the vertebral column) and the pattern of movement that results is akin to the raising and lowering of the handle on a water pump.

The other form of rib movement is vertical excursion along the side of the rib cage. This excursion involves a rotation of the rib around an axis extending between its two ends. The rotation is either upward and outward or downward and inward, the result being an increase or decrease, respectively, in the side-to-side diameter of the rib cage. Such movement is similar to the raising and lowering of the handle on a water bucket.

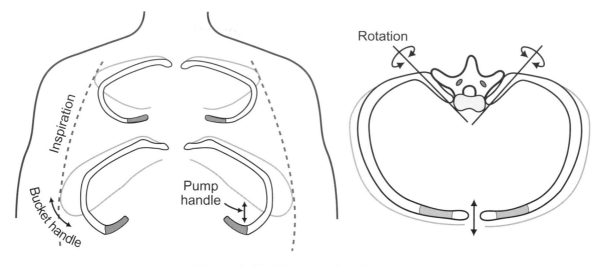

Figure 2–10. Movements of the ribs.

These two types of rib movement occur together and in phase. Thus, the circumference of the rib cage wall increases and decreases along with increases and decreases in its two diameters (front-to-back and side-to-side).

Movements of the Diaphragm. Movements of the diaphragm are hidden from view and must be inferred from movements of other structures of the chest wall. Such movements are manifested in changes in the radius of curvature of the diaphragm and depend on the relative fixation of the central tendon and lower ribs.

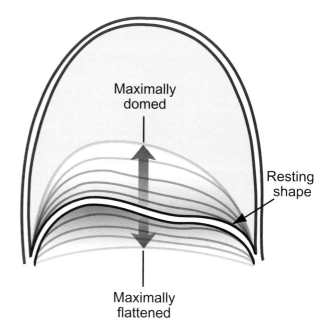

Figure 2–11. Movements of the diaphragm.

Not Doing What Comes Naturally

The initiation and execution of voluntary breathing movements comes "naturally" for most of us. But, for some individuals with maldeveloped or damaged brains, these may not be easy, or even possible, to do. Their problem is praxis or action. They have dyspraxia when they have difficulty with action, and apraxia when they are unable to carry out action at all. One of the most perplexing clients we ever encountered was a young man who showed difficulties with breathing actions following a traumatic brain injury. When he attempted to initiate voluntary inspirations or expirations on command, he often became frozen in position. Occasionally, his attempt resulted in movement in the opposite direction (he breathed in when trying to breathe out). He knew exactly what he wanted to do, but just couldn't do it. Imagine the depth of his frustration.

As depicted in Figure 2–11, the diaphragm can be made to flatten or become more highly domed. Flattening is brought about by descent of the central tendon and/or elevation of the lower ribs, and can range from slight to marked. When marked, the diaphragm assumes the shape of an inverted pie pan. Increased doming of the diaphragm results from elevation of the central tendon and/or descent of the lower ribs, and can also range from slight to marked. When marked, the diaphragm assumes the shape of a rounded bullet nose.

When the rib cage is fixed in position, the movement of the diaphragm is coextensive with the movement of the central tendon. In contrast, when the central tendon is fixed in position, the movement of the diaphragm is coextensive with the movement of the abdominal wall.

Movements of the Abdominal Wall. The configuration of the abdominal wall differs from person to person. Factors such as abdominal muscle tone and body type contribute to such differences. When standing or sitting erect, the lower abdominal wall is distended somewhat. This is because the pressure inside the abdomen is greater near the bottom than near the undersurface of the diaphragm and forces the lower abdominal wall outward. Two movements can change the configuration of the abdominal wall. These include moving the wall inward and outward.

Inward movement flattens the abdominal wall. Such flattening can range from slight to marked. When flattening is marked, the configuration of the wall is linear or may actually be curved inward slightly in someone who is exceptionally lean. More pronounced distension of the abdominal wall is accomplished by moving it outward. Outward movement increases the degree to which the wall is protruded. When such protrusion is marked, the configuration of the wall makes the torso appear much like a pear in side view.

Relative Movements of the Rib Cage Wall, Diaphragm, and Abdominal Wall. Figure 2–12 illustrates that the movements of the rib cage wall, the diaphragm, and the abdominal wall can have different functional consequences. The reason is that the rib cage wall and diaphragm-abdominal wall are in contact with different proportions of the surface of the lungs.

The rib cage wall contacts about three fourths of the surface of the lungs. Thus, its movement has a major influence on alveolar pressure and the movement of air. Even a small movement of the rib cage wall can cause a significant pressure change or move a large amount of air into or out of the pulmonary apparatus.

In contrast, the diaphragm contacts only about one-fourth of the surface of the lungs. This means that the diaphragm must go through a much greater excursion than the rib cage wall to accomplish the same alveolar pressure change or move the same amount of air into or out of the pulmonary apparatus.

The abdominal wall presents a similar situation. The abdominal wall and diaphragm are opposite surfaces of a very large chest wall part (the diaphragm-abdominal wall), with the abdominal content lying between them. Thus, the abdominal wall is indirectly in contact with the pulmonary apparatus by way of the diaphragm and has access to the same one-fourth of

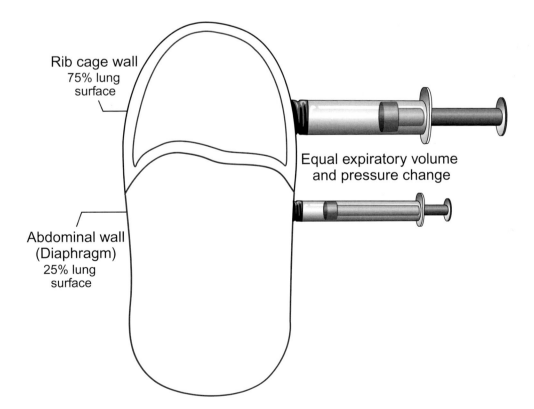

Figure 2–12. Relative movements of the rib cage wall, diaphragm, and abdominal wall.

the surface of the lungs as does the diaphragm. Like the diaphragm, then, the abdominal wall must go through a much greater excursion than the rib cage wall to effect the same alveolar pressure change or move the same amount of air into or out of the pulmonary apparatus.

Adjustments of the Breathing Apparatus

The breathing apparatus can make many adjustments. Some of these are confined to the parts of the chest wall in which they occur. Others are the result of actions between and among different parts of the chest wall. Figure 2–13 summarizes the passive and active forces that can contribute to adjustments of the breathing apparatus. These are depicted for the pulmonary apparatus, chest wall, and the three components of the chest wall individually—rib cage wall, diaphragm, and abdominal wall. Negative and positive signs in the figure represent forces that tend to inspire and expire the breathing apparatus, respectively.

Pulmonary Apparatus

The pulmonary apparatus only participates passively in adjustments of the breathing apparatus. It recoils toward a smaller size at all times, like a stretched coil spring. Thus, it operates only in the expiratory direction.

Chest Wall

The chest wall can participate both passively and actively in adjustments of the breathing apparatus. It recoils inward at large chest wall sizes and outward at small chest wall sizes. Thus, it complements the recoil of the pulmonary apparatus at large chest wall sizes

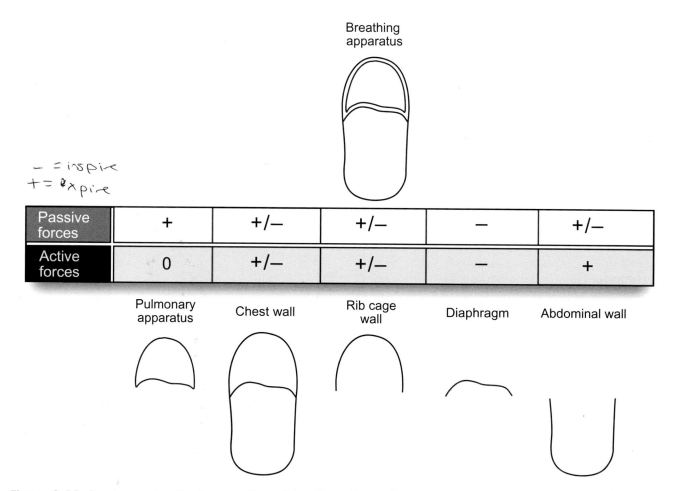

	Pulmonary apparatus	Chest wall	Rib cage wall	Diaphragm	Abdominal wall
Passive forces	+	+/−	+/−	−	+/−
Active forces	0	+/−	+/−	−	+

Figure 2–13. Passive and active forces of breathing. From *Evaluation and management of speech breathing disorders: Principles and methods* (p. 31), by T. Hixon and J. Hoit, 2005, Tucson, AZ: Redington Brown. Copyright 2005 by Thomas J. Hixon and Jeannette D. Hoit. Modified and reproduced with permission.

and opposes it at small chest wall sizes. Muscles of the chest wall can generate active force to either inspire or expire the breathing apparatus at any chest wall size. Muscles that inspire the apparatus are located in the rib cage wall and diaphragm, and muscles that expire the apparatus are located in the rib cage wall and abdominal wall. Active force available to inspire the breathing apparatus is greater at small chest wall sizes, whereas active force available to expire the apparatus is greater at large chest wall sizes. This is because the inspiratory and expiratory muscles of the chest wall are on more favorable portions of their length-force characteristics at small and large chest wall sizes, respectively.

Rib Cage Wall. The rib cage wall can contribute both passively and actively to adjustments of the breathing apparatus. It recoils inward at large sizes and outward at small sizes (except in downright body positions). Thus, it complements the recoil of the pulmonary apparatus at large rib cage sizes and opposes it at small rib cage sizes. Muscles of the rib cage wall can generate active force in both the inspiratory and expiratory directions. Those responsible for inspiratory force are located in superficial layers of the rib cage wall and those responsible for expiratory force are located in deep layers of the wall. Active force available to inspire the breathing apparatus is greater at small rib cage wall sizes, whereas active force available to expire the apparatus is greater at large rib cage wall sizes. The force advantages at different sizes of the rib cage wall relate to more favorable length-force characteristics for the inspiratory and expiratory muscles at small and large rib cage wall sizes, respectively. The smallest muscles of the breathing apparatus are located in the rib cage wall and provide it with the capability for fast and precise action.

Diaphragm. The diaphragm is capable of contributing both passively and actively to adjustments of the breathing apparatus. When displaced footward and being less highly domed, as it is at large lung volumes, it develops no recoil. In contrast, when displaced headward and being more highly domed, as it is at small lung volumes, it recoils in the inspiratory direction. Inspiratory recoil is caused by passive stretch of the muscle fibers of the diaphragm brought about by forces acting across the structure. Thus, the diaphragm opposes the recoil of the pulmonary apparatus at small lung volumes. The diaphragm can generate active force in the inspiratory direction only. The more highly domed the configuration of the diaphragm, the more active force the structure is able to exert. This is because its muscle fibers are elongated and are on more favorable portions of their length-force characteristics.

Abdominal Wall. The abdominal wall can make both passive and active contributions to adjustments of the breathing apparatus. It recoils in the expiratory direction at large abdominal wall volumes and in the inspiratory direction at small abdominal wall volumes (except in downright body positions). Thus, it complements the recoil of the pulmonary apparatus at large abdominal wall volumes and opposes it at small abdominal wall volumes. The abdominal wall can only generate active force in the expiratory direction. Such active force can be greater at large abdominal wall volumes because the abdominal wall muscles are on more favorable portions of their length-force characteristics.

Pulmonary Apparatus-Chest Wall Unit

Mechanical arrangements between different parts of the pulmonary apparatus-chest wall unit condition how actions of the breathing apparatus are manifested. Such arrangements make it possible for one part of the breathing apparatus to cause adjustments in other parts of the apparatus, as illustrated in Figure 2–14 and discussed in the following examples.

Actions of the rib cage wall can cause adjustments in both the diaphragm and abdominal wall. For example, when the rib cage wall expands and the diaphragm and abdominal wall are quiescent, pleural pressure lowers and pulls the diaphragm headward and the abdominal wall inward. This action is akin to the way in which liquid is pulled upward in a drinking straw (hence the phrase "sucking it in" when referring to the consequence on the abdominal wall). In contrast, when the rib cage wall compresses, pleural pressure rises and pushes the diaphragm footward and the abdominal wall outward.

Actions of the diaphragm can cause adjustments in both the rib cage wall and abdominal wall. The nature of these adjustments will depend on the mechanical status of the rib cage wall and abdominal wall. For example, when the rib cage wall is fixed in position, movement of the diaphragm is resolved into footward displacement and abdominal wall distention. In contrast, when the abdominal wall is fixed in position, movement of the diaphragm is resolved into headward displacement of the rib cage wall. Usually, neither the rib cage wall nor abdominal wall is rigidly positioned, so that they move in accordance with their relative compliance (floppiness).

Actions of the abdominal wall can cause adjustments in both the rib cage wall and diaphragm. For example, when the muscles of the abdominal wall contract, they force the abdominal wall inward and raise abdominal pressure. This forces the lower rib cage wall

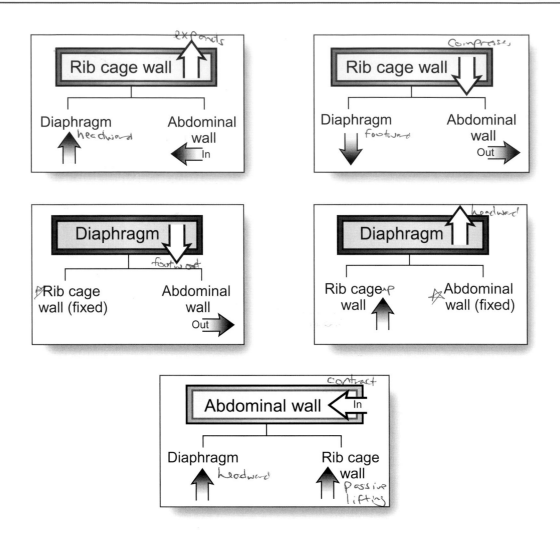

Figure 2-14. Influence of rib cage wall, diaphragm, and abdominal wall components on one another.

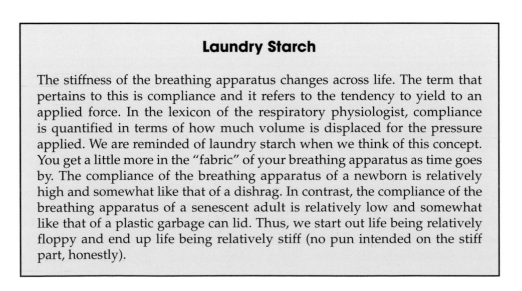

Laundry Starch

The stiffness of the breathing apparatus changes across life. The term that pertains to this is compliance and it refers to the tendency to yield to an applied force. In the lexicon of the respiratory physiologist, compliance is quantified in terms of how much volume is displaced for the pressure applied. We are reminded of laundry starch when we think of this concept. You get a little more in the "fabric" of your breathing apparatus as time goes by. The compliance of the breathing apparatus of a newborn is relatively high and somewhat like that of a dishrag. In contrast, the compliance of the breathing apparatus of a senescent adult is relatively low and somewhat like that of a plastic garbage can lid. Thus, we start out life being relatively floppy and end up life being relatively stiff (no pun intended on the stiff part, honestly).

outward and the diaphragm headward. The combination of these two effects causes a passive lifting of the rib cage wall, such that it moves higher and higher with more and more inward movement of the abdominal wall.

Actions of the breathing apparatus often seem deceptively simple and can be erroneously ascribed as being caused only by the parts of the apparatus in which they are observed. As noted above, however, the mechanical interplay between and among different parts of the breathing apparatus is significant and must be considered when trying to understand any adjustment of the breathing apparatus.

Output Variables of Breathing

The breathing apparatus controls a number of variables. Those that are important in the present context are volume, pressure, and shape.

Volume

Volume is defined as the size of a three-dimensional object or space. The volume of interest here is the volume of air inside the pulmonary apparatus. This volume is termed the lung volume and it reflects the size of the breathing apparatus. Lung volume is important because the behavior of the breathing apparatus depends on lung volume.

Movements of the breathing apparatus can cause a change in lung volume by moving air into or out of the pulmonary apparatus. Such volume change, termed volume displacement, can occur only if the larynx and upper airway are open.

The volume variable can be partitioned into what are called lung volumes and lung capacities. Volume is often displayed in a spirogram, a record of lung volume change over time obtained from a spirometer (a device that records volume displacement). A spirogram is shown in Figure 2–15.

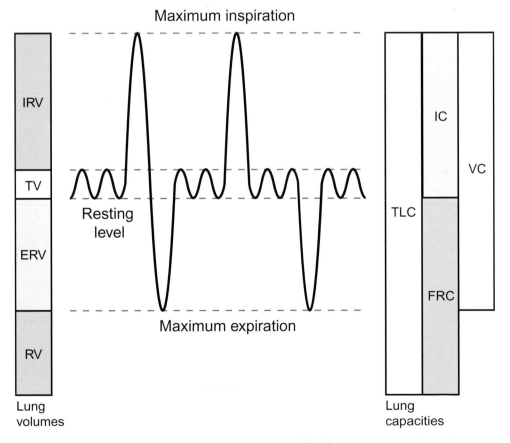

Figure 2–15. Lung volumes and lung capacities. From *Evaluation and management of speech breathing disorders: Principles and methods* (p. 36), by T. Hixon and J. Hoit, 2005, Tucson, AZ: Redington Brown. Copyright 2005 by Thomas J. Hixon and Jeannette D. Hoit. Modified and reproduced with permission.

There are four lung volumes. Each covers a portion of the lung volume range that is mutually exclusive of the others.

The *tidal volume* (TV) is the volume of air inspired or expired during the breathing cycle. When recorded in the resting individual, this volume is termed the resting tidal volume.

The *inspiratory reserve volume* (IRV) is the maximum volume of air that can be inspired from the tidal end-inspiratory level (the peak of the tidal volume cycle).

The *expiratory reserve volume* (ERV) is the maximum volume of air that can be expired from the tidal end-expiratory level (the trough of the tidal volume cycle).

The *residual volume* (RV) is the volume of air in the pulmonary apparatus at the end of a maximum expiration. This volume cannot be measured directly, because the pulmonary apparatus cannot be emptied voluntarily.

There are four lung capacities. Each includes two or more of the lung volumes discussed above.

The *inspiratory capacity* (IC) is the maximum volume of air that can be inspired from the resting tidal end-expiratory level. It is the sum of the tidal volume and the inspiratory reserve volume.

The *vital capacity* (VC) is the maximum volume of air that can be expired following a maximum inspiration. It includes the inspiratory reserve volume, the tidal volume, and the expiratory reserve volume.

The *functional residual capacity* (FRC) is the volume of air in the pulmonary apparatus at the resting tidal end-expiratory level. This capacity includes the expiratory reserve volume and the residual volume.

The *total lung capacity* (TLC) is the volume of air in the pulmonary apparatus at the end of a maximum inspiration. It includes the inspiratory reserve volume, the tidal volume, the expiratory reserve volume, and the residual volume.

Figure 2–16 depicts the range of manipulable lung volumes (in percent vital capacity, %VC) in a different graphic format than that just considered for the spirogram. This display indicates the lung volumes used in a number of everyday breathing activities. The resting level of the breathing apparatus is shown as 40 %VC in this figure.

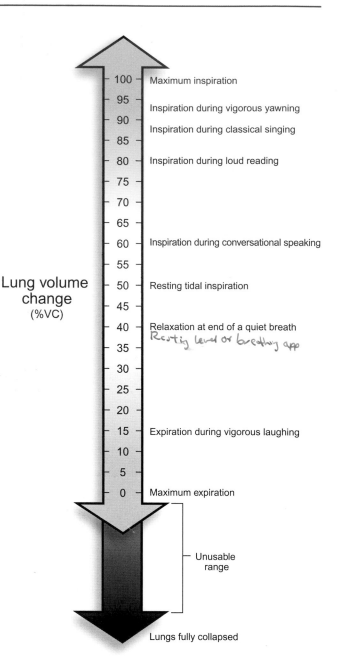

Figure 2–16. Lung volumes used in some everyday activities.

Pressure

Pressure is defined as a force distributed over a surface (pressure = force/area). The most important pressure for present purposes is the pressure inside the lungs. Recall that this pressure is termed the alveolar pressure. Alveolar pressure represents the sum of all the passive and active forces operating on the breathing apparatus.

Alveolar pressure is generated by the collision of air molecules within the lungs. When air molecules are more crowded, more collisions occur and pressure is higher. In contrast, when air molecules are less crowded, fewer collisions occur and alveolar pressure is lower. When the larynx and/or upper airway are closed, lung volume and alveolar pressure are inversely related. That is, a halving of volume causes a doubling of pressure, and a doubling of volume causes a halving of pressure (provided temperature remains constant).

One way to display alveolar pressure is in a volume-pressure diagram, such as that shown in Figure 2–17. The vertical axis of the diagram represents lung volume (in %VC) and the horizontal axis represents alveolar pressure (in centimeters of water, cmH$_2$O). The solid horizontal line represents the resting level of the breathing apparatus, shown to be 40 %VC in the diagram. The solid vertical line represents atmospheric pressure (zero, by convention). Points to the left of this line represent pressures that are below atmospheric (negative, by convention) and points to the right of this line represent pressures that are above atmospheric (positive, by convention). The three curves represent volume-pressure relations during relaxation, maximum inspiration, and maximum expiration.

The relaxation pressure is the pressure produced entirely by the passive force of the breathing apparatus. As shown in Figure 2–17, the relaxation pressure varies with lung volume. Relaxation pressure is positive at lung volumes larger than the resting level of the breathing apparatus, and negative at lung volumes smaller than the resting level. The greatest positive relaxation pressure is generated at the largest lung volume, and the greatest negative relaxation pressure is generated at the smallest lung volume. In the midrange of the vital capacity, the relaxation pressure changes nearly in direct proportion to lung volume change, whereas at the extremes of the vital capacity, pressure changes more abruptly with volume change. This is because the breathing apparatus is stiffer at very large and very small lung volumes.

Departures from the relaxation pressure require active muscular effort. A net inspiratory muscular pressure is needed to generate pressure that is lower than the relaxation pressure (to the left of the volume-pressure relaxation curve) at the prevailing lung volume. In contrast, a net expiratory muscular pressure is needed to generate pressure that is higher than the relaxation pressure (to the right of the curve) at the prevailing lung volume. When net is specified, as it

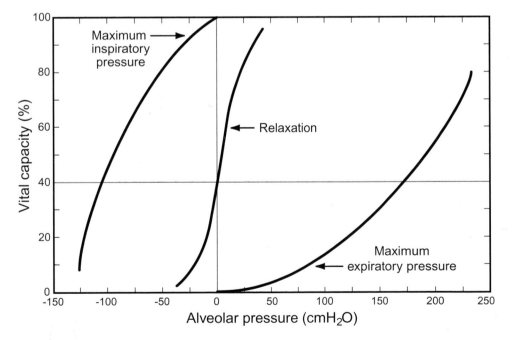

Figure 2-17. Volume-pressure diagram. From *Evaluation and management of speech breathing disorders: Principles and methods* (p. 38), by T. Hixon and J. Hoit, 2005, Tucson, AZ: Redington Brown. Copyright 2005 by Thomas J. Hixon and Jeannette D. Hoit. Modified and reproduced with permission.

Where Did That Come From?

We have seen many young children with cerebral palsy and breathing disorders. Many of these children, especially those who are quadriplegic and show major signs of spasticity, seem to have a governor on them. That is, they behave like there's a device that is limiting the degree to which they can willfully adjust the breathing apparatus. For example, when asked to perform an inspiratory capacity maneuver ("Take in all the air you can"), they may only be able to inspire to their resting tidal end-inspiratory level. Try it over and over again and the same thing happens. Then, out of the blue, the child shows you a gaping yawn of boredom and takes in an enormous breath. The breath may actually be several times the size the child could generate during voluntary inspiration. Now, you're faced with a dilemma. What do you record as the child's inspiratory capacity? Think about it, carefully.

Figure 2–18 shows the range of achievable alveolar pressures (in cmH$_2$O) in a different form of graphic display. Shown along the pressure scale is a list of activities and typical alveolar pressures associated with those activities.

is here, it means that both inspiratory and expiratory muscular pressures may be operating simultaneously, but one or the other is predominating. When pressure is equal to the relaxation pressure, this may mean that all the muscles of the breathing apparatus are relaxed, or it may mean that equal inspiratory and expiratory muscular pressures are being exerted so that they cancel one another.

The maximum inspiratory pressure that can be generated by the breathing apparatus is represented by the leftmost curve in Figure 2–17. The maximum inspiratory pressure is greater at smaller lung volumes than larger lung volumes. This is because negative relaxation pressure is more forceful at smaller lung volumes, and because the inspiratory muscles are operating under more favorable length-force conditions at smaller lung volumes.

The maximum expiratory pressure that can be generated by the breathing apparatus is represented by the rightmost curve in Figure 2–17. The maximum expiratory pressure is greater at larger lung volumes than smaller lung volumes. This is because positive relaxation pressure is more forceful at larger lung volumes, and because the expiratory muscles are operating under more favorable length-force conditions at larger lung volumes.

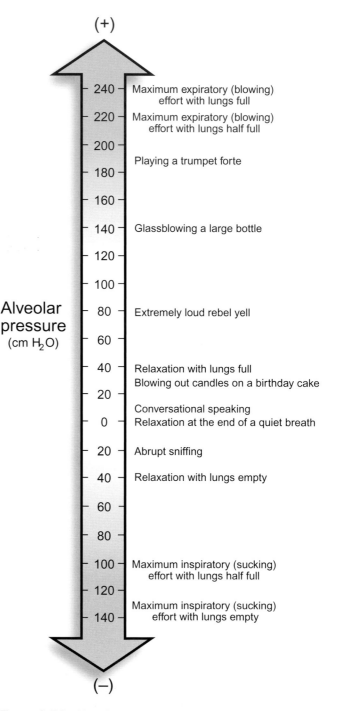

Figure 2-18. Alveolar pressures used for different activities.

Shape

Shape is the configuration of an object, independent of its size or volume. The shape of interest in the present context is the shape of the chest wall. More specifically, shape is the surface configuration of the rib cage wall and abdominal wall, the two parts of the chest wall that can be observed externally. Shape is important because it provides information about the prevailing mechanical advantages of different parts of the chest wall.

The rib cage wall and abdominal wall each usually behave with a single degree of freedom with respect to their movement. Thus, it is possible to characterize the shape of the chest wall when the relative sizes (which can be converted to volumes) of the rib cage wall and abdominal wall are monitored. One convention for illustrating shape is to display the relative sizes of the rib cage wall and abdominal wall against one another. This convention is portrayed in Figure 2–19, which displays rib cage wall anteroposterior (front-to-back) diameter (a measure of size) on the vertical axis, increasing upward, and abdominal

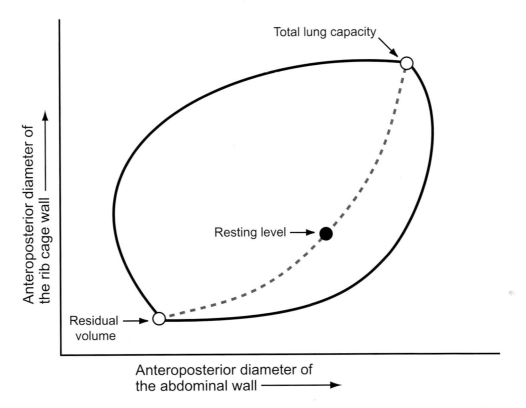

Figure 2–19. Relative diameter diagram. From *Evaluation and management of speech breathing disorders: Principles and methods* (p. 41), by T. Hixon and J. Hoit, 2005, Tucson, AZ: Redington Brown. Copyright 2005 by Thomas J. Hixon and Jeannette D. Hoit. Modified and reproduced with permission.

wall anteroposterior diameter on the horizontal axis, increasing rightward.

The dashed line in Figure 2–19 represents the relaxation characteristic of the chest wall. This is the shape assumed by the chest wall at different lung volumes when the breathing muscles are completely relaxed. The circle at the top of the relaxation characteristic represents the total lung capacity, and the circle at the bottom of the characteristic represents the residual volume. The filled circle near the middle of the characteristic represents the resting level of the breathing apparatus. The circumscribed area in the diagram depicts the full range of shapes that the chest wall can assume. The range of shapes is smaller near the diameter extremes, where both the rib cage wall and abdominal wall are very large or very small. The range of shapes is greatest in the diameter midrange.

Each point in Figure 2–19 represents a unique combination of chest wall shapes and lung volumes that can be interpreted in relation to underlying muscular mechanism. Figure 2–20 illustrates how this can be done.

Points on the relaxation characteristic in Figure 2–20 represent either complete relaxation of the muscles of the chest wall or equal and opposite muscular forces that cancel one another. Points that are not on the relaxation characteristic can only be achieved using active muscular force. Points to the left of the relaxation characteristic can be achieved using: (a) a net inspiratory

rib cage wall force, (b) an expiratory abdominal wall force, (c) a net inspiratory rib cage wall force and an expiratory abdominal wall force, or (d) a net expiratory rib cage wall force and a greater expiratory abdominal wall force. Points to the right of the relaxation characteristic can be achieved using: (a) a net expiratory rib cage wall force, or (b) a net expiratory rib cage wall force and a lesser expiratory abdominal wall force.

Figure 2–21 shows the range of achievable chest wall shapes (in relative terms) in a different form of

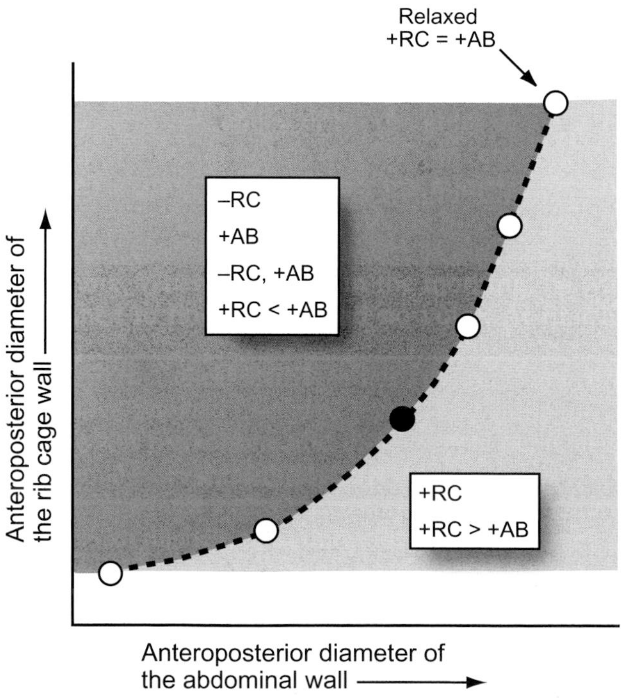

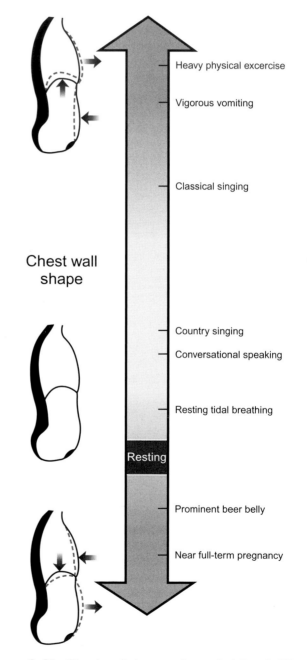

Figure 2-21. Chest wall shapes characteristic of different events and conditions.

Figure 2-20. Interpretation of muscular mechanism from the relative diameter diagram.

graphic display. Shown along the scale in the figure is a list of events and conditions and the chest wall shapes associated with them.

Neural Control of Breathing

Breathing movements are controlled by the nervous system. This section describes the neural bases of breathing with focus on its substrates and their participation in the control of tidal breathing and special acts of breathing. Detailed coverage of the nervous system is provided in Chapter 6.

Neural Substrates

Figure 2–22 depicts the structures of the nervous system that are important to the control of breathing. These structures are located in two major subdivisions

of the nervous system, the central nervous system and the peripheral nervous system.

The central nervous system includes the brain and spinal cord. The former is a mass of neural tissue within the skull and the latter is a long appendage of the brain that extends downward through the vertebral column.

The peripheral nervous system connects the central nervous system with different parts of the breathing apparatus. These connections are effected through cranial and spinal nerves. Four cranial nerves are participants in the control of breathing. These include cranial nerves IX (glossopharyngeal), X (vagus), and XII (hypoglossal), which innervate muscles that dilate the larynx and upper airway during inspiration, and cranial nerve IX (accessory), which innervates the *sternocleidomastoid* muscle that elevates the sternum, clavicle, and rib cage.

Twenty-two spinal nerves contribute to the control of breathing. These are listed in Table 2–2 along with

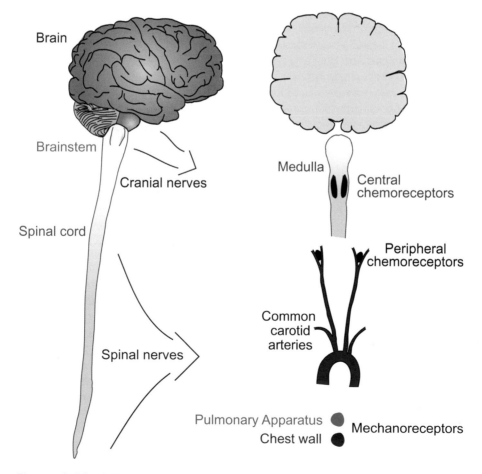

Figure 2–22. Adult nervous system. From *Evaluation and management of speech breathing disorders: Principles and methods* (p. 43), by T. Hixon and J. Hoit, 2005, Tucson, AZ: Redington Brown. Copyright 2005 by Thomas J. Hixon and Jeannette D. Hoit. Modified and reproduced with permission.

Table 2-2. Summary of the Segmental Origins of the Motor Nerve Supply to the Muscles of the Chest Wall

MUSCLE	SPINAL NERVE
RIB CAGE WALL	
Sternocleidomastoid[1]	C1–C5
Scalenus Group	C2–C8
Pectoralis Major	C5–C8
Pectoralis Minor	C5–C8
Subclavius	C5–C6
Serratus Anterior	C5–C7, T2–T3
External Intercostals	T1–T11
Internal Intercostals	T1–T11
Transversus Thoracis	T2–T6
Latissimus Dorsi	C6–C8
Serratus Posterior Superior	T2–T3
Serratus Posterior Inferior	T9–T12
Lateral Iliocostals Group	C4–T6, T1–T11, T7–L2
Levatores Costarum	C8–T11
Quadratus Lumborum	T12–L2
Subcostals	T1–T11
DIAPHRAGM	
Diaphragm	C3–C5
ABDOMINAL WALL	
Rectus Abdominis	T7–T12
External Oblique	T8–L1
Internal Oblique	T8–L1
Transversus Abdominis	T7–T12
Latissimus Dorsi	See above
Lateral Iliocostal Lumborum	See above
Quadratus Lumborum	See above

[1]Innervation of the **sternocleidomastoid** muscle comes from the spinal portion of the spinal accessory nerve, which is considered to be a cranial nerve (cranial nerve XI, see Chapter 6). The spinal accessory nerve also innervates the **trapezius** muscle; however, this muscle is not included in this chapter because it does not have a breathing function.

(C = cervical, T = thoracic, L = lumbar)

Source: Based on Dickson and Maue-Dickson (1982).

the muscles they innervate. As shown there, the spinal nerves relevant to breathing include the eight cervical (C) nerves, the twelve thoracic (T) nerves, and the first two lumbar (L) nerves. Successively lower spinal nerves generally provide motor nerve supply to successively lower regions of the breathing apparatus. An exception is the diaphragm, which derives its motor nerve supply from C3 to C5, a collection of motor nerves designated as the phrenic nerve. Table 2–2 lists only the motor nerve supply to the muscles of the chest wall. The sensory nerve supply to the chest wall is generally similar in pattern to its motor nerve supply, a notable exception being that the sensory supply of the diaphragm is vested in the phrenic nerve and lower thoracic nerves.

These neural substrates control a wide variety of breathing activities. Such activities can be associated with different states, including being awake, alert, aroused, asleep, conscious, or unconscious. Such activities can also be classified using different schemes that include terms such as automatic, metabolic, reflexive, learned, voluntary, behavioral, purposeful, or emotional. For present purposes, discussion of the control of breathing is organized around the simple dichotomy of tidal breathing and special acts of breathing.

Control of Tidal Breathing

Tidal breathing, the most common form of breathing, is sometimes called automatic breathing, metabolic breathing, or involuntary breathing. The control of tidal breathing is vested in the brainstem. Of special importance are structures located in the medulla, the region of the brainstem that is contiguous with the spinal cord. These structures include a network of neurons that are collectively designated as the lower brain center for breathing. The primary tasks of this lower brain center are to generate a rhythmic pattern of breathing and to regulate gas levels (oxygen and carbon dioxide) in arterial blood by adjusting ventilation (Feldman & McCrimmon, 1999; Lumb, 2000). The lower brain center can run breathing on its own automatically without input from higher brain centers and is often called the central pattern generator for breathing.

Signals from the brainstem travel via peripheral nerves to reach the muscles of the chest wall. For example, for inspiration, signals from the brainstem reach the **diaphragm** muscle via the phrenic nerve and cause its fibers to contract. Signals may also travel to the **external intercostal** muscles, causing them either to stiffen the rib cage wall (during resting tidal inspiration) or to assist the diaphragm as a supplemental prime mover (during more forceful tidal inspiration). Signals sent simultaneously to laryngeal and upper airway muscles increase the size of their associated airways to reduce the resistance to inspiratory airflow and stiffen the tissues that line them to reduce their chances of being sucked inward.

The breathing pattern generated by the brainstem is strongly conditioned by afferent (incoming) information from a variety of sources. Most of the time, this afferent information is received and processed unconsciously. Sometimes, however, afferent information is processed to a level of awareness (sensation) or to a level of meaning and association (perception). At such times, individuals may begin to consciously attend to their breathing and to develop breathing-related perceptions having to do with forces, movements, and feelings of breathing comfort, to give a few examples.

The most important afferent information comes from chemoreceptors and mechanoreceptors. Chemoreceptors are sensitive to chemical status and those most relevant to breathing are called central and peripheral chemoreceptors. Central chemoreceptors, which are located on the front and side surfaces of the medulla, respond primarily to changes in the amount of carbon dioxide in cerebral spinal fluid. Peripheral chemoreceptors are located in the carotid bodies at the bifurcation of the common carotid arteries, near the major blood supply to the brain. These are the primary oxygen receptors for the body, although they also respond to changes in the level of carbon dioxide and acidity-alkalinity balance in arterial blood. Central and peripheral chemoreceptors generally act synergistically to stimulate adjustments in breathing by providing moment-to-moment updates on the concentration of gas in the blood. Changes in the concentration of gas stimulate the brainstem to make appropriate adjustments in ventilation. For example, an increase in carbon dioxide or a decrease in oxygen stimulates the brainstem to send signals through the peripheral nerves to the chest wall muscles to increase breathing.

Mechanoreceptors are sensitive to mechanical changes and those of special importance to the control of tidal breathing are located in the pulmonary apparatus and chest wall. Those in the pulmonary apparatus respond to stimuli such as the stretching of smooth muscles (such as occurs with an increase in lung volume), airway irritants (such as smoke, dust, chemicals, or cold air), and distortions of the alveolar wall (such as might occur when excess fluid surrounds the alveoli). Signals from these pulmonary mechanoreceptors reach the central nervous system by way of cranial nerve X. Mechanoreceptors in the chest wall respond to changes in muscle length (such as occur with changes in rib cage wall or abdominal wall volume) or changes in force (such as occur with changes in inspiratory or expiratory muscular efforts). Their afferent signals reach the central nervous system via spinal nerves.

Other afferent input can also influence tidal breathing (Shea, Walter, Pelley, Murphy, & Guz, 1987; Wyke, 1974). For example, afferent signals from mechanoreceptors located in the larynx or upper airway and signals from cranial nerves that transmit visual and auditory information (cranial nerves II and VIII, respectively) can affect breathing. Thus, tidal breathing can be altered by the presence of an irritant in the larynx or upper airway, by the images in an action-packed movie, or by rhythms of a musical concert.

Tidal breathing can also be influenced by internally generated activity from brain areas outside the brainstem (Mador & Tobin, 1991; Shea, 1996; Shea, Murphy, Hamilton, Benchetrit, & Guz, 1988; Western & Patrick, 1988). For example, cognitive activity (originating from cortical areas), such as that associated with the performance of mental arithmetic, can change tidal breathing. In fact, merely being consciously aware of breathing can change its pattern. Emotional influences (originating from limbic areas) can also have a profound influence on tidal breathing. Feelings of excitement, anger, or fear, for example, can be associated with hyperventilation, breath holding, or erratic breathing. Changes in tidal breathing can even be a primary sign (and feelings of breathlessness a primary symptom) of certain psychogenic disorders, such as anxiety disorder or panic disorder. These types of disorders have been so strongly linked to breathing that they are sometimes classified as hyperventilation disorders (Gardner, 1996).

Control of Special Acts of Breathing

Special acts of breathing can be defined as acts of breathing that are not effected for the primary purpose of maintaining homeostasis of arterial blood gases (Shea, 1996). They are controlled by higher brain centers that either override or bypass activity of the lower (brainstem) center for breathing. Special acts of breathing can be voluntary (highly conscious), such as breath holding or performing a guided breathing exercise. Or, they can be learned, well practiced, and require little conscious control of breathing—for example, breathing associated with glass blowing, wind instrument playing, singing, or speaking. Other special acts of breathing, such as laughing or crying, are driven primarily by emotions.

As with any voluntary motor act, a voluntary act of breathing requires a motor program. Motor programs and the process of generating them are complex and only partially understood. What is known for sure is that many brain centers participate in the process, including cortical and subcortical structures. As a behavior becomes learned and less consciously

Breathing as a Laughing Matter

Breathing plays a huge role in laughter. Much of laughter, especially the hearty type, goes on within the expiratory reserve volume. Laughter also involves large movements of the abdominal wall. This is probably the reason our folk language is riddled with statements like "I busted a gut laughing," "He kept me in stitches with his jokes," and "We laughed 'til our sides hurt." The neural mechanisms that underlie laughter are different from those that underlie speech breathing. This is illustrated dramatically in persons who can't move the abdominal wall on command or use it for speech production, but show vigorous movement of the wall during involuntary laughter. Thus, even if someone appears to be paralyzed, it's always wise to ask the question, "Paralyzed for what activity?"

guided, there is likely to be less reliance on cortical participation in the development of the motor program. Commands from higher brain centers can be integrated at the brainstem level such that they override the central pattern generator for breathing. Commands can also be routed directly from the cortex to spinal nerves, bypassing the brainstem altogether (Corfield, Murphy, & Guz, 1998) and imposing cortical control over the breathing act.

Special acts of breathing that are associated with emotional expression are driven by the limbic system, a phylogenetically old part of the brain. The limbic system has a strong influence on the control of special acts of breathing such as crying and laughing. Crying and laughing can even override voluntary acts of breathing, indicating that limbic drive can prevail over cortical drive. Consider, for example, the situation of attempting to speak while sobbing.

It is common for the nervous system to manage multiple breathing-related drives simultaneously, and often these drives compete with one another. Voluntary breath holding is one example. Breath holding is controlled by the cerebral cortex and is a clear demonstration of the ability of the cortex to override the brainstem. Nevertheless, cortical control must eventually give way to brainstem control as danger signals from chemoreceptors make it impossible to continue to inhibit inspiration. Less dramatic examples of competing drives occur frequently and include situations such as attempting to speak while exercising, or playing a wind instrument while experiencing stage fright.

Ventilation and Gas Exchange During Tidal Breathing

Tidal breathing is the most common type of breathing. Its name comes from the ebb and flow of air that resembles the ebb and flow of an ocean tide. Tidal breathing is driven by the need to ventilate (to move air in and out of the pulmonary apparatus) for the purpose of gas exchange (to deliver oxygen, O_2, to the body and remove carbon dioxide, CO_2, from it).

Figure 2–23 depicts the process of gas exchange during tidal breathing. Air, which consists of approximately 21% oxygen, enters the alveoli during tidal breathing. Oxygen then leaves the alveoli and enters

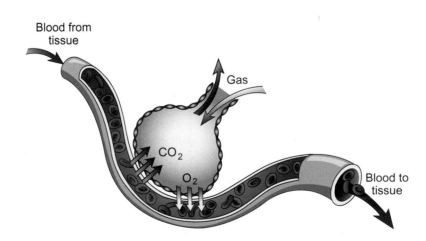

Figure 2–23. Process of gas exchange during tidal breathing.

the bloodstream to travel to tissues throughout the body. Tissues absorb oxygen from the blood and return carbon dioxide (a byproduct of metabolism) to the blood. The carbon dioxide then travels through the bloodstream and eventually reaches the alveoli where it is released. When metabolic demand increases, as with increased physical or mental activity, more oxygen is consumed and more carbon dioxide is produced.

Tidal breathing at rest is associated with a relatively regular inspiration-expiration pattern that begins and ends at the resting level of the breathing apparatus. This pattern is exemplified for lung volume (in liters, L), airflow (in liters per second, LPS), and alveolar pressure (in cmH$_2$O) in Figure 2–24. During inspiration, the chest wall expands, causing the lungs to expand and alveolar pressure to fall. This creates a pressure gradient, with the pressure inside the pulmonary apparatus being lower than that outside the apparatus. As a result, air flows into the pulmonary apparatus. When equilibration is reached (the pressure outside and inside the pulmonary apparatus are equal) inspiratory airflow ceases.

Expiratory airflow begins as the lungs compress and alveolar pressure rises. Such airflow continues until the resting level of the breathing apparatus is reached. These patterns of volume, airflow, and pressure change are generally the same across body positions, except that the absolute lung volume range differs with body position. For example, resting tidal breathing may range from 40 to 50 %VC in upright body positions and from 20 to 30 %VC in the supine body position.

Resting tidal breathing is driven by a combination of passive and active forces. These are summarized graphically in Figure 2–25 for the upright and supine body positions. During inspiration, essentially all of the active force comes from the diaphragm. The diaphragm contracts and displaces the rib cage wall and abdominal wall outward. This is true for all body positions. In the upright body position, some rib cage wall muscles and abdominal wall muscles are also active during inspiration (Hixon, Goldman, & Mead, 1973; Loring & Mead, 1982). Rib cage wall muscle activity stiffens the rib cage wall to prevent it from being sucked inward when the diaphragm contracts. Abdominal wall muscle activity usually causes the abdominal wall to move inward. When the abdominal wall moves inward, the rib cage wall is lifted and the diaphragm is pushed headward. This stretches the fibers of the diaphragm so that they are placed on more favorable portions of their length-force characteristics for contraction. In the supine body position, as in the upright body position, the rib cage wall muscles are slightly active to stiffen the

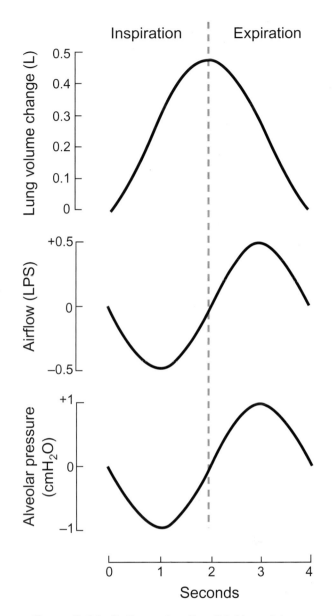

Figure 2-24. Pattern of resting tidal breathing.

rib cage wall. However, in contrast to upright body positions, the abdominal wall muscles are relaxed. This is because the abdominal wall is already pulled inward and the diaphragm is already pushed headward by the force of gravity.

During resting tidal expiration, the relaxation pressure of the breathing apparatus moves the rib cage wall and abdominal wall inward. Thus, resting tidal expiration is primarily a passive event. Nevertheless, in the upright body position, the abdominal wall muscles remain active throughout the resting tidal breathing cycle.

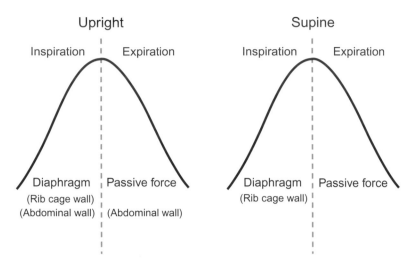

Figure 2–25. Passive and active forces of resting tidal breathing.

Although resting tidal breathing shares general features across individuals, its specific details differ from person to person. In fact, each person has what might be thought of as a signature resting tidal breathing pattern that remains relatively unchanged over the years (Benchetrit et al., 1989; Dejours, 1996; Shea & Guz, 1992; Shea, Horner, Benchetrit, & Guz, 1990; Shea, Walter, Murphy, & Guz, 1987).

Ribbit, Ribbit

Ever watch a frog breathe? Did you notice how its cheeks moved? Frogs don't have a diaphragm to pull air into their lungs. They push the air in using their mouths like pistons. Frogs are positive pressure breathers. People are negative pressure breathers. A frog doesn't have the ability to emulate us (except, perhaps, Kermit) if its positive pressure pump fails. But, we have the ability to emulate the frog if our negative pressure pump fails, by doing what is called glossopharyngeal breathing. And what would you suppose is the common name for such breathing? Well, it's "frog breathing." In frog breathing, the tongue and throat are used to pump air into the lungs. Air is gulped in small portions (mouthfuls), each held in place by closing the larynx as a one-way valve. Frog breathing isn't difficult to learn and once mastered can be used to fill the lungs in a stepwise fashion all the way to the top.

BREATHING AND SPEECH PRODUCTION

The breathing apparatus provides the driving forces that enable the generation of speech. Actions of the breathing apparatus during speech production contribute to the control of speech intensity (loudness), voice frequency (pitch), linguistic stress (emphasis), and the segmentation (division) of speech into units (syllables, words, phrases). At the same time the breathing apparatus performs these speech-related functions, it continues to serve its primary functions of ventilation and gas exchange.

This section describes two forms of speech breathing—extended steady utterances and running speech activities—as performed in the upright body position (standing or seated erect). Following these descriptions, consideration is given to speech breathing as it relates to other body positions, ventilation and gas exchange, drive to breathe, cognitive-linguistic factors, conversational interchange, body type, development, age, and sex.

Breathing in Extended Steady Utterances

Extended steady utterances are those that are produced throughout most of the vital capacity. An extended steady utterance begins after taking the deepest inspiration possible and continues until the air supply is depleted. Such an utterance might be a sustained vowel, a series of repeated syllables of equal stress, or a sung note. Extended steady utterances are considered here following the conceptualizations and elaborations of others (Hixon, 1973; Hixon & Hoit, 2005; Hixon, Mead, & Goldman, 1976; Weismer, 1985).

Figure 2–26 shows the volume, pressure, and shape events associated with a sustained vowel produced at a usual and steady loudness, pitch, and voice quality. As can be seen in the figure, lung volume decreases at a constant rate throughout the utterance. Alveolar pressure rises abruptly, remains steady throughout the utterance, and falls abruptly as the utterance ends. Rib cage wall volume and abdominal wall volume, which together reflect the shape of the chest wall, decrease at constant and similar rates.

Both relaxation pressure and muscular pressure contribute to extended steady utterance production.

This is illustrated in Figure 2–27 for the same utterance depicted in Figure 2–26. In the top panel of Figure 2–27, alveolar pressure (in cmH$_2$O) is plotted on the horizontal axis, ranging from negative (inspiratory) to positive (expiratory). Lung volume (in %VC) is plotted on the vertical axis, with 40 %VC representing the resting level of the breathing apparatus. Recall that the resting level is the level at which the breathing apparatus is in a mechanically neutral position and alveolar pressure is the same as atmospheric pressure, or zero. Note that the relaxation pressure is positive at lung volumes larger than the resting level and negative at lung volumes smaller than the resting level. The targeted alveolar pressure is shown to be constant throughout the lung volume (this is analogous to the pressure tracing from Figure 2–26, oriented vertically instead of horizontally).

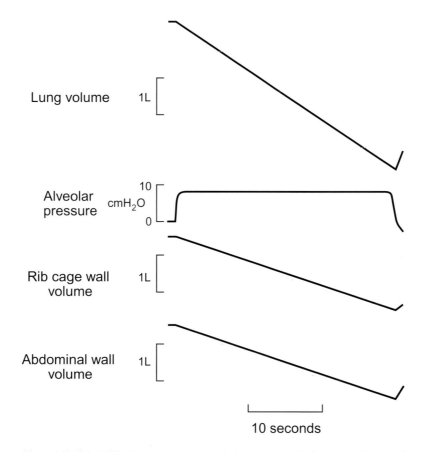

Figure 2–26. Volume, pressure, and shape events for an extended steady utterance produced in the upright body position. Only expiration (speaking) is represented. From *Evaluation and management of speech breathing disorders: Principles and methods* (p. 57), by T. Hixon and J. Hoit, 2005, Tucson, AZ: Redington Brown. Copyright 2005 by Thomas J. Hixon and Jeannette D. Hoit. Modified and reproduced with permission.

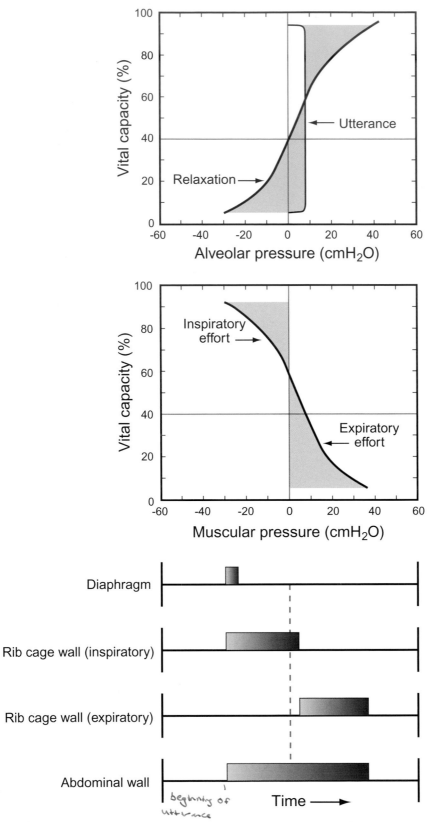

Figure 2-27. Relaxation pressure, targeted alveolar pressure, muscular pressure, and temporal activity of chest wall components for a sustained vowel produced in the upright body position. Only expiration (speaking) is represented. From *Evaluation and management of speech breathing disorders: Principles and methods* (p. 59), by T. Hixon and J. Hoit, 2005, Tucson, AZ: Redington Brown. Copyright 2005 by Thomas J. Hixon and Jeannette D. Hoit. Modified and reproduced with permission.

Complete Relaxation

Complete relaxation isn't as easy as it sounds. When you attempt to relax your breathing muscles for observations like those discussed in the text, nobody knows for sure how successful you are. Some people are able to quiet the electrical activity of their major breathing muscles. But, that isn't evidence of complete relaxation, because it's not feasible to monitor the electrical activity of all the muscles of breathing. Respiratory physiologists consider people to be "excellent relaxers" if they're able to produce repeatable relaxation pressures throughout the vital capacity without any feedback other than the usual sensations associated with the task. Such people are also thought to be excellent bets for "complete relaxation" because their data correspond well with those obtained during studies of drug-induced paralysis in humans. How would you like to be in one of those studies? Not we. We're content with not knowing if we can completely relax.

The middle panel of Figure 2–27 shows the muscular pressure required to achieve the targeted alveolar pressure. At large lung volumes (near the beginning of the utterance), a negative (inspiratory) muscular pressure is required to counteract the high positive (expiratory) relaxation pressure. In the mid-lung-volume range, a slight positive muscular pressure is required to achieve the targeted alveolar pressure. And, at small lung volumes (near the end of the utterance), increasingly greater positive muscular pressure is required. By studying the top two panels of Figure 2–27, it should be clear that it is possible to specify the required muscular pressure by knowing the targeted alveolar pressure and the relaxation pressure at the prevailing lung volume. In this example, the targeted alveolar pressure for an extended steady utterance of normal loudness is 8 cmH2O. The targeted alveolar pressure is higher for louder utterances and lower for softer utterances. For higher targeted alveolar pressures (loud speech), less negative muscular pressures are required at large lung volumes and more positive muscular pressures are required at small lung volumes. In contrast, for lower targeted alveolar pressures (soft speech), more negative muscular pressures are required at large lung volumes and less positive muscular pressures are required at small lung volumes.

The bottom panel of Figure 2–27 illustrates the activities of the different components of the breathing apparatus in the generation of muscular pressure.[1] The solid horizontal bars indicate when the different components of the chest wall are active. The darker the shading within the bars, the greater the magnitude of the muscular pressure being generated. Reading from left to right, the panel shows that the diaphragm (inspiratory), the inspiratory rib cage wall component, and the abdominal wall (expiratory) component are active at the beginning of the utterance. The diaphragm and the inspiratory rib cage wall component generate the negative pressure required to counteract the positive relaxation pressure in this large lung volume range. However, the diaphragm shuts off very quickly and the inspiratory rib cage wall component alone assumes the role of "braking" against the high expiratory relaxation pressure. At the instant the inspiratory rib cage wall component shuts off, the expiratory rib cage wall component becomes active and remains active until the end of the utterance. Note that the abdominal wall component is active throughout the utterance.

Thus, extended steady utterance is produced using a continuously changing combination of relaxation pressure and muscular pressure, and a continuously changing activation of different chest wall components. Relaxation pressure goes from substantially positive to substantially negative. Muscular pressure follows an opposite pattern, going from substantially negative to substantially positive. The inspiratory muscles of the rib cage wall do nearly all of the inspiratory work at large lung volumes and the expiratory muscles of the rib cage wall and abdominal wall muscles do all of the expiratory work. Interestingly, the abdominal wall

---

[1]This panel is based on the work of Hixon et al. (1976) and was distilled by Hixon and Hoit (2005) into the simple graphic display shown. The actions of the rib cage wall, diaphragm, and abdominal wall portrayed in the panel are based on strain-stress (volume-pressure) analyses, which enabled the determination of the individual muscular pressure contributions of different components of the chest wall. The data required for these analyses included rib cage wall volume, abdominal wall volume, and lung volume (estimated via respiratory magnetometers — devices described in this chapter), as well as pleural pressure, abdominal pressure, and transdiaphragmatic pressure (estimated from catheter-balloon devices swallowed into the esophagus and stomach and connected to pressure transducers). The data of Hixon et al. do not specify how individual muscles contribute to the muscular pressure generated by each chest wall part (except for the diaphragm, where there is only a single muscle in the part). Such data as are available on how individual muscles function have come from the use of electromyography, a method that senses the electrical activity of muscles through the use of metal electrodes placed over them or inserted directly into them. Available data of this type are piecemeal, incomplete, and, in some cases, are known to be invalid (Hixon & Weismer, 1995).

muscles are active throughout the utterance, even at times when a net negative pressure is required.

Why do the inspiratory muscles of the rib cage wall do most of the inspiratory braking rather than the diaphragm? The answer to this question is a mechanical one and is illustrated in Figure 2–28. When the inspiratory muscles of the rib cage wall contract and the diaphragm is inactive, the rib cage wall expands and pleural and abdominal pressures decrease. The decrease in abdominal pressure causes the liquid-filled abdominal content to place a downward hydraulic pull on the undersurface of the diaphragm. This hydraulic pull creates a stable base against which the inspiratory muscles of the rib cage wall can contract, without the diaphragm having to contract to stay in position. In effect, the hydraulic pull of the abdominal content enables the inspiratory muscles of the rib cage wall to simultaneously elevate the rib cage wall and pull downward on the diaphragm. There is no need to activate two sets of muscles under this circumstance, because the inspiratory muscles of the rib cage wall can effectively perform the function of two chest wall components. This mechanism works in the upright body position, but not in the supine body position, as discussed below.

Why do the muscles of the abdominal wall remain active throughout extended steady utterance, even when a net inspiratory muscular pressure is required (at large lung volumes)? The answer appears to be that activation of the abdominal wall enhances the precision and control of speech breathing. When the diaphragm

is inactive (as it is throughout almost all of extended steady utterance production), any pressure change is manifested identically across both the rib cage wall and abdominal wall (the breathing apparatus becomes a single compartment functionally). Whether such pressure resolves into movement of the rib cage wall, abdominal wall, or both, depends on the relative impedance of the two structures. If one part has relatively high impedance (due to muscle activation) and the other has relatively low impedance (due to absence of muscle activation), then alveolar pressure change will initially result in movement of the low impedance part.

Hixon and Hoit (2005) have suggested a simple analogy for the concepts just discussed. This analogy is portrayed in Figure 2–29 and discussed in the following quote from their work.

The inefficiencies that would result from not using simultaneous activity in the two parts can be appreciated by performing some simple maneuvers on a long inflated balloon (representing the breathing apparatus) containing a squeaker in its neck (representing the larynx). If the half of the balloon nearest the squeaker (representing the rib cage wall) is squeezed (to simulate a decreasing rib cage wall volume achieved by a decreasing rib cage wall inspiratory effort), pressure inside the balloon (representing alveolar pressure) will increase and cause the other half of the balloon (representing the abdominal wall) to move outward. However, if both halves of the balloon are squeezed simultaneously (representing decreases in rib cage wall volume and

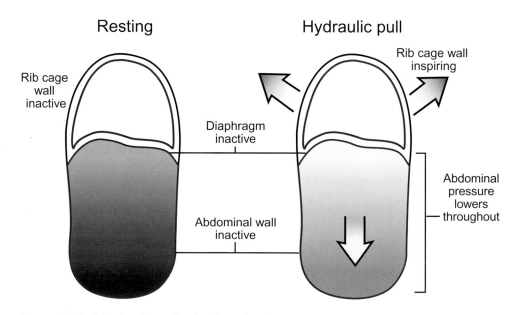

Figure 2–28. Mechanism of hydraulic pull of the abdominal content on the diaphragm.

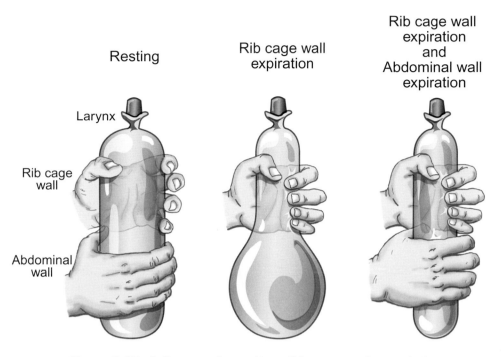

Figure 2-29. Balloon analogy of breathing apparatus control.

abdominal wall volume), less extensive and slower movement is required of the half representing the rib cage wall to achieve an equivalent pressure adjustment. This also means that an unproductive outward (paradoxical) movement of the half of the balloon representing the abdominal wall is avoided. When both halves of the balloon are moved inward simultaneously, it is possible to have greater precision of control over the pressure inside the balloon. (p. 63)

Breathing in Running Speech Activities

Running speech activities present different demands and require a different set of muscular strategies than extended steady utterances. Running speech activities include reading aloud, extemporaneous speaking, conversational speaking, and other activities that demand relatively continual utterance production. As with the discussion for extended steady utterances, running speech activities are considered here following the earlier conceptualizations and elaborations of Hixon (1973), Hixon et al. (1976), Weismer (1985), and Hixon and Hoit (2005).

Volume, pressure, and shape events associated with running speech activities are much more varied than those associated with extended steady utterances. This is because running speech is characterized by vari-

ations in phonetic content (sounds that differ in voicing and manner of production), prosody (utterances that differ in rate, intonation, loudness variation, and linguistic stress), and voice quality (utterances that differ in breathiness and timbre).

Volume events during running speech activities usually occur in the midrange of the vital capacity. As illustrated in Figure 2–30, conversational speech production generally starts at twice resting tidal breathing depth (or less) and continues to near the resting level of the breathing apparatus, although at times it may encroach upon the expiratory reserve volume. There are mechanical advantages to speaking in this lung volume range. To begin, the breathing apparatus is not as stiff and the relaxation pressure is not as extreme as at very large and very small lung volumes. Furthermore, the relaxation pressure is positive for most running speech production (because relaxation pressure is positive at lung volumes larger than the resting level of the breathing apparatus) and this positive pressure is used to supplement the positive muscular pressure required. When speech production encroaches upon the expiratory reserve volume, muscular pressure must be exerted against a negative relaxation pressure.

Alveolar pressure is relatively steady during running speech production. Small variations in pressure are typically associated with linguistic stress, wherein stressed (relatively more prominent) syllables are

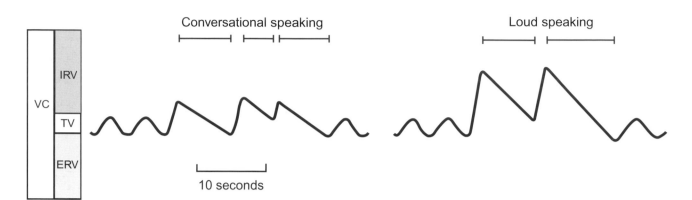

Figure 2–30. Volume events during running speech production.

What's Your Sign?

Speech is usually produced on expiration. But it's possible to produce it on inspiration. Try it. It's a bit awkward and difficult at first and your voice may sound higher in pitch and be more harsh than usual. But, you should be able to produce quite intelligible speech during inspiration, especially if you whisper. Once in a while, a person is encountered who uses inspiratory speech production. For example, we've seen people who produce voice more easily on inspiration than expiration following surgical reconstruction of a damaged larynx. Some people become so proficient at inspiratory speech production that you can be tricked into believing you're observing expiratory speech production (with a voice quality disorder). Never take a speaker's sign for granted.

generated by momentary pressure increases. Sometimes alveolar pressure declines slightly at the ends of breath groups, particularly at the ends of declarative sentences where loudness and pitch tend to decrease.

Rib cage wall and abdominal wall volumes generally decrease throughout the breath group in running speech activities. In most people, rib cage wall volume decreases at a much faster rate than abdominal wall volume. Recall that the rib cage wall covers a much larger surface of the lungs than does the abdominal wall (indirectly, through the diaphragm). Thus, the rib cage wall is well suited for effecting lung volume change for running speech activities.

Both relaxation pressure and muscular pressure contribute to the production of running speech breath-ing, as illustrated in Figure 2–31. The targeted alveolar pressure is usually higher (more positive) than the prevailing relaxation pressure (top panel of figure), so that positive muscular pressure must be added to the relaxation pressure throughout the breath group (middle panel of figure). To maintain the targeted alveolar pressure, the magnitude of the positive muscular pressure increases as the breath group proceeds because the relaxation pressure becomes increasingly less positive, and might even become negative if the breath group continues through lung volumes that are smaller than the resting level of the breathing apparatus. There is usually not a need to use inspiratory muscular pressure during running speech production, unless utterance is initiated at a larger than usual lung volume, and then inspiratory braking might be required briefly.

For running speech activities that are louder or softer than normal, targeted alveolar pressures are higher or lower, respectively, than those used to generate usual running speech. Thus, higher than normal muscular pressure is required for louder speech and lower than normal muscular pressure is required for softer speech at the prevailing lung volume. Nevertheless, it is important to note that louder speech is often initiated at larger lung volumes (see Figure 2-30), where the prevailing relaxation pressure is greater.

As depicted in the bottom panel of Figure 2–31, the expiratory phase of most running speech is produced with expiratory rib cage wall and abdominal wall muscular pressures, the latter predominating. The inspiratory phase of the running speech breathing cycle (not included in the figure) is driven by the diaphragm. Interestingly, expiratory muscles of the rib cage wall and abdominal wall maintain a low level of activity during inspiration. This enables them to be in a state of readiness to begin driving expiration (speech production) as soon as inspiration has ended.

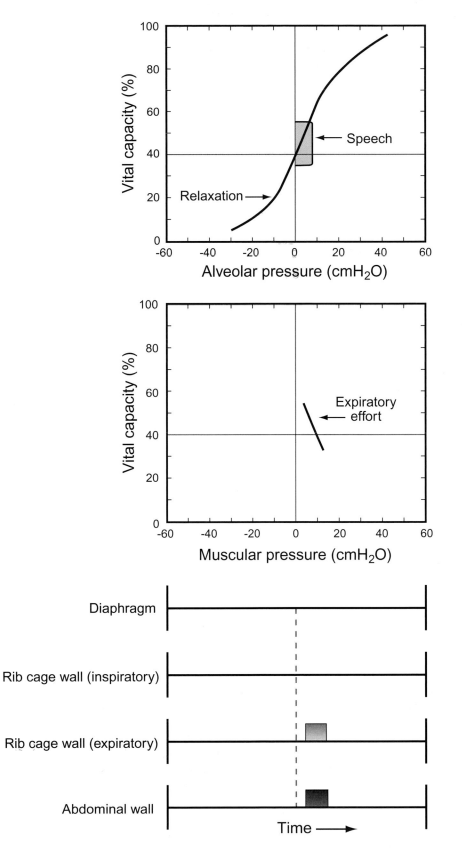

Figure 2–31. Relaxation pressure, targeted alveolar pressure, muscular pressure, and temporal activity of chest wall components for a running speech activity performed in the upright body position. Only expiration (speaking) is represented.

The abdominal wall plays an important role in running speech breathing. It generates most of the expiratory muscular pressure during speech production. It is also responsible for imposing the general background configuration assumed by the chest wall throughout the speech breathing cycle. As it turns out, there are important advantages to having the abdominal wall play such a prominent role in running speech breathing.

Figure 2–32 illustrates these advantages in the context of the shape of the chest wall for running speech activities. Inward displacement of the abdominal wall (by its own muscular action) has important consequences for the diaphragm and rib cage wall. As the abdominal wall moves inward, the diaphragm is pushed headward such that its radius of curvature increases and its principal muscle fibers elongate. This positions the diaphragm so that it can produce the quick and powerful inspirations that are critical for minimizing interruptions during running speech activities. Inward displacement of the abdominal wall also lifts the rib cage wall. This stretches the expiratory muscles of the rib cage wall, thereby increasing their potential for generating the quick expiratory pulses needed to produce linguistic stress and loudness change. Also, with the abdominal wall held firmly inward, expiratory efforts by the rib cage wall can be fully resolved into pressure change. If the abdominal wall were not held firmly in place, expiratory efforts of the rib cage wall would be resolved into outward movement of the abdominal wall before a pressure change could be effected (recall the balloon analogy provided above). Thus, the activation of abdominal wall muscles and the resultant inward displacement serve to "mechanically tune" the breathing apparatus for inspiration and expiration during running speech breathing. When the abdominal wall muscles are impaired, speech breathing is predictably impaired (recall the Scenario at the start of the chapter and see its continuation at the end of the chapter).

A good deal of information about volume, pressure, and shape events for running speech activities is carried in the speech (acoustic) signal. Thus, it is possible for a listener to gather clues about running speech breathing by just listening to a person's speech. Breath group length provides clues about volume events. In general, the longer the breath group, the larger the volume excursion. Loudness provides clues about alveolar pressure. As a general rule, the louder the speech produced, the higher the alveolar pressure. Finally, inspiratory duration and the rate of loudness change provide clues about the shape of the chest wall. When the chest wall is configured appropriately for speech production (larger than relaxed rib cage wall and smaller than relaxed abdominal wall), inspirations are short and loudness changes for linguistic stress are quick.

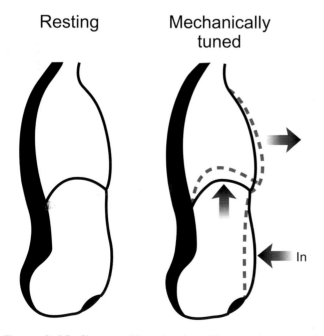

Resting   Mechanically tuned

In

Figure 2-32. Shape of the chest wall for running speech activities.

Thomas J. Hixon (1940–2009)

What is this? An author writing a sidetrack about himself? No, it's the other two authors writing about Tom Hixon, who left us too early to help with this second edition, because we want you to know something about him. At age 25, Tom burst on the scene, having already completed his master's degree (in 1 year) and his PhD (in 2 years!) from University of Iowa. His intense fascination of speech breathing led him to Harvard where, under the tutelage of Jere Mead, Tom learned about respiratory mechanics. He spent hours each day in Countway Library poring over articles on respiratory physiology and then more hours poring over data in the laboratory. He immersed himself for years, doing the experiment again and again, until he understood beyond doubt exactly how the respiratory system works for speech production. He completely revolutionized our understanding of this complicated system, and then presented it with elegant simplicity in this text. You can thank Tom for everything you know about speech breathing.

Adaptive Control of Speech Breathing

Although speech breathing is usually carried out in the ways described above, there are many other ways it can be performed. This means that speech breathing can be adapted when the circumstances call for change.

Adaptive control is not unique to speech breathing, but occurs in essentially all motor control systems. For example, if a violinist breaks a string during a performance, he may decide not to stop, but rather to continue playing by reprogramming his usual fingering (Wolff, 1979). In a skilled violinist, this reprogramming can be done instantly and without much effort. This is adaptation par excellence. The violinist adapts by allowing the "motor idea" to control the performance. The goal is the important thing, not the way it is attained.

Adaptive control is commonplace in speech breathing as well. For example, a speaker must adapt when body position changes, when ventilatory drive changes (as with exercise or a change in elevation), when a tight-fitting belt restricts chest wall movement, or when the air temperature is extremely hot or cold. Experimental work has provided interesting documentation as to how speech breathing can be changed without compromising its output goals (Bouhuys, Proctor, & Mead, 1966; Hixon et al., 1973; Hixon & Weismer, 1995; Warren, Morr, Rochet, & Dalston, 1989).

For example, by increasing the effective relaxation pressure of the breathing apparatus (by using a device to lower the pressure at the airway opening), it is possible to change the usual strategy for braking against high positive relaxation pressure at large lung volumes. Whereas a person usually brakes almost solely with the inspiratory muscles of the rib cage wall (when in an upright body position), the diaphragm supplements the braking effort of the rib cage wall when relaxation pressure is made to be abnormally high.

As another example, although the usual background shape of the chest wall is relatively constant, it is possible to produce speech with a constantly changing chest wall shape. This can be demonstrated by moving the abdominal wall in and out repeatedly while sustaining a vowel and maintaining a constant alveolar pressure (voice loudness).

Another example is one that involves interaction with another part of the speech production apparatus, the velopharynx. When a velopharyngeal leak is created experimentally (by "talking through the nose"), a person will expire more air than usual while speaking. This adaptation serves to maintain adequate levels of oral pressure to achieve suitable consonant production.

A final example is one that happens in many everyday situations. A person in an upright body posi-

tion usually performs running speech activities using a chest wall shape in which the rib cage wall is larger and the abdominal wall is smaller than their respective sizes during rest at the prevailing lung volume. However, when the arms are folded across the front of the rib cage wall, the same person will use a chest wall shape that involves a smaller than usual rib cage wall size and a larger than usual abdominal wall size. This is because the abdominal wall surrenders to the heavy mechanical load imposed by the folded arms.

Body Position and Speech Breathing

A change in body position may alter the mechanical behavior of the breathing apparatus, primarily because gravity has such a strong influence on this massive structure. Thus, with each new body position, a new mechanical solution may need to be found for speech breathing. Most of this section is devoted to discussion of the supine body position (as contrasted to the upright body position discussed above), but other body positions are considered as well. As with the sections on extended steady utterances and running speech activities, the discussion here is based on conceptualizations and elaborations of Hixon (1973), Hixon et al. (1976), and Hixon and Hoit (2005).

Figure 2–33 depicts the influence of gravity on different parts of the chest wall in the upright and supine body positions. In the upright body position,

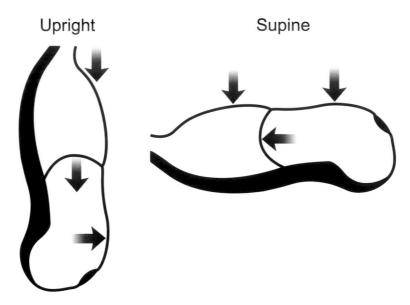

Figure 2–33. Gravitational effects on the breathing apparatus.

gravity acts in the expiratory direction on the rib cage wall, tending to reduce its size, whereas gravity acts in the inspiratory direction on the abdominal wall, tending to increase its size. When a shift is made to the supine body position, gravity acts in the expiratory direction on both the rib cage wall and abdominal wall. This causes the relaxation pressure to be greater at any given lung volume in the supine body position than in upright body position. The expiratory gravitational force exerted on the abdominal wall pushes the diaphragm headward, causing the resting level of the breathing apparatus to decrease to about 20 %VC from its upright value of about 40 %VC. These changes in the mechanical status of the breathing apparatus have an effect on speech breathing.

Extended Steady Utterances in the Supine Body Position

Figure 2–34 represents a sustained vowel of normal loudness produced throughout the vital capacity in the supine body position, and is analogous to Figure 2–27 for the upright body position. Comparison of the top panels of Figures 2–34 and 2–27 reveals that the relaxation pressure is higher (positioned more rightward on the graph) and the resting level of the breathing apparatus (the lung volume at which the relaxation pressure curve intersects zero alveolar pressure) is smaller for the supine than the upright body position.

Comparison of the middle panels of the two figures shows that, to achieve the same targeted alveolar pressure in the supine body position, a greater inspiratory effort (a greater negative muscular pressure) must be exerted at large lung volumes and that effort must be continued to a smaller lung volume than in the upright body position. Also, at small lung volumes a less substantial expiratory effort (a lower positive muscular pressure) is required in the supine body position compared to the upright body position.

Flat Out

Two terms that get more than their fair share of misuse are "supine" and "prone." Supine means lying on your back (usually face up). The easy way to remember this is to consider the spelling of supine. Take out its second letter and you have "spine." On your spine is on your back. So-called couch potatoes spend a lot of time supine in front of their television sets. Prone, also called procumbent, means lying on your front (usually face down). Take its first three letters and you have the first three letters of the word "prostrate" (as in face down submission or adoration). Shooters often spend time lying prone (on their front) when practicing with a rifle on a firing range. The confusion encountered when using the terms supine and prone arises because both involve being flat out. The memory devices suggested here should make it easy to keep the two body positions straight (pun intended).

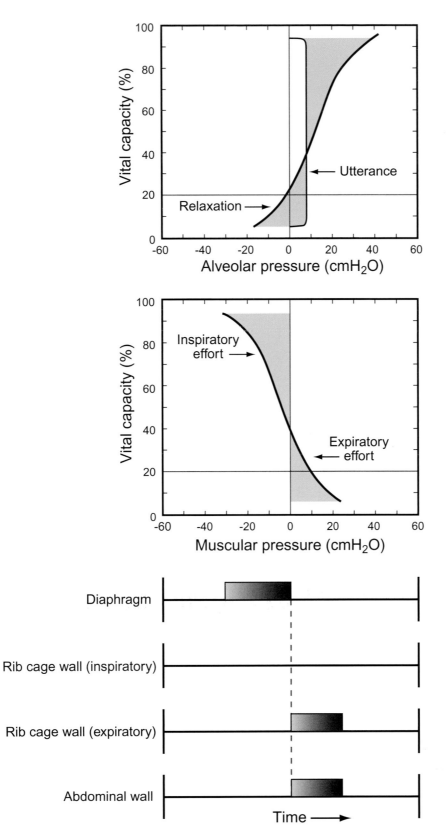

Figure 2-34. Relaxation pressure, target alveolar pressure, muscular pressure, and temporal activity of chest wall components for a sustained vowel produced in the supine body position. Only expiration (speaking) is represented. From *Evaluation and management of speech breathing disorders: Principles and methods* (p. 72), by T. Hixon and J. Hoit, 2005, Tucson, AZ: Redington Brown. Copyright 2005 by Thomas J. Hixon and Jeannette D. Hoit. Modified and reproduced with permission.

The bottom panel of Figure 2–34 depicts the activities of the different chest wall components during extended steady utterance in the supine body position. At the beginning of the utterance, the diaphragm is the only active chest wall component. It exerts a continuously decreasing inspiratory (braking) force throughout the range of lung volumes where muscular pressure is negative. At the instant the diaphragm ceases its activity, the rib cage wall and abdominal wall initiate expiratory activity and remain active in the expiratory direction throughout the remainder of the utterance. This pattern of chest wall activity is generally the same for different targeted alveolar pressures. The only differences are that for higher targeted alveolar pressures, there is less inspiratory braking and earlier and greater expiratory activity, and for lower targeted alveolar pressures, there is more inspiratory braking and later and less expiratory activity.

A major difference between extended steady utterances produced in the two body positions is that inspiratory braking is carried out solely by the diaphragm in the supine body position and primarily by the inspiratory rib cage wall muscles in the upright body position. There are mechanical reasons for this. In the supine body position, there is a substantial influence of gravity on the abdominal wall, causing abdominal pressure to be high. There is no significant hydraulic pull on the undersurface of the diaphragm, as there is in the upright body position. Without a significant hydraulic pull, the inspiratory rib cage wall muscles cannot contribute much to the lowering of alveolar pressure (because they have nothing to pull against, unless the diaphragm also activates). Thus, contracting the diaphragm is the only efficient way to break against the high relaxation pressure at large lung volumes in the supine body position.

Running Speech Activities in the Supine Body Position

Breathing during running speech activities also differs in the supine body position compared to the upright body position. Although running speech starts from about twice resting tidal depth (or less) and continues to near the resting level of the breathing apparatus, just as it does in the upright body position, the actual lung volume range is different. Lung volume events range from about 40 to 20 %VC in supine compared to about 60 to 40 %VC in upright, because the resting level of the breathing apparatus shifts with body position. Alveolar pressure events for running speech activities are the same in both body positions. In contrast, rib cage wall volume and abdominal wall volume events differ substantially, with volume change for the two chest wall parts being relatively equal in the supine body position, whereas rib cage wall volume change predominates in the upright body position.

Chest wall shape during supine running speech production is unlike that assumed in upright running speech production. Whereas speech in the upright body position is produced with the abdominal wall displaced inward and the rib cage wall elevated, the opposite chest wall shape is used in the supine body position. That is, the abdominal wall is pushed outward and the rib cage wall is smaller relative to their relaxed positions at the prevailing lung volume.

As shown in Figure 2–35, both relaxation pressure and muscular pressure contribute to running speech production in the supine body position. Relaxation pressure is slightly positive in the range of lung volumes where running speech is produced (top panel of figure), but not positive enough to achieve the targeted alveolar pressure for most speech production (generally 5 cmH$_2$O or greater; 8 cmH$_2$O in the figure). Therefore, positive muscular pressure is required throughout the breath group (middle panel of figure), the magnitude of which depends on the desired speech loudness.

In the supine body position, most running speech is produced by activation of the rib cage wall expiratory component alone. Only when loud speech is produced or when speech is produced within the expiratory reserve volume does the abdominal wall component also become active. This is illustrated in the bottom panel of Figure 2–35. Inspiration during running speech production (not shown in the figure) is driven by the diaphragm, just as it is in the upright body position. The expiratory muscles of the rib cage wall remain active during inspiration, as they do for running speech activities in the upright body position, so that no time is lost in reactivating them for expiration (speaking).

The muscular strategy for the abdominal wall is quite different for supine running speech activities compared to upright running speech activities. Whereas the abdominal wall plays a critically important role for speech produced in the upright body position, it plays little or no role for such speech produced in the supine body position. This is because in the supine body position gravity does what the abdominal wall muscles do in the upright body position. That is, in supine gravity drives the abdominal content and diaphragm headward, stretching the muscle fibers of the diaphragm and positioning them to be able to generate forceful and rapid inspirations. Gravity also forces the rib cage wall headward and positions its expiratory muscles for quick actions.

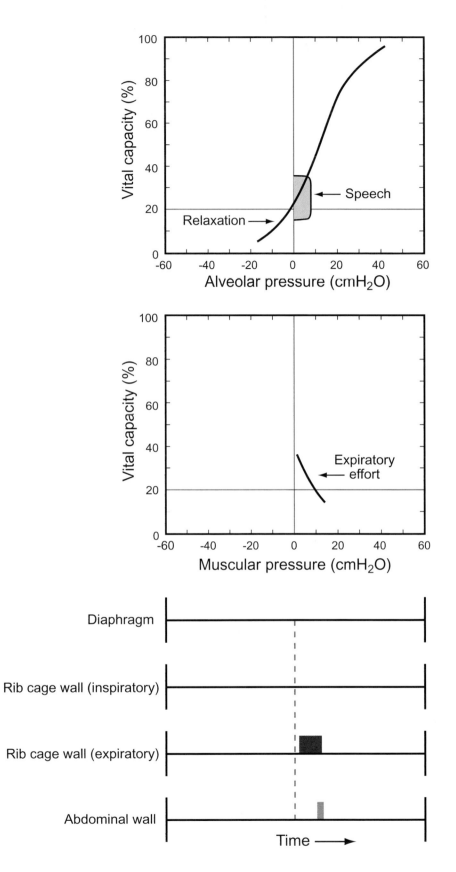

Figure 2-35. Relaxation pressure, targeted alveolar pressure, muscular pressure, and temporal activity of chest wall components for a running speech activity performed in the supine body position. Only expiration (speaking) is represented.

Speech Breathing in Other Body Positions

The number of body positions is limitless. Nevertheless, there are some overarching principles that can be used to extrapolate function to body positions that are other than upright or supine.

One principle is that the resting level of the breathing apparatus changes as body position changes. This is illustrated in Figure 2–36 for several different body positions. Much of the change in resting level can be attributed to the influence of gravity on the abdominal content and the resultant axial displacement of the diaphragm. As the diaphragm is pushed headward, air moves out of the pulmonary apparatus and shifts the resting level to a smaller lung volume. Conversely, as the diaphragm is pulled footward, air moves into the pulmonary apparatus and shifts the resting level to a larger lung volume. Of particular importance in the present context is the fact that lung volume events for running speech production are determined primarily by the resting level of the breathing apparatus (as shown by the several sets of vertical lines in Figure 2–36, each line representing a single breath group).

A second principle is that the relaxation pressure for any given lung volume increases as the body is tilted from upright toward supine. This means that a different muscular pressure is required to achieve a given alveolar pressure target at a specified lung volume.

A third principle is that different chest wall components assume different roles in generating muscular pressure as body position changes. In more upright body positions, the inspiratory muscles of the rib cage wall do most of the inspiratory braking at large lung volumes, whereas the diaphragm takes over this role as the body is tilted toward supine. Also, in more upright body positions, the abdominal wall muscles are highly active, whereas they are increasingly less active as the body is tilted toward supine.

The fourth principle is that the expiratory rib cage muscles almost always participate in running speech

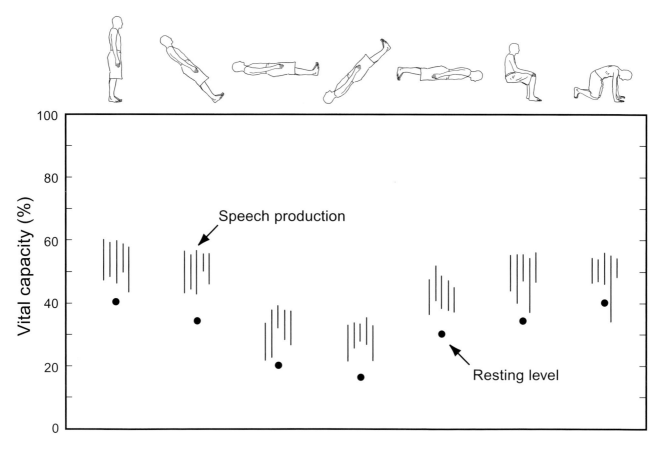

Figure 2–36. Breath groups during running speech production in different body positions. From *Evaluation and management of speech breathing disorders: Principles and methods* (p. 77), by T. Hixon and J. Hoit, 2005, Tucson, AZ: Redington Brown. Copyright 2005 by Thomas J. Hixon and Jeannette D. Hoit. Modified and reproduced with permission.

Somebody Ought To

Various kinematic aspects of speech breathing have been studied in different body positions. We know pretty much what to expect when shifting body position from upright to supine to head down and so forth. But what we don't know much about are the effects of changing body "posture." What happens when you talk with your arms folded across the front of your abdominal wall? What happens when you talk while sitting with your elbows on your desk? What happens when you talk with your feet up on the edge of your desk? What happens when you talk with your legs flexed against your chest while sitting on the floor? And what happens when you talk while wearing a heavy backpack? Somebody ought to study such things so we'll know what to say about these topics in the next edition of this book. Maybe it can be you.

production, regardless of body position. The rib cage wall has the mechanical advantage of covering a much larger area of the lungs than does the diaphragm-abdominal wall and the structural advantage of containing small and fast-acting muscles. These features make the rib cage wall well suited for generating muscular pressure change for speech production in all body positions.

Ventilation, Gas Exchange, and Speech Breathing

The main focus of this chapter is on breathing for speech production. Nevertheless, it is important to keep in mind that the primary function of the breathing apparatus is to sustain life through ventilation and gas exchange. Ventilation is the movement of air in and out of the pulmonary airways and lungs, and has as its purpose gas exchange. Gas exchange is the process of delivering oxygen to the body and releasing carbon dioxide from it. Fortunately, it is possible to speak and still maintain appropriate ventilation and gas exchange, even though the pattern of ventilation is different for speaking than resting tidal breathing (inspirations are quicker and expirations are usually slower).

Most of the time, air is moved in and out of the breathing apparatus at a rate that matches the metabolic needs of the body. For example, less air is moved

in and out when sleeping (low metabolic need) than when exercising (high metabolic need). Sometimes, however, too much or too little air may be moved in and out of the breathing apparatus, resulting in hyperventilation or hypoventilation, respectively. Because the act of speaking requires that air be moved in (inspiration) and out (expiration, during speaking) of the breathing apparatus, ventilation and gas exchange go on at the same time speech breathing does.

There have been several studies of ventilation during speaking. In some cases, these studies have measured gas exchange as well. Essentially all of these studies have shown that we tend to hyperventilate when we speak (Abel, Mottau, Klubendorf, & Koepchen, 1987; Bunn & Mead, 1971; Hoit & Lohmeier, 2000; Meanock & Nicholls, 1982; Warner, Waggener, & Kronauer, 1983). That is, we move more air in and out and we have lower carbon dioxide levels when we speak than when we sit quietly without speaking.

The degree of hyperventilation is dictated, in part, by the nature of the speaking activity. Ventilation is greater during continuous speaking (such as lecturing) than during intermittent speaking (such as conversing, wherein part of the time is spent speaking and part of the time is spent listening). In addition, ventilation is greater when the speech sample is heavily loaded with high-flow sounds (such as voiceless consonants) than if the sample contains all-voiced sounds. Greater ventilation may also be associated with a breathy voice quality compared to a pressed voice quality. Finally, ventilation is greater during loud speaking than during soft speaking (Russell, Cerny, & Stathopoulos, 1998).

Drive to Breathe and Speech Breathing

Most of the time speech breathing is so easy that it can be done without thinking about it. But there are certain times that speech breathing can become a struggle. Almost everyone can recall trying to speak at a high elevation or while exercising. What is usually easy suddenly becomes difficult. When the drive to breathe is strong, there arises an awareness of having to balance the need to breathe with the desire to speak, calling into play additional neural resources (see section on Neural Control of Breathing and Figure 2–37).

Speech breathing under conditions of high drive has been studied using two general approaches. One is to have people speak while exercising, such as walking on a treadmill or riding a stationary bicycle. The other is to alter the gas composition of the blood, usually by having people breathe air that has high concentrations of carbon dioxide in it. Studies that have used these

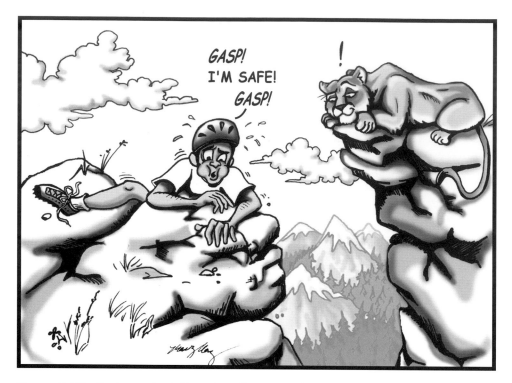

Figure 2–37. Cartoon depicting elevation, exercise, and speaking as a triple challenge to ventilation.

two approaches have yielded similar findings and have shown that speech breathing is quite different under conditions of high drive compared to usual conditions (Bailey & Hoit, 2002; Bunn & Mead, 1971; Doust & Patrick, 1981; Hale & Patrick, 1987; Hoit, Lansing, & Perona, 2007; Meanock & Nicholls, 1982; Otis & Clark, 1968; Phillipson, McClean, Sullivan, & Zamel, 1978).

The most robust finding is perhaps the least surprising—ventilation increases while speaking during exercise or when breathing high levels of carbon dioxide. That is, breathing increases when the drive to breathe increases. Increases in ventilation are accomplished by increasing tidal volume, increasing breathing frequency, or both. In general, ventilation increases as the stimulus level (exercise or carbon dioxide) increases. It is interesting to note, however, that although ventilation increases when a person is speaking under high drive, it does not increase as much as it does if the person is not speaking. This suggests that the act of speaking tends to suppress (or override) the full response to a high-drive stimulus.

Another consistent finding of these studies is that less speech is produced per breath group when speaking under high drive than when speaking under usual conditions. This may seem counterintuitive; given that

more air is expired per breath under high drive conditions (expiratory volumes typically are larger than usual). However, this is easily explained by two strategies that are commonly adopted by people so that they can ventilate more when speaking under high drive. The first strategy is to "blow off" air. When people use this strategy, they may produce a few syllables and then expire the remainder of the breath without speaking. A variation of this is to expire first and then speak and then expire again. The second strategy for ventilating more is the "breathy speech" strategy. When people use this strategy, they use high airflow while speaking so that air is expired more quickly. This usually means that the airflow through the larynx is higher during productions of voiced-speech segments and that airflow associated with voiceless consonant productions is also higher. Often, people use a combination of these two strategies.

When speaking under high drive, people tend to adjust the overall size and shape of the breathing apparatus. Regarding size, people tend to begin and end breath groups at larger than usual lung volumes, so that the breathing apparatus is larger overall than it is when they are speaking under usual conditions. Regarding shape, it is common for large shape changes to accompany speaking in high drive. These are usually in the form of <u>large rib cage wall and abdominal wall movements</u>, movements that are much larger and faster than those seen during usual speaking. These adjustments in size and shape may reflect physiological strategies to help relieve the discomfort that accompanies a high drive to breathe.

Finally, there seems to be one speech breathing behavior that is relatively resistant to change under high-drive conditions. This is the coordination of inspirations with the linguistic content of speech. Even when individuals attempt to speak while "gasping for air," they tend to pause (to blow off air, inspire, or both) at linguistically appropriate junctures, such as sentence, clause, or phrase boundaries, at least when reading aloud. This illustrates the strong influence of linguistic factors on speech breathing, even when the drive to breathe is very strong.

Cognitive-Linguistic Factors and Speech Breathing

The previous section discussed the strong influence that linguistic factors can have on speech breathing when faced with the challenge of speaking under conditions of high drive. But should it be assumed that strong linguistic influence prevails in all aspects of speech breathing? The short answer is "no." As explained below, speech breathing is influenced by what is said, but only in certain ways.

Cognitive-linguistic demands differ widely, depending on whether one recites a well-memorized poem, reads aloud a simple paragraph, converses with a friend, or delivers an extemporaneous speech on a complex topic. When reciting a poem, the linguistic content is provided and even the tempo and location of pauses are scripted. The linguistic content is also provided when reading a paragraph, but there are choices regarding how much speech to produce on a breath and where to pause for inspirations. When engaging in casual conversation, the linguistic content is free to vary and must be formulated on line, but is strongly influenced by what the conversational partner does and says. When speaking extemporaneously, the ideas and linguistic content must be formulated on line and without external cues or guidance. Of these four speaking activities, speaking extemporaneously on a complex topic generally carries the highest cognitive-linguistic load. Different studies of speech breathing have used different types of speaking activities, thereby allowing insight into how cognitive-linguistic demands might or might not influence speech breathing. As it turns out, cognitive-linguistic factors affect certain details of the speech breathing cycle, but not the general mechanical behavior of the breathing apparatus.

Inspirations, especially their timing and depth, are influenced by cognitive-linguistic factors. Inspirations are most likely to occur at linguistic structural boundaries (sentence, clause, and phrase boundaries), especially during reading aloud and, to a lesser degree, when speaking extemporaneously (Bailey & Hoit, 2002; Conrad, Thalacker, & Schonle, 1983; Grosjean & Collins, 1979; Henderson, Goldman-Eisler, & Skarbek, 1965; Hixon et al., 1973; Sugito, Ohyama, & Hirose, 1990; Winkworth, Davis, Adams, & Ellis, 1995; Winkworth, Davis, Ellis, & Adams, 1994). Also, inspirations tend to be larger (deeper) when followed by longer breath groups and smaller (shallower) when followed by shorter breath groups during reading aloud and speaking extemporaneously (Denny, 2000; Horii & Cooke, 1978; Huber & Darling, 2011; McFarland & Smith, 1992; Sperry & Klich, 1992; Whalen & Kinsella-Shaw, 1997; Winkworth et al., 1994, 1995).

Expirations, too, are influenced by cognitive-linguistic factors. The number of speech units (syllables) produced during expiration generally dictates where within the vital capacity the breath group stops. Expirations containing more speech units tend to end at smaller lung volumes and expirations containing fewer speech units tend to end at larger lung volumes (Hodge & Rochet, 1989; Wilder, 1983; Winkworth et al., 1994, 1995). However, the most powerful cognitive-linguistic influence on expirations relates to silent pausing. Silent pauses, moments of silence that last at least 200 to 250 milliseconds, are believed to reflect the time needed to formulate the upcoming spoken message (Goldman-Eisler, 1956; Greene, 1984; Greene & Cappella, 1986; Henderson et al., 1965; Lay & Paivio, 1969; Reynolds & Paivio, 1968; Rochester, 1973; Taylor, 1969). Silent pauses that are accompanied by breath holding seem to be associated with particularly high cognitive-linguistic demands, but those that are accompanied by nonspeech expirations are more common (Mitchell, Hoit, & Watson, 1996; Webb, Williams, & Minifie, 1967). Because nonspeech expirations "waste air," there tends to be less speech produced per breath when cognitive-linguistic demands are high than when they are low.

Although several features of the inspiratory and expiratory phases of speech breathing are influenced by cognitive-linguistic factors, the general mechanical behavior of the breathing apparatus does not appear to be affected. Whether reading aloud or speaking extemporaneously, speech breathing tends to be produced within the midrange of the vital capacity, at volumes larger than the resting level, using a larger than relaxed rib cage wall and smaller than relaxed abdominal wall, and engaging predictable muscular strategies (Hixon et al., 1973, 1976; Hodge & Rochet, 1989; Hoit & Hixon, 1986, 1987; Hoit, Hixon, Altman, & Morgan, 1989; Hoit, Hixon, Watson, & Morgan, 1990; Mitchell et al., 1996).

Conversational Interchange and Speech Breathing

Most speech breathing takes place during conversational interchange, such as that shown in Figure 2–38. Even people whose careers have high didactic speaking demands—teachers, newscasters, politicians, and preachers—probably spend most of their speech breathing time conversing with family, friends, and colleagues. Conversational speech breathing differs from other forms of speech breathing in important ways. This is because the behavior of one conversational partner (or partners) influences the behavior of the other conversational partner (or partners).

There are rhythmic patterns that occur during conversation. A typical conversational pattern is one in which one person speaks a while and then listens while the other person speaks. There is substantial evidence that people tend to entrain their intrinsic biological and behavioral rhythms with people with whom they are interacting and that the most enjoyable interactions are those in which individual rhythms entrain easily to one another (Chapple, 1970).

Two types of rhythms have been identified in conversational speech breathing (McFarland, 2001; Warner et al., 1983). These have been called long-term oscillations and short-term oscillations. Long-term oscillations, which range from as short as a minute to as long as several minutes, have been found in ventilation and speaking during conversation. Specifically, both ventilation and speaking activity tend to wax and wane relatively cyclically during conversation. Interestingly, the rhythmic coupling between conversational partners (in which one speaks while the other listens, and vice versa) is stronger than the coupling of speaking activity and ventilation within an individual. This suggests that social influences are more powerful than physiological constraints during conversation.

Short-term oscillations are characterized by synchrony between the breathing movements of conversational partners. This synchronicity is characterized by breathing movements during listening that resemble the speech breathing movements of the conversational partner. That is, when someone listens to another person speak during conversational interchange, inspiratory movements are quicker (more like the inspirations produced during speech breathing) than when not lis-

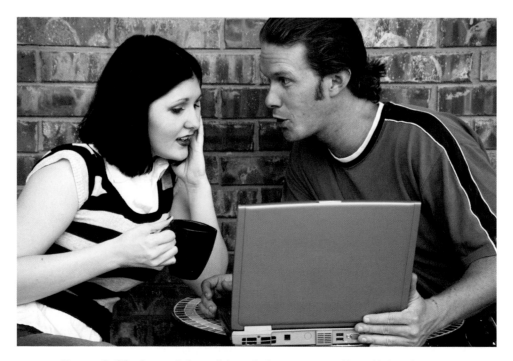

Figure 2–38. Speech breathing during conversational interchange.

tening to someone speak. Also, expiratory movements tend to be longer (more like the expirations produced during speech breathing) immediately before taking one's turn to speak. Finally, during actual turn-taking moments, the breathing movements of conversational partners tend to be correlated such that they are either simultaneous in the same direction (both inspiratory or both expiratory) or in opposite directions (one inspiratory and one expiratory).

Thus, speech breathing produced in the context of conversational interchange appears to have emergent properties. Its nature is complex and is determined by the speaker, the conversational partner(s), and interactions between the speaker and conversational partner(s).

Body Type and Speech Breathing

People come in many different sizes, shapes, and compositions, or so-called body types. Because the breathing apparatus makes up a large portion of the body, it makes sense that different body types would also be reflected in different sizes, shapes, and compositions of the breathing apparatus. It also makes sense that those differences might influence the way the breathing apparatus functions for speech breathing. This, in fact, turns out to be true.

Figure 2–39 illustrates men with three very different body types (from left to right): highly endomorphic (high in relative fatness), highly mesomorphic (high in musculoskeletal development), and highly ectomorphic (high in relative linearity). When the speech breathing of young men with these body types was studied (Hoit & Hixon, 1986), the most dramatic contrasts were found between the speech breathing of the endomorphic and ectomorphic men. Specifically, the endomorphic men tended to keep the abdominal wall held inward farther and they tended to move the abdominal wall a greater distance than did the ectomorphic men during speech breathing. The mesomorphic men generally fell between these two extremes.

There is probably good reason why people with different body types speech breathe differently. The best explanation has to do with optimizing the speed and efficiency of inspiratory efforts. Recall that to produce rapid and forceful inspiratory force, the diaphragm (the major muscle of inspiration) needs to be in a domed position so that its muscle fibers are elongated. This domed position is achieved by moving the abdominal wall inward, which, in turn, pushes the diaphragm headward. Consider the difference in the resting configuration of the diaphragm in an endomorphic person and an ectomorphic person (in an upright

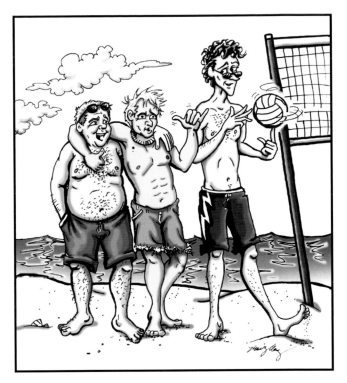

Figure 2–39. Cartoon of three teammates of different body types (endomorph, mesomorph, and ectomorph).

body position). The large abdominal mass of the endomorphic person pulls down on the diaphragm, flattens it, and shortens its muscle fibers, thus placing the diaphragm at a poor mechanical advantage for generating inspiratory force. In contrast, the flat abdominal wall of the ectomorphic person maintains the diaphragm in a domed configuration with elongated muscle fibers, even at rest. Thus, for the endomorphic person to achieve the inspiratory advantage that is maintained effortlessly by the ectomorphic person, the endomorphic person must use the abdominal wall muscles to position the abdominal wall inward. The endomorphic person must also keep the abdominal wall moving inward while speaking to prepare the diaphragm for the next inspiration.

Development and Speech Breathing

Thus far, this chapter has discussed speech breathing from the perspective of a fully developed system, an adult system. However, speech breathing does not begin this way. It develops over time, as do all other motor behaviors, and continues to change during infancy, childhood, and adolescence. The development of speech breathing can be attributed to the myriad of changes that occur during the first 2 decades of life, such as changes in the size of the breathing apparatus, musculoskeletal geometry, chest wall compliance, pressure generation capability, neural control, linguistic sophistication, and many other factors.

Breathing for vocalization and speech production has been documented throughout development, from early infancy through 16 years of age (Boliek, Hixon, Watson, & Jones, 2009; Boliek, Hixon, Watson, & Morgan, 1996, 1997; Connaghan, Moore, & Higashakawa, 2004; Hoit et al., 1990; Moore, Caulfield, & Green, 2001). Studies of breathing in infants and toddlers up to age 3 years, considered to be a period of emergence of a motor skill, have revealed some clear developmental trends (Boliek et al., 1996, 1997). For example, the amount of air expired per breath becomes increasingly larger as infants and toddlers become older and increase in size. In contrast, other features of breathing for vocalization do not change with age. For example, infants and toddlers, whether 5 weeks or 3 years of age, usually initiate breath groups within the midrange of the vital capacity. The exact nature of the syllables uttered does not appear to affect breathing behavior (Parham, Buder, Oller, & Boliek, 2011). Also, as early as 18 months of age, inspirations preceding vocalization are quicker than inspirations associated with tidal breathing, in the same way they are in adults (Boliek et al., 1997; Parham et al., 2011). Nevertheless, the most striking feature, and the feature that makes breathing for vocalization so different in infants and toddlers from speech breathing in adults, is its variability. Unlike adults, who tend to be rather consistent in their speech breathing across time, infants and toddlers seem to use a different strategy for each vocalization (different lung volumes, different chest wall shapes, and different relative volume contributions of the rib cage wall and abdominal wall to lung volume change). It is as though they are experimenting with the breathing apparatus to see what works best, just as they are experimenting with their vocal behaviors.

As the young child grows older, control of speech breathing continues through a period of refinement. Most of our knowledge of this period comes from a large-scale study of speech breathing in 4-, 5-, and 6-year-old boys and girls (Boliek et al., 2009) and from another study that included 7-year-old boys and girls (Hoit et al., 1990). During this refinement period, certain features of speech breathing are relatively stable and similar to those of adulthood. For example, inspiratory durations are relatively short and expiratory durations are relatively long compared to tidal breathing, as they are during the emergence period. Also,

breath groups tend to be initiated in the midrange of the vital capacity where recoil forces are most favorable (although the absolute volumes increase with age and breathing apparatus size). Other features of speech breathing are more immature and often quite variable (though somewhat less variable than during the emergence period). For example, relative volume contribution of the rib cage wall to lung volume change is generally smaller (until age 7 years) and less consistent than in older children and adults. Other examples are that children in this age range produce few syllables per breath group, expend a substantial volume of air per syllable, and include frequent nonvocal expirations. These speech breathing behaviors are attributed to developmental changes in the size of the breathing apparatus, speech fluency, and cognitive-linguistic skill. It is also well known that during this period of refinement children tend to use higher alveolar pressures for speech production than do adolescents and adults (Bernthal & Beukelman, 1979; Netsell, Lotz, Peters, & Schulte, 1994; Stathopoulos & Sapienza, 1993, 1997; Stathopoulos & Weismer, 1985).

As children grow older and move into adolescence, breathing for speech becomes less variable and more adult like. In fact, when volume measures are normalized to take into account age-related size differences, speech breathing is essentially adultlike in

---

Rock-a-Bye Baby

Lullabies tend to put infants to sleep and change their breathing patterns. A supine infant who is awake breathes with in-phase movements of the rib cage wall and abdominal wall. The two structures rise and fall together in a gentle rhythm. But, if the same infant falls asleep, there may be an abrupt change in breathing pattern. During rapid eye movement sleep, for example, the pattern may change to out-of-phase movements of the rib cage wall and abdominal wall. One structure rises while the other falls. The reason is that, during sleep, structures in the pharyngeal-oral airway relax and the tongue falls toward the back of the infant's throat. This increases the airway resistance through which the breathing apparatus must work. One consequence is that pleural pressure must be lowered more during each inspiration, causing the floppy rib cage wall to be "sucked" inward. So, it's rock-a-bye baby, but bye-bye in-phase movements.

most features by 10 years of age (before puberty). The only major differences seen beyond age 10 years are increases in the amount of speech per breath group, reflecting changes in linguistic skill and sophistication (Hoit et al., 1990).

Age and Speech Breathing

Growing old presumably makes people wiser. Growing old also changes the structure and function of the breathing apparatus. For example, age brings changes to the subdivisions of the lung volume, pulmonary compliance and chest wall compliance, musculoskeletal composition and configuration, and neural control. Thus, it may come as no surprise that growing old also brings on changes in speech breathing.

Studies have shown that the major changes in speech breathing occur around the seventh or eighth decade of life, at least in very healthy adults (Hoit & Hixon, 1987; Hoit et al., 1989; Huber, 2008; Sperry & Klich, 1992). The speech breathing of someone in senescence, when compared to someone in young adulthood, is found to involve breath groups that: (a) start from larger lung volumes (and rib cage volumes), (b) encompass more of the vital capacity (and rib cage capacity), and (c) entail the expenditure of more air per syllable. This suggests that senescent individuals tend to "waste air" when they speak, and that they take deeper breaths before speaking, probably to compensate for the anticipated air loss. It appears that the air loss is due to uneconomical valving by downstream structures. Subsequent research pointed to the larynx as the valve most responsible for the air wastage exhibited by senescent speakers, although the mechanism of wastage appears to differ for men and women. In men, air wastage has been attributed to an age-related decrease in laryngeal airway resistance during phonation (Melcon, Hoit, & Hixon, 1989; see Chapter 3 for details). In contrast, women do not exhibit an analogous decrease in laryngeal airway resistance during phonation (Hoit & Hixon, 1992); rather, they tend to release air (produce nonspeech expirations) before or after spoken utterances (Sperry & Klich, 1992).

It is relevant to point out that the concept of age can have more than one meaning. Although one typically thinks of age as chronological age, biological age is often more important, especially when considering physiological status. Thus, it may well be that age-related changes in speech breathing and laryngeal function are more tightly linked to biological age than chronological age.

Sex and Speech Breathing

There is a pervasive myth that males and females breathe differently. This myth might also be applied to speech breathing, except that there is substantial evidence that contradicts it (Boliek et al., 1996, 1997, 2009; Hodge & Rochet, 1989; Hoit et al., 1989, 1990). From infancy through senescence, speech breathing is generally the same in the two sexes. The one exception is that, after puberty, the absolute lung volumes associated with speech breathing are generally larger in boys than girls (and men than women) because boys are generally taller and, thus, their airways are larger. Nevertheless, when volume measures are normalized to take into account differences in size, there are no sex-related differences in speech breathing to be found.

MEASUREMENT OF BREATHING

This section considers instrumental measurements of breathing, especially those that are often encountered in clinical endeavors. The three categories of measurements highlighted here pertain to the mechanical measurement of volume, pressure, and shape.

Volume Measurement

The most important volume for speech breathing is lung volume. This volume reflects the prevailing size of the breathing apparatus and can be measured at either the airway opening or body surface.

Volume measurement at the airway opening relies on the movement of air to and from the lungs through the mouth and/or nose. The measurement device is coupled to the person by either a mouthpiece or a mask, depending on the particular application. Several devices can be used to make the desired measurement. Two of these are the wet spirometer and the pneumotachometer (with a signal integrator).

Figure 2–40 depicts a wet spirometer. This device includes a chamber containing water and a bell that floats inside the chamber. Volume displaced into and out of the bell causes it to rise and fall, respectively, the height of the bell being directly proportional to the volume of air in the spirometer. A pen fixed to the bell makes a record of volume change on paper attached to a rotating drum. Or a potentiometer driven by movement of the bell may provide an electrical signal for display on a screen.

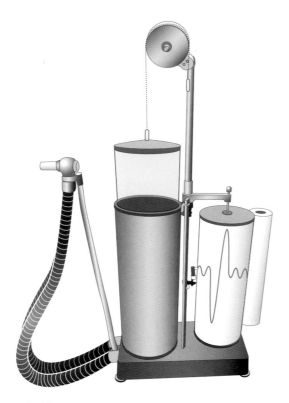

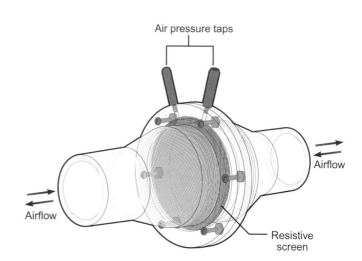

Figure 2–41. Pneumotachometer. From *Evaluation and management of speech breathing disorders: Principles and methods* (p. 162), by T. Hixon and J. Hoit, 2005, Tucson, AZ: Redington Brown. Copyright 2005 by Thomas J. Hixon and Jeannette D. Hoit. Modified and reproduced with permission.

Figure 2–40. Wet spirometer. From *Evaluation and management of speech breathing disorders: Principles and methods* (p. 160), by T. Hixon and J. Hoit, 2005, Tucson, AZ: Redington Brown. Copyright 2005 by Thomas J. Hixon and Jeannette D. Hoit. Modified and reproduced with permission.

Figure 2–41 portrays a pneumotachometer that senses airflow through it in both directions by recording the instantaneous air pressure difference across a resistive screen. The pressure difference is sensed by a differential air pressure transducer, which provides an electrical signal proportional to airflow. An electronic integrator is then used to integrate (sum) the signal to provide a measure of volume change. Airflow measurement is like reading the speedometer in an automobile and volume measurement (by airflow integration) is like reading the odometer in an automobile. The volume change signal obtained from airflow integration is analogous to that obtained by measuring movement of the bell of the wet spirometer.

Volume measurement at the body surface relies on the sensing of movements of the torso and using these as estimates of volume change. Several devices can be used to make measurements of this type. Two of these are respiratory magnetometers and respiratory inductance plethysmographs.

Figure 2–42 portrays respiratory magnetometers as they might be positioned to make volume measurements. Pairs (front and back mates) of electromagnetic coils are used to sense anteroposterior diameter changes of the rib cage wall and abdominal wall. The rib cage wall and abdominal wall each displace volume as they move and together they displace a volume equal to that displaced by the lungs. Thus, one need only sum the output signals from the two pairs of electromagnetic coils to obtain a measurement of lung volume change at the body surface. Respiratory magnetometers generate low power electromagnetic fields that are safe for clinical use. Nevertheless, it is prudent to avoid using respiratory magnetometers on pregnant women or on anyone with an implanted electronic pacemaker.

Figure 2–43 depicts respiratory inductance plethysmographs as they might be positioned to make volume measurements. Broad elastic bands with embedded electrical wires are used to sense average cross-sectional areas of the rib cage wall and abdominal wall. Again, as with respiratory magnetometers, the rib cage wall and abdominal wall each displace volume as they move and the summed displacement equals that of the lungs. One need only sum the output signals from the two elastic sensing bands (average cross-sectional areas) to arrive at a measurement of lung volume change at the body surface.

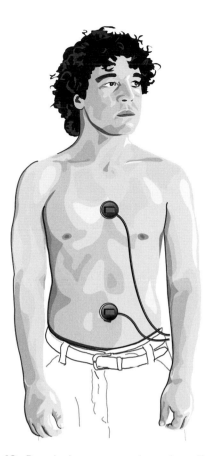

Figure 2–42. Respiratory magnetometers. From *Evaluation and management of speech breathing disorders: Principles and methods* (p. 167), by T. Hixon and J. Hoit, 2005, Tucson, AZ: Redington Brown. Copyright 2005 by Thomas J. Hixon and Jeannette D. Hoit. Modified and reproduced with permission.

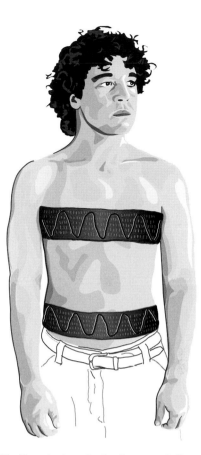

Figure 2–43. Respiratory inductance plethysmographs. From *Evaluation and management of speech breathing disorders: Principles and methods* (p. 168), by T. Hixon and J. Hoit, 2005, Tucson, AZ: Redington Brown. Copyright 2005 by Thomas J. Hixon and Jeannette D. Hoit. Modified and reproduced with permission.

Where's the Border?

Borders may or may not be important. Ride your Harley-Davidson motorcycle around the monument at the Four Corners junction from Arizona through New Mexico through Colorado to Utah (for the geographically challenged, this is a continuous left turn) without wearing a helmet and there will be times you're breaking the law and times you're not. You need to know each state's law and identify each border to know your status. But the border between the rib cage wall and the abdominal wall is another story. When the two structures move, it's hard to identify where their two edges meet. The respiratory magnetometers discussed in the text make it so that you don't have to fret such delineation. Magnetometers have the advantage that their coils can be placed at the center of the surfaces being monitored and far away from their edges. Where's the border? Who cares? It's not important to know when using respiratory magnetometers.

Pressure Measurement

The most important pressure for speech breathing is alveolar pressure. Alveolar pressure cannot be measured directly during speech production. The problem is that speech production is characterized by various obstructions and constrictions along the larynx and pharyngeal-oral apparatus that preclude access to the alveoli. Nevertheless, alveolar pressure can be estimated from oral pressure during the production of a particular type of speech sample (Hertegård, Gauffin, & Lindestad, 1995; Netsell & Hixon, 1978).

As shown in the upper panel of Figure 2–44, a small polyethylene pressure sensing tube is placed at one corner of the mouth just behind the front teeth so that one of its ends is perpendicular to the flow of air out of the mouth. The other end of the tube is connected to an air pressure transducer, which converts the pressure into an electrical equivalent.

The key is to capitalize on a period during speech production when oral pressure and alveolar pressure are equal. This period occurs during the closed phase of voiceless stop-plosive production when the oral and velopharyngeal valves are sealed airtight and the laryngeal valve is open. During this period, the pressure recorded by the oral pressure sensing tube is essentially equal to the pressure in the alveoli. When an utterance sequence is designed to include interspersed voiceless stop-plosives (/pipipipipipipi/), the peak oral pressures measured during the consonants need only be interconnected to reveal the underlying alveolar pressure contour. This is done by constructing a contour

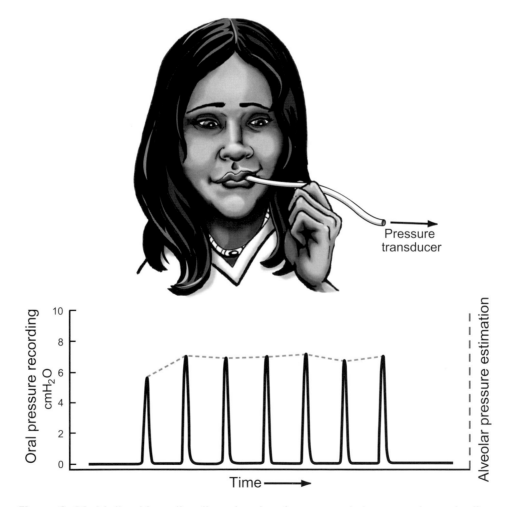

Figure 2–44. Method for estimating alveolar air pressure during speech production. Upper panel illustrates speaker-instrumentation interface. Lower panel shows underlying alveolar air pressure contour constructed from successive linear interpolations between peak oral air pressures associated with adjacent voiceless stop-plosives.

from successive linear interpolations between the peak pressures of adjacent consonants, as illustrated in the lower panel of Figure 2–44.

Shape Measurement

Shape is measured at the body surface. It is measured with the same devices, respiratory magnetometers and respiratory inductance plethysmographs, as discussed above for measuring lung volume change from the torso wall. However, the signals from the rib cage wall and abdominal wall are not summed electronically to create an estimate of lung volume change. Rather, they are displayed against one another in a manner similar to that shown in Figure 2–19, with the rib cage wall signal depicted on a vertical axis, increasing upward, and the abdominal wall signal depicted on a horizontal axis, increasing rightward. Using such a diagram, the shape of the chest wall for speaking events is revealed directly, with points in the diagram specifying the prevailing configurations of the chest wall.

SPEECH BREATHING DISORDERS

Speech breathing disorders come in many forms and can affect individuals of all ages and from all walks of life. Speech breathing disorders can be classified as having functional bases or organic bases. These can even occur together.

Speech breathing disorders of functional origin are those that have no known physical cause. Functional misuse of the breathing apparatus is sometimes observed in individuals who use speech extensively in their work, such as teachers, salespersons, preachers, newscasters, inspirational speakers, and actors. For example, a teacher might have a habit of speaking in exceptionally long breath groups and at small lung volumes, a habit that might cause breathing discomfort and fatigue. Functional speech breathing disorders can also have psychogenic bases. Examples include malingering (pretending to be ill or injured) and conversion reaction (loss of voluntary control over motor or sensory functions as a result of emotional conflict). Malingering might take the form of someone pretending to have difficulty with breathing as a ploy to win a personal injury lawsuit. Conversion reaction might take the form of an actual feeling of breathing difficulty (with no physical basis, but nonetheless real) brought on by fear of expressing negative emotions to family members.

Speech breathing disorders of organic origin are those that have identifiable physical causes. Such dis-orders can involve impairment of the chest wall and/or the pulmonary apparatus. Disorders of the chest wall may include developmental or acquired deformities of the skeletal framework, an example of which is scoliosis (an abnormal lateral curvature of the spine). Most common among chest wall disorders of organic origin are those caused by injury or disease of the nervous system. One example is spinal cord injury, which is particularly prevalent in young men. Spinal cord injury may cause paralysis of the chest wall muscles, the extent of which depends on what part of the spinal cord is injured. If only the lower part of the spinal cord is damaged, speech breathing may be adequate, but if the upper part of the spinal cord is damaged, speech breathing may be severely impaired. Other examples are cerebral palsy (a developmental neural disorder that affects muscle control) and amyotrophic lateral sclerosis (a disease in which motor nerves die). In these latter examples, and others like them, the entire speech production apparatus is often affected, not just the breathing apparatus.

Speech breathing disorders of organic origin also include those associated with diseases of the pulmonary apparatus. These include diseases that obstruct the flow of air, such as asthma and emphysema, and diseases that cause the lungs to become stiff, such as sarcoidosis. Individuals with pulmonary disease often complain of breathing discomfort (dyspnea) and may alter their speech breathing to relieve that discomfort.

Pink Puffers and Blue Bloaters

No, we're not talking about exotic tropical fish. Pink puffers and blue bloaters are terms that refer to people with chronic obstructive pulmonary disease. Pink puffers suffer mainly from emphysema. Their blood is relatively well saturated with oxygen, making their complexion pink. The puffer part comes from their compensatory expiration through pursed lips. They have decreased lung recoil, decreased vital capacity, increased residual volume, and increased total lung capacity. Blue bloaters suffer mainly from chronic bronchitis. They have associated heart problems with cyanosis and edema. Thus, their bodies turn blue and become bloated. They show decreased vital capacity and increased residual volume. Chronic obstructive pulmonary disease can be nasty and debilitating. Bronchitis may be reversible. Emphysema usually is not.

Sometimes, disorders of the chest wall or pulmonary apparatus cause such severe breathing impairment that a ventilator is required to sustain life. This can happen to individuals with high cervical spinal cord injury, those with certain progressive neuromotor diseases, or those with severe chronic obstructive pulmonary disease. In such cases, speech breathing may be driven in large part (or totally) by the ventilator. Figure 2–45 shows a person using a ventilator.

CLINICAL PROFESSIONALS AND SPEECH BREATHING DISORDERS

When an individual presents with a speech breathing disorder, or a suspected speech breathing disorder, there are several professionals who have a potential role in the evaluation and management of that disorder. Included among these are the speech-language pathologist, pulmonologist, respiratory therapist, neurologist, physical therapist, and psychologist. Usually, a person would be seen by only a subset of these professionals.

The speech-language pathologist is considered the expert in speech breathing disorders. In certain cases, the speech-language pathologist is the only professional to evaluate and manage a person with a speech breathing disorder. A good example of this is an individual with a functional-misuse disorder who exhibits inappropriate speech breathing behavior (and no signs of a physical disorder). Management in this case is behavioral therapy conducted by the speech-language pathologist alone. In many cases, however, the speech-language pathologist is only one of the professionals involved in an individual's care.

A pulmonologist is a physician with expertise in breathing disorders. Examples of the types of persons who are under the care of a pulmonologist include those with pulmonary disease, such as cystic fibrosis (a genetic disease that causes excess secretion of mucus and airway obstruction), and those with severe neuromuscular disease, such as muscular dystrophy (a genetic disease that causes weakness and degeneration of muscles). People who are supported by ventilators are always overseen by a pulmonologist. A pulmonologist has the first and last word when it comes to the care of a person with a breathing disorder, because breathing outweighs everything else in importance.

A respiratory therapist carries out specific evaluation and management procedures requested by a pulmonologist. A speech-language pathologist may work side by side with a respiratory therapist when evaluating or managing people with certain types of disorders, especially those who are supported by ventilators.

A neurologist is a physician with expertise in disorders of the nervous system. Examples of the types of individuals who are under the care of a neurologist are those with Parkinson disease (a degenerative brain disease that causes problems such as slow movement,

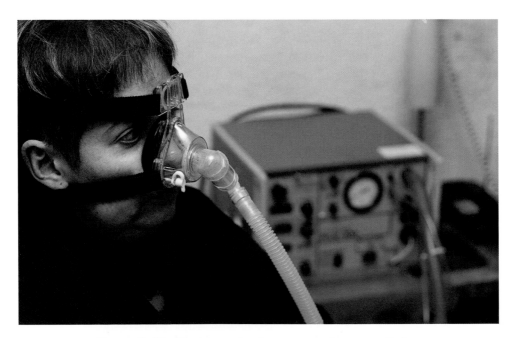

Figure 2–45. Photograph of a person using a ventilator.

rigidity, and tremor), multiple sclerosis (a disease of the myelin that surrounds axons within the central nervous system and causes problems such as muscle weakness and dyscoordination), and spinal muscular atrophy (a disease of the motor nerves in the spinal cord that causes problems with weakness or paralysis of chest wall muscles). A speech-language pathologist often sees the same people as does a neurologist, although not necessarily for speech breathing disorders exclusively. This is because such people often have speech problems related to laryngeal, velopharyngeal-nasal, and/or pharyngeal-oral function as well.

A physical therapist is a professional with expertise in the evaluation and management of body movement. Examples of the types of individuals that a physical therapist might evaluate and manage include those with structural injury or deformity, spinal cord injury, traumatic brain injury, degenerative neural disease, and vestibular (balance) disorder, among others. A speech-language pathologist might work with a physical therapist to determine optimal body positioning for an individual with a speech breathing disorder caused by a neural disease, such as cerebral palsy or muscular dystrophy.

A psychologist is a professional with expertise in the psychological bases of behavior. A psychologist sees individuals with many types of disorders, some of whom may be referred for problems related to speech breathing disorders. For example, a psychologist might evaluate and manage a person with a psychogenic speech breathing disorder, such as hyperventilation syndrome (a psychogenic disorder characterized by hyperventilation for no apparent physical reason). For another example, the services of a psychologist may be needed for an individual who has begun using a ventilator and is having difficulty dealing with the trauma of physical dependency. In both these examples, a speech-language pathologist might also be managing the individual's speech breathing behavior during the same period.

REVIEW

A speech breathing disorder may manifest as a problem of breathing movement, gas exchange, breathing comfort, or any combination of these.

The breathing apparatus is a mechanical pump that includes an energy source and passive components that couple this source to the air it moves.

The breathing apparatus is formed around a skeletal superstructure and consists of the pulmonary apparatus and chest wall (linked together as a unit), the former including the pulmonary airways and lungs and the latter including the rib cage wall, diaphragm, abdominal wall, and abdominal content.

The forces of breathing are passive and active, the former arising from the natural recoil of tissues, surface tension within alveoli, and gravity, and the latter being vested in more than 20 muscles of the chest wall.

Muscles of the rib cage wall include the *sternocleidomastoid, scalenus anterior, scalenus medius, scalenus posterior, pectoralis major, pectoralis minor, subclavius, serratus anterior, external intercostal, internal intercostal, transversus thoracis, latissimus dorsi, serratus posterior superior, serratus posterior inferior, lateral iliocostalis cervicis, lateral iliocostalis thoracis, lateral iliocostalis lumborum, levatores costarum, quadratus lumborum,* and *subcostal.*

Muscle of the diaphragm partition includes the *diaphragm.*

Muscles of the abdominal wall include the *rectus abdominis, external oblique, internal oblique, transversus abdominis, latissimus dorsi, lateral iliocostalis lumborum,* and *quadratus lumborum.*

The movements of breathing occur within the rib cage wall, diaphragm, and abdominal wall and result from forces applied to and by different parts of the breathing apparatus.

The adjustment capabilities of the breathing apparatus involve passive and active interactions within and among different parts of the apparatus and provide a challenge when attempting to specify what actions are responsible for various adjustments.

The output variables of breathing include lung volume, alveolar pressure, and chest wall shape.

The nervous system controls different acts of breathing through a group of lower and higher brain centers that mediate movement, perception of movement, and feelings about the need to breathe.

Ventilation supports the life-sustaining process of oxygen and carbon dioxide exchange and is characterized by patterns that are relatively individualized across people, and are influenced by body position.

Speech breathing is the process by which driving forces are supplied to generate the sounds of speech, while simultaneously serving the functions of ventilation and gas exchange.

Speech breathing is achieved through the combining of relaxation pressure and muscular pressure, the muscular pressure required at any moment depending on the relaxation pressure available at the prevailing lung volume and the targeted alveolar pressure of the utterance.

The activity of individual parts of the chest wall (rib cage wall, diaphragm, and abdominal wall) may change for the generation of utterances involving different alveolar pressures at different lung volumes.

The control strategy for running speech activities is distinct from that for other forms of breathing and serves to enhance function during both the inspiratory and expiratory phases of breathing to facilitate speech communication.

Speech breathing is adaptive and accommodates to changing mechanical and ventilatory demands, some predictable and some not.

Speech breathing is influenced by body position, mainly because gravity affects relaxation pressure, the resting level of the breathing apparatus, and the mechanical advantages of different parts of the chest wall.

People hyperventilate during speech breathing, as shown in measures of ventilation (more air moved in and out of the breathing apparatus than during resting tidal breathing) and in measures of gas exchange (less carbon dioxide in expired air when speaking than when resting tidal breathing).

Speech breathing becomes more difficult when the drive to breathe is strong enough to compete with the drive to speak, such as during exercise or when inspiring high levels of carbon dioxide, and is characterized by breathing apparatus adjustments that tend to relieve breathing discomfort.

Cognitive-linguistic factors influence speech breathing in ways that determine when inspirations will occur, what their depth will be, how long the subsequent expiration will be, how often pauses will occur, and how much speech will be produced per breath group.

Conversational partners influence the nature of interaction and the nature of speech breathing, with synchronies being established on both long-term and short-term bases.

Body type significantly influences speech breathing, with the most dramatic contrasts existing between people who are endomorphic (high in relative fatness) and ectomorphic (high in relative linearity), the former showing a high degree of abdominal wall participation and the latter showing a high degree of rib cage wall participation.

Speech breathing develops over time and continues to change during infancy, childhood, and adolescence, being essentially adult like by 10 years of age, except for subsequent increases in the amount of speech per breath group (reflecting changes in linguistic skill and sophistication).

Age influences speech breathing around the seventh or eighth decade of life, such that breath groups start from larger lung volumes and more of the available air is expended per utterance, factors believed to be related to laryngeal valving economy and air wastage.

Despite the pervasive myth that the two sexes breathe differently, there is no evidence to support this notion, and, in the case of speech breathing, substantial evidence to contradict it.

Instrumental methods can profitably be applied to the study of speech breathing, especially those that yield measurements of lung volume, alveolar pressure, and chest wall shape.

Speech breathing disorders come in many forms and can affect people of all ages and from all walks of life, their causes being of functional and organic origins and affecting the pulmonary apparatus and chest wall.

Various clinical professionals have roles in the evaluation and management of speech breathing disorders and include, among others, speech-language pathologists, pulmonologists, respiratory therapists, neurologists, physical therapists, and psychologists.

Scenario

An electric wheelchair was her new mode of conveyance. She had mastered it well. Her competitive drive was reemerging and the closest of her college classmates were faithfully trying to buoy her spirit through emails and an occasional group telephone call. With the help of a counselor and her priest, she was slowly coming to a realization that her career plans might need to change to more closely match her physical prognosis. She knew for sure that her continuing gregarious nature would lead her to do something that involved talking. It was with this outlook and her desire to have a service dog that she approached her speech rehabilitation.

A speech-language pathologist and a pulmonologist teamed together to stage her management. Other professionals were included as necessary. Manual bracing of her abdominal wall suggested that general breathing function and speech breathing could be improved with the abdominal wall supported inward from its usual distended position.

Improvements were sufficiently robust to encourage the fitting of an abdominal wall truss.

An orthotist was enlisted to custom fit a truss for her lower torso that resembled a tight-fitting corset with adjustable Velcro™ straps. This device could be configured to hold the abdominal wall in an inward position, even when the diaphragm was forcefully contracted. A respiratory therapist was authorized by the pulmonologist to make adjustments to the truss, which was worn only during waking hours and when tolerated. The truss was adjusted initially to position the abdominal wall inward at about the midpoint of its total range of excursion. It was worn intermittently for 10 days and then measurements were made with and without the truss in place.

Measurements without the truss were consistent with those from the initial evaluation, whereas measurements with the truss in place showed favorable changes in the inspiratory capacity (from 35% of predicted to 45% of predicted) and the maximum inspiratory pressure (from 31% of predicted to 38% of predicted). The expiratory reserve volume and maximum expiratory pressure showed no change. Speech signs changed favorably with the device in place. Breath groups were longer by two syllables, on average, and speech was louder. Inspirations for conversation were perceptibly quicker (confirmed by measurements using respiratory inductance plethysmography), but remained abnormally slow. She also reported that her breathing was more comfortable and that her speaking was "easier and less tiring."

Disuse atrophy was suspected in the inspiratory muscles of breathing and inspiratory muscle training was initiated. Training was carried out with the abdominal wall truss in place. The speech production goal of this training was to increase starting lung volumes for breath groups so that speech might last longer and be louder. With approval from the pulmonologist, the speech-language pathologist and a physical therapist designed and conducted an inspiratory muscle-training program. A spring-loaded pressure-threshold training device was used in a 6-week training program (5 days a week) with the pressure threshold reset weekly based on 75% of maximum inspiratory pressure attainable with the abdominal wall truss in place. Repeated measurements of respiratory function at the end of the 6-week training period revealed favorable results.

Maximum inspiratory pressure had increased by 54% from its pretraining value and inspiratory capacity had increased by 45% from its pretraining value. A maintenance regimen was instituted to assist in maintaining the newly gained strength and endurance.

Behavioral training was instituted once inspiratory muscle training was complete. This part of management was designed to optimize speech production against the background of gains achieved from abdominal wall trussing and inspiratory muscle training. Behavioral training focused on speech breathing during conversational interactions. Emphasis was placed on starting breath groups at large lung volumes to improve the potential for longer and louder utterances. An emphasis was also placed on changing a persistent breathy voice toward the more pressed end of the voice quality continuum. This served the purposes of making her voice louder and conserving her available air supply during utterance. By the end of behavioral training, she was able to produce breath groups that were 12 syllables in length and speech of near-normal loudness. She was also using conversational interchange strategies that enabled her to hold the floor during conversation. Specific strategies were also practiced to acquire skills to control a service dog with voice commands. These involved inspiring maximally before utterance, alerting an imaginary dog of intent to command, and the delivery of commands crisply and emphatically.

She got her service dog, Molly, and with her new companion and new confidence sought employment as a receptionist at the agency where she had trained with her dog. She got that job and a year later got a job as an assistant with a wilderness adventure company that specialized in outdoor activities and adaptive sports for persons with physical disabilities. She soon worked her way into a position in which she was responsible for the design and testing of such activities. As fate would have it, much of her job involved traveling to various locations on the Colorado Plateau, where she once again came in sight of the continental divide and the San Juan Mountains. Life was certainly different than it had been the last time she was here. She felt herself to be full of purpose and very fortunate. Molly seemed to understand.

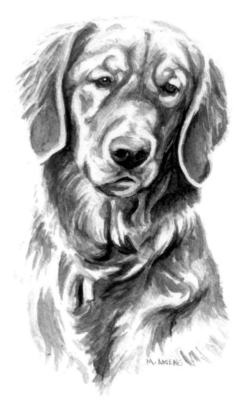

The Young and the Reckless

Young men contribute mightily to the statistics on spinal cord injury. They tend to engage in activities that involve fast movement and in which collision may occur. And they are less concerned about taking risks than are their opposite sex counterparts (many of the readers of this book) or their elders. No wonder insurance companies charge them high premiums. There are about a quarter of a million people in the United States with spinal cord injury (a number equal to the population of Rochester, New York). Each year about 10,000 new cases are added to the roll. More than 80% of people with spinal cord injury are men. Automobile crashes lead the way as the cause, followed by violent acts (such as gunshot wounds) and falls. Although not all spinal cord injury is preventable, education to alter risk-taking behavior holds the key to reducing the number of people who suffer this fate each year.

REFERENCES

Abel, H., Mottau, B. Klubendorf, D., & Koepchen, H. (1987). Pattern of different components of the respiratory cycle and autonomic parameters during speech. In G. Sieck, S. Gandevia, & W. Cameron (Eds.), *Respiratory muscles and their neuromotor control* (pp. 109–113). New York, NY: Alan R. Liss.

Bailey, E., & Hoit, J. (2002). Speaking and breathing in high respiratory drive. *Journal of Speech, Language, and Hearing Research, 45,* 89–99.

Benchetrit, G., Shea, S., Pham Dinh, T., Bodocco, S., Baconnier, P., & Guz, A. (1989). Individuality of breathing patterns in adults assessed over time. *Respiration Physiology, 75,* 199–210.

Bernthal, J., & Beukelman, D. (1978). Intraoral air pressure during the production of /p/ and /b/ by children, youths, and adults. *Journal of Speech and Hearing Research, 21,* 361–371.

Boliek, C., Hixon, T., Watson, P., & Jones, P. (2009). Refinement of speech breathing in healthy 4- to 6-year-old children. *Journal of Speech, Language, and Hearing Research, 52,* 990–1007.

Boliek, C., Hixon, T., Watson, P., & Morgan, W. (1996). Vocalization and breathing during the first year of life. *Journal of Voice, 10,* 1–22.

Boliek, C., Hixon, T., Watson, P., & Morgan, W. (1997). Vocalization and breathing during the second and third years of life. *Journal of Voice, 11,* 373–390.

Bouhuys, A., Proctor, D., & Mead, J. (1966). Kinetic aspects of singing. *Journal of Applied Physiology, 31,* 483–496.

Bunn, J., & Mead, J. (1971). Control of ventilation during speech. *Journal of Applied Physiology, 31,* 870–872.

Chapple, E. (1970). *Culture and biological man.* New York, NY: Holt, Rinehart, and Winston.

Connaghan, K., Moore, C., & Hagashakawa, M. (2004). Respiratory kinematics during vocalization and nonspeech respiration in children from 9 to 48 months. *Journal of Speech, Language, and Hearing Research, 47,* 70–84.

Conrad, B., Thalacker, S., & Schonle, P. (1983). Speech respiration as an indicator of integrative contextual processing. *Folia Phoniatrica, 35,* 220–225.

Corfield, D., Murphy, K., & Guz, A. (1998). Does the motor cortical control of the diaphragm "bypass" the brain stem respiratory centres in man? *Respiratory Physiology, 114,* 109–117.

Dejours, P. (1996). *Respiration.* New York, NY: Oxford University Press.

Denny, M. (2000). Periodic variation in inspiratory volume characterizes speech as well as inspiration. *Journal of Voice, 10,* 23–38.

Dickson, D., & Maue-Dickson, W. (1982). *Anatomical and physiological bases of speech.* Boston, MA: Little, Brown, and Company.

Doust, J., & Patrick, J. (1981). The limitation of exercise ventilation during speech. *Respiration Physiology, 46,* 137–147.

Feldman, J., & McCrimmon, D. (1999). Neural control of breathing. In M. Zigmond, F. Bloom, S. Landis, J. Roberts, & L. Squire (Eds.), *Fundamental neuroscience* (pp. 1063–1090). New York, NY: Academic Press.

Gardner, W. (1996). The pathophysiology of hyperventilation disorders. *Chest, 109,* 516–534.

Goldman-Eisler, F. (1956). The determinants of the rate of speech output and their mutual relations. *Journal of Psychosomatic Research, 1,* 137–143.

Greene, J. (1984). Speech preparation processes and verbal fluency. *Human Communication Research, 11,* 61–84.

Greene, J., & Capella, J. (1986). Cognition and talk: The relationship of semantic units to temporal patterns of fluency in spontaneous speech. *Language and Speech, 29,* 141–157.

Grosjean, F., & Collins, M. (1979). Breathing, pausing, and reading. *Phonetica, 36,* 98–114.

Hale, M., & Patrick, J. (1987). Ventilatory patterns during human speech in progressive hypercapnia. *Journal of Physiology, 394,* 60P.

Henderson, A., Goldman-Eisler, F., & Skarbek, A. (1965). Temporal patterns of cognitive activity and breath control in speech. *Language and Speech, 8,* 236–242.

Hertegård, S., Gauffin, J., & Lindestad, P-Å. (1995). A comparison of subglottal and intraoral pressure measurements during phonation. *Journal of Voice, 9,* 149–155.

Hixon, T. (1973). Respiratory function in speech. In F. Minifie, T. Hixon, & F. Williams (Eds.), *Normal aspects of speech, hearing, and language* (pp. 75–125). Englewood-Cliffs, NJ: Prentice-Hall.

Hixon, T., Goldman, M., & Mead, J. (1973). Kinematics of the chest wall during speech production: Volume displacements of the rib cage, abdomen, and lung. *Journal of Speech and Hearing Research, 16,* 78–115.

Hixon, T., & Hoit, J. (2005). *Evaluation and management of speech breathing disorders: Principles and methods.* Tucson, AZ: Redington Brown.

Hixon, T., Mead, J., & Goldman, M. (1976). Dynamics of the chest wall during speech production: Function of the thorax, rib cage, diaphragm, and abdomen. *Journal of Speech and Hearing Research, 19,* 297–356.

Hixon, T., & Weismer, G. (1995). Perspectives on the Edinburgh study of speech breathing. *Journal of Speech and Hearing Research, 38,* 42–60.

Hodge, M., & Rochet, A. (1989). Characteristics of speech breathing in young women. *Journal of Speech and Hearing Research, 32,* 466–480.

Hoit, J., & Hixon, T. (1986). Body type and speech breathing. *Journal of Speech and Hearing Research, 29,* 313–324.

Hoit, J., & Hixon, T. (1987). Age and speech breathing. *Journal of Speech and Hearing Research, 30,* 351–366.

Hoit, J., & Hixon, T. (1992). Age and laryngeal airway resistance during vowel production in women. *Journal of Speech and Hearing Research, 35,* 309–313.

Hoit, J., Hixon, T., Altman, M., & Morgan, W. (1989). Speech breathing in women. *Journal of Speech and Hearing Research, 32,* 353–365.

Hoit, J., Hixon, T., Watson, P., & Morgan, W. (1990). Speech breathing in children and adolescents. *Journal of Speech and Hearing Research, 33,* 51–69.

Hoit, J., Lansing, R., & Perona, G. (2007). Speaking-related dyspnea in healthy adults. *Journal of Speech, Language, and Hearing Research, 50,* 361–374.

Hoit, J., & Lohmeier, H. (2000). Influence of continuous speaking on ventilation. *Journal of Speech, Language, and Hearing Research, 43,* 1240–1251.

Horii, Y., & Cooke, P. (1978). Some airflow, volume, and duration characteristics of oral reading. *Journal of Speech and Hearing Research, 21,* 470–481.

Huber, J. (2008). Effects of utterance length and vocal loudness on speech breathing in older adults. *Respiratory Physiology and Neurobiology, 164,* 323–330.

Huber, J., & Darling, M. (2011). Effect of Parkinson's disease on the production of structured and unstructured speaking tasks: Respiratory physiologic and linguistic considerations. *Journal of Speech, Language, and Hearing Research, 54,* 33–46.

Lay, C., & Paivio, A. (1969). The effects of task difficulty and anxiety on hesitations in speech. *Canadian Journal of Behavioral Sciences, 1,* 25–37.

Loring, S., & Mead, J. (1982). Abdominal muscle use during quiet breathing and hyperpnea in uninformed subjects. *Journal of Applied Physiology, 52,* 700–704.

Lumb, A. (2000). Control of breathing. In A. Lumb (Ed.), *Nunn's applied respiratory physiology* (pp. 82–112). Boston, MA: Butterworth-Heinemann.

Mador, J., & Tobin, M. (1991). Effect of alterations in mental activity on the breathing pattern in healthy subjects. *American Review of Respiratory Disease, 144,* 481–487.

McFarland, D. (2001). Respiratory markers of conversational interaction. *Journal of Speech, Language, and Hearing Research, 44,* 128–143.

McFarland, D., & Smith, A. (1992). Effect of vocal task and respiratory phase on prephonatory chest wall movements. *Journal of Speech and Hearing Research, 35,* 971–982.

Meanock, C., & Nichols, A. (1982). The effect of speech on the ventilatory response to carbon dioxide or to exercise. *Journal of Physiology, 325,* 16P–17P.

Melcon, M., Hoit, J., & Hixon, T. (1989). Age and laryngeal airway resistance during vowel production. *Journal of Speech and Hearing Disorders, 54,* 282–286.

Mitchell, H., Hoit, J., & Watson, P. (1996). Cognitive-linguistic demands and speech breathing. *Journal of Speech and Hearing Research, 39,* 93–104.

Moore, C., Caulfield, T., & Green, J. (2001). Relative kinematics of the rib cage and abdomen during speech and nonspeech behaviors of 15-month-old children. *Journal of Speech, Language, and Hearing Research, 44,* 80–94.

Netsell, R., & Hixon, T. (1978). A noninvasive method for clinically estimating subglottal air pressure. *Journal of Speech and Hearing Disorders, 43,* 326–330.

Netsell, R., Lotz, W., Peters, J., & Schulte, L. (1994). Developmental patterns of laryngeal and respiratory function for speech production. *Journal of Voice, 8,* 123–131.

Otis, A., & Clark, R. (1968). Ventilatory implications of phonation and phonatory implications of ventilation. In A. Bouhuys (Ed.), *Sound production in man* (pp. 122–128). New York, NY: Annals of the New York Academy of Sciences.

Parham, D., Buder, E., Oller, D. K., & Boliek, C. (2011). Syllable-related breathing in infants in the second year of life. *Journal of Speech, Language, and Hearing Research, 54,* 1039–1050.

Phillipson, E., McClean, P., Sullivan, C., & Zamel, N. (1978). Interaction of metabolic and behavioral respiratory control during hypercapnia and speech. *American Review of Respiratory Disease, 117,* 903–909.

Reynolds, A., & Paivio, A. (1968). Cognitive and emotional determinants of speech. *Canadian Journal of Psychology, 22,* 164–175.

Rochester, S. (1973). The significance of pauses in spontaneous speech. *Journal of Psycholinguistic Research, 2,* 51–81.

Russell, B., Cerny, F., & Stathopoulos, E. (1998). Effects of varied vocal intensity on ventilation and energy expenditure in women and men. *Journal of Speech, Language, and Hearing Research, 41,* 239–248.

Shea, S. (1996). Behavioural and arousal-related influences on breathing in humans. *Experimental Physiology, 81,* 1–26.

Shea, S., & Guz, A. (1992). Personnalite ventilatoire: An overview. *Respiration Physiology, 52,* 275–291.

Shea, S., Horner, R., Benchetrit, G., & Guz, A. (1990). The persistence of a respiratory "personality" into Stage IV sleep in man. *Respiration Physiology, 80,* 33–44.

Shea, S., Murphy, K., Hamilton, R., Benchetrit, G., & Guz, A. (1988). Do the changes in respiratory pattern and ventilation seen with different behavioural situations reflect metabolic demands? In C. von Euler & M. Katz-Salamon (Eds.), *Respiratory psychophysiology* (pp. 21–28). Basingstoke, UK: MacMillan Press.

Shea, S., Walter, J., Murphy, K., & Guz, A. (1987). Evidence for individuality of breathing patterns in resting healthy men. *Respiration Physiology, 68,* 331–344.

Shea, S., Walter, J., Pelley, C., Murphy, K., & Guz, A. (1987). The effect of visual and auditory stimuli upon resting ventilation in man. *Respiration Physiology, 68,* 345–357.

Sperry, E., & Klich, R. (1992). Speech breathing in senescent and younger women during oral reading. *Journal of Speech and Hearing Research, 35,* 1246–1255.

Stathopoulos, E., & Sapienza, C. (1993). Respiratory and laryngeal measures of children during vocal intensity variation. *Journal of the Acoustical Society of America, 94,* 2531–2543.

Stathopoulos, E., & Sapienza, C. (1997). Developmental changes in laryngeal and respiratory function with variations in sound pressure level. *Journal of Speech, Language, and Hearing Research, 40,* 595–614.

Stathopoulos, E., & Weismer, G. (1985). Oral airflow and air pressure during speech production: A comparative study of children, youths, and adults. *Folia Phoniatrica, 37,* 152–159.

Sugito, M., Ohyama, G., & Hirose, H. (1990). A preliminary study on pauses and breaths in reading speech materials. *Annual Bulletin of the Research Institute of Logopedics and Phoniatrics, 24,* 121–130.

Taylor, I. (1969). Content and structure in sentence production. *Journal of Verbal Learning and Verbal Behavior, 8,* 170–175.

Warner, R., Waggener, T., & Kronauer, R. (1983). Synchronized cycles in ventilation and vocal activity during spontaneous conversational speech. *Journal of Applied Physiology, 54,* 309–317.

Warren, D., Morr, K., Rochet, A., & Dalston, R. (1989). Respiratory response to a decrease in velopharyngeal resistance. *Journal of the Acoustical Society of America, 86,* 917–924.

Webb, R., Williams, F., & Minifie, F. (1967). Effects of verbal decision behavior upon respiration during speech production. *Journal of Speech and Hearing Research, 10,* 49–56.

Weismer, G. (1985). Speech breathing: Contemporary views and findings. In R. Daniloff (Ed.), *Speech science* (pp. 47–72). San Diego, CA: College-Hill Press.

Western, P., & Patrick, J. (1988). Effects of focusing attention on breathing with and without apparatus on the face. *Respiration Physiology, 72,* 123–130.

Whalen, D., & Kinsella-Shaw, J. (1997). Exploring the relationship of inspiration duration to utterance duration. *Phonetica, 54,* 138–152.

Wilder, C. (1983). Chest wall preparation for phonation in female speakers. In D. Bless & J. Abbs (Eds.), *Vocal fold physiology: Contemporary research and clinical issues* (pp. 109–123). San Diego, CA: College-Hill Press.

Winkworth, A., Davis, P., Adams, R., & Ellis, E. (1995). Breathing patterns during spontaneous speech. *Journal of Speech and Hearing Research, 38,* 124–144.

Winkworth, A., Davis, P., Ellis, E., & Adams, R. (1994). Variability and consistency in speech breathing during reading: Lung volumes, speech intensity, and linguistic factors. *Journal of Speech and Hearing Research, 37,* 535–556.

Wolff, P. (1979). Theoretical issues in the development of motor skills. *Symposium on developmental disabilities in the pre-school child.* Chicago, IL: Johnson and Johnson Baby Products.

Wyke, B. (1974). Respiratory activity of intrinsic laryngeal muscles: An experimental study. In B. Wyke (Ed.), *Ventilatory and phonatory control systems* (pp. 408–429). New York, NY: Oxford University Press.

3

Laryngeal Function and Speech Production

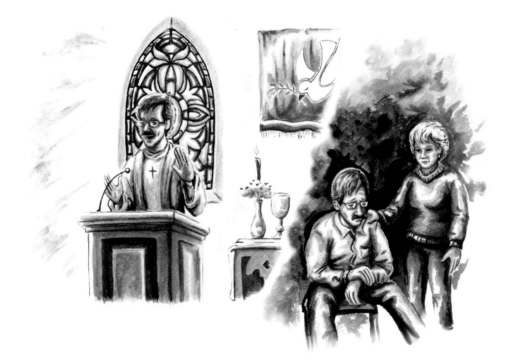

Scenario

His voice was his livelihood and in many ways his life. At age 42, he was at the top of his ecumenical game. As a member of the clergy, he was outstanding by any metric. The members of his large church were extremely fond of him and looked to him for guidance. He had a very successful weekly radio ministry that broadcasted his influence well beyond the walls of his church and the territory of his local congregation. His wife was a rock of his life. She cared for their family that included a girl 18 years old, and two boys, 16 and 15. She also was an accomplished musician and directed the church choir. The children were all interested in horses, 4-H, and music, although somewhat different from the music of their mother.

The daughter left in the fall to attend her first semester of college. She had chosen a small college with religious affiliation. The choice was at the urging of her parents. The mother was saddened by the daughter's departure, but things went on pretty much as usual. The daughter's first-semester grades were not impressive (poor would be more accurate), especially given her track record in high school. The sons had turned their interests to cars and motorcycles. The father had been hoping their interests would follow something in team sports, but this did not meet their fancy. Near the end of the year, the mother underwent surgery for breast cancer.

It was in the spring that the father received a phone call from a member of his church who had a daughter a year ahead of his daughter at the same college. It was a rather lengthy conversation and after hanging up the phone, the minister became noticeably quiet and subdued. He told his wife he was not feeling well and went to bed early that evening. When he awoke in the morning, he was stunned to find that he had no voice. At first he thought he might have a cold or flu, but there were no other symptoms. Except for having no voice, he felt physically fine. A long, hot shower didn't help, nor did gargling with salt water. His concern turned to panic when he realized the implications and approached the kitchen with dread and embarrassment at having to face his wife. When his wife saw what was going on, she immediately telephoned his physician, also a member of the church, and told him about the problem. The physician offered to see him right away, but the results of a physical examination were unremarkable. The physician told him that perhaps he was under more stress than usual and suggested he take it easy for a few days.

But the problem did not go away. The minister had to ask the assistant pastor of the church to do his radio show for the week and despite his thinking that he would somehow be able to deliver his Sunday sermon, he finally realized that he could not do it. A substitute was quickly recruited.

The situation had become desperate and the physician from his church managed to get him in to see an ear, nose, and throat specialist (otorhinolaryngologist) on short notice. No diagnosis was made, but the specialist thought there might be some sort of neurological problem and referred the minister to a neurologist. It took longer to get this appointment, but it too was not fully enlightening. The neurologist found nothing suggestive of neural disease.

What could turn the life of a healthy 42-year-old man around in such a short time and be so utterly debilitating? This once articulate, fluent, verbally engaging individual had been rendered functionally speechless, unable to administer to his congregation, completely stymied as to the cause of his problem and his fate. It was a terrible turn of events that nobody seemed to understand.

INTRODUCTION

The larynx is an air valve located within the front of the neck. This valve is positioned vertically between the trachea (windpipe) and pharynx (throat) and can be adjusted to vary the amount of coupling between the two. The larynx serves a variety of functions, including speech (inclusive of voice) production.

This chapter begins with a discussion of the fundamentals of laryngeal structure and function. This is followed by consideration of laryngeal function for speech production, measurement of laryngeal function, laryngeal disorders that affect speech production, and clinical professionals who evaluate and manage such disorders. The chapter ends with a review and a closing scenario.

FUNDAMENTALS OF LARYNGEAL FUNCTION

This section covers topics fundamental to the understanding of laryngeal function. These include: (a) anatomy of the laryngeal apparatus, (b) forces and movements associated with its actions, (c) adjustments resulting from its actions, (d) control variables involved in its behaviors, (e) neural substrates of laryngeal control, and (f) laryngeal functions.

Anatomy of the Laryngeal Apparatus

The skeleton of the larynx, its joints, and its internal topography are considered in this section. Muscular components are discussed below under the section on active forces.

Skeleton

Figure 3–1 depicts the skeletal framework of the laryngeal apparatus. This framework consists of bone, cartilage, ligament, and tendon. The flexibility of this superstructure changes with age, being soft and pliable in childhood and hard and more rigid in adulthood.

Thyroid Cartilage. The thyroid cartilage is the largest of the laryngeal cartilages and forms most of the front and sides of the laryngeal skeleton. This cartilage provides a shieldlike housing for the larynx and offers protection for many of its structures.

Figure 3–2 shows the thyroid cartilage. Two quadrilateral plates, called the thyroid laminae, are fused together at the front of the thyroid cartilage and diverge widely (more so in women than in men) toward the back. The configuration of the two thyroid

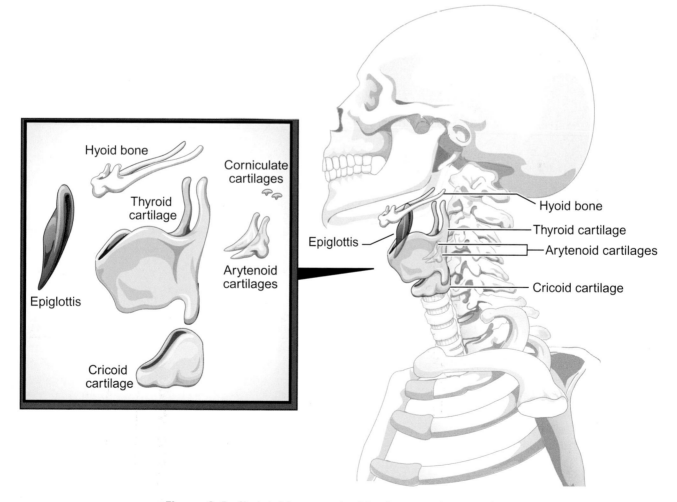

Figure 3-1. Skeletal framework of the laryngeal apparatus.

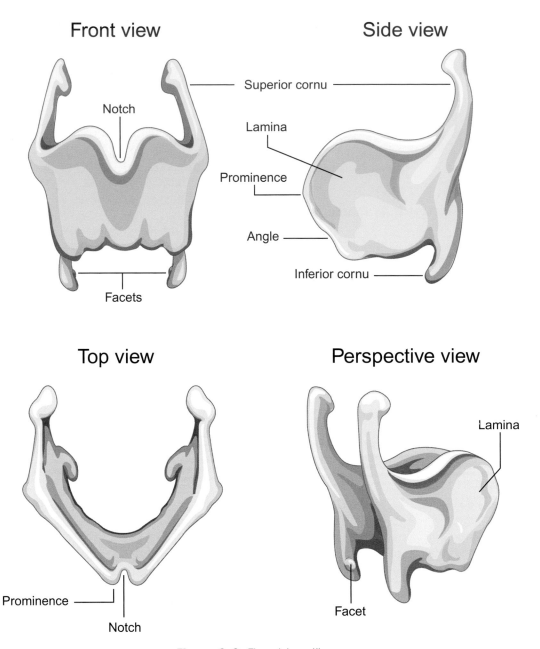

Figure 3–2. Thyroid cartilage.

laminae resembles the bow of a ship. The line of fusion between the two plates is called the angle of the thyroid. The upper part of the structure contains a prominent V-shaped depression that is termed the thyroid notch and can be palpated at the front of the neck. This notch is located just above the most forward projection of the cartilage, an outward jutting called the thyroid prominence or Adam's apple.

The back edges of the thyroid laminae extend upward into two long horns and downward into two short horns. The upper horns, called the superior cor-

nua, are coupled to the hyoid bone (discussed below). The lower horns, termed the inferior cornua, have facets (areas where other structures join) on their lower inside surfaces. These facets provide for the formation of joints with the cricoid cartilage. The inferior cornua straddle the cricoid cartilage like a pair of legs.

Cricoid Cartilage. The cricoid cartilage forms the lower part of the laryngeal skeleton. It is a ring-shaped structure located above the trachea. As shown in Figure 3–3, the cricoid cartilage has a thick plate at the back, the

Side oblique view

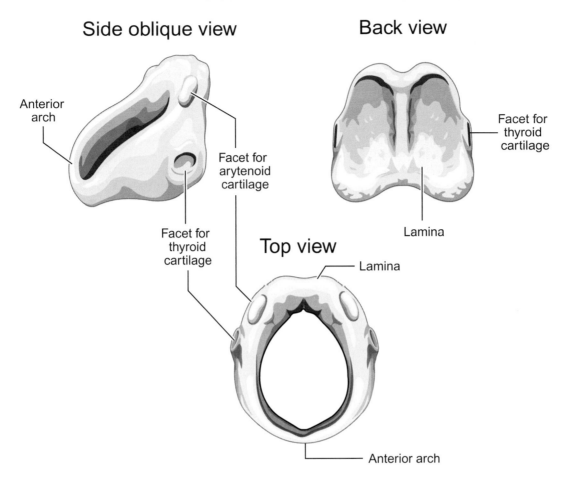

Figure 3–3. Cricoid cartilage.

Sizing Things Up

There's a tendency when viewing anatomical drawings, photographs, and video images of structures of the larynx to overestimate the size of things. The trachea looks long and large in cross-section. The glottis seems to be a big hole. The vocal folds appear to be massive lips. The vocal ligaments look like pencils. And the vibratory movements of the vocal folds (when slowed down) give the impression of a flag blowing in a stiff wind. Some calibration may be helpful. Your trachea is about as long and big around as your middle finger. Your wide-open glottis is about the size of a dime. Your approximated vocal folds have a surface area about the size of your thumbnail (well trimmed). The vocal ligaments are about as thick as wooden matchsticks. And your vocal folds only move about the length of the cuticle on your thumbnail. If you're like us, you'll find this to be surprisingly small. Yes?

---

posterior quadrate lamina, which resembles a signet on a finger ring. A semicircular structure, called the anterior arch, forms the front of the cricoid cartilage and is akin to a band on a finger ring.

Four facets are located on the cricoid cartilage. The lower two facets, one on each side at the same level, are positioned near the junction of the posterior quadrate lamina and anterior arch. Each of these facets articulates with a facet on one of the inferior cornua of the thyroid cartilage. The upper two facets of the cricoid cartilage, one on each side at the same level, are located on the sloping rim of the posterior quadrate lamina. Each of these facets articulates with a facet on the under-surface of one of the arytenoid cartilages.

Arytenoid Cartilages. There are two arytenoid cartilages. Each is located atop one side of the sloping rim of the posterior quadrate lamina of the cricoid cartilage. As shown in Figure 3–4, each arytenoid cartilage has a complex shape that includes an apex, base, and three sides. The apex of each cartilage is capped with another small cone-shaped cartilage called a corniculate cartilage that is often fused to the arytenoid cartilage. The base of each arytenoid cartilage has a flexible pointed projection that extends toward the front and is designated the vocal process. The base also includes a rounded stubby projection that extends toward the back and side and is referred to as the muscular process. The undersurface of each muscular process has a facet that articulates with one of the upper facets of the cricoid cartilage.

Epiglottis. Figure 3–5 depicts the epiglottis. The epiglottis is a single cartilage that is positioned behind the hyoid bone (discussed below) and root of the tongue. The upper part of the epiglottis, its body, is broad and resembles the distal end of a forward-curving shoehorn. The front and back surfaces of this part of the structure are referred to as its lingual (tongue) and laryngeal (larynx) surfaces, respectively. The lingual surface attaches to the hyoid bone. The lower part of the cartilage tapers downward into a stalk called the petiolus (little leg) and attaches to the inside of the thyroid cartilage just below the thyroid notch.

Hyoid Bone. Figure 3–6 depicts the hyoid bone (tongue bone). Technically, the hyoid bone is not a part of the larynx. Nevertheless, it serves as an integral component in many laryngeal functions. Thus, it is commonly afforded a prominent place in discussion of the laryngeal skeleton.

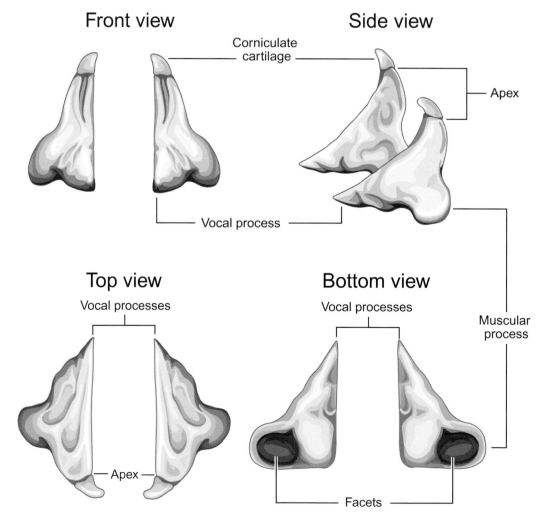

Figure 3–4. Arytenoid cartilages.

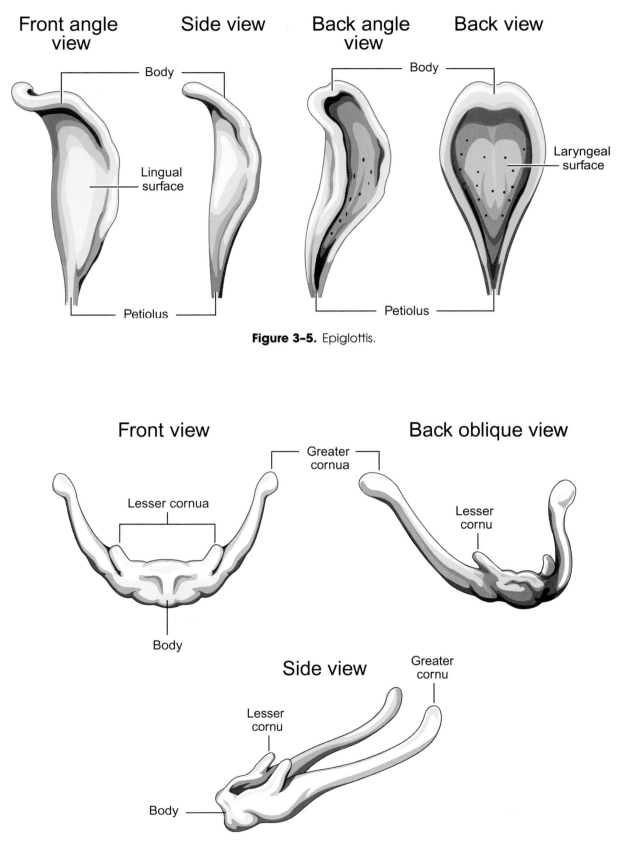

Figure 3–5. Epiglottis.

Figure 3–6. Hyoid bone.

The hyoid bone is free-floating in the sense that it is not attached to any other bone. It is a U-shaped structure that is positioned horizontally within the neck, its open end facing toward the back. The hyoid bone consists of a body and two pairs of greater and lesser horns (cornua) that project upward. The greater cornua are located toward the back of the structure and join with the superior cornua of the thyroid cartilage. The lesser cornua extend from the body of the structure and may be capped by tiny cone-shaped cartilages. The hyoid bone is positioned at the top of the larynx and suspends it from above through various connections.

Laryngeal Joints

There are two pairs of joints in the larynx. One pair is between the cricoid and thyroid cartilages on each side. The other pair is between the cricoid and arytenoid cartilages on each side. Movements at these joints are conditioned by the nature of the facets on their articulating cartilages and the arrangement of surrounding ligaments.

Cricothyroid Joints. Figure 3–7 depicts the cricothyroid joints. These joints are positioned on the sides of

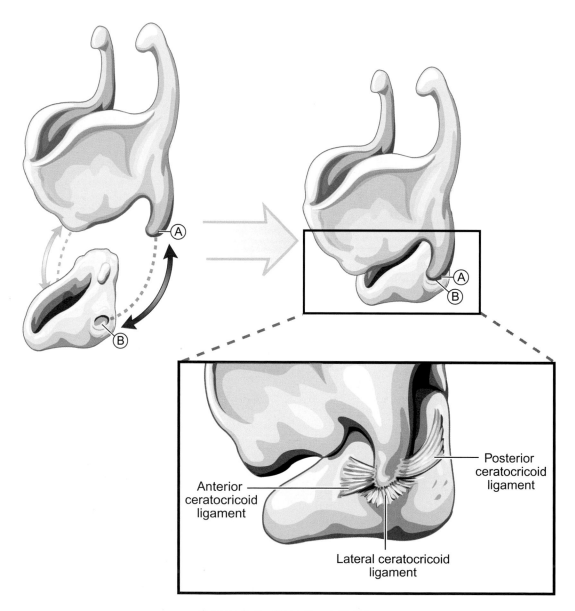

Figure 3–7. Cricothyroid joints.

the larynx and involve articulations between facets on the outer surfaces of the lower part of the cricoid cartilage and the inner surfaces of the inferior cornua of the thyroid cartilage. The cricothyroid joints are encapsulated by membranes that secrete synovial fluid. This fluid serves as a lubricant.

Facets on the cricoid and thyroid cartilages vary from larynx to larynx and from side to side within the same larynx (Dickson & Maue-Dickson, 1982). Those on the cricoid cartilage generally face upward, toward the side, and backward. They are usually round or oval in shape and are concave. Facets on the thyroid cartilage typically face downward, toward the midline, and forward. They are usually round in shape and are convex. Occasionally a larynx will have cricothyroid joint facets that are rudimentary. Then the articulation between the cricoid and thyroid surfaces is formed by fibrous connective tissue (Zemlin, 1998).

Three ligaments extend between the side and back surfaces of the cricoid cartilage and the lower outside surfaces of the inferior cornu of the thyroid cartilage on each side. These three ligaments encircle most of the corresponding cricothyroid joint and are referred to as the anterior, lateral, and posterior ceratocricoid (cerato meaning horn) ligaments. The anterior ligament extends backward into the front surface of the inferior cornu. The lateral ligament extends upward into the lower surface of the cornu. And the posterior ligament extends forward into the back surface of the cornu. Together the three ligaments bind the corresponding cricothyroid joint and place restrictions on the movements of the cricoid and thyroid cartilages.

Figure 3–8 portrays the nature of movements at the cricothyroid joints. They are of two types, rotating and sliding.

The most significant movements at the cricothyroid joints are rotational and occur about a lateral axis extending through the two joints. Either or both the cricoid and thyroid cartilages can rotate about this axis (Mayet & Muendnich, 1958; Takano & Honda, 2005; Vennard, 1967; Zemlin, 1998). One consequence of rotation is a change in the distance between the top of the anterior arch of the cricoid cartilage and the bottom of the laminae of the thyroid cartilage at the front. This change is analogous to rotating the chin guard (representing the anterior arch of the cricoid cartilage) and the visor (representing the laminae of the thyroid cartilage) on a motorcycle helmet.

Secondary movements at the cricothyroid joints are of a sliding nature and can occur in those larynges that have oval-shaped cricoid facets. These movements are small and occur along the long axes of the cricoid

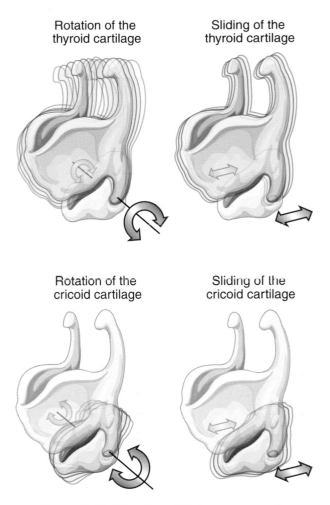

Figure 3–8. Cricothyroid joint movements.

facets (Takano & Honda, 2005; Titze, 1994; van den Berg, Vennard, Berger, & Shervanian, 1960).

Cricoarytenoid Joints. Figure 3–9 depicts the cricoarytenoid joints. These joints are positioned near the top of the larynx and involve articulations between the facets on the sloping rims of the cricoid cartilage and the undersurfaces of the arytenoid cartilages. Synovial membranes encapsulate these joints and lubricate them.

Facets on the cricoid and arytenoid cartilages are relatively uniform in characteristics from larynx to larynx and from side to side within a larynx (Dickson & Maue-Dickson, 1982). Facets on the cricoid cartilage face upward, toward the side, and forward. These facets are usually oval in shape and are convex. Facets on the arytenoid cartilages face downward, toward the midline, and backward. They are usually round in shape and are concave (Frable, 1961; Zemlin, 1998).

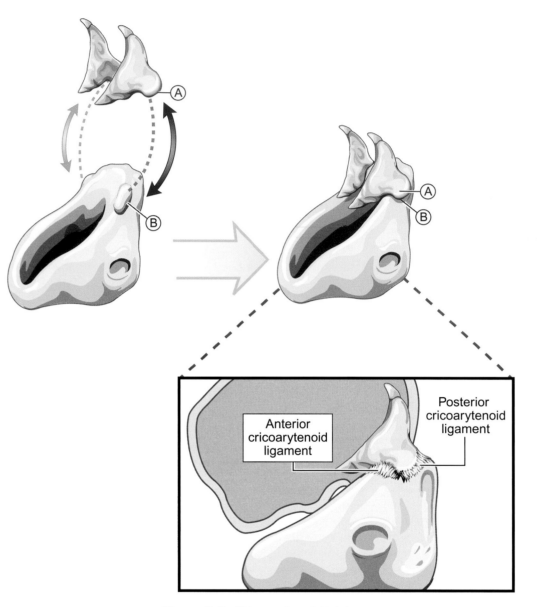

Figure 3–9. Cricoarytenoid joints.

Two ligaments influence the function of each cricoarytenoid joint by binding it and restricting its movements. These include the anterior and posterior cricoarytenoid ligaments. The anterior cricoarytenoid ligament extends from the side of the cricoid cartilage to the front and side of the arytenoid cartilage. The ligament runs upward and backward and limits the degree to which the arytenoid cartilage can be moved backward. The posterior cricoarytenoid ligament extends upward and toward the side from the back of the cricoid cartilage to the back of the arytenoid cartilage. This ligament limits the degree to which the arytenoid cartilage can be moved forward.

Figure 3–10 depicts the nature of movements at the cricoarytenoid joints. Movements at these joints can be of two types: rocking and sliding.

The most significant movements at the cricoarytenoid joints are of a rocking nature in which the arytenoid cartilages move at right angles to the long axes of their articulating cricoid facets (Ardran & Kemp, 1966; Selbie, Zhang, Levine, & Ludlow, 1998; Sellars & Keen, 1978; Sonesson, 1959; von Leden & Moore, 1961). The long axes of interest slope downward and toward the sides of the cricoids cartilage. This means that as the arytenoid cartilages rock on the cricoid cartilage their vocal processes move either upward and outward or downward and inward.

Rocking of the
arytenoid cartilages

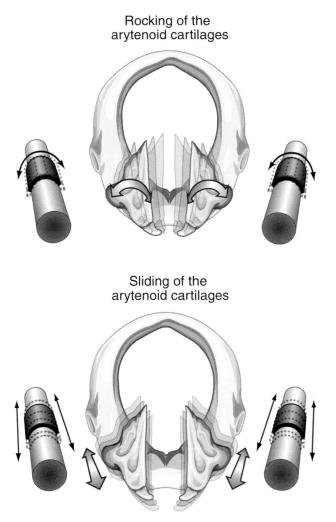

Sliding of the
arytenoid cartilages

Figure 3–10. Cricoarytenoid joint movements.

Limited sliding movements can also occur along the cricoid facets. These movements involve small upward and inward or downward and outward adjustments of the arytenoid cartilages that follow the courses of the long axes of the cricoid facets (Fink, Basek, & Epanchin, 1956; Pressman, 1942; von Leden & Moore, 1961; Wang, 1998).

Internal Topography

The interior of the larynx defines the boundaries of the laryngeal airway. Figure 3–11 depicts the structures that form these boundaries and lie immediately deep to them.

Laryngeal Cavity. The laryngeal cavity extends from a lower opening formed by the base of the cricoid cartilage to an upper opening designated as the laryngeal aditus. The laryngeal aditus forms a collar at the top of the larynx. The rim of this collar comprises the tops of the arytenoid cartilages (and corniculate cartilages), sides of the epiglottis, and the aryepiglottic folds. The aryepiglottic folds run between the arytenoid cartilages and the epiglottis and envelop the aryepiglottic muscles (discussed below) and a pair of small cuneiform (wedge-shaped) cartilages. The cuneiform cartilages stiffen the aryepiglottic folds and help to maintain the upper opening (collar entrance) into the larynx.

Subglottal and Supraglottal Regions. The lower and upper regions of the laryngeal cavity are often referred to as the subglottal and supraglottal regions, respectively. The subglottal region is bounded below by the lower margin of the cricoid cartilage and above by the vocal folds. This region is cone-shaped and converges toward the undersurface of the vocal folds.

The supraglottal region is bounded below by the ventricular folds and above by the laryngeal aditus (upper opening into the larynx). This region is also called the laryngeal vestibule (cavity approaching a cavity). The configuration of the vestibule is roughly that of a funnel, the lumen of which increases in size toward its upper end.

Vocal Folds. The vocal folds are two prominent shelf-like structures that extend from the sidewalls of the laryngeal cavity into the laryngeal airway. Each vocal fold has a front attachment near the midline of the thyroid cartilage and a rear attachment to the vocal process of the arytenoid cartilage on the same side. Much of each vocal fold consists of muscular tissue and a vocal ligament that runs through the shelflike structure near its inner edge from front to back.

The vocal folds are not structurally homogeneous, but are made up of different layers. Figure 3–12 shows a frontal section through the midlength of an adult vocal fold that exemplifies this characteristic layering. Up to five layers are recognized (Hirano, 1974; Hirano & Sato, 1993) and include: (a) a thin stiff capsule of squamous epithelium that determines the outer shape of vocal fold, (b) a superficial layer of lamina propria (subflooring) that consists of loose fibrous matrix and is akin to soft gelatin, and is anchored to the epithelium through a region called the basement membrane zone, (c) an intermediate layer of lamina propria that contains elastic fibers and is likened to a bundle of soft rubber bands, (d) a deep layer of lamina propria that contains collagen fibers and bears analogy to a bundle of cotton thread, and (e) muscle fibers that form the inner vocal fold and are the equivalent of a bundle of stiff rubber bands. These five layers are often subgrouped into a so-called body of the vocal fold and a

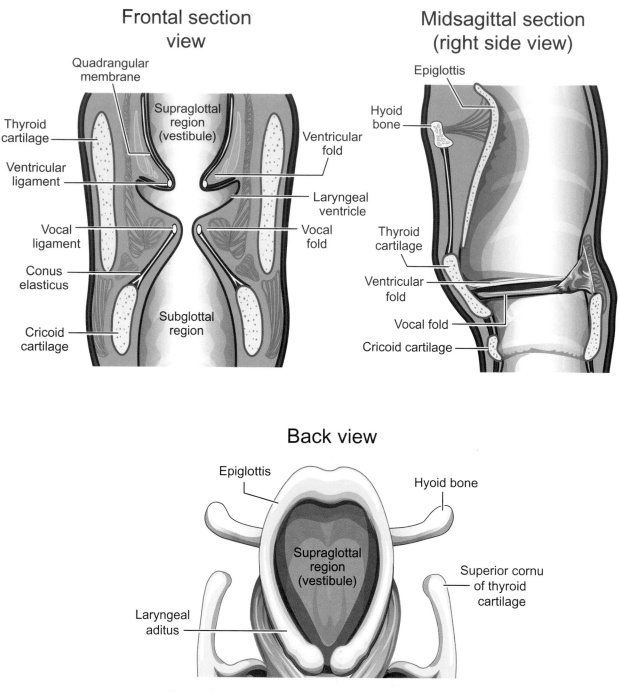

Figure 3–11. Structures of the interior of the larynx.

so-called cover, the body comprising muscle fibers and the deep layer of the lamina propria and the cover comprising the intermediate and superficial layers of the lamina propria and the epithelium.

Although the layering in Figure 3–12 is typical at the midlength of the vocal folds, the precise nature of the layering may be quite different at other locations because the layers of the lamina propria change in their relative proportions along the length of the vocal fold. For example, toward the ends of each vocal fold, elastic fibers and then collagenous fibers predominate. These masses of elastic and collagenous fibers act to cushion and protect those areas of the vocal folds from stresses. There are also differences in the cellular structure and concentration of other constituents at other locations within the lamina propria (Catten, Gray, Hammond,

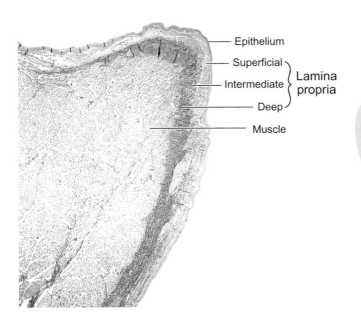

Epithelium

Superficial ⎫
Intermediate ⎬ Lamina propria
Deep ⎭

Muscle

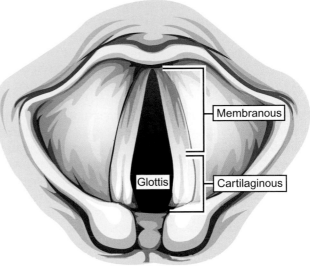

Membranous

Glottis

Cartilaginous

Figure 3–13. Glottis.

Figure 3-12. Frontal section through the midlength of the membranous adult vocal fold. From *Histological color atlas of the human larynx,* (1st ed., p. 45), by M. Hirano and K. Sato, 1993, Belmont, CA: Delmar Learning. Copyright 1993 by Delmar Learning, a Division of Thomson Learning: www.thomsonrights.com. Fax: 800-730-2215. Modified and reproduced with permission.

Zhou, & Hammond, 1998; de Melo et al., 2003; Ishii, Zhai, Akita, & Hirose, 1996; Obrebowski, Wojnowski, & Obrebowski-Karsznia, 2006; Strocchi et al., 1992).

When viewed from above, the medial borders of the vocal folds diverge from front to back, as illustrated in Figure 3–13. Between the vocal folds is a triangularly shaped opening, called the glottis. The front part of the glottis is called the membranous glottis and occupies about 60% of the length of the vocal folds. It lies between the thyroid cartilage and the tips of the vocal processes of the arytenoid cartilages and courses along the vocal ligaments. The back part of the glottis is called the cartilaginous glottis. It occupies about 40% of the length of the vocal folds and lies between the tips of the vocal processes of the arytenoid cartilages and the most rearward points on their medial surfaces.

Ventricular Folds. As shown in Figure 3–11, another set of shelflike structures also extends from the sidewalls of the laryngeal cavity into the laryngeal airway. These structures lie above the vocal folds (but are less prominent) and are referred to as the ventricular folds or false vocal folds. These folds attach to the thyroid cartilage at the front and to the fronts and sides of the arytenoid cartilages at the back. Each fold contains a ventricular ligament that runs from front to back near

its medial edge. Muscular tissue is sparse within the ventricular folds. The opening between the ventricular folds is referred to as the false glottis and is nearly always wider than the glottis between the vocal folds.

Laryngeal Ventricles. The vocal folds and ventricular folds have a sinus (depression) between them (see Figure 3–11). This sinus is termed the laryngeal ventricle

---

Two Worlds

Technical and colloquial definitions of terms can sometimes be quite different. Take, for example, the term "elastic." In a physical sense, something that's elastic returns to its original shape following deformation. Throw a golf club on the floor and it will deform and then return to its original shape. And you can predict what that shape will be. But consider the waistband of your underwear. Throw your underwear on the floor and its waistband will not assume a shape you can predict. That's because, in a physical sense, it's inelastic—it doesn't return to its original shape following deformation. So, although you might think of the waistband of your underwear as being elastic, a physicist would think just the opposite. Both of you are right in your colloquial and technical uses of the term "elastic," but you need to know which world you're talking in (colloquial or technical) before you consider something to be "elastic" or not.

and constitutes a horizontal pouch in each sidewall of the laryngeal tube. The laryngeal ventricles extend most of the length of the vocal folds. Toward the front of the larynx they course upward into saccules that are richly endowed with mucous glands. These glands can be milked to lubricate the vocal folds.

Ligaments and Membranes. Ligaments and membranes are important to laryngeal function. Ligaments that bind the joints of the larynx (the anterior, lateral, and posterior ceratocricoid ligaments, for the cricothyroid joints, and the anterior and posterior cricoarytenoid ligaments, for the cricoarytenoid joints) are discussed above and depicted in Figures 3–7 and 3–9. Most of the other intrinsic and extrinsic ligaments and membranes are depicted in Figure 3–14 and discussed below.

Intrinsic Ligaments and Membranes. The intrinsic ligaments and membranes of the larynx are those that connect laryngeal cartilages to one another. These ligaments and membranes are important in regulating the extent and direction of movement of the laryngeal cartilages in relation to one another. Most of the intrinsic ligaments and membranes of the larynx arise from a common sheet of connective tissue called the elastic membrane. This sheet lines the entire laryngeal airway, except for the part that lies between the vocal and ventricular ligaments on each side. This discontinuity enables the mucous glands in the laryngeal saccules to be expressed into the laryngeal cavity as lubricant.

The part of the elastic membrane that lines the subglottal region connects the cricoid, arytenoid, and thyroid cartilages to one another and is designated as the conus elasticus. This membrane gives rise to a middle cricothyroid ligament, two lateral cricothyroid membranes, and two vocal ligaments. The middle cricothyroid ligament extends between the top of the anterior arch of the cricoid cartilage and the bottom of the thyroid cartilage in the region of the angle of the thyroid cartilage. This ligament limits the degree to which the cricoid cartilage and thyroid cartilage can be separated vertically at the front. The two lateral cricothyroid membranes are thinner than the middle cricothyroid ligament and extend upward from the upper border of the anterior arch of the cricoid cartilage at the sides. They, like the middle cricothyroid ligament, restrict the separation of the cricoid and thyroid cartilages toward the front. The lateral cricothyroid membranes thicken significantly toward the top of the conus elasticus. These thickenings form the vocal ligaments of the larynx. The vocal ligaments extend between the angle of the thyroid cartilage and the vocal processes of the arytenoid cartilages and lie near the free margins of the vocal folds. These ligaments restrict the degree to which the thyroid and arytenoid cartilages can be separated from front to back.

The part of the elastic membrane that lines the supraglottal region connects the epiglottis, thyroid cartilage, arytenoid cartilages, and corniculate cartilages to one another and is referred to as the quadrangular membrane. This membrane is paired left and right and thickens significantly toward the bottoms of the pair to form the ventricular (false vocal fold) ligaments. These ligaments extend the length of the ventricular folds near their free margins and attached to the thyroid and arytenoid cartilages. The ventricular ligaments place limits on the degree to which the thyroid and arytenoid cartilages can be separated from front to back. The remaining intrinsic ligament of the larynx is the thyroepiglottic ligament. This ligament extends between the bottom of the epiglottis and the inside of the angle of the thyroid cartilage, just beneath the thyroid notch, and functions as a fastener.

Extrinsic Ligaments and Membranes. Extrinsic ligaments and membranes of the larynx are those that connect laryngeal cartilages to structures outside the larynx. These provide support and stability for the laryngeal housing. The cricotracheal membrane (sometimes called the cricotracheal ligament) comprises the lowermost extrinsic connection to the larynx. This membrane extends around the bottom of the larynx between the first tracheal ring and the lower margin of the cricoid cartilage. The cricotracheal membrane is somewhat more extensive than the connective tissue between successive tracheal rings, the first tracheal ring being somewhat larger than the rest. The hyoepiglottic ligament extends between the upper back surface of the body of the hyoid bone and the lingual surface of the epiglottis. This ligament limits the degree to which these two structures can be separated from front to back. The hyothyroid (also called the thyrohyoid) ligaments and membrane form a large interconnection between the hyoid bone and the upper margin of the thyroid cartilage of the larynx. This interconnection gives the appearance that the laryngeal housing proper is suspended from the hyoid bone. The hyothyroid membrane thickens toward the midline of the larynx at the front and is designated in that location as the middle hyothyroid ligament. The same membrane also thickens toward the back in the space between the greater cornua of the hyoid bone and the superior cornua of the thyroid cartilage. These thickenings are referred to as the lateral hyothyroid ligaments. Often embedded within each of these lateral ligaments is a small triticial (grain of wheat) cartilage.

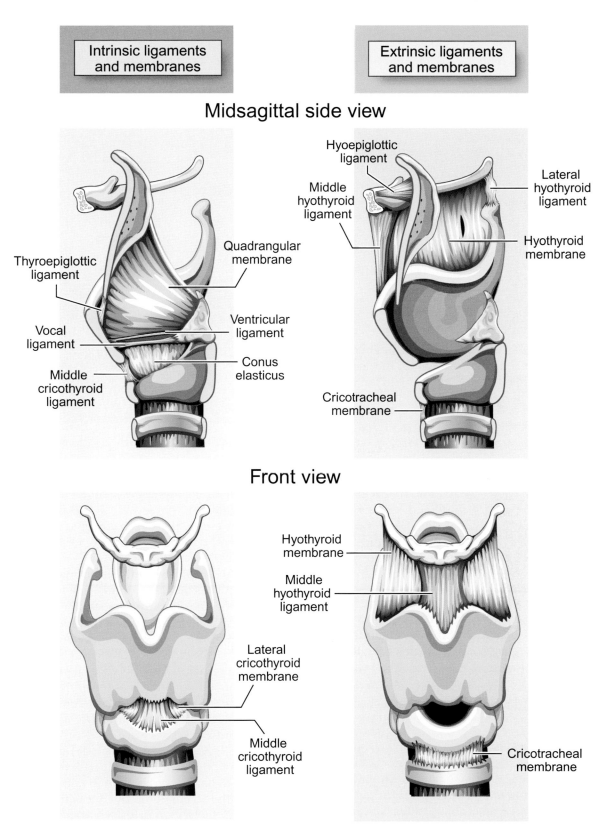

Intrinsic ligaments and membranes

Extrinsic ligaments and membranes

Midsagittal side view

Hyoepiglottic ligament

Middle hyothyroid ligament

Lateral hyothyroid ligament

Hyothyroid membrane

Thyroepiglottic ligament

Quadrangular membrane

Vocal ligament

Ventricular ligament

Middle cricothyroid ligament

Conus elasticus

Cricotracheal membrane

Front view

Hyothyroid membrane

Middle hyothyroid ligament

Lateral cricothyroid membrane

Middle cricothyroid ligament

Cricotracheal membrane

Figure 3–14. Intrinsic and extrinsic laryngeal ligaments and membranes.

Mucous Membrane. The entire internal laryngeal cavity is lined by a mucous membrane, like the trachea below it and the pharynx above it. This lining is covered by columnar epithelium, except for the inner edges of the vocal folds and ventricular folds and the upper half of the epiglottis, which are covered with squamous epithelium.

Forces and Movements of the Laryngeal Apparatus

Forces applied to and by different components of the laryngeal apparatus are responsible for its movements. Its movements contribute to the functional potential of the larynx.

Forces of the Laryngeal Apparatus

Two types of force, passive and active, operate on the larynx. Passive force is inherent within the apparatus. Active force is applied in accordance with the will and ability of the individual.

Passive Force. The passive force of the larynx comes from several sources. These include the natural recoil of muscles, cartilages, and connective tissues (ligaments and membranes), the surface tension between structures in apposition (vocal folds, ventricular folds, epiglottis and aryepiglottic folds, and/or tongue), and the pull of gravity. The distribution, sign, and magnitude of passive force depend on the mechanical milieu, including the positions, deformations, and levels of activity (if applicable) of different parts of the laryngeal apparatus.

Active Force. The active force of the laryngeal apparatus results from the contraction of muscles. Laryngeal muscles can be categorized as intrinsic, extrinsic, or supplementary. Muscles categorized as intrinsic have both ends attached within the larynx, whereas muscles categorized as extrinsic have one end attached within the larynx and one end attached outside the larynx. Muscles categorized as supplementary do not attach to the larynx directly but influence it by way of attachments to the neighboring hyoid bone.

The function described below for individual muscles assumes that the muscles of interest are engaged in shortening (concentric) contractions, unless otherwise specified as being engaged in lengthening (eccentric) contractions or fixed-length (isometric) contractions. The influence of individual muscle actions may also be conditioned by whether or not other muscles are active.

Motorboat

Probably as a child you played "motor boat" with friends by rapidly pounding your fists on their chests or backs while they sustained "ah." The variation in loudness that sounded to you like an idling motorboat was caused by rapid changes in alveolar pressure. Pound on someone's chest or back and with each blow their lungs compress a small amount and the air pressure inside them goes up momentarily. Pound at different rates and you change the perceived speed of your imaginary motor noise. The basis of all this fun is that the laryngeal apparatus and the voice are sensitive to adjustments in the breathing apparatus. You don't necessarily need to have a friend pounding on you to appreciate this sensitivity. Try to talk while driving a car down a cross-rutted dirt road or while sitting atop a trotting horse. The road and the horse will effectively do the pounding for you by bouncing your gut up and down and changing your alveolar pressure.

Intrinsic Laryngeal Muscles. Figure 3–15 depicts the intrinsic muscles of the larynx. These muscles are responsible for changing the position and mechanical status of structures that form the walls of the laryngeal cavity. They are the *thyroarytenoid, posterior cricoarytenoid, lateral cricoarytenoid, arytenoid,* and *cricothyroid* muscles.

The *thyroarytenoid* muscle forms most of each vocal fold. This muscle extends between the inside surface of the thyroid cartilage (near the angle) and the arytenoid cartilage on the corresponding side. The front attachment of the muscle lies to the side of the front attachment of the corresponding vocal ligament. Fibers run generally parallel to the vocal ligament to insert on the front and outer sides of the arytenoid cartilage. Upper fibers run a straight course from front to back, whereas lower fibers twist in their course and swing off in an outward, backward, and upward direction (Broad, 1973; Zemlin, 1998). A small number of fibers toward the side of the muscle depart from the predominant front-to-back orientation of the others and course upward to the aryepiglottic fold, the side of the epiglottis, and into the region of the ventricular fold on the same side (Zemlin, 1998). The effects of contraction of different parts of the *thyroarytenoid* muscle are portrayed in Figure 3–16. Contraction of its longitudinal fibers shortens it and reduces the distance between the

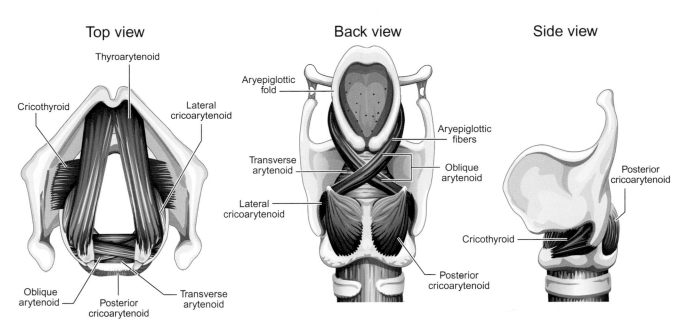

Figure 3–15. Intrinsic muscles of the larynx.

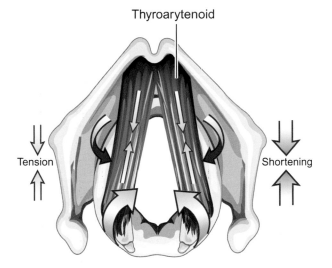

Figure 3–16. Effects of contractions of different parts of the *thyroarytenoid* muscles.

thyroid and arytenoid cartilages. The reduction in distance between the two cartilages is typically effected as a forward pull on the arytenoid cartilage that rocks it toward the midline. Fixed-length (isometric) or lengthening (eccentric) contractions of the *thyroarytenoid* muscle (with other intrinsic muscles opposing) increase its internal tension (force per unit length). Contraction of vertical fibers of the *thyroarytenoid* muscle near the sidewall of the larynx may have an influence on the position and configuration of the corresponding ventricular fold (Reidenbach, 1998).

The *thyroarytenoid* muscle is sometimes described as having two distinct parts (Dickson & Maue-Dickson, 1982; van den Berg & Moll, 1955; Wustrow, 1953), called the *external thyroarytenoid* muscle (*thyromuscularis*) and the *internal thyroarytenoid* muscle (*thyrovocalis* or *vocalis*). As depicted schematically in Figure 3–17, the *external thyroarytenoid* muscle lies nearest the laryngeal wall and to the side of the *internal thyroarytenoid* muscle. The *internal thyroarytenoid* muscle flanks the vocal ligament. The *internal thyroarytenoid* muscle and the vocal ligament are sometimes referred to as the vocal cord, as distinguished from the vocal fold, although the terms vocal cord and vocal fold are also used interchangeably. The term vocal fold is more descriptive of the entire shelflike structure and is preferred.

The notion of a two-part *thyroarytenoid* muscle, although embraced by many, is not accepted universally. Some argue that dissections have failed to reveal a separating fascial sheath within the *thyroarytenoid* muscle that would support the notion of two distinct anatomical parts (Mayet, 1955; Zemlin, 1998). Others argue that, with or without such a separating fascial sheath, the *thyroarytenoid* muscle is capable of differential actions in what is conceptualized to be its *thyromuscularis* and *thyrovocalis* subdivisions (Broad, 1973; Sonesson, 1960). These presumed differential actions (discussed below in another section) are believed by

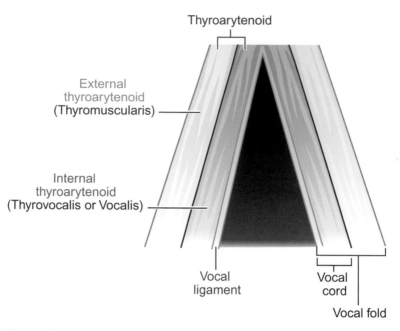

Figure 3–17. *Thyromuscularis* and *thyrovocalis* subdivisions of the *thyroarytenoid* muscles.

some to have salience in the control of voice production (Kahane, 2007; Orlikoff & Kahane, 1996; Titze, 1994).

There is some anatomical evidence to support differential actions of the two subdivisions of the *thyroarytenoid* muscle. For example, the *thyrovocalis* muscle appears to have distinct subcompartments in which muscle fibers are differentially packed, suggesting that they function independently (Sanders, Rai, Han, & Biller, 1998). And, for another example, slow tonic muscle fibers have been found within the *thyrovocalis* muscle, but not within the *thyromuscularis* muscle (Han, Wang, Fischman, Biller, & Sanders, 1999). Contractions of these muscle fibers are prolonged, stable, precisely controlled, and fatigue resistant, all desirable characteristics for adjusting the background mechanical properties of the inner part of the vocal fold. Current evidence suggests that slow tonic muscle fibers are not present in other mammals (including primates) and, therefore, may be a unique human specialization (Han et al., 1999).

The *posterior cricoarytenoid* muscle is a fan-shaped muscle located on the back surface of the cricoid cartilage. The muscle originates on the cricoid lamina and courses upward and toward the side in a converging pattern to insert on the upper and back surfaces of the muscular process of the arytenoid cartilage. As illustrated in Figure 3–18, contraction of the *posterior crico-*

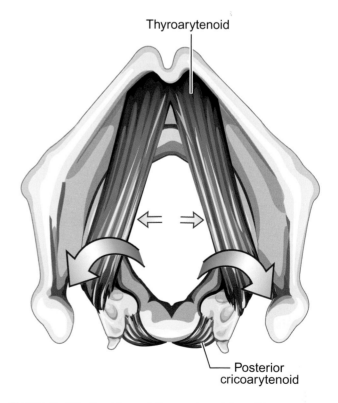

Figure 3–18. Rocking of the arytenoid cartilages away from the midline by contractions of the *posterior cricoarytenoid* muscles.

LARYNGEAL FUNCTION AND SPEECH PRODUCTION

arytenoid muscle rocks the arytenoid cartilage away from the midline. This rocking is effected mainly by fibers located laterally within the muscle and that insert on the upper surface of the muscular process. Forceful contraction of these fibers may also slide the arytenoid cartilage upward and backward along the sloping rim of the cricoid cartilage. Fibers in the medial part of the *posterior cricoarytenoid* muscle insert on the back surface of the muscular process and contract to stabilize the arytenoid cartilage against other forces that are directed forward (Zemlin, Davis, & Gaza, 1984).

The *lateral cricoarytenoid* muscle is a small fan-shaped muscle that originates from the upper rim of the cricoid cartilage. Fibers of this muscle extend upward and backward to insert on the muscular process and front surface of the arytenoid cartilage. As depicted in Figure 3–19, contraction of the *lateral cricoarytenoid* muscle rocks the arytenoid cartilage toward the midline. Activation of the *lateral cricoarytenoid* muscle may also slide the arytenoid cartilage forward and toward the side along the downward sloping path of the long axis of the cricoid facet of the cricoarytenoid joint.

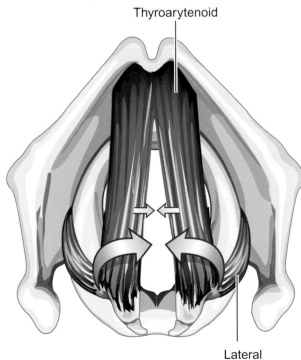

Thyroarytenoid

Lateral cricoarytenoid

Figure 3–19. Rocking of the arytenoid cartilages toward the midline by contractions of the *lateral cricoarytenoid* muscles.

The *arytenoid* muscle (also called the *interarytenoid*) extends from the back surface of one arytenoid cartilage to the back surface of the other arytenoid cartilage. The *arytenoid* muscle is a complex structure that is considered to have two distinct and separate subdivisions, one designated as the *transverse arytenoid* muscle and one designated as the *oblique arytenoid* muscle. The *transverse arytenoid* muscle arises from the back surface and side of one arytenoid cartilage and courses horizontally to insert on the back surface and side of the other arytenoid cartilage. Those muscle fibers that insert on the sides of the arytenoid cartilages interdigitate with fibers of the *thyroarytenoid* muscles. The *oblique arytenoid* muscle overlies the transverse component of the muscle and diagonally crosses the back surface of the two arytenoid cartilages. The muscle originates from the back and side surface and muscular process of one arytenoid cartilage and courses upward to insert near the apex of the other arytenoid cartilage. Some muscle fibers of the *oblique arytenoid* muscle extend around the side of the apex of the arytenoid cartilage and course upward and forward to insert into the side of the epiglottis. This part of the muscle is given its own name, the *aryepiglottic* muscle. As illustrated in Figure 3–20, contraction of different components of the *arytenoid* muscle has different effects. Contraction of the *transverse arytenoid* muscle pulls the arytenoid cartilages toward one another. This is manifested through an upward, inward, and backward sliding movement along the long axis of each cricoarytenoid joint. Contraction of the *oblique arytenoid* muscle pulls one arytenoid cartilage toward the other in a tipping action that occurs in accordance with the movement permitted at the cricoarytenoid joint. And contraction of the *aryepiglottic* muscle pulls the epiglottis backward and downward to cover the upper opening into the larynx.

The *cricothyroid* muscle extends between the outer front and side of the anterior arch of the cricoid cartilage and the outer front and side of the lower border of the lamina and inferior cornu of the thyroid cartilage. The muscle is fan-shaped with its fibers diverging as they course from the cricoid cartilage to the thyroid cartilage. Two subdivisions of the muscle are most often recognized, a vertical component toward the front, called the *par rectus*, and an upward sloping component toward the back, called the *pars oblique* (Zemlin, 1998). A third subdivision, the *pars media*, is occasionally noted. Its fibers lie underneath and closer to the midline than the fibers of the *pars rectus* (Charpied & Shapshay, 2004), although some consider the *pars media* to be an anatomical variation of the *cricothyroid* muscle proper

Back view

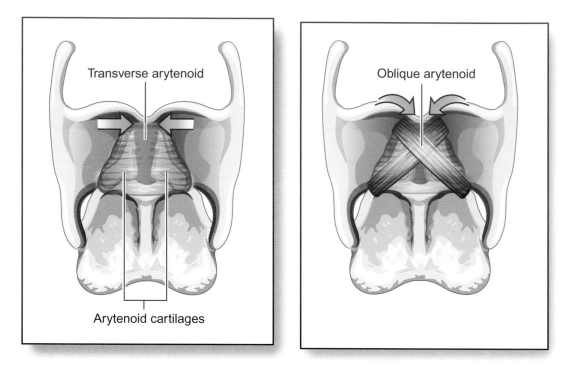

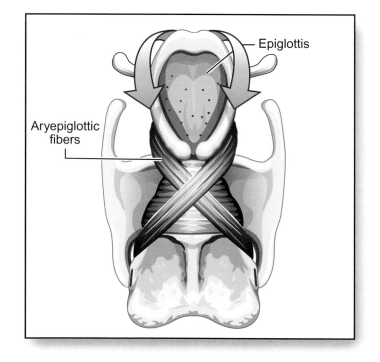

Figure 3–20. Effects of contractions of different parts of the *arytenoid* muscles.

(Kucinski, Okrazewska, & Piszcz, 1979). As illustrated in Figure 3–21, contraction of the *cricothyroid* muscle increases the distance between the thyroid and arytenoid cartilages and decreases the distance between the upper border of the cricoid cartilage and the lower border of the thyroid cartilage at the front of the larynx (decreases the visor angle formed between the two cartilages). These distance changes result from a rotation of the thyroid cartilage on the cricoid cartilage and/or a rotation of the cricoid cartilage on the thyroid cartilage. Rotation is effected through activation of both the *pars rectus* and *pars oblique* components of the *cricothyroid* muscle. Activation of the *pars oblique* component also results in a secondary movement that increases the distance between the thyroid and arytenoid cartilages. This movement amounts to a limited forward sliding of the thyroid cartilage, backward sliding of the cricoid cartilage, or both (Arnold, 1961; Takano & Honda, 2005; van den Berg et al., 1960).

Extrinsic Laryngeal Muscles. Figure 3–22 depicts the extrinsic muscles of the laryngeal apparatus. The extrinsic muscles have a role in supporting and stabilizing the larynx and in changing its position within the neck. They include the ***sternothyroid, thyrohyoid***, and ***inferior constrictor*** muscles.

The ***sternothyroid*** muscle is a long muscle located toward the front and side of the larynx. It originates from the back surface of the top of the sternum (breastbone) and the first costal (rib) cartilage. Fibers of the muscle course upward and slightly toward the side to insert on the outer surface of the thyroid cartilage. Contraction of the ***sternothyroid*** muscle pulls the thyroid cartilage downward. This action may also enlarge the pharynx by drawing the larynx forward and downward (Zemlin, 1998).

The ***thyrohyoid*** muscle is located on the front and side of the larynx. It extends between the outer surface of the thyroid cartilage and the lower edge of the greater cornu of the hyoid bone. The course of its fibers is essentially vertical. Contraction of the ***thyrohyoid*** muscle decreases the distance between the thyroid cartilage and the hyoid bone. Relative fixation of the thyroid cartilage and hyoid bone determines the extent to which the structures may move toward one another.

The ***inferior constrictor*** muscle (discussed in more detail in Chapter 4) is the lowest of the group of three muscles that forms the back and sidewalls of the pharynx (throat). Fibers of the ***inferior constrictor*** muscle extend forward from the median raphe at the back of the pharynx to insert on the sides of the cricoid and thyroid cartilages. Contraction of the ***inferior constrictor*** muscle moves the sidewall of the lower pharynx inward and decreases the size of the pharyngeal lumen. Its activation also serves to stabilize the position of the laryngeal housing.

Supplementary Muscles. Some muscles do not attach on the larynx, but are nonetheless important in influencing its position and stability. These muscles,

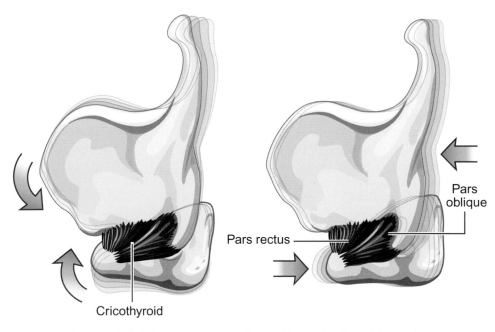

Figure 3–21. Effects of contractions of the *cricothyroid* muscles.

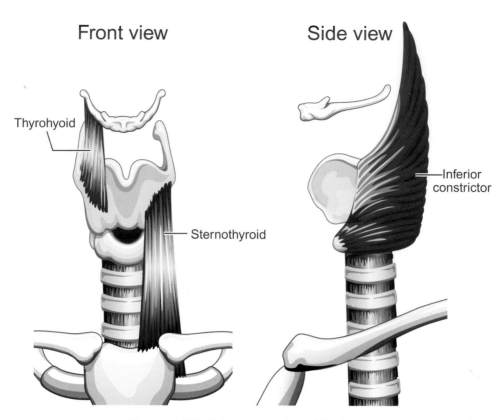

Figure 3–22. Extrinsic muscles of the larynx.

depicted in Figure 3–23, are referred to as supplementary muscles of the larynx. Most of them attach to the hyoid bone and are subdivided into those that originate below the hyoid bone, the so-called infrahyoid muscles, and those that originate above the hyoid bone, the so-called suprahyoid muscles.

Infrahyoid Muscles. The infrahyoid muscles include the *sternohyoid* and *omohyoid* muscles. These two muscles apply forces that can influence the positioning of the hyoid bone from below.

The *sternohyoid* muscle is a flat structure that courses vertically along the front surface of the neck and overlies one of the extrinsic laryngeal muscles, the *sternothyroid* muscle. The *sternohyoid* muscle originates from the back surface of top of the sternum and the inner end of the clavicle (collar bone). Fibers course upward and insert on the lower edge of the body of the hyoid bone. Contraction of the *sternohyoid* muscle places a downward pull on the hyoid bone. This downward pull lowers the hyoid bone, or it can anchor the hyoid bone in position if the downward pull is counterbalanced by other forces.

The *omohyoid* (shoulder-to-hyoid bone) muscle is located on the front and side of the neck. It is a narrow muscle that has two long bellies. The *posterior*

(lower) belly arises from the upper edge of the scapula (shoulder blade) and courses horizontally inward and forward to attach to an intermediate tendon positioned near the sternum. The *anterior* (upper) belly arises

Needing a Massage

Excess tension within the larynx can negatively influence the voice. This is not unlike excess tension that develops elsewhere in the body, tension that can often be relieved by massage. Thus, an uptight larynx that produces an uptight voice can benefit from a laryngeal massage. The essence of this form of massage is physical manipulation of the larynx back and forth in association with a kneading of its supporting muscles. The overly tense laryngeal apparatus may tend to ride high and tight within the neck. Signs of its relief from excess tension may be a lowering of its position, a more relaxed musculature, and a less pressed voice quality. Laryngeal massage is the province of the speech-language pathologist or the laryngologist and not of the routine masseuse or masseur.

Front view

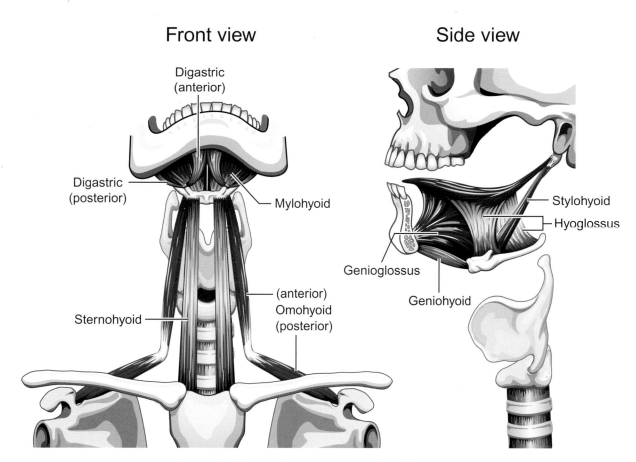

Digastric
(anterior)

Digastric
(posterior)

Mylohyoid

Sternohyoid

(anterior)
Omohyoid
(posterior)

Side view

Stylohyoid

Hyoglossus

Genioglossus

Geniohyoid

Figure 3-23. Supplementary muscles of the larynx.

from the opposite end of the same intermediate tendon and runs vertically and toward the midline to attach to the lower edge of the greater cornu of the hyoid bone. Contraction of the *omohyoid* muscle places a downward and backward pull on the hyoid bone. Contraction also tenses the supporting fascia in the region and prevents the neck from being sucked inward during forceful inspiration.

Suprahyoid Muscles. The suprahyoid muscles apply forces that can influence the positioning of the hyoid bone from above. They are the *digastric, stylohyoid, mylohyoid, geniohyoid, hyoglossus*, and *genioglossus* muscles.

The *digastric* muscle is a two-bellied sling of muscle in which the two bellies are joined end-to-end by an intermediate tendon that attaches to the top of the hyoid bone. The *anterior* belly originates inside the lower border of the mandible (jaw) and courses downward and backward to the intermediate tendon. The *posterior* belly originates from the mastoid process of the temporal bone of the skull and courses downward and forward to the intermediate tendon. Contraction of

the *digastric* muscle pulls upward on the hyoid bone and/or downward on the mandible. The relative movement of the hyoid bone and mandible is dependent on the degree to which the two structures are fixed in position by other muscles. Of interest here are influences on the hyoid bone. Contraction of the *anterior* belly of the muscle moves the hyoid bone upward and forward, whereas contraction of the *posterior* belly of the muscle moves the hyoid bone upward and backward. Contraction of the two bellies of the *digastric* muscle at the same time pulls the hyoid bone upward and forward or upward and backward at any angle, depending on the forces generated by the two bellies.

The *stylohyoid* muscle runs a course somewhat parallel to the *posterior* belly of the *digastric* muscle. The *stylohyoid* muscle originates from the back and side surfaces of the styloid process of the temporal bone of the skull and courses downward and forward to the hyoid bone. The muscle divides into two bundles that pass on either side of the intermediate tendon of the *digastric* muscle before inserting at the junction of the body and greater cornu of the hyoid bone. Contraction of the *stylohyoid* muscle places an upward and backward pull on the hyoid bone. The action is similar to that which results from contraction of the *posterior* belly of the *digastric* muscle.

The *mylohyoid* muscle contributes to the formation of the floor of the oral cavity. Fibers of this muscle originate along much of the inner surface of the body of the mandible and course inward, backward, and downward. They join with fibers of their paired mate of the opposite side at a tendinous midline raphe (running down the center of the floor of the oral cavity). Fibers toward the rear of the oral cavity attach directly into the front surface of the body of the hyoid bone. Contraction of the *mylohyoid* muscle results in an upward and forward pull on the hyoid bone. Contraction can also result in elevation of the floor of the oral cavity and tongue. With the hyoid bone fixed in position, contraction of the *mylohyoid* muscle may lower the mandible.

The *geniohyoid* muscle is a cylindrical muscle that lies above the *mylohyoid* muscle. This muscle extends from the inner surface of the front of the mandible to the front surface of the body of the hyoid bone. Its fibers extend backward and downward in a diverging pattern. The muscle bundle runs above and nearly parallel to the fiber course of the *anterior* belly of the *digastric* muscle. Contraction of the *geniohyoid* muscle pulls the hyoid bone upward and forward. Its functional potential is similar to that of the *anterior* belly of the *digastric* muscle.

The *hyoglossus* muscle is an extrinsic muscle of the tongue (having attachments within and outside the tongue) that has the potential to exert force on the hyoid bone and move the housing of the larynx. Fibers of the muscle course vertically and extend between the side of the tongue toward the back and the body and greater cornu of the hyoid bone. When the *hyoglossus* muscle contracts, it retracts and depresses the tongue and/or elevates the hyoid bone. If the tongue is relatively more fixed than the hyoid bone, the hyoid bone will rise within the neck.

The *genioglossus* muscle is also an extrinsic muscle of the tongue and is the largest and strongest of such extrinsic muscles. This muscle has the potential to exert force on both the tongue and hyoid bone. Fibers of the *genioglossus* muscle extend from the inner surface of the mandible and course complexly to insert into the entire undersurface of the tongue and body of the hyoid bone. Contraction of the *genioglossus* muscle can have a variety of influences on the positioning of the tongue and/or hyoid bone. Its major influence on the hyoid bone is to draw it upward and forward.

Summary of the Laryngeal Muscles. The laryngeal muscles are categorized as intrinsic, extrinsic,

Harry Hollien

Hollien has been a champion of the study of laryngeal function in the context of experimental phonetics for half a century. He pioneered the quantification of vocal fold correlates of voice fundamental frequency change, one of his most clever endeavors being his work on stroboscopic laminagraphy (phase-advanced frontal x-rays). He also contributed significantly to our understanding of factors influencing speech intelligibility in deep-water divers. Well known for his forensic studies on speaker identification, most consider him the most celebrated expert witness in the world in matters involving the use of voice in the commission of crime. Hollien founded the American Association of Phonetic Sciences and has fostered the careers of many outstanding speech and voice scientists. A colorful and outspoken advocate for his professional passions, Hollien is one of the key figures in the history of experimental phonetics.

and supplemental, depending on the locations of their attachments (inside or outside the larynx). Actions of the intrinsic laryngeal muscles (those with both attachments inside the larynx) have a direct and profound influence on the vocal folds. Specifically, they can abduct, adduct/compress, shorten, lengthen, and tense the vocal folds. Actions of the extrinsic and supplemental laryngeal muscles (those with at least one attachment outside the larynx) serve to stablize the larynx and can change its position within the neck. In general, contractions of muscles with attachments below the larynx can lower the larynx and contractions of those with attachments above the larynx can raise the larynx. These laryngeal movements and their associated forces are detailed in the next two sections.

Movements of the Laryngeal Apparatus

Movements of the laryngeal interior and laryngeal housing enable the laryngeal apparatus to function as a valve. These movements are discussed here apart from the forces that cause them.

Movements of the Interior of the Larynx. Movements of the interior of the larynx include those of the vocal folds, ventricular folds, and epiglottis. Each of these structures may move alone or in various combinations with the others.

Movements of the Vocal Folds. The vocal folds are movable and flexible. Changes can be effected in their vertical and side-to-side positioning and in their shape and length.

Each vocal fold can go through vertical and side-to-side position changes as its corresponding arytenoid cartilage rocks at a right angle to the long axis of its associated cricoid facet. When the rocking movement is downward and inward, the back end of the vocal fold moves downward and toward the midline. When rocking movement is upward and outward, the back end of the vocal fold moves upward and toward the side. Under normal circumstances, the two arytenoid cartilages move simultaneously and similarly so that the two vocal folds move in similar trajectories.

The cross-sectional shape of each vocal fold can change. Changes in shape mainly constitute a thinning or thickening of the vocal fold toward its free margin. Thus, the free margin may be relatively sharp or blunt in cross-section toward the airway. The vocal fold may also appear to be somewhat tilted in its configuration.

The vocal folds can be lengthened or shortened considerably. Lengthening is limited by the degree to which the covering tissue of the vocal fold, vocal ligament, and different parts of the *thyroarytenoid* muscle are distensible. Lengthening of the vocal folds is effected when either or both the thyroid and cricoid cartilages are moved away from one another. Shortening of the vocal folds is effected when either or both the thyroid and cricoid cartilages are drawn toward one another.

Movements of the Ventricular Folds. The ventricular folds, like the vocal folds, are movable and flexible. Principal changes in their position can be effected vertically and side to side. Most vertical change is found to occur in a downward direction from rest in which each ventricular fold can reach the upper surface of the vocal fold on the corresponding side of the larynx. Side-to-side positioning of the ventricular folds can range from a significantly lateral position to a midline position. The shape of the ventricular folds can be changed, but less so than is usually the case for the vocal folds.

Movements of the Epiglottis. The epiglottis is usually oriented upright. From this position, it can be moved backward and downward to horizontal or beyond. This results in a covering of the laryngeal aditus. Downward movement of the epiglottis can also be segmental, such that the upper third can be folded backward over the laryngeal aditus. Other aspects of the shape of the epiglottis are also subject to change. Most notably, the upper part of the structure can be made more convex toward the back of the pharynx by

a bending of its lateral edges toward one another (like bending the edges of a banana peel inward).

Movements of the Laryngeal Housing. The housing of the larynx is subject to movement within the neck. Although movement can be in nearly all directions, the most important movement is vertical. Thus, the larynx can be raised or lowered considerably relative to its usual resting position within the neck. Such movements have reciprocal implications for the lengths of the tracheal and pharyngeal airways, such that as one lengthens the other shortens. The housing of the larynx can also be shifted forward or backward within the neck, having a potential for greater forward than backward movement from its resting position.

Adjustments of the Laryngeal Apparatus

The laryngeal apparatus is capable of a variety of adjustments (combinations of movements of different structures). These have implications for both the laryngeal interior (vocal folds, ventricular folds, and epiglottis) and the positioning of the larynx within the neck.

Abduction of the Vocal Folds

Vocal fold abduction involves the movement of a vocal fold away from the midline. Such abduction is normally simultaneous and symmetric in the two vocal folds. As the two vocal folds move toward the side, the glottis (space between them) increases in size. As portrayed in Figure 3–24, full abduction of the vocal folds results in a wide glottis and the condition in which air

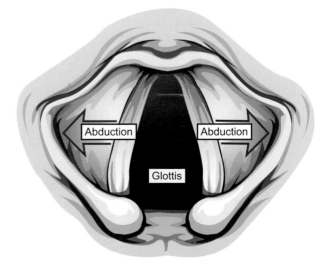

Figure 3–24. Vocal fold abduction.

flows most freely in and out of the pulmonary apparatus. Use of the term abduction in this context means lateral movements of the vocal folds (although other meanings are possible; see Figure 3–25 for an example). It is the vocal folds that abduct, not the glottis.

Abduction of the vocal folds and concomitant enlargement of the glottis are effected mainly by contractions of the *posterior cricoarytenoid* muscles. These pull on the muscular processes of the arytenoid cartilages to swing the vocal folds upward and outward.

Abduction of the vocal folds can also be the result of a passive force that tends to pull each vocal fold toward the side of the larynx and enlarge the glottis. This force is brought about by any downward pull placed on the conus elasticus (lower elastic lining of the larynx). Such a pull tends to tug the free margin of the vocal fold downward and toward the side, thus dilating the laryngeal airway (Zenker, 1964). Tracheal tug occurs, for example, when the diaphragm is displaced footward and pulls downward on the trachea.

The actions of the *posterior cricoarytenoid* muscles and of tracheal tug are complementary in that they both abduct the vocal folds and increase the size of the glottis. The contribution of the *posterior cricoary-*

tenoid muscles is almost always the more important of the two.

Adduction of the Vocal Folds

Vocal fold adduction requires the movement of a vocal fold toward the midline. The two vocal folds usually follow similar movement pathways and the glottis decreases in size. As illustrated in Figure 3–26, movement toward the midline may be sufficient to approximate the entire free margins of the two vocal folds and close the laryngeal airway. Movement toward the midline may also be limited to the membranous part of the vocal folds (front 60%), resulting in closure of only that portion of the airway, while leaving the cartilaginous portion (back 40%) of the vocal folds abducted.

Adduction resulting in full approximation of the two vocal folds is caused by the combined contraction of the *lateral cricoarytenoid* muscles and *arytenoid* muscles (*transverse* and *oblique* components), whereas adduction resulting in approximation of only the membranous portions of the vocal folds is caused by contraction of the *lateral cricoarytenoid* muscles alone. Action of the *lateral cricoarytenoid* muscles pulls for-

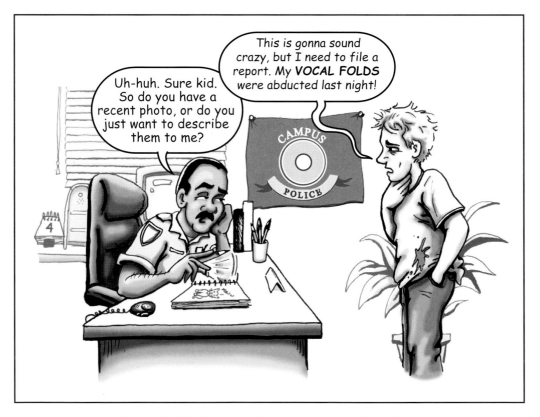

Figure 3–25. Cartoon about vocal fold abduction.

ward on the muscular processes of the arytenoid cartilages, rocking them over the cricoid cartilage and swinging the vocal folds downward and inward.

Once the vocal folds are approximated (fully adducted), the vertical extent of their approximation and the compressive force maintaining their approximation can be adjusted. That is, the amount of contact and the force of contact can be altered. Amount of contact relates to the cross-sectional thickness through the approximated surfaces, a factor that can be adjusted by the configuration of the *thyrovocalis* muscle portion of the *thyroarytenoid* muscle and by how forcefully the vocal folds are "squeezed" together by actions of the *lateral cricoarytenoid* muscles and the *arytenoid* muscles. The squeezing force exerted between the vocal processes of the arytenoid cartilages by the *lateral cricoarytenoid* muscles has been called medial compression (van den Berg et al., 1960). Medial compression can be applied even when the vocal folds are separated along their cartilaginous length.

Changing the Length of the Vocal Folds

The length of the vocal folds can be changed through a variety of external and internal adjustments. These can occur individually or in different combinations. Length changes can be mediated through either the cricoarytenoid joints or cricothyroid joints, or both.

Length changes mediated through the cricoarytenoid joints are portrayed in Figure 3–27. These are the result of rocking and sliding of the arytenoid cartilages on the cricoid cartilage, which carries the tips of the vocal processes of the arytenoid cartilages upward, backward, and outward or downward, forward, and inward. Upward, backward, and outward movement of the vocal processes abducts the vocal folds and

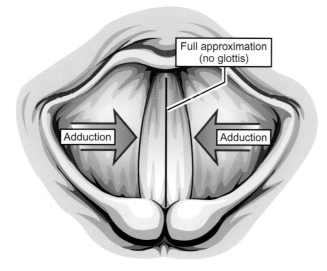

Figure 3–26. Vocal fold adduction.

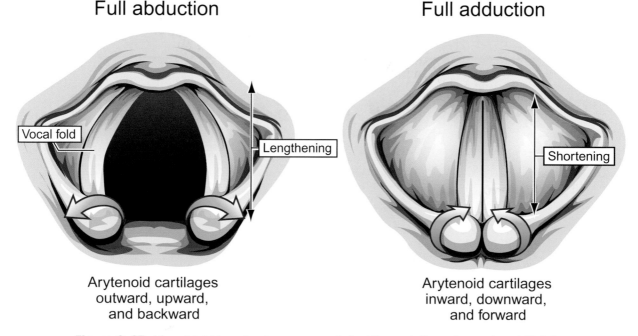

Figure 3–27. Vocal fold length changes mediated through the cricoarytenoid joints.

lengthens them, whereas downward, forward, and inward movement of the processes adducts the vocal folds and shortens them. Maximum vocal fold length is achieved at full abduction, whereas minimum vocal fold length is achieved at full adduction.

The active forces for vocal fold lengthening associated with cricoarytenoid joint actions come from the *posterior cricoarytenoid* muscles, whereas the active forces for vocal fold shortening come from the *lateral cricoarytenoid* muscles. Muscle relaxation following activation of each muscle pair results in counteractive length changes to those caused by the concentric contraction of each pair.

The mechanisms responsible for length changes of the vocal folds that are mediated through the cricothyroid joints are best understood in the context of full approximation of the vocal folds and are illustrated in Figure 3–28. Length changes of the approximated vocal folds result from forward and/or backward directed muscle forces that are produced external to the vocal folds and from concentric muscle forces that are developed internal to the vocal folds.

Vocal fold lengthening is achieved by forward directed forces pulling on the front ends of the vocal folds at their points of attachment to the inside of the thyroid cartilage and/or by backward directed forces pulling on the back ends of the vocal folds at their points of attachment to the vocal processes of the arytenoid cartilages. Forward directed forces result from contraction of the *cricothyroid* muscles, which place pulls on the front ends of the thyroid and cricoid cartilages that tend to close the visor angle of the larynx by rocking the thyroid cartilage on the cricoid cartilage and/or rocking the cricoid cartilage on the thyroid cartilage. The consequence of any combination of rocking of the front ends of these two cartilages toward one another is an increase in the distance between the front of the thyroid cartilage and the vocal processes of the arytenoid cartilages and a forward stretching of the vocal folds. Actions of the *cricothyroid* muscles (especially the *pars oblique* portions) can also cause a sliding movement at the cricothyroid joints that increases the distance between the front of the thyroid cartilage and the vocal processes of the arytenoid cartilages and contributes to vocal fold lengthening.

Actions of the *posterior cricoarytenoid* muscles are counteractive to those of the *cricothyroid* muscles and serve to anchor the arytenoid cartilages and their

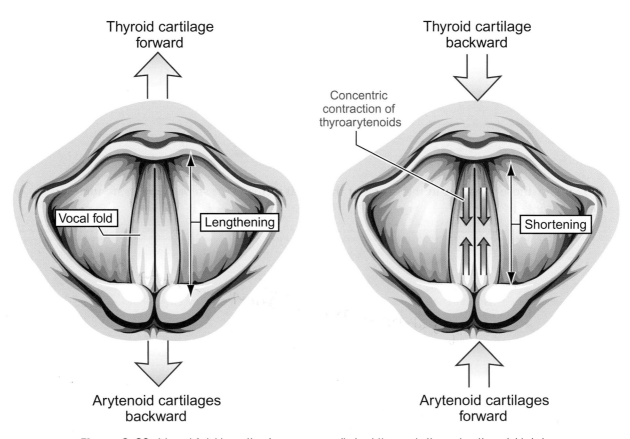

Figure 3–28. Vocal fold length changes mediated through the cricothyroid joints.

vocal processes from forward tilting and sliding during contractions of the *cricothyroid* muscles. The *posterior cricoarytenoid* muscles may also lengthen the vocal folds somewhat by pulling the arytenoid cartilages backward and upward along the facets on the slope of the cricoid rim. Thus, the *cricothyroid* muscles are responsible for stretching the vocal folds to a greater length in a forward direction, whereas the *posterior cricoarytenoid* muscles are responsible for securing the back ends of the vocal folds or for stretching them to a greater length in a rearward direction.

Shortening of the vocal folds results from relaxation of the external distending muscles just discussed or from concentric contractions of the *thyroarytenoid* muscles. Because the *thyroarytenoid* muscles constitute the main mass of the vocal folds, their contraction shortens the vocal folds and their internal fibers. If unopposed by actions of other muscles of the larynx, *thyroarytenoid* muscle contractions serve to draw the thyroid and arytenoid cartilages toward one another (pull the two ends of the vocal folds toward their respective centers lengthwise). Relaxation of such a shortening contraction is followed by a passive increase in vocal fold length.

Changing the Position and/or Configuration of the Ventricular Folds

The ventricular folds can move and change configuration. Although the ventricular folds are usually widely separated and rounded toward the airway, they sometimes adduct and change to a less rounded appearance. Under certain circumstances, they may extend well into the airway to form a roof over the vocal folds. The ventricular folds may also tilt downward toward the vocal folds and come in contact with them.

The muscular mechanisms for the adjustments described, and for those involved in the return of the ventricular folds to their usual positions and configurations, are not well understood. One suggestion is that the actions of other muscles in the vicinity of the ventricular folds combine to effect sphincter-like folding and unfolding of the interior of the larynx that moves and shapes the passive ventricular folds (Fink, 1975; Zemlin, 1998). Fibers of the *thyromuscularis* portions of *thyroarytenoid* muscles that course upward along the sidewalls of the larynx above the vocal folds may serve a special role in the enfolding influence on the ventricular folds. One study, for example, has identified muscle fibers that are coherent with the *thyromuscularis* portions of the *thyroarytenoid* muscles and appear to have significant mechanical advantages that could result in full adduction of the ventricular folds (Reidenbach, 1998).

Changing the Position and/or Configuration of the Epiglottis

The epiglottis is cartilage only and has no motive force other than its own recoil properties and gravity. The position and configuration of the epiglottis are subject to change through two main mechanisms. One mechanism relates to the contraction of the *aryepiglottic* muscles, which can lower the epiglottis and/or alter its configuration by folding it inward upon itself from top-to-bottom and/or across. The other mechanism relates to forces applied from the front surface of the epiglottis that tend to drive it backward and downward over the laryngeal aditus. These forces result mainly from elevation of the laryngeal housing. Such elevation forces the front of the epiglottis against the base of the tongue, compressing it backward and downward over the upper opening into the larynx. This action helps to protect the laryngeal airway and prevent the aspiration of food or liquid into the pulmonary apparatus during swallowing (see Chapter 13).

Changing the Position of the Laryngeal Housing

The larynx rides firmly but freely within the neck and can be repositioned from its usual position through muscular adjustments. Extrinsic and supplementary laryngeal muscles are responsible for changes in the position of the laryngeal housing. These changes result from pulls on the larynx proper as well as on the hyoid bone.

Upward movements of the laryngeal housing can be brought about by activation of one or a combination of muscles that includes the *thyrohyoid, digastric* (*anterior* and *posterior* bellies), *stylohyoid, mylohyoid, geniohyoid, hyoglossus*, and *genioglossus* muscles. Downward movements of the housing can be brought about by activation of one or a combination of muscles that includes the *sternothyroid, sternohyoid*, and *omohyoid* (*anterior* and *posterior* bellies) muscles.

Forward movements of the laryngeal housing can result from activation of one or a combination of muscles that includes the *sternothyroid, digastric* (*anterior* belly), *mylohyoid, geniohyoid*, and *genioglossus* muscles. Backward movements of the housing can be brought about through activation of one or a combination of muscles that includes the *omohyoid* (*anterior* and *posterior* bellies), *digastric* (*posterior* belly), and *stylohyoid* muscles.

The larynx can be moved or fixed in position through different combinations of counteractive forces. Fixation can also include activation of the *inferior constrictor* muscle of the pharynx, which can stabilize the larynx against forward directed forces. Figure 3–29 schematically summarizes the potential actions of the

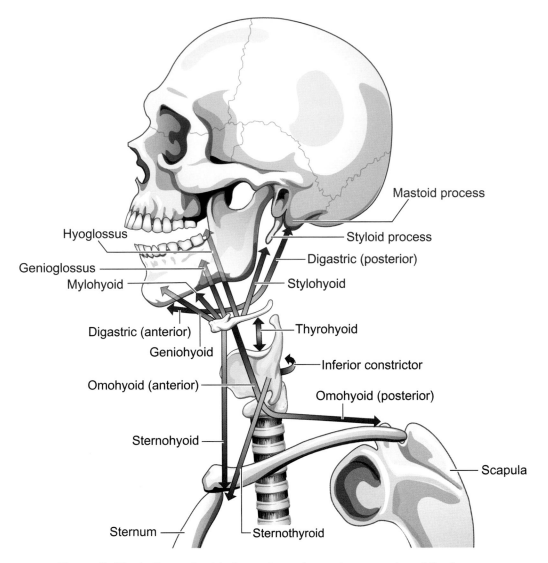

Figure 3–29. Actions of extrinsic and supplementary muscles of the larynx.

extrinsic and supplementary muscles of the larynx that may influence the positioning and stabilization of the laryngeal housing.

Control Variables of Laryngeal Function

Several control variables are important in laryngeal function. Their relative significance depends on the particular activity being performed, whether it is breathing, speaking, singing, laughing, whistling, swallowing, coughing, panting, bearing down, weight-lifting, or wind instrument playing. For example, singing requires certain adjustments based on acoustic goals, whereas swallowing does not. And, for another

example, stiffness of the vocal folds may be important for an activity such as fundamental frequency adjustment of the voice, but be inconsequential for an activity such as whistling.

For purposes of this chapter, discussion is devoted to five control variables that influence laryngeal function. These are: (a) laryngeal opposing pressure, (b) laryngeal airway resistance, (c) glottal size and configuration, (d) stiffness of the vocal folds, and (e) effective mass of the vocal folds.

Laryngeal Opposing Pressure

Laryngeal opposing pressure is a measure of the opposition provided by the larynx to translaryngeal air pressure (the air pressure difference between the trachea and pharynx) when the larynx is closed airtight (Hixon & Minifie, 1972). This opposition is represented by the force provided at the level of the larynx to maintain it in a closed configuration despite positive or negative aeromechanical forces that tend to either blow or suck it open. As illustrated in Figure 3–30, laryngeal opposing pressure is the net opposing pressure in this context and has three components. These include (a) compressive muscular pressure that "squeezes" the closed larynx and holds the vocal folds together, (b) surface tension between the apposed surfaces of the moist vocal folds that holds them together, and (c) gravity that weighs down the vocal folds and influences them differently in different body positions (or different gravity fields). Of these three, compressive muscular pressure is the greatest contributor to laryngeal opposing pressure.

The laryngeal opposing pressure required to effect airtight closure of the larynx for an activity involving minimal translaryngeal pressure may be low (a few cmH$_2$O of muscular pressure), whereas the opposing pressure must be high for an activity involving a high translaryngeal pressure (perhaps tens of cmH$_2$O of muscular pressure). The adjustment of laryngeal opposing pressure (principally through the adjustment of compressive muscular pressure) is critical to providing the opposition needed to allow tracheal air pressure to be raised for certain activities.

Laryngeal Airway Resistance

Laryngeal airway resistance is a measure of the opposition provided by the larynx to airflow through it. Such resistance is a property of the airway itself. Because the main constriction within the larynx is at the level of the vocal folds, this region of the larynx is the foremost contributor to laryngeal airway resistance. The ventricular folds are a secondary contributor. Thus, by adjusting the cross-sectional area and/or length of the internal larynx in the region of the vocal folds and ventricular folds, the laryngeal airway resistance will likely change. Resistance increases with increasing constriction and length of constriction.

It is important to note that laryngeal airway resistance is airflow dependent. This is portrayed in Figure 3–31 and means that even at fixed cross-sectional areas and/or lengths of the laryngeal airway, the value of resistance is influenced by how fast air is moving (van den Berg, Zantema, & Doornenbal, 1957). Laryngeal airway resistance is not measurable, but is calculated from the quotient of translaryngeal air pressure (in cmH$_2$O) to translaryngeal airflow (the flow of air through the larynx, in liters per second, LPS).

The range of potential airway resistance values is large and can go from a very low resistance (wide open

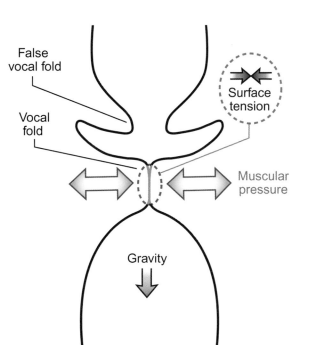

Figure 3–30. Laryngeal opposing pressure adjustment.

Opposition to Certain Terms of Opposition

Laryngeal airway resistance, discussed in the text, is opposition to the movement of air through the laryngeal airway. This resistance is often mistakenly labeled as vocal fold resistance, glottal resistance, or laryngeal resistance. It's none of these. It's not a measure of the mechanical status of the vocal folds nor is it a measure of the size of the hole designated as the glottis. Laryngeal airway resistance is a property of the airway itself. To gain a more concrete understanding (pun intended), think of a plaster cast of the inside of a larynx. Nothing in the plaster cast is adjustable. Everything is dead-stiff rigid. Yet, resistance to the flow of air through the cast is airflow dependent. Force air through the cast in either direction and you'll find that laryngeal airway resistance goes up and down as airflow goes up and down. Laryngeal airway resistance isn't something you can look at and measure. It's something you have to calculate.

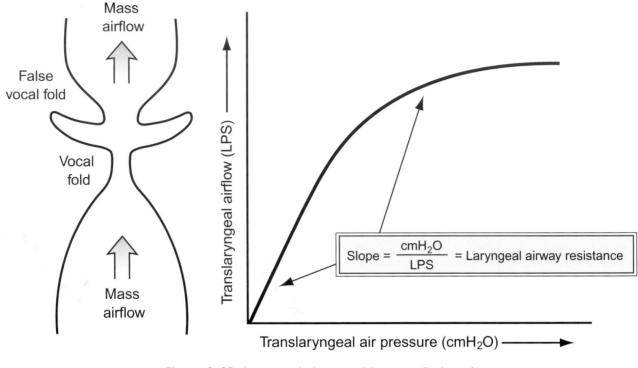

Figure 3–31. Laryngeal airway resistance adjustment.

airway) to infinity (airtight closure of the airway). It is common to conceptualize laryngeal airway resistance in terms of a value that represents the average opposition to airflow through the laryngeal valve. This average opposition is often taken to reflect the magnitude of coupling between the trachea and pharynx during the activity of interest (Smitheran & Hixon, 1981).

Glottal Size and Configuration

The size and configuration of the glottis can be adjusted in a variety of ways. Such adjustments are reflected in changes in physical dimensions such as length, diameter, area, and shape in the horizontal plane, although vertical aspects (depth and shape) are also important.

Figure 3–32 shows examples of contrasting glottal sizes and configurations. Panel A of the figure illustrates a large glottis of maximum length, diameter, and area that diverges toward the back. This glottis is attendant to full abduction of the vocal folds and a maximally opened airway. Panel B illustrates a glottis of medium size that is of lesser diameter and area than for full abduction and is typical of a glottis associated with resting tidal breathing. Panel C illustrates a small glottis compared to the diameters and areas of those portrayed in Panels A and B and shows a somewhat constricted airway. Panel D illustrates another small

glottis, this one located at the back of the larynx. And Panel E illustrates an airway that is closed airtight and has no glottis.

Abduction and adduction of the vocal folds are the main contributors to glottal size and configuration changes. When the glottis extends the entire length of the vocal folds, abduction and adduction influence glottal size mainly through side-to-side movements of the free margins of the vocal folds. During breathing, these free margins are widely separated, but typically go through an abduction-adduction cycling that corresponds to the cycling of inspiration-expiration. Maximum glottal size can be achieved during very deep inspiration following panting (Sekizawa, Sasaki, & Takishima, 1985).

Abduction of the vocal folds increases glottal size, whereas adduction of the vocal folds decreases it. Active and/or passive forces can cause abduction of the vocal folds. Active abduction of the vocal folds results mainly from contraction of the *posterior crico-arytenoid* muscles, with secondary abduction forces resulting from downward stretching of the conus elasticus. Active adduction is brought about by contraction of the *lateral cricoarytenoid* muscles and *arytenoid* muscles (*transverse* and *oblique* subdivisions). When just the *lateral cricoarytenoid* muscles are activated, the arytenoid cartilages are made to toe inward and

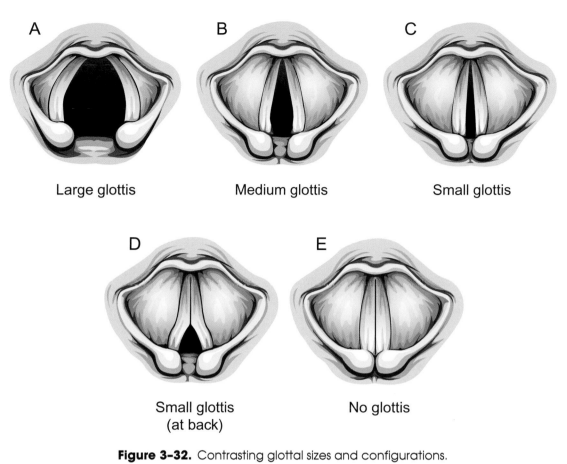

A Large glottis B Medium glottis C Small glottis

D Small glottis (at back) E No glottis

Figure 3–32. Contrasting glottal sizes and configurations.

the front portions of the vocal folds are in apposition and full adduction, whereas the back portions remain somewhat separated, such that only a small-size opening exists (see Panel D in Figure 3–32).

Stiffness of the Vocal Folds

Figure 3–33 portrays factors that can adjust the stiffness of the vocal folds. Stiffness of the vocal folds is an indication of their rigidity or tautness. Stiffness is the reciprocal of compliance and in physical terms conveys an indication of how much the vocal folds move for a given force applied to them. The stiffness of the vocal folds may differ somewhat from one location to another within the vocal folds. For example, the folds may be stiffer nearer their points of attachment to the thyroid and arytenoid cartilages than at their midpoints.

The most important component of vocal fold stiffness is manifested perpendicular to the long axes of the vocal folds (Titze, 1994). Vocal fold stiffness can be changed by contractions of muscles external to the vocal folds that tend to stretch them and/or pull them more taut from end to end and by contractions of mus-

cles internal to the vocal folds that modify their internal mechanical status.

Stretching of the vocal folds and/or pulling them more taut from end to end is accomplished by muscle actions that increase the distance between the two ends of the vocal folds (the inner surface of the thyroid cartilage and the tips of the vocal processes of the arytenoid cartilages) and/or increase the longitudinal tension operating along them lengthwise. These actions are similar to the stretching of a guitar string by the turning of its tuning peg to tighten and tense the string. The tensile strength of the vocal ligaments along the medial edges of the vocal folds is the limiting factor as to how much the vocal folds can be stretched and how much longitudinal tension can be applied. The *cricothyroid* muscles are primary contributors to this stretching action.

Contraction of muscles within the vocal folds themselves can also change their stiffness. The more forceful the contraction, the greater stiffness. Contractions of muscle fibers that lie within the lateral portions of the vocal folds (the *thyromuscularis* muscles) mainly stiffen those parts of the vocal folds, and

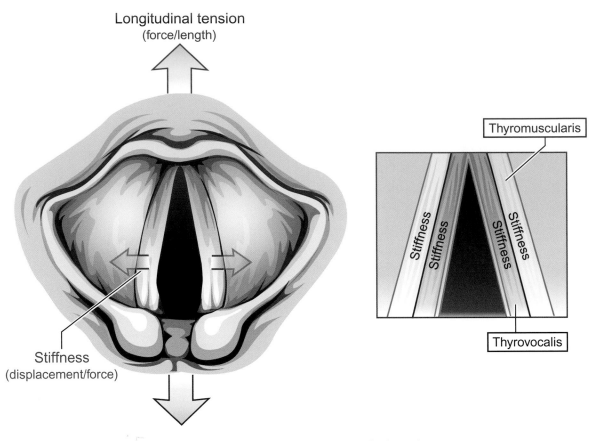

Figure 3–33. Vocal fold stiffness adjustment.

contractions of the muscle fibers that lie within the medial portions of the vocal folds (the *thyrovocalis* muscles) mainly affect those portions.

Effective Mass of the Vocal Folds

Mechanisms for changing the length of the vocal folds are discussed above. However, the length set by these mechanisms may or may not be the "effective" length employed for some activities. That is, the full mass of the vocal folds may not participate in certain activities and a lesser "effective" mass may participate.

Full mass and effective mass are the same when the vocal folds are fully abducted, maximally elongated, and have unencumbered free margins along their lengths. Full mass and effective mass are different, however, when the full mass of the vocal folds is partitioned by action that encumbers the vocal folds at some intermediate point along their lengths. An example can be seen in Figure 3–34 in the form of adductory adjustments of the vocal folds that are mediated through the cricoarytenoid joints, activated by the *lateral cricoarytenoid* muscles, and manifested as medial

compression between the tips of the vocal processes of the arytenoid cartilages. When the vocal processes of the arytenoid cartilages are made to toe inward sufficiently (see section above on glottal size and configuration), the membranous portions of the vocal folds are approximated and their cartilaginous portions remain separated. Under this circumstance, the vocal folds are partitioned longitudinally into two masses having very different functional potentials. The membranous portion of the configuration blocks the flow of air through the larynx, whereas the cartilaginous portion allows the free passage of air.

Considering this example further, different levels of activation of the *lateral cricoarytenoid* muscles generate different magnitudes of medial compression. Once the tips of the vocal processes are approximated, increasingly forceful contractions of the *lateral cricoarytenoid* muscles can further reduce the effective mass of the membranous portions of the vocal folds by forcing the tips of the vocal processes to make additional forceful and forward contact in association the downward and forward rocking of the vocal processes of the arytenoid cartilages.

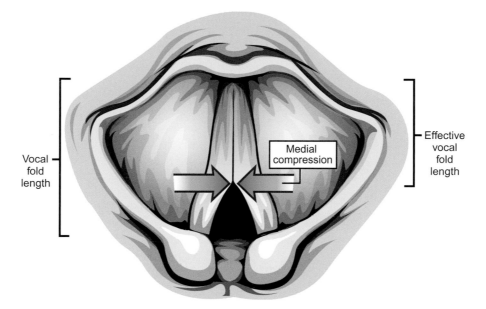

Figure 3–34. Effective vocal fold length adjustment.

Neural Substrates of Laryngeal Control

Laryngeal movement is controlled by the nervous system. The nature of such movement and the nature of its control are different for different activities. For example, control of the laryngeal apparatus is different for coughing, throat clearing, crying, singing, speaking, and swallowing. These and other activities involve a range of laryngeal adjustments, some of which are reflexive and others of which are precisely monitored and voluntarily controlled. Speaking and swallowing are the two most important activities for the purposes of this book. Control for swallowing is discussed in Chapter 13.

All control commands to the laryngeal apparatus are sent through cranial nerves and cervical spinal nerves. Cranial nerves originate in the brainstem, whereas cervical spinal nerves originate within the uppermost segments of the spinal cord. These nerves course outward to provide motor innervation to the intrinsic, extrinsic, and supplementary muscles of the laryngeal apparatus. As shown in Table 3–1, motor innervation to the laryngeal apparatus is effected by five cranial nerves and three spinal nerves. Cranial nerve innervations include cranial nerves V (trigeminal), VII (facial), X (vagus), XI (accessory), and XII (hypoglossal), and spinal nerve innervations include cervical spinal segments C1, C2, and C3.

Innervation to the five intrinsic muscles of the larynx is through cranial nerves X and XI. Some consider cranial nerve X to be primary (Zemlin, 1998), whereas others consider the bulbar branch of cranial nerve XI to be primary (Dickson & Maue-Dickson, 1982; Orlikoff & Kahane, 1996). There is general agreement that two branches of cranial nerve X are critical to vocal fold function. The recurrent laryngeal branch (also called the inferior laryngeal branch) provides motor supply to four intrinsic muscles, the *thyroarytenoid, posterior cricoarytenoid, lateral cricoarytenoid*, and *arytenoid* muscles. The remaining intrinsic muscle of the larynx, the *cricothyroid* muscle, receives its motor supply from the external branch of the superior laryngeal nerve. There is variation among larynges concerning the way specific nerves branch on their way to the larynx and how they interconnect with other nerves (Sanders, Wu, Mu, & Biller, 1993; Sanudo et al., 1999). For example, the recurrent laryngeal nerve has been shown to bifurcate or trifurcate before entering into the left or right sides of the larynx in more than one-third of larynges studied (Beneragama & Serpell, 2006).

Innervation of the three extrinsic muscles of the larynx is provided differentially via cranial nerves X, XI, and XII and cervical spinal nerves C1, C2, and C3. A mixture of cranial nerve and cervical spinal nerve supply is provided for the *sternothyroid* and *thyrohyoid* muscles, whereas the *inferior constrictor* muscle of the pharynx is supplied by cranial nerves X and XI.

The eight supplementary muscles of the laryngeal apparatus receive their motor innervation in various combinations through cranial nerves V, VII, and XII and cervical spinal nerves C1, C2, and C3. The *sternohyoid, omohyoid, geniohyoid, hyoglossus*, and

Table 3–1. Summary of the Cranial and Segmental Origins of the Motor Nerve Supply to the Muscles of the Laryngeal Apparatus

MUSCLE	INNERVATION
INTRINSIC	
Thyroarytenoid	X, XI
Posterior Cricoarytenoid	X, XI
Lateral Cricoarytenoid	X, XI
Arytenoid	X, XI
Cricothyroid	X, XI
EXTRINSIC	
Sternothyroid	XII, C1, C2, C3
Thyrohyoid	XII, C1, C2
Inferior Constrictor	X, XI
SUPPLEMENTARY	
Sternohyoid	XII, C1, C2, C3
Omohyoid	XII, C1, C2, C3
Digastric	V, VII
Stylohyoid	VII
Mylohyoid	V
Geniohyoid	XII
Hyoglossus	XII
Genioglossus	XII

Note: All of the intrinsic muscles of the larynx are innervated by the recurrent laryngeal branch (also called the inferior laryngeal branch) of cranial nerve X, except for the **cricothyroid** muscle, which is innervated by the external branch of the superior laryngeal nerve.

Cranial nerves include V (trigeminal), VII (facial), X (vagus), XI (accessory), and XII (hypoglossal). Spinal nerves include the first three cervical spinal nerves (C1, C2, C3). Muscles are categorized as intrinsic, extrinsic, or supplementary.

genioglossus muscles are supplied by cranial nerve XII, with the *sternohyoid* and *omohyoid* muscles also receiving motor supply from C1, C2, C3. The remaining three supplementary muscles are innervated by cranial nerves V and/or VII. The *digastric* muscle receives motor innervation from both cranial nerves, its *anterior* belly from cranial nerve V and its *posterior* belly from cranial nerve VII (Dickson & Maue-Dickson, 1982). The other of the remaining supplementary muscles, the *stylohyoid* and *mylohyoid* muscles, receive

motor innervation from cranial nerve VII and cranial nerve V, respectively.

Laryngeal adjustments are not executed without information about their consequences. This is especially true for activities in which rapid and precise movements are at a premium, such as those that are characteristic of vocal fold adjustments. Sensory information is critical to the control of such movements. This information comes from several sources, the relative importance of which depends on the activity being performed. These sources have in common some type of mechanoreceptor that converts a mechanical event into a neural signal that is then transmitted along a sensory nerve to the central nervous system.

Mechanoreceptors are distributed throughout the larynx in its muscles, joints, and mucosal coverings. Included among these are receptors that provide information about muscle lengths and their rates of change (Konig & von Leden, 1961b; Okamura & Katto, 1988; Sanders, Han, Wang, & Biller, 1998), joint movements (Jankovskaya, 1959; Kirchner & Wyke, 1965), and mucosal deformations (Kirchner & Suzuki, 1968; Konig & von Leden, 1961a; Sampson & Etyzaguirre, 1964). Such information is used to determine the mechanical status of the larynx and to elicit certain reflexive behaviors. There remains much to be known about the contribution of mechanoreceptors during laryngeal adjustments. Presumably they function as part of an integrated laryngeal feedback system (Orlikoff & Kahane, 1996). For laryngeal adjustments that target sound production, such a system would also have to take into account information provided by another type of mechanoreceptor, hair cells within the cochlea of the auditory system (via cranial nerve VIII).

Less than full agreement exists about which cranial and spinal nerves and branches convey sensory information from different structures of the larynx to the central nervous system (Dickson & Maue-Dickson, 1982). Most agree that the internal branch of the superior laryngeal nerve (part of cranial nerve X) carries sensory information from the mucosa that covers the supraglottal region of the laryngeal cavity, including the base of the tongue, epiglottis, aryepiglottic folds, and backs of the arytenoid cartilages. This nerve is also believed to transmit information from mechanoreceptors in the muscles of the larynx that respond to stretch (Duffy, 2005). There is general agreement that the recurrent laryngeal nerve (part of cranial nerve X) carries sensory information from the mucosa of the subglottal region of the laryngeal cavity and structures that are located below the vocal folds. Sensory information from the extrinsic and supplementary muscles travels via several different nerves. For example, the *mylo-hyoid* and *stylohyoid* muscles are served by sensory components of cranial nerves V and VII, respectively, whereas the *digastric* muscle is served by sensory components of both cranial nerves V and VII.

Laryngeal Functions

The larynx performs a variety of functions. Those considered here relate to: (a) degree of coupling between the trachea and pharynx, (b) protection of the pulmonary airways, (c) containment of the pulmonary air supply, and (d) sound generation.

Degree of Coupling Between the Trachea and Pharynx

Actions of the larynx determine the degree of coupling between the trachea (windpipe) and pharynx (throat). For the most part, changing the positions of the vocal folds changes the connectivity between these two components of the airway. For example, the laryngeal airway is open during breathing to enable the movement of air to and from the lungs (ventilation). The degree of coupling for breathing events depends on the depth of breathing, rate of breathing, force of breathing, and phase of breathing (inspiratory or expiratory).

Coupling between the trachea and pharynx is also important in certain special acts of breathing (discussed in Chapter 2). For certain of these acts, the laryngeal airway is held open so that the full force of tracheal pressure and airflow can be delivered to downstream structures (such as the tongue and lips) or to devices placed in the oral cavity or at the airway opening (such as the mouthpieces of wind instruments).

Protection of the Pulmonary Airways

The pulmonary airways are a major part of the respiratory lifeline and the maintenance of their integrity is critical. The larynx is positioned at the juncture between the pulmonary airways and the so-called upper airway (pharyngeal cavity, oral cavity, nasal cavities). As such, the larynx is strategically located as a valve to protect the pulmonary airways from the invasion of foreign matter.

The main food channel (from the mouth to the esophagus) and the main air channel (from the nose and mouth to the larynx) cross paths in the lower pharynx. Thus, the laryngeal airway must be closed during swallowing to prevent food or liquid from entering the trachea. This closure is accomplished by approximation of the vocal folds and other structures and includes a period of apnea (breath holding) during swallowing (see Chapter 13 for details).

Containment of the Pulmonary Air Supply

Closure of the laryngeal valve is important to containment of the pulmonary air supply for activities that require the generation of high pressures at different locations within the torso (abdominal, pleural, alveolar, tracheal) and/or the fixation of structures of the torso (rib cage wall, diaphragm, abdominal wall). Closure of the laryngeal valve is critical to the initiation and/or maintenance of forceful acts such as coughing, vomiting, defecation, urination, parturition (child birth), and the lifting of heavy objects.

Sound Generation

Much of the interest in the present chapter is with sound generation. Sound generation at the level of the larynx can be of several types, three of which are most relevant to the concerns of this chapter. They are: (a) transient (popping) sound, in which the airstream is momentarily obstructed and then abruptly released; (b) turbulence (hissing) sound, in which air is forced through a narrowed airway; and (c) quasi-periodic (buzzing) sound, in which the vocal folds are forced into vibration and move rapidly to and fro to interrupt the airstream repeatedly. The last of these generates voice and is what gives the larynx its popular designation as the "voice box."

LARYNGEAL FUNCTION IN SPEECH PRODUCTION

Laryngeal function in speech production is complex and takes many forms. Three of these forms are: (a) transient utterances, (b) extended sustained utterances, and (c) running speech activities. Understanding the principles that underlie these forms of laryngeal function enables extrapolation to other forms.

Transient Utterances

A transient (very brief duration) utterance can be produced at the level of the larynx in the form of a sudden explosive burst. This constitutes a glottal stop-plosive that is analogous to the downstream production of the voiceless stop-plosives consonants /p/, /t/, and /k/.

Get Thee Out

Reflexive coughing is our friend. It serves to clear the breathing airway via a powerful and violent explosion or series of such explosions. Your own experience with uncontrollable coughing is evidence of just how dedicated the pulmonary apparatus and laryngeal apparatus are to keeping things out of your lungs. Enormous air pressures and airflows are generated during reflexive coughing that cause violent movements of the vocal folds. Exces-

sive reflexive coughing can be abusive to the larynx, lead to unpleasant symptoms, and result in voice disorders. Less violent coughing done voluntarily and repeatedly over long periods can have similar cumulative effects. Then there is the equally notorious family cousin, the bad habit of continual throat clearing. Less outgoing than its other two relatives (pun intended), frequent throat clearing can be grating on the vocal folds. Abuse not thy larynx.

As depicted in Figure 3–35, glottal stop-plosive production involves an initial blockage of the laryngeal airstream by full adduction of the vocal folds. Air pressure then builds up within the tracheal space. This is followed by an abrupt release of the vocal fold adductory force and a simultaneous abrupt release of the pent-up air (Rothenberg, 1968; Stevens, 2000).

The speed with which air flows through the rapidly opening laryngeal airway is very high and gives rise to the generation of a brief burst of noise that excites the pharyngeal-oral airway. The entire act is somewhat like that of a weak voiceless cough in which the sudden release of pent-up air results in an impulse-like popping sound at the glottis (Broad, 1973). The release phase bears analogy to the discharge of an electrical capacitor through a time-varying resistance (Fant, 1960). The noise excitation during the release causes the pharyngeal-oral airway to vibrate throughout its entire length and to produce a plosive utterance that is distinctly lower in "pitch" than the pitches associated with other stop-plosives generated downstream by the tongue and lips.

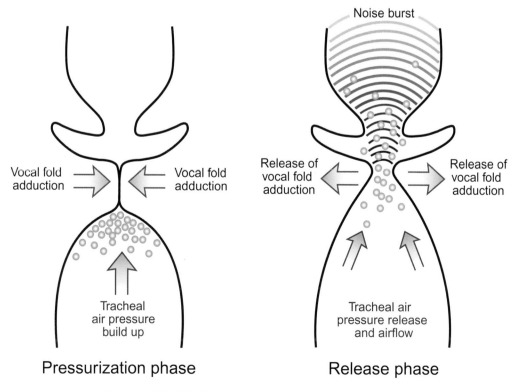

Figure 3–35. Glottal voiceless stop-plosive production.

Sustained Utterances

Two types of sustained utterances are discussed in this section. One is turbulence noise production and the other is voice production. The first relies on the flow of air through a relatively stable or slowly changing constriction, whereas the second has to do with vibration of the vocal folds that is faster than the naked eye can follow.

Turbulence Noise Production

Air flowing from the breathing apparatus may encounter constrictions within the laryngeal airway. The most important of these usually occur at the level of the glottis, where inward movements of the vocal folds reduce the size and/or change the configuration of the airway.

Major constrictions cause air to flow turbulently. This means that air tumbles on itself, forming eddies (back flows), burbles (bubbles), and other irregularities. This agitation of air results in the generation of turbulence (friction) noise that contains a broad range of frequencies. The specific spectrum (frequency and sound pressure level content) of this noise depends on the nature of the interaction between the airstream and the constriction (Fant, 1960; Hixon, 1966; Minifie, 1973; Stevens, 2000).

Sustained noise is associated with sustained voiceless sound production in the larynx. One example is the production of the glottal fricative /h/, as illustrated in Figure 3–36. Glottal fricative production is achieved by positioning the vocal folds well inward to form a long slitlike constriction.

The act of whispering is another example of sustained noise production. Whispering can also be accomplished with a long slitlike constriction, but is often accompanied by other glottal configurations. One of the most frequent of these is a rearward-facing Y configuration. In this configuration, the membranous front parts of the vocal folds are firmly approximated (as in Figure 3–34), loosely approximated, or not approximated at all (Monoson & Zemlin, 1984; Rubin, Praneetvataku, Gherson, & Moyer, 2006; Solomon, McCall, Trosset, & Gray, 1989; Zemlin,1998), and the cartilaginous rear parts of the vocal folds are relatively far apart. This configuration is achieved by contracting the *lateral cricoarytenoid* muscles so that the vocal processes of the arytenoids cartilages toe inward, while leaving the *arytenoid* muscles less active or inactive.

Quiet whispering and loud whispering (also called stage whispering) have been reported by some to be associated with different laryngeal adjustments (Monoson & Zemlin, 1984; Pressman & Keleman, 1955; Sawashima & Hirose, 1983). However, the most

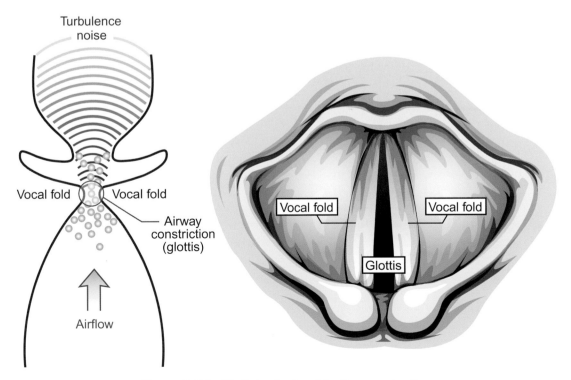

Figure 3–36. Glottal voiceless fricative production.

comprehensive study done of laryngeal configurations during whispering failed to find a consistent set of patterned adjustments for different types of whispering across speakers (Solomon et al., 1989). This suggests that the size of the glottis, rather than its specific configuration, may be the more important variable of the two (along with turbulent airflow) in the production of whispering of all types.

Under conditions of the sustained production of /h/ or whispering, the size and configuration of the glottis remain relatively fixed. Therefore, changes in the frequency content and sound pressure level of the noise are most influenced by the magnitude of the tracheal air pressure generated by the breathing apparatus and the resultant flow of air through the larynx (Hixon, Minifie, & Tait, 1967). When compared to usual voice production, quiet whispering has been shown to be produced using lower tracheal air pressure, higher translaryngeal airflow, and lower laryngeal airway resistance (Stathopoulos, Hoit, Hixon, Watson, & Solomon, 1991; Sundberg, Scherer, Hess, & Muller, 2010).

Voice Production

Voice results from vibration of the vocal folds. Such vibration modulates (chops up) the airstream into a series of air puffs. As depicted in Figure 3–37, the disturbances that constitute the voice source correspond to the series of abrupt closures of the laryngeal airway in association with the terminations of these air puffs. That is, the repeated, sudden decreases in airflow are what acoustically excite the upper airway (pharyngeal, oral, and nasal cavities) during voice production (Gauf-

fin & Sundberg, 1989; Rothenberg, 1983). This section discusses the nature of vocal fold vibration during sustained voice production, how voice production is initiated, and various other aspects of voice, including fundamental frequency, sound pressure level, fundamental frequency-sound pressure level profiles, spectrum, and registers.

Vocal Fold Vibration. Once vibration is established in the vocal folds, it proceeds in a relatively steady quasi-periodic fashion. Each vibration consists of lateral and medial excursions of the vocal folds that rapidly and repeatedly valve the expiratory airstream. Movements of the vocal folds under this condition are passive and akin to the movements of the lips when air is blown between them. (Try it. Moisten your lips, pucker up slightly, gently blow air through them, and feel them vibrate.)

Each vibration of the vocal folds (or lips) is not caused by muscular contractions that pull them apart and force them back together again. Muscular forces are important, but only in the sense that they "set" the vocal folds (or lips) in position to be able to passively move to and fro when aeromechanical forces are applied to them. Thus, a key element of the laryngeal adjustment for sustained vocal fold vibration is to position and hold the vocal folds in the airway so that vibration can be established and maintained by air pressures and airflows acting on the vocal folds (van den Berg, 1958). The conditions needed to sustain vocal fold vibration, once established, are a steady source of energy from the breathing apparatus and some form of nonlinear interaction with the structures being vibrated, namely, the vocal folds.

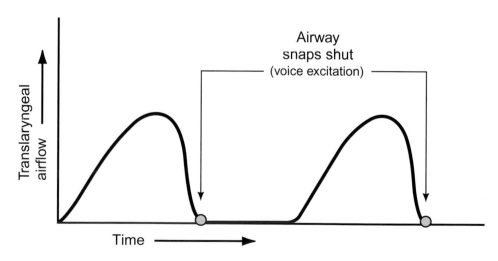

Figure 3–37. Voice source generation through abrupt closures of the laryngeal airway and sudden airflow declination.

A single cycle of vocal fold vibration is depicted in Figure 3–38. Taking closure of the larynx (full approximation of the edges of the vocal folds) as a starting point, movement begins when the air pressure below the vocal folds (tracheal air pressure) rises and forces the bottom edges of the two folds apart, followed by a forcing apart of the middle and upper parts of the folds. This pattern of lateral excursion of the vocal folds exhibits a so-called vertical phase difference in which lower points on the medial surfaces of the vocal folds are displaced earlier than points above them. A vertical phase difference is also manifested as the vocal folds move back together again. That is, lower points on the medial surfaces of the vocal folds move together before points on the upper surfaces move together (Hirano, Yoshida, & Tanaka, 1991; Schonharl, 1960; Timcke, von Leden, & Moore, 1958). These types of movements of the medial surfaces of the vocal folds occur because the covers of the vocal folds are relatively loosely coupled to their muscular bodies (Story & Titze, 1995). Such movements have been described as to and fro undulations of the surfaces of the vocal folds that are of a vertical-elliptical-horizontal nature (Baer, 1981) or as vertically propagating mucosal waves (like surface

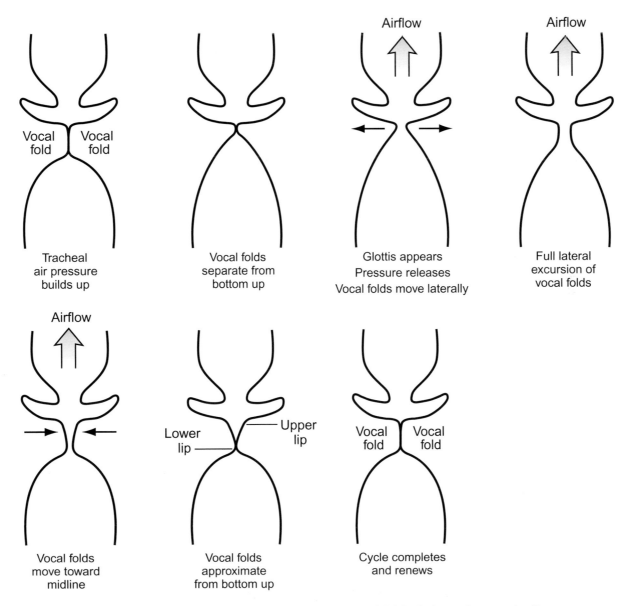

Figure 3-38. Vertical phase difference of the vocal folds during voice production.

To or Fro and To and Fro

Is this title a misprint? No. It's about oscillation and vibration. Many writers use the terms oscillation and vibration as if they were interchangeable. Some dictionaries do likewise. But, in the strictly correct use of the two terms, they are not synonymous. An oscillation is a movement in one direction (either to or fro), whereas a vibration is a double oscillation in two directions (to and fro). Consider the name of the oscilloscope, which is a device that can display signal change in one direction (or two, if you like). It's not called a vibroscope. And consider your summer electrical fan that turns side to side. Read the box it came in and you'll see that it's called a double-oscillation fan. It could just as well be called a single-vibration fan. So, the next time someone says they saw an oscillation of a vocal fold, ask which way it went, because an oscillation doesn't need to make a round trip like a vibration does.

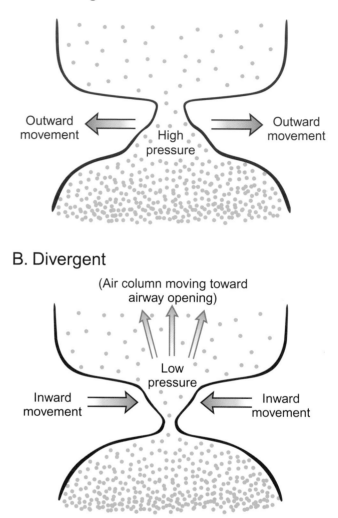

Figure 3–39. Convergent (**A**) and divergent (**B**) glottis shapes and associated intraglottal air pressure and vocal fold movements.

waves on water) that progress within the covers of the vocal folds and whose rippling effects can be seen on the top surfaces of the vocal folds (Berke & Gerratt, 1993; Hirano, Kakita, Kawasaki, Gould, & Lambiase, 1981). The vertical phase difference of vocal fold vibration has also been conceptualized as two primary modes of movement, one translational and one rotational (Berry & Titze, 1996). The translational mode is the lateral movement of the vocal folds away from the midline and back again. The rotational mode is the rotation of the vocal fold cover around a pivot point located somewhere between the bottom and top of the medial surface (the location of the pivot point depends on factors such as muscle activation levels and hydration of the tissue).

Details of the events associated with a single cycle of vocal fold vibration are illustrated in Figure 3–39. As tracheal pressure rises and pushes the lower portion of the vocal folds apart, a convergent-shaped glottis is created, as shown in Figure 3–39A. At this point in the vibratory cycle, the intraglottal air pressure (the pressure within the glottis) is relatively high, higher than the opposing recoil force being exerted by the vocal fold tissues. The intraglottal pressure pushes the vocal folds away from the midline until the restoring force exerted by the vocal folds exceeds the force exerted by the intraglottal pressure. At this point, the vocal folds begin to move inward toward the midline, starting

from the bottom and rotating into a divergent-shaped glottis, as shown in Figure 3–39B. As this divergent-shaped glottis is created, intraglottal pressure decreases rapidly because the air column above the vocal folds is continuing to flow toward the airway opening, leaving fewer air molecules within the glottis and just above it. This drop in intraglottal pressure, along with the recoil force of the vocal fold tissue, causes the vocal folds to move medially toward each other relatively rapidly.

Vibration of the vocal folds is self-sustained because the intraglottal pressure is relatively high as the vocal folds are moving outward (away from the midline), and it is relatively low as the vocal folds are moving inward (toward the midline). These conditions are created by

Every Which Way

Despite current understanding of how the vocal folds vibrate to produce voice, it was only within the earlier part of the last century that scholars were unenlightened about many aspects of the process. Some scholars argued that voice resulted from up and down movements of the two vocal folds in opposite directions. Other scholars believed that vocal fold movements during voice production were strictly horizontal and akin to stiff shutters that slid together and apart repeatedly. These incorrect "guesses" about how the vocal folds functioned during voice production were dispelled by data obtained with high-speed motion picture filming of the larynx. This technology enabled the study of the rapid movements of the vocal folds in precise detail. Thus, what earlier in the last century seemed to be "every which way" of vocal fold movement during voice production, has settled down to the way things are as described in the adjacent text.

two important factors. One factor is the dynamic nature of the glottal geometry, the alternating convergent and divergent shaped glottis. The other factor relates to the changes in air flow and air pressure just above of the glottis. As the vocal folds move outward away from midline, airflow through the glottis increases and accelerates the column of air above it. This causes the air pressure above the vocal folds to build up and increase the already high intraglottal pressure, thereby driving the vocal folds outward. When the tissue recoil forces reverse the movement of the vocal folds so that they begin to move inward, the airflow through the glottis decreases, but the accelerated air column continues to move upward. This reduces the air pressure just above the vocal folds and helps lower intraglottal air pressure to allow an unimpeded return of the tissue toward midline (see Titze [2006a] for a more detailed explanation).

Initiation of Voice. A number of events precede the sustained quasiperiodic vibrations of the vocal folds that generate voice. These include adjustments of the larynx that preset the voice production apparatus and determine the form of vibration at voice onset.

Presetting adjustments of the larynx occur in advance of actual voice production (Faaborg-Andersen, 1957; Hirano, Kiyokawa, & Kurita, 1988) and are

coordinated with adjustments of the breathing apparatus (Faaborg-Andersen, Yanagihara, & von Leden, 1967; Hixon, Watson, Harris, & Pearl, 1988). Presetting adjustments of the larynx may have influences on the laryngeal opposing pressure, laryngeal airway resistance, glottal size and/or configuration, vocal fold stiffness, and effective vocal fold mass. The adjustments chosen depend on the nature of the ensuing voice production. For example, different fundamental frequencies, sound pressure levels, and voice registers will condition the nature of the presetting adjustments. Laryngeal presetting is accomplished before any acoustic feedback having to do with the voice is available (Orlikoff & Kahane, 1996). This means that the larynx is mechanically "tuned" by the nervous system (as are other subsystems of the speech production apparatus) prior to the production of voice.

The intricate details of voice onset are manifested in the manner in which the larynx and breathing apparatus interact to generate the first few cycles of vocal fold vibration. This phase of vocal fold adjustment is often designated as the vocal attack phase (Daniloff, Schuckers, & Feth, 1980; Koike, 1967; Koike, Hirano, & von Leden, 1967; Moore, 1938). The most frequently used system for classifying vocal attack includes three different interplays between the laryngeal apparatus and the breathing apparatus. These are depicted in Figure 3–40 and include: (a) simultaneous action of the laryngeal apparatus and breathing apparatus, (b) action of the laryngeal apparatus preceding action of the breathing apparatus, and (c) action of the breathing apparatus preceding action of the laryngeal apparatus.

Simultaneous vocal attack (sometimes labeled usual or normal) is characterized by the synchronous generation of expiratory airflow and the approximation of the vocal folds along their length. This form of vocal attack is characterized by a gradual increase in tracheal air pressure and voice onset that stabilizes relatively rapidly into the quasiperiodic pattern typical of sustained vocal fold vibration.

Vocal attack in which laryngeal action precedes that of the breathing apparatus is often designated as a hard vocal (or glottal) attack or so-called coup de glotte. Laryngeal opposing pressure is very high during hard glottal attack and "squeezes" the vocal folds firmly against one another prior to any significant rise in tracheal air pressure. Action of the breathing apparatus raises tracheal air pressure to a level that is sufficient to overcome the laryngeal opposing pressure. Vibration of the vocal folds begins abruptly and with greater amplitude initially than is characteristic of simultaneous vocal attack and its accompanying lower tracheal air pressure.

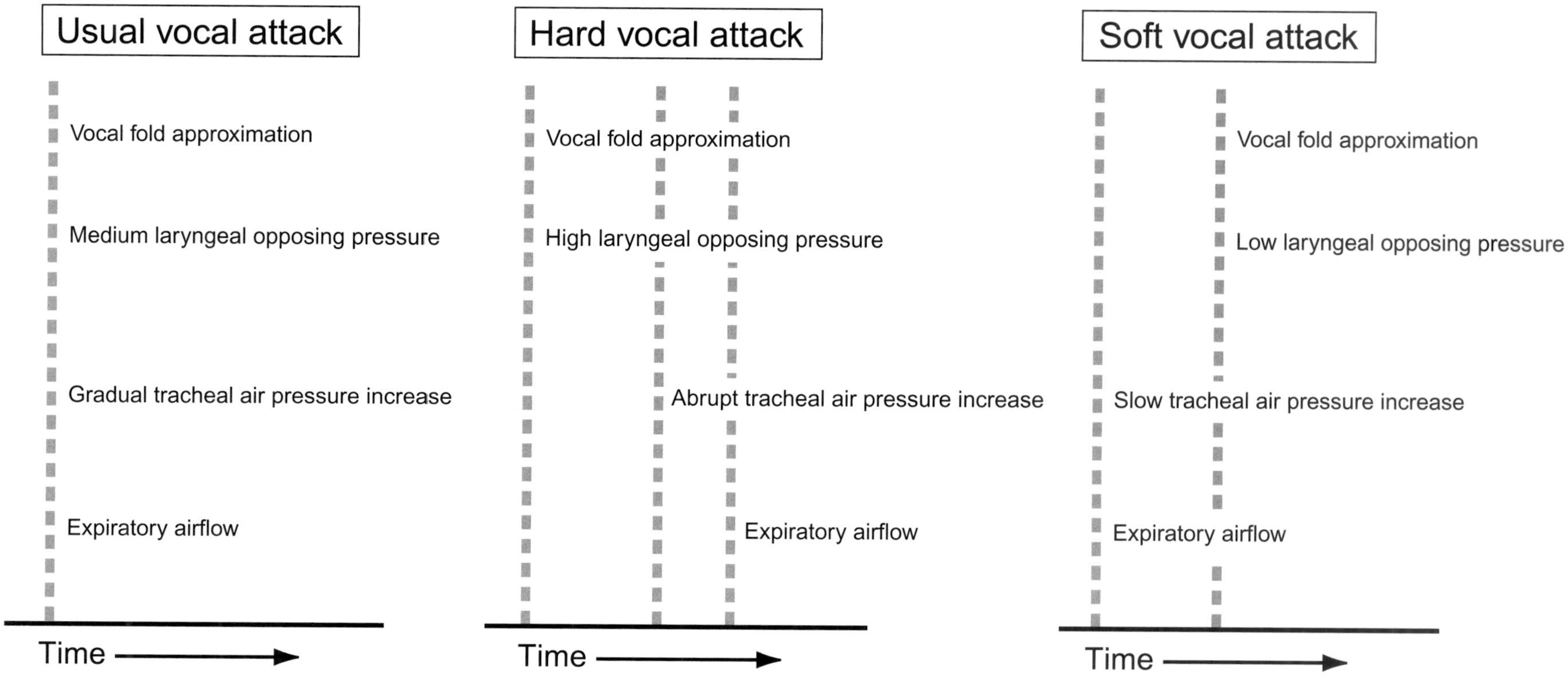

Usual vocal attack

Vocal fold approximation

Medium laryngeal opposing pressure

Gradual tracheal air pressure increase

Expiratory airflow

Time →

Hard vocal attack

Vocal fold approximation

High laryngeal opposing pressure

Abrupt tracheal air pressure increase

Expiratory airflow

Time →

Soft vocal attack

Vocal fold approximation

Low laryngeal opposing pressure

Slow tracheal air pressure increase

Expiratory airflow

Time →

Figure 3–40. Three types of vocal attack.

116

Vocal attack in which breathing action leads laryngeal action is designated as breathy (sometimes called aspirate or soft). In this form of vocal attack, expiratory airflow begins before the vocal folds are moved to the midline. Movement of the vocal folds into the airstream may cause noise to be generated initially. As the vocal folds approach one another and constrict the airway, vibration begins. Fast flowing air lowers the air pressure between the vocal folds and helps to move them inward toward the midline. This inward force is opposed by elastic recoil of the vocal folds that tends to restore their set position. These two medial-lateral forces alternate such that momentum increases with each successive vibration. The vocal folds move closer and closer together with successive vibrations until they approximate and a regular and even cycle of movement is established. An analog to this form of vocal attack can be demonstrated with the lips and an airstream. (Try it. Moisten your lips. Take a deep breath and then expire briskly through your lips while slowly moving them together. They should vibrate with increasing amplitude until a continuous steady vibratory pattern is established.)

Vocal fold vibration will not begin without sufficient drive from the breathing apparatus. The pre-set laryngeal apparatus will simply sit in position until breathing force is adequate to set the vocal folds into vibration. The onset of vibration is conditioned largely by tracheal air pressure and translaryngeal airflow. The threshold where such air pressure and airflow come into play (and voicing begins) depends on the prevailing laryngeal opposing pressure. The threshold (minimum) tracheal air pressure needed to produce voice (sometimes called the phonation threshold pressure) typically ranges in the neighborhood of 2 to 3 cmH_2O. This air pressure is required to overcome the muscular opposing pressure, surface tension, and gravitational force operating to maintain closure of the laryngeal airway at the level of the glottis. There is a slight hysteresis (force direction difference) in the rise and fall of tracheal air pressure and the threshold pressure for voice production. This is shown in a clear effect for voice production to cease at a slightly lower tracheal air pressure than the air pressure it takes to just get it started (Hixon, Klatt, & Mead, 1971; Plant, Freed, & Plant, 2004).

Fundamental Frequency. The fundamental frequency is the rate at which the vocal folds vibrate. Fundamental frequency can be changed over a very wide range, typically about three octaves (an octave is a doubling or a halving of frequency) for a young adult (Fairbanks, 1960). Fundamental frequency is usually expressed on a continuum in units of cycles per second or hertz. It can also be expressed on a musical scale in semitones (the interval between two adjacent keys on a keyboard instrument) (Baken & Orlikoff, 2000). The average fundamental frequency of the human voice depends in large part on the size of the larynx and the sex of the individual, with men having lower average fundamental frequencies than women, and women having lower average fundamendal frequencies than children. Control of change in fundamental frequency is vested primarily in adjustments of the vocal folds. Adjustments of the breathing apparatus have a supporting role in fundamental frequency control.

The strongest auditory-perceptual correlate of fundamental frequency is the pitch of the voice. Pitch is the subjective impression of the relative position of a sound along a musical scale. Sound pressure level and spectral content of the voice also influence the perception of pitch, but to far less important degrees than does the fundamental frequency. Thus, for the most part, a higher pitch is associated with a higher fundamental frequency and a lower pitch is associated with a lower fundamental frequency.

Vocal fold adjustments that influence fundamental frequency (and pitch) are those that determine the stiffness of the vocal folds and their effective vibrating mass, with stiffness generally considered to be the more

---

Needling the Teacher

One way to tap tracheal pressure is to puncture the trachea with a hypodermic needle. We know someone whose tracheal pressure was studied this way. The physician inserted the needle (attached to a syringe), but had difficulty on the first attempt. He withdrew the needle and made a successful second insertion. After the study, the subject went off to teach. Shortly into the lecture, a pea-size bump rose on his neck. As the lecture continued, the bump enlarged to walnut-size. Seeing it continue to grow, a student told the teacher what was happening. In the emergency room, it was discovered that the teacher had emphysema (air inflation) within the interstices (spaces) inside his neck. Some air had apparently been pumped into the interstices during attempts at needle insertion. When the teacher raised internal pressures to speak, this air was forced to the surface and made his neck balloon. Never again did he allow himself to be needled.

important of the two factors (Stevens, 2000). The most important mechanisms for increasing vocal fold stiffness operate through external force exerted by the *cricothyroid* muscles and internal force exerted through the *thyroarytenoid* muscles. As discussed above and illustrated in Figure 3–33, contraction of the *cricothyroid* muscles tends to stretch the vocal folds and increase the force per unit length along them, whereas activation of the *thyroarytenoid* muscles (particularly the *thyrovocalis* part) tends to increase the stiffness of the muscular part of the vibrating vocal folds while shortening the overall vocal fold length. It is the combined activities of these two pairs of muscles that are primarily responsible for setting the effective stiffness of the vocal folds and for controlling the fundamental frequency (Shipp & McGlone, 1971; Titze, 1994; Titze, Jiang, & Drucker, 1988; Titze, Luschei, & Hirano, 1989).

When moving up the musical scale from lower to higher fundamental frequencies, the relative activations of the *cricothyroid* and *thyroarytenoid* muscles tend to alternate. For example, *cricothyroid* muscle activity may increase the fundamental frequency of the voice by applying an external stretching force to the vocal folds over a limited range of fundamental frequencies and then *thyroarytenoid* muscle activity may further adjust fundamental frequency by exerting an internal force on the vocal folds. These actions modify both the effective stiffness and vibrating mass. Once the upper limit of a particular external adjustment in stiffness is reached, the *cricothyroid* muscle increases its level of activity to set the next externally generated stiffness range and the *thyroarytenoid* muscle further adjusts internally to meet the stiffness demands of the fundamental frequency target. This alternation of activity is often referred to as a stair-step adjustment of stiffness, coming partly from outside the vocal folds and partly from within the vocal folds (Hollien, 1960b). This two-part adjustment is also referred to as loading the vocal folds (from without) through isotonic or isometric *cricothyroid* muscle activity and tuning of the vocal folds (from within) through isometric *thyroarytenoid* muscle activity (Arnold, 1961).

The relative activations of the *cricothyroid* and *thyroarytenoid* muscles can vary substantially for the production of a given fundamental frequency (Titze & Story, 2002). This is represented in graphic form in Figure 3–41, with the relative activation of the *cricothyroid* muscle increasing upward and the relative activation of the *thyroarytenoid* muscle increasing rightward. This graph illustrates that a given fundamental frequency can be produced by a continuum of different combinations of muscular activities. For example, a fundamental frequency of 120 Hz can be produced by using relatively high activation of the *cricothyroid* muscles

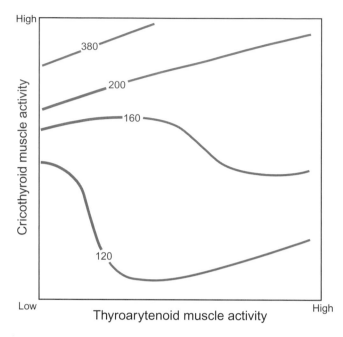

Figure 3–41. Continuum of *thyroarytenoid* and *cricothyroid* muscle activations for the production of selected fundamental frequencies (based on modeling data from Titze and Story (2002)).

combined with relatively low activation of the *thyroarytenoid* muscles; alternatively, the same 120 Hz fundamental frequency can be produced using relatively low activation of the *cricothyroid* muscles and a relatively high activation of the *thyroarytenoid* muscles. Thus, the same fundamental frequency can be produced in many different ways.

Although modification of *cricothyroid* and *thyroarytenoid* muscle activity is the primary mechanism for changing fundamental frequency, it is not the only one. The mechanism of medial compression can also effect changes in the fundamental frequency of the voice. This is done through actions of the *lateral cricoarytenoid* muscles that vary the medial compression of the vocal folds in the area of approximation of the tips of the vocal processes (illustrated in Figure 3–34). Studies of air-driven excised larynges, in which medial compression was experimentally manipulated, have shown that increases in medial compression result in increases in fundamental frequency (van den Berg & Tan; 1959; van den Berg et al., 1960). The suspected mechanism is a decrease in the effective vibrating mass of the vocal folds by stopping their vibration in the region of the tips of the arytenoid processes (Honda, 1995). This mechanism has been likened to the pressing of a guitar string against a fret so that only the part of the string nearer the sounding box of the guitar is permitted to vibrate (Broad, 1973). The action of increasing medial compression may also serve to stiffen the vocal folds in the vicinity of the forceful adduction and further shorten the vocal folds as the tips of the vocal processes are rocked inward and forward. The collective effects of stopping the vibration of the back parts of the vocal folds and shortening and stiffening the remaining front parts (the membranous parts) results in a more rapid rate of vibration of the vocal folds. Medial compression is usually considered to be a secondary or ancillary mechanism of fundamental frequency control.

Still another mechanism that influences the fundamental frequency of the voice relates to the elevation of the larynx (sometimes referred to as its vertical height). When high fundamental frequencies are generated, there is a tendency for the larynx to rise in the neck, especially near the upper extreme of the fundamental frequency range. This elevation is probably accomplished by activation of the *thyrohyoid* muscles (Faaborg-Andersen & Sonninen, 1960; Sonninen, 1968). Elevation of the larynx is believed to further increase the stiffness of the vocal folds once major effort has been exerted to increase stiffness through activation of the *thyroarytenoid* and *cricothyroid* muscles. Elevation of the larynx results in a downward pull on the under-surface of the vocal folds mediated through the conus elasticus (interior elastic lining of the larynx in the subglottal region). This pull stiffens the covers of the vocal folds (especially at the free margins of the vocal folds) by placing a vertical tug on them, and increases the rate at which the vocal folds vibrate (Ohala, 1972). This mechanism is usually the last biomechanical adjustment invoked to reach the highest fundamental frequencies possible. As with the case for changing the effective vibrating mass of the vocal folds, laryngeal elevation is considered a secondary or ancillary mechanism of fundamental frequency control.

Not all fundamental frequency control is vested in the larynx. The breathing apparatus also makes adjustments in association with changes in fundamental frequency. The most consistent of these is a tendency for tracheal air pressure to increase with increases in fundamental frequency (Shipp & McGlone, 1971). This is believed to relate to the need for a higher driving pressure in the face of both increasing laryngeal opposing pressure and laryngeal airway resistance (Kunze, 1962). This higher tracheal air pressure is needed to initiate voicing and maintain it under the conditions of increased stiffness of the vocal folds. In one sense, it is a cost placed on the breathing apparatus as a result of the laryngeal adjustment to achieve a higher fundamental frequency (Plant & Younger, 2000). The magnitude of this cost has been found to increase the most toward the upper end of the fundamental frequency range, suggesting that increments in the stiffness of the vocal folds may be especially large in that region (Kunze, 1962; Shipp & McGlone, 1971).

Adjustment of the breathing apparatus alone under conditions of a fixed laryngeal adjustment is not a very viable means of adjusting fundamental frequency of the voice (except in the loft voice register, discussed below). This is because increases in tracheal air pressure result in only small increases in fundamental frequency (Rubin, 1963; van den Berg, 1957). Typical magnitudes of change are only 2 to 4 Hz in fundamental frequency per cmH_2O of air pressure (Hixon et al., 1971; Titze, 1989). Thus, a change in fundamental frequency for a one octave change in an adult male (perhaps 120 Hz to 240 Hz) would require a 30 to 60 cmH_2O pressure change (an exorbitant cost) if effected solely through a breathing adjustment.

Mechanisms for lowering fundamental frequency, when decreases involve changes from frequencies that are above the usual fundamental frequency, are somewhat the inverse of those for raising fundamental frequency. That is, lowering fundamental frequency may be accomplished by decreasing vocal fold stiffness and/or tracheal air pressure.

To lower fundamental frequency below its usual value, other mechanisms may come into play. One mechanism is to reduce vocal fold stiffness by contraction of the *thyromuscularis* (lateral) portions of the *thyroarytenoid* muscles. This contraction shortens the

The Cattle Are Lowing

An effective method for teaching certain principles of voice production involves the use of an excised cow larynx. The cow larynx is large compared to the human larynx and is different in some respects. The cow larynx does not have false vocal folds, nor is it richly endowed with mucous glands for lubricating the vocal folds. After all, cows don't produce voice for long periods like people do. A cow larynx can be made to vibrate by attaching the blower end of a vacuum cleaner to the tracheal end of the larynx and then manually adjusting such factors as medial compression and longitudinal tension of the vocal folds. Fundamental frequency, sound pressure level, and source spectrum changes are easily made. Placing an inverted container (the size of a coffee pot) above the larynx roughly simulates the resonance contribution of the missing upper airway. When all is done right, the experience is both instructive and "moooooving" to students.

vocal folds and causes a slackening of the vocal ligaments and the *thyrovocalis* (medial) portions of the *thyroarytenoid* muscles (Zemlin, 1998). Another frequency-lowering mechanism entails a lowering of the larynx within the neck, which decreases the stiffness of the vocal folds by removing some of the usual traction placed on their undersurfaces. This is brought about through activation of the *sternothyroid* and *sternohyoid* muscles, which pull downward on the laryngeal housing (Atkinson, 1978; Honda, 1995; Ohala, 1972; Ohala & Hirose, 1970; Zemlin, 1998).

Sound Pressure Level. The sound pressure level of speech (the acoustic signal) is a measure of its physical magnitude (Baken & Orlikoff, 2000). This magnitude is related to the amplitude of the sound emanating from the upper airway and is generically referred to as the intensity of the signal (although technically sound pressure level and intensity are different quantities and the latter is more difficult to measure).

The sound pressure level (abbreviated as SPL) of speech is expressed on a continuum in ratio units of decibels (dB) and can be changed over a wide range, typically by about 40 dB for a young adult (Coleman,

Mabis, & Hinson, 1977). Sound pressure level can be measured on different physical scales that are weighted to account for the relative prominence of different concentrations of energy. The sound pressure level depends on the nature of the speech being produced and the location relative to the lips. A vowel produced at a typical level and measured 30 cm from the lips (a standard distance) might be 65 dB, whereas a vowel produced at a shouting level might be in excess of 100 dB.

The strongest auditory-perceptual correlate of sound pressure level is loudness. Loudness is the subjective sensation of the relative magnitude of sound. This perception relies mainly on sound pressure level, but is influenced to lesser degrees by the fundamental frequency and spectral content of the sound produced. Generally, the higher the sound pressure level, the greater the magnitude of the perceived loudness.

Control of the sound pressure level of speech is vested in adjustments of the breathing apparatus, laryngeal apparatus, and pharyngeal-oral apparatus. These adjustments are usually executed simultaneously across these three subsystems, as depicted in Figure 3–42.

Breathing behavior influences sound pressure level of the voice through changes in tracheal air pres-

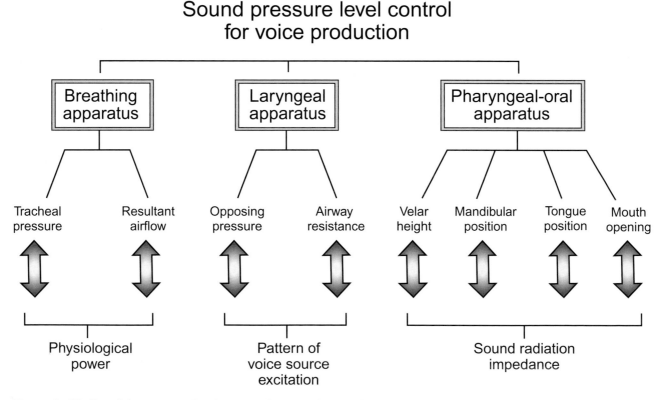

Figure 3–42. Breathing apparatus, laryngeal apparatus, and pharyngeal-oral apparatus control of sound pressure level.

sure, which correspond closely to changes in alveolar air pressure. That is, increases and decreases in tracheal air pressure cause increases and decreases in sound pressure level (Cavagna & Margaria, 1965; Hixon & Minifie, 1972; Isshiki, 1964; Ladefoged & McKinney, 1963; Titze, 1994; van den Berg, 1956). A doubling of tracheal air pressure for usual voice production might result in an increase in sound pressure level in the neighborhood of 8 to 12 dB (Broad, 1973; Daniloff et al., 1980; Stevens, 2000). The precise linkage between change in tracheal air pressure and change in sound pressure level depends on the prevailing sound pressure level of the voice. For example, a 1 cmH$_2$O change in tracheal air pressure during the production of a soft voice results in as much as a 3 dB change in sound pressure level, whereas the same change in tracheal air pressure during the production of a loud voice results in only a 0.5 dB change in sound pressure level (Hixon & Minifie, 1972).

Laryngeal opposition also plays a role in changing sound pressure level. Both laryngeal opposing pressure and laryngeal airway resistance increase with increases in the sound pressure level of the voice (Isshiki, 1964; Kunze, 1962). Increases in opposing pressure, effected by increasingly forceful contractions of the *lateral cricoarytenoid* and *arytenoid* muscles (*transverse* and *oblique* subdivisions), are needed to contain the increased tra-

---

Rest in Peace

You may wonder why we don't use the term "subglottal pressure" in the text. The reason is that we believe the term has problems. Consider the following. The "sub" part of the term isn't specific to a location. Bronchial and alveolar pressures are also "sub" glottal. The "glottal" part of the term is also troublesome. Glottis means hole. There are times during voice production when the vocal folds are in apposition and the larynx is closed. How during those times can anything be "sub" glottal. You can't be below a hole when there isn't one. Respiratory physiologists use tracheal pressure to refer to the pressure of interest. Tracheal pressure designates the site of the pressure and is accurate regardless of whether the laryngeal airway is open or closed. Using the term tracheal pressure also removes ambiguity involved in the use of "sub" as a location. The term subglottal pressure should be buried. Rest in peace.

---

cheal air pressure and prevent it from escaping uselessly (Daniloff et al., 1980). Increases in laryngeal airway resistance, also effected by contractions of the adductory muscles, relate to a reduction in average glottal size (Holmberg, Hillman, & Perkell, 1988).

The combined increase in tracheal pressure and heightened opposition provided by the larynx results in a change in the pattern of vocal fold vibration and excitation of the upper airway. For speech of higher sound pressure level, the vocal folds separate faster, return to the midline faster, and remain in approximation at the midline for a longer period during each cycle of vocal fold vibration (Minifie, 1973).

Two underlying features of laryngeal behavior are critically important to how efficiently energy from the breathing apparatus is converted into acoustic energy (Titze, 1988b, 1994, 2006b). One of these is the abruptness with which the vocal folds return to the midline and airflow declines (referred to as the airflow declination rate or glottal area declination rate). The abruptness of this decline relates to the strength of the acoustic excitation of the upper airway (Dromey, Stathopoulos, & Sapienza, 1992; Holmberg et al., 1988; Titze, 2006b). The other important feature of laryngeal behavior is the average size of the glottis during the attempt to produce a higher sound pressure level. Exploration with computer modeling suggests that the optimal acoustic power is generated when the average glottal size is about midway between that for tight adduction of the vocal folds, as associated with a pressed voice, and that for loose adduction of the vocal folds, as associated with a breathy voice (Titze, 1994).

Although the breathing apparatus and laryngeal apparatus contribute most to sound pressure level changes, the pharyngeal-oral apparatus also influences sound pressure level of the voice. In general, it tends to blossom open more and more with successive increases in sound pressure level, achieving an effect that is somewhat akin to that provided by a megaphone. The velum (soft palate and uvula) elevates, the mandible lowers, the tongue lowers, and the mouth opening increases (Netsell, 1973; Tucker, 1963), adjustments that lower the radiation impedance of the pharyngeal-oral apparatus so that the sound energy is transmitted more effectively to the atmosphere (Fant, 1960; Flanagan, 1972).

Prowess in the generation of high sound pressure level is viewed by some as a virtue and is especially prized when the voice can be used without amplification to shatter a glass goblet. There are few who can accomplish this feat, but chances of succeeding are best when following scientific principles about resonance rather than relying on brute force of the voice (Behrman, 2007; Walker, 1977).

Listen My Children and You Shall Hear

Some people are loud and then some people are really loud. The conversion of aerodynamic power to acoustic power is better in some than in others and some of the best at it have been listed as celebrities in folk sources. Different hollering, yelling, screaming, shouting, and loud voice champions have been crowned around the world. The *Guinness Book of Records* (Folkard, 2006) lists Jill Drake as the reigning screaming champion at 129 dB and Annalisa Wray as the reigning shouting champion at 121.7 dB. Alan Myatt, the town crier of Gloucester, England, once was touted in the *Guinness Book of Records* as having the world's loudest voice, an ear-piercing 112.8 dB. Had Paul Revere been so endowed as a town crier he wouldn't have had to knock on so many doors and he might have been able to awaken all of Lexington, Massachusetts on a single breath. Well, maybe not all, but at least much of the South Side.

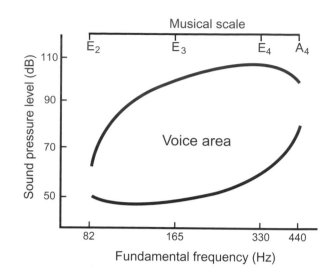

Figure 3–43. Fundamental frequency-sound pressure level profile of an adult male.

Fundamental Frequency-Sound Pressure Level Profiles. The term "voice range" is most often used when referring to the lowest and highest values that can be produced in either the fundamental frequency or sound pressure level of the voice. These two variables are not independent of one another in that the fundamental frequency has a different set of lowest and highest values at different sound pressure levels, and the sound pressure level has a different set of lowest and highest values at different fundamental frequencies (Fairbanks, 1960). These relations are illustrated in fundamental frequency-sound pressure level profiles that graphically portray fundamental frequency on a horizontal axis and sound pressure level on a vertical axis (Coleman et al., 1977; Damste, 1970; Gramming, 1991). An example profile from an adult male is shown in Figure 3–43.

Figure 3–43 depicts the lowest and highest fundamental frequencies and sound pressure levels attainable (and sustainable for brief durations) across the ranges of fundamental frequency and sound pressure level. This figure illustrates that, in general, lower fundamental frequencies and sound pressure levels can be produced at lower values of the other variable, whereas higher fundamental frequencies and sound pressure levels can be produced at higher values of the other variable. The fundamental frequency range of the voice

is greatest in the midrange of sound pressure levels. Similarly, the sound pressure level range of the voice is greatest in the midrange of fundamental frequencies.

By displaying the minimum and maximum fundamental frequencies and sound pressure levels of the voice at different values of the other variable, the capabilities of the production apparatus are revealed (Gramming & Sundberg, 1988; Titze, 1992). An important clinical implication is that when evaluating the fundamental frequency and/or sound pressure level capabilities of the voice, it is important to keep in mind that the results obtained can be greatly influenced by whether or not the other variable is controlled and, if so, at what value.

Spectrum. The spectrum of the sound generated by the vibrating larynx is complex and composed of a combination of different frequencies and sound pressure levels (Minifie, 1973; Stevens, 2000). The usual laryngeal source spectrum consists of a fundamental frequency and successive odd and even harmonics (whole number multiples of the fundamental frequency) that decrease in sound pressure level with increasing harmonic number at a rate of about 12 dB per octave (each doubling of frequency) above 1000 Hz (Fant, 1960). A wide variety of source spectra can be produced through changes in tracheal air pressure and translaryngeal airflow, and through changes in the mechanical properties of the vocal folds.

The voice source spectrum changes with fundamental frequency because the spacing of the harmonics depends on the fundamental frequency (as fundamental frequency increases, the spacing between the harmonics increases). The spectrum also changes with sound pressure level (as sound pressure level increases, the energy in the higher frequency region tends to increase). The spectral content of the voice source is also influenced by changes in the vibratory pattern of the vocal folds (Stevens, 2000) and the degree to which the laryngeal airway is constricted. The extremes are embodied in the spectra generated with pressed voice (vocal folds set to be tightly approximated) and breathy voice (vocal folds set to be easily parted and to allow continuous airflow between them). These factors are strongly conditioned by actions of the intrinsic muscles of the larynx, most notably the *thyroarytenoid, lateral cricoarytenoid,* and *arytenoid* muscles.

The voice source generated at the laryngeal level constitutes the raw material of voice production. This input from the larynx to the upper airway sounds like a coarse buzz that is further conditioned and filtered before sound is radiated from the mouth and voice quality is manifested publicly. Much more about these important factors is discussed in subsequent chapters.

Voice Registers. The nature of vocal fold vibration is strongly conditioned by so-called voice registers. Voice registers reflect different modes of vocal fold vibration that result from different mechanical conditions (Titze, 1994) and that give rise to differences in perceived voice quality (Laver, 1991). Accordingly, a voice register can be defined perceptually as a series of consecutive utterances of similar voice quality produced along a pitch scale through application of similar mechanical principles.

The topic of voice registers is controversial, especially in singing pedagogy. The number and nature of voice registers is often argued in the singing literature, as are the mechanisms involved in their generation (sometimes taken to include both laryngeal and upper airway adjustments). Far less controversy exists about the number and nature of voice registers in the speaking voice and the mechanisms of their generation. This section is limited to a discussion of voice registers that pertain to speaking.

There are three voice registers in the speaking voice. The general location of these along the fundamental frequency scale is illustrated for men and women in Figure 3–44. They are labeled as the pulse, modal, and loft voice registers and correspond to three different modes of vocal fold vibration encountered in sequence when speaking at an ascending fundamental frequency from the lowest to highest fundamental frequencies within the speaking range (Hollien, 1972, 1974). Each voice register is confined to a restricted

range of fundamental frequencies and within each register a particular mode or pattern of vocal fold vibration prevails. The boundary between adjacent registers is determined by raising and lowering the fundamental frequency and noting where an abrupt change in voice quality occurs.

The modal voice register is the middle of the three speaking voice registers and gets its name from the statistical mode, the most often occurring event (in fundamental frequency). The modal register is characteristic of the type of vocal fold vibration described thus far in this chapter and is the voice register typically used during most conversational speech production. Voice production in the modal voice register is characterized by moderate values of vocal fold length, vocal fold thickness, vocal fold stiffness, laryngeal opposing pressure, laryngeal airway resistance, tracheal air pressure, and translaryngeal airflow (Hollien, 1960a, 1960b, 1962; Hollien, Brown, & Hollien, 1971; Hollien & Colton, 1969; Hollien & Curtis, 1960; Hollien & Moore, 1960; Isshiki, 1964; Kunze, 1962; Murry & Brown, 1971b; Shipp & McGlone, 1971; van den Berg, 1956).

The pulse voice register is the lowest of the three speaking voice registers and derives its name from the nature of its pulselike voice source waveform. The quality of voice produced in this register is sometimes referred to as vocal fry, glottal fry, or creaky voice, and has a certain growl-like or popping sound to it that some have described as coarse and bubbly (Orlikoff & Kahane, 1996). Voice can be produced continuously in the pulse voice register, although this would be atypical. During usual running speech production, pulse voice register manifests intermittently at the ends of breath groups when the voice trails off in sound pressure level and drops in fundamental frequency (comes to a growling halt).

The vibration of the vocal folds in pulse voice register is distinct and is characterized by prolonged approximation of the vocal folds and brief appearances of a small glottis. The pulse produced in association with this short-lived glottis is relatively rich in harmonic structure, but low in sound pressure level. Fundamental frequency and sound pressure level tend to change together in the pulse register and do not have the relative independence found in modal voice register (Murry & Brown, 1971a, 1971b).

Voice production in the pulse voice register is generated with moderate or low values of tracheal air pressure and translaryngeal airflow (Allen & Hollien, 1973; Holmberg, Hillman, & Perkell, 1989; McGlone, 1967; McGlone & Shipp, 1971; Murry, 1971; Murry & Brown, 1971b). The vocal folds are short, thick, slack, and compliant (Allen & Hollien, 1973; Hollien, Damste,

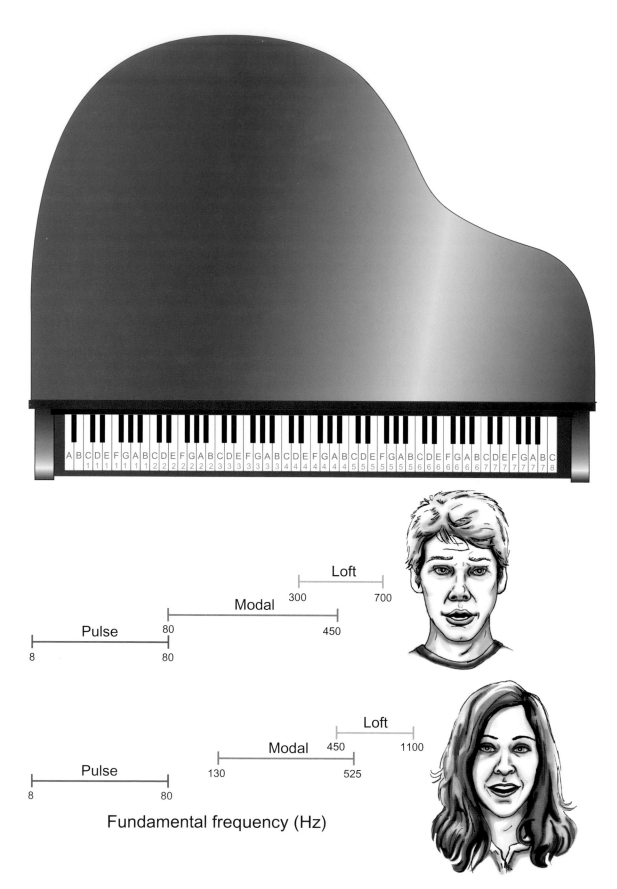

Figure 3–44. Voice registers along the fundamental frequency scale.

& Murry, 1969) and medial compression is moderate (McGlone & Shipp, 1971). Lateral vocal fold movements are moderate and usually not along the entire length of the membranous portion of the vocal folds (Orlikoff & Kahane, 1996) and there is a pronounced vertical phase difference. A prolonged approximation phase of vocal fold vibration results in a near-total damping of upper airway excitation with each pulse of activity (Coleman, 1963; Titze, 1988a; Wendahl, Moore, & Hollien, 1963). The voice source, therefore, is a series of nearly discrete excitations to the upper airway that gives the listener the perception that the voice is a string of tiny pops (like those that can be made by applying repeated bursts of pressure behind the lips when they are thickly puckered and gently held together).

The loft voice register is the highest of the three speaking voice registers and gets it name from its high placement within the fundamental frequency range. This register is also called the falsetto voice register. The quality of the voice produced in this register is sometimes described as thin, flutelike, and breathy, with acoustic characteristics that resemble a pure tone.

The vibration of the vocal folds in the loft voice register is somewhat simpler than that for the modal and pulse voice registers. Excursions of the vocal folds are relatively small and the glottis is narrow. The vibratory pattern of the vocal folds entails little or no vertical phase difference. Rather, movements are mainly horizontal and confined to the vicinity of the free margins of the vocal folds. Such movements take on the appearance of vibrating strings alternately moving horizontally away from and toward one another. Approximation of the vocal folds is not obligatory for voice production in the loft register. When the vocal folds do approximate, the contact between them is usually light (involves low adductory forces). The voice source produced in conjunction with loft voice register contains less high harmonic energy than that for modal voice register (Colton, 1972) and the sound pressure level of the voice is lower in the loft register than in the modal register (Orlikoff & Kahane, 1996).

Voice production in the loft voice register is generated with moderately high tracheal air pressure and translaryngeal airflow (Large, Iwata, & von Leden, 1970; McGlone, 1970; Shipp & McGlone, 1971; Shipp, McGlone, & Morrisey, 1972), elongated and thin vocal folds that are under great longitudinal tension (Hollien & Moore, 1960), and very high stiffness of the mucosal covers of the vocal folds (Gay, Hirose, Strome, & Sawashima, 1972; Hirano, 1974; Hirano, Vennard, & Ohala, 1970). Changes in fundamental frequency and sound pressure level in the loft register are significantly influ-

---

Not an Island Unto Itself

The behavior of the larynx is not independent of its surrounds. When transitioning back and forth across the boundary between the modal and loft voice registers, the boundary between the two registers will differ somewhat in fundamental frequency from one transition to another. This is because the larynx is coupled to the breathing apparatus and the breathing apparatus has resonance properties that interact with the mode of vibration of the vocal folds. These resonance properties change when there are different amounts of air in the lungs. Thus, transitioning back and forth across the boundary between the modal and loft voice registers occurs at different fundamental frequency breaking points when the lung volume is different. The lesson contained in this observation is that a neighbor can influence the behavior of the larynx. It is not an island unto itself.

---

enced by changes in tracheal air pressure and airflow through the larynx (Colton, 1973; Isshiki, 1964, 1965; van den Berg et al., 1960; Yanagihara & Koike, 1967), with acoustic variables following directional changes in aeromechanical variables (Hollien, 1972). For example, increases in airflow through the larynx result in increases in both fundamental frequency and sound pressure level of the resulting laryngeal tone (van den Berg et al., 1960).

Running Speech Activities

The larynx is a critical participant in running speech activities. During inspiration, the vocal folds abduct and dilate the laryngeal airway to allow air to flow freely into the pulmonary apparatus. During expiration, the vocal folds adduct to produce voice and intermittently abduct to allow air pressures and airflows to reach downstream structures for oral consonant production (Hixon & Abbs, 1980; Netsell, 1973). The vocal folds act as an articulator by moving in and out of the airway to valve the flow of air during glottal stop-plosive and fricative consonant productions (Hirose, 1977; Lofqvist & Yoshioka, 1984; Orlikoff & Kahane, 1996; Sawashima, Abramson, Cooper, & Lisker, 1970). Consideration is given to the articulatory functions of the larynx in Chapter 5 where the articulatory functions of pharyngeal-oral structures are discussed. Adjustments of the laryngeal tone are the main concern of this section.

The laryngeal tone is the carrier of speech and has an important influence on speech intelligibility. It also conveys information about the speaker's age, sex, physical stature, health status, emotional status, identity, and other factors. The laryngeal tone can be adjusted in fundamental frequency, sound pressure level, and spectrum. These adjustments can be made individually or in different combinations and may occur within individual speech sounds or extend across two or more sounds. Such adjustments are used to convey different meanings, disambiguate certain aspects of the communication, emphasize certain parts of the flow of speech over others, provide information through different voice shadings and nuances, establish certain affects (impressions), and affirm roles in relationships.

Fundamental Frequency

Fundamental frequency change is prominent during running speech activities and can range as much as two octaves (Fairbanks, 1960). Fundamental frequency is often displayed and measured in a tracing called a fundamental frequency contour, which tracks change in fundamental frequency over time. Such a contour is shown in Figure 3–45 for a spoken sentence.

Listening to fundamental frequency change in the voice evokes a perception of time-varying pitch change that is referred to as an intonation contour. Perceptions

of intonation contours are influenced by sensitivity to pitch inflections and pitch shifts. Inflections are modulations in pitch during voiced segments, whereas shifts are changes in pitch from the end of one voiced segment to the beginning of the next (Fairbanks, 1960). The intonation contour underlies what the listener comes to consider as the melody or tunefulness of speech. This contour operates around a mode (the most often sensed pitch) that determines what the listener judges to be the characteristic pitch level of the voice.

Adjustments in fundamental frequency during running speech activities are vested mainly in laryngeal actions. These laryngeal actions rely, in large part, on interplay between contractions of the *cricothyroid* and *thyroarytenoid* muscles, along with bracing actions of the *posterior cricoarytenoid* muscles, which also adjust the stiffness of the vocal folds. (Atkinson, 1978; Gay et al., 1972; Hirano, Ohala, & Vennard, 1969; Netsell, 1969). Actions of the *cricothyroid* muscles are more strongly correlated with the fundamental frequency of the voice than are the actions of other intrinsic muscles of the larynx, as long as the *cricothyroid* muscles are not functioning near their maximum output (Atkinson, 1978; Titze, 1994). Thus, as discussed above for sustained voice production, changes in the longitudinal tension of the vocal folds (via *cricothyroid* muscle activation) and change in internal stiffness of the vocal folds (via *thyroarytenoid* muscle activation) are of prime importance to the control of the fundamental frequency of the voice during running speech events.

Adjustments of the breathing apparatus in the form of changes in pressure and volume can also influence fundamental frequency. Although tracheal pressure remains relatively steady during running speech production, it does fluctuate slightly with linguistic stress. Pulsatile increases in tracheal pressure cause slight increases in the fundamental frequency of the voice (Hixon et al., 1971; Lester & Story, in press; Titze, 1989), suggesting that pressure fluctuations associated with the production of stressed syllables may contribute to momentary increases in fundamental frequency. Furthermore, although running speech is generally produced within the midrange of the vital capacity, sometimes it is produced outside this lung volume range. Running speech produced at higher than usual lung volumes may be associated with higher than usual fundamental frequencies (Watson, Ciccia, & Weismer, 2003). This may be due to higher tracheal pressures associated with higher expiratory recoil pressures at large lung volumes, or it may be due to a downward pull on the larynx (through its connections to the diaphragm) that could increase vocal fold tension, or both.

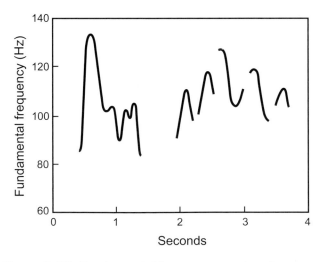

Figure 3–45. Fundamental frequency contour for a spoken sentence of an adult male. (Courtesy of Brad Story)

Sound Pressure Level

Like fundamental frequency, sound pressure level also changes significantly during running speech activities. This is true of the average sound pressure level associated with different speaking situations (soft, normal, or loud speech) and rapid variations from the average level (such as accompany varying levels of linguistic stress). A routine conversation might find the sound pressure level to swing as much as 25 to 30 dB. The magnitude of sound pressure level and its directional changes can be displayed and measured in a tracing referred to as a sound pressure level contour, one of which is shown for a sentence production in Figure 3–46.

Changes in sound pressure level over time give rise to a subjective impression of a loudness contour that embodies percepts of an average loudness and variations about it. Vowels are the main contributors to loudness judgments in running speech activities. Adjustment in vowel and consonant sound pressure levels, while usually moving in the same direction, find vowel sound pressure level to change more than consonant sound pressure level (Hixon, 1966; Stevens, 2000). This is due to a tendency to open up the pharyngeal-oral apparatus more to accomplish vowel increases, and a tendency to constrict the apparatus more to accomplish consonant increases. These two competing tendencies result in a tradeoff in sound pressure level change, in which the vowel dominates because of its more prominent carrying power (Fairbanks & Miron, 1957).

Perceived loudness contours convey what is judged to be the forcefulness or effort used to generate the acoustic product. Such contours are strongly related to actual sound pressure level contours, but do not bear a one-to-one correspondence to them. For example, when counting from one to ten, the syllables tend to sound equally loud to the listener despite the differences in sound pressure levels across the different vowels in the series. Indeed, certain sounds have intrinsically higher or lower sound pressure levels than other sounds. This is a distinction that is not usually appreciated by the casual listener.

Control of sound pressure level for running speech activities is conditioned by adjustments of the breathing apparatus, laryngeal apparatus, and pharyngeal-oral apparatus. The most important breathing apparatus adjustment has to do with changing the magnitude of the average tracheal air pressure and with effecting small increases in pressure to emphasize certain speech segments (Netsell, 1969). These background level and pulsatile tracheal air pressure events are the result of muscular pressure adjustments by the chest wall (Hixon, Mead, & Goldman, 1976).

Laryngeal participation in sound pressure level control for running speech activities usually involves heightened vocal fold adductory forces that manifest as increases in the laryngeal opposing pressure. These forces enable the buildup of tracheal air pressure and increase as speech becomes progressively louder or contrastive stress levels become greater from one syllable to another (Hirano et al., 1969; Netsell, 1969, 1973). The muscles implicated in heightening vocal fold adductory forces are primarily the *lateral cricoarytenoid* and *arytenoid* muscles, although muscles that stiffen the vocal folds (the *thyroarytenoid* and *cricothyroid* muscles) may also contribute.

Pharyngeal-oral adjustments that change the acoustic radiation impedance are often associated with changes in the sound pressure level of running speech. That is, the pharyngeal-oral apparatus tends to open more and more with successive increases in the sound pressure level to enhance transmission of acoustic energy generated at the glottis (Daniloff et al., 1980; Netsell, 1973).

Spectrum

The spectrum of the laryngeal source changes rapidly and often during running speech activities. Such changes are associated with changes in the fundamental frequency or sound pressure level of the voice and with other changes in the pattern of vocal fold vibration. Slower changes in the spectrum of the laryngeal tone may result from prolonged use of the vocal folds, transient abuse of the vocal folds, so-called laryngeal fatigue, or a reduction in hydration of the laryngeal apparatus.

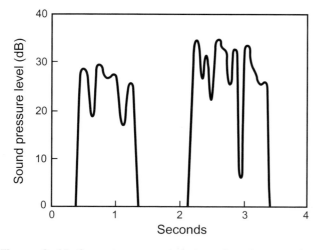

Figure 3–46. Sound pressure level contour for a spoken sentence of an adult male. (Courtesy of Brad Story)

Tick Tock

Anyone who has played music to the beat of a metronome knows how maddening it can be. When just learning the music, it's a challenge to keep up. Then, once you have the music mastered, it seems like you have to slow down to be on pace. But something has to set the pace, like a conductor of an orchestra. The larynx usually does this during speech production. It's the metronome of the speech production apparatus. The movements of other speech production structures are constrained by what the larynx does. It does no good to get to a position before the larynx because then you'll just have to wait. And, if you arrive at a position later than the time specified by the larynx, you have big problems. It's not quite as simple as we've portrayed, but it's close enough to give you the idea. Maybe you've heard the nursery rhyme "Hickory, dickory, dock, the voice box is the clock." Well, maybe not, because it was just written.

Source spectrum changes may give rise to changes in voice quality, a perceptual attribute that pertains to the sound of the voice beyond its pitch and loudness characteristics (Behrman, 2007). Depending on the speaking situation, the spectrum can change in ways that cause the listener to perceive voice qualities that range from breathy to pressed or are labeled by a great variety of other descriptors (Minifie, 1973; Stevens, 2000). The diversity of descriptors applied to different voice qualities reflects both the personal preferences of individual listeners and the difficulties involved in getting groups of listeners to arrive at a consensus.

All of the intrinsic muscles of the larynx can influence the laryngeal source spectrum during running speech activities, because all of them have influences on the nature of vocal fold vibration. Those with the most significant influence, however, are thought to be the *thyroarytenoid, lateral cricoarytenoid,* and *arytenoid* muscles.

Development and Laryngeal Function in Speech Production

Between the birth cry and adulthood, about two decades pass. During this time, laryngeal structure and function undergo significant change, as does the voice they produce. This section considers salient developmental changes and some of their influences on voice production.

The structure of the larynx undergoes relocation and remodeling during the developmental period. This includes changes in its positioning within the neck, and in its size, configuration, and mechanical properties.

The newborn larynx rides high within the neck, such that the lower edge of the cricoid cartilage is positioned between the third and fourth cervical vertebrae. The larynx and velopharynx are close companions in this arrangement. The epiglottis contacts the velum, a mechanical arrangement that facilitates the nursing needs of the infant while simultaneously ensuring an adequate airway for ventilation (Laitman & Crelin, 1976; Sasaki, Levin, Laitman, & Crelin, 1977). By 4 to 6 months of age, this arrangement begins to change and is present mainly during swallowing.

As the infant grows, the larynx descends from its initial high position (Wind, 1970). By the end of the first year of life, the lower edge of the cricoid cartilage has descended to the middle of the fourth cervical vertebra. By age 3 years, the descent has reached to the middle of the fifth cervical vertebra, and by age 5 years it has reached to the middle of the sixth cervical vertebra. Downward migration continues to the region of the seventh cervical vertebra between 10 and 20 years of age.

The framework of the larynx also undergoes significant developmental change. The thyroid cartilage, for example, is contiguous with the hyoid bone at birth and then separates from it vertically. The laminae of the thyroid cartilage form a somewhat semicircular structure in the infant larynx and proceed to a more angular form in the larynx of the older child (Kahane, 1975). The angle formed by the thyroid laminae narrows to a more prominent configuration, especially in older male children (Kahane, 1978; Malinowski, 1967).

The framework of the infant larynx is destined to triple in size during the developmental period (Bosma, 1985). Growth of the laryngeal cartilages is generally more linear in the female than the male, with the most rapid changes in the size of the male laryngeal framework occurring during the pubertal growth spurt (Dickson & Maue-Dickson, 1982; Kahane, 1978). With the exception of the front of the male thyroid cartilage, the growth of the laryngeal cartilages has been characterized as involving an increase in size and weight with configuration remaining relatively unchanged (Kahane, 1978, 1982). Structural differences in the framework of male and female larynges have been reported to exist as early as 3 years of age (Crelin, 1973). However, predominant thought has it that the most significant framework differences between male and female larynges are demonstrated somewhat later in development, with the greatest contrasts in sexual dimorphism occurring around puberty (Kahane, 1982).

The structures of the laryngeal framework are soft and pliable at the beginning of life and proceed to become firm and less flexible with age (Tucker & Tucker, 1979). Ossification (turning to bone) of the hyoid begins at about 2 years of age. Cartilages of the larynx begin to show signs of ossification much later in life, usually during the first couple of decades of adulthood (Aronson, 1990).

Structures of the laryngeal interior likewise undergo change with development. This includes enlargement and change in their relative proportions, configurations, and mechanical properties. For example, the laryngeal aditus widens and changes shape as the infant ages and the interior of the larynx becomes less pliable.

The vocal folds double their length during childhood. Puberty adds another growth spurt to the vocal folds, especially in males (Dickson & Maue-Dickson, 1982; Kahane, 1978). An important developmental change in vocal fold structure has to do with the relative lengths of the membranous and cartilaginous portions of the vocal folds. The infant larynx has a much larger cartilaginous portion than membranous portion (Tucker & Tucker, 1979). This relation changes with development, until a much larger membranous portion to cartilaginous portion exists in the adult (Zemlin, 1998). The weights of the individual intrinsic muscles of the larynx increase with age from infancy through adulthood, but remain proportional throughout the developmental period (Kahane & Kahn, 1984). The *cricothyroid* muscle is the largest of the intrinsic laryngeal muscles by weight and has been suggested as being of special importance in adjusting vocal fold length and tension (and stiffness) during vocalization in infants (Kahane & Kahn, 1984).

The composition and resulting mechanical properties of the vocal folds change significantly during development. The larynx of the newborn shows a homogeneous and undifferentiated lamina propria (Hirano & Sato, 1993). This contrasts markedly with the distinctive multilayered structure of the lamina propria of the adult vocal folds (Hirano, 1974, 1981). The vocal ligament does not develop in the child until about 4 years of age (Zemlin, 1998) and the adult-like lamina propria is not apparent until about 16 years of age (Kent, 1997). The latter occurs after the most rapid change in vocal fold length has taken place (Kazarian, Sarkissian, & Isaakian, 1978). The difference in the lamina propria between infancy and adulthood prevents the infant from achieving some of the subtle vocal fold adjustments that are a part of the adult repertoire.

These structural and functional changes, and others, contribute to voice production changes during the developmental period. Changes in the fundamental frequency of the voice are perhaps the most obvious and are portrayed in Figure 3–47. During the first decade of life, the fundamental frequency decreases in both males and females, from about 400 to 500 Hz (newborns) to about 200 to 300 Hz (10 year olds), with much of the decrease occurring during the first 3 years (Kent, 1976). Prior to the onset of puberty, males and females have a similar average fundamental frequency and a similar variation in fundamental frequency (Fairbanks, Herbert, & Hammond, 1949; Fairbanks, Wiley, & Lassman, 1949; Wilson, 1979). In cases where differences between boys and girls have been reported, they do not appear to be related to sex, per se, but rather appear to be associated with factors such as height or cultural background (Glaze, Bless, Milenkovic, & Susser, 1988; Hasek, Singh, & Murry, 1980). During and after puberty, fundamental frequency undergoes a large and rapid downward change in males to about 130 Hz, and a much less precipitous downward change in females. The greater downward change in males is a consequence of a greater growth spurt in males and is caused by a significant increase in both the length and thickness of the male vocal folds compared to the female vocal folds. The adolescent voice change that is perceptually prominent in males usually occurs between 12.5 and 14.5 years of age and may be accompanied by pitch breaks and other phenomena that reflect transient instability in the control of the voice (Hollien, Green, & Massey, 1994).

As noted above, voice change during development is the result of not only enlargement of the vocal folds, but also changes in the inner structure of the covers of the vocal folds (Hirano & Sato, 1993). Thus, it is likely that more than the fundamental frequency of the voice may be influenced by laryngeal changes associated with adolescent voice change. Hirano, Kurita, and Nakashima (1983) have suggested that the development of collagen and elastic fibers in the vocal ligaments result in the addition of mass and stiffness to the vocal folds that could lead to changes in the nature of vocal fold vibration. This may account for the observation that voice quality changes during voice mutation in adolescence. A common descriptor applied to the changing voice of the male adolescent is that it is somewhat breathy, rough, and hoarse (Curry, 1946; Kahane, 1982).

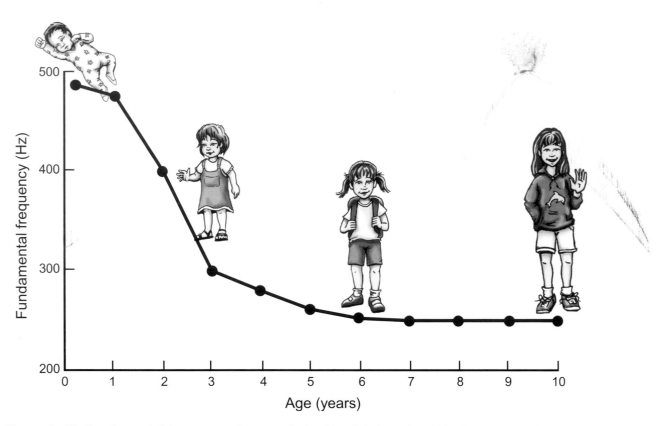

Figure 3–47. Fundamental frequency changes during the first decade of life. Based on data summarized in "Anatomical and neuromuscular maturation of the speech mechanism: Evidence from acoustic studies" (p. 423), by R. Kent, 1976, *Journal of Speech and Hearing Research, 19*, 421–447. Copyright 1976 by the American Speech and Hearing Association. Data summary reproduced with permission.

Donald Duck

Many reading this have breathed in from a helium-filled balloon and then tried to speak. The resulting sound makes people laugh because it reminds them of the voice of the cartoon character Donald Duck. What causes this? Helium is lighter than air, has a different kinematic viscosity, and effectively reduces the acoustic size of the upper airway. This makes the speech production apparatus behave acoustically as if it belonged to a smaller person. Helium results in upper airway resonances that are higher than usual in frequency. It's as if a child's upper airway were being excited by an adult's larynx. As utterance (expiration) proceeds, the inspired helium gives way to a mixture of helium and air and then just air. The sound of the voice gradually returns to normal, all the while simulating the growth of an upper airway that eventually attains its corresponding adult size to go along with its adult-size larynx.

Age and Laryngeal Function in Speech Production

Once the structure and function of the larynx are fully matured, they are subject to additional modifications throughout adulthood. Some of these changes lead to changes in the voice.

The lower edge of the cricoid cartilage has descended to the upper edge of the seventh cervical vertebra by young adulthood. Thereafter, it continues to descend to reach the middle and then the bottom of the seventh cervical vertebra as aging continues into senescence. The larynx, in fact, continues to lower slightly even throughout senescence (Wind, 1970).

The framework of the larynx also undergoes modification during the adult years. Some of the cartilages of the larynx gradually ossify (turn to bone), whereas others gradually calcify (turn to salt). These modifications make the framework of the aging adult larynx increasingly stiff and brittle as time goes on (Zemlin, 1998).

Ossification is confined to components of the framework that are constituted of a hyaline matrix and manifests sequentially in the thyroid, cricoid, and arytenoid cartilages of the larynx. Ossification begins in these three cartilages during the early decades of adulthood (a little earlier in men than in women) and is relatively complete by the time senescence begins (Hately, Evison, & Samuel, 1965; Zemlin, 1998). Calcification is confined to components of the framework that are formed by an elastic matrix. Such calcification occurs later in senescence (more pronounced in men than in women) and is exhibited in the epiglottis, corniculate cartilages, cuneiform cartilages, and parts of the arytenoid cartilages (Kent & Verporian, 1995; Malinowski, 1967). The arytenoid cartilages are unique as components of the laryngeal scaffolding because they are made of a hyaline matrix in some parts and an elastic matrix in other parts (Kahane, 1980, 1983; Sato, Kurita, Hirano, & Kiyokawa, 1990). Thus, the arytenoid cartilages are subjected to hardening twice during the aging process, early in adulthood by ossification and late in adulthood by calcification.

The joints of the larynx also change with advancing age in adulthood. The cricoarytenoid joints, for example, undergo changes in both their joint capsules and articular surfaces (Kahane & Hammons, 1987; Kahn & Kahane, 1986; Segre, 1971). Changes at the articular surfaces include abrasion, ossification, erosion, and deformation, all of which influence movements at the joints. Most important is that the movement of the arytenoid cartilages around the cricoarytenoid joints can be reduced in older individuals, which, in turn, can limit the degree to which the vocal folds can be approximated (Kahane, 1988).

The vocal folds and structures that control them also undergo change during aging in adulthood. This includes nerve fiber loss and muscle atrophy that lead to losses in mass and muscle strength (Aronson, 1990; Cooper, 1990; Ferreri, 1959). Other changes with aging include a loss of tissue elasticity in the vocal folds, dehydration of the laryngeal mucosa, edema, and alteration in the density of different fibers constituting the structural matrices of the vocal folds (Aronson, 1990; Benjamin, 1988; Kahane & Beckford, 1991; Keleman & Pressman, 1955; Kent & Vorperian, 1995; Linville, 1995; Mueller, Sweeney, & Baribeau, 1985).

Histological age-related changes in the vocal folds may have important functional consequences for voice production. With advanced age, not only is muscle tissue lost within the body of the vocal fold, connective tissue is gained (Kahane, 1983). Simultaneously, the cover of the vocal fold undergoes modification, with different layers of the lamina propria changing in different ways with advancing age (Hirano et al., 1983; Kahane, 1983; Kahane, Stadlin, & Bell, 1979). The superficial layer thickens, becomes swollen with fluid, and declines in fiber density. The intermediate layer thins out as elastic fibers wane in size and number. And the deep layer thickens (especially in males over 50 years of age) as collagenous fibers increase in size and density. These age-related changes in the lamina propria may cause the vocal folds to take on a bowed configuration (Honjo & Isshiki, 1980; Mueller et al., 1985), develop surface irregularities along their free margins (Kahane, 1983), and stiffen (Kent, 1997).

The variety of changes attendant to the aging of the framework, muscle, and fiber matrices of the larynx have implications for its function. These changes and their consequences may be somewhat different for men and women, as discussed in the section below on sex and laryngeal function in speech production.

Finally, it should be noted that nearly everything known about the influence of aging on laryngeal structure and function is based on the use of chronological age (easy to quantify) as the primary temporal marker (Shipp & Hollien, 1969). However, it may be that physiological age (more difficult to measure) is, in fact, a more relevant temporal marker. Beyond this distinction, it is also believed that health status has important implications and must be taken into account when attempting to understand voice changes across adulthood (Ramig & Ringel, 1983)

Sex and Laryngeal Function in Speech Production

The structure and function of the larynx are different in some ways between the sexes. Certain dissimilarities have an influence on voice production.

During infancy and early childhood, the structure and function of the larynx are relatively similar in males and females. Later in childhood, differences between the sexes start to emerge, especially during puberty. This period of major laryngeal mutation for males causes abrupt changes in voice that manifest as secondary sex characteristics. The most prominent of these is a lowering of the fundamental frequency of the male voice by about an octave. The sexual dimorphism in the structure and function of the larynx seen in early adolescence are maintained across the adult life span.

Ossification and calcification of the larynx occur earlier chronologically in males than in females. Ossification in males begins in the third decade of life, whereas in females it starts in the fourth decade. The female larynx may, in some cases, never completely ossify (Claassen & Kirsch, 1994).

The vocal folds also show differences in structure between the sexes across adulthood. Male vocal folds lengthen, whereas female vocal folds maintain a relatively constant length into senescence (Kazarian et al., 1978).

Men usually demonstrate full approximation of the vocal folds during voice production, whereas women usually do not. This difference is portrayed in Figure 3–48. Young women often show an opening between the vocal folds during voice production, especially in the cartilaginous segment (Behrman, 2007; Biever & Bless, 1989; Sodersten & Lindestad, 1990). Elderly women, in contrast, often show an opening during voice production in the membranous segment of the vocal folds or show a spindle-shaped opening that runs the entire length of the vocal folds (Linville, 1992; Ahmad, Yan, & Bless, in press). Reasons for male-female differences in vocal fold approximation are speculative. Factors that have been suggested include differences in the arrangement of the cricoarytenoid joints, differences in the muscle mass of the body of the vocal folds, and differences in the covers of the vocal folds (Hirano et al., 1988; Hirano, Kiyokawa, Kurita, & Sato, 1986). Cultural factors may also be at play, with a breathy voice quality being a more desirable characteristic of a female voice than a male voice (Linville, 1992).

Continuing from the adolescent period, differences in the fundamental frequencies of males and females persist throughout adulthood. However, as shown in Figure 3–49, males and females appear to evidence different patterns of age-related change across adulthood. The patterns shown from a collection of cross-sectional studies suggest that older men have a higher fundamental frequency than younger men (Hollien & Shipp, 1972; Honjo & Isshiki, 1980; Mueller et al., 1985; Stathopoulos, Huber, & Sussman, 2011), whereas older women have a lower fundamental frequency than younger women (Awan & Mueller, 1992; Benjamin, 1981; Honjo & Isshiki, 1980; Linville, 1987; Linville & Fisher, 1985; Mueller et al., 1985; Russell, Penny, & Pemberton, 1995; Stoicheff, 1981).

Menopause is one factor in the lowering of fundamental frequency in women prior to senescence. This is suggested by the fact that significantly lower fundamental frequencies have been found in women who have completed menopause than in women of the

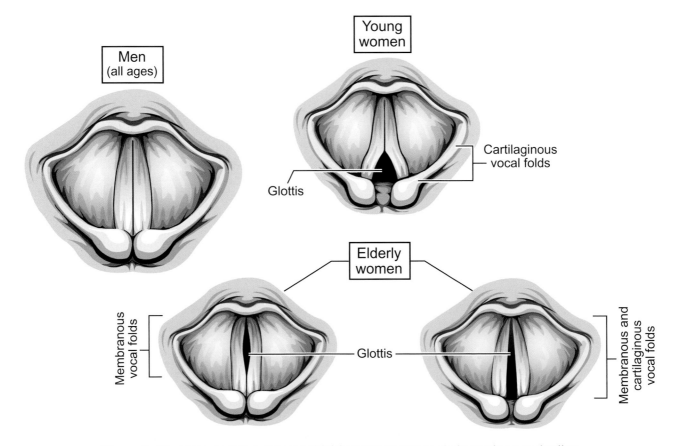

Figure 3–48. Male and female vocal fold approximations during voice production.

same age who have not completed menopause (Stoicheff, 1981). Data of this nature have prompted some to suggest that a male-female coalescence model of aging voice production may have currency (Hollien et al., 1994). In such a model, the hormone-related factors that cause differences to occur between males and females in adolescence are counteracted to some degree by hormone-related factors associated with menopause in women. The directional shift in fundamental frequency with menopause is consistent with this model.

Age effects on the larynx tend to be more significant in men than in women and to have a greater influence on function (Linville, 1995). In men, the increase in fundamental frequency may have roots in muscle atrophy, thinning of the lamina propria, and general loss of mass (Hirano, Kurita, & Sakaguchi, 1989; Kahane, 1987; Segre, 1971), factors that would tend to move the fun-

damental frequency upward. In women, the decrease in fundamental frequency (very late in life) may have roots in an age-related increase in edema (Ferreri, 1959; Honjo & Isshiki, 1980), a factor that would tend to move the fundamental frequency downward. Fundamental frequency changes with advanced age may help to explain why it is sometimes difficult to tell whether the voice on a telephone is that of a relatively high-pitched elderly man or a relatively low-pitched elderly woman. Life, as conveyed in the voice, would appear to have come full circle to anyone who has struggled to discern whether it is 6-year-old boy or a 6-year-old girl who just picked up the telephone and said "Hello."

Men and women differ in laryngeal airway resistance during voice production, due mainly to differences in the size of their laryngeal airways. A reasonable rule of thumb is that adult men and women who have

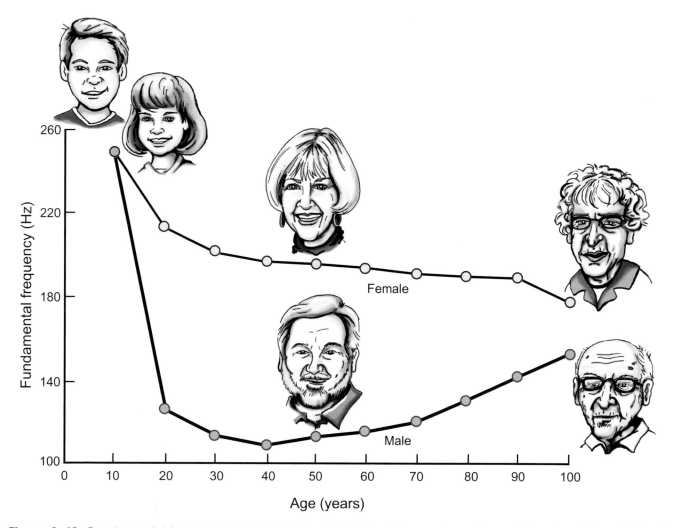

Figure 3–49. Fundamental frequency changes from ages 10 to 100 years in males and females. Data obtained from many published sources and rounded to the nearest decade for each sex.

They Didn't Quite Get It

She had a beautiful coloratura soprano voice and after years of formal training was just about to begin an operatic career. It ended abruptly on a ski slope when a careless youngster crashed into her and slammed her headfirst into a tree. She suffered facial lacerations, blunt trauma to the larynx, and temporomandibular joint damage. She never again had full singing ability. Jaw movement was especially a problem and very painful. She could no longer meet the demands of operatic roles. Forensic testimony concluded that she was 100% impaired because she could not perform a full operatic role. The career for which she had prepared was lost. The jury decided otherwise and awarded her little more than her medical expenses. The twisted logic was revealed in an interview with the foreman of the jury following the trial. "We didn't see why she couldn't just sing country songs instead. They're short and not as demanding." They didn't quite get it.

not reached senescence will demonstrate laryngeal airway resistance values during vowel production of about 35 cmH₂O/LPS and 50 cmH₂O/LPS, respectively (Hoit & Hixon, 1992; Smitheran & Hixon, 1981).

Laryngeal airway resistance remains relatively similar across adulthood for men and for women (Hoit & Hixon, 1992; Holmes, Leeper, & Nicholson, 1994; Melcon, Hoit, & Hixon, 1989) until the eighth decade of life when men begin to show a lowering of resistance compared to men of younger ages. This lowering of resistance is accompanied by a significant increase in airflow through the larynx (Melcon et al., 1989). In contrast, women in their ninth decade of life do not show a decrease in resistance compared to younger women (Hoit & Hixon, 1992). It would appear that any lessening of laryngeal valving economy, if it occurs, is significantly delayed in women compared to men.

MEASUREMENT OF LARYNGEAL FUNCTION

Laryngeal function can be measured using different types and levels of observation. This section considers four measurement approaches that are often used in clinical environments. They are endoscopy, electroglottography, aeromechanical observations, and acoustic observations.

Endoscopy

Visualization of the larynx is one of the most important tools available for determining its status and quantifying its actions. Such visualization usually entails examination of the larynx from above and may be accomplished by the insertion of a viewing device through either the oral or nasal cavities (Dailey, Spanou, & Zeitels, 2007; Sataloff et al., 1988). This method, called endoscopy, includes some form of illumination of the larynx and some form of optical device that gathers the laryngeal image (Baken & Orlikoff, 2000).

As illustrated in the upper panel of Figure 3–50, visualization via the oral route is most often done with a device called a rigid endoscope that is positioned along the upper surface of the tongue (with the tongue tip pulled forward and out of the way) and into the oropharynx. The image can be viewed through an eyepiece or recorded by one of several different optical recording systems. The rigid endoscope provides an excellent image of the larynx, but has some limitations. One limitation is that the client might find the positioning of the device to be awkward and uncomfortable. Another limitation of the rigid endoscope is that it interferes with movements of pharyngeal-oral structures so that only sustained utterances can be examined (Lofqvist & Oshima, 1993).

As illustrated in the lower panel of Figure 3–50, visualization via the nasal route is accomplished by inserting a device called a flexible endoscope through one side of the nose (usually the more open side) over the upper surface of the velum and into the pharynx. The flexible endoscope has positional controls so that its distal tip can be oriented to obtain an unobstructed view of the vocal folds (Hirano & Bless, 1993; Karnell, 1994). The image can be viewed through an eyepiece or recorded on an optical recording system. A major advantage of the flexible endoscope is that it does not encumber pharyngeal-oral structures so that the behavior of the larynx can be examined during a wide range of speech production activities (Sawashima & Hirose, 1968).

Stationary or slowly moving structures are readily observed through the use of endoscopes. However, rapid movements of the vocal folds, such as those that accompany vibration, cannot be followed with the naked eye. One way to "slow" these movements so they can be seen is by the optical illusion created with a flashing-light stroboscope. Brief flashes of light illuminate the vocal folds, with each flash being advanced slightly in time in the recurring vibratory cycle such that the phase difference between the vocal fold cycle and the flash cycle progressively increases (Baken & Orlikoff, 2000). This creates the illusion of a slowly moving vocal fold vibration that is actually a compos-

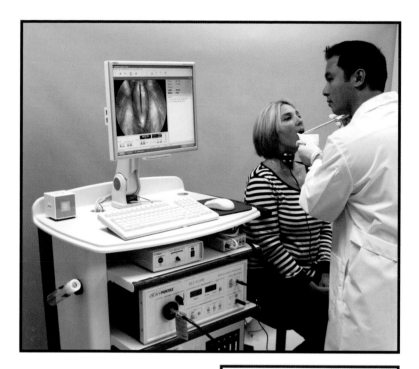

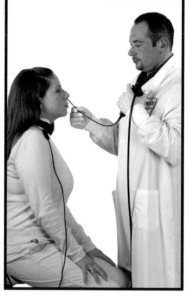

Figure 3–50. Visualization of the larynx via endoscopy. Upper panel illustrates oral approach with a rigid endoscope. Lower panel illustrates nasal approach with a flexible endoscope. Images provided courtesy of KayPENTAX, Montvale, NJ. Reproduced with permission.

ite of the sampling of successive moments throughout many cycles of vocal fold vibration (Casiano, Zaveri, & Lundy, 1992; Hirano & Bless, 1993).

A more recent application of endoscopy has incorporated high-speed digital imaging, which allows for the recording of visual images at a very rapid rate. With high-speed imaging, it is possible to capture an almost limitless number of images per vibratory cycle. A typical rate of 2000 to 8000 frames per second can usually capture at least 15 to 20 images per cycle. This allows for a detailed analysis of each cycle and offers a more complete picture of vocal fold function than does the use of stroboscopy, particularly for clients with voice disorders (Patel, Dailey, & Bless, 2008).

Being One with Your Larynx

Many aspects of laryngeal measurement show an uncanny "oneness" with the metric system. Titze (1994) suggests that this realization is helpful in making calculations off the top of your head when you don't have references at hand. A partial listing of items that he recommends be committed to memory for self-reference includes: (a) the mass of a vocal fold is about 1 g, (b) the length of a vibrating vocal fold is about 1 cm, (c) the excursion of a vibrating vocal fold is about 1 mm, (d) the shortest period of vocal fold vibration is about 1 ms, (e) the surface wave velocity on a vibrating vocal fold is about 1 m/s, (f) the maximum peak-to-peak airflow through a vibrating larynx is about 1 L/s, (g) the maximum acceleration of airflow through a vibrating larynx is about 1 m^3/s, and (h) the maximum aerodynamic power generated by a vibrating larynx is about 1 J/s. We suggest you make it a goal to memorize these before you go to sleep tonight.

Methods have been developed to quantify the images obtained through the use of endoscopy and protocols have been proposed to interpret those quantified images in ways that are relevant to clinical practice (Colton & Casper, 1996; Hirano & Bless, 1993; Kendall & Leonard, 2010). Visualization of the larynx and quantification of its image have become indispensable tools for physicians and speech-language pathologists involved in the evaluation of laryngeal disorders and voice disorders.

Electroglottography

Electroglottography is a noninvasive method for estimating the area of contact between the vocal folds (Fourcin, 1974). Electroglottography capitalizes on the electrical conduction properties of laryngeal tissues. As shown in Figure 3–51, use of an electroglottograph involves the placement of electrodes on both sides of the neck, positioned over the left and right alae of the thyroid cartilage. A weak high-frequency electrical current flows between these two electrodes and a determination is made as to the impedance (opposition) offered to that current flow by laryngeal structures.

Tissues in the vocal folds are good electrical conductors, whereas the air between the vocal folds (when a glottis exists) is an extremely poor electrical conductor. Therefore, the electrical impedance across the larynx rises when the laryngeal airway opens and falls when the vocal folds come into increasingly more extensive contact (Baken & Orlikoff, 2000). The impedance changes measured through the use of electroglottography can represent both slow laryngeal adjustments, such as those associated with general positioning of the vocal folds, and rapid changes in vocal fold contact area, such as those associated with vocal fold vibration (Childers, Hicks, Moore, Eshenazi, & Lalwani, 1990; Childers, Smith, & Moore, 1984; Titze, 1990).

The tracings in Figure 3–51 show electroglottographic recordings made during productions of ascending fundamental frequencies across three voice registers—pulse, modal, and loft. Each recording is termed an electroglottogram and reflects the time course of changes in vocal fold contact area. Recordings such as these are often interpreted in terms of the vocal fold approximation phase of the vibratory cycle, with focus on contact area change, maximum contact between the vocal folds, and other factors inferred from the waveform (Childers & Krishnamurthy, 1985; Colton & Conture, 1990; Lecluse, Brocaar, & Verschuure, 1975; Orlikoff, 1998; Rothenberg, 1981). As revealed in Figure 3–51, there are striking differences between the contact area waveforms for voice produced in the three voice registers depicted. These differences have roots in different modes of vibration of the vocal folds, as discussed above under the section on voice registers.

There are other, less commonly used applications of electroglottography. One such application involves the interpretation of certain perturbations in the electroglottographic signal to identify the onset and offset of vocal fold abduction and adduction during speech production (Rothenberg, 2009; Rothenberg & Mahshie, 1988). Another application is to track the vertical position of the larynx within the neck (Rothenberg, 1992). This application requires two pairs of electrodes, one pair placed near the lower part of the thyroid cartilage and the other placed near the upper part of the cartilage (about 0.5 cm apart). Vertical movement of the larynx is reflected in changes in the relative amplitudes of the signals generated by the upper vs lower electrode pairs.

Electroglottography has come to be used by a variety of professional disciplines concerned with understanding and altering laryngeal behavior during voice production. The popularity of this method has increased dramatically in recent years because of its simplicity and noninvasive nature and because it can be used as both an evaluation tool and a feedback device for management (Baken & Orlikoff, 2000; Kitzing, 1990; Motta, Cesari, Iengo, & Motta; 1990; Reed, 1982; Smith & Childers,

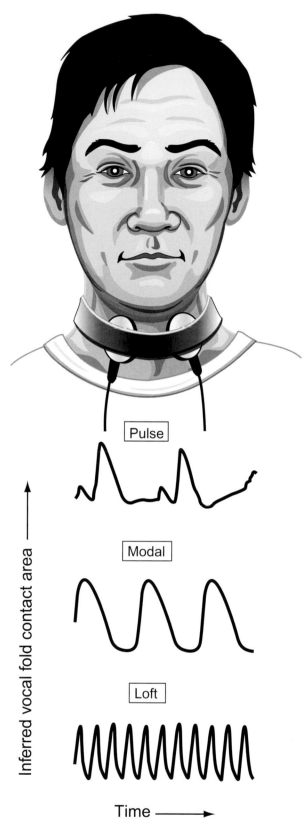

Figure 3–51. Laryngeal monitoring via electroglottography. Electrode placement is illustrated. Tracings show electroglottograms for voice produced in pulse, modal, and loft voice registers. Tracings from *Clinical measurement of speech and voice*, (2nd ed., p. 421), by R. Baken and R. Orlikoff, 2000, Belmont, CA: Delmar Learning. Clifton Park, NY: Thomson Delmar Learning. Copyright 2000 by Delmar Learning a Division of Thomson Delmar Learning: www .thomsonrights.com. Fax: 800-730-2215. Reproduced with permission.

1983). It can also be used in conjunction with other measurement methods discussed in this section because it does not interfere with the way those methods operate or with the way those methods interface with the speaker.

Aeromechanical Observations

Aeromechanical observations of laryngeal function provide information about the status of the laryngeal airway. The two most commonly used aeromechanical observations are airflow through the larynx and the calculation of resistance to airflow provided by the larynx.

Airflow through the larynx is usually measured with a pneumotachometer (air rate meter) located near the airway opening. Figure 3–52 shows a pneumotachometer attached to a facemask shaped to fit over the mouth and nose. Under certain conditions, such as during vowel production, airflow through the larynx (translaryngeal airflow) can be estimated at the airway opening because mass airflow through the larynx is continuous with that at the airway opening. Thus, airflow is an indicator of the relative openness of the larynx (providing driving pressure does not change) and the extent to which it allows air to pass between the trachea and pharynx (Isshiki & von Leden, 1964).

During voice production, the flow of air through the larynx has superimposed on it a rapidly varying component associated with vocal fold vibration. This airflow is of clinical interest because of what it reveals about the nature of vocal fold function in generating the source of laryngeal excitation to the pharyngeal-oral airway (Isshiki, 1985; Sapienza, Stathopoulos, & Dromey, 1998). The spectral content of the voice source is often derived as a reflection of the nature of the airflow pulse attendant to each cycle of vocal fold vibration.

The most common way to acquire a measurement of the airflow waveform generated at the level of the vocal folds is to record airflow changes at the airway opening with a specially designed facemask in which pneumotachometer screens are actually built into its walls (Glottal Enterprises, 2012; Rothenberg & Nezelek, 1991). This greatly improves the measurement time-constant of the flow-sensing device and enables the faithful recording of the extremely rapid airflow changes associated with vocal fold vibration. The signal obtained is then subjected to what is called inverse filtering. This filtering is designed to negate the acoustic effects that the downstream airway has on the original airflow waveform generated at the larynx. The filter network includes a circuit that is adjusted by the examiner to yield an observed minimal effect of the

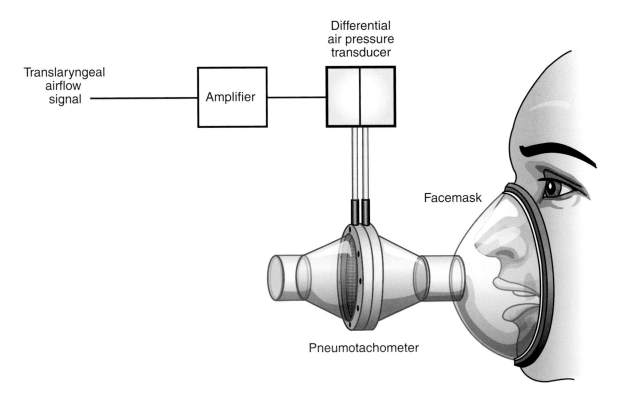

Figure 3–52. Monitoring of airflow at the airway opening as a measure of translaryngeal airflow.

acoustic properties of the downstream airway on the final airflow waveform (Rothenberg, 1973).

Airflow through the larynx is influenced not only by the openness of the larynx, but also by the forcefulness with which air is being driven through the airway (D'Antonio, Netsell, & Lotz, 1988). Thus, a better indicator of the general status of the laryngeal airway itself is an estimate of the resistance offered by the larynx to the flow of air through it (van den Berg et al., 1957). This requires knowledge of both the air pressure driving the airflow and the resultant airflow.

The most commonly used clinical method for obtaining information about laryngeal airway resistance during voice production is the method of Smitheran and Hixon (1981). This method records oral air pressure and airflow at the airway opening and uses the resultant measurements to calculate laryngeal airway resistance. As shown in Figure 3–53, measurements are taken at moments that enable estimates to be made of the air pressure difference across the larynx and the airflow through it during vowel utterances. Resistance is calculated by dividing the value for air pressure difference (estimated tracheal air pressure minus estimated pharyngeal air pressure) by the value for translaryngeal airflow (estimated from the airflow at the airway opening). Resistance determinations enable estimates of the degree of coupling between the tracheal and pharyngeal spaces and thus of laryngeal status (Holmberg et al., 1988, 1999). Accordingly, laryngeal airway resistance values that differ significantly from those of normal subjects are taken as indications of dysfunction. For example, very low resistance values during attempts to produce normal voice may reflect excessive opening of the laryngeal airway, whereas very high resistance values during such attempts may reflect excessive closing of the laryngeal airway (Leeper & Graves, 1984; Smitheran & Hixon, 1981).

The clinical measurement of laryngeal airway resistance is a powerful tool for understanding voice disorders (Kostyk & Rochet, 1998; Netsell, Lotz, & Shaughnessy, 1984; Plant & Hillel, 1998) and modifying them (D'Antonio et al., 1988; Smitheran & Hixon, 1981). Such measurements are relatively noninvasive and straightforward and may be incorporated as options in commercially available systems for making aeromechanical observations of voice production (Kay-PENTAX, 2012a).

Acoustic Observations

Acoustic observations are widely used to gain insight into voice and make inferences regarding voice produc-tion. These include observations of the fundamental frequency, sound pressure level, and spectrum of the voice as they are portrayed through the use of a variety of methods. Some measurement devices are devoted to a single acoustic variable, whereas others allow for multiple variables to be considered simultaneously.

Figure 3–54 shows a commercial device that allows for monitoring of multiple acoustic variables in clinical settings (KayPENTAX, 2012b). Such devices usually provide a visual display on a computer screen that enables perusal of the data obtained. Some devices also provide numerical displays of different statistical characteristics of the data obtained, such as mean, mode, standard deviation, and range of variable values.

Some devices may be dedicated to a particular acoustic variable. For example, sound pressure level measurements are sometimes made in clinical settings through the use of devices called sound level meters. These display sound pressure level in decibels (dB) in the form of a tracing that is calibrated to portray sound pressure level in real time, a needle deflection in which the position of the needle is calibrated against a background scale, or a digital readout on a meter face (Bruel & Kjaer, 2012).

The spectrum of the voice can be portrayed in sound spectrograms (so-called voiceprints) that provide information about the frequency, sound pressure level, and temporal events of the voice. Displays of this type are widely available and provide graphic data that can be interpreted in relation to the coordinative processes of voice production and the voice that results. For example, information is made available about voice onset and offset, temporal coordination with upper airway adjustments, and how sound energy is distributed across the overall acoustic spectrum. Sound spectrographic portrayals of this type are especially useful in characterizing patterns of energy distribution in different types of voice disorders. For example, harsh, breathy, and hoarse voices often show identifiable spectral patterns that reflect differences in laryngeal function associated with the generation of those voice qualities (Boone & McFarland, 1994; Fairbanks, 1960). Much more is said in Chapter 10 about the power of spectrographic analysis and available methods.

Fundamental frequency, sound pressure level, and voice waveform data are sometimes used clinically as feedback to help modify voice production behaviors and voice (Howard et al., 2007). They are often used in conjunction with other behavioral interventions to accelerate the rate at which change can be made. Displays of such variables can be made user friendly, attractive, and even enticing to young children in need of voice management (Patel & Salata, 2006).

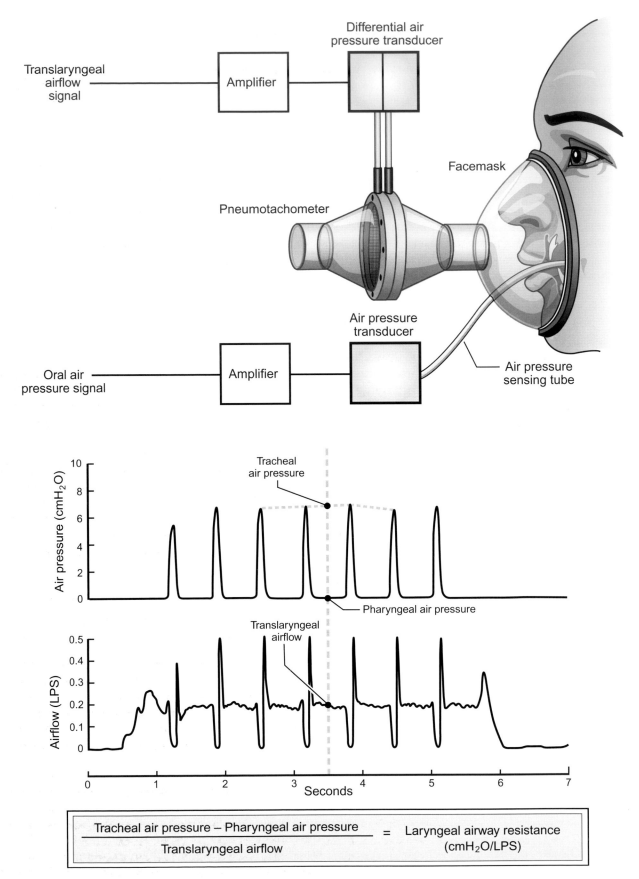

Figure 3–53. Clinical method for determining laryngeal airway resistance during voice production. Upper panel illustrates client-instrumentation interface. Lower panel shows data used for resistance calculation.

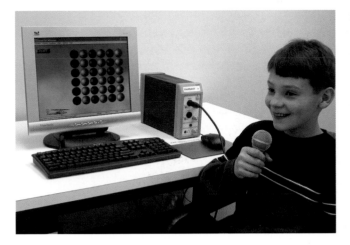

Figure 3-54. Device for monitoring multiple acoustic variables in a clinical setting. Image provided courtesy of KayPENTAX, Montvale, NJ. Reproduced with permission.

LARYNGEAL DISORDERS AND SPEECH PRODUCTION

Laryngeal disorders can result in a wide variety of speech (also meaning voice) disorders. These can have functional and/or organic bases and are found to manifest throughout the life span. Laryngeal disorders can have significant behavioral, social, and economic impacts and are among the most prevalent causes of human communication disorders.

Functional laryngeal disorders are those that do not have known physical causes. Such disorders exist despite apparently normal laryngeal structure and function and are generally ascribed to misuse of the laryngeal apparatus. Misuse in this context means that laryngeal behaviors are not effective or efficient and that they depart from what would be considered appropriate for the laryngeal apparatus. For example, individuals may use voice qualities that are deviant for no apparent physical reason, or they may use pitches that are abnormally high or low for their sex and physical stature. Any of these voice behaviors may elicit adverse attention from listeners.

The larynx can also be used in an abusive manner. Excess coughing, repeated unnecessary throat clearing, overly hard vocal attack at voice onset, and extended loud talking may result in trauma to the laryngeal mucosa and lead to swelling, inflammation, or other tissue changes in the vocal folds and associated structures. Transient abuse of the larynx, as in screaming or loud yelling at a sports event, may result in acute inflammation of the vocal folds in the form of laryngitis. The persistent use of abusive voice behaviors in speaking or singing can lead to the development of callus-like nodules on one or both vocal folds that influence their pattern of vibration. Other laryngeal pathologies that are secondary to vocal abuse may include polyps, cysts, contact ulcers, thickening of the vocal fold margins, and edema of the vocal folds.

Functional disorders of the larynx can also have psychogenic bases. Malingering (feigning illness or injury) may occur when an individual seeks personal gain through the pretense of having a voice disorder. Another form of psychogenic problem is conversion reaction (loss of voluntary laryngeal control as a result of emotional conflict) that can be manifested as a laryngeally based speech disorder, an example of which is presented in the opening and closing scenarios of this chapter. Individuals with conversion reaction voice disorders are suffering from psychic pains that somatize to the larynx rather than being handled in more conventional ways of dealing with emotional conflict.

Organically based laryngeal disorders have identifiable physical causes that can be congenital, developmental, or acquired. They are the result of medical conditions that arise because of different disease states. Included among these conditions are papilloma, a benign tumor believed to be caused by a virus, and keratosis of the vocal folds, a premalignant alteration of the laryngeal mucosa often seen in heavy cigarette smokers. Another condition is carcinoma that may require resection or radiation or chemotherapy interventions. Extensive malignant conditions may require surgical removal (amputation) of all or a part of the larynx with accompanying loss of the voice. Surgical removal of the larynx is termed laryngectomy.

Acquired structural problems of the larynx may include ankylosis (fixation) of the cricoarytenoid joints, a condition that can be caused by arthritis. Other structural problems may be the result of trauma to the larynx, through blows to the neck, penetrating neck wounds, or attempted strangulation. Such structural problems may be accompanied by fractures or displacements of laryngeal structures from their usual positions. Trauma to the larynx may also occur as a consequence of intubation (placement of a breathing tube) during surgery. A sequel to intubation may be the development of a granuloma (a fleshy beadlike surface that develops over a wound) at the site of injury, usually occurring toward the back of the larynx between the arytenoid cartilages.

Laryngeal disorders may also arise from various neuromotor diseases. Such diseases take many forms and result in paresis or paralysis of laryngeal muscles or difficulty in programming or executing movement patterns for speech production. Both central and peripheral nervous system components may be impaired. Signs may present on one or both sides of the larynx and to the same or different degrees when both sides are involved. Laryngeal disorders resulting from neuromotor disease may influence the timing of speech production due to problems in moving the vocal folds in and out of the airway. They may also result in a variety of pitch, loudness, and quality problems, often in combination. Such problems are common in cerebral palsy, traumatic brain injury, cerebral vascular accident (stroke), dystonia (sometimes focal to the larynx), Parkinson disease, amyotrophic lateral sclerosis, essential tremor, Tourette syndrome, and myasthenia gravis, among others. Certain neuromotor diseases are relatively stable, whereas others are progressive and degenerative. In the case of progressive degenerative diseases, such as Parkinson disease and amyotrophic lateral sclerosis, laryngeal impairment may increase during the course of the disease and, correspondingly, speech production capabilities that rely on the larynx may degrade. Attempts to compensate for neuromotor impairment of the larynx may also result in additional signs and symptoms beyond those that are characteristic of the disease itself.

Donation and a Growing Cause

Two recent developments hold promise for those with severe laryngeal disease. One is laryngeal transplantation in which a donor larynx from another individual is transferred to an individual whose larynx is no longer viable. The results of initial efforts in transplantation are encouraging and successful. As marvelous as transplantation is, the thought of growing a new larynx when confronted with severe laryngeal disease seems even more amazing. Tissue engineering has advanced to the stage where the successful growth of new larynges has, in fact, been accomplished in animals. Progenitor cells (precursor cells) are used to ancestrally beget other cells that grow laryngeal structures in a scaffold matrix. The new larynx slowly comes into being, approximating the structural properties of its ancestor. The thought of growing entire organs is somewhat mind boggling, but is already here for some organs and on its way for others.

CLINICAL PROFESSIONALS AND LARYNGEAL DISORDERS IN SPEECH PRODUCTION

Persons with laryngeal disorders that affect speech and/or voice production often need the evaluation and management services of clinical professionals. Some individuals can profit from behavioral treatment, some from psychological intervention, and others from surgery or other medical procedures. Prominent among the professionals who may serve people with laryngeal disorders are the speech-language pathologist, laryngologist, phonosurgeon, neurologist, and psychologist. Others, such as the voice coach and singing teacher, may play significant roles in the prevention of disorders through the use of instructional methods designed to emphasize "healthy" speaking and singing in performers.

The speech-language pathologist is the professional responsible for evaluating and managing an individual with signs and symptoms requiring behavioral intervention (following medical clearance of the client for potential organic causation of laryngeal dysfunction). An example is a person who uses abusive laryngeal behaviors extensively and has developed nodules (callus-like masses on the vocal folds). Management for such a person often entails the elimination of the abusive behaviors and instruction in the proper use of different parts of the speech production apparatus.

The speech-language pathologist is also the professional called on to quantify the status of laryngeal function and voice before and after physical or drug interventions by other professionals to help determine treatment effects. Quantification might include aeromechanical, acoustic, and auditory-perceptual measurements made before and after surgical-implant intervention to augment laryngeal closure, before and after surgical resection of a portion of a vocal fold because of cancer, and before and after the injection of botulinum toxin into the vocal folds to attempt to relieve the signs and symptoms of spasmodic dysphonia.

A laryngologist is a physician who specializes in diseases of the larynx. The laryngologist sees individuals with voice disorders to determine whether or not there is an organic basis for dysfunction. The laryngologist will usually use an endoscope to examine the larynx for possible structural problems (tumors, polyps, nodules, ulcers, fractures) and physiological dysfunction (vocal fold paralysis, tremor, joint ankylosis). The laryngologist is most often the physician who has oversight of the person with laryngeal disease and makes decisions as to the medical treatment of such an individual. The laryngologist may also counsel an individual about lifestyle habits that are harmful to the larynx, prescribe medications, perform surgical procedures, or some combination of these. It is usually the laryngologist who will give medical clearance for an individual to be managed behaviorally by the speech-language pathologist.

Some laryngologists are highly specialized in surgical procedures on the larynx that affect voice. These individuals are referred to as phonosurgeons and are called on to conduct intricate operations intended to rehabilitate, maintain, or enhance voice function. A laryngologist who specializes as a phonosurgeon might be concerned with procedures that influence the mechanical nature of vibration of the vocal fold cover, the enhancement of laryngeal closure through the implantation of different substances into the vocal folds, vascular alterations to areas of the larynx that have disrupted blood flow, and the reconstruction of parts of the larynx that are damaged or diseased. Those individuals who make their living through voice performance often turn to the skills of the phonosurgeon when their careers are threatened by laryngeal disease or injury.

The neurologist, a physician with expertise in diseases of the nervous system, may be an integral part of the evaluation and management team for persons with laryngeal problems that have a neural basis. Laryngeal dysfunction is often one of the first presenting signs of nervous system disease so that the neurologist is often among the first clinical professionals to encounter coexisting voice disorders. In some cases, the presenting signs and symptoms are relatively stable (cerebral palsy), whereas in other cases the signs and symptoms may progressively worsen (amyotrophic lateral sclerosis). A major tool of the neurologist is drug treatment.

As with the laryngologist, the neurologist will often make referrals to the speech-language pathologist for behavioral management of laryngeal dysfunction that might influence speech production and/or swallowing. The monitoring of voice by the speech-language pathologist is often valuable to the neurologist because the voice is often sensitive to subtle neurological changes that may not be detected otherwise.

A psychologist plays a significant role in the evaluation and management of individuals with laryngeal disorders that have psychogenic causes. Having expertise in the psychological bases of behavior, a psychologist might see persons with voice disorders related to malingering, conversion reaction, or other problems that appear to have no obvious physical cause. An adverse change in the voice or its loss can be associated with deterioration in psychic and/or physical wellness. The psychologist may be needed to intercede in instances of psychological depression and grief attendant to conditions that affect the voice. In many ways, the voice is an expression of the self and provides a window as to how individuals are dealing with life stresses, losses, and emotions.

Misuse and abuse of the voice production apparatus may be especially problematic in the case of heavy voice users, such as those who earn a living through use of the voice. Accordingly, those who instruct such individuals in the use of the voice, such as voice coaches and singing teachers, can have a significant influence in the prevention of voice disorders. Instruction in optimal function has many benefits, including the prevention of misuse and abuse of the voice production apparatus, the acceleration and enhancement of performance skill, the minimizing of physical work and performance effort, the reduction of performance fatigue, and the maximizing of performance endurance and comfort (Hixon, 2006).

Daniel R. Boone

The Daniel Boone you've heard of may or may not be this one. Both are pioneers. This one wrote a clinical textbook that represented the first comprehensive approach to the topic of voice disorders. He proposed a large series of facilitating techniques that were widely adopted by clinicians working with individuals with voice disorders and that remains in use today throughout the world. Boone is a master clinician and an outstanding clinical teacher. He has a knack for cutting to the heart of clinical matters quickly and few equal him in his compassion for people with serious voice disorders. Boone is a past President of the American Speech-Language-Hearing Association and was instrumental in guiding that association to prominence. He is retired and lives in Tucson, Arizona, but still travels the world lecturing about voice disorders. Boone has a wonderful sense of humor. One of his passions is the card game Hearts.

REVIEW

The larynx (voice box) is an air valve positioned between the trachea (windpipe) and the pharynx (throat) that can be adjusted to vary the amount of coupling between the two.

The skeleton of the larynx forms a superstructure consisting of bone, cartilages, ligaments, and tendons.

Major cartilages of the larynx include the thyroid, cricoid, arytenoids, and epiglottis, which function, along with the hyoid bone, as an integral unit.

Two pairs of joints mediate movements of the interior of the larynx, one between the cricoid and thyroid cartilages on each side, and one between the cricoid and arytenoid cartilages on each side.

Prominent structures within the laryngeal cavity include the vocal folds, the ventricular folds (false vocal folds), and mucous glands that lie between these two sets of folds and are milked to lubricate the vocal folds.

The vocal folds are prominent shelflike structures that have a muscular body at their core and an intricate outer covering that has distinct layers.

Two types of forces operate on the larynx, one passive that includes the natural recoil of tissues, surface tension between structures in apposition, and the pull of gravity, and one active that includes intrinsic, extrinsic, and supplementary muscles that are nearly 20 in number and are activated in accordance with will and ability.

Intrinsic muscles of the larynx include the *thyroarytenoid, posterior cricoarytenoid, lateral cricoarytenoid, arytenoid,* and *cricothyroid.*

Extrinsic muscles of the larynx include the *sternothyroid, thyrohyoid,* and *inferior constrictor.*

Supplementary muscles of the larynx include the *sternohyoid, omohyoid, digastric, stylohyoid, mylohyoid, geniohyoid, hyoglossus,* and *genioglossus.*

Movements of the larynx can result in changes in the positioning of the laryngeal housing, vocal folds, ventricular folds, and epiglottis.

Adjustments of the vocal folds include abduction, adduction, length change, and change in cross-sectional configuration.

The control variables of laryngeal function include laryngeal opposing pressure, laryngeal airway resistance, glottal size and configuration, stiffness of the vocal folds, and effective mass of the vocal folds.

The neural substrates of laryngeal control are supported by cranial nerves V, VII, X, XI, XII and cervical spinal nerves C1, C2, C3, which provide motor supply to the intrinsic, extrinsic, and supplementary muscles of the larynx and sensory supply that conveys information from mechanoreceptors about muscle lengths, rates of change in muscle length, joint movements, and mucosal deformations.

Laryngeal function is concerned mainly with the degree of coupling between the trachea and pharynx, protection of the pulmonary airways, containment of the pulmonary air supply, and sound generation.

Laryngeal function for speech production includes the generation of transient (very brief duration) utterances, extended sustained utterances (both noise and voice), and running speech activities.

Voice production relies on quasiperiodic vocal fold vibration that is governed by nonlinear interaction between an energy source (the breathing apparatus) and the structures being vibrated (the vocal folds).

Vocal fold vibration is self-sustaining because certain conditions exist, including alternations in the shape of the glottis (ranging from convergent to divergent), alternations in the intraglottal pressure (ranging from relatively high to relatively low), and the presence of vocal fold tissue recoil force (ranging from lower than intraglottal pressure to higher than the intraglottal pressure).

Presetting adjustments of the larynx occur in advance of actual voice production and in advance of any acoustic feedback having to do with the voice.

The onset of voice production (often designated as the vocal attack phase) is conditioned by the manner in which the larynx and breathing apparatus function to generate the first few cycles of vocal fold vibration.

The fundamental frequency of the voice (correlated with the pitch of the voice) is the rate of vocal fold vibration and is controlled by the stiffness, effective vibrating mass, and tautness (as vertically applied) of the vocal folds, as well as by supporting adjustments of the breathing apparatus.

The sound pressure level (intensity) of the voice (correlated with the loudness of the voice) is related to its physical magnitude and is controlled by adjustments in tracheal air pressure, laryngeal opposing pressure, laryngeal airway resistance, and laryngeal airflow (that alter the level of excitation provided to the pharyngeal-oral airway), and postural adjustments of the airway that alter radiation impedance.

The lowest and highest values that can be produced in fundamental frequency and sound pressure level of the voice are not independent of one another, with the fundamental frequency range being greatest in the midrange of sound pressure levels and the sound pressure level range being greatest in the midrange of fundamental frequencies.

The voice source (tone produced at the larynx) is complex and composed of a combination of frequencies and sound pressure levels that vary with changes in the magnitude of tracheal air pressure and airflow through the larynx and changes in the adjustment of the vocal folds, such as those that accompany changes in fundamental frequency (pitch), sound pressure level (loudness), and spectrum (quality) of the voice.

Pulse, modal, and loft are terms applied to three different voice registers that correspond to three different modes of vocal fold vibration and voice qualities encountered when speaking from the lowest to highest fundamental frequencies within the speaking range.

Laryngeal function during running speech activities is complex in that adjustments are made to control fundamental frequency, sound pressure level, and spectrum of the voice, to control abduction of the vocal folds for breathing and the delivery of forces downstream of the larynx, and to control actions of the larynx that constitute articulatory behaviors.

The larynx undergoes relocation and remodeling during a developmental period that extends into adolescence and is characterized by sexual dimorphism and a rapid growth spurt in males that lowers their fundamental frequency significantly in relation to females.

The mature larynx is subject to modification throughout adulthood as a result of aging processes that stiffen it, degrade its joints, decrease its muscle mass, alter its composition, and otherwise make its function less efficient, especially in males.

Males and females show laryngeal differences and voice production differences that have roots in different hormonal changes, different rates of ossification and calcification of laryngeal cartilages, different patterns of change in the covers of the vocal folds, different patterns of valving by the vocal folds, and different cultural expectations.

The measurement of laryngeal function incorporates many methods, including endoscopy, electroglottography, aeromechanical observations, and acoustic observations.

Laryngeal disorders can result in a wide variety of speech and voice problems that can have functional and/or organic bases, manifest throughout the life span, and result in significant impairment and a lessening of the quality of life.

Persons with laryngeal disorders that affect speech production often need the services of professionals, prominent among these being the speech-language pathologist, laryngologist, phonosurgeon, neurologist, and psychologist.

Scenario

It would take a well-trained speech-language pathologist to get to the bottom of the minister's problem and turn his life back around. Essentially unable to use his voice for any part of his work, the reverend turned to a speech-language pathologist who specialized in voice disorders.

Evaluation by the speech-language pathologist revealed no signs of organic involvement of the voice production apparatus. Diagnostic voice management was initiated and, as it turned out, brought dramatic results. By guiding the minister through a series of carefully orchestrated exercises involving activities such as humming and chanting, the speech-language pathologist was able to elicit a normal-sounding voice from the minister. He was startled by the sound of his own voice and surprised by how strange it felt to be able to speak again. Later, as the therapy session was drawing to a close, the speech-language pathologist turned to what appeared to be casual conversation, but which was motivated by other factors. When the topic got around to family and ultimately to the minister's daughter, there was a longer than usual hesitation before the father attempted to speak. Tears began to well from his eyes and he lowered his head. He managed a "She's okay," but the speech-language pathologist sensed otherwise.

It was the end of the working day, time to go home, but neither was watching the clock. The speech-language pathologist explained that life stresses sometimes show up in the voice. The minister seemed not to be listening or to be somewhere else and then the dam broke and he sobbed uncontrollably. Words were of no use and the speech-language pathologist wisely rode out the event. When the minister finally stopped crying, he seemed emotionally spent and greatly relieved. The speech-language pathologist reassured him that everything between them was confidential, and with that the minister revealed a psychic pain that was the basis for his voice problem.

As it turned out, the minister had a psychogenic voice disorder. The phonecall he had received from the parent of his daughter's friend was what had precipitated his loss of voice. The caller had told the minister that the older coed had revealed that the minister's daughter was addicted to drugs and had turned to prostitution to support her habit. The minister had withheld the information from his wife who was dealing with breast cancer at the time. He had tried to manage the daughter's problems himself, but was unsuccessful. As he expressed it, he had "enormous shame and guilt about her situation," but he felt helpless to do anything about it. He tried to get her to enroll in a counseling program at the college. She resisted. He had tried to ride out this storm alone. He had not made the connection between his psychic hurt over his daughter and his own voice problem until the speech-language pathologist had given him the information to connect the dots.

The speech-language pathologist referred the minister to a psychologist. Eventually the minister's wife was included in his readjustment. Meanwhile, the speech-language pathologist continued voice management that incorporated speaking in increasingly stressful situations, voice hygiene (reduced throat clearing and coughing, increased hydration), and proper voice production techniques. Within 2 months, the minister was able to resume his usual speaking activities. The problems with his daughter were not resolved, but he had new ways to deal with them that did not incapacitate him. Also, his wife was an effective partner in helping the two of them work through what was a major tragedy for them. As his voice returned, so did he.

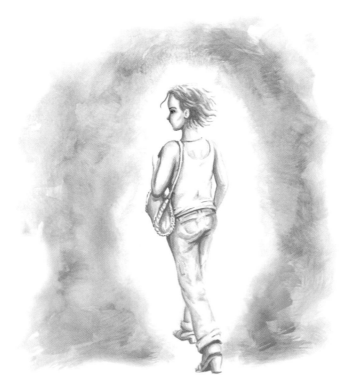

REFERENCES

Ahmad, K., Yan, Y., & Bless, D. (in press). Vocal fold vibratory characteristics of healthy geriatric females—Analysis of high-speed digital images. *Journal of Voice*.

Allen, E., & Hollien, H. (1973). Vocal fold thickness in pulse (vocal fry) register. *Folia Phoniatrica, 25*, 241–250.

Ardran, G., & Kemp, F. (1966). The mechanism of the larynx, I: The movements of the arytenoid and cricoids cartilages. *British Journal of Radiology, 39*, 641–654.

Arnold, G. (1961). Physiology and pathology of the cricothyroid muscle. *Laryngoscope, 71*, 687–753.

Aronson, A. (1990). *Clinical voice disorders: An interdisciplinary approach* (3rd ed.). New York, NY: Thieme.

Atkinson, J. (1978). Correlation analysis of the physiological factors controlling fundamental voice frequency. *Journal of the Acoustical Society of America, 63*, 211–222.

Awan, S., & Mueller, P. (1992). Speaking fundamental frequency characteristics of centenarian females. *Clinical Linguistics and Phonetics, 6*, 249–254.

Baer, T. (1981). Observation of vocal fold vibration: Measurement of excised larynges. In K. Stevens & M. Hirano (Eds.), *Vocal fold physiology* (pp. 199–233). Tokyo, Japan: University of Tokyo Press.

Baken, R., & Orlikoff, R. (2000). *Clinical measurement of speech and voice* (2nd ed.). San Diego, CA: Singular.

Behrman, A. (2007). *Speech and voice science*. San Diego, CA: Plural.

Beneragama, T., & Serpell, J. (2006). Extralaryngeal bifurcation of the recurrent laryngeal nerve: A common variation. *ANZ Journal of Surgery, 76*, 928–931.

Benjamin, B. (1981). Frequency variability in the aged voice. *Journal of Gerontology, 36*, 722–736.

Benjamin, B. (1988). Changes in speech production and linguistic behaviors with aging. In B. Shadden (Ed.), *Communication behavior and aging: A sourcebook for clinicians* (pp. 162–181). Baltimore, MD: Williams & Wilkins.

Berke, G., & Gerratt, B. (1993). Laryngeal biomechanics: An overview of mucosal wave mechanics. *Journal of Voice, 7*, 123–128.

Berry, D., & Titze, I. (1996). Normal modes in a continuum model of vocal fold tissues. *Journal of the Acoustical Society of America, 100*, 3345–3354.

Biever, D., & Bless, D. (1989). Vibratory characteristics of the vocal folds in young adult and geriatric women. *Journal of Voice, 3*, 120–131.

Boone, D., & McFarland, S. (1994). *The voice and voice therapy* (5th ed.). Englewood-Cliffs, NJ: Prentice-Hall.

Bosma, J. (1985). Postnatal ontogeny of performance of the pharynx, larynx, and mouth. *American Review of Respiratory Disease, 131*, 10–15.

Broad, D. (1973). Phonation. In F. Minifie, T. Hixon, & F. Williams (Eds.), *Normal aspects of speech, hearing, and language* (pp. 127–167). Englewood-Cliffs, NJ: Prentice-Hall.

Bruel & Kjaer, Inc. (2012). *Sound level meters and accessories*. Naerum, Denmark: Author.

Casiano, R., Zaveri, V., & Lundy, D. (1992). Efficacy of videostroboscopy in the diagnosis of voice disorders. *Otolaryngology-Head and Neck Surgery, 107*, 95–100.

Catten, M., Gray, S., Hammond, T., Zhou, R., & Hammond, E. (1998). Analysis of cellular location and concentration in vocal fold lamina propria. *Otolaryngology-Head and Neck Surgery, 118*, 663–667.

Cavagna, G., & Margaria, R. (1965). An analysis of the mechanics of phonation. *Journal of Applied Physiology, 20*, 301–307.

Charpied, G., & Shapshay, S. (2004). *Anatomy and histology of the pars media of the cricothyroid muscle: A comparative study*. Paper presented at the International Conference on Voice Physiology and Biomechanics, Marseille, France.

Childers, D., Hicks, D., Moore, G., Eshenazi, L., & Lalwani, A. (1990). Electroglottography and vocal fold physiology. *Journal of Speech and Hearing Research, 33*, 245–254.

Childers, D., & Krishnamurthy, A. (1985). A critical review of electroglottography. *Critical Review of Biomedical Engineering, 12*, 131–161.

Childers, D., Smith, A., & Moore, G. (1984). Relationships between electroglottography, speech, and vocal cord contact. *Folia Phoniatrica, 36*, 105–118.

Classen, H., & Kirsch, T. (1994). Temporal and spatial localization of type I and II collagens in human thyroid cartilage. *Anatomy and Embryology, 189*, 237–242.

Coleman, R. (1963). Decay characteristics of vocal fry. *Folia Phoniatrica, 15*, 256–263.

Coleman, R., Mabis, J., & Hinson, J. (1977). Fundamental frequency—sound pressure level profiles of adult male and female voices. *Journal of Speech and Hearing Research, 20*, 197–204.

Colton, R. (1972). Spectral characteristics of the modal and falsetto registers. *Folia Phoniatrica, 24*, 337–344.

Colton, R. (1973). Vocal intensity in the modal and falsetto registers. *Folia Phoniatrica, 25*, 62–70.

Colton, R., & Casper, J. (1996). *Understanding voice problems: A physiological perspective for diagnosis and treatment* (2nd ed.). Baltimore, MD: Williams & Wilkins.

Colton, R., & Conture, E. (1990). Problems and pitfalls of electroglottography. *Journal of Voice, 4*, 10–24.

Cooper, D. (1990). *Maturation, characteristics, and aging of laryngeal muscles*. Paper presented at the Pacific Voice Conference, San Francisco, CA.

Crelin, E. (1973). *Functional anatomy of the newborn*. New Haven, CT: Yale University Press.

Curry, E. (1946). Voice changes in male adolescents. *Laryngoscope, 56*, 795–805.

Dailey, S., Spanou, K., & Zeitels, S. (2007). The evaluation of benign glottic lesions: Rigid telescopic stroboscopy versus suspension microlaryngoscopy. *Journal of Voice, 21*, 112–118.

Damste, H. (1970). The phonetogram. *Practica Oto-Rhino-Laryngologica, 32*, 185–187.

Daniloff, R., Shuckers, G., & Feth, L. (1980). *The physiology of speech and hearing*. Englewood-Cliffs, NJ: Prentice-Hall.

D'Antonio, L., Netsell, R., & Lotz, W. (1988). Clinical aerodynamics for the evaluation and management of voice disorders. *Ear, Nose, and Throat Journal, 67*, 394–399.

de Melo, E., Lemas, M., Filho, J., Sennes, L., Saldiva, P., & Tsuji, D. (2003). Distribution of collagen in the lamina propria of the human vocal fold. *Laryngoscope, 113*, 2187–2191.

Dickson, D., & Maue-Dickson, W. (1982). *Anatomical and physiological bases of speech.* Boston, MA: Little, Brown and Company.

Dromey, C., Stathopoulos, E., & Sapienza, C. (1992). Glottal airflow and electroglottographic measures of vocal function at multiple intensities. *Journal of Voice, 6*, 44–54.

Duffy, J. (2005). *Motor speech disorders: Substrates, differential diagnosis, and management* (2nd ed.). New York, NY: Mosby.

Faaborg-Andersen, K. (1957). Electromyographic investigation of intrinsic laryngeal muscles in humans. *Acta Physiologica Scandinavica, 41*(Suppl. 140), 1–150.

Faaborg-Andersen, K., & Sonninen, A. (1960). The function of the extrinsic laryngeal muscles at different pitch: An electromyographic and roentgenologic investigation. *Acta Otolaryngologica, 51*, 89–93.

Faaborg-Andersen, K., Yanagihara, N., & von Leden, H. (1967). Vocal pitch and intensity regulation: A comparative study of electrical activity in the cricothyroid muscle and the airflow rate. *Archives of Otolaryngology, 85*, 448–454.

Fairbanks, G. (1960). *Voice and articulation drillbook.* New York, NY: Harper & Row.

Fairbanks, G., Herbert, E., & Hammond, J. (1949). An acoustical study of vocal pitch in seven- and eight-year-old girls. *Child Development, 20*, 71–78.

Fairbanks, G., & Miron, M. (1957). Effect of vocal effort upon the consonant-vowel ratio within the syllable. *Journal of the Acoustical Society of America, 29*, 621–626.

Fairbanks, G., Wiley, J., & Lassman, F. (1949). An acoustical study of vocal pitch in seven- and eight-year-old boys. *Child Development, 20*, 63–69.

Fant, G. (1960). *Acoustic theory of speech production.* Hague, Netherlands: Mouton.

Ferreri, G. (1959). Senescence of the larynx. *Italian General Review of Otorhinolaryngology, 1*, 640–709.

Fink, B. (1975). *The human larynx: A functional study.* New York, NY: Raven Press.

Fink, B., Basek, M., & Epanchin, V. (1956). The mechanism of opening of the human larynx. *Laryngoscope, 66*, 410–425.

Flanagan, J. (1972). *Speech analysis, synthesis, and perception.* New York, NY: Springer-Verlag.

Folkard, C. (2006). *Guinness world records: 2006.* New York, NY: Bantam Books.

Fourcin, A. (1974). Laryngographic examination of vocal fold vibration. In B. Wyke (Ed.), *Ventilatory and phonatory control systems* (pp. 315–326). London, UK: Oxford University Press.

Frable, M. (1961). Computation of motion at the cricoarytenoid joint. *Archives of Otolaryngology, 73*, 551–556.

Gauffin, J., & Sundberg, J. (1989). Spectral correlates of glottal voice source waveform characteristics. *Journal of Speech and Hearing Research, 32*, 556–565.

Gay, T., Hirose, H., Strome, M., & Sawashima, M. (1972). Electromyography of the intrinsic laryngeal muscles during phonation. *Annals of Otology, Rhinology, and Laryngology, 81*, 401–409.

Glaze, L., Bless, D., Milenkovic, P., & Susser, R. (1988). Acoustic characteristics of children's voice. *Journal of Voice, 2*, 312–319.

Glottal Enterprises, Inc. (2012). *Two-channel electroglottograph and microphone preamplifier, Model EG2-PCX.* Syracuse, NY.

Gramming, P. (1991). Vocal loudness and frequency capabilities of the voice. *Journal of Voice, 5*, 144–157.

Gramming, P., & Sundberg, J. (1988). Spectrum factors relevant to phonetogram measurement. *Journal of the Acoustical Society of America, 83*, 2352–2360.

Han, Y., Wang, J., Fischman, D., Biller, H., & Sanders, I. (1999). Slow tonic muscle fibers in the thyroarytenoid muscles of human vocal folds: A possible specialization for speech. *Anatomical Record, 256*, 146–157.

Hasek, C., Singh, S., & Murry, T. (1980). Acoustic attributes of children's voices. *Journal of the Acoustical Society of America, 68*, 1252–1265.

Hately, B., Evison, G., & Samuel, E. (1965). The pattern of ossification in the laryngeal cartilages: A radiological study. *British Journal of Radiology, 38*, 585–591.

Hirano, M. (1974). Morphological structures of the vocal cord as a vibrator and its variations. *Folia Phoniatrica, 26*, 89–94.

Hirano, M. (1981). *Clinical examination of voice.* New York, NY: Springer-Verlag Wien.

Hirano, M., & Bless, D. (1993). *Videostroboscopic examination of the larynx.* San Diego, CA: Singular.

Hirano, M., Kakita, Y., Kawasaki, H., Gould, W., & Lambiase, A. (1981). Data from high-speed motion picture studies. In K. Stevens & M. Hirano (Eds.), *Vocal fold physiology* (pp. 85–93). Tokyo, Japan: University of Tokyo Press.

Hirano, M., Kiyokawa, K., & Kurita, S. (1988). Laryngeal muscles and glottal shaping. In O. Fujimura (Ed.), *Vocal physiology: Voice production, mechanisms, and functions* (pp. 49–65) New York: Raven Press.

Hirano, M., Kiyokawa, K., Kurita, S., & Sato, K. (1986). Posterior glottis: Morphological study in excised larynges. *Annals of Otology, Rhinology, and Laryngology, 95*, 576–581.

Hirano, M., Kurita, S., & Nakashima, T. (1983). Growth, development and aging of human vocal folds. In D. Bless & J. Abbs (Eds.), *Vocal fold physiology: Contemporary research and clinical issues* (pp. 22–43). San Diego, CA: College-Hill Press.

Hirano, M., Kurita, S., & Sagaguchi, S. (1989). Aging of the vibratory tissue of the human vocal folds. *Acta Otolaryngologica, 107*, 428–433.

Hirano, M., Ohala, J., & Vennard, W. (1969). The function of the laryngeal muscles in regulating fundamental frequency and intensity of phonation. *Journal of Speech and Hearing Research, 12*, 616–628.

Hirano, M., & Sato, K. (1993). *Histological color atlas of the human larynx.* San Diego, CA: Singular.

Hirano, M., Vennard, W., & Ohala, J. (1970). Regulation of register, pitch and intensity of voice. *Folia Phoniatrica, 22*, 1–20.

Hirano, M., Yoshida, T., & Tanaka, S. (1991). Vibratory behavior of human vocal folds viewed from below. In J. Gauffin

& B. Hammarberg (Eds.), *Vocal fold physiology: Acoustic, perceptual, and physiological aspects of voice mechanisms* (pp. 1–6). San Diego, CA: Singular.

Hirose, H. (1977). Laryngeal adjustments in consonant production. *Phonetica, 34,* 289–294.

Hixon, T. (1966). Turbulent noise sources for speech. *Folia Phoniatrica, 18,* 168–182.

Hixon, T. (2006). *Respiratory function in singing: A primer for singers and singing teachers.* Tucson, AZ: Redington Brown.

Hixon, T., & Abbs, J. (1980). Normal speech production. In T. Hixon, L. Shriberg, & J. Saxman (Eds.), *Introduction to communication disorders* (pp. 42–87). Englewood-Cliffs, NJ: Prentice-Hall.

Hixon, T., Klatt, D., & Mead, J. (1971). Influence of forced transglottal pressure change on vocal fundamental frequency. *Journal of the Acoustical Society of America, 49,* 105.

Hixon, T., Mead, J., & Goldman, M. (1976). Dynamics of the chest wall during speech production: Function of the thorax, rib cage, diaphragm, and abdomen. *Journal of Speech and Hearing Research, 19,* 297–356.

Hixon, T., & Minifie, F. (1972). *Influence of forced transglottal pressure change on vocal sound pressure level.* Paper presented at the Convention of the American Speech and Hearing Association, San Francisco, CA.

Hixon, T., Minifie, F., & Tait, C. (1967). Correlates of turbulent noise production for speech. *Journal of Speech and Hearing Research, 10,* 133–140.

Hixon, T., Watson, P., Harris, F., & Pearl, N. (1988). Relative volume changes of the rib cage and abdomen during prephonatory chest wall posturing. *Journal of Voice, 2,* 13–19.

Hoit, J., & Hixon, T. (1992). Age and laryngeal airway resistance during vowel production in women. *Journal of Speech and Hearing Research, 35,* 309–313.

Hollien, H. (1960a). Some laryngeal correlates of vocal pitch. *Journal of Speech and Hearing Research, 3,* 52–58.

Hollien, H. (1960b). Vocal pitch variations related to changes in vocal fold length. *Journal of Speech and Hearing Research, 3,* 150–156.

Hollien, H. (1962). Vocal fold thickness and fundamental frequency of phonation. *Journal of Speech and Hearing Research, 5,* 237–243.

Hollien, H. (1972). Three major vocal registers: A proposal. In A. Rigault & R. Charbonneau (Eds.), *Proceedings of the Seventh International Congress of Phonetic Sciences* (pp. 320–331). Hague, Netherlands: Mouton.

Hollien, H. (1974). On vocal registers. *Journal of Phonetics, 2,* 125–143.

Hollien, H., Brown, W., & Hollien, K. (1971). Vocal fold length associated with modal, falsetto and varying vocal intensity phonations. *Folia Phoniatrica, 23,* 66–78.

Hollien, H., & Colton, R. (1969). Four laminagraphic studies of vocal fold thickness. *Folia Phoniatrica, 21,* 179–198.

Hollien, H., & Curtis, J. (1960). A laminagraphic study of vocal pitch. *Journal of Speech and Hearing Research, 3,* 362–371.

Hollien, H., Damste, H., & Murry, T. (1969). Vocal fold length during vocal fry phonation. *Folia Phoniatrica, 21,* 257–265.

Hollien, H., Green, R., & Massey, K. (1994). Longitudinal research on adolescent voice change in males. *Journal of the Acoustical Society of America, 34,* 80–84.

Hollien, H., & Moore, P. (1960). Measurements of the vocal folds during changes in pitch. *Journal of Speech and Hearing Research, 3,* 157–163.

Hollien, H., & Shipp, T. (1972). Speaking fundamental frequency and chronological age in males. *Journal of Speech and Hearing Research, 15,* 155–159.

Holmberg, E., Hillman, R., & Perkell, J. (1988). Glottal airflow and transglottal air pressure measurements for male and female speakers in soft, normal, and loud voice. *Journal of the Acoustical Society of America, 84,* 511–529.

Holmberg, E., Hillman, R., & Perkell, J. (1989). Glottal airflow and transglottal air pressure measurements for male and female speakers in low, normal, and high pitch. *Journal of Voice, 3,* 294–305.

Holmes, L., Leeper, H., & Nicholson, I. (1994). Laryngeal airway resistance of older men and women as a function of vocal sound pressure level. *Journal of Speech and Hearing Research, 37,* 789–799.

Honda, K. (1995). Laryngeal and extra-laryngeal mechanisms of Fo control. In F. Bell-Berti & L. Raphael (Eds.), *Producing speech: Contemporary issues — For Katherine Safford Harris* (pp. 215–245). New York, NY: American Institute of Physics.

Honjo, I., & Isshiki, N. (1980). Laryngoscopic and voice characteristics of aged persons. *Archives of Otolaryngology, 106,* 149–150.

Howard, D., Brereton, J., Welch, G., Himonides, E., DeCosta, M., Williams, J., & Howard, A. (2007). Are real-time displays of benefit in the singing studio? An exploratory study. *Journal of Voice, 21,* 20–34.

Ishii, K., Zhai, W., Akita, M., & Hirose, H. (1996). Ultra-structure of the lamina propria of the human vocal fold. *Acta Otolaryngologica, 116,* 778–782.

Isshiki, N. (1964). Regulatory mechanism of voice intensity variation. *Journal of Speech and Hearing Research, 7,* 17–29.

Isshiki, N. (1965). Vocal intensity and air flow rate. *Folia Phoniatrica, 17,* 92–104.

Isshiki, N. (1985). Clinical significance of a vocal efficiency index. In I. Titze & R. Scherer (Eds.), *Vocal fold physiology: Biomechanics, acoustics, and phonatory control* (pp. 230–238). Denver, CO: The Denver Center for the Performing Arts.

Isshiki, N., & von Leden, H. (1964). Hoarseness: Aerodynamic studies. *Archives of Otolaryngology, 80,* 206–213.

Jankovskaya, N. (1959). The receptor innervation of the perichondrium of the laryngeal cartilages. *Arkhiv Anatomii, Gistologii l'Enbriologii, 37,* 70–75.

Kahane, J. (1975). *The developmental anatomy of the human prepubertal and pubertal larynx.* Doctoral dissertation, University of Pittsburgh, Pittsburgh, PA.

Kahane, J. (1978). A morphological study of the human prepubertal and pubertal larynx. *American Journal of Anatomy, 151,* 11–20.

Kahane, J. (1980). Age related histological changes in the human male and female laryngeal cartilages: Biological and functional implications. In V. Lawrence (Ed.), *Transcripts of the Ninth Symposium: Care of the Professional Voice, Part I* (pp. 11–20). New York, NY: The Voice Foundation.

Kahane, J. (1982). Growth of the human prepubertal and pubertal larynx. *Journal of Speech and Hearing Research, 25,* 446–455.

Kahane, J. (1983). A survey of age-related changes in the connective tissue of the human adult larynx. In D. Bless & J. Abbs (Eds.), *Vocal fold physiology: Contemporary research and clinical issues* (pp. 44–49). San Diego, CA: College-Hill Press.

Kahane, J. (1987). Connective tissue changes in the larynx and their effects on voice. *Journal of Voice, 1,* 27–30.

Kahane, J. (1988). Age-related changes in the human cricoarytenoid joint. In O. Fujimura (Ed.), *Vocal physiology: Voice production, mechanisms, and functions* (pp. 145–157). New York, NY: Raven Press.

Kahane, J. (2007). *A description of regional specialization in the human thyroarytenoid muscle.* Paper presented at the 36th Annual Symposium on Care of the Professional Voice, Philadelphia, PA.

Kahane, J., & Beckford, N. (1991). The aging larynx and voice. In D. Ripich (Ed.), *Handbook of geriatric communication disorders* (pp. 165–186). Austin, TX: Pro-Ed.

Kahane, J., & Hammons, J. (1987). Developmental changes in the articular cartilage of the human cricoarytenoid joint. In T. Baer, C. Sasaki, & K. Harris (Eds.), *Laryngeal function in phonation and respiration* (pp. 14–28). San Diego, CA: College-Hill Press.

Kahane, J., & Kahn, A. (1984). Weight measurements of infant and adult intrinsic laryngeal muscles. *Folia Phoniatrica, 36,* 129–133.

Kahane, J., Stadlin, J., & Bell, J. (1979). *A histological study of the aging human larynx.* Scientific exhibit presented at the Convention of the American Speech-Language-Hearing Association, Atlanta, GA.

Kahn, A., & Kahane, J. (1986). India pin prick experiments on surface organization of cricoarytenoid joints (CAJ) articular surfaces. *Journal of Speech and Hearing Research, 29,* 536–543.

Karnell, M. (1994). *Videoendoscopy: From velopharynx to larynx.* San Diego, CA: Singular.

KayPENTAX, Inc. (2012a). *Phonatory aerodynamic system (PAS): A comprehensive airflow system for the voice laboratory.* Montvale, NJ: Author.

KayPENTAX, Inc. (2012b). *Visi-Pitch IV, Model 3950: The latest generation of the most widely used speech therapy instrument.* Montvale, NJ: Author.

Kazarian, A., Sarkissian, L., & Isaakian, D. (1978). Length of the human vocal cords by age. *Zhurnal Eksperimentalnoi I Klinicheskoi Meditsiny, 18,* 105–109.

Keleman, G., & Pressman, J. (1955). Physiology of the larynx. *Physiological Review, 35,* 506–554.

Kendall, K., & Leonard, R. (2010). *Laryngeal evaluation: Indirect laryngoscopy to high-speed digital imaging.* New York, NY: Thieme Medical.

Kent, R. (1976). Anatomical and neuromuscular maturation of the speech mechanism: Evidence from acoustic studies. *Journal of Speech and Hearing Research, 19,* 421–447.

Kent, R. (1997). *The speech sciences.* San Diego, CA: Singular.

Kent, R., & Vorperian, H. (1995). Development of the craniofacial-oral-laryngeal anatomy: A review. *Journal of Medical Speech-Language Pathology, 3,* 145–190.

Kirchner, J., & Suzuki, M. (1968). Laryngeal reflexes and voice production. *Annals of the New York Academy of Sciences, 155,* 98–109.

Kirchner, J., & Wyke, B. (1965). Articular reflex mechanisms in the larynx. *Annals of Otology, Rhinology, and Laryngology, 74,* 749–768.

Kitzing, P. (1990). Clinical applications of electroglottography. *Journal of Voice, 4,* 238–249.

Koike, Y. (1967). Experimental studies on vocal attack. *Practica Otologica Kyoto, 60,* 663–688.

Koike, Y., Hirano, M., & von Leden, H. (1967). Vocal initiation: Acoustic and aerodynamic investigations of normal subjects. *Folia Phoniatrica, 19,* 173–182.

Konig, W., & von Leden, H. (1961a). The peripheral nervous system of the human larynx, 1: The mucous membrane. *Archives of Otolaryngology, 73,* 1–14.

Konig, W., & von Leden, H. (1961b). The peripheral nervous system of the human larynx, 2: The thyroarytenoid (vocalis) muscle. *Archives of Otolaryngology, 74,* 153–163.

Kostyk, B., & Rochet, A. (1998). Laryngeal airway resistance in teachers with vocal fatigue: A preliminary study. *Journal of Voice, 12,* 287–299.

Kucinski, P., Okrazewska, E., & Piszcz, W. (1979). Variability of the course of the cricothyroid muscle in humans. *Folia Morphologica, 38,* 391–396.

Kunze, L. (1962). *An investigation of changes in sub-glottal air pressure and rate of air flow accompanying changes in fundamental frequency, intensity, vowels, and voice registers in adult male speakers.* Doctoral dissertation, University of Iowa, Iowa City.

Ladefoged, P., & McKinney, N. (1963). Loudness, sound pressure, and subglottal pressure in speech. *Journal of the Acoustical Society of America, 35,* 454–460.

Laitman, J., & Crelin, E. (1976). Postnatal development of the basiocranium and vocal tract region in man. In J. Bosma (Ed.), *Symposium on Development of the Basiocranium* (pp. 206–220). Washington, DC: Department of Health, Education, and Welfare.

Large, J., Iwata, S., & von Leden, H. (1970). The primary female register transition in singing: An aerodynamic study. *Folia Phoniatrica, 22,* 385–396.

Laver, J. (1991). The gift of speech. *Papers in the analysis of speech and voice.* Edinburgh, Scotland: Edinburgh University Press.

Lecluse, F., Brocaar, M., & Verschuure, J. (1975). The electroglottography and its relation to glottal activity. *Folia Phoniatrica, 27,* 215–224.

Leeper, H., & Graves, D. (1984). Consistency of laryngeal airway resistance in adult women. *Journal of Communication Disorders, 17,* 153–163.

Lester, R., & Story, B. (in press). Acoustic characteristics of simulated respiratory-induced vocal tremor. *American Journal of Speech-Language Pathology.*

Linville, S. (1987). Maximum phonational frequency range capabilities of women's voices with advancing age. *Folia Phoniatrica, 39,* 297–301.

Linville, S. (1992). Glottal gap configurations in two age groups of women. *Journal of Speech and Hearing Research, 35*, 1209–1215.

Linville, S. (1995). Vocal aging. *Current Opinion in Otolaryngology and Head and Neck Surgery, 3*, 183–187.

Linville, S., & Fisher, H. (1985). Acoustic characteristics of perceived versus actual age in controlled phonation by adult females. *Journal of the Acoustical Society of America, 78*, 40–48.

Lofqvist, A., & Oshima, K. (1993). Endoscopy, stoboscopy, and transillumination in speech research. *Measuring speech production, Part one: Respiration, phonation, and aerodynamics.* Woodbury, NY: Acoustical Society of America.

Lofqvist, A., & Yoshioka, H. (1984). Intrasegmental timing: Laryngeal-oral coordination in voiceless consonant production. *Speech Communication, 3*, 279–289.

Malinowski, A. (1967). Shape, dimensions, and process of calcification of the cartilaginous framework of the larynx in relation to age and sex in the Polish population. *Folia Morphologica, 26*, 118–128.

Mayet, A. (1955). Zur functionellen anatomie der men-schlichen stimmlippe. *Zeitschrift fur Anatomie und Entwicklungsgeschichte, 119*, 87–111.

Mayet, A., & Muendnich, K. (1958). Beitrag zur anatomie und zur funktion des m. cricothyroideus und der cricothyreiodgelenke. *Acta Anatomica, 33*, 273–288.

McGlone, R. (1967). Air flow during vocal fry. *Journal of Speech and Hearing Research, 10*, 299–304.

McGlone, R. (1970). Air flow in the upper register. *Folia Phoniatrica, 22*, 231–238.

McGlone, R., & Shipp, T. (1971). Some physiologic correlates of vocal fry phonation. *Journal of Speech and Hearing Research, 14*, 769–775.

Melcon, M., Hoit, J., & Hixon, T. (1989). Age and laryngeal airway resistance during vowel production. *Journal of Speech and Hearing Disorders, 54*, 282–286.

Minifie, F. (1973). Speech acoustics. In F. Minifie, T. Hixon, & F. Williams (Eds.), *Normal aspects of speech, hearing, and language* (pp. 236–284). Englewood-Cliffs, NJ: Prentice-Hall.

Monoson, P., & Zemlin, W. (1984). Quantitative study of whisper. *Folia Phoniatrica, 36*, 53–65.

Moore, P. (1938). Motion picture studies of the vocal folds and vocal attack. *Journal of Speech and Hearing Disorders, 3*, 235–238.

Motta, G., Cesari, U., Iengo, G., & Motta, G. (1990). Clinical application of electroglottography. *Folia Phoniatrica, 42*, 111–117.

Mueller, P., Sweeney, R., & Baribeau, L. (1985). Acoustic and morphologic study of the senescent voice. *Ear, Nose, and Throat Journal, 63*, 71–75.

Murry, T. (1971). Subglottal pressure and airflow measures during vocal fry phonation. *Journal of Speech and Hearing Research, 14*, 544–551.

Murry, T., & Brown, W. (1971a). Regulation of vocal intensity in vocal fry phonation. *Journal of the Acoustical Society of America, 49*, 1905–1907.

Murry, T., & Brown, W. (1971b). Subglottal air pressure during two types of vocal activity: Vocal fry and modal phonation. *Folia Phoniatrica, 23*, 440–449.

Netsell, R. (1969). *A perceptual-acoustic physiological study of syllable stress.* Doctoral dissertation, University of Iowa, Iowa City.

Netsell, R. (1973). Speech physiology. In F. Minifie, T. Hixon, & F. Williams (Eds.), *Normal aspects of speech, hearing, and language* (pp. 211–234). Englewood-Cliffs, NJ: Prentice-Hall.

Netsell, R., Lotz, W., & Shaughnessy, A. (1984). Laryngeal aerodynamics associated with selected voice disorders. *American Journal of Otolaryngology, 5*, 397–403.

Obrebowski, A., Wojnowski, W., & Obrebowski-Karsznia, Z. (2006). The characteristics of vocal fold molecular structure. *Otolaryngologia Polska, 60*, 9–14.

Ohala, J. (1972). *How is pitch lowered?* Paper presented at the Spring Meeting of the Acoustical Society of America. Buffalo, NY.

Ohala, J., & Hirose, H. (1970). The function of the sternohyoid muscle in speech. *Annual Report of the Institute of Logopedics and Phoniatrics, 4*, 41–44.

Okamura, H., & Katto, Y. (1988). Fine structure of muscle spindle in interarytenoid muscle of the human larynx. In O. Fujimura (Ed.), *Vocal fold physiology: Voice production, mechanisms, and functions* (pp. 135–143). New York, NY: Raven Press.

Orlikoff, R. (1998). Scrambled EGG: The uses and abuses of electroglottography. *Phonoscope, 1*, 37–53.

Orlikoff, R., & Kahane, J. (1996). Structure and function of the larynx. In N. Lass (Ed.), *Principles of experimental phonetics* (pp. 112–181). St. Louis, MO: Mosby.

Patel, R., Dailey, S., & Bless, D. (2008). Comparison of high-speed digital imaging with stroboscopy for laryngeal imaging of glottal disorders. *Annals of Otology, Rhinology, and Laryngology, 117*, 413–424.

Patel, R., & Salata, A. (2006). Using computer games to mediate caregiver-child communication for children with severe dysarthria. *Journal of Medical Speech-Language Pathology, 14*, 279–284.

Plant, R., Freed, G., & Plant, R. (2004). Direct measurement of onset and offset phonation threshold pressure in normal subjects. *Journal of the Acoustical Society of America, 116*, 3640–3646.

Plant, R., & Hillel, A. (1998). Direct measurement of sub-glottic pressure and laryngeal resistance in normal subjects and in spasmodic dysphonia. *Journal of Voice, 12*, 300–314.

Plant, R., & Younger, R. (2000). The interrelationship of sub-glottic air pressure, fundamental frequency, and vocal intensity during speech. *Journal of Voice, 14*, 170–177.

Pressman, J. (1942). Physiology of the vocal cords in phonation and respiration. *Archives of Otolaryngology, 35*, 355–398.

Pressman, J., & Keleman, G. (1955). Physiology of the larynx. *Physiological Reviews, 35*, 506–554.

Ramig, L., & Ringel, R. (1983). Effects of physiological aging on selected acoustic characteristics of voice. *Journal of Speech and Hearing Research, 26*, 22–30.

Reed, V. (1982). The electroglottography in voice teaching. In V. Lawrence (Ed.), *Transcripts of the Tenth Symposium on the Care of the Professional Voice* (pp. 58–65). New York, NY: The Voice Foundation.

Reidenbach, M. (1998). The muscular tissue of the vestibular folds of the larynx. *European Archives of Otorhinolaryngology, 255*, 365–367.

Rothenberg, M. (1968). The breath-stream dynamics of simple-released-plosive production. *Bibliotheca Phonetica No. 6*. Basel, Switzerland: S. Karger.

Rothenberg, M. (1973). A new inverse-filtering technique for deriving the glottal air flow waveform during voicing. *Journal of the Acoustical Society of America, 53*, 1632–1645.

Rothenberg, M. (1981). Some relations between glottal air flow and vocal fold contact area. *American Speech and Hearing Association Reports, 11*, 88–96.

Rothenberg, M. (1983). An interactive model for the voice source. In D. Bless & J. Abbs (Eds.), *Vocal fold physiology: Contemporary research and clinical issues* (pp. 155–165). San Diego, CA: College-Hill Press.

Rothenberg, M. (1992). A multichannel electroglottograph. *Journal of Voice, 6*, 36–43.

Rothenberg, M. (2009). Voice onset time versus articulatory modeling for stop consonants. *Logopedics Phoniatrics Vocology, 34*, 171–180.

Rothenberg, M., & Mahshie, J. (1988). Monitoring vocal fold abduction through vocal contact area. *Journal of Speech and Hearing Research, 31*, 338–351.

Rothenberg, M., & Nezelek, K. (1991). Airflow-based analysis of vocal function. In J. Gauffin & B. Hammarberg (Eds.), *Vocal fold physiology: Acoustic, perceptual, and physiological aspects of voice mechanisms* (pp. 139–148). San Diego, CA: Singular.

Rubin, A., Praneetvataku, V., Gherson, S., & Moyer, C. (2006). Laryngeal hyperfunction during whispering: Reality or myth? *Journal of Voice, 20*, 121–127.

Rubin, H. (1963). Experimental studies in vocal pitch and intensity in phonation. *Laryngoscope, 72*, 973–1015.

Russell, A., Penny, L., & Pemberton, C. (1995). Speaking fundamental frequency changes over time in women: A longitudinal study. *Journal of Speech and Hearing Research, 38*, 101–109.

Sampson, S., & Eyzaguirre, C. (1964). Some functional characteristics of mechanoreceptors in the larynx of the cat. *Journal of Neurophysiology, 27*, 464–480.

Sanders, I., Han, Y., Wang, J., & Biller, H. (1998). Muscle spindles are concentrated in the superior vocalis subcompartment of the human thyroarytenoid muscle. *Journal of Voice, 12*, 7–16.

Sanders, I., Rai, S., Han, Y., & Biller, H. (1998). Human vocalis contains distinct superior and inferior subcompartments: Possible candidates for the two masses of vocal fold vibration. *Annals of Otology, Rhinology, and Laryngology, 197*, 826–833.

Sanders, I., Wu, L., Mu, Y., & Biller, H. (1993). Innervation of the human larynx. *Archives of Otolaryngology-Head and Neck Surgery, 119*, 934–939.

Sanudo, J., Maranillo, E., Xavier, L., Mirapeix, R., Orus, C., & Quer, M. (1999). An anatomical study of anastomoses between the laryngeal nerves. *Laryngoscope, 109*, 983–987.

Sapienza, C., Stathopoulos, E., & Dromey, C. (1998). Approximations of open quotient and speed quotient from glottal air flow and EGG waveforms: Effects of measurement criteria and sound pressure level. *Journal of Voice, 12*, 31–43.

Sasaki, C., Levin, P., Laitman, J., & Crelin, E. (1977). Post-natal descent of the epiglottis in man: A preliminary report. *Archives of Otolaryngology, 103*, 169–171.

Sataloff, R., Spiegel, J., Carroll, L., Schiebel, B., Darby, K., & Rulnick, R. (1988). Strobovideolaryngoscopy in professional voice users: Results and clinical value. *Journal of Voice, 1*, 359–364.

Sato, K., Kurita, S., Hirano, M., & Kiyokawa, K. (1990). Distribution of elastic cartilage in the arytenoids and its physiologic significance. *Annals of Otology, Rhinology, and Laryngology, 99*, 363–368.

Sawashima, M., Abramson, A., Cooper, F., & Lisker, L. (1970). Observing laryngeal adjustments during running speech by use of a fiberoptics system. *Phonetica, 22*, 193–201.

Sawashima, M., & Hirose, H. (1968). A new laryngoscopic technique by use of fiberoptics. *Journal of the Acoustical Society of America, 43*, 168–169.

Sawashima, M., & Hirose, H. (1983). Laryngeal gestures in speech production. In P. MacNeilage (Ed.), *The production of speech* (pp. 11–38). New York, NY: Springer-Verlag.

Schonharl, E. (1960). *Die stroboskopie in der praktischen laryngologie*. Stuggart, Germany: Thieme-Verlag.

Segre, R. (1971). Senescence of the voice. *Eye, Ear, Nose, and Throat Monthly, 50*, 223–233.

Sekizawa, K., Sasaki, H., & Takishima, T. (1985). Laryngeal resistance immediately after panting in control and constricted airways. *Journal of Applied Physiology, 58*, 1164–1169.

Selbie, W., Zhang, L., Levine, W., & Ludlow, C. (1998). Using joint geometry to determine the motion of the cricoarytenoid joint. *Journal of the Acoustical Society of America, 103*, 1115–1127.

Sellars, I., & Keen, E. (1978). The anatomy and movements of the cricoarytenoid joint. *Laryngoscope, 88*, 667–674.

Shipp, T., & Hollien, H. (1969). Perception of the aging male voice. *Journal of Speech and Hearing Research, 12*, 704–710.

Shipp, T., & McGlone, R. (1971). Laryngeal dynamics associated with voice frequency change. *Journal of Speech and Hearing Research, 14*, 761–768.

Shipp, T., McGlone, R., & Morrissey, P. (1972). Some physiologic correlates of voice frequency change. In A. Rigault & R. Charbonneau (Eds.), *Proceedings of the 7th International Congress of Phonetic Sciences* (pp. 407–411). Hague, Netherlands: Mouton.

Smith, A., & Childers, D. (1983). Laryngeal evaluation using features from speech and the electroglottograph. *IEEE Transactions on Biomedical Engineering, 30*, 755–759.

Smitheran, J., & Hixon, T. (1981). A clinical method for estimating laryngeal airway resistance during vowel production. *Journal of Speech and Hearing Disorders, 46*, 138–146.

Sodersten, M., & Lindestad, P. (1990). Glottal closure and perceived breathiness during phonation in normally speaking subjects. *Journal of Speech and Hearing Research, 33*, 601–611.

Solomon, N., McCall, G., Trosset, M., & Gray, W. (1989). Laryngeal configuration and constriction during two types of whispering. *Journal of Speech and Hearing Research, 32,* 161–174.

Sonesson, B. (1959). Die funktionelle anatomie des cricoarytaenoidgelenkes. *Zeitschrift fur Anatomie und Entwicklungsgeschichte, 121,* 292–303.

Sonesson, B. (1960). On the anatomy and vibratory pattern of the human vocal folds. *Acta Otolaryngologica, Supplement 156,* 1–80.

Sonninen, A. (1968). The external frame function in the control of pitch in the human voice. *Annals of the New York Academy of Sciences, 155,* 68–90.

Stathopoulos, E., Hoit, J., Hixon, T., Watson, P., & Solomon, N. (1991). Respiratory and laryngeal function during whisper. *Journal of Speech and Hearing Research, 34,* 761–767.

Stathopoulos, E., Huber, J., & Sussman, J. (2011). Changes in acoustic characteristics of the voice across the life span: Measures from individuals 4–93 years of age. *Journal of Speech, Language, and Hearing Research, 54,* 1011–1021.

Stevens, K. (2000). *Acoustic phonetics.* Cambridge, MA: MIT Press.

Stoicheff, M. (1981). Speaking fundamental frequency characteristics of nonsmoking female adults. *Journal of Speech and Hearing Research, 24,* 437–441.

Strocchi, R., De Pasquale, V., Messerotti, G., Raspanti, M., Franchi, M., & Ruggeri, A. (1992). Particular structure of the anterior third of the human true vocal cord. *Acta Anatomica, 145,* 189–194.

Story, B., & Titze, I. (1995). Voice simulation with a body-cover model of the vocal folds. *Journal of the Acoustical Society of America, 97,* 1249–1260.

Sundberg, J., Scherer, R., Hess, M., & Muller, F. (2010). Whispering—A single-subject study of glottal configuration and aerodynamics. *Journal of Voice, 24,* 574–584.

Takano, S., & Honda, K. (2005). Observation of the cricothyroid joint by high-resolution MRI. *Japanese Journal of Logopedics and Phoniatrics, 46,* 174–178.

Timcke, R., von Leden, H., & Moore, P. (1958). Laryngeal vibrations: Measurements of the glottic wave, I: The normal vibratory cycle. *Archives of Otolaryngology, 68,* 1–19.

Titze, I. (1988a). A framework for the study of vocal registers. *Journal of Voice, 2,* 183–194.

Titze, I. (1988b). Regulation of vocal power and efficiency by subglottal pressure and glottal width. In O. Fujimura (Ed.), *Vocal fold physiology: Voice production, mechanisms, and functions* (pp. 227–238). New York, NY: Raven Press.

Titze, I. (1989). On the relation between subglottal pressure and fundmental frequency in phonation. *Journal of the Acoustical Society of America, 85,* 901–906.

Titze, I. (1990). Interpretation of the electroglottographic signal. *Journal of Voice, 4,* 1–9.

Titze, I. (1992). Acoustic interpretation of the voice range profile. *Journal of Speech and Hearing Research, 35,* 21–34.

Titze, I. (1994). *Principles of voice production.* Englewood-Cliffs, NJ: Prentice-Hall.

Titze, I. (2006a). *The myoelastic aerodynamic theory of phonation.* Iowa City, IA: National Center for Voice and Speech.

Titze, I. (2006b). Theoretical analysis of maximum flow declination rate versus maximum area declination rate in phonation. *Journal of Speech, Language, and Hearing Research, 49,* 439–447.

Titze, I., Jiang, J., & Drucker, D. (1988). Preliminaries to the body-cover theory of pitch control. *Journal of Voice, 1,* 314–319.

Titze, I., Luschei, E., & Hirano, M. (1989). Role of the thyroarytenoid muscle in regulation of fundamental frequency. *Journal of Voice, 3,* 213–224.

Titze, I., & Story, B. (2002). Rules for controlling low-dimensional vocal fold models with muscle activation. *Journal of the Acoustical Society of America, 112,* 1064–1076.

Tucker, L. (1963). *Articulatory variations in normal speakers with changes in vocal pitch and effort.* Master's thesis, University of Iowa, Iowa City.

Tucker, J., & Tucker, G. (1979). A clinical perspective on the development and anatomical aspects of the infant larynx and trachea. In G. Healy & T. McGill (Eds.), *Laryngo-tracheal problems in the pediatric patient* (pp. 3–8). Springfield, IL: Charles C. Thomas.

van den Berg, J. (1956). Direct and indirect determination of the mean subglottic pressure. *Folia Phoniatrica, 8,* 1–24.

van den Berg, J. (1957). Subglottic pressure and vibrations of the vocal folds. *Folia Phoniatrica, 9,* 64–71.

van den Berg, J. (1958). Myoelastic-aerodynamic theory of voice production. *Journal of Speech and Hearing Research, 1,* 227–244.

van den Berg, J., & Moll, J. (1955). Zur anatomie des menschlichen musculus vocalis. *Zeitschrift fur Anatomie und Entwicklungsgeschichte, 118,* 465–470.

van den Berg, J., & Tan, T. (1959). Results of experiments with human larynxes. *Practica Oto-Rhino Laryngologica, 21,* 425–450.

van den Berg, J., Vennard, W., Berger, D., & Shervanian, C. (1960). *Voice production* (Black and white 16-mm sound motion picture film). Utrecht, Netherlands: SFW-UNFI.

van den Berg, J., Zantema, J., & Doornenbal, P. (1957). On the air resistance and the Bernoulli effect of the human larynx. *Journal of the Acoustical Society of America, 29,* 626–631.

Vennard, W. (1967). *Singing: The mechanism and the technic.* New York, NY: Carl Fischer.

von Leden, H., & Moore, P. (1961). The mechanics of the cricoarytenoid joint. *Archives of Otolaryngology, 73,* 541–550.

Walker, W. (1977, May). Demonstrating resonance by shattering glass with sound. *Physics Teacher,* pp. 294–296.

Wang, R. (1998). Three-dimensional analysis of cricoarytenoid joint motion. *Laryngoscope, 108,* 1–17.

Watson, P., Ciccia, A., & Weismer, G. (2003). The relation of lung volume initiation to selected acoustic properties of speech. *Journal of the Acoustical Society of America, 113,* 2812–2819.

Wendahl, R., Moore, P., & Hollien, H. (1963). Comments on vocal fry. *Folia Phoniatrica, 15,* 251–255.

Wilson, K. (1979). *Voice disorders in children.* Baltimore, MD: Williams & Wilkins.

Wind, J. (1970). *On the phylogeny and the ontogeny of the human larynx.* Groningen, Netherlands: Wolters-Noordhoff.

Wustrow, F. (1953). Bau und funktion des menshlichne musculus vocalis. *Zeitschrift fur Anatomie und Entwick-lungsgeschichte, 116,* 506–522.

Yanagihara, N., & Koike, Y. (1967). The regulation of sustained phonation. *Folia Phoniatrica, 19,* 1–18.

Zemlin, W. (1998). *Speech and hearing science: Anatomy and physiology.* Boston, MA: Allyn & Bacon.

Zemlin, W., Davis, P., & Gaza, C. (1984). Fine morphology of the posterior cricoarytenoid muscle. *Folia Phoniatrica, 36,* 233–240.

Zenker, W. (1964). Questions regarding the function of external laryngeal muscles. In D. Brewer (Ed.), *Research potentials in voice physiology* (pp. 20–40). New York, NY: State University of New York.

Velopharyngeal-Nasal Function and Speech Production

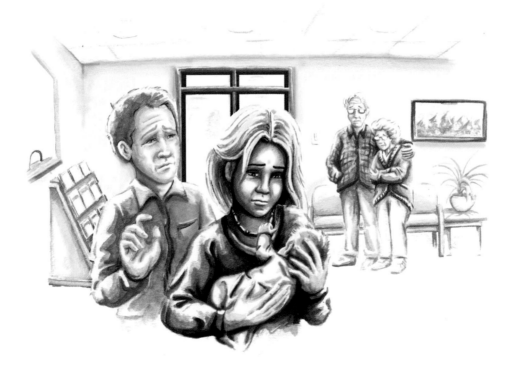

Scenario

It was to be their first baby and anticipation was running high. They were somewhat older parents who had chosen to focus initially on careers rather than on starting a family during the first decade of their marriage. The prospective grandparents (retired Ohio-Florida snowbirds) on the mother's side of the family had come south 3 weeks earlier than usual with the expectation of being helpful. A nursery was readied, routines were sketched out for a planned first month of parenthood, and the hopeful grandfather had managed to get his hands on two boxes of Cuban cigars for his son-in-law to distribute once the official celebration was begun. All was going well.

The pregnancy was full term and the delivery started out uneventfully, although labor turned out to be somewhat difficult. Finally the moment arrived and it was a boy. There was no need to elicit a cry. The new member of the family announced himself voluntarily and with intensity. However, his announcement had a bit of a strange quality to the ear of the obstetrician and other medical staff. The mother was understandably dazed and not fully cognizant, but she managed a smile at the obstetrician's declaration that it was a boy. Then she slumped into relief and exhaustion.

The obstetrician was the first to see the problem. The umbilical cord was cut and the newborn was handed to the delivery nurse. Nothing needed to be said to her. The father was comforting the mother as the obstetrician examined the baby more closely. The baby appeared to be physically normal, with one major exception. There was a cleft of both the lip and palate. The obstetrician took the father aside and explained the circumstances. A few minutes later, when the mother awoke, the same message was delivered.

The parents, especially the mother, seemed to collapse psychologically under the weight of the words. There was stunned silence and anguish. Then questions came in a flood, along with a flood of emotions. How could this be? Why did it happen? Had they done anything to cause this? Why had prenatal examinations not detected the problem? What did this mean for the baby? Was he mentally retarded? Could he go home? Would he be able to breastfeed? What should they do? Did he have to have surgery? When would it be done? Would he ever look normal? During these moments their dreams seemed shattered. It was overwhelming. Each tried to support the other, while trying to cope with feelings for each other and the baby. It was not the day they had envisioned in their rehearsals. The father talked with his wife's parents and then telephoned his own parents in Seattle.

A team of specialists in cleft palate and craniofacial disorders was called in to develop a management program. The management was expected to be lengthy. When the baby was 3 months of age, surgery was done to close the cleft of the lip. Then, when he was 12 months of age, another surgery was performed to close the cleft of the palate.

Middle ear infections proved to be a problem and were treated with antibiotics and the insertion of tubes to drain the middle-ear cavities. Speech development was monitored periodically and on the child's second birthday was found to have progressed to syllable and word utterances. Nasal emission of air could be heard during voiceless consonants and moderate hypernasality was perceived during vowels. Visualization of the velopharynx through nasoendoscopy revealed that the velopharynx was not closed for oralized speech production. This was confirmed via measures of nasal airflow. The management team recommended secondary surgery as the course to be taken. Two options were being considered, further surgery on the palate itself or the surgical construction of a pharyngeal flap. However, as it turned out, the management team did not have an opportunity to exercise either option.

Marital problems of the parents had led to divorce with the mother being awarded custody of the child. She and the child moved to another part of the country and severed ties with the child's father and the management team. She was depressed and after the move she distanced herself from her parents and friends. The mother and child lived a life of relative seclusion, his contact with other children being infrequent. Except for occasional visits to a pediatrician for earaches, his other health care needs were on hold.

INTRODUCTION

The velopharyngeal-nasal apparatus is located within the head and neck and comprises a system of valves and air passages. This system interconnects the throat and the atmosphere through the nose. Although most textbooks focus on the velopharyngeal part of this system, this chapter covers the complete velopharyngeal-nasal apparatus as a single functional entity. This leads to a more comprehensive understanding of normal and abnormal function and a fuller appreciation for the principles involved in making evaluation and management decisions.

The chapter begins by discussing the fundamentals of velopharyngeal-nasal function, and then turns to consideration of velopharyngeal-nasal function and speech production. Subsequent sections cover measurement of velopharyngeal-nasal function, velopharyngeal-nasal disorders in speech production, and clinical professionals who work with velopharyngeal-nasal disorders in speech production. The chapter concludes with a review and the completion of its opening scenario.

FUNDAMENTALS OF VELOPHARYNGEAL-NASAL FUNCTION

This section considers the fundamentals of velopharyngeal-nasal function and lays the groundwork for subsequent consideration of velopharyngeal-nasal function in speech production. Topics include the anatomy of the velopharyngeal-nasal apparatus, forces and movements of the velopharyngeal-nasal apparatus, adjustments of the velopharyngeal-nasal apparatus, control variables of velopharyngeal-nasal function, neural substrates of velopharyngeal-nasal control, and ventilation and velopharyngeal-nasal function.

Anatomy of the Velopharyngeal-Nasal Apparatus

The valves and air passages of the velopharyngeal-nasal apparatus are linked together such that some of the components are arranged in mechanical series (one after another) and some are arranged in mechanical parallel (side by side). This section begins by discussing the skeletal superstructure that supports the velopharyngeal-nasal apparatus. From there, the section proceeds to separate discussions of the anatomy of the pharynx, velum, nasal cavities, and outer nose.

Duane C. Spriestersbach (1916–2011)

Spriestersbach had a distinguished career as a clinical investigator of the communication problems of children with cleft palate and craniofacial disorders. "Sprie," as he was affectionately called, served for many years as the program director of a large federally funded research grant on cleft palate at the University of Iowa. His leadership fostered much of the research done over 2 decades on normal velopharyngeal function for speech production and on the mechanisms involved in control of the velopharyngeal apparatus in individuals with velopharyngeal incompetence. Many of the names in the reference list to this chapter cut their research teeth under his guidance. Spriestersbach was an exceptional thinker. He had an enormous impact on translating the products of research into practical clinical applications for those with speech disorders caused by cleft palate. In his spare time, he took to the stage where he performed in the Iowa City Community Theatre and to the card table where he played a legendary mean hand of poker.

Skeletal Superstructure

Figure 4–1 depicts the skeletal superstructure of the velopharyngeal-nasal apparatus. This superstructure consists of the first six cervical vertebrae and various bones of the skull. The skull bones include bones of the cranium (braincase) and facial complex (forehead, eyes, nose, mouth, and upper throat). These bones are individually intricate structures that are rigidly joined together into a unified framework. This framework contributes to the walls, floor, and roof of the velopharyngeal-nasal apparatus through a system of structural processes, plates, and projections, and provides for the attachment of muscles of the velopharyngeal-nasal apparatus. Some of the most important bony structures of the apparatus include the temporal bones (sides of the lower braincase), frontal bone (front of the upper braincase), palatine bones (back of the floor of the nasal cavities), maxillary bones (front of the floor of the nasal cavities), sphenoid bone (back wall of the nasal cavities), ethmoid bone (upper side walls of the nasal cavities and upper part of their medial wall), vomer bone (lower part of the medial wall of the nasal cavities), inferior conchae (lower side walls of the nasal cavities), and nasal bones (bridge of the outer nose). The bony structures mentioned can be seen in various perspectives

Front view

Side view

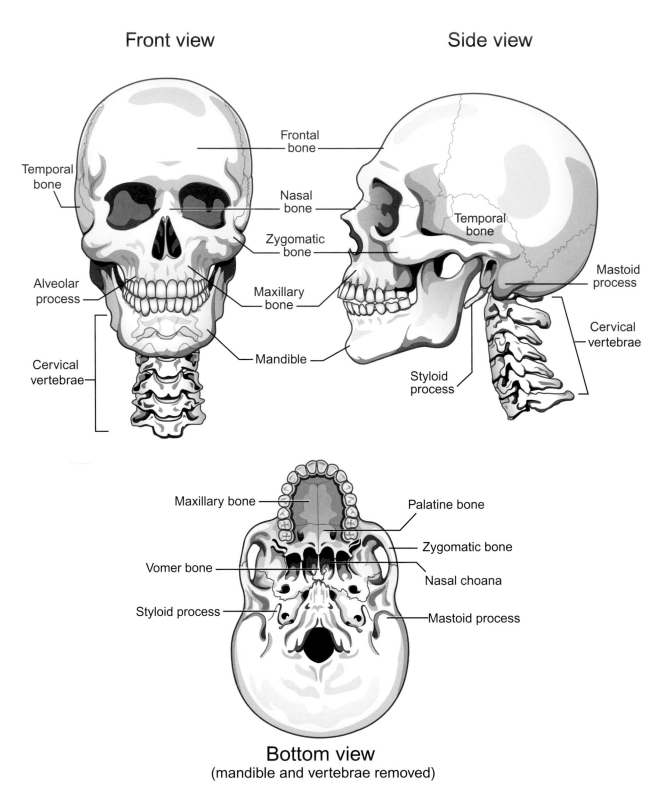

Temporal bone

Frontal bone

Nasal bone

Zygomatic bone

Temporal bone

Alveolar process

Maxillary bone

Mastoid process

Mandible

Cervical vertebrae

Cervical vertebrae

Styloid process

Maxillary bone

Palatine bone

Vomer bone

Zygomatic bone

Nasal choana

Styloid process

Mastoid process

Bottom view
(mandible and vertebrae removed)

Figure 4-1. Skeletal superstructure of the velopharyngeal-nasal apparatus. The mandible (lower jaw) is shown for reference in front and side views. The bottom view has the mandible and vertebrae removed.

in Figure 4–1, in other figures in this chapter, and in depictions of the bony skeleton of the oral apparatus in Chapter 5.

Pharynx

Figure 4–2 depicts some of the salient structural features of the pharynx (throat). The pharynx is a tube of tendon and muscle that extends from the base of the skull to the cricoid cartilage in the front and to the sixth cervical vertebra in the back. The mix of tendon and muscle varies along the length of the pharynx. At the upper end of the structure, the makeup is solely connective tissue, called the pharyngeal aponeurosis, which effectively suspends the pharyngeal tube from above (the way the rim of a basketball goal suspends the net). Muscular tissue increases in proportion down the length of the pharynx until it predominates. At the lower end, the pharynx is solely muscular and is continuous with the esophagus (gullet), where its front and back walls are in contact. This contact is broken during activities such as swallowing and regurgitation.

The pharyngeal tube is widest at the top and narrows down its length. It is oval in cross-section, being larger side to side than front to back. The front wall of the pharynx is partially formed by the back surfaces of the velum (defined below), tongue, and epiglottis. Otherwise, the structure is open at the front and connects, from top to bottom, with the nasal cavities, oral cavity, and laryngeal aditus (upper entrance to the larynx).

The pharynx comprises three cavities that are designated, from top to bottom, as the nasopharynx, oropharynx, and laryngopharynx. The boundaries of these cavities are shown in Figure 4–3. The nasopharynx lies behind the nose and above the velum. Because the velum is mobile, the lower boundary of the nasopharynx is somewhat arbitrary. Thus, a common convention is to specify this boundary operationally. For example, in midsagittal x-ray studies of the velopharyngeal-nasal apparatus, the boundary is often specified by a reference line extending between the upper surface of the hard palate and the most forward point on the uppermost vertebra.

The nasopharynx always remains patent, a feature that distinguishes it from the other subdivisions of the pharynx. The pharyngeal orifices of the eustachian (auditory) tubes are located on the lateral walls of the nasopharynx. These tubes enable pressure equilibration

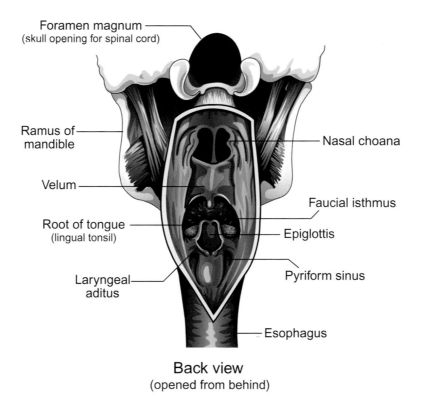

Back view
(opened from behind)

Figure 4–2. Salient features of the pharynx as revealed from a back view in which the posterior pharyngeal wall is opened from behind. The skull, mandible, and selected muscles are shown for reference.

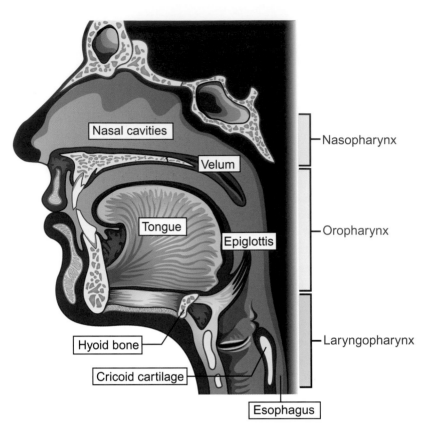

Figure 4–3. Boundaries of the nasopharynx, oropharynx, and laryngopharynx.

between the middle ears and atmosphere. Across the back surface of the nasopharynx, between the pharyngeal orifices of the eustachian tubes, lies a large mass of lymphoid tissue called the pharyngeal tonsil. This tissue is also referred to as the nasopharyngeal tonsil and, when abnormally enlarged, is designated as adenoid tissue (or just the adenoids). At the front, the nasopharynx connects to the nasal cavities through the nasal choanae (funnel-like openings). These are two oval-shaped apertures that are about twice as long (top to bottom) as they are wide (side to side) and are oriented in the vertical plane. The nasal choanae are also referred to as the posterior nares (nostrils) or internal nares and are somewhat like the breech ends of the barrels of a side-by-side double-barreled shotgun.

The oropharynx forms the middle part of the pharyngeal tube. The upper boundary of the oropharynx is coextensive with the lower boundary of the nasopharynx. The lower boundary of the oropharynx is the hyoid (tongue) bone. As shown in Figure 4–4, the front of the oropharynx opens into the oral cavity through the faucial isthmus (the narrow passage situated between the velum and the base of the tongue). This isthmus is bounded on the left and right sides by the anterior and posterior faucial pillars, pairs of muscular bands that resemble pairs of legs. The palatine tonsils are located between the anterior and posterior faucial pillars on each side of the isthmus. They are also often called the faucial tonsils and are "the" tonsils most often referred to colloquially. The back surface of the tongue is the site of still another tonsil, the so-called lingual tonsil. This tonsil is a broad aggregate of lymph glands distributed across much of the root of the tongue.

The oropharynx is the only subdivision of the pharynx that can be visualized without special equipment. The back wall of the oropharynx can be seen when looking at the pharynx through the faucial isthmus. Even more of the back wall can be observed when the velum is elevated, as in "open your mouth wide and say 'ah.'"

The laryngopharynx constitutes the lowermost part of the pharynx. The upper boundary of the laryngopharynx is the hyoid bone and the lower boundary is the base of the cricoid cartilage, where the pharynx

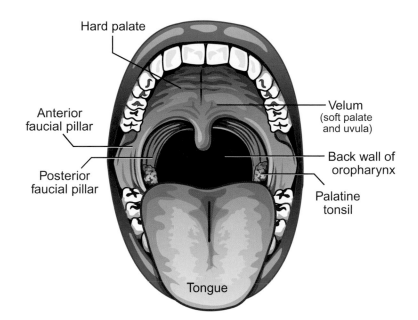

Figure 4–4. View of the oropharynx through the faucial isthmus.

is continuous with the esophagus. At the front, the laryngopharynx is bounded by the back surface of the tongue (and the lingual tonsil), the laryngeal aditus (formed by the epiglottis and aryepiglottic folds), and the pyriform sinuses (pear-shaped cavities located lateral to the aryepiglottic folds).

Muscle tissue is an important part of the pharynx and encircles it, much like bands of cord encircle the casing (tread and sidewalls) of a radial automobile tire. In effect, the pharynx is an elongated structure that has the architecture of a sphincter. Its overall arrangement is similar to that of the gut. This should come as no surprise, because one of the duties of the pharynx involves its actions as a component of the digestive system.

Velum

The velum is a pendulous flap consisting of the soft palate and uvula. The word velum means "curtain." In this case, it is the curtain that hangs down from the back of the roof of the mouth, as illustrated in Figures 4–3 and 4–4. A broad sheet of connective tissue, the palatal aponeurosis, forms a fibrous skeleton for the velum.

Despite a similar surface appearance throughout, the velum is not structurally homogeneous, but differs in composition from one region to another. These regional differences are manifested in layers of different types of tissues within the velum and differences in the distribution of muscle fibers within the structure.

Four tissue layers have been identified in the velum (Kuehn & Kahane, 1990). These include: (a) a layer toward the under surface (oral surface) that is glandular (secreting) tissue with adipose (fat) tissue at the sides, (b) a middle layer of muscle tissue in which fibers run side to side in the central portion of the structure and front to back in its more superficial portion toward the upper surface (nasal surface), (c) an upper front layer consisting of connective tissue (tendon), and (d) a lower back layer consisting largely of glandular tissue.

Patterns of muscle fiber distribution differ along the length of the velum (Kuehn & Moon, 2005). These include: (a) a front portion that is void of muscle fibers, (b) a middle one-third that is rich with muscle fibers that course in various directions (including across the midline) and include insertions into the lateral margins of the structure, (c) a proportioning of muscle fibers that tapers off toward the front and back of the structure, and (d) a uvular portion that is sparsely interspersed with muscle fibers.

In one sense, the uvula (meaning "little grape") is a pendulous structure suspended from another pendulous structure, the soft palate. One of several distinctions between the two is the nature of their blood supplies. The uvula has a richer vascular system than does the soft palate, a fact that has prompted the suggestion that this difference might serve to prevent excessive cooling of the smaller of the two structures (Moon & Kuehn, 2004).

Show Me Your Hand

They were twin girls. Each had speech that was a dead ringer for the other and was characterized by multiple misarticulations and hypernasality. What was the cause? Had they developed some sort of twin speech? Did one have a problem and the other was imitating it? Oral examinations revealed identical structural anomalies. Each girl had a short velum. Nasoendoscopic examinations further revealed that, for each girl, the velum elevated only occasionally during speech production, but never came close to the posterior pharyngeal wall. The girls' parents were with them and being interviewed by a student clinician and her supervisor. The moment the mother spoke there were suspicions. She had a severe speech disorder characterized by multiple misarticulations and hypernasality, and exhibited pronounced nasal grimacing when speaking. She allowed an oral examination. She had a short velum. It was three of a kind.

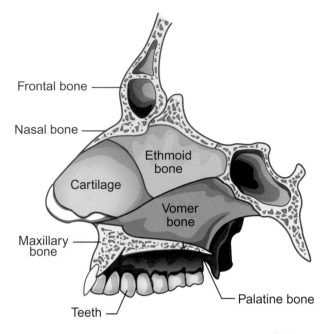

Figure 4–5. Components of the nasal septum. Selected other bones and teeth are shown for reference.

Nasal Cavities

The nasal cavities, also termed the nasal fossae (pronounced like posse), lie behind the outer nose. They constitute the inner nose and are two large chambers that run side by side (recall the double-barreled shotgun analogy suggested above). The two nasal cavities are separated from each other by the nasal septum, a partition in the midsagittal plane (although not often perfectly vertical). As shown in Figure 4–5, this partition has: (a) a front part composed of cartilage, (b) an upper back part that is the perpendicular plate of the ethmoid (sievelike) bone, and (c) a lower back part that is the vomer (ploughshare-like) bone. The floor of the nasal cavities is broad and slightly concave and formed by the hard palate. This floor consists of two sets of bones. The palatine processes of the maxillary bones (left and right upper jaws) form the front three-fourths of the hard palate, and the horizontal processes of the palatine bones form the back one-fourth of the structure (see Figure 4–1). The roof of the nasal cavities, in contrast to the floor, is quite narrow and formed by the cribriform plate of the ethmoid bone. The configuration of the two cavities is similar to the roofline of an A-frame house.

By far the most complex formations within the nasal cavities are located on its lateral walls. These formations are convoluted and labyrinthine and contain many nooks and crannies. Three shell-like structures give rise to this complexity. These structures are portrayed in Figure 4–6 and include the superior, middle, and inferior nasal conchae, formations that extend along the length of the nasal cavities. The nasal conchae, also called the nasal turbinates, have corresponding meatuses (passages) named for the conchae with which they are associated. The enfolding structure of the nasal cavities provides a large surface area to the inner nose and has a rich blood supply. A final structure of interest in each nasal cavity is the nasal vestibule, a modest dilation just inside the aperture of the anterior naris.

Outer Nose

Unlike the other components of the velopharyngeal-nasal apparatus, the parts of the outer nose are familiar to everyone, especially the surface features of the structure. The outer nose is, in fact, hard to ignore because it is in the center of the face and projects outward and downward conspicuously. The more prominent surface features of the outer nose include the root, bridge, dorsum, apex, alae, base, septum, and anterior nares, as shown in Figure 4–7.

The root (point of attachment) of the outer nose is to the bottom of the forehead. Following downward along the center line are the bridge (upper bony part),

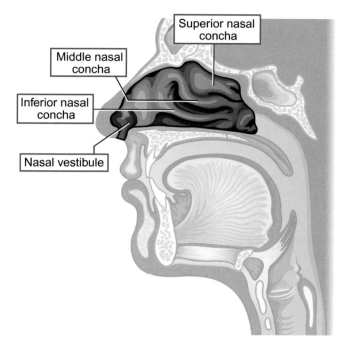

Figure 4–6. Superior, middle, and inferior nasal conchae.

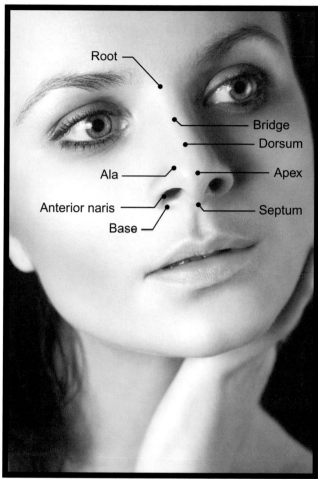

Figure 4–7. Surface features of the outer nose.

dorsum (prominent upper surface), and apex (tip). The alae (wings) form much of the sides of the nose and contribute significantly to its general shape. The base of the nose constitutes the bottom of the structure, partitioned down the middle (more or less) by the lowermost part of the nasal septum, and including the anterior nares (nostrils). The anterior nares are also referred to as the external nares and are somewhat pear-shaped apertures that are typically about twice as long (front-to-back) as they are wide (side-to-side). The orientation of the plane of the apertures of the anterior nares varies among individuals, but most often ranges from horizontal to upwardly oblique toward the side. The two anterior nares are somewhat akin to the muz-zle ends of the barrels of a side-by-side double-barreled shotgun. Margins of the anterior nares include stiff hairs, called vibrissae. These hairs arrest the passage of particles riding on air currents.

Disposing of Things

Mucus (a slimy substance) is formed in the nose to the tune of about half a pint a day (more when you have a cold). Particles filtered by the nose are collected in a blanket of mucus and moved through the nose by the action of cilia (tiny hair cells that collectively form a fringe). Things that get trapped are moved along toward the back of the throat and then swallowed into the stomach. Some material dries before reaching the back of the throat and fraction-ates into pieces containing filtered particles. This happens at different spots within the nose and in residues of various consistencies. Prim and proper folks refer to these residues as nasal exudates or pieces of dried nasal mucus. Most of us refer to them as "boogers." They are best gently blown into a tissue to rid them from the nose, but we all know other manual methods that are commonly practiced.

Forces and Movements of the Velopharyngeal-Nasal Apparatus

Much of the functional potential of the velopharyngeal-nasal apparatus lies in its capacity for movement. This movement is caused by forces applied to and by different components of the apparatus.

Forces of the Velopharyngeal-Nasal Apparatus

The forces operating on the velopharyngeal-nasal apparatus are of two types: passive and active. Passive force is inherent and always present (although subject to change), whereas active force is applied depending on the will and ability of the individual. The passive and active forces operating on the velopharyngeal-nasal apparatus make up the total force functioning at different locations.

Passive Force. The passive force of velopharyngeal-nasal function arises from several sources. These include the natural recoil of muscles, cartilages, and connective tissues, the surface tension between structures in apposition, the pull of gravity, and aeromechanical forces within the upper airway (throat, mouth, and nose).

The distribution, sign, and magnitude of passive force depend on the prevailing mechanical conditions, including the positions, deformations, and levels of activity of different components of the velopharyngeal-nasal apparatus. For example, the pull of gravity differentially influences velopharyngeal-nasal function when body position is changed. Such influences are considered in detail below in another section.

Active Force. The active force of velopharyngeal-nasal function arises from muscles distributed within different components of the velopharyngeal-nasal apparatus. This active force results from the contraction of muscle fibers. The contribution of specific muscles to such force generation is not completely understood. Nevertheless, based on individual muscle architecture, consequences of muscle activation, and observations of the electrical activity of muscles during various activities, the probable roles of specific muscles can be specified with reasonable certainty.

The function described here for individual muscles assumes that the muscle under consideration is activated and involved in a shortening (concentric) contraction. Actually, the influence of individual muscle actions depends on whether or not related muscles are active, the mechanical status of different components of the velopharyngeal-nasal apparatus, and the nature of the activity being performed. The muscles of the pharynx, velum, and outer nose are considered below.

Muscles of the Pharynx. Figure 4–8 portrays the muscles of the pharynx. Six muscles within and attached to the walls of the pharynx can influence the lumen of the pharyngeal tube (the cross-section along its length). Of course, other structures along the front side of the pharynx can also influence the lumen of the pharynx through their adjustments (velum, tongue, and epiglottis).

The *superior constrictor* muscle is located in the upper part of the pharynx. It is a complex muscle with multiple origins that arise from the front of the pharyngeal tube. Front points of attachment include the medial pterygoid plate (of the sphenoid bone), the pterygomandibular ligament (a tendinous inscription between the *superior constrictor* muscle and the *buccinator* muscle, described in Chapter 5), the mylohyoid line (site of attachment of the *mylohyoid* muscle, described in Chapter 5, on the inner surface of the body of the mandible), and the side of the back part of the tongue. These multiple points of origin are sometimes used as a basis for conceptualizing the *superior constrictor* muscle as a cluster of four individual muscles. From top to bottom, these four are designated as the *pterygopharyngeus*, *buccopharyngeus*, *mylopharyngeus*, and *glossopharyngeus*. Fibers from the multiple origins of the *superior constrictor* muscle course backward, toward the midline, and upward to insert into the fibrous median raphe (seam) of the posterior pharyngeal wall. There, they join with fibers of the paired muscle from the opposite side. The uppermost fibers of the *superior constrictor* muscle are horizontal and located at the level of the velum. When the *superior constrictor* muscle contracts, it reduces the regional cross-section of the pharyngeal lumen by forward movement of the posterior pharyngeal wall and forward and inward movement of the lateral pharyngeal wall. The paired *superior constrictor* muscles encircle the posterior and lateral walls of the upper pharynx (recall the radial tire analogy from above), so that their simultaneous contraction constricts the lumen of that part of the pharyngeal tube in the manner of a sphincter.

The *middle constrictor* muscle is a fan-shaped structure located midway along the length of the pharyngeal tube. Fibers of the muscle arise from the greater and lesser horns of the hyoid bone and the stylohyoid ligament (which runs between the downward and forward projecting styloid process of the temporal bone and the lesser horn of the hyoid bone) and radiate backward and toward the midline where they insert into the

Back view

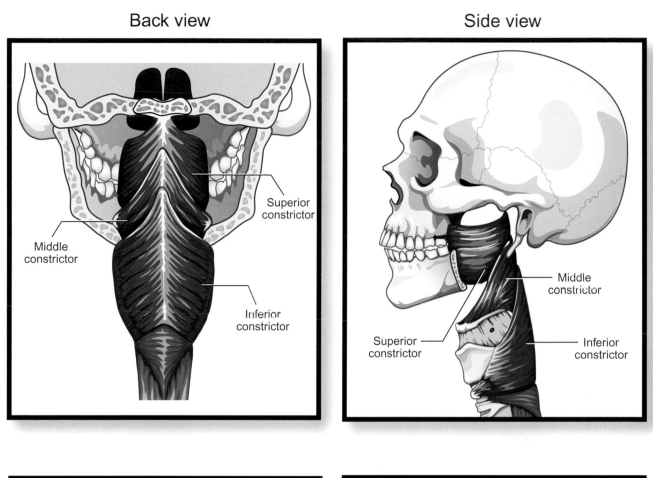

Side view

Middle
constrictor

Superior
constrictor

Inferior
constrictor

Middle
constrictor

Superior
constrictor

Inferior
constrictor

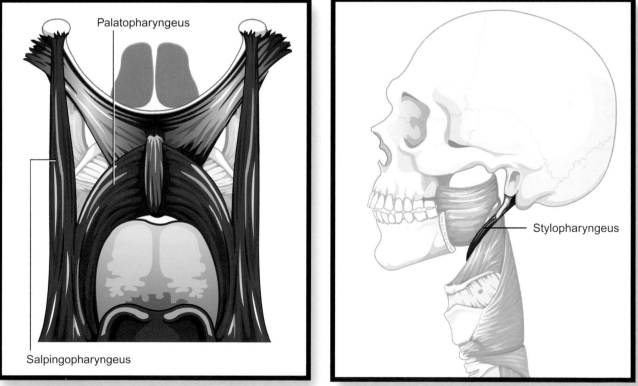

Palatopharyngeus

Salpingopharyngeus

Stylopharyngeus

Figure 4–8. Muscles of the pharynx.

median raphe of the pharynx. The *middle constrictor* muscle is also sometimes conceptualized as comprising two muscles designated as the *chondropharyngeus* and *ceratopharyngeus* muscles. The uppermost fibers of the *middle constrictor* muscle course obliquely upward and overlap the lower fibers of the *superior constrictor* muscle, whereas the lowermost fibers of the muscle run obliquely downward beneath the fibers of the *inferior constrictor* muscle (discussed below). The middle fibers of the *middle constrictor* muscle run horizontally. The overlapping arrangement of the muscle fibers between the *middle constrictor* and *superior constrictor* muscles and between the *inferior constrictor* and *middle constrictor* muscles is akin to the way in which roof shingles partially overlap. When the *middle constrictor* muscle contracts, it decreases the cross-section of the pharynx regionally, by virtue of forward movement of the posterior pharyngeal wall and forward and inward movement of the lateral pharyngeal wall. When the *middle constrictor* muscle acts in conjunction with its paired mate on the opposite side, the pharyngeal lumen is regionally constricted in the manner of a sphincter.

The *inferior constrictor* muscle is the most powerful of the three constrictor muscles of the pharynx. The fibers of this muscle arise from the sides of the thyroid and cricoid cartilages. The *inferior constrictor* muscle is sometimes thought of as consisting of two muscles. These are referred to as the *thyropharyngeus* and *cricopharyngeus* muscles. From the origins noted, fibers of the *inferior constrictor* muscle diverge in a fanlike configuration and course backward and toward the midline. There, they interdigitate with fibers from the *inferior constrictor* muscle of the opposite side at the median raphe of the pharyngeal tube. The middle and upper fibers of the *inferior constrictor* muscle ascend obliquely, whereas the lowermost fibers run horizontally and downward and are continuous with those of the esophagus. When the *inferior constrictor* muscle contracts, it draws the lower part of the posterior wall of the pharynx forward and pulls the lateral walls of the lower pharynx forward and inward. This action, in conjunction with that of the *inferior constrictor* muscle on the opposite side, constricts the lumen of the lower pharynx.

The *salpingopharyngeus* muscle is a narrow muscle that arises from near the lower border of the pharyngeal orifice of the eustachian tube. The fibers of the muscle course downward vertically and insert into the lateral wall of the lower pharynx where they blend with fibers of the *palatopharyngeus* muscle (discussed below). When the *salpingopharyngeus* muscle contracts, it pulls the lateral wall of the pharynx upward and inward. Acting simultaneously with its paired muscle from the opposite side, the effect achieved is one of decreasing the width of the pharynx.

The *stylopharyngeus* muscle is a slender muscle that runs a relatively long course. It originates from the styloid process of the temporal bone and runs downward, forward, and toward the midline. Most fibers of the muscle insert into the lateral wall of the pharynx at and near the juncture of the *superior constrictor* and *middle constrictor* muscles. Some fibers extend lower in the pharyngeal wall and insert into the thyroid cartilage. When the *stylopharyngeus* muscle contracts, it pulls upward on the pharyngeal tube and draws the lateral wall of the pharynx toward the side. Together with similar action of its paired mate from the opposite side, there results a widening of the lumen of the pharynx in the region where the muscle fibers insert into the lateral walls of the pharyngeal tube. There is also an upward pull placed on the larynx when the *stylopharyngeus* muscles contract.

The *palatopharyngeus* muscle runs the length of the pharynx and is a pharyngeal muscle. At the same time, it is also a muscle of the soft palate and in that context is called the *pharyngopalatine* muscle. The muscle is considered here from the pharyngeal perspective. The *palatopharyngeus* muscle arises mainly from the soft palate. The uppermost fibers are directed horizontally and intermingle with fibers of the *superior constrictor* muscle. A major fiber course is downward and toward the side through the posterior faucial pillar. Below the pillar, the fibers continue into the lower half of the pharynx and spread to the lateral wall of the structure and the thyroid cartilage. Some have suggested that the portion of the muscle that attaches to the thyroid cartilage be given recognition of its own as the *palatothyroideus* muscle (Cassell & Elkadi, 1995), whereas others disagree (Moon & Kuehn, 2004). When the velum is relatively stable, contraction of the *palatopharyngeus* muscle results in two movements. The uppermost fibers of the muscle draw the lateral pharyngeal wall inward to complement the action of the *superior constrictor* muscle of the pharynx, whereas the lowermost fibers of the muscle pull upward on the lateral pharyngeal wall and elevate the pharynx (attachments to the thyroid cartilage also effect an upward and forward pull on the larynx).

Figure 4–9 graphically illustrates the general force vectors for the six muscles of the pharynx discussed in this section. This illustration summarizes the potential active forces operating on the pharynx and shows the combinations of forces that could be in play at any moment to decrease or increase the lumen of the pharynx and/or change its positioning.

Side view   Front view

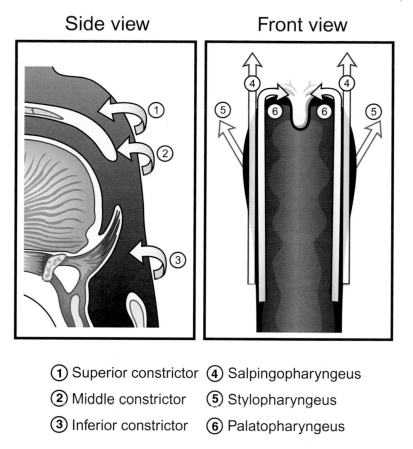

① Superior constrictor ④ Salpingopharyngeus

② Middle constrictor   ⑤ Stylopharyngeus

③ Inferior constrictor ⑥ Palatopharyngeus

Figure 4–9. Summary of force vectors of the muscles of the pharynx.

Having It Both Ways

A muscle is usually thought of as having an origin and an insertion. The origin is its anchored end and the insertion is its movable end. This is all well and good in textbooks, but in real life things are a bit more complicated. What may be the anchored end of a muscle for one activity may be the movable end of that muscle for another activity. A lot of it has to do with what neighboring muscles are doing. Thus, a muscle's function may change from time to time because various forces cause the mobility of its two ends to change in relation to one another. The convention adopted in this book is to reflect such change by alternately labeling a muscle in accordance with its perceived primary function in a given context. Some purists may not embrace this convention, but it carries instructive power and simply points out that in the busy world of the muscle, turnabout is fair play.

Muscles of the Velum. Figure 4–10 illustrates the muscles of the velum. The muscles shown can influence the positioning, configuration, and mechanical status of the structure.

The ***palatal levator*** muscle (also called the ***levator veli palatini*** muscle) forms much of the bulk of the velum. The ***palatal levator*** muscle is a flattened cylindrical structure that arises from the petrous (hard) portion of the temporal bone and from the cartilaginous portion of the eustachian tube. From there, it courses downward, forward, and toward the midline, passing on the outside of the posterior naris. Fibers of the ***palatal levator*** muscle insert into the side of the velum and spread out where they join those of the ***palatal levator*** muscle from the opposite side. The spread of muscle fibers in each of the ***palatal levator*** muscles is to the midline and beyond to the other side of the velum (Kuehn & Moon, 2005). Fibers extend from behind the hard palate to the front of the uvula, encompassing approximately the middle 40% of the velum (Boorman & Sommerlad, 1985) or more (Kuehn & Kahane, 1990). The paired ***palatal levator*** muscles form a muscular sling from their cranial attachments through the velum.

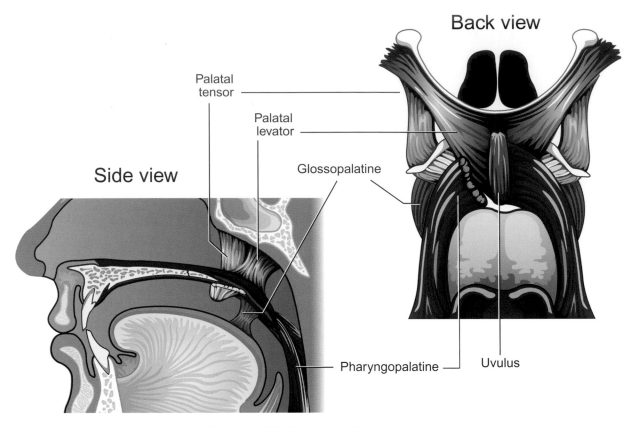

Figure 4–10. Muscles of the velum.

Each *palatal levator* muscle inserts into the velum at an angle of about 45°. When the *palatal levator* muscle contracts, it draws the velum upward and backward. Simultaneous contraction of the paired *palatal levator* muscles lifts the velum toward the posterior pharyngeal wall along an angular trajectory. Kuehn and Kahane (1990) have concluded that the force resulting from contraction of the *palatal levator* muscles is spread over a considerable distance within the soft palate. The significance of this observation is that it favors a potentially broad velum-to-pharynx contact area. Apposition between the velum and the posterior pharyngeal wall happens frequently and may involve significant contact forces. The upper surface of the velum consists of stratified squamous epithelium and is favorably composed to withstand such contact forces. Apposition between the velum and the posterior pharyngeal wall may also involve frictional forces associated with the velum sliding up and down the posterior pharyngeal wall. These forces are mitigated by glandular secretions of the velum, which lubricate the contact areas (Kuehn & Moon, 2005).

The *palatal tensor* muscle (also termed the *tensor veli palatini* muscle) lies on the outer side of the *pal-*

atal levator muscle. It arises from the pterygoid and scapular fossae and angular spine of the sphenoid bone as well as the cartilaginous portion of the eustachian tube. From there, fibers course vertically downward to terminate in a tendon and insert into the hook-shaped hamulus of the medial pterygoid plate of the sphenoid bone. The tendon of the *palatal tensor* muscle (along with a sparse number of *palatal tensor* muscle fibers) courses inward and inserts into the hard palate and the velum (Barsoumian, Kuehn, Moon, & Canady, 1998). The *palatal tensor* muscle has an important role in opening the eustachian tube. Earlier conceptions of the function of the *palatal tensor* muscle also suggested that its contraction would tense the velum, because it was thought that the muscle itself wrapped around the hamulus to contribute to the horizontal portion of the structure. However, the fact that the *palatal tensor* muscle is now known to insert on the hamulus, with only a few fibers continuing on to insert into the velum, indicates that it does not have the mechanical means to tense the velum to any significant degree. In contrast, the tendon does seem to play an important mechanical role. The prominent size of this tendon suggests that it may relieve stress at the junction between the hard and soft palates, stress induced by frequent up-and-down movements of the velum. The stress-relief function is believed to be akin to a reinforced collar at the junction between an electrical plug and the wire extending from it (Kuehn, 1990).

The *uvulus* muscle is the only intrinsic muscle of the velum. Fibers of the muscle originate to the side of the posterior nasal spine formed by the palatine bones and behind the hard palate near the sling formed by the *palatal levator* muscles and about a fourth of the way along the length of the soft palate from the front. The muscle courses downward and backward, in rope-like fashion, extending through much of the length of the soft palate. Very few fibers of the *uvulus* muscle actually enter the uvula proper, from which the muscle historically derived its name (Azzam & Kuehn, 1977; Huang, Lee, & Rajendran, 1997). This has prompted some to argue (and seemingly rightfully so) that the designation of this muscle as the *uvulus* muscle is both a misnomer and anatomically misleading (Moon & Kuehn, 2004). The location of the so-called *uvulus* muscle is above the sling formed by the *palatal levator* muscles. Structurally, the paired *uvulus* muscles account for the longitudinal convexity of the upper surface of the velum. This is true even in the region of the uvula, where muscle fibers are sparse, if they exist at all. One reason is that the encapsulating sheath that surrounds each *uvulus* muscle persists into the uvula, providing some cohesiveness between the soft palate and uvula and girdering the latter (Kuehn & Moon, 2005). When the *uvulus* muscle contracts, it has several effects that can be realized alone or in combination. These include that it (a) shortens the velum, (b) lifts the velum, and (c) increases the thickness (bulk) of the velum in the third quadrant of its length. Classic thought about the function of the paired *uvulus* muscles focused on the first of these effects, shortening of the velum. More recent conceptualizations, however, have focused on possible effects that involve the control of the stiffness of the upper part of the velum (Kuehn, Folkins, & Linville, 1988). Stiffness effected in the back part of the velum may counteract the deformation imposed on the velum by contraction of the *palatal levator* muscles. This avoids stretching of the top layer of the velum upward rather than moving the overall mass of the structure. It may also be that the *uvulus* muscles act to exert force within the upper part of the velum that causes the curvilinear structure to behave like a flexible beam that rotates the back half of the structure toward the posterior pharyngeal wall (somewhat analogous to extending flexed fingers with the palm of the hand facing downward). In this case, the *uvulus* muscles function as muscles that shorten the distance between the

velum and the posterior pharyngeal wall or facilitate contact and/or force of contact between the two.

The *glossopalatine* muscle is both a muscle of the tongue and a muscle of the velum, and is discussed here as a muscle of the velum. Fibers of the *glossopalatine* muscle arise from the side of the tongue where they are closely blended with longitudinal fibers of the dorsum of the tongue. They course upward and inward, forming the substance of the anterior faucial pillar, and insert into the lower surface of the palatal aponeurosis. The location of attachment to the soft palate is reported to vary across individuals, with some having insertions forward near the hard palate and others having insertions rearward near the uvula (Kuehn & Azzam, 1978). When the dorsum of the tongue is relatively fixed, contraction of the *glossopalatine* muscle places a downward and forward pull on the velum. Although the *glossopalatine* muscle has force potential on the velum, that potential is limited in comparison to the force potential of the *pharyngopalatine* muscle (Moon & Kuehn, 2004).

The *pharyngopalatine* muscle (discussed above as the *palatopharyngeus* muscle in the context of the pharynx) is considered here in the context of the velum. Its fibers arise from the lower half of the lateral wall of the pharynx and thyroid cartilage and course upward and toward the midline where they pass through the posterior faucial pillar and insert into the soft palate (also the *superior constrictor* muscle). Fibers do not approach or cross the midline of the soft palate, but insert more laterally within the structure (Kuehn & Kahane, 1990).

One notion of mechanical prominence is that there is a downward directed sling formed by the *pharyngopalatine* muscles that is antagonistic to the upward directed sling provided by the *palatal levator* muscles (Fritzell, 1969). This notion has intuitive appeal but has been questioned on anatomical grounds, given the observation that fibers of the *pharyngopalatine* muscles do not extend to the midline of the velum (Moon & Kuehn, 2004). Dismissal of the notion based on this criticism may be premature, however, because interconnection through other structures of the velum may still effect a functional, if not anatomical, sling that can direct force downward symmetrically as a consequence of action of the paired *pharyngopalatine* muscles. When the pharyngeal attachment of the *pharyngopalatine* muscle is relatively fixed, contraction of its fibers (especially those which are vertically oriented) pulls downward and backward on the velum. The action suggested here is founded on assumed muscle vector pulls inferred from anatomical observations. This approach may or may not be wholly correct.

Additional explanatory power seems to be gained by viewing the velum as a muscular hydrostat (the principle of muscular hydrostat is discussed in more detail in Chapter 5 in the context of the tongue). From this perspective, certain actions of the velum may be better understood as a structure that maintains a constant volume (size) but undergoes shape changes dependent on its muscle activations (Kier & Smith, 1985). The important notion is that contraction of certain muscle fibers within the velum provides a basis of support, off which other muscle fibers can achieve intricate adjustments in other parts of the structure. For

example, Ettema and Kuehn (1994) have suggested that one way the *pharyngopalatine* muscle could contribute to closure of the velopharynx (a muscle not classically considered to contribute to closure) could be by "squeezing the contents of the more posterior aspects of the velum and forcing the posterior nasal surface of the velum to conform to the concavity of the surrounding pharyngeal walls, much like forcing a water balloon to conform to the walls of a cylindrical container" (p. 311).

Figure 4–11 graphically illustrates the general force vectors for the four muscles that are known to

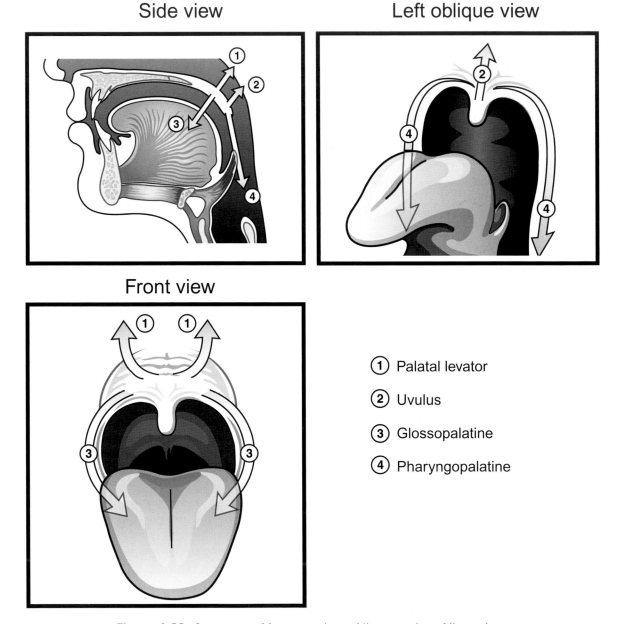

① Palatal levator

② Uvulus

③ Glossopalatine

④ Pharyngopalatine

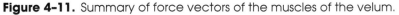

Figure 4-11. Summary of force vectors of the muscles of the velum.

operate on the velum. The *palatal tensor* muscle is not included in this figure because it does not appear to have a significant role in velar function.

Muscles of the Outer Nose. Figure 4–12 depicts selected muscles of the outer nose. All of the muscles of the outer nose can be used for facial expression to convey meaning. For the purposes of this chapter, however, interest in these muscles has to do with their potential to influence velopharyngeal-nasal function. Five muscles of the outer nose have this potential and it is these muscles that are discussed here.

The *levator labii superioris alaeque nasi* muscle (the muscle with the longest name of any muscle in animals) is a thin structure located at the side of the outer nose between the orbit of the eye and the upper lip. Its origin is from the frontal process and infraorbital margin of the maxilla. From there, the muscle courses downward and toward the side, subdividing into two muscular slips. One slip inserts into the upper lip (blending with the *orbicularis oris* muscle, described in Chapter 5) and the other slip (of more interest here) inserts into the cartilage of the nasal ala. Contraction of this latter muscular slip draws the ala upward on the same side of the outer nose (like lifting a side flap on a tent) and enlarges the corresponding anterior naris.

The *anterior nasal dilator* muscle is a small muscle positioned on the lower lateral surface of the outer nose. It arises from the lower edge of the lateral nasal cartilage and runs downward and outward. Following a short course, it inserts into the deep surface of the skin near the outer margin of the naris on the same side. Contraction of the *anterior nasal dilator* muscle enlarges the anterior naris on that side of the outer nose.

The *posterior nasal dilator* muscle is a small muscle located on the lower lateral surface of the outer nose. It lies behind the *anterior nasal dilator* muscle. Fibers of the *posterior nasal dilator* muscle originate from the nasal notch of the maxilla and adjacent sesamoid cartilages of the outer nose. From this origin, they follow a short course and insert into the skin near the lower part of the alar cartilage along the outer margin of the naris on the same side. Contraction of the *posterior nasal dilator* muscle enlarges the corresponding anterior naris.

The *nasalis* muscle is located on the side of the outer nose. It originates from the maxilla, above and lateral to the incisive fossa. Fibers run upward and toward the midline and insert into an aponeurosis that is continuous with its paired muscle from the opposite side. When the *nasalis* muscle contracts, it draws down the cartilaginous part of the outer nose on the same side (like pulling down a side flap on a tent) and decreases the aperture of the corresponding anterior naris. Under extreme action, contraction of this muscle and its counterpart from the opposite side may bring

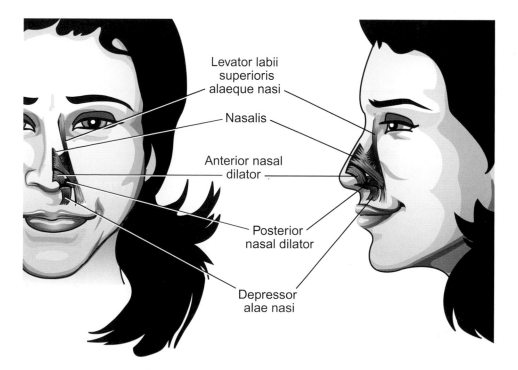

Figure 4–12. Muscles of the outer nose.

the two alae of the outer nose together or compress them against one another.

The *depressor alae nasi* muscle is a short muscle that originates from the incisive fossa of the maxilla and radiates upward to insert into the back part of the ala and the cartilaginous septum of the outer nose. When the *depressor alae nasi* muscle contracts, it draws the ala of the outer nose downward on the side of action and decreases the aperture of the corresponding naris.

Movements of the Velopharyngeal-Nasal Apparatus

Movements enable the velopharyngeal-nasal apparatus to perform many of its functions. Such movements are considered here apart from the forces that cause them. The relation of forces to movements is considered in the next section on adjustments.

Movements of the Pharynx. The pharynx is a highly mobile tube. As illustrated in Figure 4–13, this mobil-ity is vested in structures of the pharynx itself and in structures that comprise its lower and front boundaries. Four movement capabilities exist in the form of: (a) lengthening and shortening through downward and upward movements of the larynx, (b) inward and outward movements of the lateral pharyngeal walls, (c) forward and backward movements of the posterior pharyngeal wall, and (d) forward and backward movements of velum, tongue, and epiglottis. Being a hollow tube, movements of the pharynx are manifested in changes in the shape of its internal cavity. This internal cavity can be constricted or dilated at multiple sites as the result of different combinations of movements of the structure. For example, one part of the pharynx may be constricted, another part dilated, and yet another part alternately constricted and dilated during an activity.

Movements of the Velum. The velum is a fleshy flap that is largely muscular. Most of the time, it hangs pendulously in the oropharyngeal space, but for

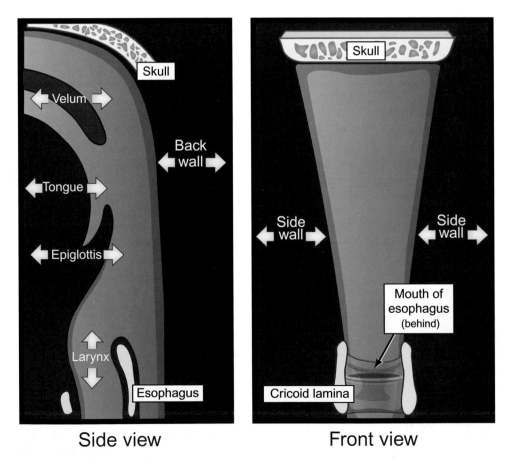

Side view   Front view

Figure 4–13. Movements of the pharynx.

many activities it moves substantially. Movements of the velum are mainly along an upward-backward or downward-forward path, in which those in one direction closely trace those in the other. The angular trajectory is reported to be slightly curvilinear (Kent, Carney, & Severeid, 1974) or linear (Kuehn, 1976). Maximum upward movement of the velum places the upper surface of the structure within the nasopharynx (above the boundary specified by convention to separate the oropharynx and nasopharynx).

Although the velum is a flap, and in some ways resembles a trapdoor, it does not move like a trapdoor. That is, it does not move as if were swinging from a hinge. Rather, as depicted in Figure 4–14, the shape of the velum actually changes when it moves. The farther up and back it moves, the more "hooked" its appearance (from the side) and the farther down and forward it moves, the more "pendulous" its appearance (from the side). This is because the major lifting force that pulls the velum upward is applied toward the middle of the velum. The hooked appearance of the velum results in identifiable landmarks during movement. The top of the hook (on the upper surface of the velum) is referred to as the velar eminence and the undersurface of the hook (on the lower surface of the velum) is designated as the dimple of the velum.

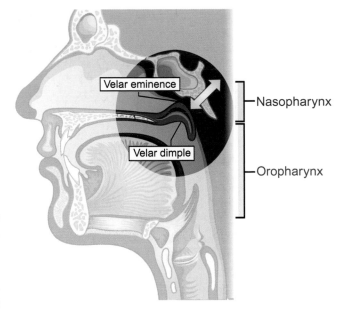

Figure 4-14. Elevated configuration of the velum.

Movements of the Outer Nose. Movements of the outer nose result mainly from outward or inward movements of the nasal alae that may change the cross-sections of the apertures of the anterior nares (nostrils). Under most circumstances, these movements are small. Exceptions occur during certain breathing events (see below), when signaling emotions (disdain, contempt, and anger), and when using the nares to slow the flow of air from the outer nose by increasing resistance at its exit ports.

Adjustments of the Velopharyngeal-Nasal Apparatus

The velopharyngeal-nasal apparatus is capable of many adjustments. The present discussion is limited to those adjustments that influence the degree of coupling between the oral and nasal cavities (through the velopharyngeal port) and between the nasal cavities and atmosphere (through the apertures of the anterior nares). Adjustments of lower parts of the pharynx are considered in Chapter 5 and Chapter 13.

Coupling Between the Oral and Nasal Cavities

The degree of coupling between the oral and nasal cavities can be adjusted. Such adjustment has a bearing on the size of the velopharyngeal port (the usual opening between the oral and nasal cavities). The range

---

Sonar in a Teacup

Early study of lateral pharyngeal wall movement was problematic because x-ray techniques of the day did not provide good frontal views of the pharynx. Two speech scientists and a medical physicist from the University of Wisconsin provided the first clean data on lateral pharyngeal wall movement through the use of pulsed ultrasound. The technique sounded the depth of a point on the pharyngeal wall (like tracking a submarine). To learn the technique, they attended a short course on obstetrics where the uses of ultrasound were being taught as a pioneering means for scanning the abdomen of pregnant women. The first monitoring of lateral pharyngeal wall movement during speech production was done at that short course on an individual immersed (except for the face) in a water-filled gunner's turret of a bomber (envision an enormous teacup). Gels were just then starting to be used to transmit ultrasound into the body for medical purposes.

of possibilities extends from a fully open port to a fully closed port.

The velopharyngeal port is open most of the time to accommodate nasal breathing. Closure of the port can be brought about through action of the velum and/or pharynx. Combined action of the two structures is often described as a flap-sphincter action, the flap being movement of the velum and the sphincter being movement of the pharynx.

There is no universal pattern for achieving velopharyngeal closure. On the contrary, several movement strategies for achieving closure of the velopharyngeal port have been identified that involve different actions or combinations of actions of the velum, lateral pharyngeal walls, and posterior pharyngeal wall (Croft, Shprintzen, & Rakoff, 1981; Finkelstein et al., 1995; Poppelreuter, Engelke, & Bruns, 2000; Shprintzen, 1992; Skolnik, McCall, & Barnes, 1973). These movement strategies are illustrated in Figure 4–15 and include: (a) elevation of the velum alone, (b) inward movement of the lateral pharyngeal walls alone, (c) elevation of the velum combined with inward movement of the lateral pharyngeal walls, and (d) elevation of the velum combined with inward movement of the lateral pharyngeal walls and forward movement of the posterior pharyngeal wall.

The prevailing wisdom is that these different movement strategies for achieving closure are rooted in differences in anatomy of the velopharyngeal region (Finkelstein et al., 1995). For example, individuals with smaller front-to-back than side-to-side dimensions to the resting velopharyngeal port are more likely to use elevation of the velum alone as the strategy for achieving closure of the port than are individuals with other port configurations. In contrast, individuals with more nearly equal front-to-back and side-to-side dimensions to the velopharyngeal port are more likely to use inward movement of the lateral walls of the pharynx alone or simultaneous elevation of the velum and inward movement of the lateral walls of the pharynx as the strategy for achieving closure.

It should also be noted that different movement strategies for achieving closure of the velopharyngeal port are not fixed within individuals, but can change over time as velopharyngeal anatomy changes. For example, the nasopharyngeal tonsil (called the adenoids when abnormally enlarged) is often large in young children and enables closure to be achieved solely by elevation of the velum against its mass. This mass atrophies with age, however, and elevation of the velum without other adjustments of the pharynx may no longer be sufficient to achieve closure of the velopharyngeal port (Finkelstein, Berger, Nachmani, & Ophir, 1996; Siegel-

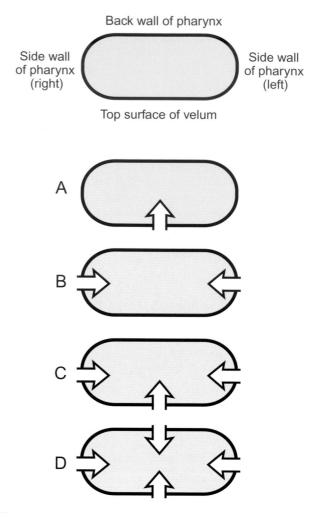

Figure 4–15. Patterns of velopharyngeal closure as seen from above.

Sadewitz, & Shprintzen, 1986). More is said about this under the section on the development of velopharyngeal-nasal function in speech production. For now, the important thing to know is that strategies for achieving velopharyngeal closure are subject to modification with changes in velopharyngeal anatomy.

The positioning of the velum in the adjustment of oral-nasal coupling is most often attributed to action of the *palatal levator* muscles (Dickson, 1972). Thought typically has been that lifting of the structure follows from the contractile force provided by these muscles and accounts for the midportion of the velum usually attaining the highest elevation during closure of the velopharyngeal port (Bell-Berti, 1976; Fritzell, 1963; Lubker, 1968; Seaver & Kuehn, 1980). Although action of the *palatal levator* muscles seems to be clearly associated with the flap component of the flap-sphincter closure adjustment, correlations between *palatal leva-*

tor activity and the elevation of the velum are weaker (albeit positive) than would be expected were the *palatal levator* muscles alone responsible for positioning the velum (Fritzell, 1979; Lubker, 1968). This suggests that other muscles must also be active in positioning the velum. Research, in fact, supports this inference.

Kuehn, Folkins, and Cutting (1982) made observations of the electrical activity of muscles of the velopharyngeal-nasal apparatus and related these observations to lateral x-ray images of the position of the velum. Muscles capable of exerting upward and downward force on the velum were among those studied. Kuehn et al. found that different combinations of activity among the *palatal levator, glossopalatine*, and *pharyngopalatine* muscles were associated with the same positioning of the velum, suggesting a trading relationship among them.

The same three muscles have also been considered as a coordinative system in which function-based interaction rules prevail. Moon, Smith, Folkins, Lemke, and Gartlan (1994b), for example, studied the relative contributions of the *palatal levator, glossopalatine*, and *pharyngopalatine* muscles to a range of voluntary adjustments of the velopharynx performed as subjects visually monitored (via a phototransduction system) the relative opening of the velopharyngeal port. Based on multivariate statistical modeling, the authors concluded that these three velar muscles form a coordinative system in which voluntary adjustments of the velopharyngeal port are flexible and allow for different combinations of muscle activation. Clearly, classical notions of the velum being controlled by the *palatal levator* muscles alone are inadequate.

Finally, it is important to note that closing and opening adjustments of the velopharyngeal port are controlled by different factors. Closing adjustments are predominated by muscular forces that must overcome the passive forces of the velopharyngeal-nasal apparatus. Opening adjustments, in contrast, also involve muscular forces, but are usually aided by passive forces, such as the natural recoil of muscle and connective tissue and the pull of gravity (in upright body positions).

Coupling Between the Nasal Cavities and Atmosphere

The degree of coupling between the nasal cavities and atmosphere can be adjusted by changing the size of the anterior nares. The range of possibilities extends from fully open nares to fully closed nares. It is also possible to have different degrees of coupling for the two nares (one being open more than the other).

The anterior nares, like the velopharynx, are relatively open most of the time to accommodate nasal breathing. Dilation or constriction of the nares can be brought about through the actions of muscles of the outer nose. Such actions can be either opposed or supplemented by aeromechanical forces associated with breathing. For example, muscles that dilate the anterior nares may activate to resist the tendency of the nares to collapse in response to low air pressures (created by high airflows) in their lumina. The need for such activation can be appreciated by sniffing briskly while watching the outer nose in a mirror. Both the nares and alae of the outer nose tend to be sucked inward by the lowering of nasal pressures. More forceful inspirations require increasingly forceful contractions of nasal dilators to maintain patent nares (Bridger, 1970).

Although dilation of the nares is more commonly associated with normal function than is constriction, there are times during expiration when constriction of the anterior nares can slow airflow through the nose. An exaggerated version of such constriction is often observed in individuals with velopharyngeal incompetence. Referred to clinically as "nares constriction," this is often taken as a cardinal sign of velopharyngeal dysfunction and is thought to represent an attempt to valve the airstream to compensate for an inability to valve it at the velopharynx (Warren, Hairfield, & Hinton, 1985).

Control Variables of Velopharyngeal-Nasal Function

Several control variables are important in velopharyngeal-nasal function. Their relative significance depends on the particular activity being performed, whether it is breathing, speaking, singing, blowing, sucking, swallowing, gagging, whistling, wind instrument playing, or glass blowing, among others. For example, speech production involves control variables based on acoustic goals, whereas tidal breathing does not. And, for another example, the force with which the velopharynx is closed may be an important variable for an activity that calls for very high oral air pressure (glass blowing), but be a less important variable for an activity with low oral air pressure demands (whispering). For persons with a normally functioning velopharyngeal-nasal apparatus, the most significant features of control pertain to the velopharyngeal portion of the apparatus. There are times, however, when control of the outer nose can become important.

For purposes of this chapter, attention is devoted to three control variables that influence aeromechanical and acoustic aspects of velopharyngeal-nasal function. These include: (a) the magnitude of the airway resistance offered by the velopharyngeal-nasal apparatus, (b) the magnitude of the muscular pressure exerted by the velopharyngeal sphincter to accomplish and maintain velopharyngeal closure, and (c) the magnitude of the acoustic impedance offered by the velopharyngeal-nasal apparatus.

Velopharyngeal-Nasal Airway Resistance

Resistance is defined, in a mechanical sense, as opposition to movement and results in a loss of energy through friction (similar to that of direct current in an electrical circuit). Velopharyngeal-nasal airway resistance has to do with opposition to the mass flow of air (the breath) through structures of the velopharyngeal-nasal airway.

Adjustments of the velopharyngeal port, nasal cavities, and/or outer nose can effect a change in airway resistance between the oral cavity and atmosphere through the nasal route, as portrayed in Figure 4–16. Thus, changing the cross-section and/or length of the velopharyngeal port, changing the engorgement of the nasal cavities, or changing the cross-section of the anterior nares can all have consequences for the airway

resistance across the velopharyngeal-nasal apparatus. Airflow also alters the resistance because resistance is airflow dependent. Specifically, resistance increases and decreases with increases and decreases in the rate at which the air moves, even when the physical dimensions of the velopharyngeal-nasal airway remain unchanged.

The range of potential airway resistance values is large and can go from less than 1.0 cmH$_2$O/LPS (following the administration of a decongestant) to infinity (completely obstructed). Infinite airway resistance is usually effected through airtight closure of the velopharyngeal port. Obviously, once airtight velopharyngeal closure is attained, adjustments of the nasal cavities and outer nose have no further influence on the value of the resistance. Infinite velopharyngeal-nasal airway resistance can also be achieved in the case of an open velopharynx under circumstances where there is complete nasal blockage.

As should be clear from this discussion, the status of all parts of the velopharyngeal-nasal apparatus needs to be known to fully understand their influences on the movement of aeromechanical energy back and forth between the oral cavity and atmosphere via the nasal route. Historically, focus has been on the status of the velopharyngeal port alone, with little or no consid-

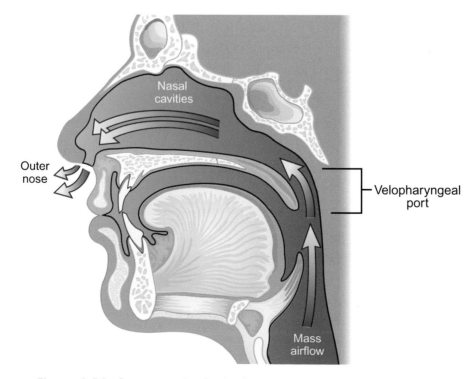

Figure 4-16. Components of velopharyngeal-nasal airway resistance.

eration given to the nasal cavities and outer nose. This limited focus is now known to have confounded certain interpretations of mechanism of velopharyngeal function and dysfunction.

Velopharyngeal Sphincter Compression

Once airtight velopharyngeal closure is attained, the force of that closure can be adjusted to meet the needs of the situation. This force, depicted in Figure 4–17, is represented by the compressive muscular pressure exerted to maintain the velopharyngeal sphincter in a closed configuration. The muscular pressure exerted at any moment must exceed the magnitude of the air pressure difference across the velopharyngeal sphincter (whether it be positive or negative) to prevent the velopharynx from being forced (blown or sucked) open. Thus, only a low compressive force is required to effect airtight velopharyngeal closure for an activity involving low oral air pressure, whereas a high compressive force is required for an activity involving high positive oral air pressure.

Certain individuals who routinely employ high oral air pressures are prone to develop stress-induced velopharyngeal incompetence. Woodwind and brass instrument players, who fall into this category, have a

---

Some Things Are Not Quite What They Seem

There seems to be a relatively large number of musicians who complain of "air leaks out the nose" during wind instrument playing. Such complaints are red flags for what might be stress velopharyngeal incompetence (discussed in the text). Sometimes physical measurements confirm that, in fact, the velopharynx is open during sound production. But sometimes physical measurements show that, surprisingly, the velopharynx is closed during sound production, despite what the musician is feeling. Why the mismatch? A study of trombonists may have found the answer. By sensing changes in air pressure at the anterior nares, Bennett and Hoit (in press) discovered that some trombonists open the velopharynx at the beginning of expiration before the sound begins, and then close the velopharynx right as the sound starts. What they felt was correct — the velopharynx was open. But it was not open while they were actually playing. Sometimes the senses play tricks on us.

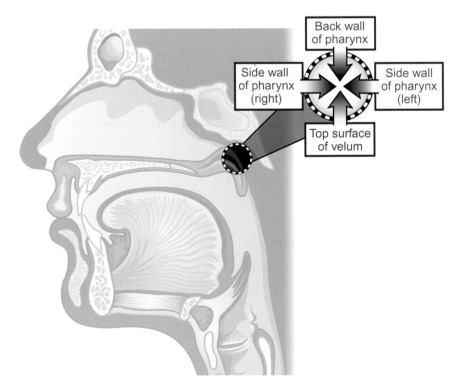

Figure 4–17. Compressive muscular pressure during velopharyngeal closure.

surprisingly high prevalence of symptoms and signs associated with velopharyngeal incompetence (Malick, Moon, & Canady, 2007; Schwab & Schulze-Florey, 2004). Most frequently affected are those who play the oboe and clarinet (instruments with high oral air pressure and high oral airflow demands, respectively). Unfortunately, velopharyngeal incompetence in performing musicians often goes undiagnosed and is mistakenly rationalized as declining performance ability rather than a curable performance problem (Klotz, Howard, Hengerer, & Slupchynskj, 2001).

Velopharyngeal-Nasal Acoustic Impedance

Certain aspects of acoustic (sound) control are made possible through actions of the velopharyngeal-nasal apparatus. These actions influence acoustic impedance, which, like airway resistance, involves opposition to flow. In the case of acoustic impedance, however, the flow is of a different type and the opposition is frequency dependent (similar to that of an alternating current in an electrical circuit). The acoustic impedance offered by the velopharyngeal-nasal apparatus does not pertain to the mass flow of air but to the rapid to-and-fro bumping of air molecules in which each stays in a very restricted region and passes energy on to its neighbors. As portrayed in Figure 4–18, acoustic impedance influences flow propagation in waves (sounds, not breath). The acoustic impedance of concern here is that distributed across the velopharyngeal port, nasal cavities, and outer nose.

As discussed above, the velopharyngeal port can be adjusted to influence the degree of coupling between the oral and nasal cavities. When the port is closed, the pharyngeal-oral airway and nasal airway are separated. Thus, nearly all of the sound energy passes through the pharyngeal-oral airway and the acoustic impedance looking into the nasal cavities from their velopharyngeal end is nearly infinite. (A small amount of sound energy may be transmitted through the closed velopharynx via sympathetic vibration, such as when the velum acts like a drumhead.)

When the velopharyngeal port is open, the oral and nasal cavities are free to exchange sound energy and interact with one another acoustically, and sound energy may pass between the outer nose and atmosphere. Changes in the size of the velopharyngeal port are important to determining how sound energy is divided between the oral and nasal cavities. Also important are configurations of the oral and nasal cavities themselves and the extent to which each impedes the flow of sound energy. In the case of the nasal part

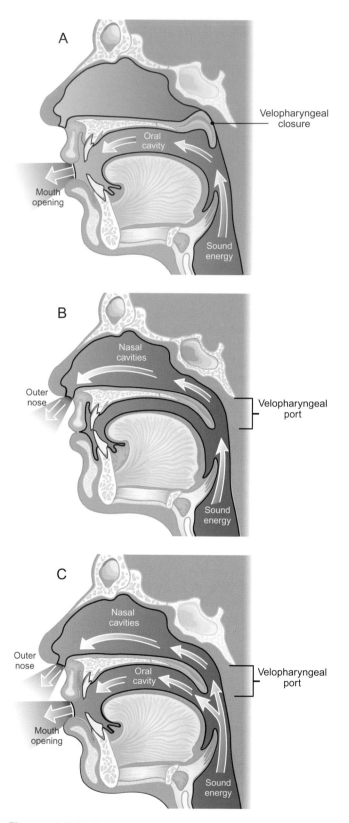

Figure 4-18. Oral-nasal sound wave propagation in relation to acoustic impedance.

<table>
<tr><td colspan="2" style="border:1px solid black; padding:8px;">

Which Hunt

It is often stated that velopharyngeal incompetence or insufficiency allows air to pass into the nasal cavities causing hypernasality. This is a misconception. Significant quantities of air can pass into the nasal cavities through the velopharynx during utterance without there being a perception of hypernasality. Also, hypernasality may be heard during utterance when no air is passing into the nasal cavities, such as when the covering tissue of a submucous cleft palate vibrates and excites the nasal cavities into sympathetic vibration. Flow of air into the nose does not cause hypernasality. In fact, hypernasality may be present when inspiratory speech is produced and airflow is passing through the nasal cavities in the opposite direction from usual. It's instructive to go through written discussions about velopharyngeal dysfunction and see which authors get it right and which authors get it wrong. Think of it as sort of a "which" hunt.

</td></tr>
</table>

of the system, degree of engorgement of the nasal cavities and status of the anterior nares are relevant factors.

The greater proportion of sound energy will be directed through the airway (oral or nasal) having the lower acoustic impedance. Thus, the distribution of sound energy between the two airways will be inversely proportional to the ratio between their respective acoustic impedances (Curtis, 1968; Fant, 1960). This ratio, of course, will differ in accordance with the prevailing configurations of the two pathways and in relation to the spectral content of the sounds passing through. Chapter 9 provides a much more detailed discussion of the effects of oral-nasal coupling on speech.

Neural Substrates of Velopharyngeal-Nasal Control

Velopharyngeal-nasal movement is controlled by the nervous system, but the nature of that movement and the nature of its control differ with the activity being performed. That is, different parts of the nervous system take charge of different components of the velopharyngeal-nasal apparatus for different types of velopharyngeal-nasal activities. For example, neural control of the apparatus is different for sneezing, blowing, swallowing, and speaking. Control of

velopharyngeal-nasal function in swallowing is covered in Chapter 13 and control of velopharyngeal-nasal function in speech production is discussed here.

Although different parts of the central nervous system are responsible for the control of different velopharyngeal-nasal activities, control commands are, nonetheless, sent through the same set of cranial nerves to muscles. These nerves originate in the brainstem and course outward to provide motor innervation to the pharynx, velum, and outer nose. As shown in Table 4–1, motor innervation of the pharynx and velum is effected through the pharyngeal plexus, a network that includes fibers from cranial nerves IX (glossopharyngeal), X (vagus), and possibly XI (accessory). An exception is found in the case of the *palatal tensor* muscle, whose motor innervation is provided by cranial nerve V (trigeminal). There may also be additional motor innervation to the pharynx and velum through cranial nerve VII (facial), especially related to the *palatal levator* and *uvulus* muscles. Motor innervation to the outer nose is effected by cranial nerve VII.

One might think that information about the motor nerve supply to different parts of the velopharyngeal-nasal apparatus would be straightforward and agreed upon. This is, indeed, the case for motor innervation to the outer nose, but not for motor innervation to the pharynx and velum. This is because the linkage between specific cranial nerves and the motor supply

Table 4–1. Summary of the Motor and Sensory Nerve Supply to the Pharynx, Velum, and Outer Nose Components of the Velopharyngeal-Nasal Apparatus

COMPONENT	INNERVATION	
	MOTOR	**SENSORY**
Pharynx	Pharyngeal Plexus	V, VII, X
Velum	Pharyngeal Plexus (except *palatal tensor* muscle, which is innervated by V)	V, VII, X
Outer Nose	VII	V

Note: There may be additional motor innervation from cranial nerve VII to certain muscles of the pharynx and velum, especially the *palatal levator* muscle and *uvulus* muscle (Shimokawa, Yi, & Tanaka, 2005).

The pharyngeal plexus is a network that includes cranial nerves IX (glossopharyngeal), X (vagus), and possibly XI (accessory). Other cranial nerves indicated in the table are V (trigeminal) and VII (facial).

to specific muscles is equivocal in some cases (Cassell & Elkadi, 1995; Dickson, 1972; Moon & Kuehn, 2004) and because conducting research on motor nerve function in the velopharyngeal-nasal region of human beings is extremely difficult (Kuehn & Perry, 2008).

Sensory innervation to the pharynx and velum is effected through cranial nerves V, VII, and X, and sensory innervation to the outer nose is effected through cranial nerve V. Neural information traveling along the sensory nerve supply from the pharynx, velum, and outer nose comes from receptors that respond to various types of stimuli, including mechanical stimuli. For example, receptors located in the mucosa of the velum and pharynx respond to light touch and receptors located in and near the velopharyngeal-nasal muscles relay information about muscle length and tension.

Much of incoming information from the velopharyngeal-nasal apparatus is not sensed or perceived. This seems to be especially true for the velopharyngeal portion of the apparatus. For example, the potential for sensing the position of the velum in space (proprioception) and its movement (kinesthesia) is believed to be rudimentary or nonexistent. Empirical evidence for this can be found in studies in which normal speakers have been shown to have difficulty controlling velopharyngeal movements voluntarily (Ruscello, 1982; Shelton, Beaumont, Trier, & Furr, 1978). Thus, it seems likely that control of the velopharyngeal apparatus relies more heavily on other types of information, such as that associated with the sensing of air pressure and airflow (Liss, Kuehn, & Hinkle, 1994; Warren, Dalston, & Dalston, 1990) and that associated with the sensing of the acoustic signal (Netsell, 1990) via cranial nerve VIII (auditory-vestibular).

Motor and sensory inputs are undoubtedly important for programming and controlling the velopharyngeal-nasal apparatus (Lubker, 1975). General models of motor skill acquisition and maintenance, in fact, rely heavily on motor and sensory substrates for control of the speech production apparatus (Kent, 1981; Schmidt, 1982). However, it is widely recognized that there is a need for additional information regarding the neural substrates of velopharyngeal-nasal control before there is a complete understanding of the motor and sensory capabilities of the normal apparatus (Kuehn & Perry, 2008; Liss, 1990).

Ventilation and Velopharyngeal-Nasal Function

Recall from Chapter 2 that ventilation is the movement of air in and out of the pulmonary apparatus for the purpose of gas exchange. This movement of air can be routed through the nose, the mouth, or both.

Resting tidal breathing usually occurs through the nose alone (unless there is obstruction in the velopharyngeal-nasal apparatus) in a rhythmical to-and-fro fashion. During inspiration, the nasal cavities function to warm, moisten, and filter air on its way from the atmosphere to the pulmonary apparatus. During expiration, the nasal cavities retain the warmth and moisture in air on its way from the pulmonary apparatus to the atmosphere. Three important aspects of velopharyngeal-nasal function for ventilation are nasal valve modulation, nasal cycling (side-to-side), and nasal-oral switching, and are discussed below.

Nasal Valve Modulation

The nose is a major source of resistance to the flow of air during breathing. This resistance is governed mainly by nasal patency and may be altered by many factors, including infection, trauma, emotion, air temperature, and eating hot food, among others (Bridger, 1970). Figure 4–19 suggests a novel solution for coping with one of the factors sometimes brought on when eating hot food, a runny nose.

In the normal upper airway, the greatest resistance to airflow occurs toward the front ends of the nasal passages in what are called the nasal valves. As portrayed in Figure 4–20, each nasal valve (left and right) comprises two components, an external valve and an internal valve.

The external nasal valve is contained in the vestibule of the nose and constitutes a vault formed by the nasal floor, nasal rim, and nasal septum. The nasal muscles can adjust the external valve in ways that dilate, constrict, and/or change its configuration, actions that can alter the (negative) pressure at which the nose is subject to collapse during high airflow events. Nasal muscles that dilate an anterior naris increase the rigidity of the external valve and change the pressure that would close it to a more negative value, whereas nasal muscles that constrict an anterior naris make the critical pressure less negative (Bridger, 1970). Active dilation of the external valve occurs with inspiration and parallels active dilation in other parts of the breathing airway, such as the pharynx and larynx (Cole, 1976; Drettner, 1979).

The internal nasal valve is an orifice that forms the transition between the vestibule and the osseous nasal cavity (fossa) on each side just in front of the inferior nasal turbinate (Stoksted, 1953). The cross-sectional area of the internal nasal valve is the smallest found in the nasal airway and accounts for up to two-thirds of

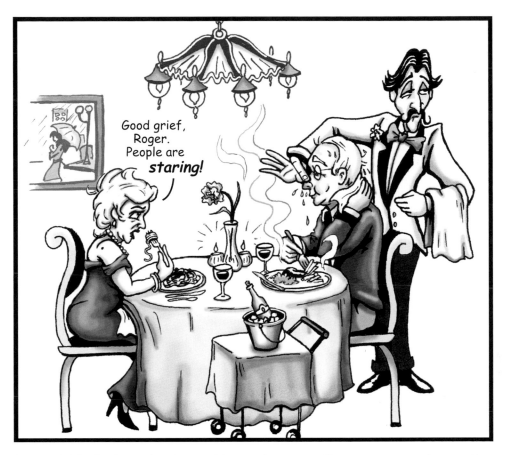

Figure 4-19. Cartoon showing a chic way to cope with a runny nose when eating hot food.

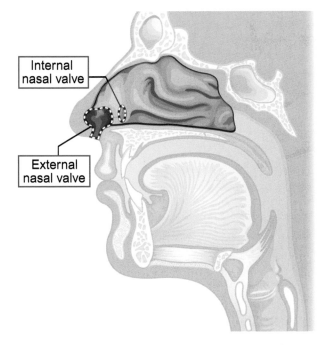

Figure 4-20. External and internal nasal valves.

the resistance to airflow through the velopharyngeal-nasal apparatus during inspiration (Foster, 1962). Based on its anatomic (Proctor, 1982) and airflow-resistive (Hairfield, Warren, Hinton, & Seaton, 1987) characteristics, this valve is considered to be the main regulator of the nasal airway. The internal nasal valve is an active participant in tidal breathing, becoming larger during inspiration and smaller during expiration (Hairfield et al., 1987). This pattern is maintained when the external nasal valve is fixed in size by the insertion of relatively rigid tubing through the anterior nares into the nasal vestibules, indicating that adjustments of the anterior nares and alae are not responsible for the effect. The precise mechanism of regulation of the internal nasal valve is unknown.

Although the effort it takes to breathe is about three times greater through the nose than through the mouth, the nasal route typically prevails. This is because it provides advantages for both inspiration and expiration. During inspiration, nasal breathing warms, humidifies, and filters the incoming air before it reaches the lungs and lower airways. During expiration, nasal breathing helps ensure adequate alveolar gas exchange (Hairfield et al., 1987). It does so by providing an in-series braking mechanism (Jackson, 1976) to accompany the laryngeal braking mechanism that serves to lengthen expiration and, thereby, enhance alveolar gas exchange (Gautier, Remmers, & Bartlett, 1973). This may help to explain the paradoxical preference people have for breathing through their nose.

Nasal Cycling (Side-to-Side)

The rhythmic exchange of resting tidal breathing usually goes unnoticed. Also usually unnoticed, and even unknown, is the fact that the two sides of the nose behave differently during breathing. The fact of the matter is, everybody has two noses (somewhat like the two barrels of a side-by-side double-barreled shotgun).

For most people (estimates range up to 80%), these two noses (one on the left side and one on the right side) go through cycles of turbinate engorgement and deflation (Principato & Ozenberger, 1970; Stoksted, 1953). As portrayed in Figure 4–21, these cycles are typically 180° out of phase between the left and right sides and have identical periods. That is, as the left side is congesting (swelling), the right side is decongesting (shrinking), and vice versa. The reciprocal alternation between the left and right sides is characterized by simi-

lar changes in nasal cavity resistance, average airflow, and volume change. Cycling time varies from person to person and can range from as short as 30 minutes to as long as 5 hours or more. These alternating blockages and returns to patency go on throughout the day and night, without awareness on the part of the person breathing, despite the fact that the effective nasal airflow is at times almost entirely a function of the patent side (Principato & Ozenberger, 1970). The explanation for this lack of awareness on the part of the breather is that the total resistance to airflow remains relatively constant (Huang et al., 2003). Thus, despite large changes in the resistance to airflow from side to side, the total nasal resistance changes little because it reflects the resistance of the more patent nasal cavity. In fact, the total nasal resistance cannot vary any more than the difference between the minimal resistances of the individual sides of the nose (Principato & Ozenberger, 1970).

The purpose of nasal cycling appears to be to permit one side of the nose to go through a period of rest from the task of conditioning inspired air. Such turn taking allows for downtime wherein "housecleaning" goes on. It has also been suggested that periodic congestion and decongestion of the nasal cavities provides a pumping mechanism for the generation of plasma exudate that serves as a vital line of defense against infection (Eccles, 1996).

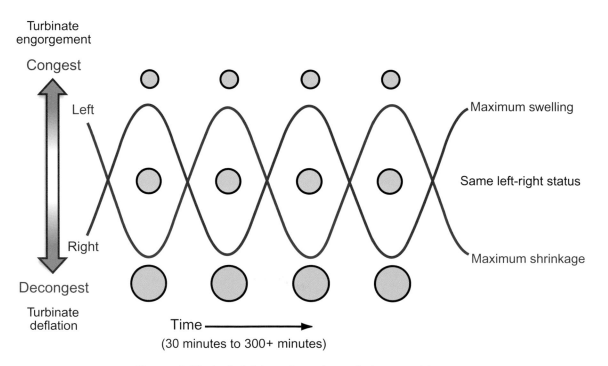

Figure 4–21. Left-right cycling of nasal airway resistance.

The pacemaker for the nasal cycle is thought to be the suprachiasmatic nucleus of the hypothalamus. This nucleus is believed to regulate autonomic tone of the left and right nasal vasculatures (Eccles & Eccles, 1981). Apparently, alternating actions by the sympathetic and parasympathetic portions of the autonomic nervous system result in vasoconstriction and decongestion, respectively. The pacemaker for the nasal cycle produces an ultradian (more frequent than once a day) rhythm that includes asymmetries in left-right cerebral electroencephalographic (EEG) activity (Werntz, Bickford, Bloom, & Shannahoff-Khalsa, 1983). This activity is such that greater EEG amplitudes are associated with decreased resistance to airflow in the nasal cavity of the opposite side.

It is interesting to note that the alternating rhythm associated with the nasal cycle is influenced by body position (Cole & Haight, 1986) and decreases with age (Mirza, Kroger, & Doty, 1997). The nasal cycle appears to be ablated in persons with high spinal cord lesions during the first year after injury. This is believed to be due to damage to the cervical sympathetic nerves supplying the nasal mucosa (Saroha, Bottrill, Saif, & Gardner, 2003). Surprisingly, individuals between 1 and 4 years out from such injuries demonstrate an irregular nasal cycle, whereas those more than 4 years out show a return to a normal alternating nasal cycle (Saroha et al., 2003). The mechanism of recovery is unknown.

Nasal-Oral Switching

Most breathing is done through the nose, for good reasons. As mentioned above, nasal breathing is desirable because it: (a) converts the temperature of incoming air to that of the body, (b) adjusts the relative humidity of incoming air to an advantageous 80%, (c) extracts dust, bacteria and other contaminants from incoming air, and (d) provides airway resistance during expiration that may aid in alveolar gas exchange.

Breathing through the mouth is much less common, but it does occur (Niinimaa, Cole, & Mintz, 1981; Saibene, Mognoni, & LaFortuna, 1978; Vig & Zajac, 1993; Warren, Drake, & Davis, 1992). However, constant mouth breathing can be problematic because it does not accomplish the warming, moistening, and filtering functions of the nose. Only a small fraction of the population breathes through the mouth routinely (Niiminaa et al., 1981; Sabiene et al., 1978), and this is usually the result of nasal obstruction. It has been estimated that about 10% of all mouth breathing is habitual rather than obligatory (Warren, Hairfield, Seaton, & Hinton, 1988).

If the tidal breathing demand exceeds that associated with rest, it may become necessary to switch to mouth breathing or mouth breathing in combination with nose breathing. The key factor in such switching appears to be the prevailing nasal resistance. Nasal resistance values for healthy adults and children range from 1.0 to 3.5 cmH$_2$O/LPS for resting tidal breathing (Warren, Duany, & Fischer, 1969; Warren, Mayo, Zajac, & Rochet, 1996). Resistance values in excess 4.5 cmH$_2$O/LPS during tidal breathing are thought to constitute impairment (McCaffrey & Kern, 1979).

The magnitude of resistance that leads to switching from solely nasal breathing to nasal-oral breathing has been found to be about 4.0 to 4.5 cmH$_2$O/LPS (Warren, Hairfield, Seaton, Morr, & Smith, 1988). This turns out to be slightly lower than the value of resistance that leads to the sensation of breathing discomfort (Warren et al., 1996). Interestingly, the switch from nasal breathing to oral-nasal breathing occurs before awareness of breathing difficulty. This observation is consistent with the established notion that physiological responses to changes in the internal environment generally occur prior to psychophysical recognition of change in all homeostatic systems (Warren, Hairfield, Seaton, & Hinton, 1987).

Who Nose?

As discussed in the text, we all have two noses that cycle side to side. We've emphasized that this involves a change in nasal resistance, but there's more to this story. Did you know that you alternate the sides you sleep on at night to alternate noses and breathe comfortably? Or did you know that nasal cycling is a marker for age-related nervous system changes? And did you know that your two noses can each sense different smells at the same time? Bet you didn't know that your spatial skills are better when you breathe through your left nostril and your verbal skills are better when you breathe through your right nostril? (Would you believe this book was written during right nostril breathing just to make it clearer? No. We didn't think you would.) Why there's even a reflex that can be elicited from your armpit (the crutch reflex) that makes your nose on the same side get congested. Isn't this amazing? Who nose what else could be going on?

The Masked Man's Nose

Nose masks are often used in research and clinical endeavors. Such masks must be sealed airtight against the face so that air doesn't leak around their edges. But therein lies a potential problem. How the face gets compressed beneath the edges of a mask can influence how air moves through the outer nose. Try the following. Breathe in and out through your nose to experience your usual nasal resistance to airflow. Next, touch your face below both your eyes and slowly slide that facial tissue toward the middle of your face—but don't touch your outer nose. Notice how it gets harder to breathe when you do this. How your facial tissue gets "scrunched" greatly influences your nasal resistance, even though you may not actually touch your outer nose. The same is true for how you position a mask on someone else. Be careful. Don't scrunch the facial tissue around the outer nose. Otherwise, you may raise nasal resistance to airflow.

VELOPHARYNGEAL-NASAL FUNCTION AND SPEECH PRODUCTION

The role of velopharyngeal-nasal function in speech production is to control the degree of coupling between the oral and nasal cavities and between the nasal cavities and atmosphere. For the production of oral speech sounds, the velopharyngeal valve is usually closed and aeromechanical and acoustic energies are channeled through the oral cavity (mouth). In contrast, for the production of nasal speech sounds, the velopharynx is open and aeromechanical and acoustic energies are channeled through the nasal cavities (nose).

Two aspects of speech production are influenced by the degree of coupling between the oral and nasal cavities. One is the ability to manage the airstream used to produce certain oral consonant sounds. Such management requires that the velopharynx be closed, or nearly so, and that aeromechanical energy be directed through the oral channel. The other aspect of production that is influenced by oral-nasal coupling is the ability to manage the flow of acoustic energy into the oral and nasal cavities. Such management is critical for the production of vowels and both oral and nasal consonants.

This section focuses on a series of topics pertinent to velopharyngeal-nasal function and speech production. These include consideration of function for sustained utterances and running speech activities, followed by separate discussions about the influences of gravity, development, age, and sex on velopharyngeal-nasal function in speech production.

Velopharyngeal-Nasal Function and Sustained Utterances

Sustained utterances of vowels and consonants that can be prolonged are usually produced with relatively stable configurations of the velopharyngeal-nasal apparatus. Observations are typically made of the velopharyngeal portion of the apparatus.

Velopharyngeal function for sustained vowels has been studied mainly through the use of x-ray and aeromechanical techniques. Observations have shown that the velum moves upward and backward toward the posterior pharyngeal wall in anticipation of vowel production (Bzoch, 1968; Lubker, 1968; Moll, 1962). At the same time, the lateral pharyngeal walls move inward[1] and the posterior pharyngeal wall may move forward slightly (Iglesias, Kuehn, & Morris, 1980). The velum is usually elevated maximally in its midportion during vowel production and contact with the posterior pharyngeal wall (if it occurs) is typically achieved by the third quadrant of the velum (Graber, Bzoch, & Aoba, 1959). There is also a tendency for the velum to be elevated to a higher position when sustained vowels are produced at higher vocal effort levels (Tucker, 1963).

---

[1]The suggestion has been made (Dickson & Dickson, 1972) that the *palatal levator* muscles are responsible for both elevation of the velum and inward movements of the lateral pharyngeal walls. Those in support of this suggestion contend that inward movements of the lateral pharyngeal walls occur in a region of the pharynx above the fiber course of the *superior constrictor* muscles (Honjo, Harada, & Kumazasa, 1976; Isshiki, Harita, & Kawano, 1985). A contrary viewpoint is that elevation of the velum and inward movements of the lateral pharyngeal walls are simply coordinated actions of the *palatal levator* muscles (to elevate the velum) and the *superior constrictor* muscles (to move the lateral pharyngeal walls inward). Those in support of this viewpoint contend that inward movements of the lateral pharyngeal walls occur below the velar eminence associated with insertion of the *palatal levator* muscles into the velum (Shprintzen, McCall, Skolnick, & Lenicone, 1975; Skolnick, 1970; Skolnick et al., 1973) and that the timing of movements of the velum and lateral pharyngeal walls are poorly correlated during speech production in normal individuals (Iglesias et al., 1980). We support this latter viewpoint in our description of velopharyngeal-nasal function and point the interested reader to Moon and Kuehn (2004) for further discussion on this topic.

Airtight closure of the velopharyngeal port may or may not occur during sustained vowel production. The probability of airtight closure favors high vowels (such as /i/ in peek) over low vowels (such as /ae/ in cat). For example, Moll (1962), in an x-ray motion picture study of the velopharynx in young adults, found some opening of the velopharyngeal port during less than 15% of high vowel utterances and nearly 40% of low vowel utterances.

Whether or not airtight velopharyngeal closure is achieved, high vowels and low vowels contrast in still other ways. Compared to low vowel production, high vowel production is associated with: (a) greater velar height, (b) greater extent of velopharyngeal contact with the posterior pharyngeal wall when the two surfaces are in apposition, and (c) smaller distance between the velum and the posterior pharyngeal wall when closure is not complete (Iglesias et al., 1980; Lubker, 1968; Moll, 1962). High vowel production also involves greater velopharyngeal sphincter compression (closing force) than low vowel production when velopharyngeal closure is complete (Gotto, 1977; Kuehn & Moon, 1998; Moon, Kuehn, & Huisman, 1994a; Nusbaum, Foly, & Wells, 1935). Velar height differences during sustained vowel productions are relatively strongly correlated with the electrical activity of the *palatal levator* muscles (Bell-Berti, 1976; Fritzell, 1969; Lubker, 1968). For example, Lubker found correlations ranging from .79 to .83 between the position of the velum and an estimate of the force of muscle contraction derived from electrical signals recorded from the *palatal levator* muscle. Less than perfect correlations may relate to partial influences of other muscles involved in trading relationships with the *palatal levator* muscle in velar height adjustments (Fritzell, 1969; Kuehn et al., 1982).

Two possible mechanisms have been proposed to account for the differences observed in velar height between high and low vowel productions. These are portrayed in Figure 4–22. One is that the velum elevates to different degrees because of anatomical constraints imposed through interconnections to structures below (Harrington, 1944; Kaltenborn, 1948; Lubker, 1968; Moll, 1962). Likely candidates include the *glossopalatine* and *pharyngopalatine* muscles that have originating attachments from below the velum. The *glossopalatine* muscle is considered to be the more important of the two candidates. The hypothesis is that the *glossopalatine* muscle tethers the velum so that low vowels (involving low tongue positions) restrict elevation of the velum and lead to lesser degrees of closure of the velopharyngeal port. The influence of tethering is less for high vowels (involving high tongue positions) because less restriction is placed on velar elevation.

The second proposed mechanism to account for velar height differences between high and low vowel productions has an acoustic basis. That is, it may be that the velum elevates to different degrees because of acoustic requirements involved in ensuring that the utterance is not perceived as nasal (Curtis, 1968; Lubker, 1968; Moll, 1962). This speculation is based on the results of electrical analog studies of the nasalization of vowels conducted by House and Stevens (1956), which demonstrated that less nasal coupling (velopharyngeal opening) is required to produce the auditory-perceptual judgment of nasal quality on high vowels than on low vowels. Thus, the velar height differences observed for high and low vowels could be purposive adjustments to control the degree of nasalization in the face of different tongue adjustments that influence the flow of acoustic energy through the oral and nasal cavities. In effect, the position of the tongue influences how the velopharynx must adjust to maintain the perception of non-nasal speech. Some have even argued that there are vowel-specific performance goals for the velopharynx and that differences in velopharyngeal function between high and low vowels is evidence in support of that specificity (Moon et al., 1994a, 1994b).

Sustained consonant utterances can include both oral and nasal speech sounds. Those most often studied with regard to velopharyngeal-nasal function have been fricatives, especially /s/ and /z/, and nasals /m/ and /n/. In their aeromechanical studies of nasal airflow during speech production, Thompson and Hixon (1979) and Hoit, Watson, Hixon, McMahon, and Johnson (1994) found airtight velopharyngeal closure on all sustained /s/ productions and essentially all sustained /z/ productions of 192 children and adults (ages 3 to 97 years). Airtight closure of the velopharyngeal port is clearly a priority on speech sounds that rely on the management of the oral airstream for their production. Support for this is also found in the x-ray study of Iglesias et al. (1980), wherein sustained production of /z/ had a higher velar elevation and more forward displacement of the posterior pharyngeal wall than did any of four sustained vowels that were studied.

Sustained nasal consonants are produced with large openings of the velopharyngeal port, as illustrated in Figure 4–23. The position of the velum is the same (or slightly higher) for /m/ productions (Lubker, 1968) and /n/ productions (Iglesias et al., 1980) compared to that observed for resting tidal breathing through the nose, and *palatal levator* muscle activity is not discernible (Lubker, 1968). Predictably, sustained nasal consonant productions are accompanied by substantial nasal airflow (Hoit et al., 1994; Thompson & Hixon, 1979).

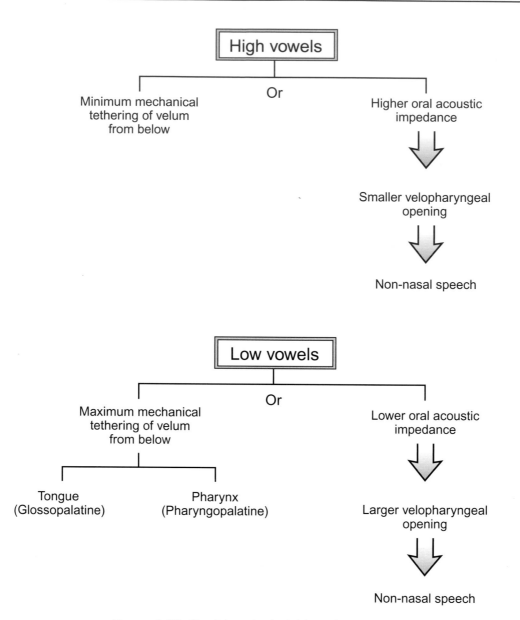

Figure 4–22. Possible velar height control mechanisms.

Activity of outer nose muscles has also been documented during sustained utterances. Lansing, Solomon, Kossev, and Andersen (1991) recorded single motor unit discharges from nasal muscles of five adults during a variety of speaking and breathing activities. They found that certain nasal motor units discharged only during speech production and not during resting tidal breathing or voluntary inspirations. Some motor units were active only during the production of sustained vowels, some during sustained nasal consonants, but none during sustained voiced fricatives. Merely thinking about the production of a speech sound did not activate these units, nor did any of them activate during solitary nonspeech movements of the breathing apparatus, larynx, tongue, or velopharynx.

Lansing et al. (1991) suggested that such nasal muscle activity is evidence that the nasal muscles assist in valving the velopharyngeal-nasal airway during speech production and that the outer nose should be considered an articulator and as part of a coordinative structure along with other components of the speech production apparatus. Two aspects of this inclusion are important. One is that the outer nose could act, along with other components of the velopharynx and the breathing apparatus, larynx, mandible (lower jaw), tongue, and lips, to control air pressures and airflows

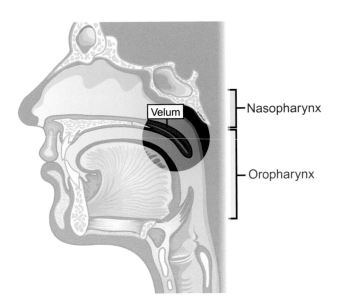

Figure 4–23. Velar position for nasal consonant production.

for speech production. The other is that the outer nose could act to change the size, shape, and stiffness of the nasal resonating cavity and its walls, thus affecting the acoustic output. The research of Lansing et al. provides convincing evidence that the outer nose is a functional component of the velopharyngeal-nasal apparatus for speech production purposes.

Velopharyngeal-Nasal Function and Running Speech Activities

Running speech activities require rapid adjustments of the velopharyngeal-nasal apparatus. A few minutes spent watching x-ray images of running speech activities reveals that velopharyngeal articulation is every bit as fast and intricate as are movements of the mandible, tongue, and lips. In fact, velar elevating and lowering gestures can each occur within a time interval of about 1/10 of a second (Kuehn, 1976). During running speech production, the velopharyngeal port closes to various degrees for oral speech sounds and opens to various degrees for nasal speech sounds. The precise pattern of opening and closing and the degree to which the velopharyngeal port is opened or closed relate to the nature of the speech sounds being spoken and the rate at which they are produced (Kent et al., 1974).

When consonants and vowels are combined as they are in running speech activities, primacy of control of the velopharyngeal-nasal apparatus is vested in consonant productions. The reason for this is that the production of many consonant elements relies heavily

on appropriate management of the airstream. Sacrificing the aeromechanical requirements of these consonants may result in sacrificing the intelligibility of speech, whereas sacrificing closure for vowel productions may increase nasalization but has only a minimal affect on speech intelligibility. Those consonant elements that rely most on aeromechanical management of the airstream are often referred to as "the pressure consonants" because they are characteristically produced with high oral air pressure and little or no velopharyngeal opening. Stop-plosive, fricative, and affricate speech sounds (see Chapter 5) are categorized as pressure consonants. In contrast, nasal consonants are produced with a low oral air pressure and a relatively wide-open velopharyngeal port.

The control of the velopharyngeal-nasal apparatus during running speech production is not simply a sequencing of separate and independent position and movement patterns for different speech sounds. To use an analogy, velopharyngeal adjustments for sequences of speech sounds are not like sequences of typewriter characters that are produced when each is called on to make an appearance (Hixon & Abbs, 1980). Rather, the position and movement patterns for two or more speech sounds may occur simultaneously, such that their productions actually overlap and intermingle. Part of this has to do with how the brain prepares in advance for velopharyngeal-nasal adjustments and

Playing by Her Own Rule

She was a young woman with a profound bilateral hearing loss. She'd received intensive behavioral therapy for imprecise articulation, but essentially no progress was being made. A puzzled speech-language pathologist made the referral. What was preventing improvement in speech? The answer was found in a recording of nasal airflow. A large burst of airflow was found to accompany each segment of speech that included a voiceless consonant. The young woman had apparently developed a production rule that said, "Only close your velopharynx for speech when your voice is on." It turned out to be a rule that could be changed by displaying nasal airflow for her to monitor on a storage oscilloscope so that she could see her rule in action and adopt a more appropriate one with some guidance. Her velopharynx cooperated and her articulation improved.

part has to do with how the mechanical-inertial properties of the velopharyngeal-nasal apparatus influence its behavior. More is said about these principles in Chapter 5.

Underlying the assembling of velopharyngeal-nasal positions and movements is the principle that consonants influence the velopharyngeal-nasal adjustments of all speech sounds (consonants and vowels) within their interval of preparation. The precise influence depends on both the type of consonant and type of vowel. For example, the preparation period for oral consonants results in smaller velopharyngeal port openings for vowels that precede them, whereas the preparation period for nasal consonants results in larger velopharyngeal port openings for vowels that precede them (Warren & DuBois, 1964). Furthermore, when a nasal consonant is preceded by two consecutive vowels, the opening of the velopharyngeal port for the nasal consonant is initiated during the production of the first vowel in the sequence (Moll & Daniloff, 1971). Even the presence of a word boundary within a sequence does not affect this observation, although velar lowering may be delayed somewhat at marked junctural boundaries (McClean, 1973). The interactions between different speech sound adjustments of the velopharyngeal-nasal apparatus condition the position and movement patterns observed such that, at any instant, the configuration of the apparatus may contain evidence of events that are coming and events that have already taken place.

Some models of velopharyngeal function have tried to account for variations in velar movement during speech production through a binary (on-off) scheme of velar function (Moll & Daniloff, 1971; Moll & Shriner, 1967). Although these models account for some of the phenomena observed in running speech activities, they do not adequately predict temporal relationships observed at the velopharyngeal-nasal periphery (Kent et al., 1974), nor do they conform to the observation that the electrical activity of muscles of the velum varies in a relatively continuous manner during speech production that correlates positively with velopharyngeal positioning (Lubker, 1968).

Adjustments of the outer nose have also been documented during running speech production in the form of single motor unit discharges from nasal muscles (Lansing et al., 1991). These motor units did not respond to large rapid, passive stretch of the skin around the mouth, cheeks, or eyes, thereby making it unlikely that the discharges during speech production were reflex responses produced by the contraction of facial muscles. Such evidence indicates that the nasal muscles play an active role in running speech production.

Some have questioned the role of the velopharyngeal apparatus as an "articulatory" structure, contending that it simply remains "on" during running speech production unless a nasal consonant or a pause occurs (Moll & Shriner, 1967). Others have contested this view and argued that the velopharynx is very much an articulator that receives its commands at the same time as do other articulatory structures (mandible, tongue, and lips), even though such commands might not always be identified as being associated with individual speech sounds (Kent et al., 1974). Now it is known that not only is the velopharynx an articulator, but so is the outer nose (Lansing et al., 1991). What remains to be known are all of the synergies between the velopharyngeal and nasal parts of the velopharyngeal-nasal apparatus.

Understandably, the study of velopharyngeal-nasal function for speech production has focused on the expiratory phase of the breathing cycle, the phase of the cycle during which speech is produced. Nevertheless, the velopharyngeal-nasal apparatus also appears to play an important role during the inspiratory phase of the speech breathing cycle. Running speech breathing usually demands quick inspirations to minimize interruptions to the flow of speech, and quick inspirations require a low resistance pathway. The best way to create such a low resistance pathway is to abduct the lips and open the velopharynx simultaneously. And this is, in fact, what people do. Thus, in contrast to resting tidal breathing, during which inspirations are typically routed through the nose exclusively, inspirations are routed through both the mouth and nose during speaking (Lester & Hoit, 2012). This not only allows for quick inspirations, but may also preserve some of the benefits of nasal inspirations, such as air filtration and humidification.

Gravity and Velopharyngeal-Nasal Function in Speech Production

Velopharyngeal-nasal function changes with changes in spatial orientation, primarily because of the influence of gravity. Each time the velopharyngeal-nasal apparatus is reoriented within a gravity field, alternate mechanical solutions are required to meet the goals for adjusting the velopharyngeal port. Reorientation in this context can result from a change in body position. For example, the usual upright (standing or seated) body position can be changed to semirecumbent, supine, prone, side-lying (left and right lateral), and head down, among others. Correspondingly, the orientation of the velopharyngeal-nasal apparatus will follow these changes.

Certain predictions can be made about the influence of body position on the velopharyngeal-nasal apparatus. These predictions are illustrated in Figure 4–24 for the upright and supine body positions. When the apparatus is in an upright position, the pull of gravity is in a direction that tends to lower the velum. This means that muscle force exerted to elevate the velum must overcome this pull, whereas muscle force exerted to lower the velum augments this pull. When in the supine body position, gravity acts to pull the velum toward the posterior pharyngeal wall and toward the nasopharynx. Thus, in supine, muscle force associated with movement of the velum toward the posterior pharyngeal wall augments the pull of gravity, and muscle force associated with moving the velum away from the posterior pharyngeal wall must overcome the pull of gravity.

Moon and Canady (1995) conducted a study of the effects of body position (and, therefore, gravity) on velopharyngeal muscle activity during speech production. They studied the activation levels (using electromyography) of the *palatal levator* and *pharyngopalatine* muscles in upright and supine body positions and hypothesized that activation would be modulated by gravitational effects. Lower peak activation levels were observed in the supine body position for the *palatal levator* muscle, suggesting that less activation was required when the pull of gravity was in the

same direction (toward the posterior pharyngeal wall). Also, the activation level of the *pharyngopalatine* muscle was usually greater in the supine body position where the pull of gravity was counter to movement of the velum away from the posterior pharyngeal wall. Overall, the observations of Moon and Canady generally support the notion that levels of muscle activity in the velum are modulated in relation to the direction of the pull of gravity, with the effect being robust in the *palatal levator* muscle.

Reorientation of the velopharyngeal-nasal apparatus in space is not restricted to changes in body position. Reorientation can also mean that the body is maintained in a fixed position and the head is moved about different axes and, thus, the spatial orientation of the velopharyngeal-nasal apparatus follows. For example, the head can be pitched about a lateral axis, rolled about a longitudinal axis, and yawed about a vertical axis. Simultaneous adjustments can also be made through more than one axis (pitching the head upward and yawing it to the right at the same time).

Rotation of the head about a lateral axis is an especially common activity that influences the spatial orientation of the velopharyngeal-nasal apparatus (nod your head yes to this statement). Full flexion and full extension of the neck (head rotated forward and backward, respectively) delimit the range of possible orientations associated with head rotation. Rotation through this

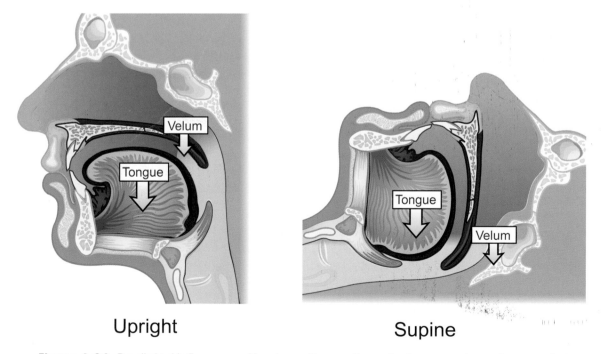

Upright　　　　　　　　　**Supine**

Figure 4–24. Predicted influences of body position on the velopharyngeal-nasal apparatus.

range places maximally contrasting gravitational forces on the velopharyngeal-nasal apparatus, especially the velum. When the head is rotated downward from its usual position (toward a position where the mandible would rest on the rib cage wall), the pull of gravity on the velum is in a direction that tends to pull it away from the posterior pharyngeal wall. In contrast, when the head is rotated upward from its usual position (toward a position where the tip of the nose is maximally elevated), the pull of gravity on the velum is in a direction that tends to pull it toward the posterior pharyngeal wall. Whereas reorientation of the velopharyngeal-nasal apparatus is not noticeable to most people, it may have a profound effect on those with borderline velopharyngeal competence. For example, in someone with a neuromotor-based weakness of the *palatal levator* muscles, rotation of the head upward may enhance movement of the velum toward the posterior pharyngeal wall and, thereby, improve velopharyngeal-nasal function for speech production. In contrast, rotation of the head downward may do just the opposite.

Finally, gravitational influences are not limited to the velopharyngeal portion of the velopharyngeal-nasal apparatus. Reorientation also affects the function of the nasal cavities. For example, it has been shown that nasal patency decreases and nasal airway resistance increases in downright as compared to upright body positions (Rudcrantz, 1969). This change in patency appears to relate to vascular changes, including increases in stroke volume, cardiac minute volume, and blood pressure associated with the assumption of downright body positions. This is followed by a baroreceptor-mediated reflex that evokes a depression in blood pressure via a decrease in heart rate and the dilation of the peripheral blood vessels (Detweiler, 1973). Such dilation in the nasal region leads to engorgement (swelling) of the nasal mucosa, reduced nasal patency, and increased nasal airway resistance. Also, because the nasal region is positioned above the heart in upright body positions and at the same level or below the heart in downright body positions, regional blood pressure changes. A higher blood pressure in downright body positions causes the blood vessels in the nasal mucosa to dilate and nasal congestion to increase (Hiyama, Ono, Ishiwata, & Kuroda, 2002).

Development of Velopharyngeal-Nasal Function in Speech Production

The infant's velopharyngeal-nasal apparatus is not just a small version of the adult's apparatus, but differs in its configuration and in its spatial relationships to surrounding structures. Several anatomical features and developmental changes in those features are relevant to how the velopharyngeal-nasal apparatus functions in infants and children (see Chapter 5 for further discussion of the development of upper airway structures).

At birth, the larynx is located high within the neck and the velum and epiglottis are approximated (Kent & Murray, 1982). Around 4 to 6 months of age, the velum and epiglottis separate (Sasaki, Levine, Laitman, & Crelin, 1977) as the larynx moves from the level of the first cervical vertebra to the level of the third cervical vertebra. This downward movement is accomplished primarily by rapid growth of the pharynx in the vertical dimension from about 4 cm in the newborn pharynx (Crelin, 1973) to approximately three times that length in the adult (Sasaki et al., 1977). During that same period, the hard and soft palates grow quickly, with the hard palate growing somewhat more quickly than the soft palate and the growth rate of both becoming more gradual after 2 years of age (Vorperian et al., 2005). These developmental changes affect the geometry and mechanical effectiveness of certain muscles. For example, as the palates grow, the orientation of the paired *palatal levator* muscles change in ways that improve their mechanical advantage for elevating the velum (Fletcher, 1973a). Another anatomical modification that can be important to velopharyngeal-nasal function is that the nasopharyngeal tonsils (the "adnoids") increase in size during infancy and childhood (Jaw, Sheu, Liu, & Lin, 1999) and then shrink during the teenage years (Subtelny & Koepp-Baker, 1956).

Because the infant velum and epiglottis are approximated early in life, it is often assumed that infants are obligate nasal breathers. However, this is not true. The preponderance of evidence indicates that most infants can breathe through the mouth when necessary. Specifically, when the anterior nares are occluded, healthy infants open the mouth and use the oral airway for breathing (Miller et al., 1985; Rodenstein, Perlmutter, & Stanescu, 1985). Therefore, the term preferential nasal breather is more appropriate to describe the predominant (rather than exclusive) use of the nasal airway for breathing in infants.

The birth cry is the first utterance for most human newborns. X-ray images of this first utterance have shown that it is made with an open velopharynx (Bosma, Truby, & Lind, 1965). Acoustic and perceptual studies of infant vocalizations during the first few months of life have suggested that the velopharynx continues to be open during cry (Wasz-Hockert, Lind, Vuorenkoski, Partanen, & Valanne, 1964) and noncry vocalizations (Buhr, 1980; Hsu, Fogel, & Cooper, 2000; Kent & Murray; 1982; Oller, 1986) up to about 4 months of age, and that the velopharynx probably closes for oral sound production sometime between 4 and 6 months of age.

However, aeromechanical data provided by Thom, Hoit, Hixon, and Smith (2006) and Bunton, Gallagher, and Hoit (2012) suggest that velopharyngeal closure for oral sound production occurs later in an infant's development.

Thom et al. (2006) studied six infants longitudinally from 2 to 6 months of age using a double-barreled nasal cannula to sense ram air pressure at the anterior nares. This device made it possible to determine the binary (open or closed) status of the velopharyngeal port during vocalization. The results showed that the velopharynx was usually open for precry windups, whimpers, and laughs, and closed for cries, screams, and raspberries at all ages studied. For nondistress vowel and syllable utterances, velopharyngeal closure increased with age, but was not complete and still undergoing development at 6 months of age (the highest age studied). Bunton et al. (2012) have continued this line of work and have shown that velopharyngeal closure for nondistress utterances occurs more frequently during the second 6 months of life than during the first 6 months, but that there is substantial variability among infants. They have also shown that the frequency of velopharyngeal closure may be conditioned by nature of the sounds being produced.

It is interesting to note that, although velopharyngeal closure for nondistress utterance is still undergoing development during the first year, infants as young as 2 months can (and do) close the velopharynx at least occasionally for nondistress utterances. Why, then, do they not consistently close the velopharynx for nondistress utterances from that time on? It is probably because velopharyngeal closure is not necessarily required for vowel production, and vowels are by far the most prevalent speech-related utterances generated by infants. Perhaps the emerging use of consonants that require high oral pressure or the purposive use of words on a regular basis constitute the critical factors influencing the consistent use of airtight velopharyngeal closure. Some evidence for this exists (Bunton et al., 2012).

More is known about velopharyngeal-nasal function during speech production in children age 3 years and older. Thompson and Hixon (1979) used nasal airflow to study the development of velopharyngeal-nasal function in children ranging in age from 3 to 18 years. Nasal airflow was found to be zero (indicating a closed velopharynx) for all of the oral utterances (simple vowels and vowel-consonant-vowel combinations) in 91 of the 92 children studied. One child, in retrospect, appeared to exhibit consonant-specific nasal airflow.

A study of velopharyngeal function in older children, 6 to 16 years, was conducted by Zajac (2000). The phonemes /m/ and /p/ were the focus of his investigation as they occurred in different syllable, word, and sentence contexts. Measurements were made of oral air pressure, nasal air pressure, and nasal airflow, and calculations were carried out to determine the minimum cross-sectional area of the velopharyngeal port for different speech segments. He interpreted his findings to be consistent with the observations of Thompson and Hixon (1979), indicating that essentially airtight velopharyngeal closure is to be expected for oral speech sounds, and significant opening of the velopharyngeal port is to be expected for nasal speech sounds regardless of age.

Aeromechanical studies have also considered the temporal characteristics of velopharyngeal-nasal function associated with speech production in children (Leeper, Tissington, & Munhall, 1998; Zajac, 2000; Zajac & Hackett, 2002). These studies have collectively considered children ranging from 3 to 16 years of age. The speech samples most often studied were nasal consonant-stop consonant combinations, which required rapid transitions between velopharyngeal opening and velopharyngeal closure. Leeper et al. reported a tendency toward shorter durations in temporal variables with increasing age, but with the children generally performing similarly to the adults studied by Warren, Dalston, Trier, and Holder (1985). Subsequently, Zajac and then Zajac and Hackett reported dissimilarities between the performances of children and adults based on their analyses. Specifically, they found differences in patterns of timing in the aeromechanical segments of speech produced by children and adults, with adults exhibiting shorter segments and less temporal variability than children.

Although airtight velopharyngeal closure is used early in childhood for oral speech sound production, the means for achieving this closure may change across childhood. One example relates to children who develop enlarged lymphoid tissue masses in the nasopharyngeal tonsils ("adenoids"). As mentioned above, these tonsils typically grow during the first decade of life and then begin to atrophy (Subtelny & Koepp-Baker, 1956), until by adulthood they have fully atrophied. Against this background of events, illustrated in Figure 4–25, velopharyngeal closure must go through a slow reorganization in those children who have been accomplishing closure through abutment of the velum and walls of the pharynx against the enlarged adenoidal tissue. This accommodation is obviously successful given the continuation of airtight velopharyngeal closure during the normal developmental schedule, but it may be interrupted if an adenoidectomy is performed in a child who is at risk for velopharyngeal problems (Andreassen, Leeper, MacRae, & Nicholson, 1994; Morris, 1975).

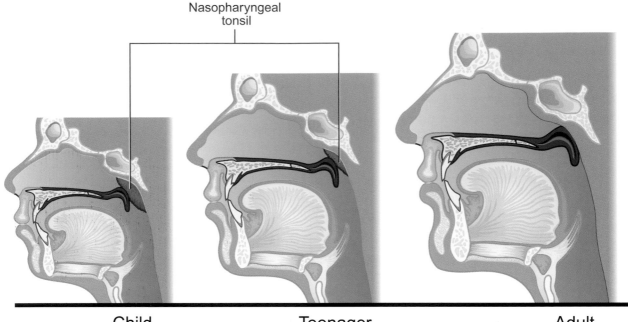

Figure 4–25. Velopharyngeal accommodation to nasopharyngeal tonsil mass.

When Is a Bad Nose Good and a Good Nose Bad?

This chapter stresses the functional unity of the normal velopharyngeal-nasal apparatus. This unity is often even better illustrated in an abnormal velopharyngeal-nasal apparatus. Not all speakers with significant velopharyngeal openings during oral consonant productions are destined to exhibit significant speech problems. With the velopharynx and nose being in mechanical series (being in line), an abnormally blocked nose may actually counteract an abnormally opened velopharynx. That is, a bad nose can be a good thing for speech, even if not for breathing. Conversely, a good nose can be a bad thing for speech when there is significant velopharyngeal impairment. The surgeon who attempts to "clean up" a bad nose and does not take into account the status of the velopharynx will sometimes figure this out after the fact when confronted with a child whose speech is worse after surgery.

Age and Velopharyngeal-Nasal Function in Speech Production

Aging affects the mature velopharyngeal-nasal apparatus as it does other parts of the body. Some age-related changes in the velopharyngeal-nasal apparatus include that the pharyngeal muscles weaken with age and the pharyngeal lumen enlarges (Zaino & Benventano, 1977), sensory innervation declines (Aviv et al., 1994), and muscle bulk and bone density decrease in this region and elsewhere (Fremont & Hoyland, 2007). Such changes would seem to have the potential to alter velopharyngeal-nasal function for activities such as speech production.

Four studies have provided information pertaining to aging of the mature velopharyngeal-nasal apparatus and speech production. Two of these made acoustic measurements and two made aeromechanical measurements.

Hutchinson, Robinson, and Nerbonne (1978) were the first to examine the potential influence of age on velopharyngeal-nasal function in speech production by making measurements of nasalance, an acoustic measurement of the quotient of nasal sound pressure level to nasal + oral sound pressure level. They studied a group of men and women ranging in age from 50 to 80 years and compared their data to those obtained from a group of men and women ranging in age from 18 to 38 years studied earlier by Fletcher (1973b). Data were collected on three different reading tasks and a sustained vowel, but only a reading passage containing all oral speech sounds revealed differences between the older and younger groups. Specifically, the older group exhibited higher average nasalance values than the younger group. Hutchinson et al. interpreted this finding as evidence that velopharyngeal function for speech production deteriorates with age such that older individuals demonstrate velopharyngeal incompetence.

Additional nasalance data bearing on this topic are embedded in a study of dialect differences reported by Seaver, Dalston, Leeper, and Adams (1991) of men and women ranging in age from 16 to 63 years. As part of their analysis, they correlated age with nasalance values for the same oral reading passage found by Hutchinson et al. (1978) to reveal a difference in nasalance values between older and younger groups. The resulting correlation indicated that age accounted for less than 10% of the variance in nasalance, and therefore did not support the earlier conclusion of Hutchinson et al.

In an aeromechanical approach was taken by Hoit et al. (1994) to determine the influence of age on velopharyngeal-nasal function during speech production. Specifically, they obtained measures of nasal airflow from men and women ranging in age from 22 to 97 years during sustained productions and vowel-consonant-vowel productions. Only very rarely were productions accompanied by nasal airflow (except those containing nasal consonants), indicating that in almost all cases the velopharynx was closed for oral sound production. Previous studies, most of which had focused on young adults, had also reported zero or minimal nasal airflow for similar types of utterances (Andreassen, Smith, & Guyette, 1992; Lubker, 1973; Lubker & Moll, 1965; Thompson & Hixon, 1979; Warren & DuBois, 1964). Hoit et al. noted that even on those few occasions when nasal airflow was observed during oral utterances, the magnitude of the flow was low. By entering such airflow values along with estimated transnasal air pressure values (taken from Arkebauer, Hixon, & Hardy, 1967) into the equation developed by Warren and Dubois (1964), Hoit et al. were able to estimate the minimal cross-sectional area of the velopharyngeal port as being less than 2 mm² and similar to area calculations reported by others for young adult speakers for occasional oral utterances that did not involve airtight velopharyngeal closure (Andreassen et al., 1992; Warren, 1964; Warren & DuBois, 1964). As expected, Hoit et al. routinely observed nasal airflow on nasal utter-

ances and on most vowel productions within nasal consonant environments, with flow magnitudes being similar to those reported by previous investigators for comparable utterance tasks (Andreassen et al., 1992; Lubker, 1973; Thompson & Hixon, 1979). Again, by entering flow values along with estimated transnasal air pressure values (taken this time from Andreassen et al.) into the Warren and DuBois (1964) equation, Hoit et al. estimated the minimal cross-sectional area of the velopharyngeal port during nasal utterances was in the range of 20 to 30 mm². The overall findings of Hoit et al. led to the conclusion that velopharyngeal function for speech production does not change with age, a conclusion that gained additional purchase when the research of Zajac (1997) is considered.

Zajac (1997) studied a group of younger adults (18 to 37 years) and older adults (68 to 83 years) using measures of oral air pressure, nasal air pressure, and nasal airflow during utterances that included repetitions of oral syllable productions and a word that contained oral and nasal sounds. He found that the data of the older adults resembled those of the younger adults and that neither group showed signs of velopharyngeal incompetence. Zajac concluded that his findings were in agreement with those of Hoit et al. (1994) and confirmed that airtight (or essentially airtight) velopharyngeal closure is to be expected in older speakers.

What could explain the lack of agreement between the conclusions of Hutchinson et al. (1978) — that velopharyngeal function for speech production deteriorates with age — and those of Hoit et al. (1994) and Zajac (1997) — that such function does not change with age? One possible explanation is that measures of nasalance do not necessarily reflect velopharyngeal function per se, but can be influenced by other factors that happen to change with age. For example, Hoit et al. have suggested that confounding variables could include: (a) an increase in the sympathetic transfer of acoustic energy from the oral cavity to the nasal cavities attendant to changes in the density of palatal structures with age (Tomoda, Morii, Yamashita, & Kumazawa, 1984), (b) a change in the spectral content of speech sounds associated with known age-related decreases in vocal tract formant frequencies (Endres, Bambach, & Flosser, 1967), and (c) the use of smaller mouth openings during oral utterances by older individuals that would be consistent with differences in characteristic mandibular movement in older compared to younger individuals (Karlsson & Carlsson, 1990). That is, it is quite possible that a senescent person could demonstrate elevated nasalance values, even when the velopharynx is closed airtight.

Thus, two conclusions can be drawn. There is no credible evidence that velopharyngeal-nasal function

He's an Old Smoothie

He was a distinguished looking white-haired grandfather. He agreed to serve as a person to be examined by graduate students learning to administer an examination for velopharyngeal-nasal function. Students had been assigned different parts of the examination and told to practice the administration of their part on at least half a dozen people so they could get "calibrated." One student who had dutifully practiced on a group of her peers, proceeded to ask the gentleman to open his mouth while she turned on a flashlight and looked in. She methodically looked at structures and made comments to the class as she went along. When she shined the light on the gentleman's hard palate, she paused briefly and said to him, "That's the smoothest hard palate I've ever seen." He smiled and said back, "That's a denture, young lady." And so it was. He took it out and showed it to the class. The moral of this story is don't just practice on your classmates.

for speech production becomes incompetent with advanced age and credible evidence that it does not. And measures of nasalance do not provide meaningful data for examining the influence of age on velopharyngeal function for speech production.

Sex and Velopharyngeal-Nasal Function in Speech Production

Sex makes a difference when it comes to the size of the velopharyngeal-nasal apparatus. For example, men, when compared to women, have longer pharynges (Fitch & Giedd, 1999), longer *palatal levator* muscles (Bae, Kuehn, Sutton, Conway, & Perry, 2011; Ettema, Kuehn, Perlman, & Alperin, 2002), longer hard palates (Bae et al. 2011), larger soft palates (Kuehn & Kahane, 1990), and longer noses (Zankl, Eberle, Molinari, & Schinzel, 2002). But do these differences influence velopharyngeal-nasal function for speech production? This question has been considered in several studies of adult speakers.

McKerns and Bzoch (1970) addressed this question through the study of lateral x-ray motion picture images of velopharyngeal movement associated with oral speech production in young men and women. The authors observed that the orientation of the velar

eminence to the uvula was an acute angle (hooklike) for men and a right angle (squared-off) for women. Detailed analysis showed that: (a) velar elevation was twice as high for men as for women, (b) the lower point of contact between the velum and posterior pharyngeal wall was above the palatal plane for men and below that plane for women, (c) the extent of contact between the velum and the posterior pharyngeal wall was half as much for men as for women, and (d) the uvula was angled much farther away from the posterior pharyngeal wall in men than in women. The authors speculated that the observed differences between the sexes could result from differences in the points of insertion of the *palatal levator, glossopalatine,* or *pharyngopalatine* muscles related to differences in skull size, orientation of the skull to the vertebral column, or oral and pharyngeal dimensions.

Kuehn (1976) provided data on velar movement trajectory differences during speech production between one young man and one young woman using lateral x-ray high-speed motion picture images. Utterances contained oral and nasal speech sounds produced at different rates. Kuehn found that the velar movement trajectory for the man was linear and formed an angle with the hard palate of approximately 60°. In contrast, the velar movement trajectory for the woman, although also linear, formed an angle with the hard palate that was less steep, approximately 50°.

Iglesias et al. (1980) studied positions of the velum, posterior pharyngeal wall, and lateral pharyngeal walls during speech production in young men and women using lateral-view and frontal-view x-ray images. Men with large head sizes and skull densities were excluded from participation because excessive radiation dosages would have been required to obtain films of acceptable quality. Five variables were evaluated during productions of oral and nasal speech sounds in different contexts: (a) displacement of the velum, (b) displacement of the posterior pharyngeal wall, (c) displacement of the lateral pharyngeal walls, (d) width of the pharynx at rest, and (e) angular trajectory of displacement of the velar eminence. No differences were found between the sexes for any of the variables. The authors noted that their findings were not consistent with those of McKerns and Bzoch (1970) and offered that their exclusion of men with large head sizes (and large velopharyngeal structures) may have resulted in the study of a less representative group of men and the obscuring of any on-average differences between the sexes.

Seaver and Kuehn (1980) conducted a study of velar position during speech production in men and women using lateral x-ray high-speed motion picture images of the velum and electrical recordings of the *palatal levator, glossopalatine*, and *pharyngopalatine* muscles. Utterances contained different oral speech sounds produced at different efforts and rates. Data plots were used to obtain information about the relations among: (a) height of the velum, (b) muscle activity of the *palatal levator, glossopalatine*, and *pharyngopalatine* muscles, and (c) height of the tongue and time delays associated with movement of the velum. The authors found that the height of the velum most strongly correlated with the height of the tongue in men and with the activity of the *pharyngopalatine* muscle in women. The authors suggested that their data did not support the general conclusions reached by McKerns and Bzoch (1970).

The nasal airflow study of Thompson and Hixon (1979) described above included some young adults. Their data indicated no sex-related differences in nasal airflow, with one exception: women were more likely to exhibit nasal airflow at the midpoint of vowels preceding nasal consonants. However, subsequent studies have not replicated this observation (Hoit et al. 1994; Zajac & Mayo, 1996).

Another aeromechanical study of young men and women, conducted by Andreassen and colleagues (1992), included simultaneous recordings of oral-nasal differential air pressure and nasal airflow, from which they calculated the minimum cross-sectional area of the velopharyngeal port for productions of oral and nasal speech sounds in different contexts. No sex differences were found for oral-nasal differential air pressure for any of the utterances studied. Significant group differences were found between the sexes for nasal airflow and the calculated minimum cross-sectional area of the velopharyngeal port, but only in the context of the utterance of the word *hamper*. In this context, the airflow and area determinations for men exceeded those for women, as would be predicted given differences in airway size between the sexes.

The nasal airflow study by Hoit et al. (1994), discussed in the previous section, included men and women of different ages and productions of oral and nasal speech sounds in different contexts. As expected, nasal airflow values were higher during nasal consonant productions for men than women due to airway size differences. However, results of eight temporal measurements showed no differences between the sexes. Hoit et al. interpreted their data to show that there was no evidence of a velopharyngeal function difference between men and women.

Zajac and Mayo (1996) conducted an investigation of aeromechanical and temporal features of velopharyngeal function during speech production in young men and women, in which they measured oral air pressure, nasal air pressure, and nasal airflow and determined nasal air volume and minimum cross-sectional area of the velopharyngeal port during productions of the word *hamper*. They found that, out of 10 aeromechanical measurements made, the only sex-related difference was that men had higher oral air pressures associated with /p/ productions, on average. Of the 15 temporal measurements made, men and women differed only with regard to how rapidly oral air pressure rose to its peak value in association with /p/ productions. Zajac and Mayo concluded that velopharyngeal function is similar in men and women, at least in terms of aeromechanical and temporal events.

Zajac (1997) studied senescent men and women and compared their data to those from the young adults of Zajac and Mayo (1996). Using the same measurements and procedures as Zajac and Mayo, Zajac found that men used higher oral air pressure than women at all ages. He also found that men and women exhibited different patterns of nasal air volume as a function of word position, supporting a possible sex-specific velopharyngeal declination effect. Declination in this context means a systematic increase in the minimum cross-sectional area of the velopharyngeal port as a function of utterance length (nasalization increases as utterance proceeds). Zajac cautioned that the effect observed was quite small. Bzoch (1968), in an x-ray

---

Lubker Bumps

Scientists often name phenomena for those who were first to describe them or figure out what they meant. In this regard, the inauguration of the term "Lubker Bumps" seems long overdue. Most who have studied velopharyngeal-nasal function using aeromechanical techniques have encountered very small variations in nasal airflow (usually oscillating around zero airflow) when the velopharynx is closed airtight. These variations, as described by James F. Lubker, result from movements of the velum up and down within a closed velopharynx, acting like a piston in a cylinder to push very small quantities of air in and out of the nasopharynx. The nasal airflow tracings that characterize such piston movements show tiny bumps up and down around zero airflow that reflect true airflows, but ones not generated by the passage of air through the velopharynx. Lubker's reputation deserves to be bumped up a notch for his astute observation.

study of velopharyngeal function in relation to syllable order in a long utterance sequence, also failed to find any evidence of a potential declination effect.

What can be concluded from this collage of findings, some of them contradictory and some of them restricted to only certain types of observations? The evidence indicates that men and women differ in certain details of velopharyngeal-nasal function in speech production, but it is not clear that these differences make a difference functionally or in their application to clinical concerns (McWilliams, Morris, & Shelton, 1990).

MEASUREMENT OF VELOPHARYNGEAL-NASAL FUNCTION

This section considers the instrumental measurement of velopharyngeal-nasal function. Focus is on selected methods that have application to the study of both normal function and function encountered in individuals with velopharyngeal-nasal disorders. Four categories of methods are highlighted. These enable measurements to be obtained from observations made through: (a) visual, (b) x-ray, (c) aeromechanical, and (d) acoustic means.

Direct Visualization

Direct visualization can be made of the outer nose, nasal cavities, velum, and pharyngeal walls. The outer nose and the vestibules of the nasal cavities can be seen with the naked eye under suitable light. The undersurface of the velum and part of the posterior pharyngeal wall can also be visualized through the oral cavity and faucial isthmus with suitable light. Other structures can be visualized using endoscopes.

As discussed in Chapter 3, endoscopes are optical instruments encased in fiberoptic conduits that can be passed through either the mouth or nose and positioned to reveal targeted internal structures. A flexible endoscope passed through the nose is the most common way of examining velopharyngeal-nasal structures (see Figure 3–50). When the distal end of the endoscope is positioned above the velum within the nasopharynx, structures of the nasopharynx and the velopharyngeal port can be visualized (Wilson, Kudryk, & Sych, 1986). The images obtained are often considered qualitatively to make global judgments about the nature of structure and function and their adequacies. Procedures have also been developed to quantify nasoendoscopic images of velopharyngeal-nasal structure and function (D'Antonio, Marsh, Province, Muntz, & Phillips, 1989; Karnell, Linville, & Edwards, 1988).

X-Ray Imaging

X-ray imaging provides shadow-cast views of the structures of the velopharyngeal-nasal apparatus through the use of ionizing radiation. The velopharyngeal-nasal apparatus is, of course, a three-dimensional structure and a complete image of its adjustments can only be revealed through the use of multiple angles. Most imaging, however, is done at the midline in what is referred to as a lateral (sagittal) view. Velopharyngeal-nasal structures are shown in such a view in Figure 4–26.

X-ray imaging of velopharyngeal-nasal structures may involve single-shot exposures in which an instant during a sustained utterance is captured (Hixon, 1949) or they may involve continuous running images in which the events of continuous speech production are viewed. The latter can be visualized on a fluoroscope or recorded through cinefluoroscopy (Moll, 1962), videofluoroscopy (McWilliams & Girdany, 1964), or through other digital recording means. X-ray imaging can also be done in other than lateral views, although the technical requirements are greater. These include frontal views that enable imaging of the lateral pharyngeal walls (Kuehn & Dolan, 1975) and multiple views that enable imaging of the velopharyngeal apparatus in lateral, frontal, and base projections (Skolnick, 1970).

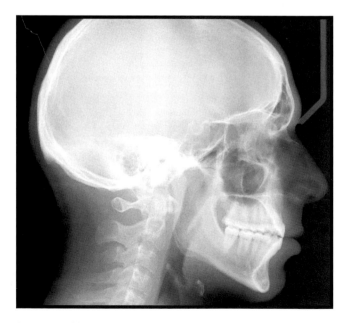

Figure 4-26. Lateral x-ray image of the velopharyngeal-nasal apparatus and other structures of the head and neck. From *Speech and voice science* (p. 266), by A. Behrman, 2007, San Diego, CA: Plural Publishing, Inc. Copyright 2007 by Plural Publishing, Inc. Image provided courtesy of David A. Behrman, D.M.D., Weill Cornell Medical Center, New York, NY. Reproduced with permission.

Don't Put Things in Your Ears

Cinefluorographic (motion picture x-ray) studies of velopharyngeal function require that the head be stabilized. Part of the instrumentation for doing this includes ear rods that fit in the ear canals (like sticking your index fingers in your ears). People aren't eager to try to turn their heads with these in place. We had occasion to see a person fall victim to a sequencing problem when a demonstration about cinefluorography was ending. The lecturer was distracted by a question and stepped on a pedal to lower a hydraulic chair in which this person was sitting before taking out the ear rods (which were bolted to the wall). It was then that the person in the chair discovered a previously unreported reflex called "grab the stabilizer frame, support your weight, and scream at the lecturer." It was do that or be hanged by your ear canals. There are two morals to this story. Don't put things in your ears and don't put things in your ears.

Aeromechanical Observations

Aeromechanical methods can provide information about the binary status of the velopharyngeal-nasal apparatus (whether it is open or closed), the sizes of different minimum cross-sectional areas, and the magnitudes of opposition to airflow through different parts of the apparatus. This is done through the measurement of airflow and/or air pressure.

Nasal airflow is a useful index for determining if the velopharynx is open or closed (Thompson & Hixon, 1979). Such airflow is usually sensed with a pneumotachometer attached to a nasal mask, as illustrated in Figure 4–27. The presence of nasal airflow during speech production indicates an open velopharynx, whereas the absence of nasal airflow during speech production indicates a closed velopharynx.

Another simple way to determine whether the velopharynx is open or closed involves monitoring nasal ram air pressure, an approach first used in a study of velopharyngeal development in infants (Thom et al., 2006). The approach requires the use of a double-barreled nasal cannula connected to a sensitive pressure transducer. Positive nasal ram pressure during

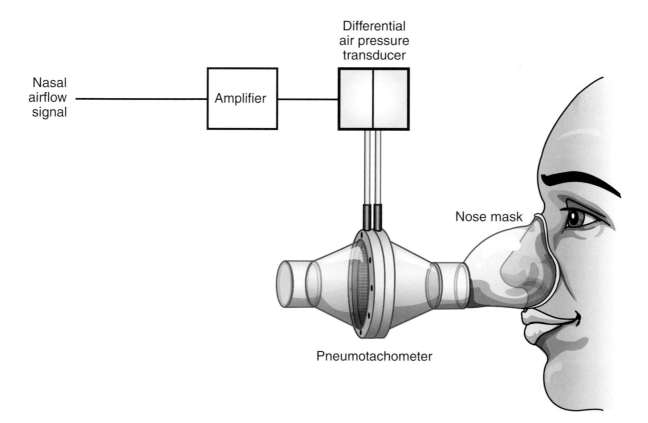

Figure 4-27. Instrumentation for measuring nasal airflow.

sound production indicates an open the velopharynx, and an atmospheric (zero) pressure during sound production indicates a closed velopharynx. This technique is easy to use and comfortable (Bunton, Hoit, & Gallagher, 2011), even for infants and toddlers, as shown in Figure 4–28.

A pressure-flow technique that is often used to calculate the minimum cross-sectional area of the velopharyngeal port during continuous speech production (Warren & DuBois, 1964) is depicted in Figure 4–29. Oral and nasal air pressures are recorded along with nasal airflow. The difference in air pressure across the velopharyngeal port and the rate of air movement through it are determined and entered into a working equation that yields the minimum cross-sectional area of the velopharyngeal port at each moment. Computer manipulations permit the prevailing size of the velopharyngeal port to be monitored continuously. Although some have proposed that nasal airflow alone is a useful measure of the degree of velopharyngeal opening (Quigley, Shiere, Webster, & Cobb, 1964), this is only true when the size of the velopharyngeal opening is small. As demonstrated by Warren (1967), the relation of nasal airflow to velopharyngeal opening is linear at small velopharyngeal orifice sizes, but the correlation between the two variables decreases as the size of the velopharyngeal orifice increases.

Pressure-flow recordings also can be used to calculate the resistance offered by the airway to the flow of air into and out of the velopharyngeal-nasal apparatus (Warren et al., 1969). Different approaches are used to partition the resistance among different segments of the apparatus (Cole & Havas, 1980). Resistance across any segment of interest is calculated from the ratio of the air pressure difference across the segment to the rate of air movement through it. Resistance values are airflow-dependent, so comparisons of resistance values are usually made at standard airflow values (Allison & Leeper, 1990).

Acoustic Observations

Speech is the acoustic product of speech production and certain acoustic observations can inform about the status of the velopharyngeal-nasal apparatus. Several acoustic approaches are available, two of which are emphasized here for illustrative purposes. Much more is said about acoustic analysis in Chapter 10.

Sound spectrography has been applied to speech events to make inferences about velopharyngeal-nasal function. The general notion underlying the use of sound spectrography is that the speech signal changes with varying degrees of velopharyngeal-nasal and pharyngeal-oral coupling and these changes can be seen in the resultant spectrogram (Curtis, 1968; Fant, 1960; Hattori, Yamamoto, & Fujimura, 1958). For example, nasalized vowels differ from nonnasalized vow-

Out Your Nose Like a Garden Hose

Some think that airflow from the nose is a measure of velopharyngeal port size. It's true that nasal airflow depends on velopharyngeal port size, but it also depends on things like the size of the nostrils and the driving pressure of the breathing apparatus. Observing airflow from the nose is like watching water flow from the end of a garden hose that is being controlled by a friend around a blind corner. Your friend may be adjusting the faucet (changing the driving pressure) or adjusting the hose (changing its cross-section). We'll exclude the possibility that you're using your thumb to adjust the "nostril" of the hose. Different actions of your friend can make the flow of water change at your end of the hose, but you can't be sure what those actions are. The same is true of airflow from the nose. It can go up or down and you don't know why. It could be because of a single adjustment or a combination of adjustments. Be safe. Don't go with the flow.

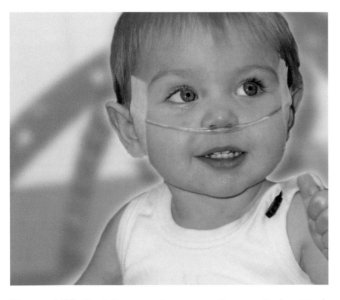

Figure 4-28. Toddler wearing a nasal cannula for monitoring nasal ram air pressure.

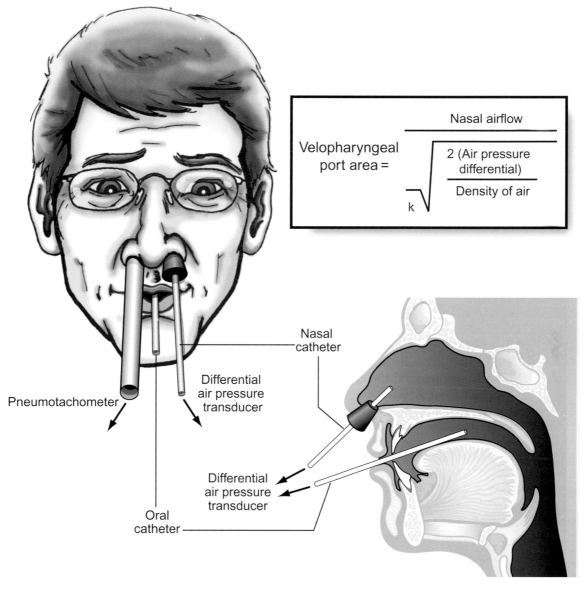

$$\text{Velopharyngeal port area} = k\sqrt{\dfrac{\dfrac{\text{Nasal airflow}}{2\,(\text{Air pressure differential})}}{\text{Density of air}}}$$

Nasal catheter

Differential air pressure transducer

Pneumotachometer

Differential air pressure transducer

Oral catheter

Figure 4–29. Pressure-flow technique for determining velopharyngeal port size.

els in that their spectrographic patterns include: (a) an absence of sound energy at certain frequencies within the sound spectrum, (b) a reduction of overall sound energy and a corresponding reduction in specific resonant (formant) peaks, (c) a broadening of the effective bandwidths around specific formant peaks, and (d) the introduction of resonances that are otherwise not present. Nasalization makes it more difficult to differentiate among vowels acoustically and spectrographic analyses sometimes help to disambiguate nasalized utterances that perplex the listener (Kent, Liss, & Philips, 1989).

Probably the most widely used acoustic approach applied to velopharyngeal-nasal function is nasalance

(Fletcher, 1976). Nasalance is an acoustic measurement based on the relative distribution of sound energy emanating from the mouth and nose. It is an expression of the root mean square amplitude of the nasal speech signal expressed as a percentage of the root mean square amplitude of the nasal and oral speech signals combined. As illustrated in Figure 4–30, the oral and nasal speech signals are recorded by separate microphones positioned on the two sides of an acoustic baffle placed between the outer nose and upper lip.

Nasalance measurements are typically taken during the production of speech samples that are loaded to different degrees with nasal consonants and comparisons

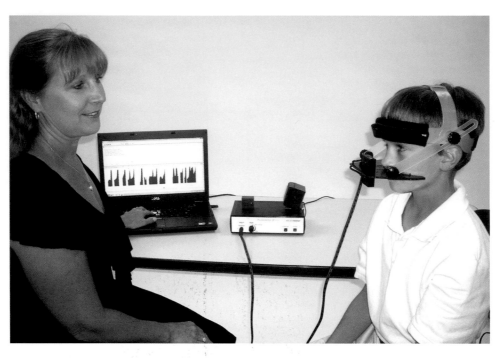

Figure 4–30. Photograph of a young boy and his clinician using instrumentation to measure nasalance. Image provided courtesy of KayPENTAX, Montvale, NJ. Reproduced with permission.

are made to databases on individuals with known velopharyngeal competence (Awan, 2001; Seaver et al., 1991). Although devices that provide information on nasalance are popular and widely used, the defined quantity itself is not a measure of velopharyngeal function given that factors other than velopharyngeal opening influence the distribution of acoustic energy between the mouth and nose (Curtis, 1968; Fant, 1960; House & Stevens, 1956).

VELOPHARYNGEAL-NASAL DISORDERS AND SPEECH PRODUCTION

Velopharyngeal-nasal disorders come in many forms and can impair speech production to different degrees. People of all ages can be affected by velopharyngeal-nasal disorders and the reasons for their disorders may have functional and/or organic bases.

Functional disorders do not have known physical causes. Such disorders exist despite the presence of an apparently capable velopharyngeal-nasal apparatus. Functional disorders are usually associated with a failure to achieve velopharyngeal closure. This may be a pervasive problem in which closure is not attained

on any speech sounds. Or it may be a more specific problem in which closure is not attained on certain oral speech sounds. For example, a child may present with a pattern in which /s/ is the only oral speech sound in which velopharyngeal incompetence is demonstrated. The /s/ in this case may be generated imprecisely, at lower than usual loudness, with audible nasal emission, and with nares constriction as a compensatory mechanism. The class of disorders to which this example belongs is called "phoneme-specific nasal emission" and sometimes masquerades as a more common developmental articulation disorder.

Velopharyngeal-nasal disorders of organic origin are those that have identifiable physical causes. Such disorders can include congenital, developmental, or acquired deformities of the velopharyngeal-nasal apparatus. An example is congenital cleft of the hard and/or soft palates and/or upper lip in which there is a separation between parts of the velopharyngeal-nasal apparatus that are normally joined at the midline. A photograph of an infant with a complete right unilateral cleft lip and palate is shown in Figure 4–31. Another example is submucous cleft of the hard palate in which unfused shelves of the hard palate are hidden from view by a covering of mucosal tissue. Other deformities may present as excesses or insuffi-

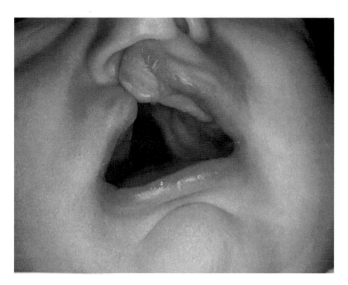

Figure 4–31. Photograph of an infant with a complete right unilateral cleft lip and palate. From *Cleft palate speech* (4th ed., p. 16), by S. Peterson-Falzone, M. Hardin-Jones, and M. Karnell, 2010. St. Louis, MO: Elsevier Mosby. Copyright 2010 by Elsevier Mosby. Reproduced with permission.

ciencies in velopharyngeal-nasal tissues. Examples of these include: (a) a velum that is abnormally short (or anatomically aberrant) and cannot make contact with the posterior pharyngeal wall, (b) a pharynx that is abnormally large and does not allow for velopharyngeal closure, and (c) blockages of the nasal cavities and outer nose that may include abnormal nasal turbinates, a deviated septum, and mishaped and/or collapsed nasal alae.

Traumas, structural disease processes, and sequelae of surgeries can also negatively influence velopharyngeal-nasal function. Surgical removal of the adenoids in children, for example, can result in velopharyngeal incompetence because the adenoids, although abnormal, may actually have been used as an assisting structure in attaining velopharyngeal closure for speech production. Surgical removal of velopharyngeal-nasal tissues, such as cancerous growths, can lead to acquired problems of velopharyngeal-nasal function in adults.

Velopharyngeal-nasal disorders that affect speech production also arise from neuromotor diseases. These most often influence the functioning of the velopharyngeal portion of the apparatus and pertain to the control of velopharyngeal closure. A variety of diseases can lead to velopharyngeal dysfunction through paresis or paralysis of the muscles of the velum and/or pharynx. Patterns of dysfunction can be distributed in different ways on one or both sides of the velopharyngeal-nasal

apparatus, depending on the nature of the disease process. Neuromotor diseases affecting velopharyngeal function include cerebral palsy, traumatic brain injury, cerebral vascular accident (stroke), Parkinson disease, amyotrophic lateral sclerosis, myasthenia gravis, and multiple sclerosis, among others.

Hixon and Netsell (1983) have summarized nine patterns of velopharyngeal dysfunction in speech production found to be associated with neuromotor disease. These include the following: (a) the velopharynx is continuously and fully open during oral speech production; (b) the velopharynx is continuously but not fully open during oral speech production; (c) the velopharynx is continuously but not fully open and varies in degree of opening during oral speech production; (d) the velopharynx demonstrates an intermittent closed-open pattern that is unpredictable during oral speech production; (e) the velopharynx demonstrates airtight closure during the first part of oral speech production and then loses its airtight seal for the remainder of the utterance; (f) the velopharynx adjusts slowly toward closure during the first part of oral speech production, closes well into the utterance, and maintains closure for the remainder of the utterance; (g) the velopharynx alternates rhythmically and predictably between moments of closure and moments of opening during oral speech production; (h) the velopharynx opens earlier than it should in anticipation of nasal

Where's the Rest?

Many studies have examined the correlation between velopharyngeal incompetence and articulation skill in children with repaired cleft palates. The highest correlation found in these studies is 0.5. Square that number and you find that velopharyngeal incompetence predicts only 25% of the variance in articulation skill. Where's the rest? Some have suggested it's to be found in "learning." We believe 75% is far too much to be attributed to such a notion. Rather, we suspect that the rest is confounded by the fact that the children studied were never categorized with regard to the magnitude of their nasal airway resistance. Not knowing or controlling for this factor would have an important influence on the strength of the correlation obtained between velopharyngeal incompetence and articulation skill. Where's the rest of the variance of interest? We think it's probably in the nose and has been overlooked.

elements in oral-nasal-oral speech production; and (i) the velopharynx retains an opening longer than it should following nasal elements in oral-nasal-oral speech production.

CLINICAL PROFESSIONALS AND VELOPHARYNGEAL-NASAL DISORDERS IN SPEECH PRODUCTION

Individuals with velopharyngeal-nasal disorders that affect speech production, or who are suspected of having such disorders, may need the services of several professionals for evaluation and management. Prominent among these are the speech-language pathologist, plastic surgeon, otorhinolaryngologist, neurologist, prosthodontist, and psychologist. Needed services might be provided by only a small subset of these professionals. Or, they might be provided by many of the professionals listed (and others) in large teams assembled to deal with complex disorders that require repeated evaluation, long-term monitoring, and inter-disciplinary approaches to management. Such teams are usually found in large medical centers and have large catchment areas. An example is a team concerned with the evaluation and management of infants and children with clefts of the palate. Another example is a team concerned with the evaluation and management of individuals with head and/or neck cancer.

The speech-language pathologist is the recognized expert on how velopharyngeal-nasal disorders influence speech production. At times, the speech-language pathologist will be the only professional to evaluate and manage velopharyngeal-nasal dysfunction in speech production. An example is with the child who presents with "phoneme-specific nasal emission" and no signs of a physical disorder of the velopharyngeal-nasal apparatus. Management in such a case could be behavioral therapy carried out by the speech-language pathologist alone.

At other times, the speech-language pathologist may evaluate velopharyngeal-nasal competence for speech production and swallowing before and after physical interventions to determine their effectiveness. Examples include: (a) before and after primary surgical repair of a cleft of the hard and soft palates in a child, (b) before and after the fitting of an obturator (a fabricated device that occludes an opening) necessitated because of surgical ablation for oral-nasal cancer in an adult, and (c) before and after the fitting of a velar-lift prostheses (a fabricated device that supports

the weight of the velum) to compensate for a paralyzed velum in a teenager.

A plastic surgeon is the physician concerned with surgical repair and/or reconstruction of deformed or destroyed parts of the body as a result of anomalous development, disease, or trauma. The plastic surgeon is responsible for performing the surgical procedures needed to provide improved structural and functional integrity to an abnormal velopharyngeal-nasal apparatus. Responsibilities of a plastic surgeon might include the primary repair of clefts of the hard and soft palates in children and any secondary surgical procedure that might be required, such as constructing a surgical flap across the velopharyngeal airway. Responsibilities of the plastic surgeon might also include surgery to remove an invading tumor from the velopharyngeal-nasal region of an adult and to reconstruct the affected area by transferring bone, cartilage, and skin from other parts of the body. Under circumstances where the outer nose is deformed as a result of anomalous development, disease, trauma, or surgical ablation, the plastic surgeon would also perform certain types of reconstructive (cosmetic) procedures to more fully normalize external appearance.

An otorhinolaryngologist is a physician who specializes in ear, nose, and throat disorders (and is, therefore, commonly referred to as an ENT) in the broad context of diseases of the head and neck. The otorhinolaryngologist may perform surgical procedures aimed at improving velophargyneal-nasal function for speech production and is often the overseeing physician for individuals with craniofacial disorders (such as cleft palate) and neoplastic (tumor) growths in the upper airway. Many of the health problems of individuals with velopharyngeal-nasal disorders are related to the condition of the upper airway and structures that connect to it. Thus, the otorhinolaryngologist is the physician responsible for managing eustachian tube dysfunction, middle ear problems, nasal obstructions, recurring tumors, and other conditions that may be related to velopharyngeal-nasal disorders.

Medical oversight of the person with a velopharyngeal-nasal disorder caused by nervous system disease is usually the province of a neurologist. The neurologist is a physician with expertise in disorders of the nervous system. The neurologist is responsible for the overall evaluation and management of the wide range of neural diseases that result in velopharyngeal-nasal dysfunction in children and adults. Many of these same neural diseases also cause problems in other subsystems of the speech production apparatus. The neurologist deals with medical concerns related to paresis and paralysis of the velopharyngeal-nasal apparatus and to involuntary movements of the apparatus. Individuals who might be under the care of a neurologist include those with a diagnosis of cerebral palsy, amyotrophic lateral sclerosis, cerebral vascular accident (stroke), nervous system tumors of various types, and Parkinson disease, among others. Some neural-based disorders of velopharyngeal-nasal function are amenable to drug treatments, although most are not. For the latter, the neurologist might consider possible mechanical interventions.

A prosthodontist is a dentist who specializes in the replacement of missing parts through artificial substitutes. These substitutes are referred to generically as prostheses and are custom fabricated to meet the needs of each individual. The prosthodontist is concerned with restoring impaired function, appearance, comfort, and health to individuals who need prosthetic devices to substitute for structures that have been affected by congenital anomalies, disease, trauma, or surgery. Individuals who require the services of a prosthodontist include those born with palatal clefts that are exceptionally wide and are managed through the fitting of a palatal obturator, a device that is fixed to the maxillary teeth and occludes the gap between the palatal shelves. Such a palatal obturator and combination denture is shown in Figure 4–32. Similarly, individuals who have large parts of the palate resected because of cancer may be fitted with an obturator as a replacement for the excised structure. A prosthodontist may fabricate customized velar-lift prostheses for persons who have paresis or paralysis of the velum. A velar-lift prosthesis consists of a plate that extends backward along the roof of the mouth to lift the velum to a horizontal plane and support its weight against the force of gravity. Persons with flaccid paresis or paralysis of the velum are often managed with this type of prosthetic device. The speech-language pathologist usually works with the prosthodontist to help evaluate the success of different prostheses on velopharyngeal-nasal function in relation to breathing, speaking, and swallowing.

A psychologist is an individual who has special expertise in helping individuals cope with significant problems of everyday living. The psychologist can play an important role for many individuals with velopharyngeal-nasal disorders that affect speech production. For example, those who have undergone surgical ablation of different parts of the head and neck or who have neural disease that has resulted in their being unable to move normally, are often in need of counseling to help them deal with the psychological processes attendant

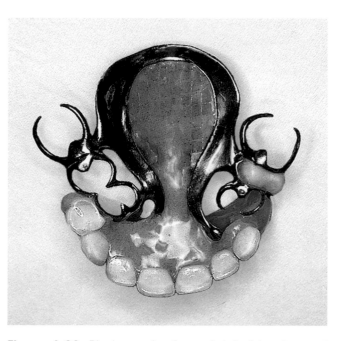

Figure 4–32. Photograph of a palatal obturator and combination denture as viewed from below. From *Cleft palate speech* (4th ed., p. 358), by S. Peterson-Falzone, M. Hardin-Jones, and M. Karnell, 2010. St. Louis, MO: Elsevier Mosby. Copyright 2010 by Elsevier Mosby. Reproduced with permission.

Wait Lifting

Occasionally a person fitted with a velar-lift prosthesis will wear it for several weeks or months and find that when it is removed the velum is able to move. Further evaluation will usually confirm that the velum is working better than it did before the prosthesis was fitted or even that it is working normally. How can this be? How can a paretic or paralyzed velum come back to life and start working again? Most likely the velum was nearly able to do its job to begin with, but its owner may have surrendered to gravity and not used whatever minimal strength was available. This, in turn, may have allowed the velum to become even weaker through disuse. Then, once in place, the prosthesis did part of the lifting work for the velum (probably the toughest part) and the velum was able to accomplish the rest on its own. Think of this as a sort of wait lifting (pun intended), if you will.

to their loss of function. Psychological depression, grief, and embarrassment are several factors often encountered in persons with acquired velopharyngeal-nasal disorders that manifest in speech production problems. In other cases, the psychologist plays an important role in helping families and loved ones cope with perceived losses or conditions surrounding velopharyngeal-nasal disorders. For example, the parents of a child born with a cleft of the palate may be overwhelmed with emotion (see the scenario at the beginning of this chapter) and need counseling and psychological support to help them deal with their situation and future.

REVIEW

The velopharyngeal-nasal apparatus is located within the head and neck and comprises a system of valves and air passages that interconnects the throat and atmosphere through the nose.

The velopharyngeal-nasal apparatus includes the pharynx, velum, nasal cavities, and outer nose.

Forces of the velopharyngeal-nasal apparatus are of two types—passive and active, the former arising from several sources and the latter arising from muscles distributed within different parts of the velopharyngeal-nasal apparatus.

Muscles of the pharynx include the *superior constrictor, middle constrictor, inferior constrictor, salpingopharyngeus, stylopharyngeus,* and *palatopharyngeus.*

Muscles of the velum include the *palatal levator, palatal tensor, uvulus, glossopalatine,* and *pharyngopalatine.*

Muscles of the outer nose include the *levator labii superioris alaeque nasi, anterior nasal dilator, posterior nasal dilator, nasalis,* and *depressor alae nasi.*

Movements of the pharynx enable its lumen to be changed along its length, either by constriction or dilation at different sites.

Movements of the velum involve shape changes of the structure and are mainly along an upward-backward or downward-forward path.

Movements of the outer nose influence the cross-sections of the anterior nares and are involved in breathing events and the signaling of emotions.

Adjustments of the velopharyngeal-nasal apparatus can influence the degree of coupling between the oral and nasal cavities and between the nasal cavities and atmosphere.

Closure of the velopharyngeal port can be achieved through a variety of movement strategies that involve different actions or combinations of actions of the velum, lateral pharyngeal walls, and posterior pharyngeal wall, strategies that are conditioned by velopharyngeal anatomy.

Closing and opening adjustments of the velopharyngeal port are controlled by different factors, with closing being controlled by muscular forces and opening being controlled by passive forces and muscular forces (in upright).

Adjustments of the anterior nares are involved in different activities and play a prominent role in breathing to resist the tendency of the outer nose to collapse in response to low pressures in its lumina.

The control variables of velopharyngeal-nasal function include airway resistance offered by the velopharyngeal-nasal apparatus, muscular pressure exerted by the velopharyngeal sphincter to maintain closure, and acoustic impedance in opposition to the flow of sound energy.

Different parts of the nervous system are responsible for the control of different components of the velopharyngeal-nasal apparatus and different activities, with motor and sensory innervation being effected mainly through cranial nerves.

Nasal airflow is modulated by the nasal valve, which consists of external and internal parts, the latter of which is primarily responsible for the governing of nasal patency.

The two sides of the nose go through changes in which their respective nasal turbinates alternately engorge and constrict in a rhythmical cycle that varies from person to person and has implications for the conditioning of inspired air and protection against infection.

The warming, moistening, and filtering aspects of nasal function are important to health, and nasal breathing prevails until airway resistance becomes excessive, whereupon a switch is made to oral-nasal breathing.

The role of velopharyngeal-nasal function in speech production is to control the degree of coupling between the oral and nasal cavities and between the nasal cavities and atmosphere.

Both the velopharynx and outer nose are active during sustained utterances, the patterning depending on the speech sound being produced, and with high vowels showing greater velar height, greater velar contact with the posterior pharyngeal wall, and greater velopharyngeal sphincter compression than low vowels.

Running speech activities involve the combining of consonants and vowels with primacy of control being vested in consonant productions, especially those that are associated with high oral pressure and little or no opening of the velopharyngeal port.

Position and movement patterns of the velopharyngeal-nasal apparatus may reflect the occurrence of two or more speech sounds simultaneously, such that their productions overlap and intermingle and show evidence of how the brain prepares in advance for velopharyngeal-nasal adjustments and how the mechanical properties of the velopharyngeal-nasal apparatus influence its behavior.

Gravity has effects on velopharyngeal-nasal function that are manifested through reorientation of the position of the body or rotation of the head about different axes, and are attributed to mechanical and cardiovascular factors.

Velopharyngeal-nasal function for speech production develops gradually, and sometime between 6 months and 3 years of age (presumably closer to the former) airtight velopharyngeal closure for oral speech sound production can be expected to occur.

There is no credible evidence that velopharyngeal-nasal function for speech production changes with age in the mature velopharyngeal-nasal apparatus.

The sex of the speaker appears to have an influence on certain details of velopharyngeal-nasal function during speech production, but it is not clear that these differences are functionally important or that they are relevant to clinical concerns.

The instrumental measurement of velopharyngeal-nasal function can be accomplished with several methods, including direct visualization, x-ray imaging, aeromechanical observations, and acoustic observations.

Velopharyngeal-nasal disorders can influence speech production to different degrees and may result from congenital, developmental, or acquired problems of the velopharyngeal-nasal apparatus that have functional or organic bases.

Different clinical professionals have roles in the evaluation and management of velopharyngeal-nasal disorders that affect speech production, including speech-language pathologists, plastic surgeons, otorhinolaryngologists, neurologists, prosthodontists, and psychologists.

Scenario

Six years had passed since that eventful morning in Florida. Time and distance had muted the mother's memories, but the realities were with her daily in the form of her son. He was about to begin an educational journey in which his mother would play a lesser role than she had to this point in his life. Others would now have things to say about the boy's welfare. The mother's inertia on health care needs for the child was about to be overturned by social forces.

It began with a first-grade teacher in conversation with the school's nurse and later in consultation with the school's psychologist. All had concerns for the child's social development and his problems with speech. He stood out among his classmates because of his shyness and reticence. The speech-language pathologist who serviced the school was asked to evaluate the boy. Her report indicated that he had speech sound misarticulations, a moderately hypernasal voice, and nares constriction on pressure consonants. She concluded that he showed signs consistent with a significant velopharyngeal leak during speech production and recommended that he be referred to the regional cleft palate and craniofacial disorders clinic for instrumental evaluation. The mother provided medical records from the previous management team at the time of clinical intake.

Evaluation showed velopharyngeal incompetence and a small anterior oronasal fistula that was difficult to discern visually because of its configuration. Measurements of the cross-sectional area of the velopharyngeal port, with and without occlusion of the fistula, indicated that the fistula contributed to the overall problem and needed to be closed along with secondary surgical management of the velopharynx. The size of the velopharyngeal port was calculated for stop-plosive sound production with the fistula occluded using aeromechanical techniques and found to be 15 mm^2. The surgical method of choice was a pharyngeal flap. Lateral pharyngeal wall movement was observed via ultrasound and found to be minimal during oral consonant productions. A relatively high-placed, broad, superiorly based pharyngeal flap was constructed. Closure of the anterior fistula and construction of the pharyngeal flap were done in one hospitalization.

Six-month follow-up evaluation of the child indicated that the closure of the anterior fistula was successful and the pharyngeal flap was functioning well. Velopharyngeal port size for stop-plosive production had reduced to 2.5 mm^2. Nasal breathing was not obstructed and the mother reported no snoring problems or sleep apnea in the child. Misarticulations persisted, hypernasality was reduced, and nares constriction was less obvious and inconsistent. The child was placed on a behavior modification program with the speech-language pathologist to deal with his remaining speech and speech production signs. He responded well and within a short period of time began to make consistent improvement.

The mother came to understand that her sheltering of the child had been detrimental, despite her protective intentions. She went through a period of self-healing that paralleled the progress made by her son. She contacted her parents and arranged a weeklong visit over the 4th of July. It was her first return to Ohio in several years and her son's first time ever to see his grandparents' horse farm. All that week he saddled up on Buster, a brown and white pony that seemed to have been waiting for him and carried a white cowboy hat on the horn of his saddle. Life was good that week in "The Buckeye State," especially in the vicinity of Canfield. There would be other fun-filled weeks in that area for years to come, including a time to show Buster at the Canfield Fair.

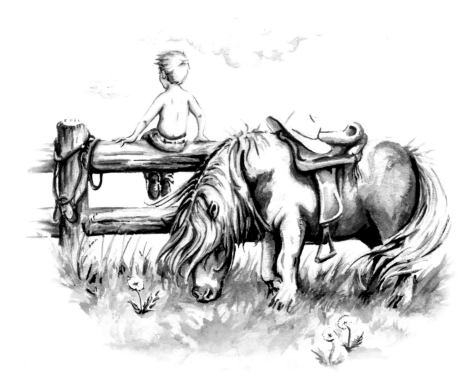

The Flap Flap

Pharyngeal flaps are secondary surgical procedures usually performed on persons with repaired cleft palates who persist with velopharyngeal incompetence or insufficiency following primary surgery. Flaps are constructed using tissue from the posterior pharyngeal wall (peeled away like the skin on a banana) and attaching it to the velum to form a bridge. Flaps have also been used in children with cerebral palsy who have paresis of the velum. They have been found to improve speech in such children, but they also have been found to have a major negative side effect. They may raise the resistance to breathing through the nose and cause some children to switch from nose breathing to mouth breathing. Mouth breathing opens the door (pun intended) to drooling. The negative social consequences of drooling are often judged to outweigh the positive social consequences of improved speech. Thus, flaps have sometimes had to be removed.

REFERENCES

Allison, D., & Leeper, H. (1990). A comparison of noninvasive procedures to assess nasal airway resistance. *Cleft Palate Journal, 27,* 40–44.

Andreassen, M., Leeper, H., MacRae, D., & Nicholson, I. (1994). Aerodynamic, acoustic, and perceptual changes following adenoidectomy. *Cleft Palate-Craniofacial Journal, 31,* 264–270.

Andreassen, M., Smith, B., & Guyette, T. (1992). Pressure-flow measurements for selected oral and nasal sound segments produced by normal adults. *Cleft Palate-Craniofacial Journal, 29,* 1–9.

Arkebauer, H., Hixon, T., & Hardy, J. (1967). Peak intra-oral air pressures during speech. *Journal of Speech and Hearing Research, 10,* 196–208.

Aviv, J., Martin, J., Jones, M., Wee, T., Diamond, B., Keen, M., & Blitzer, A. (1994). Age-related changes in pharyngeal and supraglottic sensation. *Annals of Otology, Rhinology, and Laryngology, 103,* 749–752.

Awan, S. (2001). Age and gender effects on measures of RMS nasalance. *Clinical Linguistics and Phonetics, 15,* 117–122.

Azzam, N., & Kuehn, D. (1977). The morphology of musculus uvulae. *Cleft Palate Journal, 14,* 78–87.

Bae, Y., Kuehn, D., Sutton, B., Conway, C., & Perry, J. (2011). Three-dimensional magnetic resonance imaging of velopharyngeal structures. *Journal of Speech, Language, and Hearing Research, 54,* 1538–1545.

Barsoumian, R., Kuehn, D., Moon, J., & Canady, J. (1998). An anatomic study of the tensor veli palatini and dilatator tubae muscles in relation to estachian tube and velar function. *Cleft Palate-Craniofacial Journal, 35,* 101–110.

Bell-Berti, F. (1976). An electromyographic study of velopharyngeal function in speech. *Journal of Speech and Hearing Research, 19,* 225–240.

Bennett, K., & Hoit, J. (in press). Stress velopharyngeal incompetence in collegiate trombone players. *Cleft Palate-Craniofacial Journal.*

Boorman, J., & Sommerlad, B. (1985). Levator palati and palatal dimples: Their anatomy, relationship and clinical significance. *British Journal of Plastic Surgery, 38,* 326–332.

Bosma, J., Truby, H., & Lind, J. (1965). Cry motions of the newborn infant. *Acta Paediatrica Scandinavica, 163,* 63–91.

Bridger, G. (1970). Physiology of the nasal valve. *Archives of Otolaryngology, 92,* 543–553.

Buhr, R. (1980). The emergence of vowels in an infant. *Journal of Speech and Hearing Research, 23,* 73–94.

Bunton, K., Gallagher, K., & Hoit, J. (March, 2012). *Development of velopharyngeal closure in young children: Preliminary observations.* Poster presented at the Conference on Motor Speech, Santa Rosa, CA.

Bunton, K., Hoit, J., & Gallagher, K. (2011). A simple technique for determining velopharyngeal status during speech production. *Seminars in Speech and Language, 32,* 69–80.

Bzoch, K. (1968). Variations in velar valving: The factor of vowel changes. *Cleft Palate Journal, 5,* 211–218.

Cassell, M., & Ekaldi, H. (1995). Anatomy and physiology of the palate and velopharyngeal apertures. In R. Shprintzen & J. Bardach (Eds.), *Cleft palate speech management: A multidisciplinary approach* (pp. 45–61). St. Louis, MO: Mosby.

Cole, P. (1976). The extrathoracic airways. *Journal of Otolaryngology, 5,* 74–85.

Cole, P., & Haight, J. (1986). Posture and the nasal cycle. *Annals of Otology, Rhinology, and Laryngology, 104,* 233–237.

Cole, P., & Havas, T. (1980). Resistance to respiratory airflow of the nasal passages: Comparisons between different common methods of calculation. *Rhinology, 24,* 163–173.

Crelin, E. (1973). *Functional anatomy of the newborn.* New Haven, CT: Yale University Press.

Croft, C., Shprintzen, R., & Rakoff, S. (1981). Patterns of velopharyngeal valving in normal and cleft palate subjects: A multiview videofluoroscopic and nasendoscopic study. *Laryngoscope, 91,* 265–271.

Curtis, J. (1968). Acoustics of speech production and nasalization. In D. Spriestersbach & D. Sherman (Eds.), *Cleft palate and communication* (pp. 27–60). New York, NY: Academic Press.

D'Antonio, L., Marsh, J., Province, M., Muntz, H., & Phillips, C. (1989). Reliability of flexible fiberoptic nasopharyngoscopy for evaluation of velopharyngeal function in a clinical population. *Cleft Palate Journal, 26,* 217–225.

Detweiler, D. (1973). Regulation of systemic and pulmonary circulation. In J. Brobeck (Ed.), *Best and Taylor's physiological basis of medical practice* (9th ed., pp. 3–189). Baltimore, MD: Williams & Wilkins.

Dickson, D. (1972). Normal and cleft palate anatomy. *Cleft Palate Journal, 9,* 280–293.

Dickson, D., & Dickson, W. (1972). Velopharyngeal anatomy. *Journal of Speech and Hearing Research, 15,* 372–381.

Drettner, B. (1979). The role of the nose in the functional unity of the respiratory system. *Rhinology, 17,* 3–11.

Eccles, R. (1996). A role for the nasal cycle in respiratory defence. *European Respiratory Journal, 9,* 371–376.

Eccles, R., & Eccles, K. (1981). Asymmetry in the autonomic nervous system with reference to the nasal cycle, migraine, anisocoria and Meniere's syndrome. *Rhinology, 19,* 121–125.

Endres, W., Bambach, W., & Flosser, G. (1967). Voice spectrograms as a function of age, voice disguise, and voice imitation. *Journal of the Acoustical Society of America, 49,* 1842–1848.

Ettema, S., & Kuehn, D. (1994). A quantitative histologic study of the normal human adult soft palate. *Journal of Speech and Hearing Research, 37,* 303–313.

Ettema, S., Kuehn, D., Perlman, A., & Alperin, N. (2002). Magnetic resonance imaging of the levator veli palatini muscle during speech. *Cleft-Palate-Craniofacial Journal, 39,* 130–144.

Fant, G. (1960). *Acoustic theory of speech production.* Hague, Netherlands: Mouton.

Finkelstein, Y., Berger, G., Nachmani, A., & Ophir, D. (1996). The functional role of the adenoids in speech. *International Journal of Pediatric Otorhinolaryngology, 34,* 61–74.

Finkelstein, Y., Shapiro-Feinberg, M., Talmi, Y., Nachmani, A., DeRowe, A., & Ophir, D. (1995). Axial configuration of the velopharyngeal valve and its valving mechanism. *Cleft Palate-Craniofacial Journal, 32,* 299–305.

Fitch, W., & Giedd, J. (1999). Morphology and development of the human vocal tract: A study using magnetic resonance imaging. *Journal of the Acoustical Society of America, 106,* 1511–1522.

Fletcher, S. (1973a). Maturation of the speech mechanism. *Folia Phoniatrica, 25,* 161–172.

Fletcher, S. (1973b). *Manual for measurement and modification of nasality with TONAR II.* Birmingham, AL: University of Alabama.

Fletcher, S. (1976). "Nasalance" vs. listener judgments of nasality. *Cleft Palate Journal, 13,* 31– 44.

Foster, T. (1962). Maxillary deformities in repaired clefts of lip and palate. *British Journal of Plastic Surgery, 15,* 182–190.

Fremont, A., & Hoyland, J. (2007). Morphology, mechanisms and pathology of musculoskeletal ageing. *Journal of Pathology, 211,* 252–259.

Fritzell, B. (1963). An electromyographic study of the movements of the soft palate in speech. *Folia Phoniatrica, 15,* 307–311.

Fritzell, B. (1969). The velopharyngeal muscles in speech. *Acta Otolaryngologica, Supplement 250,* 1–81.

Fritzell, B. (1979). Electromyography in the study of the velopharyngeal function—A review. *Folia Phoniatrica, 31,* 93–102.

Gautier, H., Remmers, J., & Bartlett, D. (1973). Control of the duration of expiration. *Respiration Physiology, 18,* 205–221.

Gotto, T. (1977). Tightness in velopharyngeal closure and its regulatory mechanism. *Journal of the Osaka University Dental Society, 22,* 1–19.

Graber, T., Bzoch, K., & Aoba, T. (1959). A functional study of the palatal and pharyngeal structures. *Angle Orthodontist, 29,* 30–40.

Hairfield, W., Warren, D., Hinton, V., & Seaton, D. (1987). Inspiratory and expiratory effects of nasal breathing. *Cleft Palate Journal, 24,* 183–189.

Harrington, R. (1944). A study of the mechanism of velopharyngeal closure. *Journal of Speech Disorders, 9,* 325–345.

Hattori, S., Yamamoto, K., & Fujimura, O. (1958). Nasalization of vowels in relation to nasals. *Journal of the Acoustical Society of America, 30,* 267–274.

Hixon, E. (1949). *An x-ray study comparing oral and pharyngeal structures of individuals with nasal voices and individuals with superior voices.* Master 's thesis, University of Iowa, Iowa City.

Hixon, T., & Abbs, J. (1980). Normal speech production. In T. Hixon, L. Shriberg, & J. Saxman (Eds.), *Introduction to communication disorders* (pp. 42–87). Englewood-Cliffs, NJ: Prentice-Hall.

Hixon, T., & Netsell, R. (1983). *Velopharyngeal physiopathy in dysarthria.* Paper presented at the Boys Town National Institute Symposium on Treatment of the Velopharynx for Individuals with Dysarthria, Omaha, NE.

Hiyama, S., Ono, T., Ishiwata, Y., & Kuroda, T. (2002). Effects of mandibular position and body posture on nasal patency in normal awake subjects. *Angle Orthodontist, 72,* 547–553.

Hoit, J., Watson, P., Hixon, K., McMahon, P., & Johnson, C. (1994). Age and velopharyngeal function during speech production. *Journal of Speech and Hearing Research, 37,* 295–302.

Honjo, I., Harada, H., & Kumazasa. T. (1976). Role of the levator veli palatini muscle in movement of the lateral pharyn-geal wall. *Archives of Otology, Rhinology, and Laryngology, 212,* 93–98.

House, A., & Stevens, K. (1956). Analog studies of the nasalization of vowels. *Journal of Speech and Hearing Disorders, 21,* 218–232.

Hsu, H., Fogel, A., & Cooper, R. (2000). Infant vocal development during the first 6 months: Speech quality and melodic complexity. *Infant and Child Development, 9,* 1–16.

Huang, Z., Lee, S., & Rajendran, K. (1997). Structure of the musculus uvulae: Functional and surgical implications of an anatomic study. *Cleft Palate-Craniofacial Journal, 34,* 466–474.

Huang, Z., Ong, K., Goh, S., Liew, H., Yeoh, K., & Wang, D. (2003). Assessment of nasal cycle by acoustic rhinometry and rhinomamometry. *Otolaryngology-Head and Neck Surgery, 128,* 510–516.

Hutchinson, J., Robinson, K., & Nerbonne, M. (1978). Patterns of nasalance in a sample of normal gerontologic subjects. *Journal of Communication Disorders, 11,* 469–481.

Iglesias, A., Kuehn, D., & Morris, H. (1980). Simultaneous assessment of pharyngeal wall and velar displacement for selected speech sounds. *Journal of Speech and Hearing Research, 23,* 429–446.

Isshiki, N., Harita, Y., & Kawano, M. (1985). What muscle is responsible for lateral pharyngeal wall movement? *Annals of Plastic Surgery, 14,* 224–227.

Jackson, R. (1976). Nasal-cardiopulmonary reflexes: A role of the larynx. *Annals of Otology, Rhinology, and Laryngology, 85,* 65–70.

Jaw, T., Sheu, R., Liu, G., & Lin, W. (1999). Development of adenoids: A study by measurement with MR images. *Kaohsiung Journal of Medical Sciences, 15,* 12–18.

Kaltenborn, A. (1948). *An x-ray study of velopharyngeal closure in nasal and non-nasal speakers.* Master 's thesis, Northwestern University, Evanston, IL.

Karlsson, S., & Carlsson, G. (1990). Characteristics of mandibular movement in young and elderly dentate subjects. *Journal of Dental Research, 69,* 473–476.

Karnell, M., Linville, R., & Edwards, B. (1988). Variations in velar position over time: A nasal videoendoscopic study. *Journal of Speech and Hearing Research, 31,* 417–424.

Kent, R. (1981). Articulatory-acoustic perspectives on speech development. In R. Stark (Ed.), *Language behavior in infancy and early childhood* (pp. 105–126). Amsterdam, Netherlands: Elsevier-North Holland.

Kent, R., Carney, P., & Severeid, L. (1974). Velar movement and timing: Evaluation of a model for binary control. *Journal of Speech and Hearing Research, 17,* 470–488.

Kent, R., Liss, J., & Philips, B. (1989). Acoustic analysis of velopharyngeal dysfunction in speech. In K. Bzoch (Ed.), *Communicative disorders related to cleft lip and palate* (3rd ed., pp. 258–270). Boston, MA: College-Hill Press.

Kent, R., & Murray, A. (1982). Acoustic features of infant vocalic utterances at 3, 6, and 9 months. *Journal of the Acoustical Society of America, 72,* 353–365.

Kier, W., & Smith, K. (1985). Tongues, tentacles, and trunks: The biomechanics of movement in muscular-hydrostats. *Zoological Journal of the Linnean Society, 83,* 307–324.

Klotz, D., Howard, J., Hengerer, A., & Slupchynskj, O. (2001). Lipoinjection augmentation of the soft palate for velopharyngeal stress incompetence. *Laryngoscope, 111*, 2157–2161.

Kuehn, D. (1976). A cineradiographic investigation of velar movement variables in two normals. *Cleft Palate Journal, 13*, 88–103.

Kuehn, D. (1990). Commentary on Doyle, Casselbrandt, Swarts, and Bluestone (1990): Observations on a role for the tensor veli palatini in intrinsic palatal function. *Cleft Palate Journal, 27*, 318–319.

Kuehn, D., & Azzam, N. (1978). Anatomical characteristics of palatoglossus and the anterior faucial pillar. *Cleft Palate Journal, 15*, 349–359.

Kuehn, D., & Dolan, K. (1975). A tomographic technique of assessing lateral pharyngeal wall displacement. *Cleft Palate Journal, 12*, 200–209.

Kuehn, D., Folkins, J., & Cutting, C. (1982). Relationships between muscle activity and velar position. *Cleft Palate Journal, 19*, 25–35.

Kuehn, D., Folkins, J., & Linville, R. (1988). An electromyographic study of the musculus uvulae. *Cleft Palate Journal, 25*, 348–355.

Kuehn, D., & Kahane, J. (1990). Histologic study of the normal human adult soft palate. *Cleft Palate Journal, 27*, 26–34.

Kuehn, D., & Moon, J. (1998). Velopharyngeal closure force and levator veli palatini activation levels in varying phonetic contexts. *Journal of Speech, Language, and Hearing Research, 41*, 51–62.

Kuehn, D., & Moon, J. (2005). Histologic study of intravelar structures in normal human adult specimens. *Cleft Palate-Craniofacial Journal, 42*, 481–489.

Kuehn, D., & Perry, J. (2008). Anatomy and physiology of the velopharynx. In J. Losee & R. Kirschner (Eds.), *Comprehensive cleft care*. New York, NY: McGraw-Hill Medical.

Lansing, R., Solomon, N., Kossev, A., & Andersen, A. (1991). Recording single motor unit activity of human nasal muscles with surface electrodes: Applications for respiration and speech. *Electroencephalography and Clinical Neurophysiology, 81*, 167–175.

Leeper, H., Tissington, M., & Munhall, K. (1998). Temporal aspects of velopharyngeal function in children. *Cleft Palate-Craniofacial Journal, 35*, 215–221.

Lester, R., & Hoit, J. (April, 2012). *Oral vs. nasal breathing during natural speech production*. Poster presented at the Arizona Speech-Language-Hearing Association Convention, Phoenix, AZ.

Liss, J. (1990). Muscle spindles in the human levator veli palatini and palatoglossus muscles. *Journal of Speech and Hearing Research, 33*, 736–746.

Liss, J., Kuehn, D., & Hinkle, K. (1994). Direct training of velopharyngeal musculature. *Journal of Medical Speech-Language Pathology, 2*, 243–249.

Lubker, J. (1968). An electromyographic-cinefluorographic investigation of velar function during normal speech production. *Cleft Palate Journal, 5*, 1–18.

Lubker, J. (1973). Transglottal airflow during stop consonant production. *Journal of the Acoustical Society of America, 53*, 212–215.

Lubker, J. (1975). Normal velopharyngeal function in speech. *Clinics in Plastic Surgery, 2*, 249–259.

Lubker, J., & Moll, K. (1965). Simultaneous oral-nasal air flow measurements and cinefluorographic observations during speech production. *Cleft Palate Journal, 2*, 257–272.

Malick, D., Moon, J., & Canady, J. (2007). Stress velopharyngeal incompetence: Prevalence, treatment, and management practices. *Cleft Palate Journal, 44*, 424–433.

McCaffrey, T., & Kern, E. (1979). Clinical evaluation of nasal obstruction: A study of 1000 patients. *Archives of Otolaryngology-Head and Neck Surgery, 105*, 542–545.

McClean, M. (1973). Forward coarticulation of velar movement at marked junctural boundaries. *Journal of Speech and Hearing Research, 16*, 286–296.

McKerns, D., & Bzoch, K. (1970). Variations in velopharyngeal valving: The factor of sex. *Cleft Palate Journal, 7*, 652–662.

McWilliams, B., & Girdany, B. (1964). The use of Televex in cleft palate research. *Cleft Palate Journal, 1*, 398–401.

McWilliams, B., Morris, H., & Shelton, R. (1990). *Cleft palate speech* (2nd ed.). Philadelphia, PA: B. C. Decker.

Miller, M., Martin, R., Waldemar, A., Fouke, J., Strohl, K., & Fanaroff, M. (1985). Oral breathing in newborn infants. *Journal of Pediatrics, 107*, 465–469.

Mirza, N., Kroger, H., & Doty, R. (1997). Influence of age on the 'nasal cycle.' *Laryngoscope, 107*, 62–66.

Moll, K. (1962). Velopharyngeal closure on vowels. *Journal of Speech and Hearing Research, 5*, 30–37.

Moll, K., & Daniloff, R. (1971). Investigation of the timing of velar movements during speech. *Journal of Speech and Hearing Research, 50*, 678–684.

Moll, K., & Shriner, T. (1967). Preliminary investigation of a new concept of velar activity during speech. *Cleft Palate Journal, 4*, 58–69.

Moon, J., & Canady, J. (1995). Effects of gravity on velopharyngeal muscle activity during speech. *Cleft Palate-Craniofacial Journal, 32*, 371–375.

Moon, J., & Kuehn, D. (2004). Anatomy and physiology of normal and disordered velopharyngeal function for speech. In K. Bzoch (Ed.), *Communicative disorders related to cleft lip and palate* (5th ed., pp. 67–98). Austin, TX: Pro-Ed.

Moon, J., Kuehn, D., & Huisman, J. (1994a). Measurement of velopharyngeal closure force during vowel production. *Cleft Palate-Craniofacial Journal, 31*, 356–363.

Moon, J., Smith, A., Folkins, J., Lemke, J., & Gartlan, M. (1994b). Coordination of velopharyngeal muscle activity during positioning of the soft palate. *Cleft Palate-Craniofacial Journal, 31*, 45–55.

Morris, H. (1975). The speech pathologist looks at the tonsils and the adenoids. *Annals of Otology, Rhinology, and Laryngology, 84*, 63–66.

Netsell, R. (1990). Commentary. *Cleft Palate Journal, 27*, 58–60.

Niinimaa, V., Cole, P., & Mintz, S. (1981). Oronasal distribution of respiratory airflow. *Respiratory Physiology, 43*, 69–75.

Nusbaum, E., Foly, L., & Wells, C. (1935). Experimental studies of the firmness of the velar-pharyngeal occlusion during the production of the English vowels. *Speech Monographs, 2*, 71–80.

Oller, K. (1986). Metaphonology and infant vocalizations. In B. Lindblom & R. Zetterstrom (Eds.), *Precursors of early speech* (pp. 21–36). New York, NY: Stockton Press.

Poppelreuter, S., Engelke, W., & Bruns, T. (2000). Quantitative analysis of the velopharyngeal sphincter function during speech. *Cleft Palate-Craniofacial Journal, 37,* 157–165.

Principato, J., & Ozenberger, J. (1970). Cyclical changes in nasal resistance. *Archives of Otolaryngology, 91,* 71–77.

Proctor, D. (1982). The upper airway. In D. Proctor & I. Andersen (Eds.), *The nose—upper airway physiology and the atmospheric environment* (pp. 23–44). Amsterdam, Netherlands: Elsevier Biomedical Press.

Quigley, L., Shiere, F., Webster, R., & Cobb, C. (1964). Measuring palatopharyngeal competence with the nasal anemometer. *Cleft Palate Journal, 1,* 304–313.

Rodenstein, D., Perlmutter, N., & Stanescu, D. (1985). Infants are not obligatory nasal breathers. *American Review of Respiratory Disease, 131,* 343–347.

Rudcrantz, H. (1969). Postural variations of nasal patency. *Acta Otolaryngologica, 68,* 435–443.

Ruscello, D. (1982). A selected review of palatal training procedures. *Cleft Palate Journal, 19,* 181–193.

Saibene, F., Mognoni, P., & LaFortuna, C. (1978). Oronasal breathing during exercise. *Pleugers Archives, 378,* 65–69.

Saroha, D., Bottrill, I., Saif, M., & Gardner, B. (2003). Is the nasal cycle ablated in patients with high spinal cord trauma? *Clinical Otolaryngology and Allied Sciences, 28,* 142–145.

Sasaki, C., Levine, P., Laitman, J., & Crelin, E. (1977). Postnatal descent of the epiglottis in man. *Archives of Otolaryngology, 103,* 169–171.

Schmidt, R. (1982). The schema concept. In J. Kelso (Ed.), *Human motor behavior: An introduction* (pp. 219–235). Hillsdale, NJ: Lawrence Erlbaum.

Schwab, B., & Schulze-Florey, A. (2004). Velopharyngeal insufficiency in woodwind and brass players. *Medical Problems of Performing Artists, 19,* 21–25.

Seaver, E., Dalston, R., Leeper, H., & Adams, L. (1991). A study of nasometric values for normal nasal resonance. *Journal of Speech and Hearing Research, 34,* 715–721.

Seaver, E., & Kuehn, D. (1980). A cineradiographic and electromyographic investigation of velar positioning in nonnasal speech. *Cleft Palate Journal, 17,* 216–226.

Shelton, R., Beaumont, K., Trier, W., & Furr, M. (1978). Videopanendoscopic feedback in training velopharyngeal closure. *Cleft Palate Journal, 15,* 6–12.

Shimokawa, T., Yi, S., & Tanaka, S. (2005). Nerve supply to the soft palate muscles with special reference to the distribution of the lesser palatine nerves. *Cleft Palate-Craniofacial Journal, 42,* 495–500.

Shprintzen, R. (1992). Assessment of velopharyngeal function: Nasopharyngoscopy and multiview videofluoroscopy. In L. Brodsky, L. Holt, & D. Ritter-Schmidt (Eds.), *Craniofacial anomalies: An interdisciplinary approach* (pp. 196–207). St. Louis, MO: Mosby.

Shprintzen, R., McCall, G., Skolnick, L., & Lenicone, R. (1975). Selective movement of the lateral aspects of the pharyngeal walls during velopharyngeal closure for speech, blowing, and whistling in normals. *Cleft Palate Journal, 12,* 51–58.

Siegel-Sadewitz, V., & Shprintzen, R. (1986). Changes in velopharyngeal valving with age. *International Journal of Pediatric Otorhinolaryngology, 11,* 171–182.

Skolnick, M. (1970). Videofluoroscopic examination of the velopharyngeal portal during phonation in lateral and base projections—A new technique for studying the mechanics of closure. *Cleft Palate Journal, 7,* 803–816.

Skolnick, M., McCall, G., & Barnes, M. (1973). The sphincteric mechanism of velopharyngeal closure. *Cleft Palate Journal, 10,* 286–305.

Stoksted, P. (1953). Rhinometric measurements for determination of the nasal cycle. *Acta Otolaryngologica, Supplement 109,* 1–159.

Subtelny, J., & Koepp-Baker, H. (1956). The significance of adenoid tissue in velopharyngeal function. *Plastic and Reconstructive Surgery, 12,* 235–250.

Thom, S., Hoit, J., Hixon, T., & Smith, A. (2006). Velopharyngeal function during vocalization in infants. *Cleft Palate-Craniofacial Journal, 43,* 539–546.

Thompson, A., & Hixon, T. (1979). Nasal air flow during normal speech production. *Cleft Palate Journal, 16,* 412–420.

Tomoda, T., Morii, S., Yamashita, T., & Kumazawa, T. (1984). Histology of human eustachian tube muscles: Effect of aging. *Annals of Otology, Rhinology, and Laryngology, 93,* 17–24.

Tucker, L. (1963). *Articulatory variations in normal speakers with changes in vocal pitch and effort.* Master's thesis, University of Iowa, Iowa City.

Vig, P., & Zajac, D. (1993). Age and gender effects on nasal respiratory function in normal subjects. *Cleft Palate-Craniofacial Journal, 30,* 279–284.

Vorperian, H., Kent, R., Lindstrom, M., Kalina, C., Gentry, L., & Yandell, B. (2005). Development of vocal tract length during childhood: A magnetic resonance imaging study. *Journal of the Acoustical Society of America, 117,* 338–350.

Warren, D. (1964). Velopharyngeal orifice size and upper pharyngeal pressure-flow patterns in normal speech. *Plastic and Reconstructive Surgery, 33,* 148–162.

Warren, D. (1967). Nasal emission of air and velopharyngeal function. *Cleft Palate Journal, 4,* 148–156.

Warren, D., Dalston, R., & Dalston, E. (1990). Maintaining speech pressures in the presence of velopharyngeal impairment. *Cleft Palate Journal, 27,* 53–58.

Warren, D., Dalston, R., Trier, W., & Holder, M. (1985). A pressure-flow technique for quantifying temporal patterns of palatopharyngeal closure. *Cleft Palate Journal, 22,* 11–19.

Warren, D., Drake, A., & Davis, J. (1992). Nasal airway in breathing and speech. *Cleft Palate-Craniofacial Journal, 29,* 511–519.

Warren, D., Duany, L., & Fischer, N. (1969). Nasal pathway resistance in normal and cleft lip and palate subjects. *Cleft Palate Journal, 6,* 134–140.

Warren, D., & DuBois, A. (1964). A pressure-flow technique for measuring velopharyngeal orifice area during continuous speech. *Cleft Palate Journal, 1,* 52–71.

Warren, D., Hairfield, W., & Hinton, V. (1985). The respiratory significance of the nasal grimace. *ASHA, 27,* 82.

Warren, D., Hairfield, W., Seaton, D., & Hinton, V. (1987). The relationship between nasal airway cross-sectional area and nasal resistance. *American Journal of Orthodontics and Dentofacial Orothopedics, 92*, 390–395.

Warren, D., Hairfield, W., Seaton, D., & Hinton, V. (1988). Relationship between the size of the nasal airway and nasal-oral breathing. *American Journal of Orthodontics and Dentofacial Orthopedics, 93*, 289–293.

Warren, D., Hairfield, W., Seaton, D., Morr, K., & Smith, L. (1988). The relationship between nasal airway size and nasal-oral breathing. *American Journal of Orthodontics and Dentofacial Orthopedics, 93*, 289–293.

Warren, D., Mayo, R., Zajac, D., & Rochet, A. (1996). Dyspnea following experimentally induced increased nasal airway resistance. *Cleft Palate-Craniofacial Journal, 33*, 231–235.

Wasz-Hockert, O., Lind, J., Vuorenkoski, V., Partanen, T., & Valanne, E. (1964). The infant cry: A spectrographic and auditory analysis. *Clinics in Developmental Medicine, Supplement 29*. London, UK: Heinemann.

Werntz, D., Bickford, R., Bloom, F., & Shannahoff-Khalsa, D. (1983). Alternating cerebral hemispheric activity and the lateralization of autonomic nervous function. *Human Neurobiology, 2*, 39–43.

Wilson, F., Kudryk, W., & Sych, J. (1986). The development of flexible fiberoptic video nasendoscopy (FFVN) clinical-teaching-research applications. *ASHA, 28*, 25–30.

Zaino, C., & Benventano, T. (1977). Functional, involutional, and degenerative disorders. In C. Zaino & T. Benventano (Eds.), *Radiologic examination of the oropharynx and esophagus* (pp. 141–170). New York, NY: Springer-Verlag.

Zajac, D. (1997). Velopharyngeal function in young and older adult speakers: Evidence from aerodynamic studies. *Journal of the Acoustical Society of America, 102*, 1846–1852.

Zajac, D. (2000). Pressure-flow characteristics of /m/ and /p/ production in speakers without cleft palate: Developmental findings. *Cleft Palate-Craniofacial Journal, 37*, 468–477.

Zajac, D., & Hackett, A. (2002). Temporal characteristics of aerodynamic segments in the speech of children and adults. *Cleft Palate-Craniofacial Journal, 39*, 432–438.

Zajac, D., & Mayo, R. (1996). Aerodynamic and temporal aspects of velopharyngeal function in normal speakers. *Journal of Speech and Hearing Research, 39*, 1199–1207.

Zankl, A., Eberle, L., Molinari, L., & Schinzel, A. (2002). Growth charts for nose length, nasal protrusion, and philtrum length from birth to 97 years. *American Journal of Medical Genetic, 111*, 388–391.

Pharyngeal-Oral Function and Speech Production

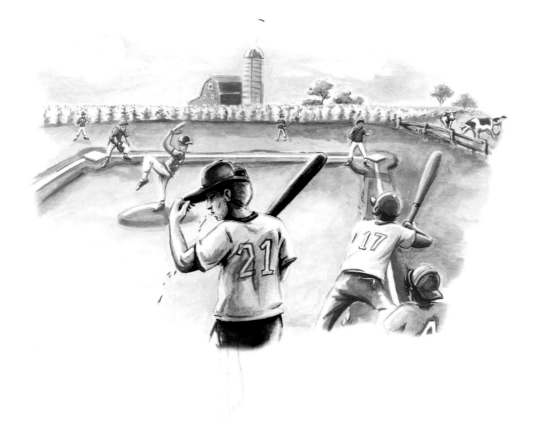

Scenario

His early life was good. He graduated from high school and was the first in his family to attend college. He made it through his sophomore year in agriculture and then his funds were drawn down. His parents were not people of means and could not help him. He took a job in a feed store to try to make enough money to continue his education. His intentions were good, but he never again saw the inside of a college classroom. It was partly because of the need to work and partly because a young woman captured his heart. After that, it was two children. He rose to become the manager at work.

One of his passions was baseball and he was very good at it. So good, in fact, that he once was given a tryout for a major-league farm team. He didn't make the team, but he was good enough to play during summers in a first-rate amateur baseball league in a nearby city. He could chew tobacco and spit with the best of them and the fans called him the vacuum cleaner because he would suck up any ball hit in the vicinity of third base. Little did he know, at the time, that his baseball habits would turn on him.

It was about a decade after his wedding that his life's burden fell on him. There was a feeling of fullness along the left side of his tongue. When he touched that side it felt different from the right side. He thought it might be the beginnings of a canker sore. He tried to look in his mouth with a mirror but he couldn't see anything special. It just felt different. He gargled with salt water, but his symptoms persisted. He thought they might eventually go away and so he procrastinated. It did him no good. The fullness remained.

He mentioned the problem to his wife and she insisted that he see a physician. The physician was suspicious. They discussed his history with chewing tobacco and she referred him to an otolaryngologist who performed a biopsy and did other tests that revealed cancer in his tongue. The problem was thought to be widespread and would require surgery to excise the cancerous tissue. The procedure would be extensive and had uncertainties that could only be resolved during the surgery itself. The waiting carried its own pain, took away sleep, and instilled increasing fear.

As he succumbed to anesthesia, his thoughts were pessimistic. When he awoke, it was worse than he had imagined. Spread of the cancer was such that his surgeon had to perform a total glossectomy (complete tongue removal) and also remove parts of his cheek and mandible on the left side. His oral cavity was empty down to the muscles that ran along the bottom of his mandible. His larynx was in clear view when he opened his mouth. The left side of his face was markedly disfigured. When he tried to speak to his wife, both were in disbelief. His voice sounded hollow and bizarre and his speech was unintelligible. He couldn't eat by mouth.

He came to feel desperate and sometimes cried when alone. He fell into psychological depression and lost a significant amount of weight. His spirit was broken. Physical recovery was painful and he felt embarrassment in front of his family and friends because of the way he looked and sounded. He came to believe that he would never again be able to speak in a social situation or be able to return to work. Life was grim for him and he felt isolated. He considered suicide on several occasions. His wife was also under stress. Fortunately, what seemed to be a certain dark future, turned out to have some bright spots.

Gone But Not Forgotten

Arm and leg amputations occurred in large numbers during the Civil War. Amputees from this era reported that pain or other sensations continued to arise from where their missing limbs had been. Some described them as sensory ghosts and many doctors of the time thought that those who reported them had mental problems. Not so. Phantom limb pain or other sensations are now recognized to be common following amputation of any body part and scientists have embraced a number of theories about their origins. Those who have had their tongues amputated (usually surgically and because of cancer) also report tongue pain or other sensations that are analogous to those associated with their better known phantom-limb counterpart. Ghost tongues are most prominent right after surgery and tend to fade away with time, although they are known to abruptly reappear on occasion. All of this is really quite haunting when you think about it.

HALF PRICE BOOKS ®

Half Price Books
1835 Forms Drive
Carrollton, TX 75006
OFS OrderID   18003142

SKU	ISBN/UPC	Title & Author/Artist		Shelf ID	Qty	OrderSKU
S31643474	9781597565202	Preclinical Speech Science: Anatomy, Physi.... Jeannette D. Holt;Gary Weismer,Thomas J. H.	-	26--12--3	1	

Thank you for your order, Halo Books BHW_AG115506-1823POBHW_!

Thank you for shopping with Half Price Books! Please contact Support@hpb.com. if you have any questions, comments or concerns about your order (113-9316446-2977065)

SHIPPED STANDARD TO:
Halo Books BHW_AG115506-1823POBHW_
2711 West Ash Street
AG115506-1823-1
Columbia MO 65203
zd5jwiw1h58cz0g@marketplace.amazon.com

ORDER# 113-9316446-2977065
AmazonMarketplaceUS

INTRODUCTION

The pharyngeal-oral apparatus, together with the velopharyngeal-nasal apparatus (discussed in Chapter 4), forms the upper airway. The pharyngeal-oral part of this airway is critical to various activities. Especially important in the present context are its functions during speaking and swallowing.

This chapter considers the fundamentals of pharyngeal-oral function, followed by a discussion of speech production. Also discussed are methods for measuring pharyngeal-oral function, pharyngeal-oral disorders, and the clinical professionals who are concerned with such disorders. The chapter then proceeds to a review and the presentation of a closing scenario. The function of the pharyngeal-oral apparatus during swallowing is discussed in Chapter 13.

FUNDAMENTALS OF PHARYNGEAL-ORAL FUNCTION

This section is concerned with the principles underlying pharyngeal-oral function. It includes a discussion of the anatomy of the pharyngeal-oral apparatus,

the forces and movements of the apparatus, potential adjustments of the apparatus, control variables of pharyngeal-oral function, and neural substrates of pharyngeal-oral control. Finally, attention is directed toward the range of functions that are performed by the pharyngeal-oral apparatus.

Anatomy of the Pharyngeal-Oral Apparatus

The pharyngeal-oral apparatus is a flexible tube that extends from the larynx to the lips. The fabric of this tube is formed mainly of bone and muscle. The apparatus undergoes an approximate 90-degree bend (like a plumber's elbow joint) at the level of the oropharynx. There, the shorter and vertical pharyngeal portion communicates through the oropharyngeal (faucial) isthmus with the longer and horizontal oral portion. Skeletal structure supports the pharyngeal-oral apparatus and provides the framework around which its internal topography is organized. Both this skeletal structure and its associated internal topography are considered below.

Skeleton

Figure 5–1 shows the skeletal superstructure of the pharyngeal-oral apparatus. This framework comprises

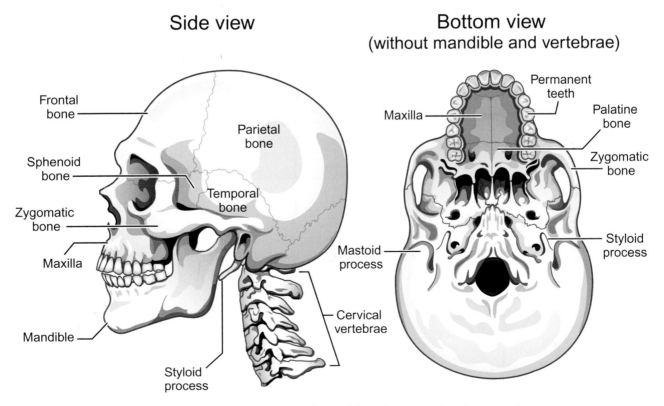

Side view

Bottom view
(without mandible and vertebrae)

Figure 5–1. Skeletal superstructure of the pharyngeal-oral apparatus.

the upper portion of the vertebral column and various bones of the skull.

Cervical Vertebrae. The upper portion of the vertebral column supports the skull and provides a scaffold for the neck. The cervical (neck) segments of the vertebral column lie behind the three subdivisions of the pharynx—laryngopharynx, oropharynx, and nasopharynx—and form part of the substance of their back walls (see Chapter 4).

Skull. The skull forms the framework of the head and comprises a large number of irregularly shaped bones. These are distributed in two major subdivisions. One is the cranium (braincase), which houses and protects the brain, and the other is the facial skeleton, which provides an underlying superstructure for much of the pharyngeal-oral apparatus. Certain parts of the facial skeleton are discussed in Chapter 4, in the context of the velopharyngeal-nasal apparatus, and are given further consideration here, along with other parts introduced below. The bones of the facial skeleton are especially important to the pharyngeal-oral apparatus in that they contribute to the formation of the roof, floor, and sides of the oral cavity.

Maxilla. Figure 5–2 depicts the maxilla. The maxilla forms the upper jaw and most of the hard palate. It consists of two complex bones (one on the left and one on the right) that combine at the midline. The maxilla lends strength to the roof of the oral cavity (as well as to the floor of the nasal cavities) and provides a buttress for the facial skeleton. Each bone of the maxilla has a palatine process that extends horizontally to the midline and joins with the palatine process from the opposite side to form the front three-fourths of the hard palate. The back one-fourth of the hard palate is formed by the much smaller palatine bones, which are closely associated with the palatine processes of the maxilla, and have horizontal processes that extend to the midline from each side to complete that part of the hard palate.

Other processes project from the maxilla. One of the most important of these is the alveolar process (sometimes called the alveolar arch). The alveolar process of the maxilla is a thick spongy projection that extends downward and houses the upper teeth. This process accommodates 16 permanent teeth (8 on each side): 6 molars, 4 premolars, 2 canines, and 4 incisors. Ten deciduous teeth (baby teeth or milk teeth) are typically found in infants and young children and are later replaced by the permanent teeth.

Mandible. Figure 5–3 shows the salient features of the mandible. The mandible (lower jaw) is a large horseshoe-shaped structure when viewed from above or below. Its open end faces toward the back. The front and sides of the mandible together form what is termed the body of the structure. The left and right halves of the mandible join at the front through a fibrous symphysis (line of union) that ossifies (turns to bone) during the first year of life. The tooth-bearing upper surface of the body of the mandible is termed its alveolar process (a counterpart to the lower surface of the maxilla). In the adult, the alveolar process of the mandible, like the alveolar process of the maxilla, accommodates 16 permanent teeth: 6 molars, 4 premolars, 2 canines, and 4 incisors. Also, like the alveolar process of the max-

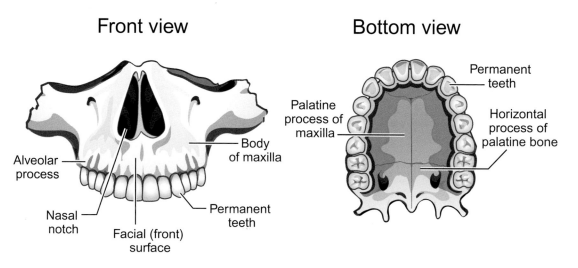

Figure 5–2. Maxilla.

illa, the alveolar process of the mandible usually holds 10 deciduous teeth (baby teeth or milk teeth) in infants and young children that are later replaced by permanent teeth.

On each side of the mandible toward the back, there is an upward projection. This part of the mandible is referred to as the ramus (meaning a branch from the body). The location along the bottom of the mandible where each ramus diverges upward is designated as the angle. The upper part of each ramus has two projections, one at the front called the coronoid process and one at the back called the condylar process (also called the condyle). The coronoid process is somewhat rounded, whereas the condylar process has a neck and a prominent head.

Other Bones of the Skull. Other bones of the skull form important components of the pharyngeal-oral apparatus. These bones are some 20 in number and are individually complex structures joined together by immovable fibrous joints (sutures). These bones present a wide array of processes, plates, projections, and air chambers that provide for the purchase of muscles and for the formation of sinuses within the head. The sinuses are hollows within the skull that have connections to the nasal cavities, the most important of which are the so-called paranasal sinuses (frontal, maxillary, ethmoid, and sphenoid).

In addition to the maxilla and mandible, some of the most important bony structures of the skull include the frontal bone (front of the upper braincase), parietal bones (sides of the upper braincase), temporal bones (sides of the lower braincase), sphenoid bone (base of the front of the cranium), palatine bones (back of the roof of the mouth), and zygomatic bones (part of the bony cheeks). Bony structures associated with the velopharyngeal-nasal apparatus are discussed in Chapter 4. The cartoon in Figure 5–4 illustrates that the link between bony structures and physiology has been understood for a long time.

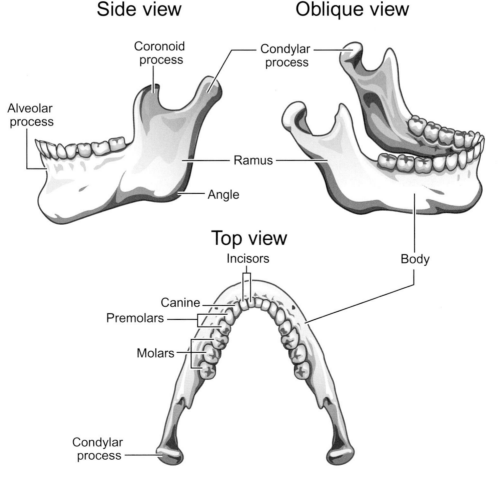

Figure 5-3. Mandible.

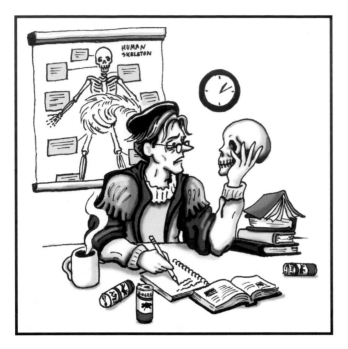

Figure 5-4. "That skull had a tongue in it, and could sing once." (Hamlet in *Hamlet*, Act 5, Scene 1, William Shakespeare).

Grant Fairbanks (1910–1964)

Fairbanks was a giant in speech science. He also trained others who became distinguished scientists. Fairbanks was a key figure in the development of speech science as a discipline and had a major influence in bringing it to the fore as an integrated science. One of his best-known works was the development of the notion that speech production was controlled in the manner of a servomechanism that relied on sensory feedback. His book titled *Voice and Articulation Drillbook* (Fairbanks, 1960) is a classic and contains the famous *Rainbow Passage* that has been used in more speech research studies than any other reading. Fairbanks died while on a flight between Chicago and San Francisco. The flight was diverted to Denver where the coroner ruled that he had choked to death while eating. Fairbanks was greatly admired as a scientist. The three of us are honored to be able to directly trace our professional lineages to him.

Temporomandibular Joints

The mandible (lower jaw) articulates with the left and right temporal bones along the sides of the skull

to form the temporomandibular joints. As illustrated in Figure 5–5, these joints are located just in front of and below the ear canals. They can be palpated when the mandible is alternately raised and lowered. The temporomandibular joints are enclosed by a fibrous capsule and lubricated by synovial fluid. Each joint is of the condyloid variety in that it consists of an ovoid (egg-shaped) process (the head of the condyle) that fits into an elliptical-shaped cavity within the temporal bone on the corresponding side (Dickson & Maue-Dickson, 1982).

The anatomical arrangement of each temporomandibular joint is such that the condyle of the mandible (the more rearward of its two processes) is separated from its receiving cavity by a cartilaginous meniscus (crescent) called the articular disk. The surfaces of the condyle and the temporal bone are themselves covered with fibrocartilage that is devoid of vascular tissue (Sicher & DuBrul, 1975).

Three ligaments influence the function of each temporomandibular joint (see Figure 5–5). These are the temporomandibular ligament, the sphenomandibular ligament, and the stylomandibular ligament. The temporomandibular ligament extends between the outer surface of the zygomatic arch and the outer and back surfaces of the neck of the condyle. This ligament limits the degree to which the condyle can be displaced downward and backward. The sphenomandibular ligament extends between the angular spine of the sphenoid bone and the inner surface of the ramus below the condyle. It limits downward and backward displacement of the mandible. The stylomandibular ligament extends between the styloid process of the temporal bone to near the angle of the mandible. This ligament limits downward and forward displacement of the mandible.

Temporomandibular Joint Movements

Movements at the temporomandibular joints are conditioned by the physical arrangements of the joints and their binding ligaments (both discussed above). The skull and mandible represent the articulating structures of the joint and the relative movement of these two dictates the nature of the action possible. For most activities, the skull is considered to be the more rigidly fixed member of the pair. Under some circumstances, however, the opposite is true. An example is when the chin is rested on the top of a table and the jaws are separated, such that the skull rotates upward and backward. Excluding such circumstances, movements at the temporomandibular joints are routinely conceptualized as movements of the mandible relative to a stabilized skull. This convention is followed here.

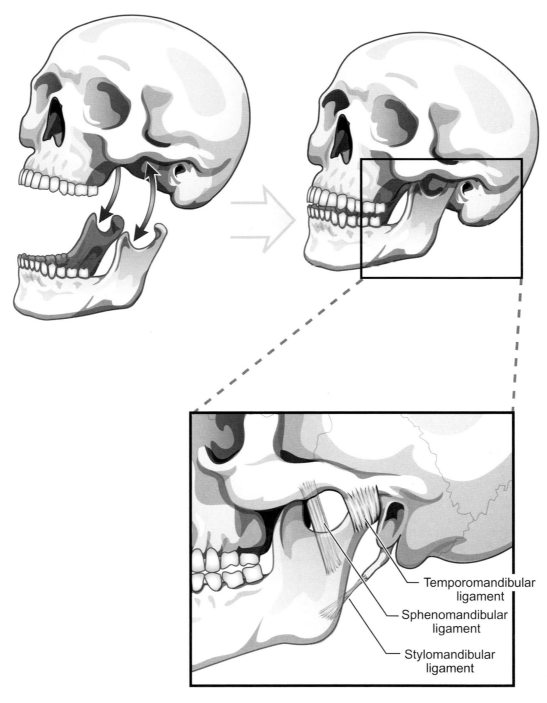

Figure 5–5. Temporomandibular joints and ligaments.

Movements of the mandible are mediated through its condyloid processes and are determined by how these processes are oriented within the elliptical-shaped receiving cavities of the temporal bones. The mandible can be moved in several ways relative to the skull. As shown in Figure 5–6, it can be displaced upward and downward, forward and backward, and side to side. These three displacement possibilities are made possible by a hingelike action, a forward and backward gliding action, and a side-to-side gliding action, respectively. The displacement possibilities depicted in Figure 5–6 are portrayed individually. This portrayal belies the fact that the movements at the temporomandibular joints are often multidimensional and very complex. This complexity is discussed below in other sections.

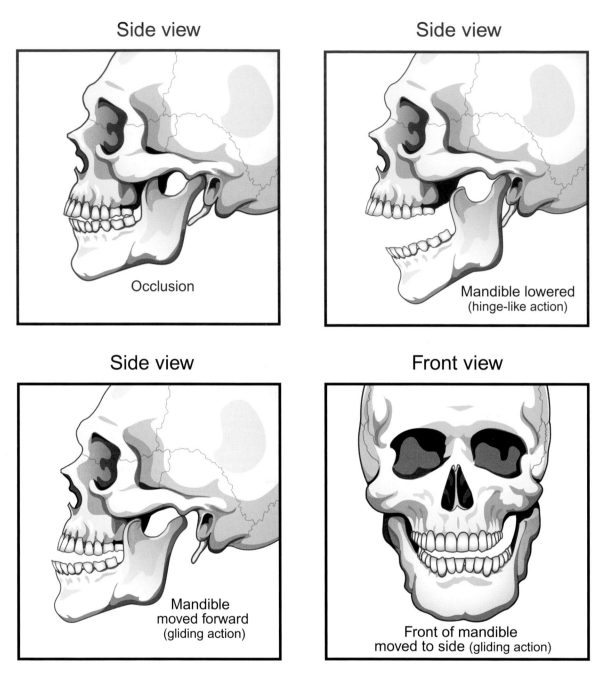

Side view

Occlusion

Side view

Mandible lowered
(hinge-like action)

Side view

Mandible
moved forward
(gliding action)

Front view

Front of mandible
moved to side (gliding action)

Figure 5–6. Temporomandibular joint movements.

Internal Topography

The internal topography of the pharyngeal-oral apparatus is fashioned around a hollow tube that bends at a right angle at the junction between the pharyngeal and oral portions of the structure. The pharyngeal, oral, and buccal cavities and their mucous lining deserve individual consideration.

Pharyngeal Cavity. Recall from Chapter 4 that the pharynx (throat) is a tube of tendon and muscle that extends from the base of the skull to the larynx. This tube is widest at the top and narrows down its length and is larger side to side than front to back. The lower and middle parts of the pharyngeal tube are designated as the laryngopharynx and oropharynx, respectively, and are the parts of greatest interest in this chapter.

Pharyngeal muscles ring the back and sides of the laryngopharynx and oropharynx. The lower part of the oropharynx is bounded by the tongue and epiglottis, whereas the upper part of the structure opens into the mouth at the front through the anterior faucial pillars (palatoglossal arch). The back wall of the upper part of the oropharynx can be seen when looking back through the faucial isthmus (see Figure 4–4).

Oral Cavity. Figure 5–7 depicts the oral cavity (mouth cavity). The oral cavity is bounded at the front and sides by the lips, teeth, and alveolar processes of the maxilla and mandible, above by the hard palate and velum, below by the floor of the mouth (mainly the tongue), and at the back by the anterior faucial pillars (palatoglossal arch). The front entryway to the oral cavity is designated as the oral vestibule and is defined to include the lips, cheeks, front teeth, and forward-most segments of the alveolar processes of the maxilla and mandible. The lips and/or front teeth form the front orifice of the oral cavity (oral airway opening). The palatoglossal arch forms an orifice at the back of the cavity.

The tongue is, of course, a prominent feature of the oral cavity. Although unitary in nature, it is sometimes subdivided into different regions. The subdivisions chosen may have either anatomical or functional bases,

depending on their purpose. Anatomical schemes usually recognize a root and a blade to the tongue, the former pertaining to the vertically oriented back wall of the structure (front wall of the laryngopharynx and oropharynx) and the latter pertaining to the horizontally oriented upper surface of the structure (floor of the oral cavity) (Zemlin, 1998). In contrast, functional schemes usually recognize regions of the tongue that are considered important to the behavior of the structure (Kent, 1997). Figure 5–8 adopts a scheme that has relevance to the purposes of this chapter and those of Chapter 13 (Swallowing).

Figure 5–8 shows the tongue as consisting of five different components, termed the tip, blade, dorsum, root, and body. The tip of the tongue is the part of its surface nearest the front teeth at rest. The blade is the part of its surface that lies behind the tip and below the alveolar ridge of the maxilla and the front part of the hard palate. The dorsum of the tongue constitutes the surface that lies behind the blade and below the back part of the hard palate and the velum. The root of the tongue designates the part of the surface of the structure that faces the back of the pharynx and the front of the epiglottis. And, the body of the tongue represents its central mass, which underlies the other four surface features discussed.

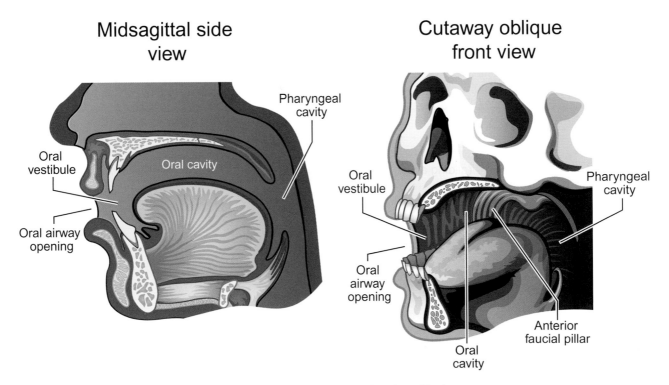

Figure 5–7. Oral cavity and oral vestibule.

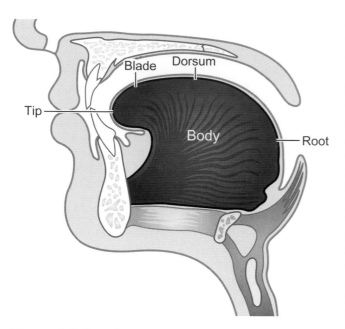

Figure 5–8. Functional scheme showing five components of the tongue.

Buccal Cavity. The buccal cavity lies to the sides of the oral cavity. This cavity constitutes the small space between the gums (gingivae) and teeth internally and the lips and cheeks (buccae) externally. The buccal cavity connects to the oral cavity through spaces between the teeth and behind the last molars. The status of the lips and cheeks are major determinants of the size of the buccal cavity.

Mucous Lining. The pharyngeal-oral apparatus contains a mucous lining on its internal surfaces. This lining consists of an outer layer of epithelium and an inner layer of connective tissue (lamina propria). The details of this layering differ at different locations within the pharyngeal-oral apparatus, especially the outer layer of epithelium (Dickson & Maue-Dickson, 1982). The most prominent mucosa lining has a shiny appearance and covers all of the soft tissues of the apparatus except the gums, hard palate, and tongue. A so-called masticatory mucosa covers the gums and the hard palate and has a collagen subflooring that causes its epithelium to hold firmly against adjacent bone. The upper surface of the tongue is covered with what is termed a specialized mucosa. This mucosa contains an array of small pockets and crypts that house taste buds.

Forces and Movements of the Pharyngeal-Oral Apparatus

Forces are responsible for movements of the pharyngeal-oral apparatus. Such forces and movements constitute the mechanical level of function of the apparatus.

Forces of the Pharyngeal-Oral Apparatus

Two types of forces are applied to the pharyngeal-oral apparatus, passive and active. Passive force is inherent and always present, but subject to change. Active force is applied in accordance with the will and ability of the individual.

Passive Force. The passive force of the pharyngeal-oral apparatus arises from several sources. These include the natural recoil of structures that line its walls, the surface tension between structures in apposition (lips, tongue, gums, hard palate, velum), the pull of gravity, and aeromechanical forces within the pharyngeal and oral portions of the apparatus (throat, mouth, oral vestibule). The distribution, sign, and magnitude of passive force depend on mechanical circumstances, including the positions, deformations, and levels of activity (if pertinent) of different components of the pharyngeal-oral apparatus.

Active Force. The active force of pharyngeal-oral function comes from the contraction of muscles. Some muscles are intrinsic, meaning that they have both ends

---

Dancing in the Moonlight

He was a pleasant young man who was honorably discharged after serving in the military. He had made his way to a large Veterans Administration Medical Center. His only complaint was hearing loss, but the audiologist thought his speech was inconsistent with his hearing test results. The moment he said his name to the speech-language pathologist, there was suspicion that he had impairment of one or both cranial nerves serving the tongue. When asked to open his mouth, the beam of a flashlight revealed a shrunken and wrinkled tongue that seemed to dance around under the surface like a bagful of jumping beans. The signs were classic of lower motor neuron disease and a neurologist reported presumptive bilateral congenital agenesis (failure to develop) of the hypoglossal nerves (motor nerves to the tongue). How had this escaped detection during his physical examination for the military? Perhaps he was only asked to say "ah."

attached within a component, and some are extrinsic, meaning that they have one end attached within a component and one end attached outside the component. Muscle actions within the pharyngeal-oral apparatus are not fully understood, but are known with reasonable certainty based on their architectures, the consequences of muscle activations, and observations of electrical activities.

The function portrayed here for individual muscles assumes that the muscle of interest is engaged in a shortening (concentric) contraction, unless otherwise specified as being involved in a lengthening (eccentric) contraction or a fixed-length (isometric) contraction. The tongue presents a somewhat more complex situation because of its special status as a muscular hydrostat (see below). The influence of individual muscle actions also depends on whether other muscles are active simultaneously, the mechanical status of different components of the apparatus, and the nature of the activity being performed.

Muscles of the Pharynx. The muscles of the pharynx are discussed in detail and portrayed in Chapter 4. These are located within the laryngopharynx, oropharynx, and nasopharynx. For the purposes of this chapter, those within the laryngopharynx and oropharynx are of primary interest and are reviewed here briefly.

Muscles of the laryngopharynx and oropharynx can influence the lumen of the pharynx (the cross-section along its length) in the region that lies behind the tongue, epiglottis, and oral cavity (the back wall of which is easily visualized through the faucial isthmus). The lumen of the pharynx in this region can also be influenced by adjustments of the tongue and epiglottis. Muscles that attach to the laryngopharynx and oropharynx fabric proper (within the posterior and lateral pharyngeal walls) are revisited here. These include the *inferior constrictor* muscle, *middle constrictor* muscle, and *stylopharyngeus* muscle (see Figure 4–8).

The *inferior constrictor* muscle of the pharynx is located toward the bottom of the structure. Fibers of the muscle arise from the sides of the thyroid and cricoid cartilages and diverge in a fanlike configuration as they course backward and toward the midline. There they interdigitate with fibers of the paired mate from the opposite side. The middle and upper fibers of the muscle ascend obliquely, whereas the lowermost fibers run horizontally and downward and are continuous with those of the esophagus. When the *inferior constrictor* muscle contracts, it pulls the lower part of the back wall of the pharynx forward and draws the sidewalls of the lower pharynx forward and inward. These actions cause the lumen of the lower pharynx to reduce in cross-section.

The *middle constrictor* muscle of the pharynx is located midway along the length of the pharyngeal tube. Fibers of the muscle arise from the greater and lesser horns of the hyoid bone and the stylohyoid ligament and course backward and toward the midline where they insert into the median raphe of the pharynx. The uppermost fibers of the *middle constrictor* muscle course obliquely upward and overlap the lower fibers of the *superior constrictor* muscle, whereas the lowermost fibers of the muscle run obliquely downward beneath the fibers of the *inferior constrictor* muscle. Recall that this fiber arrangement is akin to the way in which roof shingles partially overlap. When the *middle constrictor* muscle contracts, it decreases the cross-sectional area of the oropharynx by pulling forward on the posterior pharyngeal wall and forward and inward on the lateral pharyngeal wall. Simultaneous contraction of the left and right *middle constrictor* muscles causes the pharyngeal lumen to constrict regionally in the manner of a sphincter.

The *stylopharyngeus* muscle extends between the styloid process of the temporal bone and the lateral wall of the pharynx near the juncture of the *superior constrictor* and *middle constrictor* muscles of the pharynx. Its fibers run downward, forward, and toward the midline. When the *stylopharyngeus* muscle contracts, it pulls the pharyngeal tube upward and draws the lateral wall of the pharynx toward the side. Together with similar action of its paired mate from the opposite side, there results a widening or dilation of the lumen of the pharynx, especially in the region of the oropharynx, but also elsewhere along the length of the pharyngeal tube.

Muscles of the Mandible. Seven muscles provide active forces that operate on the mandible. These muscles are depicted in Figure 5–9 and are responsible for positioning the mandible in accordance with the movements allowed by the temporomandibular joints. Included among these muscles are the *masseter, temporalis, internal pterygoid, external pterygoid, digastric, mylohyoid,* and *geniohyoid.*

The *masseter* muscle is a flat, quadrilateral structure that covers much of the outer surface of the ramus of the mandible. Fibers of the muscle are in two layers. An outer layer forms the bulk of the muscle and courses from an aponeurosis along the front two-thirds of the zygomatic arch downward and backward to insert on the angle and nearby outer surface of the ramus of the mandible. An inner layer of fibers courses from the entire length of the zygomatic arch downward and forward to insert into the outer surface of the upper half of the ramus and its coronoid process. Contraction of the outer layer of the *masseter* muscle results

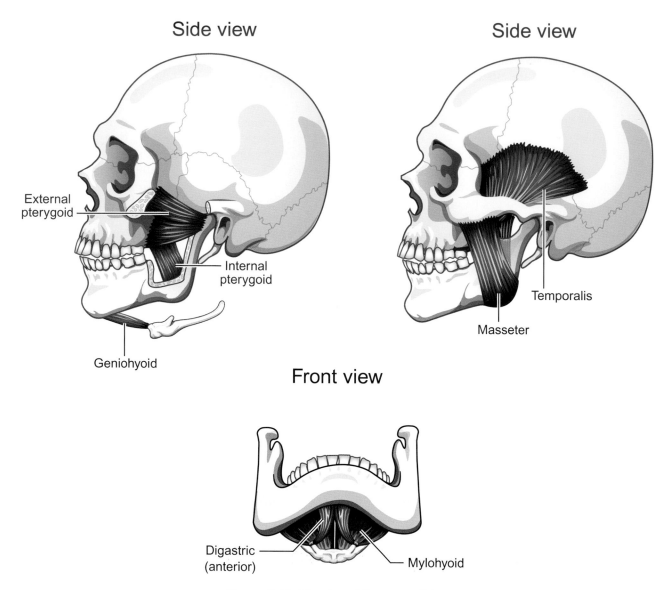

Figure 5–9. Muscles of the mandible.

in elevation of the mandible and approximation of the mandible and maxilla. The elevation is along a path that is at a right angle to the plane of occlusion of the molars. If the elevation is sufficient, pressure is brought to bear on the molars. Contraction of the inner layer of the muscle also results in elevation of the mandible and additionally exerts a force on the mandible that pulls it backward and aids in approximating the jaws.

The *temporalis* muscle is a broad, fanshaped muscle that covers much of the side of the cranium. Fibers of the muscle originate from the inferior temporal line of the parietal bone and the greater wing of the sphenoid bone. These converge as they course downward under the zygomatic arch and insert on the inner surface and front

border of the coronoid process and the front surface of the ramus of the mandible. Fibers toward the front and middle of the muscle course vertically, whereas those toward the back of the muscle have a more horizontal orientation. Contraction of the *temporalis* muscle results in an upward and backward pull on the mandible, with vertically oriented fibers contributing to the upward component and horizontally oriented fibers contributing to the backward component. Activation of the *temporalis* muscle on only one side may result in retraction of the mandible on the same side and movement of the front of the mandible toward the activated side.

The *internal pterygoid* muscle is a quadrilateral structure that follows an orientation that generally parallels that of the *masseter* muscle. Fibers of the *internal pterygoid* muscle originate from the lateral pterygoid plate and the perpendicular plate of the palatine bone. From there, they course downward, backward, and outward to insert on the inner surface of the angle and ramus of the mandible. Contraction of the *internal pterygoid* muscle results in elevation of the mandible. Sufficient elevation causes pressure to be placed on the opposing teeth of the mandible and maxilla. Activation of the muscle on only one side may result in slight movement of the corresponding condyle toward the opposite side.

The *internal pterygoid* muscle has a special relationship with the *masseter* muscle (already discussed). Together these two muscles form a muscular sling that surrounds the angle of the mandible. This anatomical sling holds the angle from above and effectively straps the ramus to the skull. The result is a functional articulation between the mandible and the maxilla, with the temporomandibular joint acting as an enabling guide for movements of the mandible (Zemlin, 1998).

The *external pterygoid* muscle is one of the smaller muscles of the mandible. Fibers of the *external pterygoid* muscle have two origins toward the front, one from the greater wing of the sphenoid bone and one from the lateral pterygoid plate. Fibers from these two points of origin tend to converge as they run generally horizontally backward to insert into the neck of the condyle of the mandible. Contraction of the *external pterygoid* muscle causes the condyle to slide downward and forward. Contraction of the *external pterygoid* muscle on only one side tends to move the front of the mandible toward the opposite side.

Three other muscles have a role in actions of the mandible. These are the *digastric* (*anterior* belly), *mylohyoid*, and *geniohyoid* muscles, all supplementary muscles of the laryngeal apparatus. The structure and function of these muscles are presented in detail in Chapter 3 and are reviewed here only briefly.

The *digastric* muscle is a two-bellied muscle arranged such that it can pull upward on the hyoid bone and/or downward on the mandible. Its action is dependent on the degree to which either or both of these structures are fixed in position by other muscles. With greater relative fixation of the hyoid bone, contraction of the *anterior* belly of the *digastric* muscle results in a lowering of the mandible. This increases the distance between the jaws.

The *mylohyoid* muscle is positioned along the floor of the oral cavity. It is oriented such that its fibers can exert an upward and forward pull on the hyoid bone or a downward pull on the mandible. With greater relative fixation of the hyoid bone, contraction of the *mylohyoid* muscle brings about a lowering of the mandible. Thus, the jaws will separate.

The *geniohyoid* muscle is a cylindrical muscle that lies above the *mylohyoid* muscle. The course of its muscle fibers is essentially parallel to the fiber course of the *anterior digastric* muscle (just discussed). Orientation of the muscle is such that it can pull upward and forward on the hyoid bone or downward on the mandible. As with the other two supplementary muscles discussed here, relative fixation of the hyoid bone and mandible by other muscles determines the consequence of action by the *geniohyoid* muscle. With greater relative fixation of the hyoid bone, contraction of the *geniohyoid* muscle results in a lowering of the mandible and an increase in the distance between the jaws, a functional consequence similar to that provided by the *anterior* belly of the *digastric* muscle.

Figure 5–10 schematically summarizes the potential actions of the muscles of the mandible that may influence the positioning and stabilization of the structure. General force vectors are depicted for the seven muscles of the mandible. These muscles, used in various combinations, can adjust the position of mandible up and down, front to back, and side to side.

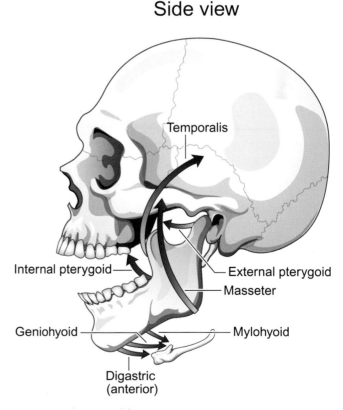

Side view

Figure 5–10. Actions of muscles of the mandible.

Muscles of the Tongue. The pharyngeal-oral apparatus receives skeletal support from the upper portion of the vertebral column and various bones of the skull. The tongue is additionally endowed with a special "soft skeleton" of its own. This personal skeleton of the tongue is largely connective tissue and serves to both surround and separate different components of the structure, including left and right halves (Dickson & Maue-Dickson, 1982). This skeleton also provides a confining "hide" in the form of a dense feltlike network of fibrous elastic tissue that lies below the epidermis and constitutes an encapsulating structural bag around the tongue (Zemlin, 1998). It is through this special soft skeleton of the tongue that various muscles are able to bring about the wide variety of tongue movements that are possible (see discussion below).

Eight muscles are responsible for movements of the tongue. These include four intrinsic muscles (having both their origins and insertions within the tongue) and four extrinsic muscles (having their origins in adjacent structures and their insertions in the tongue).

The intrinsic muscles of the tongue include the ***superior longitudinal, inferior longitudinal, vertical,*** and ***transverse*** muscles. These muscles are depicted in Figure 5–11.

The ***superior longitudinal*** muscle is a broad, flat muscle that lies just beneath the expansive upper surface (dorsum) of the tongue. Fibers originate within the root of the tongue from the hyoid bone and course forward in an imbricated pattern (like overlapping fish scales) along the long axis of the tongue. Forward attachments of the muscle are in the region of the front edges of the tongue and the upper surface of the tongue tip. Fibers near the midline course downward to their attachments, whereas fibers toward the side course obliquely toward the lateral boundary of the tongue. Contraction of the entire ***superior longitudinal*** muscle can shorten the tongue and increase its convexity from front to back. Because the muscle is composed of a series of short imbricated fibers, it can also activate in patterns that differentially affect the regional configuration of the tongue. For example, contraction of fibers toward the front of the tongue can pull the tongue tip upward and toward the side of muscle activation. Simultaneous contractions of comparable fibers in the paired ***superior longitudinal*** muscles elevate the tongue tip without deviation to either side. For another example, contraction of fibers that insert obliquely into the edges of the tongue can pull the lateral margins of the structure upward to create a longitudinal trough down the center of the tongue toward the front.

The ***inferior longitudinal*** muscle is positioned near the undersurface of the tongue somewhat toward the side. It arises from the body of the hyoid bone at the root of the tongue and courses forward through the body of the tongue to insert near the lower surface of the tongue tip. Fibers of the ***inferior longitudinal*** muscle blend with the fibers of different extrinsic muscles of the tongue (discussed below) within the body of the tongue. Contraction of the ***inferior longitudinal*** muscle shortens the tongue and pulls the tip of the structure downward and toward the same side. Simultaneous

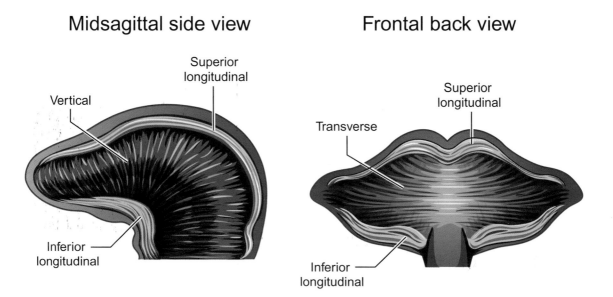

Midsagittal side view

Vertical

Superior
longitudinal

Inferior
longitudinal

Frontal back view

Superior
longitudinal

Transverse

Inferior
longitudinal

Figure 5-11. Intrinsic muscles of the tongue.

contraction of comparable fibers in the paired *inferior longitudinal* muscles pulls the tongue tip downward symmetrically.

The *vertical* muscle originates from just beneath the dorsum of the tongue and courses downward vertically and toward the side through the body of the tongue. Fibers of the *vertical* muscle terminate near the sides of the tongue along its lower surface. There is some suggestion that not all fibers follow a course through the entire body of the tongue, but rather are found only in the upper half of the tongue (Miyawaki, 1974), or that there is a mixture of short and long fibers, some of which course only through the upper half of the tongue and some of which course all the way to the lower part of the tongue (Abd-El-Malek, 1939). Contraction of the *vertical* muscle results in a flattening of the tongue on the side of action, especially toward its lateral margins. More midline parts of the upper tongue surface may also be lowered on the side of action as a result of pull exerted during the contraction of this muscle.

The *transverse* muscle, as its name implies, courses side to side within the tongue. Fibers of the muscle arise mainly from the median fibrous skeleton of the tongue and course laterally, where they terminate in fibrous tissue along the side of the tongue. Upper fibers fan out in an upward direction, whereas lower fibers fan out in a downward direction. The intermingling of *transverse* muscle fibers with those of other intrinsic and extrinsic tongue muscles is extensive and makes it hard to determine their precise course and location within different parts of the tongue. Some fibers may not extend all the way to the sides of the tongue (Miyawaki, 1974) and the extent to which fibers are located at the back of the tongue is in question (Abd-El-Malek, 1939). The *transverse* muscle is, however, a major constituent in the mass of interwoven muscle fibers that comprise the bulk of the tongue. Contraction of the *transverse* muscle results in a narrowing of the tongue from side to side and an elongation of the tongue.

The extrinsic muscles of the tongue include the *styloglossus, palatoglossus, hyoglossus,* and *genioglossus* muscles. These are depicted in Figure 5–12.

The *styloglossus* muscle originates from the front and side of the styloid process of the temporal bone and the stylomandibular ligament. Fibers of the muscle course forward, downward, and toward the midline to insert into the sides of the root of the tongue. From there, they run in various directions, but primarily toward the midline and forward within the body of the tongue. Some fibers of the *styloglossus* muscle interdigitate with fibers of the *inferior longitudinal* muscle, whereas others interdigitate with fibers of the *hyoglossus* muscle (discussed below and in Chapter 3). Ultimate blending of different fibers makes it difficult to distinguish those of one muscle from another. Contraction of the *styloglossus*

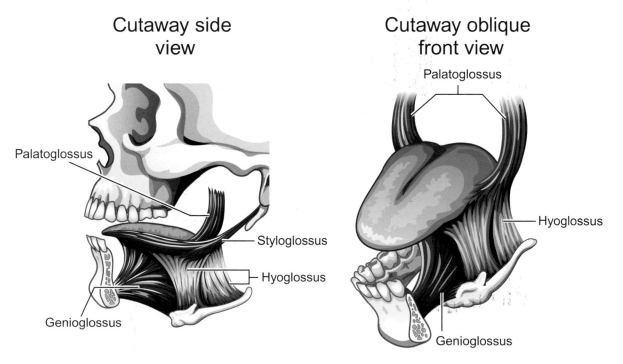

Figure 5-12. Extrinsic muscles of the tongue.

Early X-Games

This isn't about sports, but about x-rays. Early uses of x-rays to study structures of the upper airway during speech production were quite interesting. A few tidbits should give you an appreciation. A narrow gold chain was often placed down the midline of the tongue to make its longitudinal configuration easy to visualize on single shot lateral head x-rays. Some of the first findings from different laboratories were not in agreement concerning tongue positions during vowel productions. Despite public arguments about linguistic bases for the differences, it turned out that the head had not been fixed in position and variation was related to its rotation from one exposure to another. Then, there were dangers. A pioneer in the use of x-rays for speech research entered old age unable to grow a beard on one side of his face, the side he had frequently bombarded with x-rays to get the view of the speech production apparatus he wanted to study.

muscle can have multiple consequences. These include that: (a) the body of the tongue can be drawn upward and backward, (b) the side of the tongue can be pulled upward to influence the structure's concavity, (c) the tongue can be shortened, and (d) the tongue tip can be pulled toward the side.

The *palatoglossus* muscle is discussed in Chapter 4 as a part of the velopharyngeal-nasal apparatus. There it is referred to as the *glossopalatine* muscle (its origin and insertion being reversed in that context). For present purposes, the *palatoglossus* muscle can be thought of as originating from the lower surface of the palatal aponeurosis. Fibers from the muscle course downward, forward, and toward the side (forming the anterior faucial pillar) and insert into the side of the root of the tongue. There the fibers of the *palatoglossus* muscle blend with those of the *transverse*, *styloglossus*, and *hyoglossus* muscles of the tongue. When the *palatoglossus* muscle contracts, it pulls upward, backward, and inward on the root of the tongue. Through its action, the muscle can displace the tongue mass backward in the oral cavity and increase the concavity of its upper surface. When the left and right *palatoglossus* muscles contract simultaneously, the result is a lengthwise grooving of the upper surface of the tongue.

The *hyoglossus* muscle (see also Chapter 3) is a quadrilateral structure that originates from the upper border of the body and greater cornua of the hyoid bone and extends upward and forward to insert into the side of the tongue toward the rear. Fibers of the *hyoglossus* muscle intermingle with those of the *styloglossus* and *palatoglossus* muscles. Some authors consider one particular bundle of fibers within the *hyoglossus* muscle to be a separate muscle (Zemlin, 1998). This bundle is identified as the *chondroglossus* muscle and has fibers that extend from the hyoid bone farther forward into the tip of the tongue where they intermingle with fibers from intrinsic tongue muscles such as the *inferior longitudinal* muscle. Contraction of the *hyoglossus* (and *chondroglossus*) muscle results in a lowering of the body of the tongue and a backward displacement of its mass. The lowering effect is most pronounced along the sides of the tongue (Dickson & Maue-Dickson, 1982).

The *genioglossus* muscle is a complex muscle that makes up a large portion of the tongue. This muscle is fanshaped and originates as three groups of fibers from the inner surface of the body of the mandible near the midline. The lower fibers course backward to insert into the root of the tongue. The middle fibers course backward and extend upward into the tongue in the region of the juncture between the dorsum and blade of the structure. The upper fibers run vertically and forward to insert into the tip of the tongue (Langdon, Klueber, & Barnwell, 1978), although some authors report that fibers stop short of the tongue tip itself (Doran & Baggett, 1972; Miyawaki, 1974). Collectively, fibers of the *genioglossus* muscle travel through the body of the tongue between layers of muscle fibers formed by the *vertical*, *transverse*, and *superior longitudinal* muscles of the structure (Dickson & Maue-Dickson, 1982). Contraction of the *genioglossus* muscle can have a diverse set of consequences, depending on which particular fibers of the muscle are activated and in what patterns. Possible outcomes are that: (a) the root of the tongue can be moved forward so as to force the tip of the tongue against the teeth or out of the mouth, (b) the front of the tongue can be pulled backward, and (c) the center line of the tongue can be pulled downward so as to form a troughlike depression along the length of the upper surface of the structure.

Figure 5–13 depicts the general force vectors associated with actions of the eight muscles of the tongue. This illustration summarizes the potential active forces that could be in play at any moment to change the configuration of the tongue and its positioning within the pharyngeal-oral apparatus.

The discussion to this juncture about the individual capabilities of intrinsic and extrinsic tongue muscles is linear in nature and, although instructive, does

Combined side and sagittal view

Combined front and frontal view

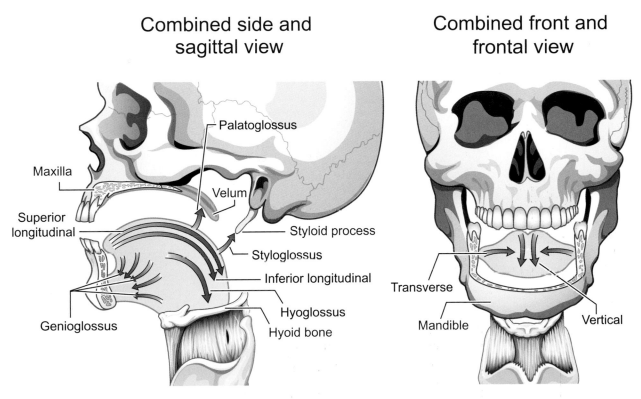

Figure 5–13. Actions of the muscles of the tongue.

not do justice to the intricate and interacting forces that can operate on and within the tongue to move it in different ways. Much of this has to do with special properties of the tongue that qualify it as a muscular hydrostat. These properties and the remarkable range of tongue movements are discussed below in the context of adjustment capabilities of the pharyngeal-oral apparatus.

Muscles of the Lips. The muscles of the lips are a subset of the muscles of the face. These muscles are more than a dozen in number and are portrayed in Figure 5–14 from different perspectives. The muscles of the lips include both intrinsic (contained within) and extrinsic (one attachment within) components. These muscles include the *orbicularis oris, buccinator, risorius, levator labii superioris, levator labii superioris aleque nasi, zygomatic major, zygomatic minor, depressor labii inferioris, mentalis, levator anguli oris, depressor anguli oris, incisivus labii superioris, incisivus labii inferioris,* and *platysma*.

The *orbicularis oris* muscle is a ring of muscle within the lips that forms a sphincter at the oral end (mouth opening) of the pharyngeal-oral apparatus. The ring of muscle is complex and is constituted of fibers from both intrinsic and extrinsic sources that intertwine to form an airway valve and the most mobile part of the face. Fibers of the *orbicularis oris* muscle that are exclusive to the lips (intrinsic) are arranged in concentric rings around the border of the sphincter. These rings follow the outer contour of the upper and lower lips. The course of the intrinsic fibers of the *orbicularis oris* muscle changes with changes in the angular circumference of the mouth opening. Contraction of the *orbicularis oris* muscle can result in several positional changes of the lips. These include movements of the lips toward one another and forward, which, if extensive enough, can result in closure of the mouth and a forcing together of the lips. The corners of the mouth may also move as a result of activation of the *orbicularis oris* muscle. Such movement can be upward, downward, toward the side, or toward the midline. Action of the muscle may also force the lips and/or corners of the mouth against the teeth.

Those lip muscles that are extrinsic are sometimes subgrouped into sets that follow fiber courses that are transverse (horizontal), angular (oblique to the corners of the mouth), vertical (from above or below), and parallel (adjacent to and alongside the lips). These subsets are considered, in turn, below. An additional muscle is

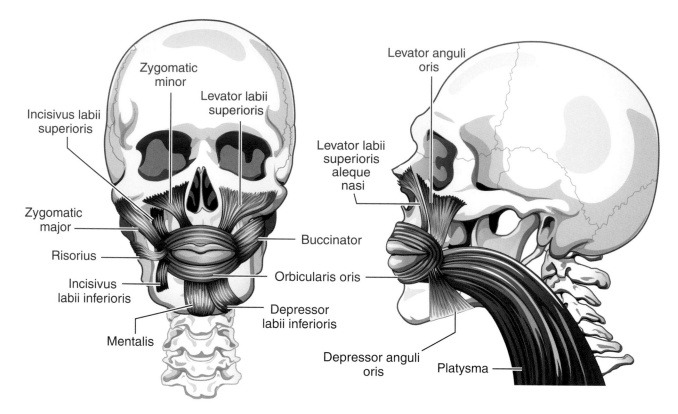

Figure 5–14. Muscles of the lips.

also discussed at the end of this section. This muscle, the *platysma*, is classified as a cervical (neck) muscle, but is included as a special case because it has extrinsic influences on the lower lip.

The transverse facial muscles that influence the lips are the *buccinator* muscle and the *risorius* muscle. The former is sometimes called the bugler's muscle and the latter is often referred to as the laughter muscle.

The *buccinator* muscle is a broad muscle that forms part of the cheek. It originates from the pterygomandibular ligament, the outer surface of the alveolar process of the maxilla, and the mandible from the region of the last molars. Fibers course horizontally forward and toward the midline to insert into the upper and lower lips near the corner of the mouth. Uppermost fibers of the muscle enter the upper lip, whereas lowermost fibers enter the lower lip. Fibers of the central part of the muscle converge near the corner of the mouth and cross such that the lower fibers of that part of the muscle insert into the upper lip and the upper fibers insert into the lower lip. Contraction of the *buccinator* muscle can pull the corner of the mouth backward and toward the side. It can also force the lips and cheek against adjacent teeth.

The *risorius* muscle is a small muscle located within the cheek, but closer to the surface than the

buccinator muscle. It arises from fascia of the *masseter* muscle and courses horizontally forward and toward the midline to insert into the corner of the mouth and the lower lip. Contraction of the *risorius* muscle draws the corner of the mouth backward and toward the side. Contraction of the muscle may also force the lips against adjacent teeth.

The angular muscle group includes five muscles. These are the *levator labii superioris* muscle, *levator labii superioris aleque nasi* muscle, *zygomatic major* muscle, *zygomatic minor* muscle, and the *depressor labii inferioris* muscle.

The *levator labii superioris* muscle has a broad origin from below the orbit of the eye, the front of the maxillary bone, and the zygomatic bone. Its fibers course downward and slightly inward and insert into the upper lip. Contraction of the *levator labii superioris* muscle results in elevation of the upper lip. Contraction may also cause an outward turning (eversion) of the upper lip.

The *levator labii superioris aleque nasi* muscle originates as a slender slip from the front of the maxilla and courses vertically downward and slightly toward the side. The muscle divides into a nasal segment and a lip segment. Fibers from the lip segment of the muscle insert into the upper lip where they intermingle with

---

Street Talk About Talking

The folk language is filled with indications that the person on the street knows something about pharyngeal-oral function in speech production. Below are some expressions that we generated off the tops of our heads. Look at these and then try to add to the list from your own knowledge of the folk language. Our favorite from the list below is the last one, used during World War II to mean be careful to whom you are talking. Here goes. "That's a real tongue twister." "We were just jawing it." "He's bumping his gums." "They were flapping their cheeks." "She's lying through her teeth." "Don't give me any of your lip." "I don't chew my cabbage twice." "He's running off at the mouth again." "Hold your tongue, young man." "She's a big loudmouth." "His father told him to cork it." And our favorite, "Loose lips sink ships."

---

fibers of the *orbicularis oris* muscle. Contraction of the lip segment of the *levator labii superioris aleque nasi* muscle causes elevation of the upper lip. Contraction of the nasal segment of the muscle dilates the anterior naris on the corresponding side, as described in Chapter 4.

The *zygomatic major* muscle has its origin on the side of the zygomatic bone and runs down and toward the midline where it inserts into the corner of the mouth. Fibers associated with its insertion intermingle with those of the *orbicularis oris* muscle. Contraction of the *zygomatic major* muscle pulls backward on the corner of the mouth. At the same time, action of the muscle lifts the corner of the mouth upward and toward the side.

The *zygomatic minor* muscle originates from the inner surface of the zygomatic bone. Its fibers course downward and toward the midline where they insert into the upper lip and interweave with fibers of the *orbicularis oris* muscle. Contraction of the *zygomatic minor* muscle results in elevation of the upper lip. It also pulls the corner of the mouth upward.

The *depressor labii inferioris* muscle is a small, flat muscle located off the midline of the lower lip. Fibers of the muscle originate from the front surface of the mandible and course upward and inward to insert into the lower lip from near the midline to the corner of the mouth. Contraction of the *depressor labii inferioris* muscle pulls the lower lip downward and toward the side. It may also cause the lower lip to turn outward.

The vertical facial muscles are three in number. They include the *mentalis* muscle, *levator anguli oris* muscle, and the *depressor anguli oris* muscle.

The *mentalis* muscle lies on the front of the chin. It is a small muscle that arises from the front and side of the mandible near the midline and inserts into the *orbicularis oris* muscle and the skin overlying the chin. Contraction of the *mentalis* muscle results in upward displacement of the soft tissue of the chin, a forcing of the lower part of the lower lip against the alveolar process of the mandible, and an outward curling of the lower lip. The lower lip may also elevate somewhat during contraction of the *mentalis* muscle. The functional potentials described are consistent with the familiar signs of pouting and, indeed, the *mentalis* muscle is sometimes called the "pouting muscle."

The *levator anguli oris* muscle (also referred to as the *caninus* muscle) originates from the front of the maxilla and courses downward and forward to insert into both the upper lip and the lower lip near the corner of the mouth. There, its fibers intermingle with those of the *orbicularis oris* muscle. Contraction of the *levator anguli oris* muscle draws the corner of the mouth upward and toward the side. Activation of the muscle can also elevate the lower lip against the upper lip and force the lips together.

The *depressor anguli oris* muscle is also sometimes referred to as the *triangularis* muscle. As its alternate name implies, the muscle is roughly triangular in form. This muscle has a broad origin from the outer surface of the mandible. Its fibers course upward and converge before inserting into the *orbicularis oris* muscle at the corner of the mouth and into the upper lip. Contraction of the *depressor anguli oris* muscle pulls the corner of the mouth downward. It also forces the lips together by drawing the upper lip downward against the lower lip.

There are two parallel facial muscles. These are the *incisivus labii superioris* muscle and the *incisivus labii inferioris* muscle.

The *incisivus labii superioris* muscle is a small, narrow muscle that lies beneath the *levator labii superioris* muscle. Fibers of the *incisivus labii superioris* muscle originate from the maxilla in the region of the canine tooth and course parallel to the transverse fibers of the *orbicularis oris* muscle of the upper lip. Insertion of the muscle is in the region of the corner of the mouth where its fibers intermingle with the fibers of other muscles. Contraction of the *incisivus labii superioris* muscle pulls the corner of the mouth upward and toward the midline.

The *incisivus labii inferioris* muscle constitutes the lower lip counterpart of the *incisivus labii superioris* muscle. The *incisivus labii inferioris* muscle lies below the corner of the mouth and underneath the *depressor labii superioris* muscle. The muscle originates on the mandible in the region of lateral incisor tooth and courses parallel to the transverse fibers of the *orbicularis oris* muscle of the lower lip. The insertion of the *incisivus labii inferioris* muscle is into the region of the corner of the mouth. Contraction of the muscle results in a downward and inward pull on the corner of the mouth. The downward component of this action is antagonistic to the upward pull provided by the *incisivus labii superioris* muscle.

The *platysma* muscle is a very board muscle that covers most of the front and side of the neck and much of the side of the face. The muscle has an extensive origin from a sheet of connective tissue within the neck above the clavicle and may even extend from as far below as the front of the chest wall and regions of the back of the torso. Fibers of the *platysma* muscle run upward and forward to attach to the lower edge of the mandible along the side and interweave with fibers of the opposite side at the front of the mandible. Its fibers have a broad distribution about the face, which

includes a blending of fibers associated with different muscles of the lower lip and the corner of the mouth. Contraction of the *platysma* muscle draws the skin of the neck toward the mandible. It may also pull the lower lip and corner of the mouth to the side and downward and/or force the lower lip against the lower teeth and the alveolar process of the mandible.

Figure 5–15 portrays the general force vectors for the 14 muscles of the lips. These vectors summarize the active forces operating on the lips and their consequences on the positioning of the lips and corners of the mouth up and down, side to side, and with regard to compression against the teeth and/or alveolar processes of the maxilla and mandible. Figure 5–15 evokes images about the seeming infinite variety of lips adjustments that are possible and how those adjustments are intricately involved in human expression. Figure 5–16 offers a humorous view of how the lips can be involved in expression.

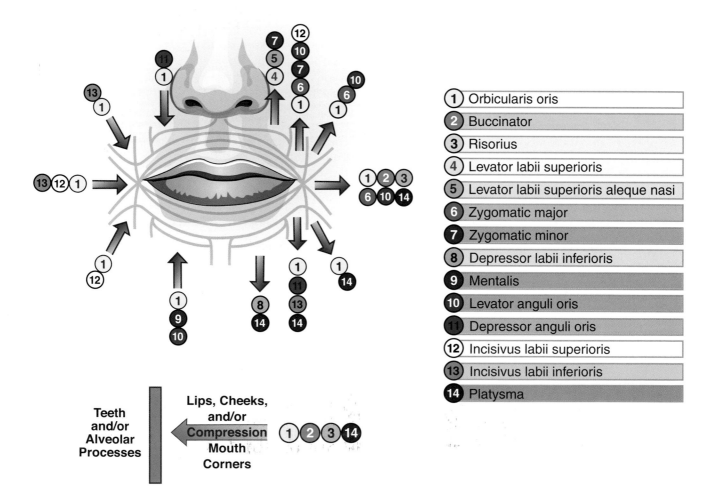

(1)	Orbicularis oris
(2)	Buccinator
(3)	Risorius
(4)	Levator labii superioris
(5)	Levator labii superioris aleque nasi
(6)	Zygomatic major
(7)	Zygomatic minor
(8)	Depressor labii inferioris
(9)	Mentalis
(10)	Levator anguli oris
(11)	Depressor anguli oris
(12)	Incisivus labii superioris
(13)	Incisivus labii inferioris
(14)	Platysma

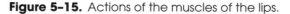

Figure 5–15. Actions of the muscles of the lips.

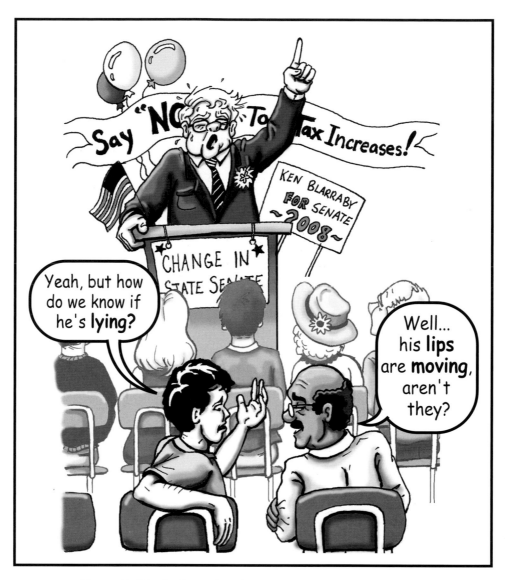

Figure 5–16. Cartoon showing a discerning potential voter.

The Cold War

With prolonged exposure to very cold weather, your face tightens up and your speech slows down. Certain parts of your speech production apparatus actually get stiffer as you chill down. You can live with this because your body, although coping with change at the periphery, is still winning the cold war. Should things get worse, however, such that hypothermia sets in, you'll be in trouble. Hypothermia occurs when your body can't replace heat lost to its surroundings and your core temperature begins to drop. From the usual 98.6°F down to 95°F, your speech will continue to sound normal. Below 95°F down to 90°F, your speech will become slurred and progressively more so as temperature decreases. Once your core temperature passes below 90°F, your speech will be unintelligible. The cooling of the body is simply too much for the nervous system to handle and all remaining resources are devoted to preserving the organism.

Movements of the Pharyngeal-Oral Apparatus

Movements are important to many functions of the pharyngeal-oral apparatus. Potential movements are considered below apart from the forces that cause them. The relation of forces to movements is discussed in the section on adjustments.

Movements of the Pharynx. The potential movements of the overall pharynx are discussed in detail in Chapter 4 and illustrated there (see Figure 4–13). Focus here is on potential movements of the laryngopharynx and oropharynx. These portions of the pharyngeal tube are relatively mobile and present three movement capabilities. These include: (a) inward and outward movement of their sidewalls, (b) forward and backward movement of their back wall, and (c) forward and backward movement of their front wall (tongue and/or epiglottis). These movements enable the lumen of the laryngopharynx and oropharynx to be changed in size and shape.

Movements of the Mandible. The mandible is capable of a wide range of movements in three-dimensional space. Complex movements of the structure derive from its potential to move upward and downward, forward and backward, and side to side through the different hingelike and gliding actions of the temporomandibular joints described above (see Figure 5–6).

Upward and downward and forward and backward movements of the mandible often include both rotational and translational components (Zemlin, 1998). Rotational movements are hingelike and resemble the swinging of a two-hinged trap door about an axis that extends through the center pins of its hinges. Such movements of the mandible take place about a lateral axis that passes through the condyloid processes on the left and right sides of the skull. Translational movements, in contrast, involve downward and forward or upward and backward displacements of the mandible along the rear slopes of the articular facets of the temporomandibular joints. These movements are of the nature observed when the mandible is moved forward or backward without an accompanying hingelike rotational component and are based on the forward and backward gliding potential at the temporomandibular joints. Side-to-side movements of the mandible provide for additional complexity by taking advantage of the to-and-fro gliding action at the temporomandibular joints that enable the mandible to be moved from left to right or vice versa.

The multiple movement possibilities of the mandible can combine to pitch the structure upward or downward about a lateral axis, roll it to one side or the other about a longitudinal axis, and yaw it to the left or right about a vertical axis. An example where the three movements combine is seen in the crushing and grinding associated with chewing. The movements of boats and airplanes are also good examples of how a structure can pitch, roll, and yaw all at the same time.

Movements of the Tongue. The tongue is a fleshy muscular structure that is exceedingly mobile. Its mobility derives from the fact that: (a) it rides with the mandible and floor of the oral cavity and goes as a whole where they go (see section below on adjustments), (b) its position within the oral cavity can be shifted en masse as a body (akin to moving a closed fist around in space), and (c) its shape can be changed markedly and relatively independently of the first two sources of mobility.

Movements of the tongue are often segmental and differ along its major and minor axes. Thus, one part of the structure may move more or less than another or even in a different direction than another. Movements of different points on the surface of the structure can be upward and downward, forward and backward, side to side, or different combinations of these. Vertical movements can extend from the trough of the mouth to the roof of the oral cavity. Front-to-back movements can range from a maximally forward displacement of the tongue out of the mouth to a maximally rearward displacement of the structure against the back wall of the pharynx. Side-to-side movements can range from the stretchable limits of one cheek to the other.

Movements of the Lips. The mobility of the face in the region of the lips rivals that of the fine movements of the fingers. Movements of the lips can occur along vertical, side-to-side, and front-to-back dimensions. Each lip can be moved independently of the other or the two lips can be coordinated in their movements. The upper lip is fixed in spatial coordinates to the fixed position of the maxilla, whereas the lower lip rides with the mandible and the consequences of its positional changes are dictated, in part, by the prevailing position of the mandible. The juncture of the two lips at the corners of the mouth can entail movements of both the upper and lower lips and is influenced by both intrinsic and extrinsic forces imparted by the facial muscles. The wide range of possible lip movements implicates a complex array of combinations of muscle forces operating on the lips. Experimenting with lip movements in front of a mirror gives one an almost awesome appreciation for the degrees of freedom of movement in the region of the mouth opening.

Adjustments of the Pharyngeal-Oral Apparatus

Adjustments of the pharyngeal-oral apparatus reflect the potential configurations that can be assumed by the overall apparatus and its component parts. Such adjustments involve combinations of the movements discussed in sections above.

Adjustments of the Pharynx

The pharynx is capable of many adjustments. Chapter 4 includes a discussion of adjustment capabilities within the upper part of the pharynx (nasopharynx) and their roles in adjusting the degree of coupling between the oral and nasal cavities through the velopharyngeal port. Interest here is in adjustment capabilities of the lower and middle parts of the pharynx (the laryngopharynx and oropharynx, respectively) and their roles in changing the regional lumen of the pharynx and the degree of coupling between the oropharynx and the oral cavity through the palatoglossal arch (anterior faucial pillars).

Recall that the lumen of the pharynx is oval in cross-section, being larger side to side than front to back. This lumen can be adjusted so as to change both its size and/or shape. Adjustments in size can range from a maximally enlarged pharyngeal airway to one that is fully obstructed. In the case of complete obstruction, the walls of the pharynx may not only come in contact, but may also undergo forceful compression against one another. When a pharyngeal lumen exists, it can be changed in both size and shape. Shape adjustments may range from elliptical to circular or otherwise.

Certain pharyngeal adjustments, or components of them, can result from the actions of other structures. For example, lowering of the mandible results in an inward pull on the sides of the pharynx that causes a reduction in its side-to-side diameter and a smaller and more circular lumen (Minifie, Hixon, Kelsey, & Woodhouse, 1970). Thus, simply raising and lowering the mandible, without the activation of muscles in the pharyngeal region, results in significant changes in the size and/or shape of the pharyngeal airway.

Passive influences notwithstanding, more purposeful adjustments of the pharynx are effected by the actions of muscles that attach to and directly influence the positioning of the four walls of the structure. Inward movements of the sides of the structure are effected mainly through contractions of the *inferior* and *middle constrictor* muscles and outward movements are effected through contractions of the *stylopharyngeus*

muscle. Forward and backward movements of the back wall of the pharynx figure into certain adjustments of the airway, whereas forward and backward movements of its front wall (tongue and epiglottis) are prominent contributors to many adjustments. The velum may also be involved in actively adjusting the lumen of the oropharynx. When at rest, the velum hangs pendulously and its upper surface forms the upper front wall of the oropharynx. As the velum moves, it changes the upper front-to-back diameter of the oropharynx. This is true until its elevation is sufficient to carry it out of the oropharynx and into the nasopharynx, whereupon its lower surface then forms the approximate upper boundary of the oropharynx.

Adjustment of the degree of coupling between the pharyngeal cavity and oral cavity is influenced by: (a) upward and downward movements of the tongue, (b) upward and downward movements of the velum, and (c) side-to-side movements of the pillars of the palatoglossal arch (anterior faucial pillars). Decreases in the degree of coupling through the oropharyngeal isthmus are achieved through one or any combination of upward movement of the tongue, downward movement of the velum, and inward movement of the palatoglossal arch. Conversely, increases in the degree of coupling through the oropharyngeal isthmus are accomplished through one or any combination of opposite movements of these three components. Maximum coupling is brought about by a combined maximum elevation of the velum and maximum depression of the tongue. Decoupling results when the undersurface of the velum and the upper surface of the tongue are placed in full apposition and the oropharyngeal airway is occluded. When contact between the tongue and the velum occurs, it is also possible to have left- and right-side openings through which the pharynx and oral cavity are coupled.

Adjustments of the Mandible

The mandible can be adjusted in position, but not in shape. Such adjustment is usually considered in relation to some fixed structure of the skull. Most often that structure is the maxilla because it constitutes the opposing jaw for the mandible and is critical to functions that the two structures carry out collaboratively, such as chewing and speech production. Adjustments of the mandible result from individual actions or combinations of actions that displace the structure downward or upward, forward or backward, and toward one side or the other. Adjustments that involve lowering of the mandible result from the action of one or more muscles that include the *external pterygoid* muscle, *digastric* (*anterior* belly) muscle, *mylohyoid* muscle, and *geniohyoid* muscle. In contrast, adjustments that involve elevation of the mandible result from the action of one or more muscles that include the *masseter* muscle, *temporalis* muscle, and *internal pterygoid* muscle. Side-to-side movements are the domain of four muscles that include the *masseter* muscle, *temporalis* muscle, *internal pterygoid* muscle, and *external pterygoid* muscle. And forward and backward movements are caused by the actions of the *external pterygoid* muscle and the *masseter* muscle and/or *temporalis* muscle, respectively.

Using different combinations of muscular contractions, the mandible can be protruded, retracted, lateralized, or centralized. These adjustments may be made singly or in certain combinations, except where contradictory (simultaneous protrusion and retraction), and are limited only by constraints imposed by the temporomandibular joints and the forces that can be applied to the mandible through muscle activations. Combinations of adjustments of the mandible can result in marked changes in its positioning relative to when the upper and lower teeth are in contact along their opposing surfaces. For example, a combined adjustment in which the mandible is maximally lowered and maximally protruded might entail more than a 2-inch downward excursion of the front of the structure and a 0.5–inch forward excursion.

Adjustments of the Tongue

The enormous variety of possible tongue adjustments is truly amazing. What seems to be a near infinite array of adjustments has to do with the special mechanical endowment of the tongue that sets it apart from other components of the pharyngeal-oral apparatus. That endowment is that the tongue is a muscular hydrostat that can perform its functions while maintaining its overall volume (Kier & Smith, 1985; Smith & Kier, 1989). This capability is somewhat akin to adjustments that can be made in a balloon filled with water, in which the balloon, like the tongue, does not have a rigid underlying skeleton against which purchase can be gained.

The tongue can protrude, retract, lateralize, centralize, curl, point, lick, bulge, groove, flatten, rotate, and do many other things. Consider for a moment the range of adjustments the tongue goes through in "picking between one's teeth" one at a time from the outside, inside, and bottom, both the uppers and lowers, after eating something like corn on the cob. The series of adjustments that characterize some of the daily activities of the tongue has been described as paralleling the adjustments of the tentacles of an octopus or the trunk of an elephant (Kier & Smith, 1985; Smith & Kier, 1989).

These adjustments are made possible by the biomechanical property of the tongue that enables it to function like a liquid-filled, pliable structure that is incompressible. This special property of the structure, along with its personal soft skeleton that encapsulates it (see above), provides leverages for the eight muscles that give rise to its motive force. These leverages enable the tongue muscles to work off one another and its connective tissue to achieve its variety of adjustments (Miller, Watkin, & Chen, 2002). Because of its hydrostatic properties, inward displacement of one part of the tongue brings about outward displacement

---

Take It Away

The tongue rides with the mandible and goes where it goes. Thus, when trying to interpret changes in the configuration of the tongue surface, it's necessary to determine how much is attributable to adjustment of the tongue and how much is attributable to adjustment of the mandible. Suppose you had a client with a hyperkinetic disease in which both the tongue and mandible went through adventitious involuntary excursions. How could you go about parsing them in your evaluation? Not to worry! Have the client speak through clenched teeth or while biting down on a small stack of tongue depressors. Then, the abnormal movements of the tongue are on their own and not confounded by the abnormal movements of the mandible. It's called removing a degree of freedom of performance, and the principle can be applied in many ways when analyzing different structures involved in speech production.

of another part (like squeezing one part of a water-filled balloon and seeing another part bulge outward). Through the selective contraction of different muscle fibers, a relatively rigid but changing support system is created in the tongue. This changing support system provides a changing base from which the contraction of different muscle fibers can accomplish adjustments of other parts of the tongue. Thus, conceptualizing the consequences of tongue muscle actions in a classical sense is limiting and problematic. Rather, it is better to conceptualize the tongue as a mechanical platform that can change in accordance with the collective activations of the muscles within and attached to it. Because this platform maintains its overall volume, its adjustments in free space (when not contacting other structures in opposition) are best conceptualized in terms of its nature as a hydrostat.

Before the properties of muscular hydrostats were understood, a question like "How do you stick out your tongue?" would evoke an answer that usually involved a complex geometric explanation about muscle force vectors. The simple answer to this question with today's knowledge is that "You squeeze it out."

Adjustments of the Lips

The lips are highly mobile and can be moved independently or in a coordinated fashion. The forces that enable adjustments of the lips derive from the many facial muscles that surround the mouth opening. Adjustments of the lips can be viewed from a variety of perspectives, such as in relation to influences on: (a) the position and shape of each lip, (b) the position and shape of the corners of the mouth, (c) the resultant compression between the lips and/or between one or both lips and the teeth and gums, and (d) the resultant configuration (cross-section and length) of the channel that forms the airway opening.

Frequently recognized positional adjustments of the lips include puckering, protruding, retracting, spreading, pointing, curling (inward and outward), groping, rounding, and plumping (other than with supplemental collagen). Common compressions may involve forceful airtight seals between the lips, the pushing around of one lip by the other, the thinning or thickening of the contact area between the two lips, and the placement of different parts of the lips against the maxillary and/or mandibular arches and teeth. The channel that forms the airway opening is, of course, frequently adjusted such that it can be lengthened or shortened, changed in shape, and moved from side to side (consider talking out one side of the mouth, the so-called sidewinder). The lips may even be in apposition on one side and be parted on the other, as in the dying breed of the smoker who talks with a cigarette hanging from one side of the mouth.

The multitude of possible lip adjustments are effected by a large variety of muscle activations in the facial region involving different combinations of the more than dozen muscles that impart forces to the lips. These adjustments also include those associated with a host of facial expressions, such as smiling, smirking, sulking, and sneering.

Control Variables of Pharyngeal-Oral Function

Several control variables are important in pharyngeal-oral function. Their relative importance depends on the activity being performed, whether it is breathing, speaking, singing, whistling, wind instrument playing, blowing, sucking, chewing, or swallowing, among others. For the purposes of this chapter, discussion is devoted to four control variables: (a) pharyngeal-oral lumen size and configuration, (b) pharyngeal-oral contact pressure, (c) pharyngeal-oral airway resistance, and (d) pharyngeal-oral acoustic impedance.

Pharyngeal-Oral Lumen Size and Configuration

The lumen of the pharyngeal-oral apparatus (its inner open space) can be changed in both size and configuration. Such changes are the result of adjustments in the positions of structures that line the pharyngeal-oral airway. Adjustments can be manifested in physical dimensions such as length, longitudinal configuration (midsaggital outline), diameter, cross-sectional area, and cross-sectional configuration.

The open space that constitutes the pharyngeal-oral lumen can be either increased or decreased from the resting configuration of the pharyngeal-oral apparatus. Figure 5–17 summarizes the structures that may contribute individually or in combination to changing the lumen of the airway in the pharyngeal cavity, the oral cavity, and the oral vestibule.

As indicated in Figure 5–17, the dimensions of the pharyngeal-oral lumen can be changed in a variety of ways. Length changes can be achieved: (a) within the pharyngeal cavity, by different combinations of adjustments of the velum and larynx, (b) within the oral cavity, by different combinations of adjustments of the tongue and mandible, and (c) within the oral vestibule, by different combinations of adjustments of the upper lip, lower lip, and mandible. Cross-sectional changes can be achieved: (a) within the pharynx, by different

Pharyngeal-oral lumen adjustments

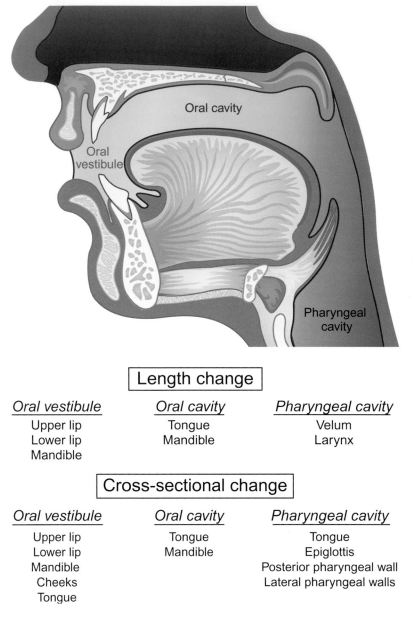

Length change

Oral vestibule	Oral cavity	Pharyngeal cavity
Upper lip	Tongue	Velum
Lower lip	Mandible	Larynx
Mandible		

Cross-sectional change

Oral vestibule	Oral cavity	Pharyngeal cavity
Upper lip	Tongue	Tongue
Lower lip	Mandible	Epiglottis
Mandible		Posterior pharyngeal wall
Cheeks		Lateral pharyngeal walls
Tongue		

Figure 5-17. Regional structures contributing to adjustments of the pharyngeal-oral lumen.

combinations of adjustments of the tongue, epiglottis, posterior pharyngeal wall, and lateral pharyngeal walls, (b) within the oral cavity, by different combinations of adjustments of the tongue and mandible, and (c) within the oral vestibule, by different combinations of adjustments of the lips, mandible, cheeks, and tongue.

Given the lengthwise and cross-sectional adjustment possibilities noted, the number of options for luminal changes in the pharyngeal-oral apparatus is exceedingly large. This fact underpins the fact that the acoustic products that emanate from the pharyngeal-oral apparatus can be richly variable, as is discussed in detail in subsequent chapters.

Open Wide

Your mandible and maxilla are separated by only a small distance when you produce speech. Activities such as calling your dog, yelling at a football game, or singing often get you to open up more. Classical (opera) singing is one activity that gets people to open very wide. One form of classical singing teaches what is referred to as a four-finger jaw position. Try it. Place the four fingers of one hand together and then, with your thumb on that hand pointing upward, insert your fingers vertically at the midline between your upper and lower front teeth. Quite a stretch, isn't it? It comes close to maximum separation between your mandible and maxilla and gives you nearly as large a mouth opening as you can achieve (or tolerate). What a great way to get that beautiful singing voice to radiate outward from the singer to the audience.

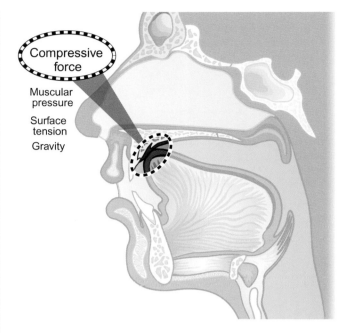

Figure 5–18. Structural contact pressure between the tongue and alveolar process of the maxilla.

Pharyngeal-Oral Structural Contact Pressure

Adjustments of the pharyngeal-oral apparatus can result in full obstruction of the pharyngeal-oral lumen at different locations. This is accomplished through structural contact between components that comprise the boundaries of the airway. Structures in apposition may include: (a) the tongue against the pharynx, velum, hard palate, alveolar process of the maxilla, teeth, and lips, and (b) the lips against the teeth and one another. Once two structures are in apposition, the structural contact pressure between them can be adjusted to meet the needs of the situation. This is manifested as a compressive force between the two structures and can be changed in accordance with the pressure needed to maintain the contact or to increase it in magnitude. Figure 5–18 portrays structural contact and its resultant compressive force between the tongue and the alveolar process of the maxilla.

Structural contact pressure can be influenced by several factors. These include: (a) muscular pressure exerted by muscular components of the contacting surfaces (tongue against alveolar ridge or two lips against one another), (b) surface tension between apposed surfaces that are moist (tongue against hard palate) and hold them together, and (c) gravity that weighs down structures and acts on them differently in different body positions (or gravity fields). The most sig-

nificant of these three is usually the muscular pressure exerted by one or more structures. Contact pressure for an activity may require low-level muscular exertion for soft contact between structures or it may require high contact pressure when it is necessary to fortify the contact in the face of high air pressures in the vicinity.

Pharyngeal-Oral Airway Resistance

Pharyngeal-oral airway resistance is a measure of the opposition provided by the pharyngeal-oral apparatus to airflow through it. As portrayed in Figure 5–19, this opposition pertains to the mass flow of air in and out of the apparatus. Pharyngeal-oral airway resistance is a property of the airway itself and is airflow dependent. This means that it increases or decreases with increases or decreases in the rate at which air moves, even without changes in the physical dimensions of the pharyngeal-oral airway. However, it is the change in the cross-section of the airway that causes the greatest change in pharyngeal-oral airway resistance. Such change can occur anywhere along the length of the pharyngeal-oral apparatus, from larynx to lips, but is most prominently the result of adjustments within the oropharynx, oral cavity, and oral vestibule. By decreasing the cross-sectional area of the airway anywhere within these regions, the airway resistance will likely increase.

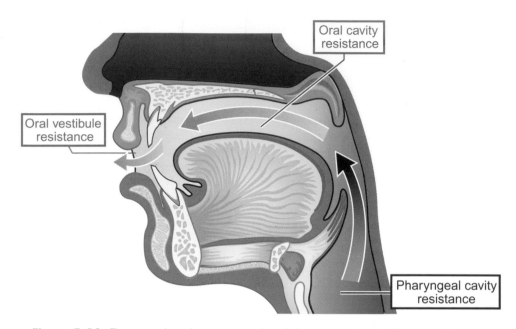

Figure 5–19. Three regional components of pharyngeal-oral airway resistance.

Airway resistance is calculated from the quotient of the pressure drop across any segment of interest and the airflow through that segment. For the entire pharyngeal-oral apparatus, airway resistance is represented by the pressure difference (in cmH_2O) between the laryngopharynx and the atmosphere divided by the airflow (in LPS) at the airway opening. The range of potential airway resistance values is from a fraction of a cmH_2O/LPS (associated with a wide open pharyngeal-oral apparatus) to infinity (associated with a closed pharyngeal-oral apparatus). The distribution of resistance along the pharyngeal-oral airway can be determined by partitioning the total resistance. All that is required is that appropriate pressure measurements be made at the two ends of each segment of interest along the airway.

Pharyngeal-Oral Acoustic Impedance

The pharyngeal-oral apparatus plays an important role in the control of acoustic impedance, which, like airway resistance, involves opposition to flow. As portrayed in Figure 5–20, this opposition is not to mass airflow, but to the movement of energy in the form of sound waves through the apparatus. These waves function like an alternating current in which adjacent air molecules collide with each other and pass energy on to their neighbors. Acoustic impedance influences how well sound waves propagate through the pharyngeal-oral airway.

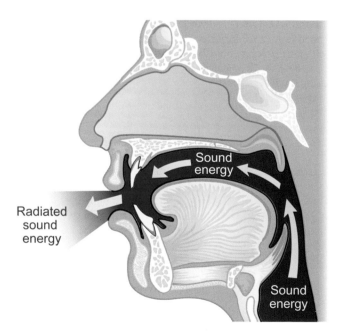

Figure 5–20. Pharyngeal-oral sound wave propagation in the presence of velopharyngeal closure.

Acoustic impedance is determined to a great extent by cross-sectional adjustments of the pharyngeal-oral airway. These adjustments influence the degree of coupling between different segments of the pharyngeal-oral apparatus. When the adjustments create a relative increase in the cross-section of the lumen of the pharyngeal-oral airway, sound waves pass relatively freely along the airway. In contrast, when the adjustments create a relative decrease in the cross-section of the lumen of the airway, sound energy does not pass as freely along the airway. Relative decreases in the cross-section of the lumen at different locations simultaneously may also influence the degree to which different segments of the pharyngeal-oral airway interact with one another acoustically. This topic is discussed in detail in subsequent chapters.

Neural Substrates of Pharyngeal-Oral Control

Pharyngeal-oral movements are controlled by the nervous system and differ with the activity being performed. Thus, speaking and swallowing, while engaging the same structures of the pharyngeal-oral apparatus, are controlled by different neural substrates and mechanisms. Control of the pharyngeal-oral apparatus during swallowing is discussed in Chapter 13, whereas control of the apparatus during speech production is discussed here.

Although different parts of the central nervous system participate in the control of different pharyngeal-oral activities, the final forms of the control commands are sent through the same set of cranial nerves. These nerves have their origins in the brainstem and course from there to provide motor innervation to the muscles of the pharynx, mandible, tongue, and lips. As shown in Table 5–1, motor innervation of the pharynx is effected through the pharyngeal plexus, which includes fibers from cranial nerves IX (glossopharyngeal), X (vagus), and possibly XI (accessory). Motor

Table 5–1. Summary of Motor and Sensory Nerve Supply to the Pharynx, Mandible, Tongue, and Lips

COMPONENT	INNERVATION	
	MOTOR	SENSORY
Pharynx	Pharyngeal Plexus	V, VII, X
Mandible	V, XII	V
Tongue	X, XII	V, VII, X
Lips	VII	V, VII

Note: The pharyngeal plexus is a network that includes cranial nerves IX, X, and possibly XI. All of the muscles of the mandible have motor and sensory nerve supply through cranial nerve V, except the **geniohyoid** muscle, which has motor and sensory nerve supply through cranial nerve XII.

All muscles of the tongue have motor nerve supply through cranial nerve XII, except the **palatoglossus** muscle, which has motor nerve supply through cranial nerve X.

Cranial nerves indicated in the table and notes are V (trigeminal), VII (facial), IX (glossopharyngeal), X (vagus), XI (accessory), and XII (hypoglossal).

innervation to the mandible is effected through cranial nerves V (trigeminal) and XII (hypoglossal). Motor innervation of the tongue includes cranial nerves X and XII, whereas motor innervation of the lips is effected through cranial nerve VII (facial).

Sensory innervation to the pharynx is carried by cranial nerves V, VII, and X. Sensory innervation to the mandible is supplied by cranial nerve V. The tongue receives sensory supply from cranial nerves V, VII, and X, whereas supply to the lips is from cranial nerves V

Low Energy Physics

Speech is clearly an energy producing enterprise. But just how much energy is involved? One scientist has calculated that 300 to 400 ergs of energy is expended in the resultant sound wave when the sentence "Joe took father's shoe-bench out" is produced at usual loudness (Fletcher, 1953). That's not a sentence that most people run around saying and many readers might not have an appreciation for how 300 to 400 ergs relates to their everyday lives. Perhaps we can help a bit. You and 499 of your closest friends (that's a Boeing-747 aircraft with all the seats filled) would have to say "Joe took father's shoe-bench out" together at your usual loudness continuously for a year to produce enough energy to heat a cup of coffee. Holy Starbucks! That's a lot of talking. It would undoubtedly contend for a Guiness World Record, but on nature's energy scale it wouldn't amount to much.

Ten Four, Good Buddy

Bell's palsy is a relatively common condition that affects cranial nerve VII, the nerve that innervates the muscles of the face. Upper and lower facial muscles can become weak or paralyzed and speech production can be impaired. Most often the cause is unknown and the problem is on one side. It may involve an autoimmune inflammatory response, a herpes viral infection, or a swelling of the nerve because of allergy. Most people who get Bell's palsy make a full recovery, especially if they're young. Exposure to cold can be a factor in Bell's palsy. Truck drivers who keep the driver's-side window down may contract Bell's palsy from the cold. Wind chill for a prolonged period across the side of the face near the window is believed to be a contributing factor to onset of the problem. Which side depends on the country in which you're driving. What's the prevention? Close the window and turn on the air conditioner.

Gumming Things Up

Some antipsychotic drugs can have a nasty side effect called by the imposing name of tardive dyskinesia (meaning after-the-fact adventitious movement). Signs of tardive dyskinesia can include involuntary movement of the mandible, tongue, and lips and can manifest in such strange actions as lip smacking and puffing. In some individuals, these signs are permanent. However, another condition may masquerade as tardive dyskinesia. Persons with poorly fitting dentures also may present with adventitious movement. The source of the problem is a changing sensory feedback from the gums caused by movement of the denture. The result is a disorganized background template of the oral cavity. This effectively gums up the control circuits for movement. Take out the denture or secure it in position and the problem will go away. When confronted with the signs of tardive dyskinesia, always check for loose-fitting dentures.

and VII. Neural information traveling along the sensory nerves supplying the pharynx, mandible, tongue, and lips results from the activation of receptors of various types within those structures. These receptors include an array of mechanoreceptors that are differentially distributed (some occurring in certain locations more than others) throughout the tissues of the pharyngeal-oral apparatus. When sound results from pharyngeal-oral activity, mechanoreceptors formed by hair cells within the cochlea (end organ of the auditory system) may be activated. Sensory information from the auditory system is effected via cranial nerve VIII (auditory-vestibular nerve).

The mechanoreceptors within the pharyngeal-oral apparatus are sensitive to a variety of stimuli and are capable of providing the nervous system with many types of information, including information about: (a) muscle length, (b) rate of change in muscle length, (c) muscle tension, (d) joint position, (e) joint movement, (f) touch, (g) surface pressure, (h) deep pressure, (i) surface deformation, (j) temperature, (k) vibration, and (l) hair deflection, among others. Mechanoreceptors within the fabric of the pharyngeal-oral apparatus and within the auditory system provide the central nervous system with information that is used to guide anticipated actions of the pharyngeal-oral apparatus and to keep track of the recent status of the pharyngeal-

oral apparatus. Recent in this case means that the information conveyed is delayed by at least the amount of time it takes to transmit signals from mechanoreceptors to centers within the brain where they are processed. This processing may include the integration of various inputs coming from the periphery and the use of this collective information to execute ongoing commands from the motor side of the system.

Pharyngeal-Oral Functions

The pharyngeal-oral apparatus performs many functions. Those of interest here relate to: (a) degree of coupling between the oral cavity and atmosphere, (b) chewing, (c) swallowing, and (d) sound generation and filtering.

Degree of Coupling Between the Oral Cavity and Atmosphere

Actions of the pharyngeal-oral apparatus determine the degree of coupling between the pharyngeal-oral apparatus and atmosphere. The coupling pathway in this case is through the oral vestibule. Changes in the positions of lips, cheeks, and alveolar process of the mandible influence such coupling. When breathing through the pharyngeal-oral apparatus, the oral vestibule is open, whereas when breathing through the velopharyngeal-nasal port, the oral vestibule may be closed. The lips are especially important in changing the degree of coupling between the oral cavity and atmosphere and can influence it not only in cross-section but also by adjusting the length of the channel formed between the oral cavity and the airway opening.

Chewing

Chewing (mastication) is the process of grinding, mashing, gnawing, crushing, and kneading food (nutriment in solid form) with the teeth. This process is aimed at the alteration of food into smaller particle sizes that can be prepared to a swallow-ready consistency. The alignment of the maxilla, mandible, and teeth is important in this process to ensure that proper biting forces can be exerted. Chewing entails extensive movement of the mandible that may have significant vertical, side-to-side, and elliptical components. These depend, in part, on the consistency of the food being manipulated.

Swallowing

Swallowing (deglutition) is a life-sustaining function of the pharyngeal-oral apparatus. Actions of the oral cavity and oral vestibule prepare food or liquid for swallowing and then propel it backward into the oropharynx (the velopharynx being closed). Thereafter, muscles of the oropharynx and laryngopharynx act to further propel the prepared substances downward through the pharyngeal tube and into the esophagus. Chapter 13 provides a comprehensive discussion about the swallowing process that includes consideration of the role played by the pharyngeal-oral apparatus.

Sound Generation and Filtering

Much of the interest in the present chapter is with sound generation and filtering by the pharyngeal-oral apparatus. Sound generation in the apparatus can be of several types. The two of these that are most important to this book are: (a) transient (popping) sounds, in which the oral airstream is momentarily interrupted and then released, and (b) turbulence (hissing) sounds, in which air is forced through a narrow constriction within the airway. Sound generated within the pharyngeal-oral apparatus or generated at the larynx and passed through the pharyngeal-oral apparatus undergoes a sound-filtering process in which its characteristics can be modified through enhancement or attenuation before becoming public at the airway opening (for details, see Chapters 8 and 9).

PHARYNGEAL-ORAL FUNCTION IN SPEECH PRODUCTION

The pharyngeal-oral apparatus is of great importance in speech production. This section and various sections of Chapters 8 and 9 emphasize this importance by stressing its role in the generation and filtering of speech sounds. Two aspects of pharyngeal-oral function are discussed here. The first is how the pharyngeal-oral apparatus makes coded adjustments that constitute the physiological bases of speech production. The second is how these coded adjustments become elaborated in real time by the pharyngeal-oral apparatus and other subsystems of the speech production apparatus.

The Speech Production Code

Previous sections have discussed the variety of adjustments that can be made by individual components of the pharyngeal-oral apparatus. Chapters 3 and 4 do likewise for the laryngeal apparatus and velopharyngeal-nasal apparatus, respectively. Adjustments across the

---

Myth Conceptions

The history of speech-language pathology is rich with clinical theories and methods that don't actually involve speech production directly. These have taken many forms. One early one took the point of view that language had its beginnings in chewing and that chewing exercises had a prominent role in the evaluation and management of speech and voice disorders. The originator of this idea said that he conceived the notion when confronted with two Egyptian hieroglyphic scripts that showed a similar sign for eating and speaking. Despite using some of the same pharyngeal-oral structures, chewing and speaking are controlled differently by the nervous system and one is not a precursor or analog of the other. Other forms of nonspeech activities and devices continue to be used even today as if they were somehow beneficial to speech production. We don't subscribe to any of these misconceptions. You shouldn't either.

Duck and Cover

Aeromechanical and acoustic energies come out of your mouth during speech production. Other things also make their way out. One of these is saliva. Today your salivary glands might produce up to a quart of liquid. The usually slippery oral cavity dries out when you talk, especially when the humidity is low. Tiny drops of saliva spew from your mouth when you speak. These are usually invisible and emerge as wet clouds that can hang around an hour or more and settle on nearby listeners. Each word spoken sends about 2.5 droplets of saliva into the atmosphere (Bodanis, 1995). Read this sidetrack aloud and you'll expel about 400 droplets of saliva. Do the same with the Gettysburg Address and the number will reach 700. The United States Constitution would get you about 11,000 droplets. And what would an assembly of 500 people reciting the Pledge of Allegiance get you? 40,000 droplets dispersed in 500 wet clouds.

different subsystems of the speech production apparatus comprise a phonetic code that specifies the positions and movements of structures. This code consists of groupings of adjustments that are associated with the generation of different speech sounds, each grouping being one component of an organized system of sounds in a language. Such a code contains a series of elements that differ from one another in one or more aspects that enable them to be distinguished from other elements. Coding schemes for vowels, diphthongs, and consonants of American English are considered here.

Vowel-Coding Scheme

Vowels are usually produced with voicing by the larynx (although they can be whispered) and with velopharyngeal closure (although they can be nasalized). They demonstrate different combinations of positions and movements by the pharynx, mandible, tongue, and lips. Whatever the pattern of adjustments, vowel productions involve relatively unconstricted configurations of the pharyngeal-oral airway. Laryngeal and velopharyngeal actions notwithstanding, the positions and movements of structures within the pharyngeal-oral apparatus are of foremost importance in the vowel-coding scheme. Figure 5–21 shows how vowels can be coded using the three dimensions of *place of major con-*

striction within the pharyngeal-oral apparatus, *degree of major constriction* within the apparatus, and *degree of lip rounding*.

Place of Major Constriction. *Place of major constriction* specifies the location at which the pharyngeal-oral airway is maximally constricted during vowel production. Three locations are coded for vowels. These include *front*, *central*, and *back*. The term *front* is used to designate constrictions formed between the tongue and the alveolar process of the maxilla. The term *central* is used to indicate constrictions formed between the tongue and the hard palate, or when no obvious constriction exists. And the term *back* designates constrictions formed between the tongue and the velum, or between the tongue and the posterior pharyngeal wall. Five vowels fall under the rubric *front* vowels, four are classified as *central* vowels, and five are considered *back* vowels. Changes across the *place of major constriction* dimension can be viewed as shifts in the position of the tongue along the length coordinate of the pharyngeal-oral apparatus.

Degree of Major Constriction. *Degree of major constriction* designates the cross-sectional size of the constricted region of the airway. Coding along this dimension typically specifies a *high*, *mid*, or *low* degree of major constriction and corresponds, in most circumstances, to the location of the highest point of the tongue surface in relation to the roof of the mouth. Exceptions occur when the major constriction is formed between the back of the tongue and the posterior pharyngeal wall. *High* degrees of constriction correspond to small cross-sectional areas at the major constriction. *Mid* degrees of constriction are associated with intermediate size cross-sections. And *low* degrees of constriction involve large cross-sectional areas. At times, *low* degrees of constriction may actually have larger cross-sectional areas than those associated with relaxation of the pharyngeal-oral apparatus. Four vowels are classified within the *high* degree of constriction category, eight within the *mid* constriction category, and two within the *low* constriction category. Changes across the *high* to *mid* to *low* degree of constriction categories correspond to lower and lower positioning of the highest point on the dorsal surface of the tongue.

Lip Rounding. *Lip rounding* designates the degree to which the lips are protruded. Such protrusion correlates directly with the size of the airway opening. Thus, an increase in lip rounding signifies a simultaneous lengthening and narrowing of the lip channel along the oral vestibule, whereas a decrease in lip round-

Place of major constriction

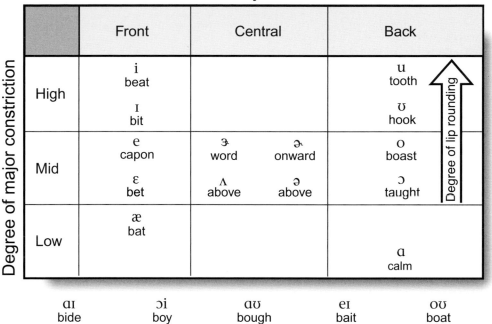

Figure 5–21. Production coding scheme for American English vowels and diphthongs coded in terms of place of major constriction, degree of major constriction, and degree of lip rounding. Physiological clusters are based on the coding scheme advocated by Hixon and Abbs (1980). Vowel symbols are from the International Phonetic Alphabet. Word exemplars are primarily from Fairbanks (1960).

ing indicates a simultaneous shortening and opening up of the lip channel. In American English, lip rounding is a coding factor on only *mid*-constriction and *high*-constriction *back* vowels. For these vowels, lip rounding increases across the *mid* to *high* categories of constriction.

Diphthong-Coding Scheme

Diphthongs (pronounced DIFF-thongs) are speech sounds that are vowel-like in nature. The classic phonetic view is that they are transitional hybrids of vowels that are formed by rapidly changing from one vowel adjustment to another. Thus, they are transcribed as pairs of vowels, there being five such pairs in American English (see row of symbols below the chart in Figure 5–21). Each diphthong is formed of a vowel pair in which the first vowel is characterized by a lesser degree of major constriction than the second vowel. Diphthongs may combine vowel pairs that transition: (a) within the same place of major constriction, (b) from back to front places of constriction, and (c) from mid to high degrees of constriction that include increases

in lip rounding. Given that diphthongs are transitional hybrids of vowel pairs in the classic phonetic view, their production coding may be conceptualized in terms of their vowel beginning and ending points and nearly continuous adjustments in between. This usual phonetic conceptualization of diphthongs is not without controversy. Acoustic studies of diphthong formation have suggested that they have unique features that are different from "pure" vowels and that their transitional components contain defining features that show them to be a different sound class than vowels. This topic is discussed in detail in Chapter 11.

Consonant-Coding Scheme

Consonants, unlike vowels and diphthongs, are usually produced with a substantially constricted or obstructed airway. Some are produced with voicing by the larynx and some are not. And some are produced with velopharyngeal closure and some are not. As shown in Figure 5–22, adjustments for consonant productions are coded along three dimensions. These include *manner of production* (five categories), *place of production* (seven

Manner of production

Place of production	Stop-plosive −	Stop-plosive +	Fricative −	Fricative +	Affricate −	Affricate +	Nasal −	Nasal +	Semivowel −	Semivowel +
Labial (lips)	p pole	b bowl						m sum		w watt
Labiodental (lip–teeth)			f fat	v vat						
Dental (tongue–teeth)			θ thigh	ð thy						
Alveolar (tongue–gum)	t toll	d dole	s seal	z zeal				n sun		l lot
Palatal (tongue–hard palate)			ʃ ash	ʒ azure	tʃ choke	dʒ joke				j,r yacht, rot
Velar (tongue–velum)	k coal	g goal						ŋ sung		
Glottal (vocal folds)			h hot							

Figure 5–22. Production coding scheme for American English consonants coded in terms of manner of production, place of production, and voicing. Voiceless and voiced elements are designated by – and + signs, respectively. Physiological clusters are based on the coding scheme advocated by Hixon and Abbs (1980). Consonant symbols are from the International Phonetic Alphabet. Word exemplars are from Fairbanks (1960).

categories), and *voicing* (two categories). These three dimensions yield 70 (5 × 7 × 2) unique coding possibilities. About one-third of these are used in American English.

Manner of Production. *Manner of production* specifies the way in which structures of the laryngeal apparatus, velopharyngeal-nasal apparatus, and pharyngeal-oral apparatus constrict or obstruct the airway during consonant generation. The manner of production dimension includes five adjustments, referred to as *stop-plosive, fricative, affricate, nasal,* and *semivowel.* Each of these adjustments is described here and considered further in Chapter 9.

Stop-plosive consonants begin with occlusion of the oral airway and a buildup of oral air pressure behind the occlusion. The airway is then abruptly opened and a burst of airflow is released. Such actions are generated in association with airtight closure of the velopharynx. Not all stop consonants demonstrate a burst of airflow following occlusion of the oral airway. Some release the pent-up air through a lowering of the velum.

This allows air to escape inaudibly through the nasal cavities. Stop consonants produced in this fashion are referred to as imploded stop consonants. This type of stop consonant occurs in American English but is not phonemically distinctive.

Fricative consonants are generated when air is forced at high velocity through a narrowly constricted laryngeal or pharyngeal-oral airway. Such sounds derive their acoustic energy from turbulent airflow near their constrictions and from airflow striking nearby obstacles such as the teeth. Fricative consonants are usually produced with a closed velopharynx, although this is not obligatory if the constriction is upstream of the velopharynx, as in a fricative produced within the larynx.

Affricate consonants are usually produced with a closed velopharynx. Such consonants start out much like stop-plosive consonants in that the oral airway is occluded and air pressure builds up behind the occlusion. However, the occlusion for affricate consonants is released less abruptly than for stop-plosive consonants and the burst of airflow that follows is less vigorous.

These characteristics of the release phase of affricate consonants are the main features that distinguish their productions from those of stop-plosives.

Nasal consonants are produced with an occluded oral airway and an open velopharyngeal airway. The aeromechanical and acoustic energy associated with their production is transmitted through the nasopharynx and nasal cavities and is emitted from the external nares.

Semivowel sounds are consonant sounds produced with a constricted oral airway. The constriction involved is greater than that for vowel sounds, but less than that for other consonant sounds. Semivowels are generated with the velopharynx closed and the aeromechanical and acoustic energy associated with their production passes through the pharyngeal-oral airway.

The five manners of production just discussed are differentially represented across the consonants of American English. The *fricative* manner of production is a feature in more than one-third of American English consonants, and the *stop-plosive* manner of production is a feature in one-fourth of such consonants. *Semivowel*, *nasal*, and *affricate* manners of production are successively less prominent in proportion within the overall coding scheme.

Place of Production. *Place of production* codes for where a consonant constriction or occlusion occurs

along the laryngeal and pharyngeal-oral airway. This dimension encompasses seven sites. Places of production include *labial*, *labiodental*, *dental*, *alveolar*, *palatal*, *velar*, and *glottal*. In the order listed, these constriction or occlusion sites lie progressively farther inward along the combined pharyngeal-oral and laryngeal airways.

Labial means that only the two lips participate in the primary action having to do with place of production. An exception exists for the semivowel /w/ which is also specified as requiring a high-back tongue configuration. *Labiodental* indicates that the place of production is between the lower lip and the upper teeth. *Dental*, *alveolar*, *palatal*, and *velar* places of production designate locations where the tongue contacts or comes very close to contacting the teeth, upper gum ridge (inside the teeth), hard palate, and velum (soft palate and uvula), respectively. The *glottal* place of production entails primary action of the two vocal folds.

The places of production are differentially represented across the consonants of American English. The *alveolar* and *palatal* places of production are equally prominent and one or the other of them is a feature in half of the consonants of American English. *Labial*, *labiodental*, *dental*, and *velar* places of production are less prominent than *alveolar* and *palatal* places, with the *glottal* place being a feature of only a single consonant of American English.

Voicing. The *voicing* dimension in the consonant-coding scheme is binary. That is, voice is either on or off for consonant productions, so consonants are categorized as either *voiced* (+) or *voiceless* (−). The majority of consonant sounds are *voiced*. Many of the consonants of American English form cognate pairs that differ only on the voicing dimension. Thus, two consonants in a cognate pair match one another in their manner of production and place of production, but differ from one another because one is *voiced* and the other is *voiceless*. Cognate pairs occur within the stop-plosive, fricative, and affricate manners of production and at nearly all places of production, the glottal site being the exception. The nasal and semivowel manners of production are *voiced*.

The Speech Production Stream

The previous section describes the nature of the phonetic code for producing the sounds of speech. This code considers each vowel, diphthong, and consonant as a discrete physiological entity that can be specified in terms of articulatory descriptions related to place-constriction-lip rounding for vowels and place-manner-voicing for

---

Raspberries

Raspberries (also called Bronx cheers) are sounds that resemble sustained flatulence (farting). Raspberries are made by blowing air between a protruded tongue and the lips. Adults use raspberries to indicate derision, sarcasm, or silliness. All cultures seem to have a fondness for them. Infants especially like them and use them in their early sound play. Raspberries aren't used as sounds in human languages. Thus, they fade from the repertoire of experimental noises as the infant figures out that they're not an important part of the linguistic code. Nevertheless, the skill acquired is not wasted. They return later on as full-blown Bronx cheers to be used to put someone down, sarcastically cheer a poor sports performance, or be the final gesture after a lost argument. Blow a raspberry the next time you see a primate at a zoo. Most primates make raspberries. You'll either get one back or get a weird look from a resident.

consonants. This type of phonetic code is didactically convenient and serves the useful role of idealizing important aspects about the production of speech sounds. A limitation of this code, however, is that the descriptors are timeless. The speech production process is not a linear assemblage of a series of idealized physiological packets (speech sounds), nor is it a series of invariant positions and movement sequences strung together like beads on a string (MacNeilage, 1970).

Studies of movements of the speech production apparatus, especially of the pharyngeal-oral subsystem, reveal the limitations of a phonetic code. X-ray images, obtained from speakers of several different languages, show the mandible, tongue, velum, and lips to undergo continuous movement throughout even the simplest sequence of sounds (Munhall, Vatikiotis-Bateson, & Tohkura, 1995). Such x-ray images reveal the sequencing and coordination of articulatory events to be far more complex than a series of discrete speech sounds abutted to one another. Rather, the speech stream, as visualized at the level of articulatory movement, appears to be fluid and continuous and to show no obvious boundaries between successive sounds. Moreover, examination of x-ray images suggests that very different movements can be associated with a single speech sound (such as a vowel), depending on the identity of the surrounding consonants. It is no exaggeration to say that the continuous and changeable movements of the articulators correspond poorly with the discrete symbols of the phonetic transcription code. The poor relationship between articulatory movements and the symbol code implies a poor relationship with the idealized descriptors of place-constriction-lip rounding for vowels and place-manner-voicing for consonants. Speech scientists have spent the last 50 years attempting to determine the relationship between articulatory movements and the intuitively appealing idea of speech production being guided by a set of discrete symbols such as phonemes or a phonetic transcription of an actual utterance.

A Primer on Theories of Speech Production

The examination of x-ray images of articulatory movements within the pharyngeal-oral apparatus during speech production shows clearly how the articulatory movements for one sound influence the movements for another sound. This mutual influence is most apparent between adjacent sounds, but there is also evidence that it can extend across several sounds. For example, in both the words "Sue" [su] and "stew" [stu], the lip rounding that is a part of the phonetic code for /u/ is observed during the [s] part of the articulatory sequence. The same thing happens when the sequence is reversed, as in "twos" [tuz] and "toots" [tuts]. In both cases, the lip rounding for the /u/ extends to the lingua-alveolar fricative /z/ or /s/, even when the fricative is separated from the /u/ by a stop consonant. These are examples of the articulatory phenomenon known as coarticulation, defined as "the influence of one sound on another" (Daniloff & Hammarberg, 1973). These mutual influences of immediately adjacent and nonadjacent sounds on one another explain, in part, why the articulators undergo continuous movement through a sound sequence and why it is so hard to identify clear sound boundaries from records of articulatory movement.

Speech scientists typically agree on two kinds of coarticulation. Forward coarticulation (also called right-to-left coarticulation) occurs when the articulatory characteristics of an upcoming sound influence the characteristics of a currently produced sound. For example, the production of lip rounding during the [s] of the word "Sue" is an example of an upcoming articulatory requirement (the lip rounding for /u/) occurring during the current /s/ articulation. The "forward" and "right-to-left" descriptions are meant to convey the idea that articulatory characteristics ahead in the speech production stream influence currently articulated sounds. Backward coarticulation (also called left-to-right coarticulation) occurs when a currently articulated sound is influenced by the articulatory characteristics of a previous sound in the speech production stream. For example, in the word "toots" [tuts], the articulatory characteristics of the /s/ include some lip rounding because of the previously articulated [u]. The "backward" and "left-to-right" descriptions suggest the idea of the currently articulated sound being influenced by a preceding articulatory event. A schematic illustration of forward and backward coarticulation (and their synonyms) is provided in Figure 5–23.

Figure 5–23 also contains terms that pertain to hypothesized mechanisms for the two types of coarticulation. Early findings that coarticulation could be right-to-left or left-to-right prompted speech scientists to hypothesize about the underlying mechanisms of these effects. Right-to-left coarticulation was hypothesized to reflect anticipatory processes (anticipatory coarticulation) and left-to-right coarticulation was hypothesized to reflect inertial properties of the articulators (carryover coarticulation). These hypothesized mechanisms are associated with what is called the traditional theory of coarticulation. This theory is based on the idea of feature spreading.

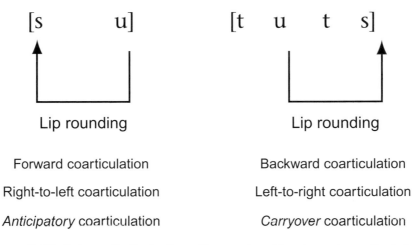

Figure 5–23. Schematic illustration of forward and backward coarticulation.

Traditional Theory of Feature Spreading

Speech sounds are often conceptualized as consisting of a small set of features, consistent with the phonetic code discussed above. Many speech scientists combine linguistic theory with the problem of speech motor control by specifying the plan for an articulatory sequence as a string of phonemes, each of which is composed of a "bundle of features" that form the phonetic code. A small-scale example of this is shown in Figure 5–24, where the words "stew" /stu/, "used" /just/ (as in "used to it"), "bomb" /bɑm/, and "mob" /mɑb/ are shown as phonemic representations specified by a set of features. The features listed in Figure 5–24 are not the complete set for each phoneme, but they suffice to illustrate the concept of feature spreading. Four features are shown, including sonorant (sounds made with a relatively open pharyngeal-oral airway or free passage through the nasal cavities), coronal (consonant sounds made by raising the tongue tip or blade toward the teeth or hard palate), lip rounding (vowels or consonants in which rounding of the lips is an integral feature), and nasal (sounds made with an open velopharyngeal port). Each of the four features in a phoneme column can be specified as "+," "–," or left blank. A feature specified as "+" means the phoneme is produced with that feature, a specification of "–" indicates the explicit absence of that feature from the phoneme's production, and a blank means that the phoneme is not specified one way or the other for the feature.

Consider the phoneme /s/ for an example of articulatory feature specification. /s/ is "–" for sonorant (not produced with an open pharyngeal-oral airway), "+" for coronal (produced by raising the tongue blade

to the front of the hard palate), blank (unspecified) for lip rounding, and "–" for nasal (because fricatives are produced with a closed velopharynx). In the traditional theory of coarticulation, the unspecified entries are of great interest because they allow a feature (or features) associated with an upcoming sound to migrate or spread to a currently articulated sound. For example, in the word "stew" /stu/, the unspecified lip rounding feature for /s/ allows the upcoming lip rounding feature for /u/ to be anticipated and produced during the /s/. The same set of conditions applies to the /t/ in "stew." Thus, when the word is articulated, lip rounding shows up on the two sounds prior to /u/. That is, [stu] shows coarticulation in the form of anticipatory lip rounding on the two consonants preceding the vowel for which lip rounding is required. Lip rounding associated with the vowel spreads to the preceding two consonants because it does not compromise their articulatory characteristics. An /s/ or /t/ can be articulated with the lips rounded or spread without changing the phonemic value of the sound. The flip side of this is that conflicting feature specifications cannot be spread through anticipation, because this would compromise the phonemic value of a sound. As an example, the /s/ and /t/ in "stew" are both specified as "–" for sonorant, whereas the vowel /u/ is specified as "+" for this feature. The "+" sonorant specification for /u/ cannot be anticipated for the /s/ and /t/ articulations because it would compromise their articulatory requirement for a nearly complete constriction (/s/) or obstruction (/t/) of the airway.

A different example of anticipatory (forward) coarticulation is given in the lower left part of Figure 5–24. There, the feature specifications for the phoneme

	/s	t	u/	/u	s	t/
Sonorant	–	–	+	+	–	–
Coronal	+	+	–	–	+	+
Lip rounding			+	+		
Nasal	–	–			–	–

	/b	ɑ	m/	/m	ɑ	b/
Sonorant	–	+	+	+	+	–
Coronal	–	–	–	–	–	–
Lip rounding	–	–	–	–	–	–
Nasal	–		+	+		–

Figure 5–24. Plans for articulatory sequences as strings of phonemes composed of bundles of features, with only selected features represented.

sequence /bɑm/ "bomb" show that all features are specified except the nasal feature for the vowel /ɑ/. The "+" nasal specification for the upcoming /m/ can, therefore, be spread to /ɑ/, resulting in a partially or completely nasalized vowel. In English, nasalization of vowels has no effect on phonemic status, so the feature spreading does not compromise the integrity of the speaker's articulatory intent or the listener's ability to recover the spoken word.

Explanations and mechanisms have been proposed to account for anticipatory coarticulation (Farnetani, 1997; Kent, 1976b). One explanation is that anticipatory coarticulation constitutes the ability to anticipate articulatory features before they are needed and is one of the ways in which speech production movements are smoothed out and made continuous across a sequence of sounds. This avoids the obviously inefficient situation of having to articulate each phoneme's "bundle of features" in discrete and successive chunks. Thus, the continuous articulation observed in x-ray studies of the movement of the pharyngeal-oral apparatus is an expression of speech motor efficiency.

A proposed mechanism for anticipatory coarticulation is one in which the plan for articulatory behavior is in the form of a sequence of phonemes and their respective feature specifications, such as depicted in Figure 5–24. Quite literally, the phoneme sequence and component features are believed to be represented somewhere in the brain. A programming operation, often referred to as a "look-ahead" operator (Daniloff & Hammarberg, 1973; Henke, 1966) supposedly scans the phoneme sequence from left to right—the intended output order—and finds features that can be anticipated without compromising the articulatory identity of a sound. In a sense, the look-ahead operator is the mechanism of anticipatory coarticulation and has the task of identifying features that can be spread from a later to an earlier occurring phoneme.

Explanations and mechanisms have also been proposed for carryover (backward) coarticulation. Carryover coarticulation is believed to be the result of articulators being unable to move immediately from one position to the next because they have mass and demonstrate inertia. The right side of Figure 5–24 contains two examples illustrative of this explanation. In the upper right sequence, the "+" for the /u/ in "used" specifies rounded lips, which not only occur when the [u] is produced, but remain to some extent during the [s] and possibly even the [t] because the lips cannot move instantaneously from a rounded to an unrounded configuration. Similarly, the example in the lower right part of Figure 5–24 indicates an open velopharyngeal port for the [m] in "mob" which cannot be closed instantaneously for the following [ɑ]. In both cases, an articulatory feature of one sound is carried over to a following sound because the articulators are subject to inertial laws.

Anticipatory and carryover coarticulation are viewed to be very different phenomena, even though they both involve feature spreading. Anticipatory coarticulation is thought of as a planning or programming phenomenon, whereas carryover coarticulation is thought to be the result of the physical characteristics of the speech production apparatus. A more general model of speech production, in which the notion of feature spreading is incorporated, is depicted in Figure 5–25. This model shows an input to the speech production apparatus, which, in this case, is the phonemic representation and feature components of the utterance "no seat" (as in "There is no seat in the auditorium"). Figure 5–25 suggests a cognitive representation of a yet-to-be discovered neural code. As in Figure 5–24, some of the features are specified and some are not. The input is delivered to a programming module, where the look-ahead operator determines the available forward coarticulations. The phonemic input with coarticulatory modifications is translated into a form suitable for speech production. This translation takes the form of motor commands to the different articulators, including the timing and strength of contraction of the many muscles that are used in speech production. These commands are sent to a production module, which implements them in the form of movements of the articulators. Carryover coarticulation occurs at this stage of production, allowing features to spread from left to right as a result of the inertial properties of the articulators.

This view of articulatory production, although greatly simplified, is accepted by most speech-language pathologists. For example, whenever a client

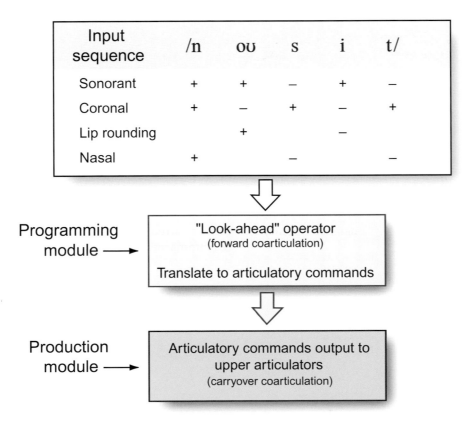

Input sequence	/n	ou	s	i	t/
Sonorant	+	+	–	+	–
Coronal	+	–	+	–	+
Lip rounding		+		–	
Nasal	+		–		–

Programming module ⟶ "Look-ahead" operator (forward coarticulation)

Translate to articulatory commands

Production module ⟶ Articulatory commands output to upper articulators (carryover coarticulation)

Figure 5–25. General model of speech production in which phonemic representation and feature spreading are elements.

is diagnosed with apraxia of speech, either in the adult or child form, there is an assumption of dysfunction in the programming component of the speech production process. Such programming dysfunction is believed to operate on input units that are very much like the phoneme representations portrayed in Figures 5–24 and 5–25. The details of these units or how they enter into the actual articulatory errors observed in apraxia of speech may vary from explanation to explanation, but the basic structure of the underlying theory is much like the one described in this section. McNeil, Pratt, and Fosset (2004), for example, have provided a detailed account of how errors in apraxia of speech can be accounted for by various speech production models that are all variants of the one depicted in Figure 5–25.

Articulatory Phonology or Gesture Theory

The application of the traditional theory of coarticulation to explanations of speech disorders such as apraxia of speech does not mean the theory is universally accepted. In fact, soon after the theory was developed and publicized in the late 1960s and early 1970s, some of its problems became apparent.

The biggest problem, according to critics of the traditional theory, is the requirement of an input representation (phonemes) that may have no reality, as well as a step that translates this representation into a form appropriate to real motor behavior. Critics of the traditional theory of coarticulation argue that it is awkward and unnecessary to imagine a speech production process in which a "digital" representation of speech (discrete phonemes) must be translated to an "analog" form (the smooth and continuous movements of the articulators). In other words, the traditional theory lacks any representation of the time element of articulatory behavior. The alternative proposed by these critics is an input to the speech production process that represents articulatory behavior as it unfolds over time.

Theories that reject the ideas of phonemes and their translation to speech motor behavior are variously called articulatory phonology (Browman & Goldstein, 1992) or gesture theories (Byrd, 1996; Saltzman & Munhall, 1989). The details of these different approaches to the production of articulatory behavior are less important than is a broad understanding of how these theories differ from the traditional theory of coarticulation. Figure 5–26 presents a model of the speech production process in which the focus is entirely on articulatory gestures (movements). There the identity and timing of selected gestures are shown for production of the word "sinew" [sinju]. Five gestures are idealized, including

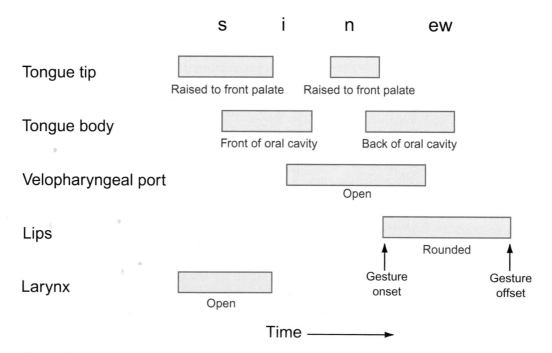

Figure 5-26. General model of speech production in which there is no phonemic representation and focus is entirely on articulatory gestures (movements). Selected articulators are represented. Rectangles delimit the time course of individual gestures.

those of the tongue tip, tongue body, velopharyngeal port, lips, and larynx. These gestures unfold in time, from left to right, just as the sounds for the word "sinew" occur in sequence. The time course of each gesture is indicated by the length of its associated narrow rectangle. The onset and offset of the lip rounding gesture are shown to illustrate how the timing of each rectangle should be interpreted.

The primary impression from this display is of the different articulatory gestures occurring at different onsets and offsets throughout the utterance and of gestures overlapping in time. For example, in addition to the overlap between the open velopharyngeal port gesture and the tongue tip-raising gesture for [n], the open port gesture also overlaps with the tongue body gestures for both the preceding [i] and the following [ju]. Thus, the vocalic sounds preceding and following the nasal sound are produced with a somewhat open velopharyngeal port. In articulatory phonology or gesture theories, this phenomenon is called coproduction, to indicate that two or more gestures are produced at the same time and overlap to some degree. In the traditional theory, the partial nasalization of [i] is an example of anticipatory coarticulation, and the partial nasalization of [ju] is an example of carryover coarticulation. Articulatory phonology or gesture theorists use the term coproduction, rather than coarticulation, to avoid

the phoneme representation implications of the traditional theory. The overlap of the open velopharyngeal port gesture with the tongue body gestures for the two flanking vowels is just that—overlap—and does not reflect the operation of an extra programming process (anticipatory coarticulation) or the physical limitation of articulatory movement (carryover coarticulation).

A criticism of the traditional theory of coarticulation is that it does not account for the timing details of articulatory behavior (Kent & Minifie, 1977). For example, x-ray images of articulatory sequences such as [bɑmz] "bums" reveal that the velopharyngeal port is actually closing during the lip closure portion of the [m], apparently in anticipation of the fricative requirement of a closed velopharynx. Two questions to be asked are, "How does the traditional theory account for this timing?" and "Why is the nasal "+" specification for [m] contradicted by a closing velopharyngeal port (like a "−" specification) when the lips gesture for the nasal is active?" Articulatory phonology or gesture theories address these two questions by eliminating the plus, minus, or unspecified feature characteristics of sounds and the need for them to have phonemic representation. The closing velopharyngeal port during the lip seal for [m] simply reflects the particular degree of overlap between gestures of the lips and velopharynx.

In articulatory phonology or gesture theories, it is the sequencing and overlapping of multiple gestures that results in articulatory sequences. An examination of the gestures portrayed in Figure 5–26 suggests that the timing component is complicated. Somehow, the gestures have to be specified for their duration and for their phasing. Phasing is a term that indicates when one gesture begins relative to another gesture. For example, the first tongue tip gesture (raised to front palate) begins earlier in time than the first tongue body gesture (front of oral cavity). These precise phasings, or timings, of successive articulatory gestures are very important because incorrect phasing can result in poorly formed (and hard-to-understand) articulatory sequences. An example of this is the larynx gesture (open), which represents the abduction of the vocal folds required for the voiceless fricative [s] at the beginning of the word. If this gesture is phased later relative to the tongue tip gesture and nothing else is changed, a good portion of the vowel [i] could be devoiced and might be difficult to understand. In articulatory phonology or gesture theories, each gesture is allowed to move or slide in time relative to other gestures. This is a very attractive feature of these theories for certain speech disorders such as so-called ataxic dysarthria (a speech problem caused by dysfunction of the cerebellum), in which articulatory gestures seem to be

Faster Than a Herd of Turtles

When you watch someone reading aloud, things are moving all over the place. The mandible, tongue, and lips can all be seen to move from here to there and back and then off again to somewhere else. The coordination among these structures is exquisite and the speech sounds come so fast that they blend together into a beautiful constant stream that flows quickly after the thoughts of the speaker. Running speech production is truly a marvelous thing to watch. The speed of articulatory movements is what impresses many observers. Look at those structures go. But just how fast are they moving? What would you guess? Put it in miles per hour. 500? 250? 125? Or would you guess 65 like a car traveling along a freeway? Well, things aren't always what they seem. The actual speed is less than 1 mile per hour. That's not much faster than a thundering herd of turtles and probably considerably less than your usual walking speed.

pulled apart (not overlapped correctly). The pulling apart of articulatory gestures could be the result of improper phasing, or gestures that are allowed to slide too much with respect to each other. The basic structure of articulatory phonology or gesture theories seems to have more potential for application to speech disorders than the traditional theory of coarticulation.

Development and Pharyngeal-Oral Function in Speech Production

The pharyngeal-oral apparatus undergoes significant change between birth and adulthood. This change involves a gradual unfolding of anatomical and physiological substrates that support breathing, chewing, swallowing, speaking, and sound filtering activities. The nature of the pharyngeal-oral apparatus at birth is a far cry (pun intended) from that in adulthood. The skeletal framework and soft tissue components of the pharyngeal-oral apparatus in the newborn infant differ from that of the adult in the relative size among their components, in configuration, and in composition.

Figure 5–27 illustrates several contrastive features of the skeletal framework of the pharyngeal-oral apparatus of the newborn infant and the adult. At birth, the skull of the newborn is relatively large compared to the body. The facial part of the skull is small, being about one-eighth of the bulk of the cranium of the newborn as opposed to about one-half of the bulk of the cranium in the adult (Zemlin, 1998). After the first year of life, the facial skeleton grows at a much faster rate than the cranial skeleton. A major feature of this development is a downward and forward growth of the face that progresses differently in different structures.

Although the cranium approximates adult size relatively early in childhood, perhaps as early as 6 years of age (Melsen & Melsen, 1982), the facial skeleton continues to grow into adolescence and possibly adulthood (Kent & Vorperian, 1995; Richtsmeier & Cheverud, 1986). During this growth period, the front-to-back depth of the bony palate nearly doubles, whereas the side-to-side expansion of the structure increases significantly less (Zemlin, 1998). The mandible also grows in size and changes in shape during its growth period (Scott, 1976). The body of the mandible increases in length to accommodate the addition of three permanent teeth on each side, and the angle between the ramus and body of the mandible becomes less obtuse (Zemlin, 1998). Growth of the mandible continues until near adulthood and progresses relatively steadily with occasional growth spurts at certain ages (Walker

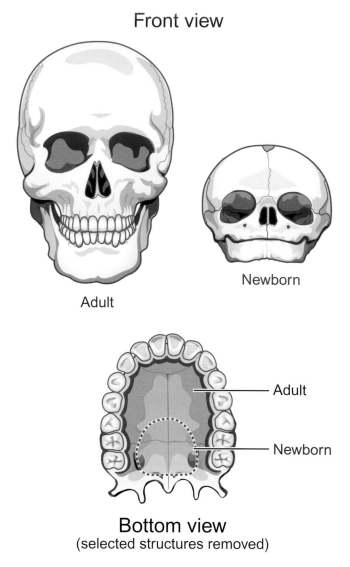

Front view

Adult

Newborn

Adult

Newborn

Bottom view
(selected structures removed)

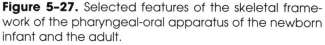

Figure 5–27. Selected features of the skeletal framework of the pharyngeal-oral apparatus of the newborn infant and the adult.

& Kowalski, 1972). Dental development is subject to significant individual variation, its consistent hallmark being the loss of deciduous teeth and their replacement with permanent teeth (Scott, 1976).

Soft tissues of the pharyngeal-oral apparatus also undergo developmental change. The pharyngeal cavity of the newborn infant is about 4 cm in length and appreciably shorter than the oral cavity (Crelin, 1973). The contour of the junction between the pharyngeal and oral parts of the pharyngeal-oral apparatus is rounded in the newborn infant rather than having the approximate right-angle sharp line of demarcation of the adult apparatus. At about 5 years of age, the two parts of the apparatus are joined at an oblique angle, whereas at puberty they approximate the right-angle configuration of the adult (Kent & Vorperian, 1995). The predominant feature of developmental growth of the pharynx is its vertical enlargement (Vorperian et al., 2005, 2009), with the pharynx tripling in length to become about 12 cm long by adulthood (Tourne, 1991).

The tongue of the newborn infant essentially fills the oral cavity (Crelin, 1976). During the first year of life the structure begins to descend within the neck and continues to do so until about 5 years of age (Laitman & Crelin, 1976). Growth of the tongue is relatively continual throughout childhood and on through puberty, showing occasional growth spurts along the way (Kerr, Kelly, & Geddes, 1991). The patterning of growth of the tongue tends to be in general harmony with the patterning of growth of the mandible (Kent & Vorperian, 1995).

The lips undergo significant developmental change between birth and adulthood. They form a near circular sphincter in the newborn infant, whereas they form a transverse, elliptical sphincter in the adult. Major reconfiguration of the lips occurs during the first 2 years of life (Burke, 1980). Thereafter, lip size changes, with forward growth of the lower lip exceeding that of the upper lip. Rapid growth of the lips is reported to occur between 10 and 17 years of age (Vig & Cohen, 1979). Growth spurts of the lips appear to be correlated with those occurring in the mandible (Walker & Kowalski, 1972).

Root of the Problem

Because the normal tongue functions as a muscular hydrostat, and therefore as a unit, its differential impairment in nervous system disease can lead to limitations imposed by one part on other parts. An example of this can be found in differential impairment of the tongue in children with cerebral palsy. Those children who have significant impairment of the root of the tongue often demonstrate inadequate movement in other parts of the tongue. When the root of the tongue does not move normally, the rest of the tongue does not have a normal base off which to work. Thus, actions of the blade and tip of the tongue may not achieve their goals because the root has failed to position them appropriately to carry out their missions. They themselves may not be at fault. They just have to put up with a bad root and make the best of it.

Raymond D. Kent

Kent has been one of the leading speech scientists in the world for over three decades. He has written extensively on a variety of topics, including speech development, normal speech acoustics, and the acoustics of speech associated with neuromotor speech disorders. His work, along with colleagues, has elucidated much of what is known about speech acoustics and inferred articulatory dynamics in speakers with dysarthria. A distinguishing feature of Kent's work is its multidisciplinary nature. Those who read his articles and books come away with an appreciation for his ability to integrate diverse literatures and bring them to bear on issues in his own discipline. Few can match him and those who know him well affectionately refer to him as "Clark Kent," the character of Superman fame, because of their awe for his powerful influence in speech science. He is retired and lives in Madison, Wisconsin.

Along with the anatomical changes described above, various aspects of the nervous system also undergo change. Neural development follows a protracted time course that extends well into adolescence. This development reflects change in cognition, memory, motor control, and other nervous system functions that are relevant to the encoding of movement by the pharyngeal-oral apparatus. Such development is conditioned by nervous system change that involves maturation in synaptic connections, axon diameters, dendrite branching, myelination of motor and sensory pathways, and the establishment of more ingrained neural networks for preferred activities (Benes, Turtle, Khan, & Farol, 1994; Huttenlocher, 1990; Lecours, 1975; Netsell, 1986; Paus et al., 2001).

Characteristic of the development of movement control of the pharyngeal-oral apparatus are sensitive periods in which skill acquisition is continuous but nonlinear and during which incremental increases in performance take what appear to be jumps forward (Netsell, 1986). Certain changes in the development of movement control appear to be governed by factors operating over long periods and involving persistent effects, whereas others occur over shorter periods (Newell, Liu, & Meyer-Kress, 2001). Motor commands to the muscles of the developing pharyngeal-oral apparatus are generated through a background of "neural noise" that may be unrelated to a movement goal (Crossman & Szafran, 1956; Schmidt, Zelaznik, Hawkins, Frank, & Quinn, 1979; Welford, 1956). Such noise influences movement proficiency and is thought to be of major significance, but to decrease in importance over the course of development (Jones, Hamilton, & Wolpert, 2002; Smits-Engelsman & Van Galen, 1997; Yan, Thomas, Stelmach, & Thomas, 2000). In short, decrease in neural noise is associated with progression toward motor performance that is more and more like that observed in adults.

Studies of speech production in children have revealed differences in pharyngeal-oral control when compared to speech production in adults. For example, children speak more slowly than adults (Kent & Forner, 1980; Nittrouer, 1993; Smith & McLean-Muse, 1986; Smith, Sugarman, & Long, 1983; Sturm & Seery, 2007) and with greater variability. Such variability is manifested in amplitude, velocity, timing, and general patterning of pharyngeal-oral movements during speech production (Goffman & Smith, 1999; Green, Moore, Higashikawa, & Steeve, 2000; Green, Moore, & Reilly, 2002; Grigos, 2009; Maner, Smith, & Grayson, 2000; Sharkey & Folkins, 1985; Smith & Goffman, 1998; Smith & McLean-Muse, 1986; Steeve, Moore, Green, Reilly, & McMurtrey, 2008; Watkin & Fromm, 1984).

Transition to faster and more stable speech production is gradual across childhood. Acoustic observations, from which inferences are made concerning the stability of motor control, suggest that adult-like performance may not occur until as late as 12 years of age (Kent, 1976a), whereas direct observations of pharyngeal-oral movements indicate that adult-like performance is not reached until near the end of the teenage years (Murdoch, Cheng, & Goozée, 2012; Smith & Zelaznik, 2004; Walsh & Smith, 2002). Other studies of the development of the vowel acoustic space (positioning of airway resonances in relation to one another) in children suggests nonlinear changes with age, with jumps in vowel space changes corresponding to anatomical growth spurts in all or part of the pharyngeal-oral apparatus (Vorperian & Kent, 2007).

Pharyngeal-oral movements must be intricately coordinated to produce intelligible speech. Coordinative movement patterns also undergo development across childhood and adolescence in the form of changes in muscle synergies that influence how different structures become functionally coupled to one another during speech performance. An example is how the upper lip, lower lip, and mandible can be variously adjusted to bring about a resultant opening or closing of the lip aperture (Smith & Zelaznik, 2004). While muscle synergies are developing, the diversity

of movement routines is also undergoing change. As a child develops, a wider range of movements can be generated, greater variation is possible in the combination of different movements, and the order in which movements can be combined becomes less rigid (Menn, 1983; Nittrouer, 1993). Beyond this, the pace at which speech production skills are acquired and the nature of the developmental trajectory are not uniform across children or structures (Nittrouer, 1993), and may even be manifested in clusters of different developmental profiles (Vick et al., 2012).

Of final interest is emerging evidence for short-term plasticity in movement of the pharyngeal-oral apparatus during speech production in school-aged children. In a study of coordinative patterns among the upper lip, lower lip, and mandible during novel word productions, Walsh, Smith, and Weber-Fox (2006) demonstrated that children's speech motor control processes adaptively change to improve performance during the course of repeated trials. This is manifested in the form of significantly less variable coupling between the upper lip, lower lip, and mandible during later productions of sequential utterances. This short-term plastic nature of speech production performance in children reveals a strong practice effect and suggests a high degree of flexibility in pharyngeal-oral function. Such flexibility may be advantageous in second language acquisition, and may explain, in part why children are less likely to have foreign accents than adults who learn a second language.

Age and Pharyngeal-Oral Function in Speech Production

Speech production is a motor skill that is functional throughout much of life and is preserved even in the oldest of the old. Once this skill is fully mature, it gives the appearance of involving little effort, proceeding automatically, and being highly ingrained. Most elderly people use this practiced motor skill exceedingly well and produce fully intelligible speech. This does not mean, however, that their speech production is unchanged from what it was decades earlier. As time passes, the structures and processes involved in speech production undergo change. Although the features of interest are subject to change on different schedules and to different degrees in different parts of the apparatus, the majority of age-related changes manifest after the 5th decade of life (Kahane, 1990). Such changes tend to be gradual and progressive, but the greatest alterations, diminutions, and functional consequences occur in elderly individuals.

The structure of the pharyngeal part of the pharyngeal-oral apparatus changes in several ways during adulthood. To begin, it gets larger. In young adults, the lower edge of the cricoid cartilage is positioned at the upper edge of the 7th cervical vertebra. This positioning lowers during adulthood until, by senescence, the lower edge of the cricoid cartilage reaches the bottom of the 7th cervical vertebra. Continuing through senescence, the cricoid cartilage descends even farther (Wind, 1970). One result of this lowering of the laryngeal framework is that the pharynx lengthens downward. At the same time the pharynx is lengthening, it is also changing in cross-section. The muscles of the pharynx tend to weaken and atrophy with age and the pharyngeal lumen widens and dilates (Linville & Fisher, 1985; Zaino & Benventano, 1977).

Other features of pharyngeal structure and function also change with age. The epithelial lining of the pharynx undergoes progressive thinning (Ferreri, 1959). Sensory innervation in the pharyngeal region decreases and sensory discrimination goes through a significant decline (Aviv et al., 1994; Ferreri, 1959). The compliance (relatively floppiness) of the pharyngeal tube increases with age (Huang et al., 1998). And the capacity to voluntarily move the pharynx progressively decreases with age (Sonies, Stone, & Shawker, 1984).

The oral part of the pharyngeal-oral apparatus (defined here to include the oral cavity and the oral vestibule) also changes in several ways during adulthood. The oral airway undergoes a gradual increase in size with age, probably in both length and cross-section. This is believed to continue even into senescence (Israel, 1968, 1973). It is uncertain, however, whether or not this trend applies to very old individuals (Kahane, 1990).

The oral epithelium thins, loses some of its elasticity, and becomes less firmly attached to adjacent bone and connective tissue (Squire, Johnson, & Hoops, 1976). Salivary function also changes, causing a tendency for saliva to thicken and alter in composition in older individuals (Chauncey, Borkan, Wayler, Feller, & Kapur, 1981). Reduced amounts of saliva result in dryness in the oral mucosa. Such change may result from structural changes of the salivary glands and/or from endocrine changes attendant to aging (Baum, 1981). These changes may be a factor in why elderly individuals have more oral infections, more oral lesions (sores), and more loose teeth than their younger counterparts (Sonies, 1991).

In those individuals who lose teeth with age, alveolar bone may be resorbed (dissolved), sometimes significantly so (Klein, 1980), although this is less of a problem with current high-quality dental care than in the past (Zemlin, 1998). Overall, bones of the oral cavity and oral vestibule may become more fragile, cartilages may lose some of their resiliency, ligaments may lose some of their elasticity, fat may get redistributed, and muscle bulk and power may wane with aging (Fremont & Hoyland, 2007).

Sensory and motor capabilities of the oral part of the pharyngeal-oral apparatus also decrease with age. For example, oral form, pressure, and touch discrimination are poorer in elderly adults than in young adults (Canetta, 1977). Spatial acuity on the surface of the lips also declines significantly in old age, especially in men (Wohlert, 1996c). The tongue may lose mobility with age (Amerman & Parnell, 1982) and its range of motion may decrease (Sonies, Baum, & Shawker, 1984). The ability to seal the lips may also decline with age (Hixon & Hoit, 2005). Reflex responses of lip muscles are significantly lower in amplitude and longer in latency in elderly individuals compared to young individuals (Wohlert, 1996b).

Other aspects of the nervous system go through changes with aging that affect both the pharyngeal and oral parts of the pharyngeal-oral apparatus. These include, among others, that cortical cells controlling the apparatus may atrophy, neurotransmitter production may decrease, blood flow may diminish, nerve-firing rates may decrease, and nerve conduction velocities may reduce (Kenney, 1982; Lexell, Taylor, & Sjostrom, 1988; Luschei, Ramig, Baker, & Smith, 1999; McGeer, Fibiger, McGeer, & Wiskson, 1971; Valenstein, 1981).

Some of the age-related changes discussed to this juncture may affect speech production. Three prominently discussed manifestations of aging are changes that affect the resonance properties of the pharyngeal-oral airway, durational features of speech production, and variability of speech production. Changes in factors such as cognition, memory, and linguistic processing may also affect speech production, but they are beyond the scope of emphasis in this introductory presentation.

As described above, the length and cross-section of the pharyngeal and oral airways increase with age during adulthood. As considered in detail in subsequent chapters, the size of these airways influences the resonant properties of the pharyngeal-oral apparatus. For example, larger airways tend to have acoustic resonances that are lower in frequency. Thus, it is unsurprising that the frequencies of vowel formants (major energy concentrations in the acoustic speech signal; see Chapter 8) have been reported to be lower in elderly individuals than in younger individuals (Linville & Fisher, 1985; Liss, Weismer, & Rosenbek, 1990; Watson & Munson, 2007). This age-related lowering is especially prominent in the first formant, the lowest resonance (Endres, Bambach, & Flosser, 1971; Linville, 2001; Linville & Fisher, 1985; Scukanec, Petrosino, & Squibb, 1991). The second and third formants (higher frequency resonances) are also documented to be lower in frequency in older individuals, but the effect is smaller than for the first formant (Linville & Fisher, 1985; Linville & Rens, 2001). Although there is general agreement that the age effect in vowel acoustics is related to enlargement of the pharyngeal-oral airway, there is some question concerning how the relative changes of the pharyngeal and oral parts of the apparatus contribute to the acoustic changes observed (Xue & Hao, 2003). Additional research using advanced technologies for measuring the three-dimensional configuration of the pharyngeal-oral lumen should be helpful in sorting out the details of this age effect.

Slowing is a hallmark of aging and is viewed as the most pervasive motor characteristic of getting older (Fremont & Hoyland, 2007; Welford, 1982). Slowing in the pharyngeal-oral apparatus is no exception and can be attributed to changes in parts of the nervous system that control the peripheral machinery of the apparatus, as well as to changes in the peripheral machinery itself (Fozard, Vercruyssen, Reynolds, Hancock, & Quilter, 1994; Kahane, 1990; Kent & Burkard, 1981; Ulatowska, 1985; Weismer & Liss, 1991). The influences of age on breathing, laryngeal, and velopharyngeal-nasal function in speech production (described in Chapters 2, 3, and 4) combine with those of the pharyngeal-oral apparatus to produce a general slowing of speech production with advanced age. This slowing has two bases, one being that articulatory rate slows and the other that older speakers pause more often during running speech production (Hartman & Danhauer, 1976; Hoit & Hixon, 1987; Ryan, 1972).

Measurements of the temporal characteristics of the speech of normal elderly adults shed light on how the slowing of speech is spread across the speech production stream (Liss et al., 1990; Smith, Wasowicz, & Preston, 1987). Smith and colleagues, for example, studied young adults (24 to 27 years of age) and elderly adults (66 to 75 years of age) producing a variety of words and sentences at normal and fast speaking rates. They measured the durations of phonetic segments (consonants and vowels), syllables, and sentences and found that the durations for each of these measures were an average of 20 to 25% longer for elderly speakers than for young speakers at both the normal and fast speaking rates. Liss and colleagues also studied a group of elderly individuals for segment durations in sentences, but in their case the participants were from among the oldest of the old (87 to 93 years of age). They found that the segment durations they measured in these very old

participants were longer than those reported in the literature for young adult speakers, but relatively similar to those produced by younger elderly speakers (65 to 82 years of age) studied by Weismer (1984).

Longer durations for speech segments in normal-speaking old and very old adults, in comparison to young adults, beg comparison to other speakers who use longer durations during speech production. Once such group is young children. For all duration comparisons with such young children, the production of elderly speakers tend to be in the range of durations exhibited by 6- and 7-year-old children (Kent & Forner, 1980; Smith et al., 1983). Thus, life would appear to go full circle from young childhood to senescence, picking up speed in early life and slowing back down in later life.

The variability of movement also undergoes change with age across adulthood. Such variability tends to increase with age and is often considered to be a measure of motor control integrity in general (Nelson, Soderberg, & Urbsheit, 1984; Weismer & Liss, 1991). Studies to determine whether or not such variability is also manifested in speech production with aging have included both physiological and acoustic observations.

Wohlert and Smith (1998) studied the spatiotemporal stability of lip movements in old adult and young adult speakers. Lip displacement waveforms were recorded for different rates of speech production and subjected to sophisticated analyses that captured information about variability of performance. Despite producing clear and fully intelligible speech, elderly adults spoke more slowly than their young adult counterparts and demonstrated less spatiotemporal (position and time) stability in lip movement. Findings of this nature imply that normal aging alters the fine motor control required for speech production.

A study of lip muscle activity in young and old adults during different activities, including speech production, was concerned with the complexity of motor patterns and whether or not they become less flexible with age (Wohlert, 1996a). Patterns of muscle activation were compared among different quadrants of the lips and were found not to differ with age for tasks such as lip protrusion and chewing. In contrast, during speech production, patterns of muscle coupling among different quadrants of the lips (inferred from correlations of myoelectric measurements of muscle activities) showed a tendency for coupling (coactivation across quadrants) to be greater in elderly individuals than in young individuals. Presumably, elderly individuals adopt an increased coupling strategy among quadrants of the lips as their fine motor control wanes with age and they are unable to use the lips in the variety of ways they could at younger years. Loss of fine motor control may require a reorganization of speech movements and one consequence may be an increase in their variability as the elderly adult attempts to cope with a changing nervous system.

Acoustic studies of speech also show greater age-related variability in measures such as sound and syllable durations (Smith et al., 1987; Weismer, 1984; Weismer & Fromm, 1983). In their study of the oldest of the old, Liss et al. (1990) determined that the variability in performance of the very old is even greater than the variability among younger elderly and much greater than among young adults. This is true not only for sound durations, but also for vowel formant (resonance) midpoints and formant transitions.

The process of aging imposes a slowing and reduction of precision on the pharyngeal-oral apparatus. Liss et al. (1990) noted that data on the acoustic characteristics of very old speakers show striking similarities to data obtained from speakers with Parkinson disease (Weismer, 1984). They interpreted this similarity to suggest a speech production analog to assertions that aging may involve processes similar to those seen in neural disease (Morgan & Finch, 1988). This is not to say that the very old are Parkinson-like, but that the speech motor performance of very old persons may be related, in part, to the deterioration of brain circuits that are affected in similar ways to those affected by Parkinson disease.

The Father Who Grew Younger

One of us had a father who had Parkinson disease. He looked younger and younger as he got older and older because increasing stiffness in his face fought off the usual wrinkling process that comes with time. Repeated muscle actions lead to the formation of the wrinkles in our faces as we age. Then there is everyday wear and tear and loss of collagen that causes sagging here and there. We wouldn't show our age so dramatically if we didn't use our facial muscles as much throughout our lives. If we never smiled or frowned or puckered up we might look younger than we are. But as Kent (1997) so aptly put it, "our social worlds would be much poorer for the loss of animated faces. And perhaps we would feel older while looking younger." So rather than hiding your facial expressions, cultivate them so that others will get a true sense of what you are all about. Smile.

Sex and Pharyngeal-Oral Function in Speech Production

Everyone knows that speech usually sounds different when produced by men and women. From discussion in previous chapters, it is clear that sex-related differences in speech production and speech are strongly associated with sex-related differences in laryngeal structure and function, but that structure and function of the breathing apparatus and velopharyngeal-nasal apparatus are only minimally different between the sexes (see Chapters 2, 3, and 4). Here, attention turns to the potential contribution of pharyngeal-oral structure and function to sex-related differences in speech production and speech.

Perhaps the most obvious structural difference between men and women is size. Men tend to be larger than women overall, and this size difference is also reflected in the pharyngeal-oral apparatus. For example, the skull is larger (Zemlin, 1998) and the vocal tract (from larynx to lips) is longer in men than women (Fitch & Giedd, 1999). One of the most important sex-related differences for speech production is that the pharynx is longer by about 22% (in the resting state) in men compared to women (Fitch & Giedd, 1999). Although sex-related size differences emerge strongly at puberty and continue to become more prominent until early adulthood (Fitch & Giedd, 1999; Goldstein, 1980), there are sex-related size differences in selected regions of the pharyngeal-oral apparatus even prior to puberty (Vorperian et al., 2011).

Men tend to be stronger than women. This also holds true for the strength of structures within the pharyngeal-oral apparatus. For example, men produce greater maximum lip forces (Barlow & Rath, 1985) and tongue forces (Youmans & Stierwalt, 2006) than women. Nevertheless, it is interesting to note that when maximum tongue force production is normalized to body muscle mass, sex-related differences disappear (Mortimore, Fiddes, Stephens, & Douglas, 1999). When considering fine force control of the lips and tongue, men generate higher velocities of force change and are more accurate in holding a target force compared to women (Gentil & Tournier, 1998).

Pharyngeal-oral function during speech production has also been shown to differ somewhat between the sexes. For example, men produce syllable-, word-, and sentence-level utterances (Smith et al., 1987) and repetitions of speech movements (Nicholson & Kimura, 1996) at faster rates than women. Examination of a single structure, the tongue, during speech production, also shows the same sex-related pattern for speed. Specifically, during diphthong productions and productions of two consecutive vowels, the posterior tongue moves faster in men than women (Simpson, 2001, 2002). This difference in speed has been attributed to the fact that the male tongue must move a greater distance than the female tongue, particularly in the posterior region of the oral cavity where the palate is domed and the pharynx is large in men.

Sex-related differences in the size of the pharyngeal-oral apparatus are reflected in speech (the acoustic product) in a number of ways. For example, the frequency spectrum of certain fricative consonants is lower in men than women due to size differences in the resonating cavities (Schwartz, 1968). Perhaps one of the most puzzling differences between the speech of men and women relates to the formant patterns (patterns of energy concentration) associated with vowel production. Although men have lower frequency vowel formants than women (as would be expected from the fact that men are larger than women), the differences in formant values are not what would be expected from size differences alone. Other factors must be also contributing.

One such factor is that men have proportionally longer pharyngeal cavities than women (Fant, 1975). Nevertheless, even this is not sufficient to explain the nonuniform differences in formants between men and women, leaving open the possibility that sex-related differences in articulatory behavior may account for at least some of the remaining variance. One suggestion is that women use smaller and longer constrictions than men in their vowel productions and these constrictions contribute to the creation of different formant patterns (Fant, 1975). Another suggestion is that women articulate in ways that create larger acoustic differences among vowels as a means of compensating for the wider distribution of energy across frequency provided by the voice source (Ryalls & Lieberman, 1982). That is, because women have higher voice fundamental frequencies than men, their harmonics are more widely spaced and there is less acoustic energy in each formant frequency region, thereby making it more difficult to distinguish among vowels. Thus, women may compensate in ways that exaggerate the acoustic and perceptual differences among vowels. Using magnetic resonance imaging, Story, Hoffman, and Titze (1997) found the female pharynx to be about 37% shorter than the male pharynx during the production of three cardinal vowels. They concluded that the female pharyngeal-oral airway shape "contains unique qualities that cannot be explained by a simple uniform compression of the male vocal tract" (p. 36) and that the shortened pharynx in the female pharyngeal-oral apparatus may be a key factor in distinguishing between male and female voice qualities during speech production.

MEASUREMENT OF PHARYNGEAL-ORAL FUNCTION

This section considers the instrumental measurement of pharyngeal-oral function. Attention is directed to selected methods that have application to the study of normal and abnormal function. Six categories of methods are discussed, including those that take advantage of: (a) x-ray imaging, (b) strain-gauge monitoring, (c) articulatory tracking, (d) magnetic resonance imaging, (e) ultrasonic imaging, (f) aeromechanical observations, and (g) acoustic observations.

X-ray Imaging

X-ray imaging is a powerful method for studying the pharyngeal-oral apparatus. Such imaging has provided much of the early data on the positions and movements of structures of the pharyngeal-oral apparatus during speech production. These data are in the forms of lateral still x-rays and cinefluorography (motion picture x-rays).

Lateral still x-rays provide images like that shown in Chapter 4 (Figure 4–26). These are most often obtained in the midsagittal plane and provide a shadow-cast "snapshot" of the pharyngeal-oral apparatus at a moment in time. Lateral still x-rays are useful for examining structures that are stationary. For example, they can be used to determine the midline positions of the lips, mandible, tongue, velum, posterior pharyngeal wall, and hyoid bone in relation to one another during sustained speech sounds where such structures are relatively fixed in position. Thus, vowels, fricative consonants, and nasal consonants are prime candidates for study using lateral still x-rays.

Cinefluorography (or videofluorography) enables the x-ray study of structures in motion (McWilliams & Girdany, 1964; Moll, 1960). Fluorographic methods, and other forms of cineradiography, provide for the monitoring of the spatial and temporal coordination among pharyngeal-oral structures. Images obtained through the use of cineflourography (or videofluorography) can be analyzed qualitatively or quantitatively. Quantitative analysis often entails a series of stop-frame observations in which the positions of structures are measured in a two-dimensional coordinate system. Such measurements are tedious and time intensive, even when semiautomated. They are, however, extremely instructive with regard to speech production behaviors of the pharyngeal-oral apparatus in that they enable visualization of the entire apparatus in one plane. A great deal of knowledge about normal and abnormal speech production has been obtained using such methodology (Kent & Moll, 1975; Magen, Kang, Tiede, & Whalen, 2003; Netsell & Kent, 1976).

Although x-ray imaging has provided valuable information about speech production, it has significant drawbacks. Most importantly, it is now known that exposure to x-ray poses serious health risks, and regulations are in place to restrict the amount of exposure allowed. In addition, x-ray imaging presents major complexities for measurement. To address these problems, a method was developed that limited x-ray exposure and simplified the quantification of the complex geometry of the pharyngeal-oral airway. This method involved fixing markers at strategic locations on pharyngeal-oral structures so that specific points and their movements could be tracked. This method is described below in the section on Articulatory Tracking.

Strain-Gauge Monitoring

Strain-gauge monitoring has been used to study both movements and forces associated with pharyngeal-oral function. Strain gauges are devices that respond to the bend placed on metal beams to which they are attached. Most often they are bonded to both sides of such beams and form two arms of an electrical circuit called a Wheatstone bridge. Bending forces on the beams cause resistance changes in the strain gauges that are converted into proportional voltage changes for monitoring.

The widest use of strain-gauge technology in the pharyngeal-oral apparatus related to measurement of structural position and movement (Hixon, 1972). For example, strain-gauge technology has been used to measure the positions and movements of the velum (Moller, Martin, & Christiansen, 1971) and the mandible and lips (Barlow, Cole, & Abbs, 1983; Muller & Abbs, 1979; Sussman & Smith, 1971). Strain-gauge systems have yielded a large amount of data on movements of the mandible and lips during speech production and their temporal and spatial coordination (Gracco, 1994; Shaiman, Adams, & Kimelman, 1997; Smith & McClean-Muse, 1987).

Different arrangements of deflection beams and strain gauges have made it possible to measure force production of pharyngeal-oral structures (Hixon, 1972). Included among these are circular or straight beam configurations using strain gauges to measure the adductory force of the two lips combined (Kim, 1971), adductory forces of the upper and lower lips separately (Barlow & Burton, 1990; Barlow & Netsell, 1986; Bar-

low & Rath, 1985), and thrusting force of the tip of the tongue in a vector toward the alveolar process of the maxilla (Barlow & Abbs, 1983). Measurements of these types have been found to be helpful in elucidating both normal behavior and the behavior of individuals with pharyngeal-oral control problems related to cerebral palsy, Parkinson disease, and traumatic brain injury (Barlow & Abbs, 1983; Barlow & Burton, 1990). Although historically important, strain-gauge monitoring has been superseded by more sophisticated approaches, such as articulatory tracking and magnetic resonance imaging.

Articulatory Tracking

Articulatory tracking in this context means the tracking of specific points on pharyngeal-oral structures during activities such as speech production. There are various methods of articulatory tracking that involve different technologies, including x-ray imaging, electromagnetic sensing, and optoelectronic tracking. These operate on the principle of flesh-point tracking, wherein positions and movements of small markers fixed to surface tissue are tracked across time. One exception to this is electro-palatography, which is discussed last.

X-ray Microbeam Imaging

X-ray studies of pharyngeal-oral function pose radiation risks; thus, limits are placed on the extent to which x-ray observations can be made in both research and clinical studies. One attempt to address this problem was the x-ray microbeam system. X-ray microbeam technology was developed at the University of Tokyo (Kiritani, Itoh, & Fujimura, 1975), and a microbeam system was installed at the University of Wisconsin-Madison in a facility supported as a national resource by the National Institutes of Health (Westbury, 1991).

The x-ray microbeam system was designed to track small pellets adhered to pharyngeal-oral structures using an extremely thin x-ray beam. The beam was focused on the pellets so that surrounding tissue received minimal radiation. Two-dimensional positions of multiple pellets could be tracked simultaneously. For example, multiple pellets could be affixed to the dorsal surface of the tongue to track the movement of different points (pellets) along its surface. The tracking of specific fleshpoints removes some of the ambiguities of studying complex gestures, especially those involved in tongue movements (Honda, 2002; Kent, 1972; Wood, 1979). Fortunately, acoustic measures of segment durations, vowel formant frequencies, and formant transitions, as well as perceptual measures, suggest that patterns of tongue movement are not appreciably changed with the pellets in place (Weismer & Bunton, 1999).

Figure 5–28A shows a midsagittal view of the pharyngeal-oral structures with pellets fixed to the outside of the upper and lower lips, on the mandible near the incisors, and at four locations on the dorsal surface of the tongue. Figure 5–28B provides a graphic representation of the movements of the flesh point pellets in two-dimensional space. The graph is oriented to indicate upward movement (toward the palate) when moving vertically along the ordinate and forward movement (toward the lips and beyond) when moving rightward along the abscissa. The tracings were generated with x-ray microbeam data recorded during production of the vowel sequence /iaui/. The movements of the pellets can be "relived" by following the tracings from the black dot (where the production of the first /i/ begins) along the trajectory of the blue line (during the movements associated with /a/ and /u/), to the red dot (the termination of the second /i/). X-ray microbeam data such as these have been exceptionally useful in elucidating kinematic behavior of structures of the pharyngeal-oral apparatus in both individuals with normal speech production (e.g., Green & Wang, 2003; Nittrouer, 1991) and individuals with neuromotor-based speech disorders (e.g., Weismer, Yunusova, & Westbury, 2003; Yunusova, Weismer, & Lindstrom, 2011). Although the x-ray microbeam system was disassembled in 2010, the data that were generated with it continue to undergo analysis.

Electromagnetic Sensing

Electromagnetic sensing also provides a means for tracking the movements of multiple points on pharyngeal-oral structures, but without the use of x-ray. Such sensing relies on the use of a generator coil (or coils) and several sensor coils. The voltage induced in the receiving coils is inversely proportional to the distance between them and the generating coil(s). Suitable electronic manipulations provide a measure of the position of the receiving coils in one-, two-, or three-dimensional space.

Electromagnetic sensing was first applied to the pharyngeal-oral apparatus in studies of one- and two-dimensional movements of a point on the mandible (Hixon, 1971). Since then, more complex systems have been developed with applications to the study of multiple points on different structures on the inside and outside of the pharyngeal-oral apparatus (Perkell et al., 1992;

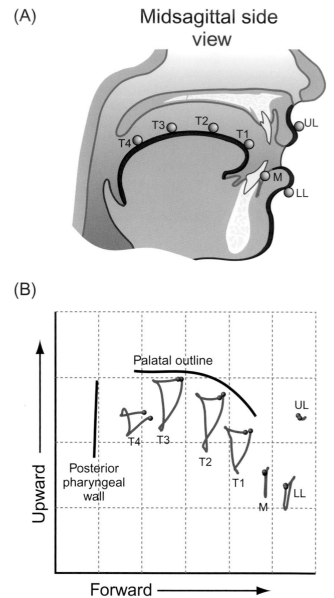

Figure 5–28. Flesh-point pellet locations (**A**) for recording x-ray microbeam data and sample tracings (**B**) representing movements during the production of the vowel sequence /iaui/. The movement sequence begins at the black dot and ends at the red dot. (Graphic data provided courtesy of Brad Story)

Schonle et al., 1987; van der Giet, 1977). The most often studied points are on the mandible, lips, and tongue (usually at multiple sites). The tracking of multiple points enables determinations to be made concerning the spatial and temporal coordination within and between different parts of the pharyngeal-oral apparatus.

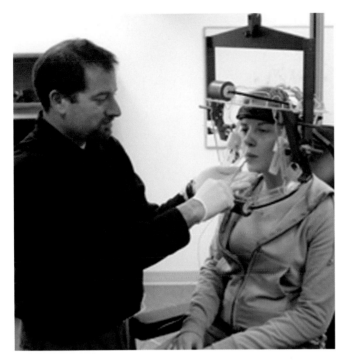

Figure 5–29. An electromagnetic articulograph. (Photograph provided courtesy of Jordan Green)

jaw. An optoelectronic tracking system requires fixing small markers (either light-emitting or reflective) on the surface of the structures of interest and the positioning of several cameras in different locations. The cameras record the position of the markers and their change in position (movements) in three dimensions. Optoelectronic tracking has been used to investigate lip and jaw movments to address questions related to topics such as normal speech development in children (e.g., Nip, Green, & Marx, 2011; Smith & Goffman, 1998) and speech disorders (e.g., MacPherson & Smith, in press). An advantage of optoelectrical tracking systems is that speech can be produced with minimal encumbrance to speech structures. A disadvantage is that only movements of externally visible structures can be tracked.

Electropalatographic Monitoring

Electropalatographic monitoring differs from the other articulatory tracking systems discussed in this section in that it does not use markers to track specific locations and movements of structures. Instead, electropalatography is designed to sense the contact of the tongue against an artificial palate. This form of sensing relies on the construction of an acrylic plate molded to fit against the hard palate of a specific individual. Within

Figure 5–29 shows a multiple-coil system called an electromagnetic articulograph. This type of system uses a computer algorithm to calculate the distance between generating (transmitting) and receiving coils as the receiving coils move through three-dimensional space over time. The resultant data can be displayed in different ways, including displacement-time plots (showing movement of flesh points over time) or x-y plots (showing the relative movements of flesh points in two-dimentional space, such as that shown in Figure 5–28B). The use of electromagnetic articulography in research and clinical studies is becoming increasingly popular and data from such use appears to be driving a more comprehensive understanding of normal speech production and certain disorders of speech production and swallowing (e.g., Katz, Bharadwaj, & Stettler, 2006; Matthies, Svirsky, Perkell, & Lane, 1996; Perkell et al., 2001; Steele & Van Lieshout, 2004).

Optoelectronic Tracking

Optoelectronic tracking is another technology that can be useful for observing movements of selected pharyngeal-oral structures, specifically those structures that are visible externally, such as the lips and

---

Cornstarch

Modern systems are available that make it possible to determine the location of tongue contact with the palate. These take advantage of sensors embedded in an acrylic device that is worn like an upper denture. Signals from these sensors are displayed in a computer array that portrays the pattern of contact. The precursor to this electronic means of observation was cornstarch. The roof of the mouth was dusted white with cornstarch and then the articulatory action of interest was executed immediately. A quick look at the roof of the mouth right afterward would reveal where the tongue had made contact with the palate. The resulting pattern could be drawn on paper or photographed from a mirror reflection of the area on the palate where the tongue contact had wiped the cornstarch away. The method was crude in comparison to today's sophisticated techniques, but it worked nonetheless.

the plate are housed dozens of small electrodes, each of which responds (lights up) when the tongue touches it. During speaking, the electrodes are activated in patterns that reflect the contact of the tongue against the artificial palate at each moment. Electropalatography has been used to study the behavior of the tongue during speech production in children and adults (e.g., Gibbon, Lee, & Yuen, 2010; Hardcastle, Barry, & Clark, 1987; Timmins, Hardcastle, Wood, & Cleland, 2011). Nevertheless, electropalatographic monitoring is less than ideal in that it requires a custom constructed appliance, has the potential to alter usual articulatory behavior by the presence of the appliance, and reflects only one aspect of upper airway articulatory behavior (tongue contact with the palate).

Magnetic Resonance Imaging

Magnetic resonance (MR) imaging offers a particularly effective way to observe pharyngeal-oral structures and their movements during speech production. MR imaging is based on the fact that protons (specifically, the nuclei of hydrogen molecules, which are abundant in the body) tend to line up when exposed to a magnetic field (induced by the MR scanner), and then tend to reorient themselves when hit with radio waves to create a signal of their own. The strength of this signal is proportional to the number of protons in a "slice" of body material. The body material in this case consists of the tissue, bone, and cartilage of the pharyngeal-oral apparatus.

Figure 5–30 is a static MR image of the head and neck in which the pharyngeal-oral structures are clearly visible. Technological advances now make it possible to capture high-quality images at a fast sampling rate so that the movements of speech production can be recorded and analyzed (Bresch, Kim, Nayak, Byrd, & Narayanan, 2008). Studies have been conducted using MR imaging to elucidate articulatory behavior during activities such as speaking (e.g., Bae, Kuehn, Conway, & Sutton, 2011), singing (e.g., Bresch & Narayanan, 2010), and yodeling (Echternach, Markl, & Richter, 2011).

Ultrasonic Imaging

Ultrasonic methods provide another means for observing pharyngeal-oral function (Kelsey, Minifie, & Hixon, 1969; Stone, 1996). Such methods rely on the use of high-frequency sound waves (above the range that humans can hear) to map the positions and

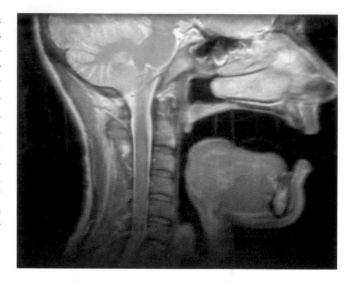

Figure 5–30. Magnetic resonance image of a sagittal view of the head and neck. (Courtesy of Brad Story)

movements of internal structures. A combined sound generator-sound receiver is placed on the outer surface of the pharyngeal-oral apparatus. Ultrasonic waves are generated and directed inward through body tissues. These waves propagate until they encounter the internal airway. Because ultrasonic energy does not travel well through air, the traveling sound waves are reflected back through the same tissues and are picked up by the sound receiver. The time it takes for ultrasonic energy to make its round trip provides a measure of how far away the reflecting airway is from the sound generator and whether or not the airway boundary is moving toward or away from the generator.

The pharyngeal-oral structures that are most easily imaged with ultrasonic techniques are the dorsal surface of the tongue (Minifie, Kelsey, Zagzebski, & King, 1971; Stone, 2005; Watkin & Rubin, 1989) and the surfaces of the lateral pharyngeal walls (Miller, 2004; Minifie et al., 1970; Zagzebski, 1975). When imaging the surface of the tongue, the ultrasonic generator and receiver are positioned below the chin and oriented so that the sound beam can be swept to scan the interface between the airway and the surface of the tongue (Stone, 1996). Figure 5–31 contains midsagittal and frontal scans of the surface of the tongue. Visualization of the tongue from one or both of these perspectives makes it possible to track the position and configuration of the surface of the tongue over time (Davidson, 2005; Stone, Epstein, & Kskarous, 2004). Ultrasonic imaging has been used to investigate aspects of normal

Midsagittal scan

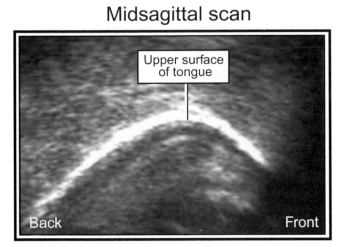

Frontal scan

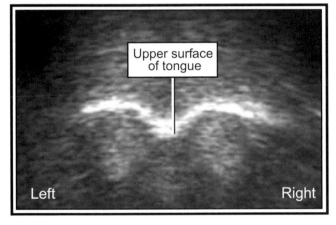

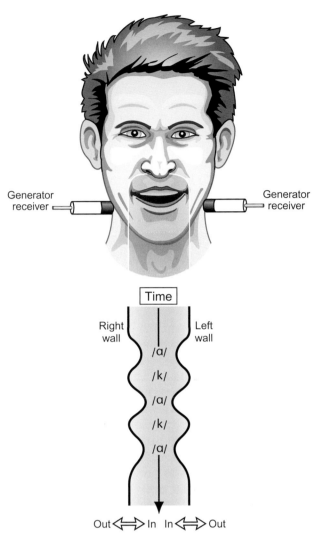

Figure 5–31. Ultrasonic images of the upper surface of the tongue in midsagittal and frontal perspectives, illustrating lengthwise dorsal configuration and midline grooving, respectively. (Images provided courtesy of Maureen Stone)

Figure 5–32. Ultrasonic monitoring of the positions of points on the left and right lateral pharyngeal walls during speech production. In and out movements are associated with /ɑ/ and /k/ elements, respectively.

speech production (e.g., Stone et al., 2007) and disordered speech production (e.g., Bressman, Radovanovic, Kulkarni, Klaiman, & Fisher, 2011).

Ultrasonic monitoring of the lateral walls of the pharynx involves placing the sound generator and sound receiver on the side of the neck corresponding to the lateral pharyngeal wall of interest (Kelsey, Ewanowski, Hixon, & Minifie, 1968). As portrayed in upper part of Figure 5–32, ultrasonic energy is beamed through the neck and travels until it strikes the pharyngeal airspace and bounces back to the receiver. More than one generator-receiver unit can be placed along

the neck to sample different vertical locations along the lateral pharyngeal wall (Miller, 2004; Zagsebski, 1975). Monitoring at the level of the oropharynx provides information about vowel and consonant adjustments of the lateral pharyngeal walls (Minifie et al., 1970; see lower part of Figure 5–32), whereas monitoring at the level of the nasopharynx provides information about velopharyngeal port adjustments involving the walls (Parush & Ostry, 1986). Such monitoring is useful in making management decisions about individuals with velopharyngeal incompetence (Kelsey et al., 1968).

Aeromechanical Observations

Aeromechanical observations provide different insights into the function of the pharyngeal-oral apparatus than do the structural-level observations discussed above. Two common types of aeromechanical observations are oral air pressure and oral airflow. Each is informative in its own right, and the two together are even more telling.

Oral air pressure is most often measured using a sensing tube attached to an air pressure transducer. One end of the tube is placed in the oral cavity in the region of interest. To measure air pressure behind the lips, the tube might be inserted between the lips and into the oral vestibule (see Figure 2–44). To measure air pressures behind constrictions formed between the tongue and roof of the oral cavity, the end of the tube is positioned farther back in the oral cavity and might be configured to run between the upper cheek and gum and curve into the airway behind the teeth (Hardy, 1965).

Measures of oral air pressure provide an indication of the force responsible for driving airflow through the pharyngeal-oral airway. Oral air pressure may differ from the pressure delivered by the breathing apparatus when there is a velopharyngeal leak (see Chapter 4) or when the vocal folds offer a significant resistance to airflow (Arkebauer, Hixon, & Hardy, 1967; Bernthal & Beukelman, 1978; Stathopoulos & Weismer, 1985). Oral air pressure may provide information about whether or not the pharyngeal-oral airstream is being adequately managed during speech production. For example, lower-than-normal oral air pressure may be an indication of poor valving because of slow and/or insufficient movements of structures of the pharyngeal-oral apparatus. Such low pressure may be accompanied by weak-sounding voiceless stop, fricative, and affricate productions and the perception that speech lacks adequate forcefulness and crispness.

Oral airflow is usually measured at the airway opening. Such airflow is most often channeled through a mouthpiece or facemask to a pneumotachometer. The arrangement shown in Figure 3–52 for measuring translaryngeal airflow is the same arrangement used to measure oral airflow. Airflow through the pharyngeal-oral apparatus is influenced by the openness of the airway and by the forcefulness with which air is being driven through the airway (Warren, 1996). Higher oral air pressures result in higher oral airflows. Measures of oral airflow are instructive regarding the status of the pharyngeal-oral airway (Gilbert, 1973; Isshiki & Ringel, 1964; Trullinger & Emanuel, 1983) and, like oral air pressure measures, provide information from which inferences can be made concerning valving adjustments and their integrity (Warren, Hall, & Davis, 1981).

Oral air pressure and oral airflow measures can be combined to calculate airway resistance along different segments of the pharyngeal-oral apparatus. This is done by dividing the air pressure difference between the two ends of a segment by the rate at which air is flowing through the segment. For example, this method can be used to determine the resistance offered by an airway constriction used to produce a fricative consonant (Warren, 1996).

Oral air pressure and oral airflow measures can also be combined to calculate the cross-sectional area of the airway at different locations along the pharyngeal-oral apparatus. For example, oral air pressure and oral airflow data can be used to calculate changes in the size of the minimum cross-section (maximum constriction) along the airway during consonant productions (Hixon, 1966; Smith, Allen, Warren, & Hall, 1978; Warren et al., 1981). Calculation is based on an aeromechanical equation similar to the one used to calculate the area of the velopharyngeal port (see Chapter 4). Figure 5–33 depicts one application of this method. Shown there are data on the minimum cross-section within the oral cavity during an /s/ production in a consonant-vowel syllable. As can be seen, the cross-section of the airway decreases significantly during the early part of the /s/, reaches its smallest value coincident with the maximum sound pressure level for the consonant, and then abruptly enlarges as the syllable transitions into the following vowel. Data of this type can be used to define the size of airway constrictions and the precision of their control in both normal individuals and in individuals with structural or neuromotor problems influencing speech production (Warren et al., 1981).

Acoustic Observations

Acoustic observations are often used to gain understanding of the function of the pharyngeal-oral apparatus. Chapters that follow, especially Chapters 8, 9, 10, and 11, make a strong case for the expanded use of such observations, particularly in clinical settings where there is interest in trying to evaluate and manage speech production disorders.

Acoustic observations applied to the pharyngeal-oral apparatus reveal information about both sound generation and sound filtering. The acoustic spectrum of speech contains information about possible positions and movements of pharyngeal-oral structures toward and away from constrictions and obstructions and how the sounds generated in the pharyngeal-oral apparatus and elsewhere are filtered by different segments of the airway. Most the adjustments that make

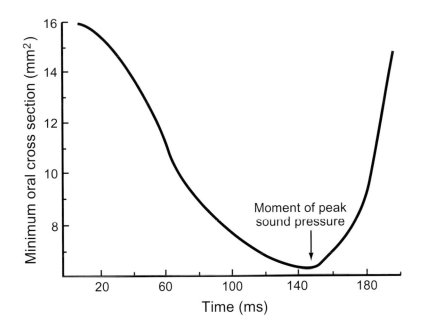

Figure 5–33. Change in the cross section of the oral airway during /s/ production in a syllable as determined through the use of an aeromechanical equation employing oral air pressure and oral airflow measurements.

speech sounds distinctive from one another have their origins in actions of the pharyngeal-oral apparatus. Thus, understanding the transform between speech physiology and speech acoustics is critically important, whether interest is in normal or abnormal speech production. Sound spectrographic portrayals of speech events are, therefore, especially useful in enabling the quantification and characterization of energy distributions in the speech acoustics waveform and in allowing one to make logical inferences about the temporal and spatial coordination of underlying adjustments (Weismer, 1984). The instrumental methods used to acquire and display acoustic observations are relevant to such analyses and are considered in detail in Chapter 10.

PHARYNGEAL-ORAL DISORDERS AND SPEECH PRODUCTION

Pharyngeal-oral disorders come in a variety of forms and can affect people of all ages. Their influence on speech production can range from mild to profound and they can have a significant impact on the quality of life because of behavioral, social, health, and economic consequences. Pharyngeal-oral disorders can have functional and/or organic bases.

Functional disorders of the pharyngeal-oral apparatus do not have known physical causes. They manifest as behavioral problems in controlling pharyngeal-oral structures for speech production. The most prevalent of such disorders are developmental speech sound articulation problems. These include sound productions that can be either delayed in their emergence or deviant in their form once they emerge. Most functional disorders of the pharyngeal-oral apparatus may actually be related to sensory, motor, and/or learning difficulties that impair the ability to acquire the movements required for normal speech articulation. Functional disorders of the types discussed here may resolve or be responsive to clinical management. Some of them will persist into late childhood, adolescence, or adulthood.

Pharyngeal-oral disorders of organic origin have identifiable physical causes that can have structural and/or physiological bases. Structural problems of the oral-pharyngeal apparatus can be congenital or acquired. A wide array of congenital craniofacial anomalies result in pharyngeal-oral deformities that can lead to speech production (and swallowing) problems. These include excesses and insufficiencies in pharyngeal-oral tissues, clefts of the oral cavity and face, mishaped and disproportioned pharyngeal-oral structures, malformed temporomandibular joints, and various misalignments

Eye Eye Eye Eye Eye

This title should catch your eye (pun intended). As a clinician you need to develop a good eye for eyes. Eyes can be an eye opener for identifying syndromes that include pharyngeal-oral problems. We can bear eyewitness to this from our own experiences. Consider the physical spacing of the eyes. Most faces are five-eyes wide at eye level (note the title of this sidetrack). This means that a space the width of one eye should fit between the two eyes and another eye should fit between the outside corner of each eye and the side of the face. Departures from this pattern come in several forms, the most common being that the two eyes are too widely spaced or too narrowly spaced. Any abnormal pattern should catch your eye and immediately cause you to eye the pharyngeal-oral apparatus for frank and subtle abnormalities. Hopefully, we see eye to eye on this. Work on developing your eye for eyes.

of structures. Hearing loss and cognitive disorders may also be concomitant problems.

Two relatively well-known congenital syndromes that may have speech production problems associated with them are Pierre Robin syndrome and Treacher Collins syndrome. Pierre Robin syndrome often includes an unusually small mandible, shortened floor of the mouth, downward positioning of the tongue, and high-arched or cleft palate. Treacher Collins syndrome often includes a small mandible, dental malocclusion, large mouth opening, sunken zygomatic arches (cheekbones), high-arched or cleft palate, significant facial deformity, and significant hearing impairment.

Acquired structural problems of the pharyngeal-oral apparatus can result from trauma, disease processes, or surgery. Traumatic injuries can result from blows to the face, penetrating orofacial wounds, and oral cavity insults that cause fractures or displacements of structures. Disease processes include tumors, premalignant alteration of mucosa, bone infiltration and alteration, joint ankylosis, and soft-tissue inflammation. Pharyngeal-oral carcinoma may require surgical resection of tissue or other interventions that include radiation or chemical therapies. When tumors are extensive they may necessitate surgical removal of a part or all of a structure, such as the tongue. Complete removal (amputation) of the tongue is referred to as a

glossectomy (see the opening and closing scenarios of this chapter).

Diseases of the nervous system cause many pharyngeal-oral problems. These may be congenital, acquired, or sequelae of surgery. Children and adults of all ages may be affected. Both central and/or peripheral components of the nervous system may be involved. Signs may be present on one or both sides of the pharyngeal-oral apparatus and to the same or different degrees when both sides are impaired. Patterns of impairment may differ significantly across different components of the apparatus, depending on the nature of the disease process.

Neuromotor disease may influence the timing of speech production, the attainment of spatial targets for articulation, and the forces applied by different components. Consequences may include inadequate valving of the airstream and inappropriate filtering of the acoustic input, resulting in consonant imprecision and vowel distortion. A wide range of neuromotor diseases can affect the pharyngeal-oral apparatus, including cerebral palsy, muscular dystrophy, multiple sclerosis, cerebral vascular accident (stroke), Bell's palsy, Parkinson disease, tumor, dyskinesia, postpolio syndrome, Guillain-Barré syndrome, myasthenia gravis, amyotrophic lateral sclerosis, Tourette syndrome, traumatic brain injury, essential tremor, and lesions to certain cranial nerves, among others. Among the diseases listed, some are transient, some stable, and some progressive. When progressive, such as in Parkinson disease and amyotrophic lateral sclerosis, pharyngeal-oral impaiment may increase during the course of the disease. Neuromotor impairment as a result of surgical interventions can be diverse and involve both the central and peripheral parts of the nervous system. Damage to the brain, such as that resulting from a cerebral vascular accident or traumatic injury, can result in an impairment in the ability to program the movements of speech production, called apraxia (or dyspraxia) of speech. Sometimes, apraxia of speech is found in children with no documented brain damage and may, in such cases, be caused by developmental brain dysfunction.

Sensory problems may also influence the control of the pharyngeal-oral apparatus for speech production. Hearing loss is the most well known of these. Congenital profound hearing loss (deafness) in both ears significantly impairs the ability to appropriately adjust the movement and positioning of pharyngeal-oral structures. Profound hearing loss denies access to the speech output signal (acoustic) in sufficient fidelity and disables the monitoring needed for normal control of speech production.

Coming and Going

He could feel when it was coming. It would come on slowly, be there for a while, and then go away slowly. When it was gone, the speech sounded normal. But, when it was there, his speech sounded as if he were drunk. We studied him, using him as his own control. What could be better? He perfectly matched himself. The psychiatrist thought the problem was all in his mind. But it turned out otherwise. What made his speech alternately normal and abnormal was a condition called paroxysmal ataxia, an uncontrollable physiological change in the ability to transmit neural signals within the cerebellum. The neurologist who diagnosed the problem was concerned. Paroxysmal ataxia can be a harbinger of another diagnosis to come, multiple sclerosis. The unwanted coming and going of speech signs can mean the ultimate coming of something else unwanted. And, as it turned out, this was the fate for this middle-aged man.

CLINICAL PROFESSIONALS AND PHARYNGEAL-ORAL DISORDERS IN SPEECH PRODUCTION

Many different clinical professionals contribute to the evaluation and management of pharyngeal-oral problems that influence speech production. Prominent among these are the speech-language pathologist, otorhinolaryngologist, plastic surgeon, neurologist, dentist, prosthodontist, and psychologist. Most clients will be seen by a subset of these professionals. Which subset will depend on the nature and severity of the problem.

The speech-language pathologist is considered the expert on how pharyngeal-oral disorders influence speech production. As well, the speech-language pathologist is the recognized expert on how such disorders influence swallowing (see Chapter 13). The speech-language pathologist may be the only professional to evaluate and manage certain individuals with speech disorders involving the pharyngeal-oral apparatus. An example is the child who presents with a speech sound disorder that reflects some delay in acquisition. Such a child might be managed through behavioral therapy conducted by the speech-language pathologist alone.

At other times, the speech-language pathologist may be engaged in the team management of an individual with major structural problems attendant to pharyngeal-oral surgery for cancer. Then, a broader array of the speech-language pathologist's skills might be called on to deal with speech, voice, and swallowing disorders. The speech-language pathologist may also assist other clinical professionals working with a client to determine the effectiveness of certain of their interventions (such as surgical or prosthetic interventions) by performing "before" and "after" measurements of speech production and swallowing.

The otorhinolaryngologist is the physician specialist concerned with ear, nose, and throat disorders and is often the first physician encountered by clients with diseases of the head and neck. This physician is intimately concerned with the evaluation and management of problems of the pharyngeal-oral apparatus and is most likely the person to have general medical oversight of clients with organically based problems that influence speech production and swallowing. The otorhinolaryngologist may perform surgical procedures aimed at improving hearing or removing tumors of the pharyngeal-oral apparatus and otherwise maintaining health of the upper airway. Of all the clinical professionals dealing with problems of the pharyngeal-oral apparatus, the otorhinolaryngologist is usually the one most closely allied with the speech-language pathologist.

The plastic surgeon is the physician who engages in surgical repair and/or reconstruction of deformed or destroyed parts of the body that result from anomalous development, disease, or trauma. The same surgeon may be called on to remove tumors from the pharyngeal-oral apparatus or perform resection or amputation of parts of the apparatus that are cancerous. Following such procedures, the plastic surgeon may also be engaged in performing reconstructive surgery to restore function or cosmetic surgery to improve appearance. The plastic surgeon may have extensive long-term care responsibilities for clients with major disorders of the pharyngeal-oral apparatus. These may include a series of surgical procedures on children with developmental craniofacial disorders or a series of surgical procedures on children or adults who have incurred major trauma to the oral and/or facial areas.

Individuals who present with neural disorders that influence the pharyngeal-oral apparatus fall under the care of a neurologist. The neurologist is a physician who is expert in matters having to do with diseases of the nervous system. Many such diseases can be manifest in the pharyngeal-oral apparatus, ranging from paresis or paralysis of muscles of the pharynx, mandible, tongue, and/or lips to involuntary movements of these structures. In addition to having a critical diagnostic role in nervous system disorders of the pharyngeal-oral apparatus, the neurologist often has a critical role in the drug management of such disorders. As noted in several previous chapters, neural disorders can influence other subsystems of the speech production apparatus, individually or in different combinations. Their role in pharyngeal-oral disorders may have important implications for speech intelligibility and swallowing because of potential impairments in movements of the pharynx, mandible, tongue, and lips. Thus, problems such as cerebral palsy, amyotrophic lateral sclerosis, cerebral vascular accidents, and certain cranial nerve lesions require the attention of the neurologist.

The dentist is the specialist responsible for the care and repair of teeth and for surgical procedures associated with the teeth and gums and certain other aspects of the oral cavity. The dentist plays a prominent role in the management of individuals with significant dental problems. Some congenital anomalies of craniofacial structures present significant dental deviations, including supernumery teeth, misaligned teeth, jumbled teeth, and the abnormal projection of teeth from and through malformed structures (such as from the shelves of a cleft hard palate) that may require dental surgery to remove, repair, or alter dental structures. Subspecialties of dentistry may be involved in such management, including the orthodontist (who corrects tooth irregularities) or the pedodontist (who is concerned with the dental problems of children). The dentist may also be called on to handle dental problems associated with traumatic injury to craniofacial structures or sequelae to the surgical resection of parts of the mandible and other structures of the facial skeleton. At times, the dentist and the plastic surgeon work closely together in planning a course of management for a client. Along with these two, the prosthodontist, another dental specialist, may be involved.

The prosthodontist is a specialist in the replacement of missing parts using oral prostheses that are fabricated to meet the individual needs of the client. Work of the prosthodontist is concerned with restoring function, appearance, and health to those who have abnormal structures caused by congenital anomaly, disease, trauma, or surgery. The role of the prosthodontist in relation to velopharyngeal-nasal disorders is considered in Chapter 4. In the context of pharyngeal-oral disorders, the prosthodontist might customize devices for the mandible, maxilla, other facial bones, and muscular tissues that have been ablated in large quantities because of injury or disease. Part of the work of the prosthodontist may be related to resizing of the oral apparatus following significant removal of tissue.

Persons with oral and facial cancers sometimes have needs for prosthetic devices to close major openings in the face and oral cavity.

Many people with pharyngeal-oral disorders (and their families) are in need of the services of a psychologist to help them cope with problems of everyday living. Trauma or surgery that results in deformity may have profound psychological effects that include depression and grief. Often clients (and their families) are unable to cope with their situation on their own and require professional intervention. The psychologist, who has knowledge about mental processes and the bases of behavior, is often a critical professional in an adult client's adjustment to loss of function. And the psychologist may be an important part of the support needed by a family of a child born with orofacial anomalies that cause abnormalities in appearance, speech development, and/or swallowing. Families can become emotionally paralyzed and may need counseling and psychological support from a psychologist to help them cope with their situation and address the future. The speech-language pathologist may also be a part of the counseling process.

REVIEW

The pharyngeal-oral apparatus forms the upper airway, except for the velopharyngeal-nasal apparatus.

The pharyngeal-oral apparatus is a flexible tube that extends from the larynx to the lips and undergoes an approximate 90-degree forward bend within the oropharynx.

The skeleton of the pharyngeal-oral apparatus consists of the cervical vertebrae and various bones of the skull, especially those of the face.

The maxilla consists of two complexly shaped bones that combine at the midline to form the upper jaw, most of the hard palate, and the alveolar process that houses the upper teeth.

The mandible is a large horseshoe-shaped bone that forms the lower jaw and holds the lower teeth.

The mandible articulates with the left and right temporal bones along the sides of skull to form the temporomandibular joints, the only freely movable joints of the skull.

Movements of the mandible are conditioned by the mechanical arrangements of the temporomandibular joints, which allow a hinge action of the mandible in relation to the temporal bone, a front-to-back gliding action, and a side-to-side gliding action.

The oropharynx is located midway along the pharyngeal cavity and is the part of the pharynx of greatest importance to function of the pharyngeal-oral apparatus for speech production.

The oral cavity is formed by the teeth, alveolar processes of the maxilla and mandible, hard palate, velum, floor of the mouth (mainly the tongue), and the anterior faucial pillars, and a forward vestibule (entryway) that is formed by the lips, cheeks, teeth, and alveolar processes of the maxilla and mandible.

The buccal (cheek) cavity constitutes the small space between the gums and teeth internally and the lips and cheeks externally and connects to the oral cavity through spaces between the teeth and behind the last molars.

The pharyngeal-oral apparatus contains a mucous lining that consists of epithelium and connective tissues that are different at different locations within the apparatus and includes a general lining mucosa, a masticatory mucosa, and a specialized mucosa.

Passive force of the pharyngeal-oral apparatus arises from the natural recoil of structures that line the walls of the apparatus, surface tension between structures in apposition (lips, tongue, gums, hard palate, velum), the pull of gravity, and aeromechanical forces within the airway.

Active force of the pharyngeal-oral apparatus comes from the contraction of muscles distributed within different components of the apparatus, including the pharynx, mandible, tongue, and lips.

Muscles of the pharynx include the *middle constrictor, inferior constrictor,* and *stylopharyngeus.*

Muscles of the mandible include the *masseter, temporalis, internal pterygoid, external pterygoid, digastric, mylohyoid,* and *geniohyoid.*

Muscles of the tongue include the *superior longitudinal, inferior longitudinal, vertical, transverse, styloglossus, palatoglossus, hyoglossus,* and *genioglossus.*

Muscles of the lips include the *orbicularis oris, buccinator, risorius, levator labii superioris, levator labii superioris aleque nasi, zygomatic major, zygomatic minor, depressor labii inferioris, mentalis, levator anguli oris, depressor anguli oris, incisivus labii superioris, incisivus labii inferioris,* and *platysma.*

Movements of the pharynx are vested in its sidewalls, back wall, and front wall and enable the lumen of the pharynx to be adjusted in size and shape, and the degree of coupling between the oropharynx and the oral cavity (through the palatoglossal arch) to be modified.

Movements of the mandible are conditioned by the physical arrangements of the temporomandibular joints and can involve both rotation and translation that combine to provide for vertical, front-to-back, and side-to-side adjustments of the structure.

Movements of the tongue derive from movements of the mandible, shifting of the tongue mass within the oral cavity, and changing of the shape of the tongue in various dimensions, all of which are facilitated by the biomechanical property of the tongue that enables it to function like a liquid-filled, incompressible, and pliable structure (a muscular hydrostat).

Movements of the lips are exceptionally versatile, with each lip being able to move independently or with the two lips coordinated in their movements, and with the range of possible adjustments including puckering, protruding, retracting, spreading, pointing, curling, groping, rounding, and plumping, among others.

The control variables of pharyngeal-oral function include pharyngeal-oral lumen size and configuration, pharyngeal-oral structural contact pressure, pharyngeal-oral airway resistance, and pharyngeal-oral acoustic impedance.

Pharyngeal-oral movements are controlled by the nervous system, with the final forms of control commands sent through cranial nerves to muscles, and with sensory innervation provided through cranial nerves to guide anticipated actions of the pharyngeal-oral apparatus and to keep track of its recent status.

Pharyngeal-oral functions of importance to this text include changing the degree of coupling between the oral cavity and atmosphere, chewing, swallowing, and sound generation and filtering.

Pharyngeal-oral function in speech production involves adjustments that physiologically code the positions and movements of structures into the formation of different speech sounds.

Vowel sounds and diphthongs are usually produced with voicing by the larynx, exclusion of nasal participation by velopharyngeal closure, and using combinations of structural positions and movements that result in relatively unconstricted configurations of the pharyngeal-oral airway that are coded along the dimensions of place of major constriction, degree of major constriction, and degree of lip rounding.

Consonant sounds are usually produced with a relatively constricted or obstructed airway, with or without voicing by the larynx, and/or with or without velopharyngeal closure, and using combinations of structural positions and movements that are coded along the dimensions of manner of production, place of production, and voicing.

The speech production stream is fluid and ongoing and structures of the pharyngeal-oral apparatus move smoothly and nearly continuously from one position to another.

Traditional theory about speech production proposes that sounds in the speech production stream influence their neighbors through processes that are anticipatory and scan ahead and processes that are a reflection of the inertial properties of the speech production apparatus.

More recent articulatory phonology or gesture theories about speech production propose that sounds in the speech production stream are assembled by the phasing of overlapping movement gestures of different structures and do not require schemes of phoneme representation to account for speech production behavior.

The development of pharyngeal-oral function in speech production involves a transition to faster speech production rates and more stable speech production movements across childhood, along with the development of muscle synergies and movement routines.

The influence of age on pharyngeal-oral function is manifested in resonances of the pharyngeal-oral airway that are lower, temporal aspects of speech production that become protracted, and variability of performance that increases in elderly individuals compared to young individuals.

Sex has certain influences on pharyngeal-oral function in speech production and speech that are related to faster utterance rates and movements in men than women and a longer pharyngeal airway in men than women that results in nonuniform differences in formants (resonances) between the sexes.

Common measurements of pharyngeal-oral function include the use of x-ray imaging, strain-gauge monitoring, articulatory tracking (using x-ray microbeam imaging, electromagnetic sensing, optoelectronic tracking, and electropalatographic monitoring), magnetic resonance imaging, ultrasonic imaging, and aeromechanical and acoustic observations.

Pharyngeal-oral disorders come in many forms, affect people of all ages, may be of functional and/or organic origin, and have a significant influence on the quality of life because of their behavioral, social, health, and economic consequences.

Many clinical professionals contribute to the evaluation and management of individuals with pharyngeal-oral disorders that influence speech production, including the speech-language pathologist, otorhinolaryngologist, plastic surgeon, neurologist, dentist, prosthodontist, and psychologist.

Scenario

Time has a way of healing things and it worked to his advantage. He had to learn the boundaries of a vastly altered pharyngeal-oral apparatus that was missing a tongue and some of the left side of his oral cavity. He had also lost some sensation. Chewing, swallowing, and speaking were three of his continual challenges and none of these was going well through the use of his own devices.

Once he had recovered from surgery, he was referred to a regional maxillofacial clinic that specialized in reconstructive and prosthetic treatments for people who had undergone ablative surgeries for cancer. There, a team of experts worked on his problems. When first seen at the clinic, he was struggling to meet his nutritional needs and his speech was severely wanting. Eating was difficult and largely restricted to liquids and very soft foods that he managed to move backward in his mouth by rotating his head upward. His speech was relatively unintelligible, except to his wife. His speech intelligibility for sentences was 47%, whereas intelligibility for single words was 32%. His voice was mildly hypernasal. Detailed phonetic analysis of his speech revealed that he had imprecise productions of vowels, diphthongs, semivowels, and other consonants, especially those that normally require tongue adjustments.

A prosthetic tongue was fabricated and fitted to his remaining lower teeth. This structure covered the floor of his mouth and had two prominent elevations on its upper surface, one located toward the front of his mouth and one located toward the back. A groove was included in the prosthesis that ran along the intact right side of his oral cavity so that liquid and thin, pureed foods could be channeled to the pharynx. The prosthesis was initially uncomfortable to him and created excessive saliva. These problems resolved after several days of using the device.

A speech-language pathologist worked on the design of programs to enhance drinking and eating and speech production. The prosthesis was worn during most daily activities and training was provided in its use with liquids and pureed substances. Slight upward rotation of the head was combined with slight rightward tiling of the head and elevation of the mandible. This moved substances to the right and backward within the oral cavity into the pharynx. Cheek activity on the right was also encouraged to help with rearward propulsion of substances. For meals at home, the prosthesis was sometimes removed so that semisolid substances could be handled through other mechanical compensations and propelled to the esophagus by sips of water.

An intensive speech management program was undertaken that focused on the development of compensations for a missing tongue. This program included strategies for using new places of production for certain speech sounds and capitalizing on differential actions involving the positioning of the larynx (to effect pharyngeal length changes), positioning of the lateral pharyngeal walls (to effect cross-sectional changes in the pharynx), positioning of the mandible (to effect cross-sectional changes in the oral cavity and oral vestibule), and positioning of the lips (to effect cross-sectional changes in the oral vestibule and oral airway length changes). Consonant speech sounds that had previously been produced at velar, palatal, alveolar, and dental sites of production were moved forward to be produced at labiodental and labial sites. Vowel, diphthong, and semivowel speech sounds that had previously relied on tongue adjustments to help form major constrictions at different locations along the pharyngeal-oral airway were made to rely on new positioning of the larynx, mandible, cheeks, and lips. Both consonant and vowels segments were adjusted in relative durations to maximize durational cues to enhance intelligibility.

Finally, other global strategies included a general slowing of speech production, a general increase in speech loudness, and using gestures to enhance intelligibility. Testing following a management program of several months duration yielded a sentence intelligibility score of 72% (up 25% from the start of the program) and a single word intelligibility score of 52% (up 20%). Self-report indicated significant satisfaction with his gains, although there was still substantial room for improvement.

A return to work followed his rehabilitation. The small group of coworkers in his environment quickly adapted to the nature of his speech communication and came to be able to understand most of what he said. Over time, the same came to be true for regular customers. He continued to have some difficulty in telephone conversations and tended to avoid these at work. Try as he may, he could not shake his fear of cancer returning, something that haunted him during quiet moments. Nonetheless, he found himself able to live a productive working life and was grateful for the understanding and love of his family and close friends. Little things didn't bother him any more. His ordeal had strengthened him and forever altered his view of what was important in life. It was time again to "Play ball."

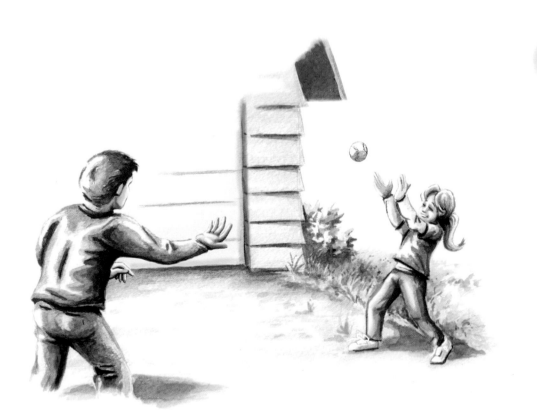

Look Away?

When engaged in a face-to-face conversation with someone, you both listen and watch. The sounds generated are made by movements you're accustomed to seeing. Things are different, however, if you're listening to and watching a good ventriloquist. Then you hear normal speech, but with hardly any movements. Even more disconcerting is the situation in which you listen to and watch a person speak who has a severe neuromotor speech disorder. Then, both the speech and the speech movements may be disordered, but the movements may contain compensations that make the speaker's tongue, lips, and face move abnormally and be incongruent with what you expect to see. Under such circumstances, looking at the speaker may be confusing and make it harder to understand the message. Not watching the speaker may actually reduce the confusion and enable you to get more of the message. So, look away momentarily or close your eyes briefly.

REFERENCES

Abd-El-Malek, S. (1939). Observations on the morphology of the human tongue. *Journal of Anatomy, 73,* 201–210.

Amerman, J., & Parnell, M. (1982). Oral motor precision in older adults. *Journal of the National Student Speech-Language-Hearing Association, 10,* 55–67.

Arkebauer, H., Hixon, T., & Hardy, J. (1967). Peak intra-oral air pressure during speech. *Journal of Speech and Hearing Research, 10,* 196–208.

Aviv, J., Martin, J., Jones, M., Wee, T., Diamond, B., Keen, M., & Blitzer, A. (1994). Age-related changes in pharyngeal and supraglottic sensation. *Annals of Otology, Rhinology, and Laryngology, 103,* 749–752.

Bae, Y., Kuehn, D., Conway, C., & Sutton, B. (2011). Real-time magnetic resonance imaging of velopharyngeal activities with simultaneous speech recordings. *Cleft-Palate Craniofacial Journal, 48,* 695–707.

Barlow, S., & Abbs, J. (1983). Force transducers for the evaluation of labial, lingual, and mandibular motor impairments. *Journal of Speech and Hearing Research, 26,* 616–621.

Barlow, S., & Burton, M. (1990). Ramp-and-hold force control in the upper and lower lips: Developing new neuromotor assessment applications in traumatically brain injured adults. *Journal of Speech and Hearing Research, 33,* 660–675.

Barlow, S., Cole, K., & Abbs, J. (1983). A new head-mounted lip-jaw movement transduction system for the study of motor speech disorders. *Journal of Speech and Hearing Research, 26,* 283–288.

Barlow, S., & Netsell, R. (1986). Differential fine force control of the upper and lower lips. *Journal of Speech and Hearing Research, 29,* 163–169.

Barlow, S., & Rath, E. (1985). Maximum voluntary closing forces in the upper and lower lips of humans. *Journal of Speech and Hearing Research, 28,* 373–376.

Baum, B. (1981). Evaluation of stimulated parotid saliva flow rate in different age groups. *Journal of Dental Research, 60,* 1292–1296.

Benes, F., Turtle, M., Khan, Y., & Farol, P. (1994). Myelination of a key relay zone in the hippocampal formation occurs in the human brain during childhood, adolescence, and adulthood. *Archives of General Psychiatry, 51,* 477–484.

Bernthal, J., & Beukelman, D. (1978). Intraoral air pressure during the production of /p/ and /b/ by children, youths, and adults. *Journal of Speech and Hearing Research, 21,* 361–371.

Bodanis, D. (1995). It's in the air: Skin, stardust, radio waves, vitamins, spider legs. *Smithsonian, 26,* 76–81.

Bresch, E., Kim, Y-C., Nayak, K., Byrd, D., & Narayanan, S. (May, 2008). Seeing speech: Capturing vocal tract shaping using real-time magnetic resonance imaging. *IEEE Signal Processing Magazine,* pp. 123–132.

Bresch, E., & Narayanan, S. (2010). Real-time magnetic resonance imaging investigation of resonance tuning in soprano singing. *Journal of the Acoustical Society of America, 128,* EL335–EL341.

Bressmann, T., Radovanovic, B., Kulkarni, G., Klaiman, P., & Fisher, D. (2011). An ultrasonic investigation of cleft-type compensatory articulations of voiceless velar stops. *Clinical Linguistics and Phonetics, 25,* 1028–1033.

Browman, C., & Goldstein, L. (1992). Articulatory phonology: An overview. *Phonetica, 49,* 155–180.

Burke, P. (1980). Serial growth changes in the lips. *British Journal of Orthodontics, 7,* 17–30.

Byrd, D. (1996). A phase window framework for articulatory timing. *Phonology, 13,* 139–169.

Canetta, R. (1977). Decline in oral perception from 20 to 70 years. *Perceptual Motor Skills, 45,* 1028–1030.

Chauncey, H., Borkan, G., Wayler, A., Feller, R., & Kapur, K. (1981). Parotid fluid composition in healthy young males. *Advances in Physiological Sciences, 28,* 323–328.

Crelin, E. (1973). *Functional anatomy of the newborn.* New Haven, CT: Yale University Press.

Crelin, E. (1976). Development of the upper respiratory system. *Clinical Symposia, 28*, 1–30.

Crossman, E., & Szafran, J. (1956). Changes with age in the speed of information-intake and discrimination. *Experientia, 4*, 128–134.

Daniloff, R., & Hammarberg, R. (1973). On defining coarticulation. *Journal of Phonetics, 1*, 239–248.

Davidson, L. (2005). Addressing phonological questions with ultrasound. *Clinical Linguistics and Phonetics, 19*, 619–633.

Dickson, D., & Maue-Dickson, W. (1982). *Anatomical and physiological bases of speech.* Boston, MA: Little, Brown and Company.

Doran, G., & Baggett, H. (1972). The genioglossus muscle: A reassessment of its anatomy in some mammals including man. *Acta Anatomica, 83*, 403–410.

Echternach, M., Markl, M., & Richter, B. (2011). Vocal tract configurations in yodelling—Prospective comparison of two Swiss yodeller and two non-yodeller subjects. *Logopedics Phoniatrics Vocology, 36*, 109–113.

Endres, W., Bambach, W., & Flosser, G. (1971). Voice spectrographs as a function of age, voice disguise, and vocal imitation. *Journal of the Acoustical Society of America, 49*, 1842–1848.

Fairbanks, G. (1960). *Voice and articulation drillbook.* New York, NY: Harper & Row.

Fant, G. (1975). Non-uniform vowel normalization. *Speech Transmission Laboratory—Quarterly Progress and Status Report, 2–3*, 1–19.

Farnetani, E. (1997). Coarticulation and connected speech processes. In W. Hardcastle & J. Laver (Eds.), *The handbook of phonetic sciences* (pp. 371–404). Oxford, UK: Blackwell.

Ferreri, G. (1959). Senescence of the larynx. *Italian General Review of Oto-Rhino-Laryngology, 1*, 640–709.

Fitch, W., & Giedd, J. (1999). Morphology and development of the human vocal tract: A study using magnetic resonance imaging. *Journal of the Acoustical Society of America, 106*, 1511–1522.

Fletcher, H. (1953). *Speech and hearing in communication.* New York, NY: Van Nostrand.

Fozard, J., Vercruyssen, M., Reynolds, S., Hancock, P., & Quilter, R. (1994). Age differences and changes in reaction time. *Journal of Gerontology: Psychological Sciences, 49*, 179–189.

Fremont, A., & Hoyland, J. (2007). Morphology, mechanisms and pathology of musculoskeletal ageing. *Journal of Pathology, 211*, 252–259.

Gentil, M., & Tournier, C. (1998). Differences in fine control of forces generated by the tongue, lips, and fingers in humans. *Archives of Oral Biology, 43*, 517–523.

Gibbon, F., Lee, A., & Yuen, I. (2010) Tongue-palate contact during selected vowels in normal speech. *Cleft Palate-Craniofacial Journal, 47*, 405–412.

Gilbert, H. (1973). Oral airflow during stop consonant production. *Folia Phoniatrica, 25*, 288–301.

Goffman, L., & Smith, A. (1999). Development and differentiation of speech movement patterns. *Human Perception and Performance, 25*, 1–12.

Goldstein, U. (1980). *An articulatory model for the vocal tracts of growing children.* Doctoral dissertation, Massachusetts Institute of Technology, Cambridge, MA.

Gracco, V. (1994). Some organizational characteristics of speech movement control. *Journal of Speech and Hearing Research, 37*, 4–27.

Green, J., Moore, C., Higashikawa, M., & Steeve, R. (2000). The physiological development of speech motor control: Lip and jaw coordination. *Journal of Speech, Language, and Hearing Research, 43*, 239–255.

Green, J., Moore, C., & Reilly, K. (2002). The sequential development of jaw and lip control for speech. *Journal of Speech, Language, and Hearing Research, 45*, 66–79.

Green, J., & Wang, Y. (2003). Tongue-surface movement patterns during speech and swallowing. *Journal of the Acoustical Society of America, 113*, 2820–2833.

Grigos, M. (2009). Changes in articulator movement variability during phonemic development: A longitudinal study. *Journal of Speech, Language, and Hearing Research, 52*, 164–177.

Hardcastle, W., Barry, R., & Clark, C. (1987). An instrumental phonetic study of lingual activity in articulation-disordered children. *Journal of Speech and Hearing Research, 30*, 171–184.

Hardy, J. (1965). Air flow and air pressure studies. *ASHA Reports, 1*, 141–152.

Hartman, D., & Danhauer, J. (1976). Perceptual features of speech for males in four perceived age categories. *Journal of the Acoustical Society of America, 59*, 713–715.

Henke, W. (1966). *Dynamic articulatory model of speech production using computer simulation.* Doctoral dissertation, Massachusetts Institute of Technology. Cambridge, MA.

Hixon, T., (1966). Turbulent noise sources for speech. *Folia Phoniatrica, 18*, 168–182.

Hixon, T. (1971). An electromagnetic method for transducing jaw movements during speech. *Journal of the Acoustical Society of America, 49*, 603–606.

Hixon, T. (1972). Some new techniques for measuring the biomechanical events of speech production: One laboratory's experiences. *ASHA Reports, 7*, 68–103.

Hixon, T., & Abbs, J. (1980). Normal speech production. In T. Hixon, L. Shriberg, & J. Saxman (Eds.), *Introduction to communication disorders* (pp. 42–87). Englewood-Cliffs, NJ: Prentice-Hall.

Hixon, T., & Hoit, J. (2005). *Evaluation and management of speech breathing disorders: Principles and methods.* Tucson, AZ: Redington Brown.

Hoit, J., & Hixon, T. (1987). Age and speech breathing. *Journal of Speech and Hearing Research, 30*, 351–366.

Honda, K. (2002). Evolution of vowel production studies and observation techniques. *Acoustical Science and Technology, 23*, 189–194.

Huang, J., Shen, H., Takahashi, M., Fukunaga, T., Toga, H., Takahashi, K., & Ohya, N. (1998). Pharyngeal cross-sectional area and pharyngeal compliance in normal males and females. *Respiration, 65*, 458–468.

Huttenlocher, P. (1990). Morphometric study of human cerebral cortex development. *Neuropsychologia, 28*, 517–527.

Israel, H. (1968). Continuing growth in the human cranial skeleton. *Archives of Oral Biology, 13,* 133–137.

Israel, H. (1973). Age factor and the pattern of change in craniofacial structures. *American Journal of Physical Anthropology, 39,* 111–128.

Isshiki, N., & Ringel, R. (1964). Air flow during production of selected consonants. *Journal of Speech and Hearing Research, 7,* 233–244.

Jones, K., Hamilton, A., & Wolpert, D. (2002). Sources of signal-dependent noise during isometric force production. *Journal of Neurophysiology, 88,* 1533–1544.

Kahane, J. (1990). Age-related changes in the peripheral speech mechanism: Structural and physiological changes. *ASHA Reports, 19,* 75–87.

Katz, W., Bharadwaj, S., & Stettler, M. (2006). Influences of electromagnetic articulography sensors on speech produced by healthy adults and individuals with aphasia and apraxia. *Journal of Speech, Language, and Hearing Research, 49,* 645–659.

Kelsey, C., Ewanowski, S., Hixon, T., & Minifie, F. (1968). Determination of lateral pharyngeal wall motion during connected speech by use of pulsed ultrasound. *Science, 161,* 1259–1260.

Kelsey, C., Minifie, F., & Hixon, T. (1969). Applications of ultrasound in speech research. *Journal of Speech and Hearing Research, 12,* 564–575.

Kenney, R. (1982). *Physiology of aging: A synopsis.* Chicago, IL: Year Book Medical.

Kent, R. (1972). Some considerations in the cineradiographic analysis of tongue movements during speech. *Phonetica, 26,* 293–306.

Kent, R. (1976a). Anatomical and neuromuscular maturation of the speech mechanism: Evidence from acoustic studies. *Journal of Speech and Hearing Research, 19,* 421–447.

Kent, R. (1976b). Models of speech production. In N. Lass (Ed.), *Contemporary issues in experimental phonetics* (pp. 79–104). New York, NY: Academic Press.

Kent, R. (1997). *The speech sciences.* San Diego, CA: Singular.

Kent, R., & Burkard, R. (1981). Changes in the acoustic correlates of speech production. In D. Beasley & G. Davis (Eds.), *Aging: Communication processes and disorders* (pp. 47–62). New York, NY: Grune and Stratton.

Kent, R., & Forner, L. (1980). Speech segment durations in sentence recitations by children and adults. *Journal of Phonetics, 8,* 157–168.

Kent, R., & Minifie, F. (1977). Coarticulation in recent speech production models. *Journal of Phonetics, 5,* 115–133.

Kent, R., & Moll, K. (1975). Articulatory timing in selected consonant sequences. *Brain and Language, 2,* 304–323.

Kent, R., & Vorperian, H. (1995). Development of the craniofacial-oral-laryngeal anatomy: A review. *Journal of Medical Speech-Language Pathology, 3,* 149–190.

Kerr, W., Kelly, J., & Geddes, D. (1991). The areas of various surfaces in the human mouth from nine years to adulthood. *Journal of Dental Research, 70,* 1528–1530.

Kier, W., & Smith, K. (1985). Tongues, tentacles, and trunks: The biomechanics of movement in muscular hydrostats. *Zoological Journal of the Linnean Society, 83,* 307–324.

Kim, B. (1971). *A physiological study of the production mechanisms of Korean stop consonants.* Doctoral dissertation, University of Wisconsin. Madison.

Kiritani, S., Itoh, K., & Fujimura, O. (1975). Tongue-pellet tracking by a computer-controlled x-ray microbeam system. *Journal of the Acoustical Society of America, 57,* 1516–1520.

Klein, D. (1980). Oral soft tissue changes in geriatric patients. *Bulletin of the New York Academy of Medicine, 56,* 721–727.

Laitman, J., & Crelin, E. (1976). Postnatal development of the basicranium and vocal tract region in man. In J. Bosma (Ed.), *Symposium on the development of the basicranium* (pp. 206–220). Bethesda, MD: Department of Health, Education, and Welfare Publication No. 76–989, Public Health Service, National Institutes of Health.

Langdon, H., Klueber, K., & Barnwell, Y. (1978). The anatomy of m. genioglossus in the 15-week human fetus. *Anatomy and Embryology, 155,* 107–113.

Lecours, A. (1975). Myelogenetic correlates of the development of speech and language. In E. Lenneberg & E. Lenneberg (Eds.), *Foundations of language development: A multidisciplinary approach* (Vol. 1, pp. 121–136). New York, NY: Academic Press.

Lexell, J., Taylor, C., & Sjostrom, M. (1988). What is the cause of ageing atrophy?: Total number, size, and proportion of different fiber types studied in whole vastus lateralis muscle from 15- to 83-year-old men. *Journal of Neurological Science, 84,* 275–294.

Linville, S. (2001). *Vocal aging.* San Diego, CA: Singular-Thomson Learning.

Linville, S., & Fisher, H. (1985). Acoustic characteristics of women's voices with advanced age. *Journal of Gerontology, 3,* 324–330.

Linville, S., & Rens, R. (2001). Vocal tract resonance analysis of aging voice using long-term average spectra. *Journal of Voice, 15,* 323–330.

Liss, J., Weismer, G., & Rosenbek, J. (1990). Selected acoustic characteristics of speech production in very old males. *Journal of Gerontology, 45,* 35–45.

Luschei, E., Ramig, L., Baker, K., & Smith, M. (1999). Discharge characteristics of laryngeal single motor units during phonation in young and older adults and in persons with Parkinson disease. *Journal of Neurophysiology, 81,* 2131–2139.

MacNeilage, P. (1970). Motor control of serial ordering of speech. *Psychological Review, 77,* 182–196.

MacPherson, M., & Smith, A. (in press). Influences of sentence length and syntactic complexity on the speech motor control of children who stutter. *Journal of Speech, Language, and Hearing Research.*

Magen, H., Kang, A., Tiede, M., & Whalen, D. (2003). Posterior pharyngeal wall position in the production of speech. *Journal of Speech, Language, and Hearing Research, 46,* 241–251.

Maner, K., Smith, A., & Grayson, L. (2000). Influences of utterance length and complexity on speech motor performance in children and adults. *Journal of Speech, Language, and Hearing Research, 43,* 560–573.

Matthies, M., Svirsky, M., Perkell, J., & Lane, H. (1996). Acoustic and articulatory measures of sibilant production with and without auditory feedback from a cochlear implant. *Journal of Speech and Hearing Research*, *39*, 916–946.

McGeer, E., Fibiger, H., McGeer, P., & Wiskson, V. (1971). Aging and brain enzymes. *Experimental Gerontology*, *6*, 391–396.

McNeil, M., Pratt, S., & Fosset T. (2004). The differential diagnosis of apraxia of speech. In B. Maassen, R. Kent, H. Peters, P. Van Lieshout, & W. Hultstijn (Eds.), *Speech motor control in normal and disordered speech* (pp. 389–413). Oxford, UK: Oxford University Press.

McWilliams, B., & Girdany, B. (1964). The use of Televex in cleft palate research. *Cleft Palate Journal*, *1*, 398–401.

Melsen, B., & Melsen, F. (1982). The postnatal development of the palatomaxillary region studied on human autopsy material. *American Journal of Orthodontics*, *82*, 329–342.

Menn, L. (1983). Development of articulatory, phonetic, and phonological capabilities. In B. Butterworth (Ed.), *Language production* (pp. 3–50). Cambridge, UK: Cambridge University Press.

Miller, J. (2004). Lateral pharyngeal wall motion during swallowing using real time ultrasound. *Dysphagia*, *12*, 125–132.

Miller, J., Watkin, K., & Chen, M. (2002). Muscle, adipose, and connective tissue variations in intrinsic musculature of the adult human tongue. *Journal of Speech, Language, and Hearing Research*, *45*, 51–65.

Minifie, F., Hixon, T., Kelsey, C., & Woodhouse, R. (1970). Lateral pharyngeal wall movement during speech production. *Journal of Speech and Hearing Research*, *13*, 584–594.

Minifie, F., Kelsey, C., Zagzebski, J., & King, T. (1971). Ultrasonic scans of the dorsal surface of the tongue. *Journal of the Acoustical Society of America*, *49*, 1857–1860.

Miyawaki, K. (1974). A study of the musculature of the human tongue. *Bulletin of the Research Institute of Logopedics and Phoniatrics, University of Tokyo*, *8*, 23–50.

Moll, K. (1960). Cinefluorographic techniques in speech research. *Journal of Speech and Hearing Research*, *3*, 227–241.

Moller, K., Martin, R., & Christiansen, R. (1971). A technique for recording velar movement. *Cleft Palate Journal*, *8*, 263–276.

Morgan, D., & Finch, C. (1988). Dopaminergic changes in the basal ganglia: A generalized phenomenon of aging in mammals. *Annals of the New York Academy of Sciences*, *515*, 145–160.

Mortimore, I., Fiddes, P., Stephens, S., & Douglas, N. (1999). Tongue protrusion force and fatiguability in male and female subjects. *European Respiratory Journal*, *14*, 191–195.

Muller, E., & Abbs, J. (1979). Strain gauge transduction of lip and jaw motion in the midsagittal plane: Refinement of a prototype system. *Journal of the Acoustical Society of America*, *65*, 481–486.

Munhall, K., Vatikiotis-Bateson, E., & Tohkura, Y. (1995). X-ray film database for speech research. *Journal of the Acoustical Society of America*, *98*, 1222–1224.

Murdoch, B., Cheng, H-Y., & Goozée, J. (2012). Developmental changes in variability of tongue and lip movements during speech from childhood to adulthood: An EMA study. *Clinical Linguistics and Phonetics, 26*, 216–231.

Nelson, R., Soderberg, G., & Urbsheit, M. (1984). Alteration of motor-unit discharge characteristics in aged humans. *Physical Therapy*, *64*, 29–34.

Netsell, R. (1986). *A neurobiologic view of speech production and the dysarthrias*. San Diego, CA: College-Hill Press.

Netsell, R., & Kent, R. (1976). Paroxysmal ataxic dysarthria. *Journal of Speech and Hearing Disorders*, *41*, 93–109.

Newell, K., Liu, Y., & Mayer-Kress, G. (2001). Time scales in learning and development. *Psychological Review*, *108*, 57–82.

Nicholson, K., & Kimura, D. (1996). Sex differences for speech and manual skill. *Perceptual and Motor Skills*, *82*, 3–13.

Nittrouer, S. (1991). Phase relations of jaw and tongue tip movements in the production of VCV utterances. *Journal of the Acoustical Society of America*, *90*, 1806–1815.

Nittrouer, S. (1993). The emergence of mature gestural patterns is not uniform: Evidence from an acoustic study. *Journal of Speech and Hearing Research*, *36*, 959–972.

Nip, I., Green, J., & Marx, D. (2011). The co-emergence of cognition, language, and speech motor control in early development: A longitudinal correlational study. *Journal of Communication Disorders*, *44*, 149–160.

Parush, A, & Ostry, D. (1986). Superior lateral pharyngeal wall movements in speech. *Journal of the Acoustical Society of America*, *80*, 749–756.

Paus, T., Zijdenbos, A., Worsley, K., Collins, D., Blumenthal, J., Giedd, J., Rapoport, J., & Evans, A. (2001). Structural maturation of neural pathways in children and adolescents: In vivo study. *Science*, *19*, 1908–1911.

Perkell, J., Cohen, M., Svirsky, M., Matthies, M., Garabieta, I., & Jackson, M. (1992). Electromagnetic midsagittal articulometer systems for transducing speech articulatory movements. *Journal of the Acoustical Society of America*, *92*, 3078–3096.

Perkell, J., Guenther, F., Lane, H., Matthies, M., Payan, Y., Perrier, P., Vick, J., Wilhelms-Tricarico, R., & Zandipour, M. (2001). The sensorimotor control of speech production. *Proceedings of the International Symposium on Measurement, Analysis, and Modeling of Human Function* (pp. 359–365). Sapporo, Japan: Hokkaido University.

Richtsmeier, J., & Cheverud, J. (1986). Finite element scaling analysis of human craniofacial growth. *Journal of Craniofacial Genetics and Developmental Biology*, *6*, 289–323.

Ryalls, J., & Lieberman, P. (1982). Fundamental frequency and vowel perception. *Journal of the Acoustical Society of America*, *72*, 1631–1634.

Ryan, W. (1972). Acoustic aspects of the aging voice. *Journal of Gerontology*, *27*, 265–268.

Saltzman, E., & Munhall, K. (1989). A dynamical approach to gestural patterning in speech production. *Ecological Psychology*, *1*, 333–382.

Schmidt, R., Zelaznik, H., Hawkins, B., Frank, J., & Quinn, J. (1979). Motor-output variability: A theory for the accuracy of rapid motor acts. *Psychological Review*, *47*, 415–451.

Schonle, P., Grabe, K., Wenig, P., Hohne, J., Schrader, J., & Conrad, B. (1987). Electromagnetic articulography: Use of alternating magnetic fields for tracking movements of multiple points inside and outside the vocal tract. *Brain and Language*, *31*, 26–35.

Schwartz, M. (1968). Identification of speaker sex from isolated, voiceless fricatives. *Journal of the Acoustical Society of America, 43,* 1178–1179.

Scott, J. (1976). *Dentofacial development and growth.* Oxford, UK: Pergamon Press.

Scukanec, G., Petrosino, L., & Squibb, K. (1991). Formant frequency characteristics of children, young adult, and aged female speakers. *Perceptual and Motor Skills, 73,* 203–208.

Shaiman, S., Adams, S., & Kimelman, M. (1997). Velocity profiles of lip protrusion across changes in speaking rate. *Journal of Speech, Language, and Hearing Research, 40,* 144–158.

Sharkey, S., & Folkins, J. (1985). Variability of lip and jaw movements in children and adults: Implications for the development of speech motor control. *Journal of Speech and Hearing Research, 28,* 8–15.

Sicher, H., & DuBrul, E. (1975). *Oral anatomy* (2nd ed.). St Louis, MO: C. V. Mosby.

Simpson, A. (2001). Dynamic consequences of differences in male and female vocal tract dimensions. *Journal of the Acoustical Society of America, 109,* 2153–2164.

Simpson, A. (2002). Gender-specific articulatory-acoustic relations in vowel sequences. *Journal of Phonetics, 30,* 417–435.

Smith, A., & Goffman, L. (1998). Stability and patterning of speech movement sequences in children and adults. *Journal of Speech, Language, and Hearing Research, 41,* 18–30.

Smith, A., & Zelaznik, H. (2004). Development of functional synergies for speech motor coordination in childhood and adolescence. *Developmental Psychobiology, 45,* 22–33.

Smith, B., & McLean-Muse, A. (1986). Articulatory movement characteristics of labial consonant productions by children. *Journal of the Acoustical Society of America, 80,* 1321–1327.

Smith, B., & McLean-Muse, A. (1987). An investigation of motor equivalence in the speech of children and adults. *Journal of the Acoustical Society of America, 82,* 837–842.

Smith, B., Sugarman, M., & Long, S. (1983). Experimental manipulation of speaking rate for studying temporal variability in children's speech. *Journal of the Acoustical Society of America, 74,* 744–748.

Smith, B., Wasowicz, J., & Preston, J. (1987). Temporal characteristics of the speech of normal elderly adults. *Journal of Speech and Hearing Research, 30,* 522–529.

Smith, H., Allen, G., Warren, D., & Hall, D. (1978). The consistency of the pressure-flow technique for assessing oral port size. *Journal of the Acoustical Society of America, 64,* 1203–1206.

Smith, K., & Kier, W. (1989). Trunks, tongues, and tentacles: Moving with skeletons of muscle. *American Scientist, 77,* 28–35.

Smits-Engelsman, B., & Van Galen, G. (1997). Dysgraphia in children: Lasting psychomotor deficiency or transient developmental delay? *Journal of Experimental Child Psychology, 67,* 164–184.

Sonies, B. (1991). The aging oropharyngeal system. In D. Ripich (Ed.), *Handbook of geriatric communication disorders* (pp. 187–203). Austin, TX: Pro-Ed.

Sonies, B., Baum, B., & Shawker, T. (1984). Tongue motion in the elderly: Initial in situ observation. *Journal of Gerontology, 39,* 279–283.

Sonies, B., Stone, M., & Shawker, T. (1984). Speech and swallowing in the elderly. *Gerontology, 3,* 279–283.

Squire, C., Johnson, N., & Hoops, R. (1976). *Human oral mucosa.* London, UK: Blackwell Scientific Publications.

Stathopoulos, E., & Weismer, G. (1985). Oral airflow and intraoral air pressure: A comparative study of children, youths and adults. *Folia Phoniatrica, 37,* 152–159.

Steele, C., & Van Lieshout, P. (2004). Use of electromagnetic midsagittal articulography in the study of swallowing. *Journal of Speech, Language, and Hearing Research, 47,* 342–352.

Steeve, R., Moore, C., Green, J., Reilly, K., & McMurtrey, J. (2008). Babbling, chewing, and sucking: Oromandibular coordination at 9 months. *Journal of Speech, Language, and Hearing Research, 51,* 1390–1404.

Stone, M. (1996). Instrumentation for the study of speech physiology. In N. Lass (Ed.), *Principles of experimental phonetics* (pp. 495–524). St. Louis, MO: Mosby-Year Book.

Stone, M. (2005). A guide to analyzing tongue motion from ultrasound images. *Clinical Linguistics and Phonetics, 19,* 455–501.

Stone, M., Epstein, M., & Kskarous, K. (2004). Functional segments in tongue movement. *Clinical Linguistics and Phonetics, 18,* 507–521.

Stone, M. Stock, G., Bunin, K., Kumar, K., Epstein, M., Kambhamettu, C., . . . Prince, J. (2007). Comparison of speech production in upright and supine position. *Journal of the Aeoustical Society of America, 122,* 532–541.

Story, B., Hoffman, E., & Titze, I. (February, 1997). Volumetric image-based comparison of male and female vocal tract shapes. *Proceedings of the International Society of Optical Engineering* (pp. 25–37). Bellingham, WA: International Society of Optical Engineering.

Sturm, J., & Seery, C. (2007). Speech and articulatory rates of school-age children in conversation and narrative contexts. *Language, Speech, and Hearing Services in Schools, 38,* 47–59.

Sussman, H., & Smith, K. (1970). Transducer for measuring mandibular movements. *Journal of the Acoustical Society of America, 48,* 857–858.

Timmins, C., Hardcastle, W., Wood, S., & Cleland, J. (2011). An EPG analysis of /t/ in young people with Down's syndrom. *Clinical Linguistics and Phonetics, 25,* 1022–1027.

Tourne, L. (1991). Growth of the pharynx and its physiologic implications. *American Journal of Orthodontics and Dentofacial Orthopedics, 99,* 129–139.

Trullinger, R., & Emanuel, F. (1983). Airflow characteristics of stop-plosive consonant production of normal-speaking children. *Journal of Speech and Hearing Research, 26,* 202–208.

Ulatowska, H. (1985). *The aging brain: Communication in the elderly.* San Diego, CA: College-Hill Press.

Valenstein, E. (1981). Age-related changes in the human central nervous system. In D. Beasley & G. Davis (Eds.),

Aging: Communication processes and disorders (pp. 47–62). New York, NY: Grune & Stratton.

van der Giet, G. (1977). Computer controlled method for measuring articulatory activities. *Journal of the Acoustical Society of America, 61*, 1072–1076.

Vick, J., Campbell, T., Shriberg, L., Green, J., Abdi, H., Rusiewicz, H., Venkatesh, L., & Moore, C. (2012). Distinct developmental profiles in typical speech acquisition. *Journal of Neurophysiology, 107*, 2885–2900.

Vig, P., & Cohen, A. (1979). Vertical growth of the lips: A serial cephalometric study. *American Journal of Orthodontics, 75*, 405–415.

Vorperian, H., & Kent, R. (2007). Vowel acoustic space development in children: A synthesis of acoustic and anatomic data. *Journal of Speech, Language, and Hearing Research, 50*, 1510–1545.

Vorperian, H., Kent, R., Lindstrom, M., Kalina, C., Gentry, L., & Yandell, B. (2005). Development of vocal tract length during early childhood: A magnetic resonance imaging study. *Journal of the Acoustical Society of America, 117*, 338–350.

Vorperian, H., Wang, S., Chung, M., Schimek, E., Durtschi, R., Kent, R., Ziegert, A., & Gentry, L. (2009). Anatomic development of the oral and pharyngeal portions of the vocal tract: An imaging study. *Journal of the Acoustical Society of America, 125*, 1666–1678.

Vorperian, H., Wang, S., Schimek, E., Durtschi, R., Kent, R., Gentry, L., & Chung, M. (2011). Developmental sexual dimorphism of the oral and pharyngeal portions of the vocal tract: An imaging study. *Journal of Speech, Language, and Hearing Research, 54*, 995–1010.

Walker, G., & Kowalski, C. (1972). On the growth of the mandible. *American Journal of Physical Anthropology, 36*, 111–118.

Walsh, B., & Smith, A. (2002). Articulatory movements in adolescents: Evidence for protracted development of speech motor control processes. *Journal of Speech, Language, and Hearing Research, 45*, 1119–1133.

Walsh, B., Smith, A., & Weber-Fox, C. (2006). Short-term plasticity in children's speech motor systems. *Developmental Psychobiology, 48*, 660–674.

Warren, D. (1996). Regulation of speech aerodynamics. In N. Lass (Ed.), *Principles of experimental phonetics* (pp. 46–92). St. Louis, MO: Mosby-Year Book.

Warren, D., Hall, D., & Davis, J. (1981). Oral port constriction and pressure-flow relationships during sibilant productions. *Folia Phoniatrica, 33*, 380–394.

Watkin, K., & Fromm, D. (1984). Labial coordination in children: Preliminary considerations. *Journal of the Acoustical Society of America, 75*, 629–632.

Watkin, K., & Rubin, J. (1989). Pseudo-three-dimensional reconstruction of ultrasound images of the tongue. *Journal of the Acoustical Society of America, 85*, 496–499.

Watson, P., & Munson, B. (August, 2007). A comparison of vowel acoustics between older and younger adults. *Proceedings of the International Congress of Phonetic Sciences* (pp. 561–564). Saarbrucken, Germany: University of Saarland.

Weismer, G. (1984). Articulatory characteristics of parkinsonian dysarthria: Segmental and phrase-level timing, spirantization, and glottal-supraglottal coordination. In M. McNeil, J. Rosenbek, & A. Aronson (Eds.), *The dysarthrias: Physiology, acoustics, perception, management* (pp. 101–130). San Diego, CA: College-Hill Press.

Weismer, G., & Bunton, K. (1999). Influences of pellet markers on speech production behavior: Acoustical and perceptual measures. *Journal of the Acoustical Society of America, 105*, 2882–2894.

Weismer, G., & Fromm, D. (1983). Acoustic analysis of geriatric utterances: Segmental and nonsegmental characteristics that relate to laryngeal function. In D. Bless & J. Abbs (Eds.), *Vocal fold physiology: Contemporary research and clinical issues* (pp. 317–322). San Diego, CA: College-Hill Press.

Weismer, G., & Liss, J. (1991). Speech motor control and aging. In D. Ripich (Ed.), *Handbook of geriatric communication disorders* (pp. 205–226). Austin, TX: Pro-Ed.

Weismer, G., Yunusova, Y., & Westbury, J. (2003). Interarticulator coordination in dysarthria: An x-ray microbeam study. *Journal of Speech, Language, and Hearing Research, 46*, 1247–1261.

Welford, A. (1956). Age and learning: Theory and needed research. *Experientia, 4*, 136–144.

Welford, A. (1982). Motor skills and aging. In J. Mortimer, F. Pirozzolo, & G. Maletta (Eds.), *The aging motor system* (pp. 152–187). New York, NY: Preager.

Westbury, J. (1991). The significance and measurement of head position during speech production experiments using the x-ray microbeam system. *Journal of the Acoustical Society of America, 89*, 1782–1791.

Wind, J. (1970). *On the phylogeny and ontogeny of the human larynx.* Groningen, Netherlands: Wolters-Noordhoff.

Wohlert, A. (1996a). Perioral muscle activity in young and older adults during speech and nonspeech tasks. *Journal of Speech and Hearing Research, 39*, 761–770.

Wohlert, A. (1996b). Reflex responses of lip muscles in young and older women. *Journal of Speech and Hearing Research, 39*, 578–589.

Wohlert, A. (1996c). Tactile perception of spatial stimuli on the lip surface by young and older adults. *Journal of Speech and Hearing Research, 39*, 1191–1198.

Wohlert, A., & Smith, A. (1998). Spatiotemporal stability of lip movements in older adult speakers. *Journal of Speech, Language, and Hearing Research, 41*, 41–50.

Wood, S. (1979). A radiographic analysis of constriction locations for vowels. *Journal of Phonetics, 7*, 25–43.

Xue, S., & Hao, G. (2003). Changes in the human vocal tract due to aging and the acoustic correlates of speech production: A pilot study. *Journal of Speech, Language, and Hearing Research, 46*, 689–701.

Yan, J., Thomas, J., Stelmach, G., & Thomas, K. (2000). Developmental features of rapid aiming arm movements across the lifespan. *Journal of Motor Behavior, 32*, 121–140.

Youmans, S., & Stierwalt, J. (2006). Measures of tongue function related to normal swallowing. *Dysphagia, 21*, 102–111.

Yunusova, Y., Weismer, G., & Lindstrom, M. (2011). Classifications of vocalic segments from articulatory kinematics: Healthy controls and speakers with dysarthria. *Journal of Speech, Language, and Hearing Research, 54,* 1302–1311.

Zagzebski, J. (1975). Ultrasonic measurement of lateral pharyngeal wall motion at two levels in the vocal tract. *Journal of Speech and Hearing Research, 18,* 308–318.

Zaino, C., & Benventano, T. (1977). Functional, involutional, and degenerative disorders. In C. Zaino & T. Benventano (Eds.), *Radiologic examination of the oropharynx and esophagus* (pp. 141–170). New York, NY: Springer-Verlag.

Zemlin, W. (1998). *Speech and hearing science: Anatomy and physiology* (4th ed.). Boston, MA: Allyn & Bacon.

6

Brain Structures and Mechanisms for Speech, Language, and Hearing

INTRODUCTION

The purpose of this chapter is to introduce the role of the central and peripheral nervous systems in speech, language, and hearing. Although other chapters in this text are focused on the speech apparatus (Chapters 2–5), the speech signal it produces (Chapters 7–11), and the perception of that signal (Chapter 12), the perspective is broadened somewhat in the current chapter to include aspects of language and production and perception. This recognizes the role of the nervous system in all of normal and disordered communication, as well as to emphasize the likelihood of overlap and interactions between speech, language, and hearing functions of the brain. Also, the current chapter makes direct reference to the early studies of the brain and human communication, which were primarily concerned with aphasia, the loss of language performance (and possibly competence) as a result of brain damage in specific brain locations.

The chapter begins with an overview in which major concepts are introduced. Next, gross neuroanatomy is presented for the cerebral hemispheres and cerebral white matter, subcortical nuclei (e.g, basal ganglia and thalamus), cerebellum, the brainstem and cranial nerves, cortical innervation patterns, and the spinal cord and its peripheral nerves. Next, cells within the nervous system and selected aspects of their function are discussed, followed by descriptions of meninges, ventricles, and the blood supply to the brain. Aspects of neurophysiology are interwoven throughout the chapter, along with selected clinical implications for the speech-language pathologist. The chapter concludes with presentation of a well-known, contemporary model of speech motor control, and some consideration of why this and other similar models are relevant to a speech-language pathologist's view of the diagnostic and therapeutic process.

THE NERVOUS SYSTEM: AN OVERVIEW AND CONCEPTS

This chapter provides an account of brain structures and brain mechanisms. The term "brain structures" refers to the anatomy of the nervous system. In this chapter, coverage of nervous system anatomy is focused primarily on gross anatomy—structures easily observable when handling and dissecting a whole brain, or when viewed using modern imaging techniques. More limited information is provided on cellular, and even molecular anatomical levels, to provide a foundation for understanding neurological diseases affecting these fine-structure components of the nervous system and, ultimately, speech and language functions of the brain. The term "brain mechanisms" is used to mean the physiology of the brain, at the molecular, cellular, neurochemical, and system levels. "System" levels of brain function are presumably the ones associated with observable *behaviors*, such as producing a sentence or providing behavioral evidence for understanding spoken language (as in following an instruction).

Selected, important concepts are provided in this section. These concepts provide a framework and set of reference terms that can be consulted throughout a reading of the chapter. They include central versus peripheral nervous system, anatomical planes and directions, white versus gray matter, tracts versus nuclei, nerves versus ganglia, efferent and afferent, and lateralization and specialization of function.

Central Versus Peripheral Nervous System

The concept of *central nervous system* (CNS) versus *peripheral nervous system* (PNS) is familiar to most readers of this textbook. The distinction between the two is simple: the CNS includes the cerebral hemispheres and its contents, the brainstem, and the spinal cord; the PNS includes the nerves issued from the brainstem and spinal cord, plus clusters of sensory nerve cells, called ganglia, located in close proximity to, but outside, the brainstem and spinal cord. In Figure 6–1, the major components of the CNS are labeled, and nerves of the PNS are shown extending from the brainstem and spinal cord.

Later in this chapter the structure of nerve cells is presented in some detail. For the current discussion of CNS versus PNS, it can be stated that nerve cells —neurons—consist of a cell body and an axon. The axon conducts electrical impulses away from the cell body to its endpoint where the electrical energy is converted into chemical energy. Bundles of these axons are

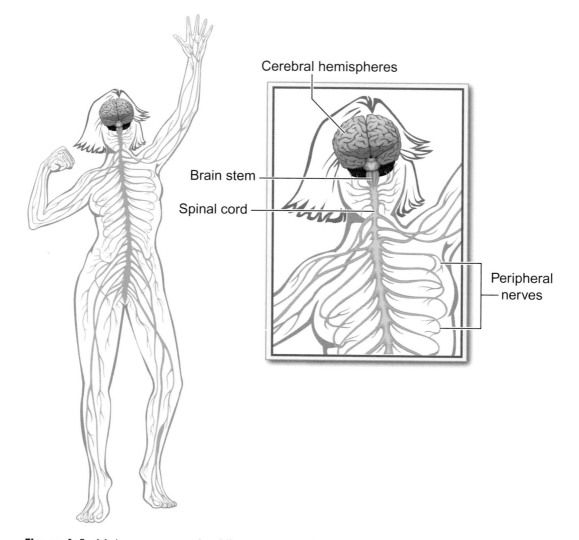

Figure 6–1. Major components of the nervous system, including three major subdivisions of the CNS (cerebral hemispheres, brainstem, spinal cord), and the major components of the PNS (peripheral nerves).

found in abundance in both the CNS and PNS. A bundle of axons in the CNS is called a *tract*; a bundle of axons in the PNS is called a *nerve*.

Anatomical Planes and Directions

The terminology for planes and directions varies depending on the part of the CNS under discussion. The left part of Figure 6–2 shows an artist's rendition of three anatomical planes as they are applied to the cerebral hemispheres. The *coronal plane* cuts the cerebral hemispheres into front and back sections, the *sagittal plane* into left and right sections, and the *horizontal plane* (also called *axial* or *transverse*) into upper and lower sections. Each of these planes can be moved along an axis perpendicular to the plane to "cut" the cerebral

hemispheres at different locations. For example, the horizontal plane can be moved up and down to obtain higher or lower "cuts." Similarly, the sagittal plane can be moved left or right, away from the midline (called the midsagittal plane) that divides the brain into equal left and right halves. Sagittal cuts away from the midline are referred to as *parasagittal* planes.

Several structures within the cerebral hemispheres have complex, curved shapes. Some structures are buried within the cerebral hemispheres and are difficult to visualize without multiplane views. Views of the brain in all three of the "standard" planes—coronal, sagittal, horizontal—are necessary to appreciate the form of these structures. A good example of the varying appearance of a single structure, the corpus callosum, is shown on the right side of Figure 6–2, where coronal (top), sagittal (middle), and horizontal (bottom) cuts

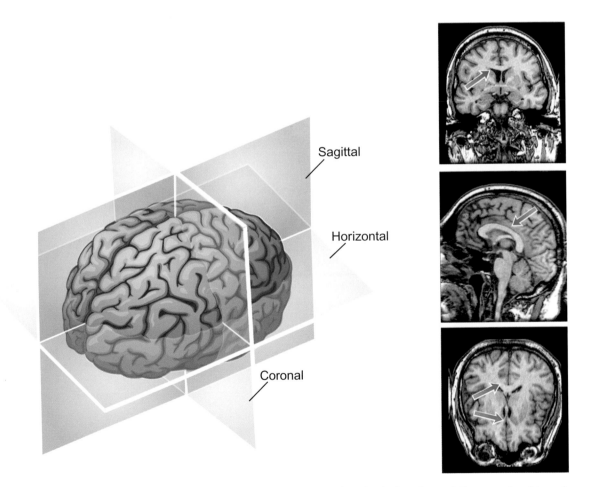

Figure 6–2. Left, major anatomical planes as seen in an anatomical drawing of the cerebral hemispheres, viewed from slightly above the hemispheres and in the sagittal plane; right, three MR images shown in the coronal (*top*), sagittal (*middle*), and horizontal (*bottom*) planes. In each of the MR images the red arrows point to the corpus callosum.

through the structure are shown as magnetic resonance (MR) images (MRI). The corpus callosum is a massive bundle of fibers (a tract) linking structures in the left and right cerebral hemispheres. The top MR image is a coronal slice, roughly at the midway point between the front and back of the brain. The red arrow points to a gently concave, white band of tissue located above two black "horns." This coronal plane image intersects the corpus callosum at a single location, where the structure extends laterally from the midline into the two hemispheres (the arrow is just off the midline, in the right hemisphere, which appears on the left from the reader's view). The appearance of the corpus callosum in the coronal plane varies depending on where the coronal slice is located along the front-to-back extent of the brain. This is better appreciated by examining the midsagittal plane MR image (Figure 6–2, middle). The white band of callosal ("callosal" = of the corpus callosum) tissue extends along the front-to-back length of the brain, and has a flattened, archlike shape with relatively complex form at its front and back ends. The coronal slice shown above the sagittal slice was taken just in front of the red arrow on the sagittal slice; this

slice interrupts the corpus callosum more or less in the middle of the flattened arch. Clearly, the appearance of the corpus callosum in a coronal section depends on where the slice is taken along the front-to-back axis of the cerebral hemispheres. The bottom MR image in Figure 6–2 shows a horizontal slice in which the white bands of corpus callosum tissue are indicated by two red arrows, one toward the front (lower part of image) and one toward the back (upper part of image) of the brain, connecting the two hemispheres. Between these two obvious areas of corpus callosum tissue, other callosal fibers are not apparent. This is because the horizontal slice is placed below the highest point of the arch seen in the midsagittal slice, which means it does not intersect this part of the corpus callosum tissue.

Locations of brain structures are often identified relative to locations of other brain structures. Figure 6–3 shows an MR image in the coronal plane, slightly posterior to the halfway point between the anterior and posterior "poles" of the cerebral hemispheres. Along the right-hand side of the image is a vertical dimension labeled *dorsal* at the top of the section, and *ventral* at the bottom; across the left-to-right extent of the image

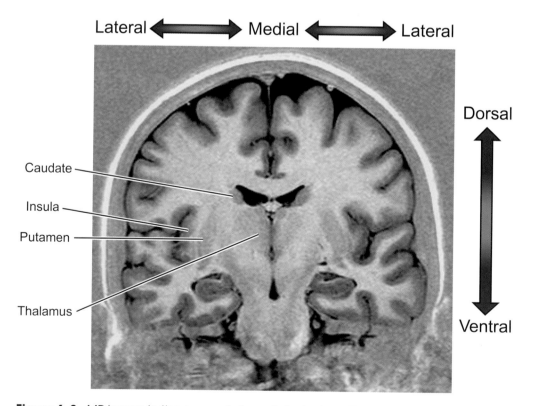

Figure 6–3. MR image in the coronal plane. Labels along the top and side axes of the image show directional terms. Selected structures within the cerebral hemispheres are labeled to illustrate the use of combined directional terms discussed in the text.

is a dimension labeled *lateral* (left), *medial* (center), and *lateral* (right). Within the cerebral hemispheres, dorsal means toward the top and ventral toward the bottom; therefore, the dorsal surface of the brain is the top surface and the ventral surface the underside of the brain. The side-to-side dimension within the cerebral hemispheres uses the term medial for the midline of the coronal view, and lateral for the sides of the brain, away from this midline.

These terms are also used, as suggested above, to locate one structure relative to another. In Figure 6–3, the cortex is the outermost tissue layer of the cerebral hemispheres, shown as a dark "rind" of tissue around the edge of the coronal image. Inside the cortical layer there is a good deal of white tissue, as well as several clusters of grayish tissue. Three of these grayish masses are labeled here—the *putamen*, *caudate*, and *thalamus*. In addition, the *insula*, a "hidden" part of the cortex beneath the lateral surface of either cerebral hemisphere, is labeled in the image (note how the insula is covered by two folds of the outer rind of cortex).

These four labeled structures are described more specifically below; here they are included to show how the terms dorsal, ventral, medial, and lateral are used to locate one structure relative to another within the cerebral hemispheres. For example, in the coronal section shown in Figure 6–3, the insula is lateral to the puta-men, and the caudate is dorsal to both the putamen and the thalamus. The position of the caudate relative to the thalamus and putamen, however, is somewhat more complex than simply "dorsal." The caudate is dorsal to the putamen, but also medial to it (closer to the midline), so a more precise statement is that the caudate is dorsomedial to the putamen. Similarly, the caudate is not only dorsal to the thalamus, but somewhat lateral as well. The caudate is therefore dorsolateral to the thalamus (or, reversing the reference structure, the thalamus is ventromedial to the caudate). This directional terminology is important because of its frequent use in descriptions of neuroanatomical structures, both in basic anatomical study and imaging studies performed for diagnostic purposes.

Figure 6–4 shows a horizontal MR image on the left, and a sagittal image on the right. Toward the top of the horizontal image—the front of the cerebral hemispheres—is the anterior direction, toward the bottom the posterior direction. The anterior-posterior dimension is also shown in the sagittal image on the right of Figure 6–4; here the directions are obvious because of the clarity of the facial features. This sagittal image introduces an interesting complication in the use of direction terms. Note the distinction between the dorsal-ventral and anterior-posterior dimensions: dorsal means toward the top of the cerebral hemispheres,

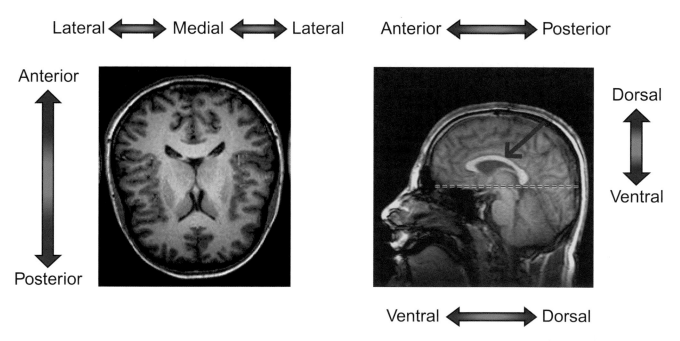

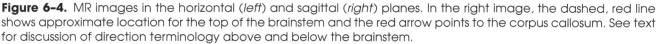

Figure 6–4. MR images in the horizontal (*left*) and sagittal (*right*) planes. In the right image, the dashed, red line shows approximate location for the top of the brainstem and the red arrow points to the corpus callosum. See text for discussion of direction terminology above and below the brainstem.

posterior toward the back of the cerebral hemispheres. For neuroanatomical structures below the top of the brainstem, however, the dorsal-ventral and posterior-anterior dimensions are one and the same. The top of the brainstem is indicated in the sagittal image by a horizontal dashed line. Below this line, dorsal and posterior indicate the same direction—toward the back of the body—and ventral and anterior both indicate toward the front of the body. The identity between the terms dorsal/posterior and ventral/anterior applies to spinal cord structures as well.

The terms *deep* and *superficial* are also used to locate one structure relative to another. These terms are typically used to designate the relative locations of structures as a path is followed from "outside to inside" (or the reverse). When the question is asked, "What is beneath this surface?" it is equivalent to asking, "What is deep to this surface?" For example, the white matter of the cerebral hemispheres is deep to the cortex (or the cortex is superficial to the white matter).

White Versus Gray Matter, Tracts Versus Nuclei, Nerves Versus Ganglia

When a brain is removed from the skull with the intention of preserving it for later study, it is "fixed" in a solution of formalin, a fluid that hardens biological tissue. A formalin-preserved brain shows certain regions having a grayish-brown appearance, and other regions with a pale, near-white appearance. Similarly, in conventional MR images of the brain there are regions that appear more grayish, and regions that appear more whitish. The coronal plane MR images in Figures 6–2 through 6–4 show both *gray* and *white matter*. Gray matter consists of clusters of neuron cell bodies (*somata*, the plural of *soma*, which means cell body); white matter is formed from myelinated axons issued by those cell bodies (neurons are discussed in detail below).

Gray Matter and Nuclei

The cortex, the outermost thick covering of the cerebral hemispheres, consists of densely packed cell bodies; the cortex is a major part of gray matter in the cerebral hemispheres. Figure 6–3 shows the cortical "rind" of gray matter enclosing extensive white matter. Within this white matter are several regions of additional gray matter (e.g., the structures labeled "caudate," "puta-

men," and "thalamus"). A specific cluster of cell bodies inside the cerebral hemispheres, or within the brainstem or spinal cord, is referred to in the singular as a *nucleus* (as in "caudate nucleus") or in some cases as a group as nuclei (as in "cranial nerve nuclei,"clusters of cell bodies within the brain stem). The clusters of cell bodies deep to the cortex but within the cerebral hemispheres, such as the caudate, putamen, and thalamus, are referred to as *subcortical nuclei*. Some subcortical nuclei, such as the thalamus, are collections of many smaller nuclei but are referred to jointly as a single structure. The term *subcortical nuclei* does not include nuclei within the brainstem and spinal cord, but is reserved for clusters of cell bodies within the cerebral hemispheres and above the brainstem. Nuclei are also found in the cerebellum; these are referred to as cerebellar nuclei.[1]

Neuronal cell bodies, whether in the cortex, subcortical region, brainstem, cerebellum, or spinal cord, most often cluster together for a common purpose; they do not aggregate randomly. In a given region of cortex, for example, cell bodies related to eye movements, or to auditory perception, are likely to cluster together. Within a particular, region of cortex, or within a subcortical or brainstem nucleus in which the cells have a common function, there is likely to be an even more fine-grained, systematic aggregation. For example, the most posterior gyrus (where gyrus = a hill of tissue on the cortical surface, separated from other gyri by deep fissures or sulci) of the frontal lobe is the primary motor cortex, containing cells that have more or less direct control over the timing, force, and duration of muscle contractions. Within this primary motor cortex, cells associated with particular parts of the body aggregate together. Hand and finger cells, for example, are found in close proximity in the primary motor cortex. The cellular representation within a specific cortical area (such as primary motor cortex) according to body part (as a maplike reflection of the body plan) is called *somatotopic organization*. Somatotopic organization is not only a feature of cortical tissue, but is also found in subcortical, cerebellar, brainstem, and spinal cord nuclei. Moreover, somatotopic organization is present in the brain for both motor and sensory systems. The primary sensory cortex, the gyrus immediately posterior to the primary motor cortex and the most anterior gyrus of the parietal lobe, is also arranged somatotopically, as are spinal cord, brainstem, and subcortical sensory nuclei. Other organizational schemes are found in

---

[1]The terms "nucleus" and "nuclei" are not used when referring to clusters of cell bodies in the cortex; these organizations of cell bodies are referred to as cortex, cortical region, cortical tissue, and so forth. Similarly, the term "nucleus" is used only sparingly when referring to gray matter in the spinal cord.

Somatotopic Representation Is Not Always "Clean"

Many studies have demonstrated the "truth" of somatotopic representation in primary motor and sensory cortices. These studies include correlations between highly localized lesions and affected body parts, electrical stimulation of very discrete locations along the cortex and observation of the resulting movements or reported sensations, and functional magnetic resonance imaging (fMRI) studies in which very local movements, as in raising of a single finger, result in the "lighting up" of a small region of the primary motor cortex. Somatotopy, however, is not always neat and clean. For example, fMRI studies of representation of speech apparatus structures in the primary motor cortex have revealed that cells for muscles of the pharynx, tongue, and lips "share" space close to the bottom of the central fissure, where the primary motor cortex meets the sylvian fissure (Takai, Brown, & Liotti, 2010). These cortical cells are not perfectly segregated by structure as might be expected by a strict somatotopy. Takai and colleagues call the mixing of cells for these three speech apparatus structures "somatotopy with overlap," meaning there is a body part ordering of orofacial cells but some overlap as well. As argued by these authors, perhaps such overlap makes functional sense for the control of coordinated behaviors such as swallowing and speaking.

the nervous system as well, such as tonotopicity, where the CNS structures associated with audition aggregate cells according to acoustic signal frequency.

The concept of somatotopic representation of cells within the brain is important not only for understanding brain anatomy, but also for gaining clinical perspectives on the effects of lesion location on function. For example, somatotopic organization explains (in part) how a stroke can affect a client's ability to walk but leave speech and language unaffected; or how a stroke can affect speech and language in the absence of other obvious problems.

White Matter and Fiber Tracts

Neurons have a cell body, an axon, and a terminal (end) structure. The primary function of a neuron is to conduct electrical impulses from the cell body along the axon to the terminal structure, also called the terminal segment or button. As discussed in more detail below, the majority of axons in the brain are wrapped in a fatty substance called *myelin*. Myelin insulates axons and in so doing makes neuronal conduction of electrical impulses faster and more efficient. Myelin gives axons the whitish appearance in fixed brains and brain images. The coronal section shown in Figure 6–3 shows a good deal of white matter, and therefore many, many axons.

Axons connect different areas of gray matter. These connections are referred to as pathways, fiber tracts, fiber bundles, fasciculi (singular = fasciculus), and lemnisci (singular = lemniscus). Bundles of axons connect different cortical regions to one another, cortical cells to subcortical and brainstem nuclei, spinal nuclei to brainstem and subcortical nuclei, cerebellar nuclei to many different nuclei in the brain—in short, myelinated pathways are everywhere in the brain, connecting and interconnecting different masses of gray matter. These pathways are typically organized in much the same way as the areas of gray matter they are connecting. In other words, fiber tracts also have somatotopic organization.

Ganglia

The term "ganglia" (singular = ganglion) is typically reserved for clusters of nerve cell bodies located *outside* the CNS. Ganglia are technically part of the PNS. They receive sensory fibers coming from receptors in the body (such as tactile receptors, or from the cochlea or retina) where a first synapse (connection with another neuron) is made prior to entry of the information into the CNS. For example, a tactile receptor in the hand is a special end organ of the PNS, embedded in skin or muscle and connected by a sensory fiber to the CNS. When the end organ is stimulated (e.g., by the compression of touch), it "fires," sending an electrical impulse to the nervous system via the sensory fiber. This fiber makes first contact—that is, makes a first synapse—with a cell in a ganglion immediately outside the spinal cord. The ganglion cell receiving this information delivers it, via its own axon, to sensory cells in the spinal cord. Similar receptors are found in muscles of the speech apparatus, including muscles of the respiratory system, larynx, and upper airway (vocal tract).

The spinal cord is associated with a series of *dorsal root ganglia*, arranged from the top to bottom segments of the cord, that serve as the first synapses for much of the sensory information delivered from the limbs and trunk to the CNS. There are also ganglia immediately outside the brainstem that serve as the first synapses for sensory information from head and neck structures. For example, the hair cells of the cochlea are the specialized sensory endings for hearing, and when they are deformed by motion of the basilar membrane they fire, sending impulses to the spiral ganglion, a bundle of nerve cells outside the brainstem where the first synapses for hearing take place. Cell bodies in the spiral ganglion then send axons into the brainstem to make synapses within the first set of nuclei along the auditory pathways.

Efferent and Afferent

The terms efferent and afferent are used in two different ways to describe information flow in the nervous system. The first use of the terms concerns overall information flow for the production of muscular effort (efferent) in contrast to the information flow for the sensation of an environmental event (afferent). When motor commands are issued from cortical tissue and travel along descending pathways through one or more motor nuclei before eventually being directed by peripheral nerves to muscles, the pathways are referred to as efferent. Sometimes the term *efference* is equated with the basic components—brain-directed muscle contractions and their patterns in space and time—of motor control. In contrast, when a sensory receptor (such as a tactile receptor in a finger, or the hair cells of the cochlea) is stimulated and the resulting signal travels via peripheral nerves to the spinal cord and then through ascending pathways to a final destination in the cortex, the pathways are said to be afferent. *Afference* is often taken to mean "sensory."

A second use of the terms efferent and afferent indicates the inputs and outputs of nuclei *within* the CNS. This usage does not imply a motor act or sensation to or from a body structure, but rather the flow of information from one nucleus to another (or one cluster of cell bodies to another cluster of cell bodies or nucleus). For example, a nucleus at the top of the brainstem, in the midbrain, is called the *substantia nigra* (SN). The SN produces an important neurotransmitter called dopamine and is interconnected with several subcortical and brainstem nuclei. The cells of the SN send information via a fiber tract to the striatum, a subcortical nucleus group made up of the caudate and putamen. One output of the SN is therefore to the striatum, or in the language of neuroscientists the striatum is one of the *efferent projections* of the SN. Note the parallel to the first use of the term efferent—both terms refer to outputs. On the other hand, the SN receives efferent pro-

jections from the *subthalamic nucleus* (STN), another subcortical nucleus; these are inputs to the SN from the STN. The SN therefore has efferent projections to the striatum, and afferent projections from the STN.

For the present purposes, the particular structures sending information to, or receiving information from, different structures are not important. Rather, the concept of efferent and afferent projections within the CNS is the point (the interconnections between SN, STN, and the cortex, as well as with other subcortical nuclei, are presented later in the chapter). Note the importance of a reference structure in naming the efferent and afferent projections of a nucleus: a nucleus' efferent projections are pathways sent to another nucleus (or the cortex), whereas the nucleus' afferent projections are pathways received from other nuclei (or the cortex). A single nucleus, such as the STN, typically has both efferent and afferent projections—the nucleus influences other cell bodies, and is influenced by other cell bodies. Sometimes these influences are in a loop, so two nuclei may communicate with each other via both efferent and afferent projections.

Most nuclei, and cortical cells as well, receive and send information to multiple locations within the brain. Each cortical region or nucleus is therefore likely to have multiple efferent and afferent projections. The dense and overlapping interconnections within the brain, including the efferent projections of a single nucleus (or cortical area) to many different nuclei (or areas), plus the variety of afferent inputs to a single nucleus (or cortical area), make the simple distinction of efferent versus afferent less useful than once thought. Clearly, motor systems are not isolated from, or independent of, sensory systems. In fact, motor and sensory systems are highly interdependent, with certain brain "circuits"—interconnected nuclei—performing sensorimotor integration for the most efficient and skilled actions. The term *sensorimotor control* is often the preferred term to represent action such as the coordinated motions of the articulators (pharyngeal-oral and velopharyngeal-nasal structures), larynx, and breathing system to produce the acoustic signal we call speech.

Lateralization and Specialization of Function

"Lateralization" and "specialization" may sometimes be used interchangeably, but the terms have different technical meanings. When a function is said to be "lateralized" in the brain, the technical meaning is that the function is primarily controlled by one hemisphere relative to the other. Good examples of lateralized functions include (of course) speech and language (thought to be controlled by left hemisphere structures in about 95% of the population), handedness (also controlled by the left hemisphere in about 95% of the population), and emotions (thought to be controlled primarily by right hemisphere structures). Lateralization of speech and language function to the left hemisphere has been demonstrated by clinical cases and research studies, including the common observation of disrupted speech and language function when a stroke affects the blood supply to the left hemisphere, but not the right hemisphere. Lateralization of speech and language has also been shown by the ability to elicit speech and language behaviors during surgical procedures, when an electrical current stimulates certain regions of the left hemisphere's cortical surface; stimulation in the same cortical regions of the right hemisphere does not elicit these speech and language behaviors.

A standard test of brain lateralization of speech and language functions is to inject a drug, called amobarbital, into either the left or right carotid artery so that the left or right hemisphere is more or less anesthetized for a brief period of time. The carotid arteries are the main source of blood flowing from the heart to the cerebral hemispheres. An injection of amobarbital into the left carotid artery initially distributes the drug to the left hemisphere, leaving the right hemisphere unaffected for at least a short time. The drug temporarily blocks neural activity in the cerebral hemisphere chosen for the test, and therefore provides a technique to determine which hemisphere has lateralized speech and language function. If injection into the left carotid artery results in speech and language deficits, but injection into the right carotid artery does not, this is good evidence for lateralization of speech and language functions to the left hemisphere.

The amobarbital test, called the *Wada* test after the Japanese-Canadian neurologist Juhn Wada who developed the procedure in the late 1940s, is used in patients undergoing resection (extraction) of parts of the brain to relieve chronic, severe epilepsy. Before the Wada test, clinical cases of stroke affecting either the left or right cerebral hemispheres led physicians and scientists to regard speech and language functions of the brain as lateralized to the left hemisphere in the vast majority of neurologically normal individuals. In epilepsy, however, there was (and is) the sense that a seizure-causing lesion in the left hemisphere may result in speech and language functions being "transferred" to the right hemisphere, or to be split more equally between the two hemispheres. The Wada test is used in these patients to identify the hemisphere to which speech and language function is lateralized, and there-

fore to indicate areas where surgical resection should be avoided or minimized for maximal preservation of communication ability.

Many studies using the Wada test have been reported in the clinical literature (for two good examples, both of which contain reviews of much of the pertinent literature, see Lee et al. [2008], and Springer et al. [1999]). Use of the Wada test in neurologically normal individuals to determine if laterality varies by handedness has been challenged by the difficulty of assembling a large enough group of left-handers to compare to more easily recruited right-handers. When the Wada test has been used to compare laterality of left- and right-handers, it is usually among presurgical patients with epilepsy. This work shows about 96% of right-handed people to have left hemisphere lateralization for speech and language, compared to 85% of left-handers (or "mixed" handers: see Rasmussen & Milner, 1977). When contemporary brain imaging methods are used to estimate lateralization of speech and language, the estimates for right-handers are almost exactly consistent with the data from Rasmussen and Milner, but more left-handers show lateralization of speech and language to the right hemisphere (Swanson, Sabsevitz, Hammeke, & Binder, 2007). Using an imaging technique similar to functional magnetic resonance imaging (fMRI), Knecht et al. (2000) obtained results showing a relationship between degree of left-handedness and the likelihood of speech and language being lateralized to the *right* hemisphere. Hard-core righties were almost all left-lateralized (~96%), whereas only about 73% of hard-core southpaws were left-lateralized; the sample of people with various degrees of "mixed" handedness fell, as a group, between these two numbers.

This very brief review of the literature on lateralization of speech and language function suggests at least two broad conclusions, as well as one additional thought concerning the concept of lateralization. First, most people, either left or right handed, have speech and language lateralized to the left hemisphere; this is what most clinicians and scientists have suspected for many years. Second, there is a greater chance for language to be lateralized to the right hemisphere, or for its representation to be split between the hemispheres, in people who are clearly left handed. Still, the majority of left-handers are "left-dominant" for speech and language, even though they are "right-dominant" for handedness. Finally, the concept of lateralization for speech and language to one hemisphere or the other is not an absolute, either-or concept. Lateralization for speech and language appears to be a continuous phenomenon, not only because of the demonstration of greater likelihood for right-hemisphere dominance

fMRI

Magnetic resonance images (MRI) are obtained by placing a body structure within a strong magnetic field and then, by application and withdrawal of a second magnetic field, causing cell nuclei to generate magnetic properties that are sensed by a coil. The coil detects different amounts of energy generated by the cells, depending on cell properties, cell locations, and other factors. Software takes the signals generated by all those cells and assembles them into an image of the target structure (for example, see right side of Figure 6–2). fMRI, or functional magnetic resonance imaging, makes use of the same general principle, but with a twist (that's a pun for those of you familiar with the magnetized behavior of brain cell nuclei). When neurons are active, the active region attracts blood flow from arteries; such arterial blood flow is oxygen rich, and oxygen-rich blood has different magnetic properties than run-of-the-mill blood. When an area of the brain is being used for a specific task, like speaking, that area generates a different signal than an area not being used for that task. The software is designed to make that active area "light up" because of increased blood flow. So, now you know that you can actually light up a room when you speak words of cheer!

with increasing left-handedness (Knecht et al., 2000), but also because certain aspects of speech and language —such as prosody—have been shown to be represented primarily in the right hemisphere. When the term "dominant hemisphere for speech and language" is used, these qualifying thoughts should be kept in mind.

How is "specialization" different from "lateralization"? Although it may seem reasonable to say that the left hemisphere is specialized for speech and language (in the same way it is lateralized for speech and language), the term "specialization" is used in a more specific—pun intended—sense. Specialization means that certain brain regions have evolved to serve distinct functions, whether lateralized or not. For example, a well-known claim for specialization is that portions of the frontal lobe are specialized for executive function (see Alvarez and Emory [2006] for a review of evidence for and against this claim). "Executive function" is, broadly speaking, the ability to organize behavior

to achieve a goal or set of goals. If the brain is a movie in production, executive function is the director of the production; executive function coordinates brain function, matches behaviors to desired outcomes, and regulates actions. In neurologically intact individuals, tasks requiring organization of complex material to achieve a certain outcome often cause parts of the frontal lobes to "light up" in fMRI studies, and people with damage to the frontal lobes are likely to show an impaired ability to deal with complex decision making and demonstrate poor regulation of behavior. Some scientists and clinicians therefore regard the frontal lobes *of both hemispheres*, or at least certain parts of them, to be specialized for executive function. Here we have a case of specialization without obvious lateralization.

Another example of hypothesized specialization is in regions of the brain thought to be critical for the representation and programming of articulatory gestures for speech. Some scientists place these two processes in a very small portion of the posterior, ventral edge of the left frontal lobe (more is said about this below). The actual neural tissue for the *execution* of speech sounds—where execution means transforming the represented and programmed sounds into movements —is thought to be located slightly posterior to this programming tissue, but still in the frontal lobe. This is an example of specialization within lateralization: speech is left-lateralized, and within this lateralized function there are finer degrees of specialization for the various components of producing speech and language.

A popular view of specialization, one that takes the concept to a logical (but in some views, extreme) conclusion is found in the idea of brain modules. Modules are thought to be regions of brain tissue that are specialized for particular tasks—"dedicated," in computer terminology—and in fact insulated from other tasks. Some scientists and clinicians believe, for example, that in humans a very specific region on the underside of the temporal lobe contains a module for human face recognition (matching a person's identity with his or her face: see Said, Haxby, and Todorov [2011]); this brain region is thought to be "insulated" from other tasks because it does not seem to be active for recognition of nonhuman/nonface objects such as cars, dogs, and so forth. Closer to our intellectual home, some speech scientists believe there is a module for speech perception in the left hemisphere, a species-specific (human) collection of neural tissue activated only by human speech or simulations of it (i.e., computer-generated speech) (see history of, and arguments for and against, the motor theory of speech perception in Galantucci, Fowler, and Turvey [2006]).

CEREBRAL HEMISPHERES AND WHITE MATTER

The cerebral hemispheres are part of the CNS (see Figure 6–1). Each hemisphere is divided into lobes and contains gray and white matter.

Cerebral Hemispheres

Figure 6–5 shows the cerebral hemispheres in four views. The top-left view is from above the brain, looking down to the dorsal surfaces of the two hemispheres. The front of the brain is toward the top of the image. This view shows the left and right cerebral hemispheres, separated by a long, front-to-back fissure called the *longitudinal fissure* (also called the *interhemispheric* or *sagittal fissure*). The visible surface tissue is *cortex*, regarded as the most complex and "sophisticated" part of the brain. Note the ridges or "hills" of the cortex, and the "dips" between them. The ridges are called *gyri* (singular = *gyrus*) and the "dips" *sulci* (singular = *sulcus*) or *fissures* (the term "fissure" is typically used to mean a particularly deep sulcus, such as the longitudinal fissure). One notable difference between the human brain and the brain of animals such as sheep, cats, and dogs, is that humans have relatively deep and numerous sulci defining the cortical surface. These deep sulci are infoldings of cortical surface forming unseen "walls" of tissue that contribute to a greater volume of cortical cells in the human brain, relative to other animals. This hidden cortical surface area and its corresponding thickness add to the cognitive and performance power of humans. By gently separating any sulcus on the surface of a prepared (formalin-hardened) brain, these walls of hidden cortical tissue can be revealed. Some authors have estimated that close to two-thirds of the human cortex is hidden inside sulcal walls (Zilles, Armstrong, Schleicher, & Kretschmann, 1988). This unique feature of the human brain appears to be an evolutionary solution to packing lots of cortical tissue into a container—the skull—of limited size.

A dramatic view of "hidden" cortical tissue can be gained by putting your thumbs inside the longitudinal fissure of a prepared brain, your two hands resting on the two hemispheres, and gently separating the hemispheres without tearing the tissue. This exposes the deep inside (medial) walls of the two hemispheres. A view of the medial wall of the right cerebral hemisphere is shown in the top-right view of Figure 6–5. A prominent feature of this midsagittal view of the cerebral hemispheres is the *corpus callosum*, the massive bundle of tissue that connects structures across the two hemispheres.

Figure 6–5, bottom-right, shows a side view of the left hemisphere of the brain. The front of the brain is toward the left of the image. This view shows the four lobes of the brain, their boundary landmarks, plus additional regions important to the discussion of the brain in speech, language, and hearing. The four lobes are the frontal (green), parietal (brown), temporal (blue), and occipital (purple) lobes. This color code is modified at specific locations to highlight important cortical regions within the hemisphere. What follows is a more detailed consideration of each of these lobes, and two additional cerebral regions (the insula and limbic system), their functions, and when relevant their assumed function for speech and language.

Frontal Lobe

The frontal lobe (green in Figure 6–5) is bounded at the back by the *central fissure* (also called the *fissure of Rolando*), and below by the front part of the *lateral sulcus* or *sylvian fissure* (see Figure 6–5, top left and right, and bottom right). The gyrus immediately in front of the central sulcus, and therefore within the frontal lobe, is the *primary motor cortex* (shown as a lighter shade of green in Figure 6–5). The primary motor cortex contains cells, called motor neurons, that send signals to motor neurons in the brainstem and spinal cord, which, in turn, send axons to muscles to control their contraction patterns. The pathway: primary motor cortex neurons→brainstem/spinal cord motor neurons→muscles, can be thought of as the route of direct nervous system control of the timing, strength, and speed of muscle contractions for head and neck and limb and torso structures. As discussed later in this chapter, this direct route to muscle control is modulated and fine-tuned by activity in several different parts of the CNS, including other cortical regions (such as the supplementary motor area, primary somatosensory cortex, and Broca's area, shown in Figure 6–5, top and bottom right), the basal ganglia, and the cerebellum, to produce everyday movement and highly skilled, specialized movement.

Primary Motor Cortex. The cells (motor neurons) of the primary motor cortex are arranged along the precentral gyrus in a *somatotopic* fashion. Imagine drawing a map of the body parts represented along the primary cortex, starting at the top of the brain (at the longitudinal fissure) and working your way down the lateral surface of

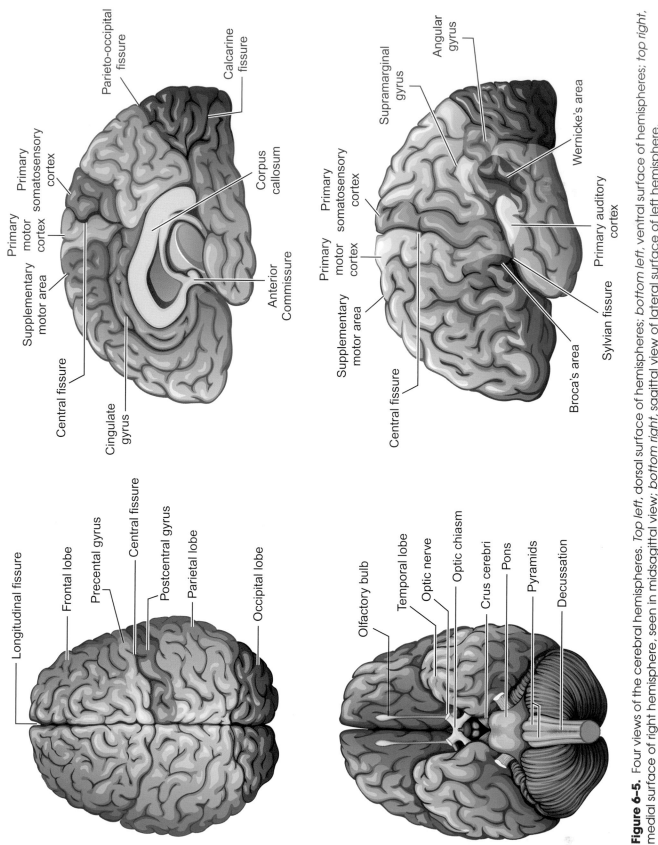

Figure 6-5. Four views of the cerebral hemispheres. *Top left,* dorsal surface of hemispheres; *bottom left,* ventral surface of hemispheres; *top right,* medial surface of right hemisphere, seen in midsagittal view; *bottom right,* sagittal view of lateral surface of left hemisphere.

either hemisphere to the sylvian fissure. If the map reflected not only *which* body parts are represented in a specific region of the primary motor cortex, but the *amount* of cortex devoted to the control of specific body parts, the result is similar to the image shown on the bottom left of Figure 6–6. The primary motor cortex (light green) is a slab of tissue that when "mapped" for body part representation shows the general somatotopic plan of cortical motor cells and the muscles they control. The most obvious characteristic of this map is the upside-down representation of the body along the primary motor cortex. Cells that control muscles of the lower part of the body (such as muscles of the hip and knee) are at the top of the primary motor cortex (or even along the medial wall of the cortex—note the location of cells for muscles of the feet), whereas control of muscles of the face, tongue, and larynx are toward the bottom of the gyrus, just above the sylvian fissure. In the drawing, the size of the body part represents how much cortical tissue is devoted to the part; the bigger the drawing of the body part, the greater the number of cells devoted to its control. Note the very

large size of the face and its associated structures (the tongue, lips, larynx), compared to the size of the feet, or even the trunk. A disproportionate number of cells in the primary motor cortex are devoted to control of the structures speech-language pathologists are most concerned with.

The disproportionate representation of cells that control movements of orofacial structures (jaw, tongue, lips) and laryngeal structures suggests the great relevance of these structures to the lives of humans. No great imagination is required to make the case for the centrality of eating and breathing in human function, and the need for sophisticated muscular control to support these behaviors. The same case can be made, of course, for any mammal, but the disproportionate representation of these structures within the primary motor cortex of humans is very much a function of our unique ability to generate spoken language. Notice the phrase "spoken *language*"; it is not just the production of sounds—many animals do this for simple communicative purposes—but the extensive use of a signal system (the acoustic signal emerging from the vocal

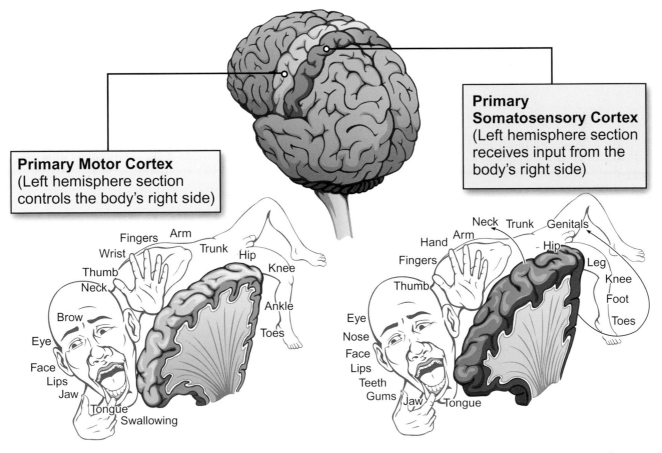

Figure 6–6. Somatotopic representations along the primary motor (*green*) and sensory (*orange*) cortices.

tract) to give meaning to abstract, complex ideas, to convey the same idea in many different ways, even to *create* ideas (Deacon, 1997).

The location of orofacial and laryngeal cells at the "bottom" (ventral aspect) of the primary motor cortex is even more interesting when considering that the premotor cortical region called Broca's area is located on the ventrolateral surface of the left hemisphere (see Figure 6–5, bottom right). Broca's area is immediately adjacent to the primary motor cortex representation of orofacial and laryngeal control. Surely this is not a coincidence.

Broca's Area. The inferior frontal gyrus, on the lateral surface of the *left* frontal lobe and immediately above the front end of the sylvian fissure, is called *Broca's area*. Broca's area is shown in Figure 6–5, bottom right, as the frontal lobe region that is colored dark green. Broca's area, along with several other areas of the frontal lobe, is *premotor cortex*, the latter term indicating a role in motor control different from direct control of muscles exerted by cells in the primary motor cortex. Broca's area is often said to have a central role in the planning and organization of motor behavior required for speech production. In the classical understanding of brain regions and their role in speech and language performance, Broca's area was considered to be the site where speech expression is controlled. This conclusion was formulated by Paul Broca (1824–1880), the famous French physician who between 1861 and 1865 reported on a few patients with primarily expressive speech-language disorders resulting from neurological disease. On autopsy of the patients' whole brains (that is, brains not subjected to dissection), Broca noted fairly distinct lesions in and around the third frontal gyrus of the left hemisphere. If this gyrus was damaged in patients who exhibited speech-language disorders largely of an expressive nature, with minimal problems in language comprehension, the function of the gyrus in healthy individuals as the center of speech expression seemed to be a logical conclusion. The conclusion was reinforced by the observations that lesions in the inferior gyrus of the right frontal lobe did not produce speech or language disorders. The emerging picture was of specialization for expressive control of speech and language in the left hemisphere, in the region of the frontal lobe where Broca had identified lesions in the brains of his patients.

We know now that historical and even some contemporary interpretations of Broca's observations are far too simplistic. First, damage to the brains of people with expressive disorders like those described by Broca (often called "Broca's aphasia" in modern textbooks) typically extends to regions well beyond the third frontal gyrus (Keller, Crow, Foundas, Amunts, & Roberts, 2009). In fact, the actual brains autopsied by Broca were recently examined using imaging techniques and shown to have widespread brain damage in addition to the obvious lesion to the inferior convolution of the left frontal lobe (Dronkers, Plaisant, Ibas-Zisen, & Cabanis, 2007). Second, there is evidence that Broca's area is involved in language *comprehension*, specifically of utterances with relatively complicated syntax (Grodzinsky & Santi, 2008) and semantics (Willems & Hagoort, 2009). Third, tissue in and around Broca's area has been shown to respond to nonlinguistic functions, one of which is *watching* finger and/or mouth movements (i.e., Broca's area "lights up" when participants *observe* these movements: see Lindenberg, Fangerau, & Seitz [2007]). Finally, for the great majority of people, speech and language control is *lateralized* to one hemisphere—neural tissue is specialized for speech and language in one hemisphere, so there is an asymmetry of function—but not everyone has lateralization to the left hemisphere. Estimates vary across studies, but right hemisphere lateralization of speech and language skills probably occurs in about 5–10% of the healthy, right-handed population; a higher percentage of right- or "mixed"-hemisphere specialization for speech and language seems to occur for left-handers and persons with epilepsy (Swanson et al., 2007).

Broca's area is clearly important for speech and language behavior, but it is not devoted exclusively to speech expression. Instead, Broca's area is part of a *network* involving extensive interconnections and shared functions, serving the complexity of all aspects of human communication. In this view it is not productive to expect simple matches between damage to particular areas of the brain and specific functions.

Premotor and Supplementary Motor Area. The gyrus just forward of, and more or less parallel to, the primary motor cortex is called *premotor cortex* (often called PMA, for "Premotor Area," not labeled in Figure 6–5; see the darker green gyrus immediately anterior to the lighter green gyrus in Figure 6–5, bottom right). Broca's area, colored dark green, is part of the premotor cortex. On the medial wall of the cortex the tissue in front of the primary motor cortex is labeled *supplementary motor cortex* (SMA) (see Figure 6–5, top and bottom right); the SMA is also part of the PMA. Note the distinction between the presumed functions of the PMA/SMA versus the primary motor cortex: PMA/SMA *plans* movement whereas primary motor cortex issues commands to *perform* movement. This distinction is important to the speech-language pathologist, who is often asked to make a diagnostic judgment of whether a speech motor control disorder is one of execution or planning (or both!). Execution disorders of speech motor control are called *dysarthrias*; planning disorders are called *apraxias*.

Prefrontal Cortex. The large mass of frontal lobe tissue anterior to the primary motor cortex and PMA/SMA is called *prefrontal cortex*. Many scientists (see, for example, Ridderinkhof, Ullsperger, Crone, & Nieuwenhuis, 2004) believe that this part of the frontal lobe performs *executive function* in the brain. Executive function, in a broad sense, is the guidance of all cognitive (and perhaps lower-level) brain functions; executive function is the brain's monitoring, selecting, and "tuning" its own, higher-level actions and behavioral goals. In a more narrow sense, executive function guides decisions such as when it is "okay" to use certain words or drink certain beverages, why it is not okay to employ violence as a reaction to situations, whether or not a certain behavior may have a profound effect on your own or someone else's life in the future, how the tuning of your sensory systems (like hearing and vision) changes from situation to situation to be sensitive to stimuli that have current or future importance, and so forth. Based on this short list it is easy to understand why scientists have connected prefrontal cortex with aspects of personality. This may have direct relevance to speech-language pathologists who work with brain-injured patients having personality changes as a consequence of injury to the frontal lobes, as well as patients with dementia due (in part) to deterioration of frontal lobe tissue.

Parietal Lobe

The parietal lobe (shown in light brown in Figure 6–5 except for its most anterior gyrus which is colored orange) is bounded at the front by the *central fissure* (or *sulcus*) or *fissure of Rolando*, below by the back part of the *sylvian fissure* (or *lateral sulcus*), and toward the back of the brain by the *parieto-occipital fissure*. The parieto-occipital fissure, which is the boundary between the parietal and occipital lobes, is easy to see on the medial wall of the cerebral hemisphere (see Figure 6–5, top right) but is only partially visible when viewing the external surface of the hemisphere. The boundary shown between the parietal and occipital lobes in the bottom right view of Figure 6–5 is therefore approximate. Similarly, the boundary between the lower part of the parietal lobe and the back of the temporal lobe is not clearly marked in bottom right view of Figure 6–5.

The gyrus immediately in back of the central (Rolandic) fissure—the most forward gyrus of the parietal lobe—is the *primary somatosensory cortex*. The primary somatosensory cortex, colored orange in Figure 6–5, runs more or less parallel to the primary motor cortex. Like the primary motor cortex, the primary somatosensory cortex is organized somatotopically, although not in precisely the same way as the motor cortex (see sidetrack on "Somatotopic Representation Is Not Always 'Clean,'" and Figure 6–6).

Stated broadly, cells in the primary somatosensory cortex respond to touch and pain stimuli from all body locations. The primary somatosensory cortex is, in fact, a good deal more complicated than this broad view. There are extensive interconnections among different cell types within the somatosensory cortex. Some cortical cells receive basic touch information from lower parts of the brain (that is, subcortical and brainstem nuclei), some use this basic information to encode information on the texture or shape of touched objects, and some may respond to the magnitude and direction of a tactile stimulus (Bear, Connors, & Paradiso, 2007). Some of the cells in primary somatosensory cortex are even interconnected with cells in primary motor cortex.

The parietal cortex posterior to the primary somatosensory cortex and anterior to the occipital lobe as well as the portion sharing a boundary with the temporal lobe is called the *posterior parietal cortex* (PPC). The PPC contains cell groups that integrate and process different sensory stimuli to create complex sensory experiences; these cells are also involved in the planning of complex motor acts such as reaching, grasping, and tool use (Culham & Valyear, 2006). Recall that primary somatosensory cortex receives information on touch and certain types of pain; what of other sensations and combinations of sensations we experience? For example, the experience of taking care to cross a street when hearing an ambulance siren and then seeing the rapidly approaching vehicle involves an integration of (at least) auditory and visual sensations with the action plan of stepping backward to the curb or sprinting across the street. Discussion of auditory and visual cortex follows below, but here it can be stated that the "primary" information on auditory and visual stimuli arrives in the temporal and occipital lobes, respectively. This information is sent to the PPC where it is analyzed and integrated into increasingly more complex perceptual and action forms. In this sense, the PPC functions as *association cortex*, literally associating different types of sensory stimuli and directing action plans on the basis of this integration.

Two examples of the integrative function of PPC are noteworthy. First, object recognition by the hand requires the ability to identify size, shape, texture, hardness/softness, and other object characteristics.

Activity in primary somatosensory cortex related to these "simple"characteristics of an object is sent to PPC for association and integration, and ultimately recognition of the object. Recognition of an object requires an attachment of meaning to the object's properties. Individuals with damage to PPC may experience *agnosia*, which is the inability to recognize objects even though basic sensory skills (as revealed by a simple test of tactition) appear to be normal. Agnosias may also occur in the visual and auditory modalities. Although basic tests of visual and auditory sensitivity reveal "normal" abilities, the person with damage to PPC may not be able to connect meaning to visual or auditory input.

The second example illustrates the complexity of PPC function in representing the sensations around us. The PPC is a major player in the creation of proper spatial relationships between our bodies and the world. The absence of such relationships can play havoc with our concept of body image and the ability to produce coordinated movements to negotiate or influence an environment. People with damage to PPC in one hemisphere experience a neurological symptom called *hemineglect*, where one side of the body or one-half of the environment is treated as if it doesn't exist. People with hemineglect may dress themselves on only one side of the body, or even reject one of their limbs as belonging to their body. Clinical observations such as these, when a patient is known to have brain damage in PPC, illustrate the complex role of the parietal lobe in the integration and even construction of perceptions.

Two other landmarks on the parietal lobe are shown in Figure 6–5. These are specific regions of parietal association cortex involved in high-level language function. The *angular gyrus* is shown as the dark turquoise region immediately behind and slightly above the back end of the sylvian fissure (see Figure 6–5, lower right). Note the location of the angular gyrus at the boundaries of the parietal, occipital, and temporal lobes. Clinically, lesions of the angular gyrus result in higher-order language deficits (such as the understanding of metaphor) and difficulty with mathematical concepts and performance. An older theory of language and brain functioning imagined the angular gyrus as the site where written language was transformed into an auditory code (Geschwind, 1965). Immediately above and slightly in front of the angular gyrus is the *supramarginal gyrus*, shown in Figure 6–5 (lower right) as a yellow region of PPC. The supramarginal gyrus is thought to be involved in word meaning, the relation of individual speech sounds to the formation of words, and the ability to connect word meanings with action patterns (i.e., to enable the performance of action on verbal command, such as, "Show me how you whistle").

Temporal Lobe

The temporal lobe, shown in blue in Figure 6–5, is located on the lower side of each cerebral hemisphere. Toward the front of each cerebral hemisphere, the sylvian fissure is the boundary between the temporal lobe and the frontal lobe above; toward the back the same fissure separates the temporal lobe from the parietal lobe. The upper part of the temporal lobe has a back boundary with the lower parietal lobe, and the lower parts of the temporal lobe have a boundary with the occipital lobe. These back boundaries are not always clearly defined by prominent fissures on the lateral surface of the hemispheres; the color scheme for the different lobes in Figure 6–5 shows approximate temporal-parietal and temporal-occipital boundaries.

The surface of the temporal lobe visible from the side has three major gyri—superior, medial, and inferior. Immediately below the sylvian fissure is the prominent superior temporal gyrus. As shown in the light blue area of Figure 6–5 (lower right), the upper lip and some surrounding tissue of the superior temporal gyrus is called *primary auditory cortex* or *Heschl's gyrus*. The primary auditory cortex is the first cortical location for processing of auditory signals; more complex processing follows when this initial analysis is forwarded to other locations within the temporal lobe.

The anatomy of primary auditory cortex—Heschel's gyrus—requires additional description with the assistance of a different view of the brain. Imagine drawing an oblique line parallel to and slightly above the sylvian fissure, as shown by the "cut line" in the upper image of Figure 6–7. Think of this line as one edge of a plane cutting through the cerebral hemispheres, dividing them into upper and lower halves. Specifically, this is a horizontal (axial) section angled to follow the "pitch" of the sylvian fissure. Looking down on the cerebral hemispheres from above, when this cut is made and the top half of the hemispheres removed, the top (dorsal) surface of the temporal lobes can be seen (along with the dorsal surfaces of medial structures, not discussed here). This view is shown in the bottom image of Figure 6–7. Recall that the superior temporal gyrus extends medially from its upper lip, like a "shelf" of cortex. This "shelf," previously hidden inside the sylvian fissure, is an important part of the auditory cortex; it is a continuation of the superior temporal gyrus toward the center of the brain. A part of this surface, exposed by the horizontal cut and removal of the top half of the hemispheres, is called the *planum temporale*. The lower image in Figure 6–7 shows, for both hemispheres, the primary auditory cortex (colored salmon) as well as the planum temporale (colored

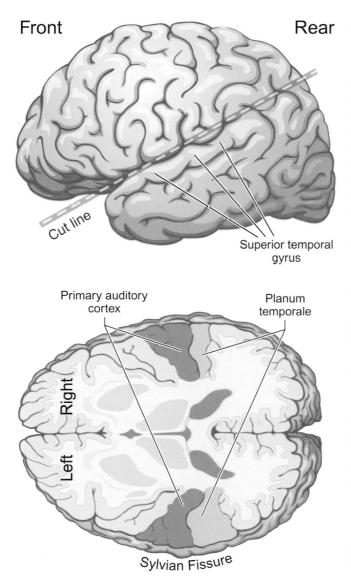

Figure 6–7. Top, lateral surface of left hemisphere, showing an oblique plane whose edge follows the upward tilt of the sylvian fissure; bottom, a view of the dorsal surface of the brain cut into upper and lower parts along this oblique plane. This section shows the "shelf" of auditory cortex inside the sylvian fissure, including the more anterior, primary auditory cortex (*colored salmon*) and the more posterior planum temporale (*colored blue*). Note the larger area of the planum temporale in the left, as compared to right, hemisphere.

blue). In both hemispheres the primary auditory cortex is anterior to the planum temporale. Note the markedly larger surface area of the planum temporale in the left, as compared to right, hemisphere.

The primary auditory cortex and planum temporale have interesting features. First, the cells in primary auditory cortex are arranged systematically with respect to auditory signal frequency; this does not seem to be the case for the planum temporale (Langers, Backe, & van Dijk, 2007). A fundamental aspect of *peripheral* auditory anatomy is the systematic frequency map of sensory receptors embedded within the organ of corti along the extent of the basilar membrane. The basilar membrane is a ribbonlike membrane housed inside the cochlea, the snail shell–like structure in the inner ear. The sensory receptors along the basilar membrane, and specifically within the organ of corti, are called hair cells (because on high-magnification imaging they appear as hairlike structures) and are analogous, as peripheral sensory cells, to rods and cones in the retina. The cochlea spirals from its base to its tip, and the basilar membrane follows this spiral. The systematic frequency map along the basilar membrane can be described in simple terms: the highest frequencies (~20,000 cycles per second) heard by humans are sensed by hair cells at the base of the basilar membrane; moving from the base toward the tip of the membrane the hair cells are sensitive to increasingly lower frequencies. At the tip of the basilar membrane the hair cells are sensitive to the lowest frequency (~20 cycles per second) heard by humans. This systematic frequency representation along the basilar membrane is referred to as *tonotopic representation*.

The tonotopic representation of the basilar membrane is, as suggested above, projected onto the primary auditory cortex. Careful research has shown that, moving in a roughly straight line across cell groups within the primary auditory cortex, cells change their responsiveness from very high frequencies to very low frequencies with the same orderly progression found from base to tip of the basilar membrane. Note the conceptual similarity between the somatotopic representation in primary motor and sensory cortex, and tonotopic representation within the primary auditory cortex. Cells in certain parts of the brain are not jumbled together in a random fashion; rather, they "map" the body (e.g., head to toe) or external stimuli (e.g., high to low frequencies) in an orderly way.

Kandel, Schwartz, and Jessel (2000) have described the primary auditory cortex as a core of cells surrounded by cortical tissue devoted to increasingly higher-level processing of auditory information. This surrounding cortical tissue is called secondary auditory cortex, and the planum temporale falls into this category. The basic characteristics of acoustic signals, such as frequency, intensity, and duration, are analyzed in primary auditory cortex. This basic analysis is sent to surrounding temporal lobe tissue (secondary auditory cortex) for higher-level analyses. A form of higher-level auditory analysis of interest to readers of this chapter is speech and language perception and understanding. The planum temporale is thought to be important to perceptual analysis of speech and language, and the evidence of anatomical asymmetries for this part of the temporal lobe have encouraged the view of this cortical region as important to the natural aptitude among humans to develop and use speech and language. Just posterior to the primary auditory cortex, along the back portion of the superior temporal gyrus, is a region of the temporal lobe (and perhaps the lateroventral portion of the parietal lobe) called *Wernicke's area* (see lower right image in Figure 6–5, dark blue area toward back of the sylvian fissure).

Wernicke's area was originally defined as the brain region associated with speech and language comprehension because postmortem examination of the brains of several patients with a lesion in this area were known, in life, to have had difficulty comprehending spoken language, even though they *produced* speech in a more or less normal way. These patients had what

---

Planum Temporale

The planum temporale has a lofty-sounding name (the *temporal plane*) and a scientific history as murky as lofty ideas tend to be. This wedge of brain tissue (see Figure 6–7) tends to be larger in the left than the right hemisphere in most people, including preverbal infants (Tervaniemi & Hugdahl, 2003). Unfortunately, at least for scientists who enjoy equating size differences with functional differences, chimps also have a larger left than right planum temporale. If only chimps communicated like humans this would not be a theoretical problem. "Oh bother," as Winnie the Pooh might say, if bears could actually talk. In fMRI studies the planum temporale tends to light up on the left side for speech sounds, and on the right side for tones. Some scientists argue that lateralization to the left hemisphere for *detection* of speech sounds can be found in the planum temporale, but that the broader needs of speech processing (extracting meaning from sound sequences) are accomplished bilaterally (Hickok, 2009). Maybe more chimp research can resolve the true role of the planum temporale in human communication: According to Winnie the Pooh, "Some people talk to animals. Not many listen though. That's the problem."

---

appeared to be well-defined lesions at the very back of the sylvian fissure, in the superior temporal gyrus. Dr. Carl Wernicke, a Prussian physician, examined one famous patient when he was alive and on postmortem examination of the brain located the region named for him.

Recent imaging work of the perisylvian (surrounding the sylvian fissure) language areas, and the temporal lobe specifically, during speech perception and language comprehension tasks supports the general ideas outlined above. The primary auditory cortex, roughly in the middle of the upper lip of the superior temporal gyrus, is very active when a person is required to make decisions concerning individual speech sounds, and especially when these decisions do not require word, sentence, or discourse meaning. It is as if this kind of task activates the part of the auditory cortex devoted to analysis of basic signal characteristics. When a person is required to make language input decisions involving meaning, more widespread regions of the temporal lobe are activated. Single word meaning, meaning tied to different levels of grammatical complexity, and very abstract meaning (as in metaphor) engage many different regions of the temporal lobe, as well as regions of the parietal, frontal, and occipital lobes (see Price [2010] for an excellent review of brain imaging and speech and language perception/comprehension).

The anterior part of the temporal lobe and the middle and inferior temporal gyri also seem to play a role in *naming* of objects or actions. Almost certainly, the idea of Wernicke's area as the important temporal lobe location for speech understanding is an oversimplification of the role of the temporal lobe in human communication. More is said about cortical activity in speech and language later in this chapter.

Occipital Lobe

The occipital lobes (colored purple in Figure 6–5) comprise the posterior parts of the cerebral hemispheres; they are the smallest among the four lobes of the brain. The occipital lobes contain primary visual cortex, whose tissue processes information entering the brain through the eyes. Like the auditory cortex, the occipital lobes contain cells that perform basic analysis of visual signals, as well as cells that perform more abstract, elaborate visual processing. The top right image of Figure 6–5 shows the medial wall of one hemisphere, where the *calcarine fissure* divides the occipital lobe into an upper (*cuneus*) and lower (*lingual gyrus*) portion. Primary visual processing is performed by cortical tissue deep within the calcarine fissure. Extensive connections between cells in the calcarine fissure and other cells within the occipital cortex power the more elaborate processing referred to above.

Insula

In Figure 6–8 the left cerebral hemisphere is shown with the lower "lips" of the frontal and parietal lobes and the upper lip of the temporal lobe pulled away to reveal underlying gyri and sulci. The retractable "lips" of the frontal, parietal, and temporal lobes are referred to as *opercula* (singular = *operculum*, from the Latin word for "lid"). The cortex that is revealed when the opercula are retracted is called the *insula* or *insular cortex*. Sometimes the insula is described as part of a fifth hemispheric lobe, the *limbic lobe* (see below). In this chapter the terms insula and insular cortex are used to denote this cortical region without commitment to the notion of the insula as part of a fifth lobe.

The insula appears to be a critical part of cortical tissue engaged in speech and language functions (Ackermann & Riecker, 2010). Clinical cases (where patients with known lesions in and around the insula exhibit certain speech and language difficulties), surgical cases (brain tumors requiring resection of insular tis-

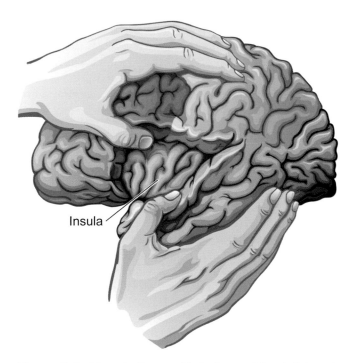

Figure 6–8. View in the sagittal plane of the left hemisphere, showing how the opercula ("lips") of the frontal, parietal, and temporal lobes can be pulled apart to reveal the underlying insula.

Insula

sue), electrical stimulation of exposed brain (in patients who are undergoing brain resections for severe epileptic seizures), and fMRI studies of healthy individuals point to a role for the front part of the insula in speech motor control and possibly in speech perception. These speech functions of the insula appear to be lateralized to the left hemisphere, in much the same way as speech and language functions are lateralized to Broca's and Wernicke's regions in an overwhelming majority of individuals.

The insula also seems to play a role in swallowing, self-awareness, control of heart rate, blood pressure, perception of pain and possibly temperature, unpleasantness of dyspnea (breathing discomfort), as well as other functions related to emotions and general body awareness. As pointed out by Ackermann and Riecker (2010), clinical cases involving isolated lesions of the insula (e.g., as a result of stroke, or surgical resection of a tumor) are very, very rare. Generally, when a stroke or surgical removal of brain tissue involves insular tissue, other nearby areas of the brain (such as regions in and around Broca's area, or parts of the primary auditory cortex, or even fiber tracts below the cortical tissue) are also affected.

Limbic System (Limbic Lobe)

Heimer and Van Hoesen (2006) recommend the term *limbic lobe* to designate the collection of structures within the cerebral hemispheres involved in emotions, motivation, memory, and adaptive functions. Not all authors assign limbic structures the status of a lobe of the cerebral hemispheres, at least in the same sense as the frontal, parietal, temporal, and occipital lobes. In fact, some authors refer to a limbic *system* to reflect a collection of structures within the brain, all of which play an important role, broadly speaking, in emotional and motivational aspects of behavior. Even authors who have argued persuasively for the existence of a limbic lobe, based on similarities in anatomical characteristics and physiological functions of its component structures, say the "system" versus "lobe" debate is not likely to be settled soon (Heimer & Van Hoesen, 2006). For the following brief discussion, the term limbic system is used.

The most easily visualized structures of the limbic system are seen on the medial surface of a hemisphere (see Figure 6–5, top right). The *cingulate gyrus* is one of these structures, forming an incomplete ring above and around the corpus callosum. The ring is partially completed on the lower side of the hemisphere by the upper gyrus of the medial temporal lobe, called the *parahippocampal gyrus* (unlabeled in Figure 6–5, top right: locate the most superior blue gyrus to identify the parahippocampal gyrus). The cingulate and para-hippocampal gyri are part of the cortex, but their cell structure is different from (for example) cells found in the primary motor, primary somatosensory, or association cortex (Heimer & Van Hoesen, 2006). The cell structure of limbic cortical areas in humans may be described as more primitive than the cell structure in many other cortical areas.

Deep within the parahippocampal gyrus of the temporal lobe is a cell group called the *hippocampus*, and another cell cluster called the *amygdala*. These structures are part of the limbic system. In addition, parts of the insula and basal ganglia, as well as cortical structures related to olfaction (sense of smell), and the ventral gyri of the frontal lobe (shown in Figure 6–5, bottom left image) are considered components of the limbic system. These structures are all interconnected, and make connections with the more "sophisticated" parts of the cortex mentioned above as well as with subcortical and brainstem structures.

The sketch presented here of structures and connections of and within the limbic system seems complicated, and also may seem far removed from the concerns of the speech-language pathologist. Nevertheless, its relevance becomes clear when considering disorders such as dementia, a behavioral syndrome characterized by memory loss, behavioral change, and communication impairment. Dementia has a neurobiological basis that largely originates in structures of the limbic system. In addition, limbic structures are often compromised by brain damage sustained in traumatic brain injury (TBI). Communication problems in persons with TBI often include difficulties with social communication (pragmatics) that can be traced at least partially if not largely to limbic system damage.

Cerebral White Matter

The surface of the cerebral hemispheres is made up of many gyri and sulci, some of which have been identified above. This surface topography is composed of gray matter, formed by densely packed clusters of neuronal cell bodies. Cut into the cerebral hemispheres, either by dividing them into left and right halves (a sagittal cut), front and back parts (a coronal cut), or top and bottom parts (a horizontal or transverse cut) and a tremendous volume of white matter is revealed. White matter consists of bundles of myelinated axons running from one group of cell bodies to another group of cell bodies. White matter connects nearby and distant cell groups within the brain.

As described above, a coronal section of the cerebral hemispheres (see Figure 6–3) shows extensive white matter. At any location within the white matter, there are fibers running in many different directions, to and from many different cell groups. Even though fiber tracts are typically "bundled" together, with a given bundle running from a specific group of cell bodies to another specific group of cell bodies, a particular volume of white matter reflects an intermixing of several such bundles. A relatively new brain imaging technique called diffusion tensor imaging (DTI) allows scientists to establish the origin, course, and termination of major fiber tracts in the human brain (see sidetrack on DTI).

DTI research has established a fairly detailed account of fiber bundles within the brain. Much of the following information, including an organizational scheme for classifying fiber bundles within the cerebral hemispheres, is adapted from a review article by Schmahmann, Smith, Eichler, and Filley (2008). Table 6–1 outlines this classification system.

Association Tracts

Association tracts connect one part of the cortex to another, *within the same hemisphere (intrahemispheric)*. These *ipsilateral* connections may consist of small groups of fibers running between adjacent gyri, or between more distantly separated gyri within the same lobe. Of greater importance for the current discussion are several association tracts that are tightly organized, large bundles of axons connecting cortical areas in one lobe to cortical areas in a different lobe. Table 6–2 lists some of these major ipsilateral, interlobe tracts; these tracts are found in both hemispheres, but may have slightly different forms depending on which hemisphere is being examined (see below). The listing of these tracts highlights the extensive interconnectedness of lobes within a single hemisphere; clearly the capability exists for a great deal of information to be shuttled between different parts of the cortex. As discussed toward the end of the chapter, increasing knowledge of the interconnectedness of intrahemispheric lobes (as well as interhemispheric connections, meaning between the hemispheres) is leading scientists away from a "center" oriented view of human behavior (e.g., a focus on Broca's and Wernicke's areas in speech and language performance) to a "network" view, wherein multiple brain locations and pathways are involved as a system to generate complex human behaviors such as speech and language.

Arcuate Fasciculus and Speech and Language Functions. Further consideration of one particular associa-

Table 6–1. A Simple Organizational Scheme for Classifying Tracts (fiber bundles), and Their Principal Connections

FIBER BUNDLE TYPE	CONNECTIONS
Association tracts	*Intra*hemispheric, both within and between lobes
Striatal tracts	From cortex to basal ganglia (principally to caudate and putamen, but also to claustrum), and from cortex to subthalamic nucleus
Commissural tracts	*Inter*hemispheric, from area of one hemisphere to similar area of the other hemisphere
Descending projection tracts	
Corticobulbar	Cortex to cell groups in brainstem
Corticospinal	Cortex to cell groups in spinal cord
Corticothalamic	Widepsread regions of the cortex to cell groups in the thalamus
Ascending projection tracts	
Posterior column medial lemniscal	Spinal cord to brainstem nuclei and thalamus
Anterolateral	Spinal cord to thalamus
Thalamocortical	Cell groups in the thalamus to widespread regions of the cortex

Source: Adapted and modified from Schmahmann et al. (2008).

Table 6–2. Some Association Fiber Tracts and the Lobes They Connect

TRACT	CONNECTIONS
Middle longitudinal fasciculus	Parietal to temporal and frontal lobes Parietal, temporal, and frontal lobes to limbic areas
Inferior longitudinal fasciculus	Occipital to temporal and parietal lobes
Fronto-occipital fasciculus	Occipital and parietal lobes to frontal lobe
Uncinate fasciculus	Temporal to frontal lobes
Superior longitudinal fasciculus (Arcuate fasciculus)	Parietal to frontal lobe (Wernicke-angular-supramarginal-Broca)

Note: In the "connections" column, a description such as "Parietal to Temporal Lobe" does not necessarily mean the fibers go in only one direction.

tion (intrahemispheric) tract is warranted because of its historical and contemporary importance in speech and language functions of the brain. Table 6–2 lists a tract called the *superior longitudinal fasciculus*, the main part of which is the *arcuate fasciculus* (AF) (see Bernal & Ardila, 2009). Figure 6–9 is a DTI reconstruction of the AF, as well as of the inferior longitudinal fasciculus and uncinate fasciculus (compare the course of these latter

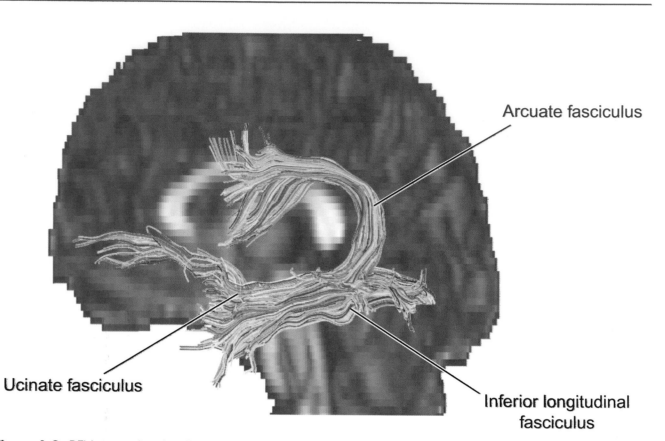

Arcuate fasciculus

Ucinate fasciculus

Inferior longitudinal fasciculus

Figure 6–9. DTI image showing the arcuate fasciculus (the "arched" fiber tract contained within the superior longitudinal fasciculus, which runs from the parietal to the frontal lobe), inferior longitudinal fasciculus (which runs from the occipital to the temporal to the parietal lobe), and the uncinate fasciculus (which runs from the temporal to the frontal lobe).

DTI

Because fiber tracts within the cerebral hemispheres are intermixed and so densely packed, it is difficult to establish the origins, pathways, and destinations of connections between cell groups. Techniques used in animal research, such as introducing certain chemicals into the brain which "label" specific fiber tracts are mostly not usable in human research. Fortunately, a relatively new technique called diffusion tensor imaging (DTI) makes it possible to monitor selected pathways without posing danger to humans. Water molecules move along specific pathways (fiber tracts) in ways that can be identified by proper computer settings of a brain scanner. In region-of-interest techniques, the brain-scanning instrument is directed at the presumed location of specific pathways, and computer reconstructions of the pathways show their extent, volume, and orientation. Conturo et al. (2008) provide an explanation of the DTI technique, and Saur et al. (2008) show how it can be used to understand speech and language connectivity of the brain.

two tracts to the information provided in Table 6–2). The AF is the arched pathway (hence "arcuate") with the one leg of the "bottom" of the arch in the temporal lobe, from which fibers run slightly back and up into the patietal lobe before turning forward to end as the other leg of the arch in the back part of the frontal lobe. Table 6–2 lists four cortical areas connected by the AF, including Wernicke's area (temporal lobe), the angular and supramarginal gyri (parietal lobe), and Broca's area (frontal lobe). This is a more or less standard way to describe the AF, as a fiber tract connecting the receptive language areas (Wernicke's area and possibly parts of the angular and supramarginal gyri) to the expressive area (Broca's area). In fact, the connections as well as the notion of "receptive" and "expressive" language areas of the brain are much more complicated than this simple but appealing picture (Bernal & Ardila, 2009; Catani & Mesulam, 2008).

The AF is emphasized because of its prominent role in theories of speech and language functions in healthy and diseased brains. The most prominent and influential of these theories has been referred to as the Wernicke-Geschwind model (Geschwind, 1965), in which the comprehension area of the brain (Wernicke's area) is connected to the expressive region (Broca's area) by means of the AF. In this model, acoustic properties of spoken words are first analyzed by the listener in the primary auditory cortex, then sent to Wernicke's area to convert this "raw" auditory analysis into meaning. The meaningful phonetic sequences thus identified—the words—can be transferred to Broca's area for production via the AF. In the Wernicke-Geschwind model, this sequence of processing centers (cortical cell bodies) and pathways (fiber tracts) is fully engaged when a person is asked to repeat a word or series of words. The neurologically intact individual has no problem with this task, because she can comprehend meaning (has a healthy primary auditory cortex and Wernicke's area) and transfer the comprehended phonetic information via the AF to the brain region specialized for speech production. Within the context of the repetition task, the model predicts that a damaged Wernicke's area impairs repetition as a result of failure to comprehend; that is, the patient cannot generate a proper, phonetically based "word image" to repeat, even though her brain center for production is perfectly intact (and, even if the primary auditory cortex performs an accurate analysis of the acoustic properties of the incoming speech). A patient with damage to Wernicke's area who is asked to repeat a fairly simple, short sentence may have normal-sounding articulation (consistent with a "healthy" Broca's area) but exchange sounds ("take" instead of "cake"or "burzday" for "birthday") and even make a sentence more complex by adding words and/or additional phrases not included in the target sentence. These errors and complications do not seem to be recognized by the patient, as if she is not monitoring or comprehending what she is saying. On the other hand, the limitation on repetition ability in patients with damage to Broca's area is explained strictly on the basis of impaired pro-

duction skills. Asked to repeat a short sentence including words such as "cake" and "birthday," the patient may struggle to produce the words with hesitations, labored dysfluencies, and an unusually slow speaking rate as evidenced by abnormally long speech sounds. Despite this poor production in the repetition task, the patient demonstrates through comprehension tasks that she knows the words she is supposed to produce.

What are the repetition problems in a patient with undamaged Wernicke's and Broca's areas, but a damaged AF? This patient can, according to the Wernicke-Geschwind model, comprehend and produce speech in a nearly normal way, but cannot transfer the comprehended message between these two cortical "centers." The patient can be shown to have normal comprehension, using nonverbal comprehension tasks such as, "Point to the picture of a dog" (this seems to be a very simple task but in the Wernicke-Geschwind model it is challenging to the patient with damage to Wernicke's area.) The patient with damage isolated to the AF has fluent speech, but within this fluent stream may have numerous sound exchange errors ("take" for "cake") recognized by the patient as mistakes, as revealed by successive attempts to repeat the target utterance to "get it right." What is unique about the patient's repetition performance is her inability to repeat, on command, words and sentences when intact comprehension skills are demonstrated. The patient's spontaneous, conversational speech is likely to be better than her repetition performance.

The speech-language profile of (a) normal spoken language comprehension demonstrated by nonverbal comprehension tests, (b) normal articulation, (c) phonetic errors recognized by the patient when they occur, and (d) poor performance on repetition tasks and especially when repetition involves complex phonetic material such as long (versus short) target utterances, or differences in syllable structure (for example, the word-initial, multiconsonant cluster in the word "struck" makes it more phonetically complex than the word-initial singleton consonant in "tuck"), is thought by many scientists and clinicians to be a result of a *disconnection syndrome*. In this specific case, the disconnection is of Wernicke's from Broca's areas, and the resulting aphasia is called *conduction aphasia*. Several other disconnection syndromes have been discussed in the literature for their potential to disrupt speech and spoken or written language performance. For example, disconnection of the occipital from temporal and parietal cortex, resulting from damage to the inferior longitudinal fasciculus (see Table 6–2; Figure 6–9), may impair the ability to read words even though the cortical tissue is healthy (Epelbaum et al., 2008). More generally, a wide range of white matter diseases, in which fiber tracts are damaged but cortical regions are spared, appears to play a major role in dementia (Schmahmann et al., 2008). Dementia, a disorder of cognition and more specifically of memory and its use in complex tasks such as speech and language, has a high prevalence within the aging population. With respect to speech and language function, white matter clearly matters.

Striatal Tracts

Deep within the cerebral hemispheres there are several clusters of cell bodies, collectively referred to as subcortical nuclei. One group of these nuclei comprise components of the *basal ganglia* (sometimes called *basal nuclei*). The *thalamus*, itself a collection of many nuclei, is another major subcortical nucleus. Beneath the cortical rind of gray matter, these nuclei appear as collections of gray matter within the extensive white matter of the cerebral hemispheres. *Striatal tracts* are fiber tracts connecting the cortical gray matter and these subcortical nuclei. It is useful to think of these fiber tracts as forming a connection loop between cortical and subcortical gray matter structures. This loop plays an important role in motor control, and in speech motor control in particular (and possibly aspects of language production). Also, there are fiber tracts that connect individual nuclei of the basal ganglia, as well as components of the basal ganglia and the thalamus; these also fall under the general category of striatal tracts. Additional detail on the cortical-basal ganglia-thalamus-cortical loop is provided below.

Commissural Tracts

Commissural tracts typically connect a specific region of one hemisphere with its similar topographical region in the other hemisphere. The wording of this description is purposely careful, because of the notion of *lateralization of function*. Brain regions having the same locations in the two hemispheres most likely do not have the same function. For example, Broca's area has a sister region in the right hemisphere, but it is not called Broca's area. Speech and language are assumed to be lateralized to the left hemisphere in about 95% of the population, so at least in the case of human communication the same topographical regions in the two hemispheres do not usually share the same functions. Nevertheless, these two frontal lobe regions are connected across the hemispheres by fibers running in the corpus callosum. The same can be said for the other cortical regions described above — they are all connected across the hemispheres by the corpus callosum,

but the connection does not imply connection for identical function.

The corpus callosum is a massive and complex bundle of fibers. A classic view of the corpus callosum is the one viewed in the midsagittal plane (see Figure 6–5, top right), where the front-to-back extent of the tract appears as a thick length of arched white matter, shaped somewhat like flattened letter "C" turned on its right side. The front-most and back-most parts of the corpus callosum are the *genu* and *splenium*, respectively. Between the genu and splenium is the central, main bulk of the corpus callosum, called the *body*. At the genu, the corpus callosum has a curl of fibers (one end of the "C") pointing slightly downward and toward the back of the cerebral hemispheres; this backward-directed curl is called the *rostrum*.

The front and back reaches of the corpus callosum, as seen in the midsagittal section of the cerebral hemispheres, do not extend to the front and back "poles" (end points) of the hemispheres. Nevertheless, fiber tracts extend from the corpus callosum forward and backward into the most anterior regions of the frontal lobe and most posterior regions of the occipital lobes, connecting these regions across the hemispheres. Finally, although in the midsagittal plane the body of the corpus callosum is beneath cortical tissue, the connecting fibers project upward to reach cortical layers at the top of the hemispheres. The extension of corpus callosum fibers into the front and back parts of the hemispheres, as well as to the top of the cortex, is shown in the sagittal plane, DTI image of Figure 6–10. The "flat" part of the tract, corresponding to the view in Figure 6–5 of the medial part of the corpus callosum, is seen toward the front of the brain in Figure 6–10, and the upcurled fibers reaching to cortical layers are seen all along the length of the tract.

The many millions of fibers (about 200,000,000!) in the corpus callosum have a topographical arrangement. The term *topographical* in this context implies both somatotopicity and systematic fiber arrangement for external signal properties (as in audition and vision). The details of the precise mapping between body parts and/or characteristics of external stimuli and fibers within the corpus callosum are still being worked out (see, for example, Wahl et al. [2007] and Doron and Gazzaniga [2008]), but like the rest of the brain the mapping is orderly.

As shown in Figure 6–5, top right, the rostrum of the corpus callosum terminates its backward path immediately in front of a structure identified as the *anterior commissure*. The anterior commissure is an interhemispheric (commissural) pathway that connects the orbital cortex (frontal lobe) and parts of the tempo-

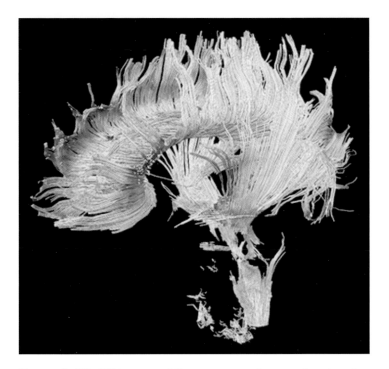

Figure 6–10. DTI image of the corpus callosum, showing the fibers extending up toward the dorsal surface of the hemispheres as well as into anterior and posterior parts of the hemispheres.

ral lobe cortex across the two hemispheres. If a pencil point is placed on the anterior commissure and moved toward the back of the brain along a straight line angled very slightly downward, the pencil line intersects the *posterior commissure* (not shown in Figure 6–5). The posterior commissure is an interhemisphereric (commissural) pathway connecting parts of the brain involved in the reflex response of the eye's pupil to light. The line connecting the anterior and posterior commissures is often used to define a surgical reference plane, especially for the therapeutic placement of intracranial electrodes.

The corpus callosum plays a storied role in the history of disconnection syndromes. As reviewed by Gazzaniga (2000) and Doron and Gazzaniga (2008), various parts of, and in many cases the entire corpus callosum, have been surgically cut to relieve chronic epileptic seizures that cannot be controlled by drugs. Many of these "split-brain" patients, when tested under controlled laboratory conditions, have provided evidence of the different abilities of the two hemispheres and the consequences of not having communication between the hemispheres. In some cases, one side of the brain literally does not know what is going on in the other side of the brain.

Descending Projection Tracts

Descending projection tracts include the descending corticobulbar and corticospinal tracts, as well as tracts running from many cortical regions to the thalamus (corticothalamic tracts, see Table 6–1). Figure 6–11 shows in a schematic coronal view the descending corticobulbar and cotricospinal fiber tracts. The corticobulbar tract ("bulbar" is a term used to indicate the brainstem), represented in Figure 6–11 by the solid pinkish-red and orange lines, includes fibers originating in cortical neuronal cell bodies and making a first synapse in one of the several brainstem motor nuclei; in short, this tract connects cortical neurons to neurons in the brainstem. The corticospinal tract, represented in Figure 6–11 by the dashed blue lines, includes fibers originating in the cortex and making a first synapse in motor cells of the spinal cord; this tract connects neurons in the cortex to the motor neurons in the ventral spinal cord. Many of these brainstem nuclei and cells in the spinal cord issue axons that leave the CNS to innervate the many muscles of the body.

As the corticobulbar and corticospinal tracts descend from the cortex to lower regions of the CNS their *location* within the brain is designated by use of

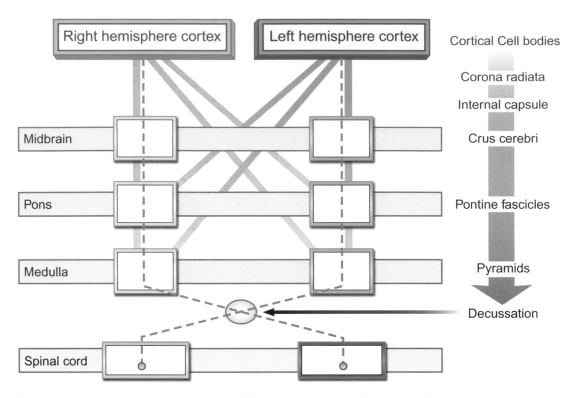

Figure 6–11. Schematic coronal view of the descending corticobulbar (*thicker pink and orange lines*) and corticospinal (*dashed blue lines*). The corticobulbar tracts are both ipsilateral and contralateral, sending axons to brainstem nuclei on the same and opposite side as their cortical origin. The corticospinal tract is primarily contralateral, crossing at the decussation of the pyramids and sending axons to ventral horn nuclei in the spinal cord on the side opposite the cortical origin.

different terms. For example, fibers of the two tracts issue from cell bodies all over the cortex and form a fanlike pattern called the *corona radiata*. The fibers of the corona radiata contribute to a good portion of the white matter immediately below the cortex. The corona radiata are represented schematically in Figure 6–11, and in the more anatomically correct image of Figure 6–12. As the fibers in the corona radiata descend they gather into a relatively tight bundle that passes between subcortical nuclei to reach the more inferior brainstem. The sagittal view in Figure 6–12 shows the corona radiata merging into this tight bundle. This part of the descending tracts, where the corticobulbar and corticospinal tracts pass between the medial thalamus and caudate nucleus, and the lateral lentiform (globus pallidus and putamen) nucleus, is called the *internal capsule* (see Figure 6–11 for location of internal capsule as the tract descends the brain).

The coronal slices in previous figures show the internal capsule at a single location along the front-to-back extent of the cerebral hemispheres (e.g., top right of Figures 6–2 and 6–3, not labeled in the figures). A greater appreciation for the distribution of these fiber

tracts is gained from careful examination of Figure 6–12 (upper left), where the front of the head is toward the left of the image. Here the cortical tissue has been stripped away to reveal the fibers of the corona radiata and internal capsule. Even though the internal capsule is the tightly focused merger of the many fibers of the corona radiata, the internal capsule can be described as having an anterior, middle, and posterior part (IC = internal capsule in Figure 6–12). The precise location of a coronal slice therefore determines which part of the internal capsule is displayed. Like so many other parts of the brain, the internal capsule is not a random jumble of fibers, but rather is arranged systematically based on the cortical origin of the fibers. In a horizontal (axial) slice (inset, lower right of Figure 6–12; the anterior part of the brain is toward the top of the image) the internal capsule in each hemisphere has a boomerang shape with the "angle" of the boomerang most medial and the two arms extending away from this angle anterolaterally and posterolaterally. To provide a rough idea of the systematic arrangement of fibers within the internal capsule, most corticobulbar fibers associated with control of facial, jaw, tongue, velopharyngeal, and

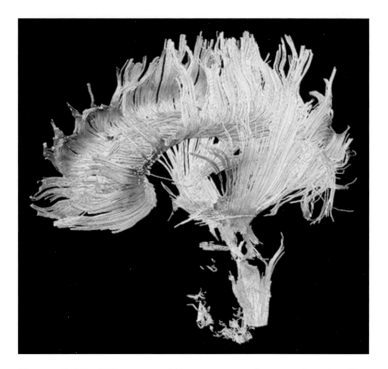

Figure 6-10. DTI image of the corpus callosum, showing the fibers extending up toward the dorsal surface of the hemispheres as well as into anterior and posterior parts of the hemispheres.

ral lobe cortex across the two hemispheres. If a pencil point is placed on the anterior commissure and moved toward the back of the brain along a straight line angled very slightly downward, the pencil line intersects the *posterior commissure* (not shown in Figure 6–5). The posterior commissure is an interhemisphereric (commissural) pathway connecting parts of the brain involved in the reflex response of the eye's pupil to light. The line connecting the anterior and posterior commissures is often used to define a surgical reference plane, especially for the therapeutic placement of intracranial electrodes.

The corpus callosum plays a storied role in the history of disconnection syndromes. As reviewed by Gazzaniga (2000) and Doron and Gazzaniga (2008), various parts of, and in many cases the entire corpus callosum, have been surgically cut to relieve chronic epileptic seizures that cannot be controlled by drugs. Many of these "split-brain" patients, when tested under controlled laboratory conditions, have provided evidence of the different abilities of the two hemispheres and the consequences of not having communication between the hemispheres. In some cases, one side of the brain literally does not know what is going on in the other side of the brain.

Descending Projection Tracts

Descending projection tracts include the descending corticobulbar and corticospinal tracts, as well as tracts running from many cortical regions to the thalamus (corticothalamic tracts, see Table 6–1). Figure 6–11 shows in a schematic coronal view the descending corticobulbar and cotricospinal fiber tracts. The corticobulbar tract ("bulbar" is a term used to indicate the brainstem), represented in Figure 6–11 by the solid pinkish-red and orange lines, includes fibers originating in cortical neuronal cell bodies and making a first synapse in one of the several brainstem motor nuclei; in short, this tract connects cortical neurons to neurons in the brainstem. The corticospinal tract, represented in Figure 6–11 by the dashed blue lines, includes fibers originating in the cortex and making a first synapse in motor cells of the spinal cord; this tract connects neurons in the cortex to the motor neurons in the ventral spinal cord. Many of these brainstem nuclei and cells in the spinal cord issue axons that leave the CNS to innervate the many muscles of the body.

As the corticobulbar and corticospinal tracts descend from the cortex to lower regions of the CNS their *location* within the brain is designated by use of

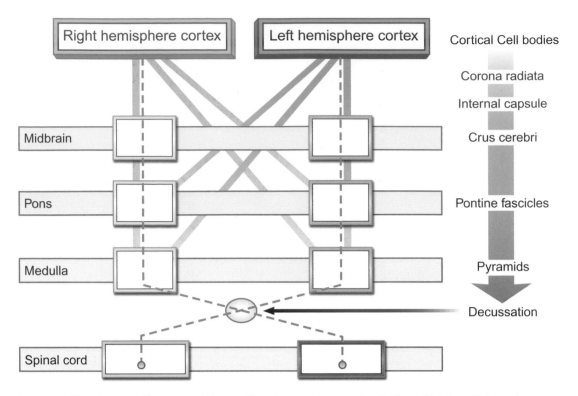

Figure 6–11. Schematic coronal view of the descending corticobulbar (*thicker pink and orange lines*) and corticospinal (*dashed blue lines*). The corticobulbar tracts are both ipsilateral and contralateral, sending axons to brainstem nuclei on the same and opposite side as their cortical origin. The corticospinal tract is primarily contralateral, crossing at the decussation of the pyramids and sending axons to ventral horn nuclei in the spinal cord on the side opposite the cortical origin.

different terms. For example, fibers of the two tracts issue from cell bodies all over the cortex and form a fanlike pattern called the *corona radiata*. The fibers of the corona radiata contribute to a good portion of the white matter immediately below the cortex. The corona radiata are represented schematically in Figure 6–11, and in the more anatomically correct image of Figure 6–12. As the fibers in the corona radiata descend they gather into a relatively tight bundle that passes between subcortical nuclei to reach the more inferior brainstem. The sagittal view in Figure 6–12 shows the corona radiata merging into this tight bundle. This part of the descending tracts, where the corticobulbar and corticospinal tracts pass between the medial thalamus and caudate nucleus, and the lateral lentiform (globus pallidus and putamen) nucleus, is called the *internal capsule* (see Figure 6–11 for location of internal capsule as the tract descends the brain).

The coronal slices in previous figures show the internal capsule at a single location along the front-to-back extent of the cerebral hemispheres (e.g., top right of Figures 6–2 and 6–3, not labeled in the figures). A greater appreciation for the distribution of these fiber tracts is gained from careful examination of Figure 6–12 (upper left), where the front of the head is toward the left of the image. Here the cortical tissue has been stripped away to reveal the fibers of the corona radiata and internal capsule. Even though the internal capsule is the tightly focused merger of the many fibers of the corona radiata, the internal capsule can be described as having an anterior, middle, and posterior part (IC = internal capsule in Figure 6–12). The precise location of a coronal slice therefore determines which part of the internal capsule is displayed. Like so many other parts of the brain, the internal capsule is not a random jumble of fibers, but rather is arranged systematically based on the cortical origin of the fibers. In a horizontal (axial) slice (inset, lower right of Figure 6–12; the anterior part of the brain is toward the top of the image) the internal capsule in each hemisphere has a boomerang shape with the "angle" of the boomerang most medial and the two arms extending away from this angle anterolaterally and posterolaterally. To provide a rough idea of the systematic arrangement of fibers within the internal capsule, most corticobulbar fibers associated with control of facial, jaw, tongue, velopharyngeal, and

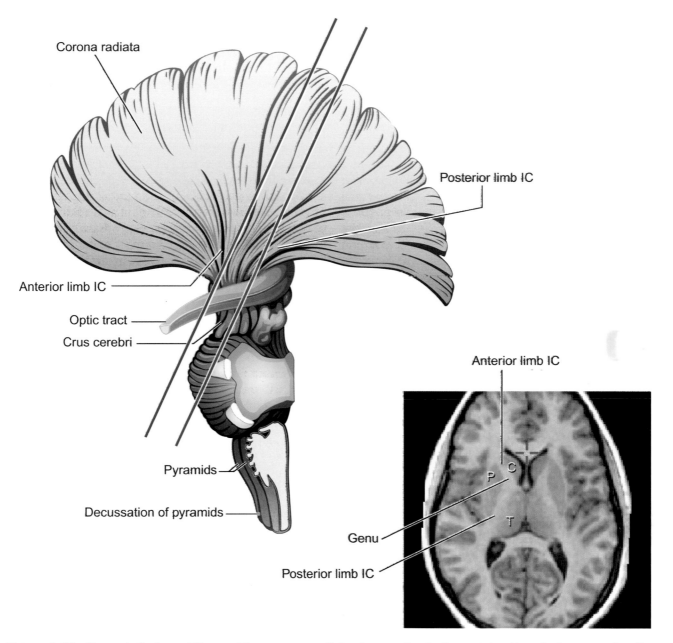

Figure 6-12. *Upper left*, view of fibers of the corona radiata descending in the cerebral hemispheres and gathering into a narrow bundle called the internal capsule (IC) to pass between several subcortical nuclei, en route to the brainstem. *Lower right*, horizontal section of cerebral hemispheres showing the "boomerang" shape of the internal capsule. The anterior and posterior limbs plus the genu of the internal capsule are labeled. C = caudate nucleus; P = putamen; T = thalamus.

laryngeal muscles run through a compact bundle close to or within the angle (called the genu) of the internal capsule. On the other hand, fibers descending to motorneurons in the spinal cord are mostly located in the posterior arm (called the "posterior limb") of the internal capsule, and within that limb the fibers for the legs are most posterior, and those for the arms are closer to the angle. These are illustrations of the systematic arrangement of fibers within the internal capsule, and are not meant to be exhaustive. For example, fibers running to the cortex from the thalamus also form parts of the internal capsule (see section below on Ascending Projection Tracts).

Descending fibers leave the internal capsule and continue their downward path in the *cerebral peduncles*, a tract in the central part of the midbrain. The largest portion of these fibers runs in the *crus cerebri*, an anterior part of the cerebral peduncles (the terms "cerebral peduncles" and "crus cerebri" are occasionally used interchangeably; see Figure 6–12). The fibers then continue through the pons in small bundles, or fascicles, and are gathered back together in the medulla as the pyramids. Some descending fibers in the cerebral peduncles, pontine fascicles, and medulla leave the descending tract to make synapses with motor nuclei in the midbrain, pons, and medulla; these fibers belong to the corticobulbar tract and the synapses they make within the brainstem define the termination of this tract. The fibers continuing into the spinal cord belong to the corticospinal tract; these make synapses in the ventral gray matter of the spinal cord, where spinal motorneurons are found.

The general routes of the corticobulbar and corticospinal tracts are summarized in Figure 6–11; a slightly more detailed representation of the corticobulbar tract is provided in Figure 6–13. For the sake of simplicity, Figure 6–13 shows connections originating from only a single hemisphere (the right hemisphere; the connections for the left would be a mirror image of the ones shown; the view is as if you are looking at a person's ventral surface). The lines are shown terminating at each of the three levels of the brainstem (midbrain, pons, medulla), indicating the presence of motor nuclei at each level (see section below on Cranial Nerves and Associated Brainstem Nuclei).

In Figure 6–13, the solid pink lines represent *bilateral* innervation of cell bodies in the brainstem by cortical cell bodies. In other words, cells in the cortex of one hemisphere—say, those controlling contraction of the *palatal levator* muscle, the muscle that lifts the soft palate and pulls it back toward the posterior pharyngeal wall—are connected by corticobulbar fibers to the nucleus containing palatal levator motoneurons on *both* sides of the brainstem. Bilateral innervation means

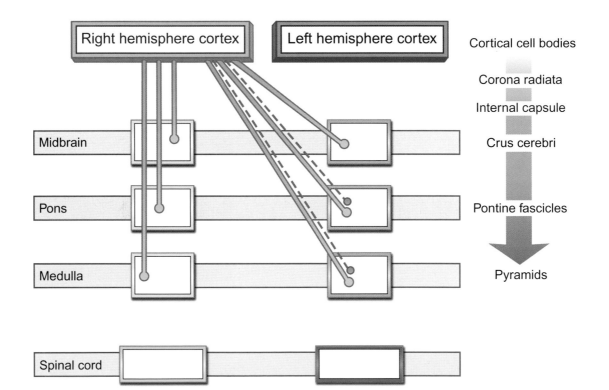

Figure 6-13. Schematic coronal view of the descending corticobulbar tracts, showing patterns of ipsilateral and contralateral connections from cortex to levels of the brainstem. Only the connections from the right hemisphere are shown; connections from the left hemisphere are mirror images of these. Bilateral connections (both ipsilateral and contralateral connections) are indicated by the solid pink lines; these are made from cortex to all three levels of the brainstem (midbrain, pons, medulla). Exclusively contralateral connections are indicated by the dashed lines; these are made from the cortex to nuclei in the pons and medulla. See Table 6–5 for specific details.

that there is an ipsilateral (same side) and contralateral (opposite side) connection. This is shown in Figure 6–13 by solid lines extending from the right hemisphere to the right (ipsilateral) and left (contralateral) sides of the brainstem, at all three levels.

The overall innervation pattern in the corticobulbar tract is mostly, but not exclusively, bilateral. Figure 6–13 shows by dashed lines exclusively contralateral connections between cortical cells in the right hemisphere and the pons and medulla levels of the *left* brainstem. Certain brainstem nuclei, or parts of nuclei, are innervated only by fibers arising in the cortex of the opposite hemisphere. These general facts concerning the connection patterns in the corticobulbar tract are considered in greater detail below in the section on cranial nerves. As explained in that section, knowledge of the bilateral and contralateral connection pattern in the corticobulbar tract has substantial value to the practicing speech-language pathologist.

The paths of the corticospinal tracts are shown in the schematic drawing of Figure 6–11, and in Figure 6–14 for one side of the brain. Fibers from each hemisphere run on their respective sides until the majority of fibers from one side (about 80%) cross to the other side at the decussation of the pyramids, a landmark on the ventral surface of the medulla created by the crossing fibers (see below, Figure 6–20). The fact that so many fibers from one cerebral hemisphere eventually travel in the spinal cord on the side opposite to their cortical origin, and innervate motor neurons on that opposite side, accounts for the well-known fact that the left hemisphere controls limbs on the right side, and the right hemisphere controls limbs on the left side. In Figure 6–14, the descent of the corticospinal tract through the internal capsule and to its crossover point within the inferior medulla is summarized by the pathway of the green line.

Ascending Projection Tracts

Ascending fiber tracts are typically associated with sensory pathways, which can be thought of as projection tracts from points below to points above. Sensory events begin in some end organ of the body, which may include touch, pressure, vibration, pain, temperature, taste, odor, light, and sound receptors. When these receptors are stimulated, an impulse is sent from them to a ganglion (a first synapse along a sensory pathway located outside the CNS but close to the entry point near the spinal cord or brainstem).

The somatosensory pathways constitute a major portion of the ascending projection tracts. These tracts run in the opposite direction from the descending pro-

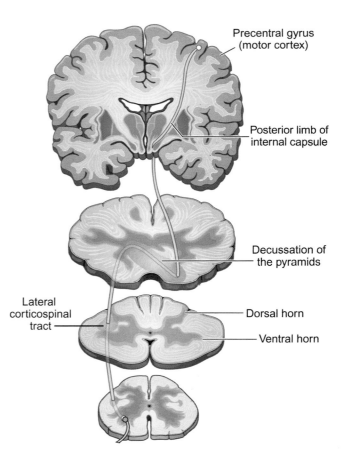

Figure 6–14. Pathway of corticospinal tract. The green pathway shows the tract originating in the cortex of one hemisphere and descending on the same side until it reaches the medulla where about 80% of the fibers cross over to the opposite side to descend in the lateral corticospinal tract. The pathway on the other side of the hemisphere is a mirror image of the one shown. Descending fibers leave the corticospinal tract at all segments of the spinal cord to make synapses with ventral horn cells (spinal motor neurons). The purple fiber shown leaving the spinal cord at the lowest level represents axons sent via peripheral nerves to muscles.

jection tracts. The "points below" mentioned in the preceding paragraph are the end organs, where stimuli are sensed, and the "points above" include several synapses along the ascending pathway with a final destination in the cortex.

There are two major somatosensory pathways for stimuli sensed below the neck (that is, on the torso or limbs). One of these, the posterior column-medial lemniscal tract (Blumenfeld, 2010), carries sensory information from one side of the body. This sensory information enters the spinal cord after making a first synapse in a dorsal root ganglion. The fibers entering the spinal cord run up the same side of the body until reaching the dorsal part of the medulla (the lowest part of the brainstem, at the top of the spinal cord) where the fibers make a synapse and then cross to the opposite side to run up through the brainstem and thalamus before terminating in the primary sensory cortex and surrounding areas. This means that sensation from one side of the body is processed in the cortex on the opposite side of the brain. Note the parallel to the corticospinal tract, one of the major descending projection tracts described above. The descending corticospinal tract crosses over on the ventral surface of the medulla whereas the ascending posterior column-medial lemniscus tract crosses over in the dorsal (posterior) part of the medulla. This ascending tract carries information on fine touch, vibration, and joint position.

A second ascending pathway for sensory stimuli entering the spinal cord is called the anterolateral tract. This tract carries information on pain, temperature, and "crude" touch (Blumenfeld, 2010), and, like the posterior column-medial lemniscus tract, conveys this information to the cortex on the side opposite to the stimulation. An important difference from the posterior column-medial lemniscus tract is the crossover point—the decussation—for pain/temperature/crude touch fibers entering the spinal cord. These latter fibers cross over to the other side of the spinal cord almost immediately after entering the cord, roughly at the level of entry; the fibers then ascend in the anterolateral tract on the side opposite their entry point. Recall that the posterior column-medial lemniscus fibers ascend in the spinal cord on the *same* side of entry before crossing over in the posterior medulla. The difference in decussation points for these two major ascending tracts has important clinical implications when trying to localize a lesion.

Both the posterior column-medial lemniscus and anterolateral tracts eventually send their information to the thalamus, where synapses are made and fibers sent to the cortex. In addition, visual and auditory ascending fibers, carrying information from the retina (vision) and hair cells (audition), also make a final synapse in the thalamus before projecting to the visual and auditory cortical areas. This mass of thalamocortical fibers, or projections, are given special note in the current discussion because they are part of the white matter seen within the cerebral hemispheres. The internal capsule and the corona radiata include these ascending fibers. Typically, then, any region of white matter in the cerebral hemispheres includes a mix of descending and ascending pathways as well as fibers running to and from the cortex and striatum, and cortex and cerebellum. The interwined, dense, multimillion fiber nature of the white matter requires special techniques to determine where fibers originate, and where they

end (see sidetrack on "DTI"). This mixing of so many fiber types within any given region of white matter also means that white matter disease, such as occurs in certain dementias, is likely to produce multiple symptoms associated with multiple "systems" within the brain that send and receive axon bundles for transmission of important information.

SUBCORTICAL NUCLEI AND CEREBELLUM

The subcortical nuclei include the various structures of the basal ganglia (also referred to as the basal nuclei), the thalamus, the hypothalamus, and other structures of the limbic system (such as the amygdala and septal nuclei). The cerebellum is subcortical, but is typically discussed separately from subcortical structures. In this section the focus is on the basal ganglia, thalamus, and cerebellum.

Basal Ganglia

The basal ganglia include the caudate and putamen nuclei (which together constitute the striatum), the globus pallidus (which paired with the putamen is referred to as the lenticular or lentiform nucleus), the subthalamic nucleus, and the substantia nigra. Technically, the substantia nigra is not a subcortical nucleus (that is, below the cortex but within the cerebral hemispheres) but rather a brainstem nucleus, because it is located in the ventral midbrain (see below, Figure 6–23). The substantia nigra is included here as a subcortical nucleus because of its close anatomical and functional connection with the striatum and subthalamic nucleus. Although different texts may include different combinations of structures within the basal ganglia, the nuclei described here as basal ganglia structures are fairly "standard" in the sense of their consistent inclusion in anatomical and functional accounts of this important sensorimotor *system*.

The gross anatomy of the basal ganglia is best appreciated in two views, one coronal and the other sagittal. Figure 6–15 (left) shows a coronal slice of a fixed human brain, the slice roughly midway between the front and back of the brain. The fixing technique shows the traditional shading difference between nuclei and tracts, with nuclei appearing darker and fiber tracts lighter. The caudate, putamen, globus pallidus, substantia nigra, and subthalamic nucleus are labeled on the left side of the brain, as is the thalamus (the same structures are labeled on the right side image

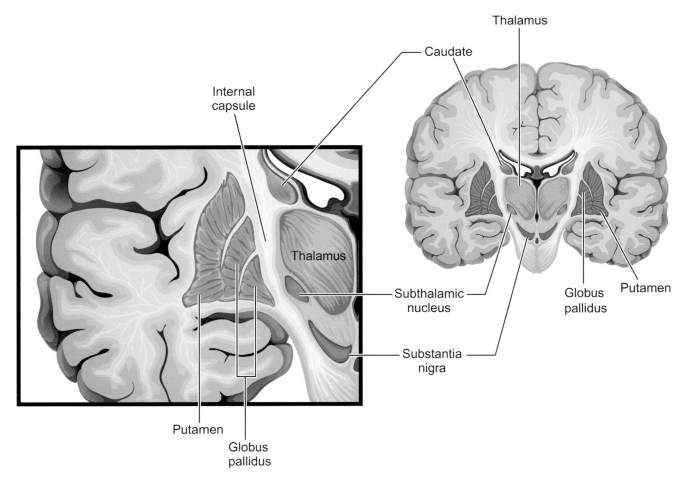

Figure 6–15. Structures of the basal ganglia shown in a coronal slice of a fixed human brain.

in Figure 6–15 in the artists's rendition of the slice). The thalamus is not considered a basal ganglia structure but is shown here for orientation purposes and because of its role in the processing of basal ganglia function (see below). Note the location of the putamen, deep to the insula; in this coronal slice the putamen is the most lateral of the basal ganglia structures. Just medial to the putamen is the globus pallidus, and together these two structures form a curved, lenslike mass of cells, explaining why the combined nuclei are called the lentiform or lenticular nucleus. Superior and medial to the lentiform nucleus and just lateral to the lateral ventricle is the caudate nucleus, which appears in this slice as a small, oval mass. Recall that the caudate and putamen are together called the striatum—note how the superior tip of the putamen is "pointing" toward the caudate (the significance of the caudate-putamen proximity is explained in the next paragraph). Inferior and medial to the lentiform nucleus is the aptly named subthalamic nucleus (note its position relative to the

massive thalamus). Inferior to the subthalamic nucleus, the relatively long, oblique strip of darkened tissue is the substantia nigra, located ventrally in the superior part of the midbrain.

Also not labeled in Figure 6–15 is a pale white strip of tissue—a fiber tract— separating the lentiform nucleus from the more medial caudate, thalamus, subthalamic nucleus and substantia nigra. Much of this fiber tract is composed of the corticospinal and corticobulbar tracts, in which information from cortical cells is conveyed to nuclei in the brainstem and spinal cord as well as to structures of the basal ganglia. The tract also includes fibers carrying sensory information from the thalamus to the cortex, and from brainstem structures to structures of the basal ganglia. The part of this tract running through the basal ganglia structures is the internal capsule (see Figure 6–12). The internal capsule is an important anatomical landmark, and often figures prominently in deficits resulting from stroke (see below, Blood Supply of the Brain).

Basal Ganglia or Basal Nuclei?

Language usage is *conventional*. If a sufficient number of people agree on the meaning of a word or phrase, its meaning is established, and technical analysis of language is, well, meaningless. This textbook is about speech; in German speech is *sprache*, in French *parle*, in Mandarin Chinese *yanyu*, in Korean *mal*, in Russian *rech*. No one of these words captures the idea of "speech" more accurately than any other, no one of the words is intrinsically "right." The words mean "speech" because speakers of the languages agree on the meaning. So it is with the term "basal ganglia." However, this is a more delicate example of the conventional nature of language usage, because it is confined to one language, English. "Basal ganglia" is technically a misnomer because a ganglion is a cluster of cell bodies just outside of the CNS, and the components of the basal ganglia (caudate, putamen, and so forth) are within the CNS. In a grave statement issued in 1998, the International Federation of Associations of Anatomists (IFAA) declared that the term basal *nuclei* should be used for this collection of structures due to the obvious error of referring to these cell groups as *ganglia* (Sarikcioglu, Altun, Suzen, & Oguz, 2008). Unfortunately for the IFAA, most scientists do not seem to be paying attention: in a PubMed search done by one of your authors on July 30, 2012, using the keywords "basal ganglia" and restricting the search from 2000 to the present (giving the scientific community plenty of time to respect the 1998 proclamation by IFAA), 12,956 "hits" were registered. In contrast, the keywords "basal nuclei" produced only 180 hits. In this text, we side with the majority, choosing convention over technical accuracy. We choose and use the term "basal ganglia."

The specific appearance of basal ganglia structures, and in some cases the presence of a structure in a particular coronal slice, depends substantially on the location of the slice along the anteroposterior axis of the cerebral hemispheres. A conceptual appreciation for this dependency can be gained by studying Figure 6–16 (the front of the brain is to the left), a sagittal-view drawing of the complex configuration of basal ganglia structures. Cerebral cortex and cerebral white matter have been eliminated from the figure,

leaving the structures of the basal ganglia "floating" free from their moorings within the cerebral hemispheres. Note the "C"-shaped form of the caudate nucleus, how the nucleus is quite massive toward the front of the hemispheres and narrows as it curls toward the back of the brain and turns around to point forward. The tail of the caudate nucleus points so far forward it terminates ventral to the globus pallidus. The image also shows the caudate and putamen nuclei joined at the anterior end of the nuclei, and splitting apart as the image is viewed from right to left (that is, from anterior to posterior within the cerebral hemispheres). The channel between the caudate and putamen, created as they separate, is the internal capsule. Note the strands of light pink tissue "bridging" the spaces between the caudate and putamen, running across the region where the descending and ascending fibers of the internal capsule are located. Especially in coronal slices taken near the anterior edge of the basal ganglia, these strands appear as gray streaks across the white matter of the internal capsule. This streaked or striated appearance of the internal capsule gives the name striatum to the putamen and caudate nuclei. The sagittal view also shows the globus pallidus in relation to the more lateral putamen, and the complex spatial configurations of the other nuclei discussed above.

The complexity of basal ganglia structures extends to their interconnections, as well as their connections to other parts of the CNS. These connections are shown schematically, and in a simplified way, in Figure 6–17. The boxes containing structure names represent nuclei (clusters of cell bodies) and the arrows represent fiber tracts connecting nuclei or cell groups in the cortex to other nuclei or cortical cell groups. The thick purple arrows show the main loop by which information is delivered from the cortex to the striatum, through the globus pallidus. The globus pallidus is the primary "output" of the basal ganglia, integrating all the processing done in this group of subcortical nuclei and sending it to the thalamus. The thalamus returns the information received from the globus pallidus to the cortical areas from which the input to the striatum was derived, completing what is often referred to as the cortico-striatal-cortical loop.

Cortical input to the striatum includes not only motor areas of the frontal cortex (both primary and premotor cortex, as well as the supplementary motor area), but also limbic cortex and occipital cortex. Note also in Figure 6–17 the direct connection between the cortex and the subthalamic nucleus. An interesting feature of the basal ganglia is that there are no direct projections—that is, no direct pathways—connecting

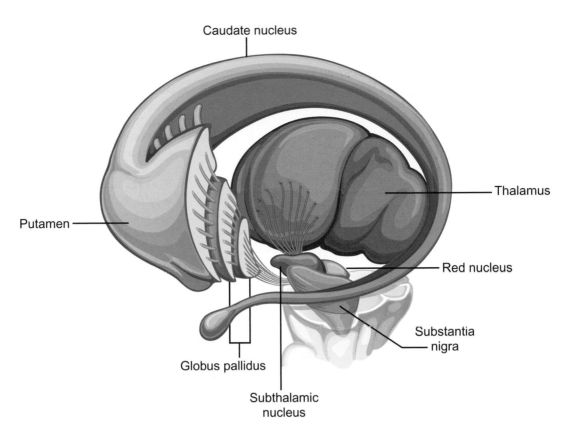

Figure 6-16. Sagittal-view drawing of the complex configuration of basal ganglia and adjacent structures. Front is to the left, green lines show fiber tracts running between the nuclei. The light pink strands toward the front of the basal ganglia structures show cell body connections between the anterior caudate and putamen.

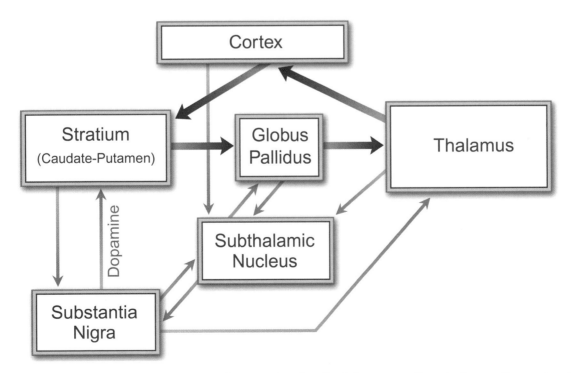

Figure 6-17. Schematic box-and-arrows diagram showing the interconnections between the cortex, basal ganglia structures, and thalamus. The boxes represent cortical cells and subcortical nuclei, the arrows represent fiber tracts. The major cortico-striatal-cortical loop is shown by structures connected by thick, purple arrows.

these subcortical nuclei to the motor nuclei of the brainstem of the spinal cord. The role of the basal ganglia in motor behavior is best thought of as one of modifying the eventual code issued from the motor cortex to the motor neurons of the brainstem and spinal cord, via the corticobulbar and corticspinal tracts.

Figure 6–17, even as a simplified version of connections among basal ganglia nuclei, and from them to other parts of the brain, appears complicated. However, several basic statements can be made to clarify the anatomical facts and functional roles of the basal ganglia in both limb and speech motor control. First, the cortico-striatal-cortical loop provides a pathway to "cycle" movement information between the cortex and basal ganglia, and in so doing refines the selection, activation, and timing of motor programs and direct commands from cells in the primary motor cortex. The concept of a "motor program" is of a *plan* for the activation of muscles, both over time and in terms of force of activation. Such a plan or program (much like a computer program) can exist without being put into action (see the concluding section of the chapter for more on speech motor programs versus execution of speech gestures). The idea of activity in the loop refining a motor program, and especially a program with a fair degree of complexity, is important because many authors have argued for the critical role of the basal ganglia in learning skilled movement and in packaging these skills as efficient units to be "turned on" or "turned off" at appropriate times (see Nambu, 2008). In fact, a very broad description of the role of the basal ganglia in motor control is that it facilitates or inhibits motor activity, depending on the nature of neuronal activity in the loop (Obeso & Lanciego, 2011).

Second, there are several bidirectional connections between nuclei of the basal ganglia, including two-way connections between the subthalamic nucleus and substantia nigra, the striatum and substantia nigra, and globus pallidus and subthalamuc nucleus. Moreover, information not only flows from the basal ganglia to the thalamus and then to the cortex, but from the thalamus to the basal ganglia (see arrow in Figure 6–17 from thalamus to subthalamic nucleus). The bidirectionality of connections is therefore not only found within the basal ganglia, but between the basal ganglia and its main output "target" (that is, the thalamus). The extensive, bidirectional connections within the basal ganglia and the potential influence of the thalamus on basal ganglia activity emphasize the difficulty of assigning a particular function to a particular structure within the basal ganglia. Thus, it is difficult to say that a lesion in a particular structure of the basal ganglia results in a very specific and unique motor deficit. The basal ganglia are a highly integrated system in which different lesion locations may produce very similar symptoms and signs. A good example of this is the difficulty of isolating separate lesion correlates of signs such as dystonia, athetosis, tics, and myoclonic jerks, all of which are involuntary movements that have been attributed to basal ganglia disease.

Third, several neurotransmitters are important for normal basal ganglia function, the best-known of which is dopamine. Dopamine is manufactured by cells in the substantia nigra, and conveyed to the striatum via the nigrostriatal pathway (in Figure 6–17 this pathway is labeled "Dopamine"). The neuropathology of Parkinson disease includes, as a major component, the death of dopamine-producing cells in the substantia nigra. The loss of dopamine production in the substantia nigra results in a deficit of usable dopamine in the striatum. Interestingly, more than half of the dopamine-producing cells of the substantia nigra can be lost before the typical signs and symptoms of Parkinson disease first appear. The signs include tremor, slowness and reduction of movement, and stiff limbs (in Parkinson disease the stiffness is referred to by the term "rigidity," which is a type of elevated muscle tone). The loss of dopamine is clearly connected with these signs, but the precise effect of dopamine reduction on the occurrence and severity of the signs is not fully understood. Generally, the presence of dopamine in the striatum is thought to control the excitability of striatal neurons (how easily they are depolarized by afferent connections from the cortex). A deficit in this excitability makes the striatum less "active," which may partially explain why people with Parkinson disease move less and more slowly, and why dopamine-replacement therapy relieves these signs (and the symptoms, as well).

Fourth, and finally, much is known about the basal ganglia and its role in motor behavior, but much is unknown as well. For example, Figure 6–17 shows a *direct* projection from the motor cortex to the subthalamic nucleus but little is known about the functional significance of this connection. Scientists are very interested in this connection because the subthalamic nucleus is the preferred insertion target for electrodes used in deep brain stimulation (DBS), a surgical approach to relieving some of the signs and symptoms of Parkinson disease. Obeso and Lanciego (2011), Nambu (2008), and Postuma and Dagher (2006) provide excellent reviews of the anatomical and functional connections of basal ganglia structures.

Lesions of basal ganglia structures are known to produce speech disorders. These are speech disorders included under the larger category of "motor speech disorders," and in the case of basal ganglia damage may include hypokinetic dysarthria (a form of dysarthria thought to be the result of small and slow move-

Deep Brain Stimulation

Deep brain stimulation (DBS) is one therapeutic approach to relieving the symptoms and signs of Parkinson disease. Neurosurgeons implant an electrode in a selected basal ganglia structure and attach the electrode to an external stimulator that is under the control of the doctor and patient. In Parkinson disease, the typical (but certainly not the only) sites for implantation of the electrode are the subthalamic nucleus or globus pallidus (see Figure 6–17). The idea is that these nuclei are overactive in Parkinson disease, producing an inhibitory effect on the output of the basal ganglia which results in the slow, small movements associated with the disease. Electrical stimulation of an implanted electrode acts like a lesion, calming down the activity of the cells and reducing the amount of inhibition of motor behavior. The good news is that there is ample evidence that DBS improves limb function in Parkinson disease. The not-so-good news is that DBS comes with a host of negative side effects, including (possibly) depression, cognitive decline, sleep problems, anxiety, and *worsening* of the dysarthria associated with Parkinson disease. See Fasano, Daniele, and Albanese (2012) for an excellent review of all these issues.

ments of speech structures, such as the tongue, lips, and jaw; hypokinetic dysarthria is usually associated with Parkinson disease), hyperkinetic dysarthria (a form of dysarthria thought to be the result of uncontrolled muscle tone or excessive, sudden, and/or rhythmic contraction of muscle groups within the speech apparatus), and possibly even apraxia of speech (a disorder in which the programming of speech sequences is disturbed, even though the speech muscles are able to perform normally in oromotor, nonverbal tasks such as maximum strength efforts). Textbooks including Duffy (2005) and Weismer (2006a) provide full introductions to motor speech disorders, including those associated with basal ganglia lesions.

Thalamus

Figure 6–15 shows the thalamus as a massive group of nuclei on either side of the midline of the hemispheres (the two thalami surround the third ventricle, as described below); in the sagittal plane (see Figure 6–16) the thalamus appears as an egg-shaped structure. The thalamus is a collection of specialized nuclei, many of which relay a specific type of sensory information from lower parts of the brain to specific cortical areas. For example, auditory and visual nuclei within the brainstem send information to specialized nuclei within the thalamus, which in turn relay this information to auditory and visual cortical areas. Similarly, tactile information from the limbs and torso ascends the dorsal columns within the spinal cord, makes synapses within dorsal column nuclei, and is relayed through the thalamus to the somatosensory regions of the cortex. Tactile information from the head and neck travels via brainstem nuclei to the thalamus before delivery to appropriate cortical areas. Taste information (but not smell) is also relayed through the thalamus.

The thalamus is the main sensory relay of the brain; all sensory roads (with the exception of olfaction, colloquially known as smell) connecting the outside world to the cortex go through the thalamus. As discussed above, the thalamus is also clearly involved in sensorimotor control.

Cerebellum

The cerebellum is located below the occipital lobe and posterior to the brainstem. The cerebellum has two lobes, and is easily distinguished from other parts of the brain due to its unique appearance which has been likened to a cauliflower (see Figure 6–19, lower image). The surface of the cerebellum is composed of a series of very slim tissue slabs, separated from each other by parallel, narrow fissures. In a prepared (fixed) brain, these tissue slabs, sometimes called *folia* (folium = a thin layer, or leaf), can be separated from one another with the careful use of dissecting instruments. In principle, this is similar to separating adjacent gyri of the cerebral cortex to look into the sulci between them, but cerebellar folia are much more tightly packed and difficult to separate by hand.

Like the cerebral hemispheres, the cerebellar lobes have an outer cortex (gray matter), as well as white matter and nuclei deep within the cortical mantle. The structure and function of the cerebellum are exceedingly complex. For the purposes of the present chapter several general observations are presented for relevance to general and speech motor control.

First, the cerebellum is connected via fiber tracts to the spinal cord, brainstem, and cortex. The cerebellar peduncles, massive bundles of axons seen on the ventral and lateral surfaces of the brainstem (see Figures 6–20 and 6–21 below), are the connections between the cerebellum and the rest of the CNS. The inferior cerebellar peduncle contains fibers running both to and from the cerebellum. In general, fibers running to the cerebellum in the inferior cerebellar peduncle carry sensory information on position and movement of body structures, whereas fibers running from the cerebellum to brainstem nuclei are associated with balance mechanisms. The middle cerebellar peduncle, the most massive of these fiber tracts, conveys information from the pontine nuclei to the cerebellum; the pontine nuclei whose axons form the middle cerebellar peduncle receive information from the motor cortex. Finally, the superior cerebellar peduncle carries fibers from the deep cerebellar nuclei to nuclei in the midbrain and pons, and most importantly (for the current purposes)

to a nucleus in the thalamus. This thalamic nucleus relays cerebellar information to the cortex.

Second, the cerebellum, like the basal ganglia, is connected to the cortex by means of a loop that runs from cortex, to cerebellum, and back to the cortex as illustrated schematically in Figure 6–18. Corticobulbar fibers from many areas of the cortex travel to the pontine nuclei, where synapses are made and information is forwarded to the cerebellum via the middle cerebellar peduncle. This information crosses the midline and enters the cerebellar cortex on the side opposite the cortical origin of this part of the loop (that is, the corticobulbar tract on the right side of the brain makes synapses with pontine cells whose output is directed to the

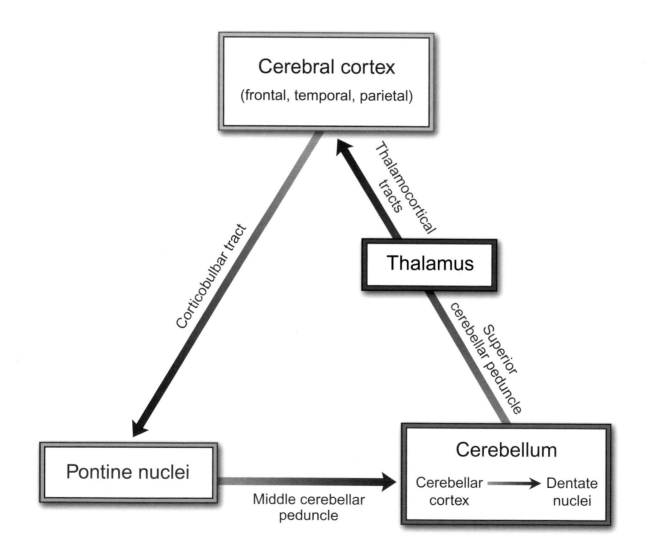

Figure 6–18. Schematic box-and-arrows diagram showing the interconnections between the cortex and the cerebellum. The cortico-cerebello-cortical loop shown here is simplified by not depicting the two fiber tract crossovers in this loop. One crossover is in the pons as fibers descend from cortex to cerebellum, the other is in the midbrain as the fibers ascend from the cerebellum on their way to the cortex via the thalamus.

left cerebellar hemisphere, and vice versa). The input to the cerebellum, delivered by the middle cerebellar peduncle, is directed to cells of the cerebellar cortex and then the dentate nuclei, which are cell bodies deep within the lateral cerebellar hemispheres. The dentate nuclei send processed information out of the lateral cerebellum to the thalamus on the opposite side of the brain, via the superior cerebellar peduncle that crosses the midline in the midbrain. The cortico-cerebello-cortical loop therefore crosses once on the way "down" from cortex to cerebellum, and then again on the way "up" from cerebellum to cortex. Finally, information received in the thalamus is processed (that is, synapses are made) and returned, via thalamocortical fibers in the internal capsule and corona radiata, to the cortical areas where the information originated.

Because the cerebellum is connected via the cortico-cerebello-cortical loop to so many parts of the cerebral cortex, as well as to the brainstem and spinal cord, it is difficult to specify its one main function. Traditionally, though, the cerebellum has been regarded as critical to motor control, and specifically to coordination of the many muscles involved in any skilled action, including speech production. People with cerebellar lesions, which may occur as a result of stroke, tumors, degenerative disease, and penetrating head injuries, often demonstrate coordination difficulties. For example, on gross visual observation, people with cerebellar lesions produce what appear to be jerky movements, lacking the smooth and integrated motions of the neurologically healthy individual. They have difficulty controlling the precision and force of muscular efforts, as evidence by their inability (for example) to point to a target or generate a specific degree of effort (such as lifting a weight to a prespecified height). In the traditional neurological test of "close your eyes and touch your nose with your index finger," people with cerebellar lesions may miss the tip of their nose and hit their face with too much (or too little) force. Finally, someone with a cerebellar lesion may demonstrate disproportionately impaired movement deficits as task complexity is increased. Tasks requiring very carefully coordinated movements are likely to be performed with a dramatic degree of impairment compared to the performance of more simple tasks.

Cerebellum and Basal Ganglia: New Concepts

A traditional view of the cortico-striatal-cortical loop (see Figure 6–17) and cortico-cerebellar-cortical loop (see Figure 6–18) is one in which cortical motor output, specifically the output of cortical cells in the primary motor cortex, is modulated by information circulating in these loops. In anatomical terms, the idea has been that both loops deliver information to the cortex via the thalamus (the globus pallidus is the basal ganglia output to the thalamus, and the dentate nucleus is the cerebellar output to the thalamus). The thalamic information, having already been modulated by both the basal ganglia and cerebellar processing, is sent back to the cortex by means of the loops. In recent years the role of these loops in brain function is being rethought to include not only aspects of motor control, but more global cognitive functions such as the planning of actions and the learning of skilled behavior. As reviewed by Middleton and Strick (2000) and Bostan and Strick (2010), both loops send distinct projections to the *prefrontal* cortex via the thalamus, not just to the primary motor cortex. Because the prefrontal cortex is known to play an important role in cognitive aspects of action planning and learning, the existence of anatomical connections between the two loops and this part of the frontal lobe implicates the basal ganglia and cerebellum as more than simply motor control structures in the strict sense of motor execution. It is relevant to note that diseases of the basal ganglia, such as Parkinson disease and Huntington's disease, and cerebellar disease, are known to include deficits of action sequence planning and action learning.

The scientific literature on the role of the basal ganglia and cerebellum in higher-order cognitive performance is enormous and is far too voluminous to cover here in proper detail. The information in this section is included to emphasize the challenges with a view of the brain as a segregated group of structures, each structure having separate and possibly exclusive functions. Such a view is not defensible in light of recent scientific advances. "Programming disorders," for example, which are quite popular as an explanation for the speech disorder called "apraxia of speech," cannot easily be assigned to a single brain location (such as the premotor cortex). Many brain structures may play a role in the same function, and when damaged may produce the same signs and symptoms.

BRAINSTEM AND CRANIAL NERVES

The brainstem can be thought of as stalk of nervous system tissue, connected above to the cerebral hemispheres and its contents, and connected below to the spinal cord. The top part of the brainstem stalk is more or less surrounded by overhanging tissue of the hemispheres. Refer again to Figure 6–4, where the midsagittal MR image (right image) shows a dotted red line separating the top of the brainstem from the bulk of the cerebral hemispheres. In this midsagittal view, identification of the major components of the brainstem is made easy by the bulging, middle part of the brainstem called the *pons*. If a horizontal line is drawn lower and parallel to the red dotted line in Figure 6–4, through the nose of the imaged person, it intersects the pons in the middle of its bulge. The smaller, narrower structure above the pons, the midbrain (mesencephalon), is the most superior component of the brainstem; its top end extends to the dotted red line. Below the pons is a short, narrow substalk of tissue called the *medulla* (sometimes referred to as the *medulla oblongata*). The medulla is the most inferior component of the brainstem and its lower border is continuous with the superior boundary of the spinal cord.

An artist's rendition of the brainstem and nearby structures in the sagittal plane is shown in the lower part of Figure 6–19. Note the location of the cerebellum, posterior to the pons and medulla and beneath the occipital lobe of the cerebral hemispheres. Note at the top of the brainstem the narrow, dark brown canal running through the midbrain and posterior to the superior part of the pons. This canal expands into a larger cavity separating the cerebellum from the pons and medulla. The narrow canal is the *cerebral aqueduct*

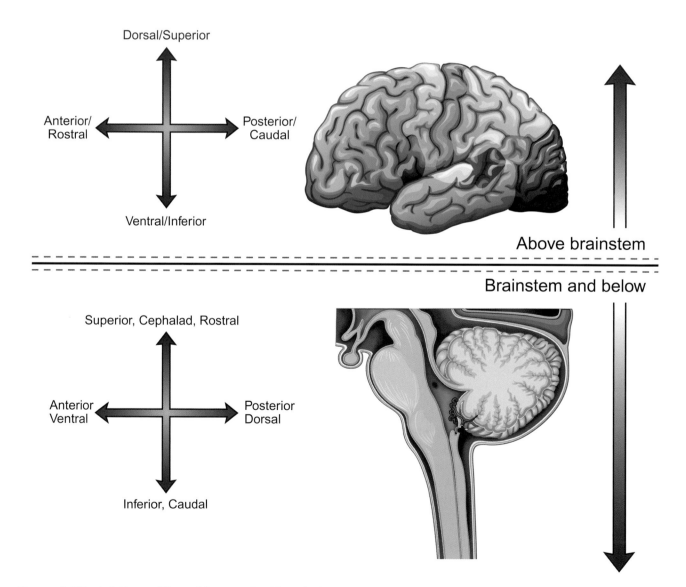

Figure 6–19. Artist's rendition of the cerebral hemispheres (*top image*) and the brainstem, cerebellum, and upper part of spinal cord (*bottom image*). Both images are shown in the sagittal plane.

and the cavity into which it expands is the *fourth ventricle*. These cavities are part of the ventricular system through which cerebrospinal fluid (CSF) flows.

The brainstem is small in comparison to the cerebral hemispheres but contains cells and tracts critical to a wide variety of sensorimotor behaviors, as well as to consciousness, mood, and basic vegetative functions. A great deal of nervous system tissue with a broad range of functions is packed into the small volume of the brainstem, and it is precisely these close quarters that explain why blood deprivation to the brainstem—as in the case of brainstem strokes—can have such devastating consequences. Of special interest to the speech-language pathologist and audiologist are the nuclei and fiber tracts of the brainstem associated with a subset of the 12 paired cranial nerves. These brainstem structures and the nerves associated with them control muscles of the head and neck and sensation (including hearing) from the same structures. Speech, swallowing, and hearing function are very much dependent on the integrity of brainstem structures and the cranial nerves.

In this section, surface features of the brainstem are reviewed first, followed by consideration of each of the 12 cranial nerves and their associated brainstem nuclei. The cranial nerves are introduced as surface features of the brainstem, and later, their anatomy and functions are presented, with special emphasis given to those nerves serving motor and sensory functions of head and neck structures important for speech, swallowing, and hearing. Within the discussion of each cranial nerve, an overview is provided of typical clinical tests used to evaluate its functional integrity.

Surface Features of the Brainstem: Ventral View

A ventral view of the brainstem, plus the thalamus above it, is shown in Figure 6–20. Recall that "ventral"

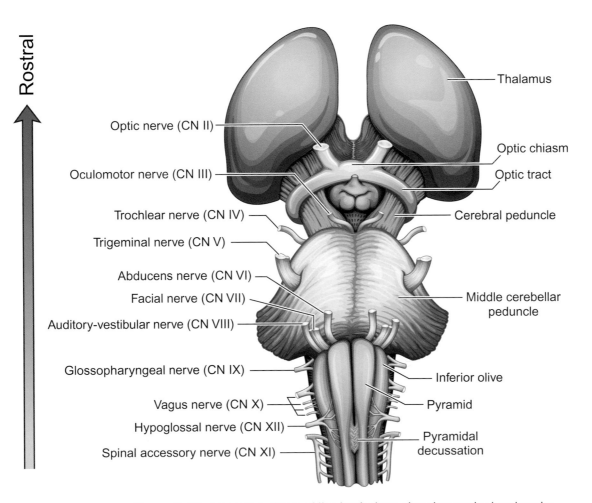

Figure 6–20. Ventral surface of the brainstem, showing major landmarks.

and "anterior" imply the same direction or surface when referring to structures from the top of the brainstem down through the spinal cord. The view in Figure 6–20 is therefore the one obtained if the midsagittal views of Figures 6–4 and 6–19 are rotated counterclockwise 90 degrees, resulting in the observer looking at the front, or ventral/anterior surface, of the brainstem.

Ventral Surface of Midbrain

Prominent surface features of the ventral midbrain include the *cerebral peduncles* (often called the *crus cerebri*, even if this term is not technically equivalent to the cerebral peduncles). The cerebral peduncles are the midbrain component of the massive, long fiber tract running from cortical motor cells to motor nuclei in both the brainstem (corticobulbar tract) and spinal cord (corticospinal tract). Figure 6–20 labels the cerebral peduncle on the left side of the midbrain (right side from the reader's point of view); of course, there is a matching peduncle on the right side of the brain because both hemispheres issue a descending tract to motor nuclei in the brainstem and spinal cord. As shown in Figure 6–20, the cerebral peduncles enter the pons and continue though the middle part of the brainstem below the ventral surface.

The *optic chiasm* is located at the midline of the ventral surface of the midbrain. The optic chiasm is the location where the two optic nerves (paired cranial nerve II) meet before continuing into the cerebral hemispheres as the optic tracts. In Figure 6–20 the optic nerves have been cut because this view of the brainstem is drawn with more anterior structures—principally the face and neck—removed. The optic nerves originate at the retinas, and the destination of the optic tracts (which originate at the optic chiasm) is the occipital lobes of the cerebral hemispheres. Figure 6–20 shows the optic nerves entering the chiasm, where about half the fibers from each eye continue to the hemisphere on the same side as the eye, and the other half crosses over to the opposite hemisphere. Each optic tract therefore carries fibers from both eyes, and a visual "field" from each eye is represented in both hemispheres.

Two additional features on the ventral surface of the midbrain are cranial nerves III (oculomotor nerve) and IV (trochlear nerve). The oculomotor nerve emerges from the midbrain at its junction with the pons, and the trochlear nerve exits the brainstem on its dorsal surface and circles around to be visible on the ventrolateral aspect of the brainstem, as shown in Figure 6–20. These cranial nerves are critical to the control of eye movements.

Ventral Surface of Pons

The anatomical structures that define the ventral surface of the pons are the thick bands of fibers running more or less laterally across this surface (see Figure 6–20). These fiber tracts create the "bulge" of the pons, and consist of three separate tracts called the *superior, middle*, and *inferior cerebellar peduncles*. The middle cerebellar peduncle (labeled in Figure 6–20) is the largest of these tracts and forms the bulk of the ventral surface of the pons. Collectively the three cerebellar peduncles connect the cerebellum to the spinal cord, brainstem, and thalamus. Pons is a word meaning "bridge," and this component of the brainstem is well named because it serves as a bridge from the cerebellum to each major part of the CNS.

The other major landmarks on the ventral surface of the pons include the roots of four cranial nerves. Figure 6–20 shows these four nerves cut shortly after emerging from the brainstem; they include cranial nerves V (trigeminal), VI (abducens), VII (facial), and VIII (auditory-vestibular). Cranial nerve V emerges as a large root from the middle of the pons, on its ventrolateral aspect. Cranial nerves VI, VII, and VIII emerge between the lower edge of the pons and upper edge of the medulla, in a medial-to-lateral order with VI being most medial and VIII most lateral. The roots of these three cranial nerves are included as surface features of the ventral pons because the nuclei to which they are attached are completely (VI, VII) or partially (VIII) within the pons (see Figure 6–22).

Ventral Surface of Medulla

The ventral surface of the medulla shows two pairs of prominent "columns." The two most medial columns are called the *pyramids*; Figure 6–20 labels the left medullary pyramid. The pyramids are the continuation into the medulla of the corticobulbar and corticospinal tracts. As noted above, these tracts descend in the midbrain as the crus cerebri and in the pons below its ventral surface (that is, inside the pons) as pontine fascicles. The pyramids are formed from the corticobulbar and corticobulbar fibers emerging from inside the pons and organized in the medulla as the relatively long, medial columns on its ventral surface. Toward the inferior border of the medulla, Figure 6–20 shows a landmark labeled "Pyramidal decussation." This is where the large majority of corticospinal fibers (roughly, 80%) from one pyramid cross over to the other pyramid before continuing their descent into the spinal cord. Fibers originating in the left cerebral hemisphere descend in the brain on the left side until crossing to the other side via the pyramidal decussation. Fibers from the right hemisphere descend in the brain on the right side, before crossing to the left side via the decussation. The fibers from both hemispheres form an "X"-like pattern as they cross at the bottom of the medulla; in fact, the word "decussate" means a crossing pattern that forms an "X." The boundary between the medulla and the spinal cord is at the inferior edge of the pyramidal decussation.

Just lateral to each pyramid, and separated from it by a groove or fissure (called the anterolateral fissure, not labeled in Figure 6–20), is a swelling of the ventral medulla due to an underlying nucleus called the *inferior olive*. The inferior olive is a nucleus that delivers information coming from the spinal cord to the cerebellum. For the current purposes it is important to recognize these columns lateral to the pyramids as landmarks on the ventrolateral surface of the medulla, and especially for locating the cranial nerves attached to the medulla.

Four cranial nerves are attached to the medulla and can be seen on its ventral and ventrolateral surface. The most superior of these is cranial nerve IX (glossopharyngeal), shown exiting the right side of the medulla just lateral to the olive. Just inferior to the exit point of cranial nerve IX is cranial nerve X (vagus), attached to the medulla as a group of rootlets just lateral to the olive. Cranial nerve XII (hypoglossal) is inferior to the exit point of cranial nerve X, but more medial, exiting the medulla in the anterolateral fissure that separates the pyramid from the olive. Finally, the most inferior of the nerves exiting the ventral surface of the medulla is cranial nerve XI (spinal accessory nerve, sometimes called the accessory nerve), which like cranial nerves IX and X emerges lateral to the olive.

Surface Features of the Brainstem: Dorsal View

A dorsal view of the brainstem, plus the thalamus above it, is shown in Figure 6–21. Recall that "dorsal" and "posterior" imply the same direction or surface when referring to structures from the top of the brainstem down through the spinal cord. The view in Figure 6–21 is the one obtained if the midsagittal views of Figures 6–4 and 6–5 are rotated clockwise 90 degrees, so that the back—the dorsal/posterior surface—of the brainstem is facing the observer. The cerebellum has also been removed from this figure, as the clockwise rotation of the intact brain would block a clear view of the dorsal surface of the brainstem with the cerebellum

in place. The cranial nerves attached to the medulla can also be seen in this dorsal view (as well the attachment point of cranial nerve IV, see the next section on "Dorsal Surface of Midbrain"), but these have been described above as ventral surface features.

Dorsal Surface of Midbrain

Prominent surface features of the dorsal midbrain include the *superior* and *inferior colliculi* and the root of cranial nerve IV (trochlear) as shown in Figure 6–21. The superior and inferior colliculi are paired "bumps" forming the roof of the midbrain, and jointly are referred to as the *corpora quadrigemina*. If the midsagittal MR image (see Figure 6–4, right) and artist's rendition (see Figure 6–5, lower left) of the midbrain are re-examined, these "bumps" can be seen on the small island of tissue that is separated from, and dorsal to, the bulk of the midbrain. The narrow channel separating the bulk of the midbrain from these dorsal bumps is the cerebral aqueduct, one of the series of cavities in the brain through which CSF is circulated.

The superior and inferior colliculi are nuclei along the visual and auditory pathways of the brain, respectively. These nuclei relay visual (superior colliculus) and auditory (inferior colliculus) information from more inferior nuclei in the brainstem to nuclei in the thalamus. Note the pathways labeled "Brachium of superior colliculus" and "Brachium of inferior colliculus" in Figure 6–21. These are fiber bundles emerging from the colliculi and terminating in thalamic nuclei (the lateral geniculate nucleus [vision] and the medial geniculate nucleus [audition]). The lateral geniculate nucleus sends its output to the visual auditory cortex on the same side, and the medial geniculate nucleus sends its output to the auditory cortex on the same side.

The root of cranial nerve IV (trochlear) emerges from the inferior border of the dorsal midbrain, close to the midline. Figure 6–21 shows the paired nerves running laterally from their roots; in fact the nerves wrap around the brainstem and can be seen in the ventral view as well (see Figure 6–20). Cranial nerve IV is distinct among the 12 cranial nerves as the only one with a root emerging from the dorsal surface of the brainstem.

Dorsal Surface of Pons

Recall that the ventral surface of the pons is formed by fibers of the three cerebellar peduncles, which connect regions of the cerebral hemispheres, the brainstem, and the spinal cord to the cerebellum. These fiber tracts wrap around the brainstem to get to the cerebellum,

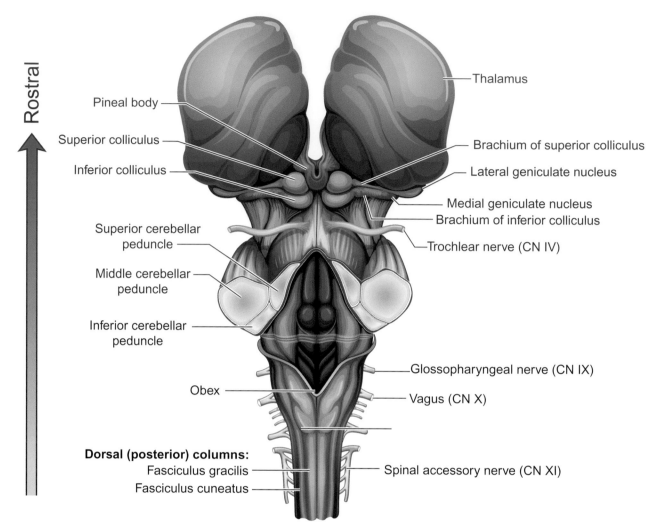

Figure 6–21. Dorsal surface of the brainstem, showing major landmarks. Cerebellum has been removed for this view and the cerebellar peduncles are shown with cuts prior to their entry point to the cerebellum.

What's Your Peduncle's Name?

Brain anatomy is complicated. It is made more complicated (and confusing!) by the naming of some of its parts. Particularly confusing is when the same term is used for different parts or when the same part is given several different names. For example, the terms crus cerebri and cerebral peduncles are often used interchangeably to denote the portion of the corticobulbar and corticospinal tracts that passes through the midbrain and defines a good deal of the midbrain's ventral surface. The term peduncle is also used to refer to *cerebellar* peduncles, which connect the cerebellum to various parts of the brain. "Peduncle" means stalk or stem, and is used widely in anatomy, botany, and any other field in which objects are attached to other objects by means of a short stalk, stem, or base. To keep the brain anatomy structures straight, focus on the adjectives: the cerebral peduncles connect the cerebrum (cerebral hemispheres) with structures in the brainstem and spinal cord, whereas the cerebellar peduncles connect the cerebellum with parts of the spinal cord, brainstem, and thalamus.

and the dorsal view of the brainstem in Figure 6–21 shows the peduncles cut, because the cerebellum has been removed from this view. The superior cerebellar peduncle primarily connects the cerebellum to the thalamus, the middle cerebellar peduncle connects the brainstem to the cerebellum, and the inferior cerebellar peduncle connects the cerebellum to the spinal cord. Note the diamond-shaped cavity surrounded superiorly and laterally by the cerebellar peduncles and laterally and inferiorly by the medulla. This cavity is the *fourth ventricle*, which can also be seen in the midsagittal images of Figure 6–4 and 6–5. The obex, at the inferior edge of the fourth ventricle, is where the fourth ventricle narrows down to continue as the central canal of the spinal cord, the spinal conduit for CSF.

Dorsal Surface of Medulla

Several bumps and bands of tissue can be seen in the "floor" of the fourth ventricle (colored brown in Figure 6–21), especially below the cut level of the inferior cerebellar peduncle. The floor of the fourth ventricle is its ventral wall, as seen from the dorsal view of Figure 6–21; the "roof" of the fourth ventricle is its dorsal wall, formed largely by the cerebellum, especially along or close to the midline. The bumps and bands are swellings of nuclei and fiber tracts that give the floor of the fourth ventricle its distinctive topography. Similar topographical features are also seen in the floor of the fourth ventricle at the level of the pons.

At the bottom of the dorsal surface of the medulla two pairs of columnlike landmarks can be seen rising superiorly to the fourth ventricle. The columns on either side of the midline are called the *fasciculi gracilis*, the columns just lateral to them are the *fasciculi cuneatus*. Collectively, these four columns are called the posterior columns, and they are fiber tracts carrying sensory information on touch, vibration, and proprioception (position and movement sensation of body parts relative to each other) up the spinal cord to the medulla where they synapse in the paired *nucleus gracilis* and *nucleus cuneatus*. These two nuclei are located in the caudal medulla, along its dorsal border (that is, right in line with the respective fasciculi identified above). These nuclei are revealed on the dorsal surface of the medulla as the slight swellings at the superior termination the fasciculi gracilis and cuneatis (see Figure 6–21, just above the level of the spinal accessory nerve). Fibers leaving the nucleus gracilis and nucleus cuneatus cross to the other side and travel up to make synapses with thalamic nuclei before traveling in fiber tracts to the cortex.

Cranial Nerves and Associated Brainstem Nuclei

Table 6–3 lists the 12 cranial nerves, their associated nuclei, which are primarily in the brainstem, and their major function(s). Figure 6–22 is a dorsal view of the brainstem showing the medio-lateral locations and superior-inferior extents of the cranial nerve nuclei. The drawing does not indicate the position of the nuclei along the ventral-to-dorsal (anterior-to-posterior) dimension of the brainstem, as would be seen in a transverse section. Each cranial nerve and its associated nucleus (or nuclei) is (are) discussed below, but emphasis is given to cranial nerves V, VII, VIII, IX, X, XI, and XII because of their relevance for speech and hearing control and disorders. Table 6–3 and Figure 6–22 should be consulted frequently throughout this discussion.

Some of the cranial nerves have purely sensory function, some purely motor function, and some have both sensory and motor functions. In Table 6–3 those cranial nerves with purely sensory function (CN I, II, VIII) are listed in normal font and those with purely motor function (CN III, IV, VI, XI, XII) in bold font. Those having both motor and sensory function are called mixed nerves and are listed in italicized font.

Two of the cranial nerves (I and II) are not directly associated with nuclei in the brainstem. Cranial nerves I and II are both sensory, and have their cell bodies in ganglia outside the brainstem, close to their specialized receptors. One cranial nerve with purely motor function, cranial nerve XI, has its nuclei in the upper part of the cervical spinal cord. The remaining cranial nerves all have motor nuclei within the brainstem, or in the case of sensory components, ganglia whose projections are to nuclei within the brainstem.

Cranial Nerve I (Olfactory)

The sensory receptors for olfaction are embedded within the cribriform plate at the top of the ethmoid bone (Chapter 4). These receptors send axons to the olfactory bulbs, where they make a first synapse in what is essentially an olfactory nucleus. As seen in the lower left image of Figure 6–5, the olfactory bulbs are located on the base of the frontal lobes. These bulbs (typically intact and available for naked-eye inspection in a fixed brain when it is turned upside down for examination of the ventral surface of the cerebral hemispheres) are swellings at the end of long, thin bands of tissue that disappear into the cortex close to the adjacent boundaries of

Table 6–3. Cranial Nerves, Their Associated Brainstem Nuclei, and General Function(s)

NERVE (NAME)	NUCLEI	FUNCTION(S)
I (Olfactory)	Olfactory Bulb[a]	Olfaction
II (Optic)	Midbrain[b]	Vision
III (Oculomotor)	**Oculomotor; Edinger-Westphal**	**Eye movement, pupil size and accommodation**
IV (Trochlear)	**Trochlear**	**Eye movement (one muscle)**
V (Trigeminal)	*Motor n. of V;*	*Control of jaw muscles (closers and opener), myloyoid m., tensor veli palatine m., tensor tympani m.*
	Sensory n. of V	*Sensation from entire face, teeth, palate, gums, anterior two-thirds of tongue*
VI (Abducens)	**Abducens**	**Eye movement (single muscle)**
VII (Facial)	*Facial motor n.*	*Control of muscles of facial expression and stapedius m.*
	Sup. Salivatory n.;	*Control of salivary glands*
	Sensory n. of V;	*Possible sensation from parts of external ear and parts of tonsils*
	N. solitarius	*Taste from anterior two-thirds of tongue*
VIII (Auditory-vestibular)	Cochlear n.,	Audition
	Vestibular n.	Balance
IX (Glossopharyngeal)	*N. ambiguus;*	*Control of stylopharyngeus m.*
	Sensory n. of V;	*Sensation from parts of external ear, medial surface of eardrum, upper pharynx, posterior one-third of tongue*
	Salivatory n.;	*Control of salivatory glands*
	N. solitarius	*Detection of chemical and pressure changes in blood; taste to posterior one-third of tongue*
X (Vagus)	*N. ambiguus;*	*Control of velopharyngeal, pharyngeal, & laryngeal muscles*
	Sensory n. of V;	*Sensation from meninges, parts of external ear and ear canal, external surface of eardrum, pharynx and larynx*
	Dorsal motor n.;	*Control of smooth muscle and glands of pharynx, larynx, heart and digestive system*
	N. solitarius	*Sensation from heart, digestive system, esophagus and trachea*
XI (Accessory)	**Accessory spinal n. (upper cervical cord)**	**Control of sternocleidomastoid and trapezius m.**
XII (Hypoglossal)	**Hypoglossal n.**	**Control of three of the four muscles of the tongue and all intrinsic muscles**

[a]The olfactory nerve has sensory receptors embedded within the cribriform plate of the ethmoid bone, and the "nuclei" are in the olfactory bulbs (Figure 6–5, lower left image) which are located on the base of the frontal lobe, external to the brainstem. The olfactory "nerve" is therefore really the olfactory "tract" but is typically called a "nerve" (see text).

[b]The optic nerve does not make connections with brainstem nuclei in the sense of cranial nerves III-XII, but rather sends fibers from the retina (the sensory receptors) to the lateral geniculate nucleus of the thalamus, which "forwards" this information to the visual cortex. Some optic nerve fibers go to the midbrain where information is used by cranial nerves III, IV, and VI to control eye movements.

Note: Nerves that are purely sensory are in regular font, nerves that are purely motor in bold font, and mixed nerves (with both sensory and motor function) are in italicized font.

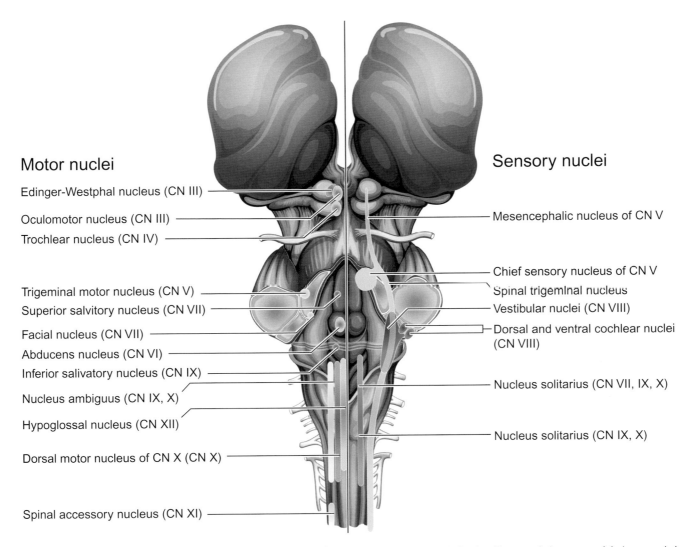

Motor nuclei

Edinger-Westphal nucleus (CN III)

Oculomotor nucleus (CN III)

Trochlear nucleus (CN IV)

Trigeminal motor nucleus (CN V)

Superior salvitory nucleus (CN VII)

Facial nucleus (CN VII)

Abducens nucleus (CN VI)

Inferior salivatory nucleus (CN IX)

Nucleus ambiguus (CN IX, X)

Hypoglossal nucleus (CN XII)

Dorsal motor nucleus of CN X (CN X)

Spinal accessory nucleus (CN XI)

Sensory nuclei

Mesencephalic nucleus of CN V

Chief sensory nucleus of CN V

Spinal trigeminal nucleus

Vestibular nuclei (CN VIII)

Dorsal and ventral cochlear nuclei (CN VIII)

Nucleus solitarius (CN VII, IX, X)

Nucleus solitarius (CN IX, X)

Figure 6–22. Dorsal view of brainstem showing locations of nuclei associated with cranial nerves. Motor nuclei are shown on the left side of the brainstem, sensory nuclei on the right side. This view allows an estimate of the location of nuclei along the medial-to-lateral plane of the brainstem, as well as the length of nuclei along the inferior-superior dimension of the brainstem, but does not provide information on nuclei location along the anterior-posterior (that is, ventral-dorsal) dimensions.

the frontal and temporal lobes. The thin bands of tissue running posteriorly, into the cortex, are called the olfactory nerves, or the paired cranial nerve I. Most of the fibers from the olfactory nerves enter the cortex and other parts of the temporal lobes. The ventromedial portions of the temporal lobe that serve olfaction are closely associated with memory mechanisms of the temporal lobe.

The olfactory nerves can be tested clinically with known odors. *Anosmia*, the disorder of lacking the sense of smell, is seen frequently in fractures of the skull base (e.g., in TBI) as well as in certain degenerative neurological diseases such as Alzheimer's disease.

Cranial Nerve II (Optic)

The sensory receptors associated with the optic nerves are the rods and cones in the retina. Rods and cones are the photocells of the retina, sensitive to light and color. When light strikes the photocells, they transform the photon energy ("photon energy" is technically a redundant term because photons are packets of light energy) to electrical impulses. These impulses are sent to ganglia within the retina where the first synapse is made. Axons emerging from the ganglia form the optic nerves, which exit each retina and run posteriorly and medially, toward the optic chiasm.

The bottom, left image of Figure 6–5 shows the cut optic nerves entering the optic chiasm. The continuation of the optic pathway beyond the chiasm is called the optic tract (see Figure 6–20). Fibers from both retinas travel through the optic chiasm and continue via the optic tracts to visual cortex in the occipital lobes.

The mapping from the external world to retina, and from retina to cerebral hemispheres is orderly, but complex. For example, fibers of the optic nerve are arranged retinotopically, and the retina is arranged so its rods and cones respond to specific regions of the visual field. As stated above, both retinas are represented in both hemispheres. Because of the way images from the external world are projected onto the retina, the left visual field is represented in the right visual cortex, and the right visual field is represented in the left visual cortex. Neurologists exploit these orderly but complex mappings between the external world, the retina, and the visual cortex in the two hemispheres to localize lesions when a patient demonstrates a specific visual field deficit. The interested reader is encouraged to consult Wilson-Pauwels, Akesson, Stewart, and Spacey (2002) and Bear et al. (2007) for details on visual field testing.

Cranial Nerve III (Oculomotor)

Figure 6–22 shows two motor nuclei (left side of figure) in close proximity near the midline of the midbrain, one the oculomotor nucleus (blue), the other the Edinger-Westphal nucleus (brown). These nuclei are roughly at the level of the superior colliculus, but when viewed in a transverse section are ventral to the colliculi, just anterior to the cerebral aqueduct (the dorsal view of Figure 6–22 cannot show the location of these nuclei along the ventrodorsal dimension of the midbrain). These two nuclei contribute fibers to cranial nerve III, a motor nerve containing two types of fibers. The oculomotor nucleus contributes fibers to innervate four extrinsic muscles that move the eyeball up, down, and toward the nose, as well as fibers to the muscle that raises the eyelid. The muscles that attach to the eyeball have their origin outside the eyeball, from a ring of tendinous tissue surrounding the inner eye socket. The Edinger-Westphal nucleus innervates intrinsic muscles of the eye that control the size of the pupil and the shape of the lens. The extrinsic muscles are "voluntary," the intrinsic "involuntary." As shown in Figures 6–20, fibers from both the oculomotor and Edinger-Westphal nuclei run together and exit the brainstem at the inferior edge of the ventral surface of the midbrain.

Neurologists perform specific tests to evaluate the integrity of the voluntary and involuntary components of cranial nerve III. When a patient is asked to follow a light without moving her head, the extrinsic (voluntary) muscles innervated by cranial nerve III are evaluated. When a neurologist asks a patient to look straight ahead while she shines a bright light into the patient's eye, and moves the light toward and away from the pupil, the intrinsic (involuntary) muscles are evaluated.

Cranial Nerve IV (Trochlear)

In Figure 6–22 the trochlear nucleus is shown slightly inferior to the oculomotor nucleus, roughly at the level of the inferior colliculus. In a horizontal section of the midbrain through the level of the inferior colliculus, shown in Figure 6–23, the trochlear nucleus can be seen ventral to the cerebral aqueduct. This nucleus is the origin of cranial nerve IV, and serves a purely motor function by innervating a single, extrinsic muscle of the eye that produces upward, downward, rotary, and side-to-side movements of the eyeball. The eye movements

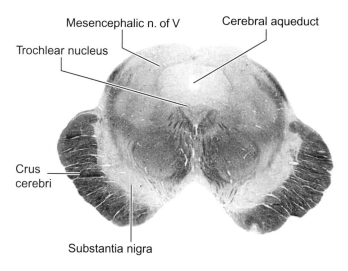

Figure 6–23. Horizontal section through a human midbrain, roughly halfway between its superior and inferior boundaries. The slice (and those in Figures 6–24, and 6–26 through 6–28) is prepared with a process that stains fiber tracts dark (note the crus cerebri at the anterior (ventral) edge of the slice) and nuclei light (note the substantia nigra, just posterior to the crus cerebri). The small hole in the center and somewhat posterior part of the section is the cerebral aqueduct, the passageway through which CSF flows from the third to fourth ventricles (see Figure 6–38).

resulting from contraction of this muscle are complex and depend on the position of the eyeball when the muscle contracts.

Cranial nerve IV is unique among the cranial nerves for two reasons. First, the trochlear nerve is the only cranial nerve that emerges from the dorsal surface of the brainstem. As described above, this paired nerve exits the dorsal surface of the midbrain and curl around the cerebral peduncles to run anteriorly in the cranial cavity, on their way to the eyes. Second, fibers emerging from the trochlear nuclei run dorsomedially within the midbrain and cross at the midline before exiting, as cranial nerve IV, from the dorsal surface of the brainstem. The trochlear nerve emerging from the right side of the brainstem (and innervating the muscle in the right eye) is therefore from the left trochlear nucleus (and the left trochlear nerve is from the right trochlear nucleus). All other motor nuclei in the brainstem, including the ones associated with cranial nerve III, emerge on the same side of the brainstem as their originating nuclei.

Neurological testing of cranial nerve IV can be challenging, but a typical assessment of the trochlear nerve asks the patient to move the eye inward (adducted, i.e., toward the nose) and down. Inabililty to produce downward gaze with the eye adducted suggests damage to the nucleus on the opposite side, or to the nerve issued by the nucleus (on the same side as the affected eye).

Cranial Nerve V (Trigeminal)

Cranial nerve V is a mixed nerve (both sensory and motor function) with three major divisions—ophthalmic, maxillary, and mandibular. The trigeminal nerve emerges from the ventrolateral surface of the pons as a large root (see Figure 6–20) containing sensory and motor fibers. A short distance away from the brainstem the root separates into three major branches. The ophthalmic and maxillary divisions are purely sensory, carrying information on touch, pressure, and pain from the mid and upper face (including the forehead, front part of the scalp, and eyeball), maxillary teeth, sinuses, and meninges of the anterior and middle cranial fossa. The mandibular division contains both sensory and motor fibers. The sensory fibers of the mandibular division carry information on touch, pressure, and pain from the lower teeth, the skin of the lower face, the anterior two-thirds of the tongue, the external auditory meatus and parts of the external ear. In addition, the sensory division carries information from specialized organs in the jaw-closing muscles to a sensory nucleus in the brainstem. These specialized organs are called muscle spindles and are an important component of the jaw-jerk reflex (described below). The motor part of the mandibular division innervates the jaw closing muscles and the single jaw-opener (anterior belly of the *digastric* muscle), the *palatal tensor* muscle, the *tensor tympani* muscle, and the *mylohyoid* muscle (see Chapters 3, 4, and 5).

The motor fibers of cranial nerve V are derived from the trigeminal motor nucleus (also called the motor nucleus of V), located in the pons roughly midway between its superior and inferior borders (see Figure 6–22, left side). In a transverse section of the pons, the trigeminal motor nuclei are found ventral to the floor of the fourth ventricle and somewhat lateral to the midline, as can be seen in Figure 6–24. The motor fibers run laterally from the two nuclei, exit the pons on the same side as the nuclei (that is, the left motor nucleus generates a motor tract on the left side of the pons) and innervate muscles on the same side of the head (that is, ipsilaterally).

As shown in light green on the right side of Figure 6–22, the sensory nucleus of V runs the entire length of the brainstem, from midbrain to medulla. The sensory nucleus of V is separated into three main parts, including the mesencephalic nucleus of V in the midbrain, the chief (or principal) sensory nucleus in the pons, and the spinal trigeminal nucleus in the lower pons and length of the medulla. Throughout the brainstem the sensory nucleus of V changes it position somewhat along the ventrodorsal dimension, but generally it is well lateral to the midline, and lateral to the trigeminal motor nucleus in the mid-pons.

Here is a simple account of the functions of the three parts of the sensory nucleus of V. The chief (principal) sensory nucleus in the pons receives information on touch and pressure from the face, tongue, teeth, and other facial structures whose sensory function is served by the trigeminal nerve. The spinal trigeminal nucleus receives information on pain and temperature from these same areas, as well as touch and pressure information from small regions of the head and neck. The mesencephalic nucleus of V, in the midbrain, is specialized for receiving fibers originating in the muscle spindles of the jaw closing muscles; these sensory fibers are part of the stretch reflex of the jaw.

Neurological evaluation of the integrity of cranial nerve V is fairly straightforward. Sensory function is evaluated through simple touch tests on the face, with care taken to stimulate gently with the edge of a tissue or perhaps a Q-tip the different regions of the face served by one of the three sensory divisions of the nerve.

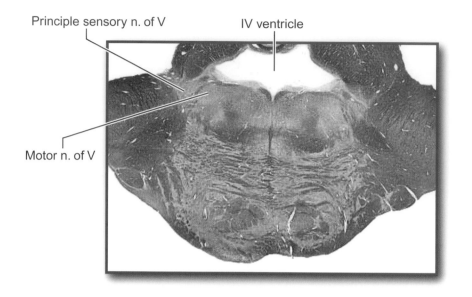

Figure 6–24. Horizontal section through a human pons, roughly halfway between its superior and inferior boundaries; the section was made in the inferior-superior dimension to intersect the motor nucleus of V (see relative inferior-superior location of motor nucleus of V in Figure 6–22).

For example, touch on the upper bridge of the nose or on the forehead stimulates sensory fibers of the ophthalmic division of the nerve, and touch on the upper and lower lips stimulate sensory fibers of the maxillary and mandibular divisions, respectively. A common evaluation of motor function of the trigeminal nerve is the masseter bulge test. Recall from Chapter 5 that the *masseter* muscle overlays the ramus of the mandible, and runs in a vertical and slightly posterior direction from its origin on the zygomatic arch to its insertion at the angle of the mandible. If an examiner places her fingers in flight attendant configuration (middle and index fingers extended) and places them at the corners of the mouth, moving them slowly back along the sides of the face while applying a small amount of pressure so the teeth can be felt through the cheeks, a ridge is encountered slightly more than halfway to the ears (try it on a friend!). This ridge is the anterior edge of the masseter muscle. Press gently against the ridges on both sides of the face and ask the person to clench her teeth together; the normal effect should be a bulge of the anterior edges of the paired muscle, reflecting its contraction (hence, "masseter bulge" test) to produce the clench. The contraction of the masseter, in the neurologically normal individual, should actually push the examiner's fingers forward (toward the examiner). If one side is weak, the examiner feels the difference in strength between the sides as one pair of fingers pushed forward, the other pair less so (or not at all).

Weakness on both sides can be inferred from a lack of finger movement during the clench.

Other evaluations of the motor function of cranial nerve V involve asking a client to open and shut the jaw rapidly or slowly, or to move the jaw side to side. Especially in the case of the open-and-shut movement, asymmetries in the pathway followed by the mandible may suggest weakness of the jaw opener and/or closers on one side.

A sensorimotor evaluation of cranial nerve V is the jaw-jerk reflex. The anatomical and physiological basis of the reflex is described in the next section, and provides a good model of how artificial the separation of sensory from motor functions may be for even simple actions.

Jaw Jerk Reflex (Stretch Reflex of the Jaw). Figure 6–25 presents an anatomical model of the stretch reflex in the jaw closing muscles. The stretch reflex is not limited to jaw closing muscles, but is a feature of virtually all striated (voluntary) muscle. The CNS mechanisms for the jaw stretch reflex are located in the brainstem, whereas central mechanisms for limb stretch reflexes are in the spinal cord. Muscles of the arms, legs, and trunk (including muscles of breathing—see Chapter 2) have a stretch reflex whose mechanisms are essentially the same as the one described here for the jaw stretch reflex.

The jaw stretch reflex (in clinical settings often called the jaw-jerk reflex) can be elicited by tapping

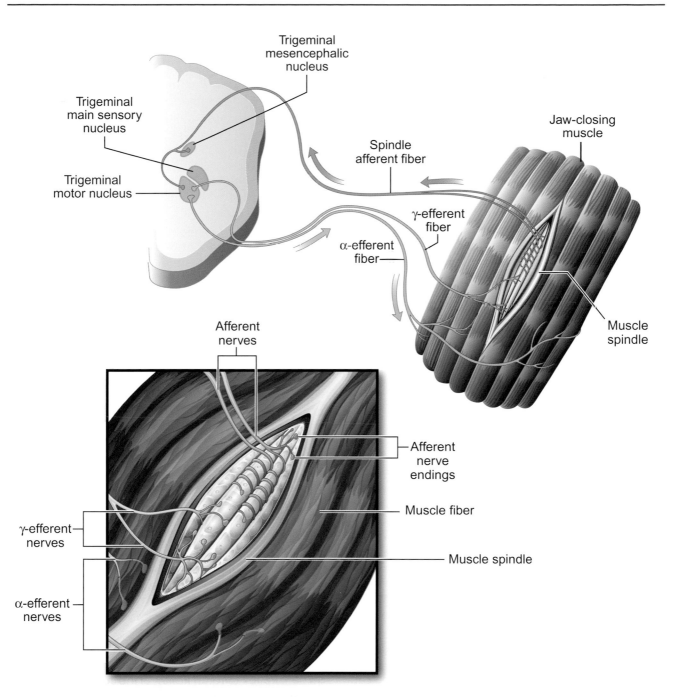

Figure 6–25. Anatomical model of the stretch reflex for jaw closing muscles. Upper part of figure shows muscle fibers (on right) containing a muscle spindle. Blue axons (spindle afferent fibers) carry sensory information from spindle to the sensory cells in the mesencephalic nucleus of V and, importantly, directly to the motor nucleus of V. Green fibers carry motor impulses (α-efferent fiber) to muscle containing the muscle spindle. Bottom part of image shows a zoom view of a muscle spindle embedded in muscle fibers, showing afferent nerves leading away from the muscle spindle to brainstem, as well as α-efferent fibers to control contraction of the jaw muscle fibers and γ-efferent fibers to control tension on spindle fibers.

down on the jaw with a reflex hammer as the patient relaxes her jaw with a slightly open mouth. A normal response to this downward tap is a slight upward movement of the jaw, or no movement at all. Readers may be more familiar with a limb reflex—the patellar reflex—involving the same mechanism. This is elicited by tapping a reflex hammer against the lower part of knee with the legs dangling; a normal response to the tap is a slight, upward "kick" of the lower leg.

In Figure 6–25, a section of muscle tissue from one of the jaw closers (e.g., the *masseter* muscle) is shown schematically. Individual fibers are depicted within the section of striated muscle as longitudinal bundles of red tissue, with nerves running to and from the midbrain (upper left part of figure); a "zoom" view of the muscle fibers and a muscle spindle is shown in the lower part of the figure. As seen in the zoom view, the muscle spindle is embedded within the muscle fibers, and attached to the fibers at both its ends. The muscle spindle, so named because of its spindlelike shape, is a specialized, sensory end organ. The muscle spindle has internal fibers of its own (shown in Figure 6–25 as whitish fibers), which are stretched when the striated muscle fiber to which it is attached is stretched. A whole muscle contains many muscle spindles connected to the individual muscle fibers forming the overall muscle, so when a whole muscle is stretched—think of the stretch as a lengthening of the whole muscle—all attached muscle spindles are stretched as well. The opposite case is also true: contraction (shortening) of a whole muscle "takes the stretch off" the fibers of the muscle spindle. The sensitivity of the muscle spindle fibers to stretch of the main muscle can also be controlled by a separate motor system called the γ-efferent (gamma-efferent) system, whose nerves are labeled in Figure 6–25. When γ-efferent nerves make the muscle spindle fibers more tense, they are much more sensitive to stretch of the whole muscle in which the spindles are embedded.

The key to understanding the stretch reflex is to appreciate what happens when muscle spindle fibers are stretched by the stretching of striated muscle fibers. The stretched muscle spindle fibers cause a sensory ending within the center of the spindle (see Figure 6–25, "afferent nerve endings") to generate an action potential and conduct an impulse away from the muscle in the direction of the brainstem. The fiber carrying this impulse is an afferent one, traveling from the sensory end organ to the CNS (see Figure 6–25, blue arrows). In the case of the jaw-jerk reflex, the afferent signal enters the brainstem via cranial nerve V *without making a first synapse outside the brainstem*; that is, there is no synapse in a ganglion cell. The afferent fiber from the muscle spindle goes directly to the mesencephalic nucleus of V where it makes a first synapse with a sensory cell. This sensory cell sends an impulse to a cell in the trigeminal motor nucleus that controls muscle contraction of precisely the section of muscle that was stretched. The cell in the trigeminal motor nucleus fires, sending a signal to the main muscle fibers to contract, via what is called the α-efferent (alpha-efferent) system (see Figure 6–25, green arrows).

The sequence of events described in the preceding paragraph and summarized in Table 6–4 is the stretch reflex. The primary mechanisms of the stretch reflex include the specialized, sensory end organ of the muscle spindle, exquisitely sensitive to stretch of the muscle in which it is embedded, and the fast "loop" linking the muscle spindle and the muscle fibers in which it is embedded. The quickness of this mechanism is underscored by the direct connection to a sensory nucleus inside the brainstem, avoiding a "stop" in a ganglion. The depolarized sensory end organ sends a signal to the brainstem when the muscle is stretched that, in effect, tells the mesencephalic nucleus of V and the trigeminal motor nucleus to "correct" the stretch with an opposing muscle contraction. This opposing muscle contraction is commanded from cells in the trigeminal motor nucleus stimulated by input from the mesencephalic nucleus of V.

The stretch reflex is a basic example of a sensorimotor loop. When neurologists test reflex loops such as the one described above, they are concerned with *signs* that reflect integrity or disease of the nervous system. A slight jaw jerk, or no upward jaw movement in response to the downward hammer tap, reflects a normally functioning stretch reflex, as does the little leg kick when the hammer tap is delivered just below the knee. On the other hand, exaggerated reflexes of the jaw or lower leg might indicate neurological disease.

When neuroscientists describe loops in the nervous system, they refer to mechanisms whereby infor-

Table 6–4. Summary of Events, in Sequence, That Constitute the Stretch Reflex for Jaw Closing Muscles

stretching of the striated muscle fiber →
stretching of the muscle spindle fiber →
firing of the sensory end organ of the muscle spindle →
conduction of the afferent impulse directly to the mesencephalic nucleus of V where a synapse is made with a sensory cell →
conduction of an impulse from a cell in the mesencephalic nucleus of V to a cell in the trigeminal motor nucleus that controls part of the muscle that was initially stretched →
conduction of an impulse from this motor cell to the muscle fiber that was stretched, which causes the muscle fiber to contract

mation generated in one part of the nervous system is sent to other parts of the nervous system for processing and then returned to the origin of the information, presumably for refinement of performance. The refinement of performance is due to processing done through the loop. In the case of the jaw stretch reflex, information generated by the muscle spindles is "processed" through the brainstem and delivered back to the jaw closing muscles. A reasonable question is, what possible refinement in performance of jaw motions is facilitated by the jaw stretch reflex?

Imagine you shell an exotic nut, place it in your mouth and, with maneuvers of your tongue, lips, and jaw, relocate the delicacy between your molars for initial crushing prior to a few rounds of chewing in advance of swallowing. Because this is an unfamiliar nut, one with which you have no previous experience, you have no knowledge of its resistance to bite force — you don't know how hard it is. With the nut between your molars you contract your jaw closers — we'll use the *masseter* muscle as the main representative of the jaw closers (Chapter 5) — to crush the nut. The magnitude of contractile force commanded by the brain for this task is speculative — there is no "contractile-force template" for crushing this particular nut because it is exotic and new. The speculation is not completely random, however, because other nuts have been crushed by action of your jaw-closing muscles and their required crushing forces have been stored in long-term memory. The speculative, "ballpark" force is commanded, which involves a specific contraction (shortening) of the muscle, at some specific rate, over the short time interval required to complete the initial crush. The nut is harder than expected, however, and the commanded shortening of the muscle is effectively interrupted when the nut's greater-than-expected resistance is encountered. The interruption of the commanded shortening is just like an unexpected stretch of the *masseter* muscle — that is, unexpected relative to the commanded shortening of the muscle. What happens? The slight stretch of the *masseter* muscle resulting from the unexpected hardness and resistance of the nut interrupts the planned shortening of the muscle and initiates a stretch reflex in the jaw closing muscles. Afferent signals from the many muscle spindles in the *masseter* muscle are triggered and travel along the spindle afferent fibers (see Figure 6–25) to the mesencephalic nucleus of V, and then to the trigeminal motor nucleus which generates a signal to "correct" the stretch with additional and perhaps more forceful contractile shortening. The correction is made and the nut is crushed with additional, proper biting force. The loop depicted in Figure 6–25, from muscle spindle to mesencephalic nucleus of V, to

the trigeminal motor nucleus and back to the muscle in which the spindle is embedded, is the pathway of this reflex arc.

Upon reflection, there is something very interesting in this account of the simple act of biting. The correction of biting force is made without additional processing above the brainstem — there is no explicit adjustment of *cortical* commands that initiated the process of biting the unknown nut. The fact that the jaw stretch reflex does not, like most other sensory information arising from sensory receptors (such as touch, pressure, or vibration receptors in the skin of the face, also carried by cranial nerve V), make an initial synapse in a ganglion outside the brainstem makes this particular reflex very fast. Reflex loops that avoid an initial synapse in a ganglion outside the CNS have the property of being very fast. In the case of the jaw jerk reflex, the direct pathway to the mesencephalic nucleus of V results in a very short amount of time from stimulus (the downward tap on the chin) to the contraction of the muscle — typically 10 ms or less! Corrections can be made rapidly, without explicit intervention of cortical mechanisms to reset muscle contraction specifications.

The jaw jerk reflex is unique among stretch reflexes because the first synapse is made in a sensory nucleus of the brainstem. All other stretch reflexes are associated with spinal cord mechanisms (with some possible exceptions). Muscle spindles embedded within striated muscles of the limb operate similarly to the spindles in jaw muscles: they send afferent fibers to the spinal cord, bypassing the ganglia to make first synapses in the sensory cells found in the dorsal horn of the central gray matter of the cord. As in the jaw jerk reflex, the dorsal horn cells of the spinal cord send fibers to the motor cells in the ventral horn of the spinal cord; these motor cells control the same muscle from which the spindle signal was sent.

Muscle spindles play an obvious role in diagnostic neurology. The absence or exaggeration of a stretch reflex can be useful in identifying and in some cases localizing neurological disease. A more important question is if, and how muscle spindles contribute to speech motor control (or motor control in general). This question is too involved for the scope of this chapter, but some appreciation of the complexity of this issue can be gained from the following. First, muscle spindles are not found in high numbers, or possibly not at all, in several important muscles of the speech apparatus. They are abundantly present in jaw muscles, as described above, but not so abundant in the tongue where they may be distributed only in conjunction with attachment to muscles of the pharynx (Saigusa, Yamashita, Tanuma, Saigusa, & Niimi, 2004). Spindles are rarely found in labial muscles or muscles of the lower face (Ito & Gomi, 2007), and are found in relatively low numbers in velopharyngeal tissue, and have been reported as absent in the *palatal levator*, a critical muscle for closure of the velopharyngeal port (Kuehn, Templeton, & Maynard, 1990). Muscle spindles have been found in the larynx, but only in specific regions of the vocal fold (Sanders, Han, Wang, & Biller, 1998). In contrast, muscle spindles are present in almost all limb musculature, and are assumed to play an important role in automatic adjustments and fine tuning of goal-directed motor control. More specifically, muscle spindles are linked to the concept of *proprioception*, the ability to sense the position of a body structure in space, the speed and force with which the structure is moving through space or against a resistance, and the positions of body structures relative to one another. Muscle spindles, by virtue of their ability to sense muscle stretch and transmit this information to the brainstem and spinal cord for quick corrective action, are much more than participants in simple reflex arcs; they play an important role in the moment-to-moment regulation of skilled body movement (Bear et al., 2007). In the case of structures of the speech apparatus, if spindles are present only in *some* head and neck muscles, and when present only in relatively sparse numbers,[2] how can their role in speech motor control be imagined? After all, the precision of articulatory motions and the underlying force of the muscles that create those motions, plus the movement coordination of multiple articulatory structures, are thought to be no less intricate and demanding than the precision of motor control required for effective grasp and use of, say, a screwdriver. Speech scientists have puzzled for many years over the potential role of muscle spindles in speech motor control, and for good reason. Sense of articulator position, magnitude of articulatory motion, and coordination between two or more moving articulators are aspects of speech motor control often addressed in clinical settings. The interested reader is referred to Kent, Martin, and Sufit (1990) for a review of some relevant literature.

Cranial Nerve VI (Abducens)

The abducens nerve originates in the abducens nucleus, which as shown in Figure 6–22 is close to the midline of the brainstem, roughly midway between the superior and inferior borders of the pons. The abducens nucleus and abducens nerve control the lateral rectus muscle of the eye. This muscle attaches to the side of the eyeball and when it contracts causes movement consistent with the name of the nucleus and nerve—it abducts the eyeball, turning it away from the nose toward the lateral surface of the head.

A transverse section of the pons at the level of the abducens nucleus shows the paired nuclei in the floor of the upper part of the fourth ventricle, close to the midline as shown in Figure 6–26. This section was prepared with a stain showing nuclei as lighter areas and fiber tracts as darker areas (the two dark, round structures at the ventral edge of the image, just lateral to the midline, show the corticospinal tract as it passes through this level of the pons). Axons exit the nuclei, run ventrally and slightly laterally to emerge from the ventral surface of the brainstem, at the junction of the pons and medulla (see Figure 6–20).

Cranial nerve VI is often considered together with cranial nerves III (oculomotor) and IV (trochlear), the two other nerves (and their associated nuclei) responsible for control of eye movement. In Figure 6–22, note how the motor nuclei for the extrinsic muscles of the eye (colored blue on the left side of the brainstem) line up along the midline. The two nuclei in the midbrain and the one in the pons are derived from the same cells during embryological development of the brain, and are interconnected to produce the complex and rapid motions of the eyeballs.

Cranial nerve VI is tested together with cranial nerves III and IV by asking a patient to follow a moving target or move the eyes in a specific direction on command. These visual tracking or movement tests are done with the head fixed in position. Problems with visual tracking or movement of the eyes in specific directions may suggest a problem with one or all of these cranial nerves or the nuclei from which they originate.

Cranial Nerve VII (Facial)

The facial nerve is a mixed nerve. The fibers exiting the brainstem as the facial nerve originate in the facial motor nucleus, located in the mid-pons. This nucleus

---

[2]The issue of numbers of muscle spindles per unit volume of muscle tissue is raised in connection with skilled movement for the following reasons. In striated muscles innervated by ventral horn cells of the spinal cord, structures involved in fine motor control are typically endowed with a higher density of muscle spindles as compared to structures involved in gross motor control. Muscles of the fingers, for example, have a much higher density of muscle spindles as compared to muscles of the abdomen. Speech is often described as requiring extremely precise motor control, which might lead to an expectation of a high density of muscle spindles in the tongue, arguably the articulator with the greatest demands for control precision in producing speech. As noted in the text, muscle spindles are found in tongue tissue, but seem to be localized to certain regions of the tongue and even then do not have a high density.

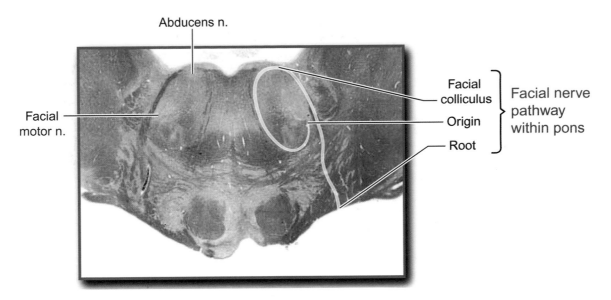

Figure 6–26. Horizontal section through a human pons, inferior to the cut shown in Figure 6–24. The section was made to intersect the facial motor nuclei and the abducens nuclei (see relative inferior-superior location of these two motor nuclei in Figure 6–22). On the right side of the section is drawn the pathway of the tract leading from the facial motor nucleus to the exit of cranial nerve VII on the ventral surface of the brainstem, at the junction between the medulla and pons. Note the "looping" of the pathway around the abducens nucleus, in the floor of the fourth ventricle, before the tract turns anteriorly toward its exit point from the brainstem.

is slightly ventral and lateral to the abducens nucleus, as labeled on the left side of Figure 6–26.

The tract issuing from the facial motor nucleus follows an interesting course within the pons before emerging from the brainstem. In Figure 6–26, right side, this tract has been outlined and labeled in three locations. The origin of the tract is where axons emerge from the facial motor nucleus. This tract runs dorsally, toward the floor of the fourth ventricle, and loops around the abducens nucleus before heading ventrally to exit from the brainstem (the exit is labeled "root" in Figure 6–26; see the ventral surface of the brainstem in Figure 6–20 for the exit point of the facial nerve, immediately lateral to the exit point for cranial nerve VI). Within the pons, the loop of fibers around the abducens nucleus is called the internal genu of the facial nerve, and the bump created in the floor of the fourth ventricle by this genu and the immediately ventral abducens nucleus is the *facial colliculus.*

Virtually all muscles of facial expression (see Chapter 5) are innervated by the voluntary motor component of the facial nerve, issued from the facial motor nucleus. The facial nerve also innervates the stapedius muscle, which attaches to the neck of the stapes in the middle ear and pulls on it reflexively, in response to acoustic events having extremely high sound energy. The acoustic (stapedius) reflex protects hair cells in the

cochlea, the end organ of hearing, from extremely loud sounds. The innervation of the stapedius muscle from the same pool of fibers supplying muscles of facial expression is a useful anatomical datum when a clinical profile includes both facial paralysis and absence of the acoustic reflex.

Cranial nerve VII also carries autonomic motor fibers to glands that secrete tears and saliva. The term "autonomic" is reserved for nervous system function that is not voluntary (such as production of saliva, regulation of blood pressure, sweat glands, and so forth). The motor cells for this part of the nerve are found in the superior salivatory nucleus (see Figure 6–22, left side, small nucleus colored brown in pons, superior to the abducens nucleus). The salivatory axons exit the brainstem with the rest of the facial nerve fibers.

The sensory component of cranial nerve VII includes general touch and pressure, and taste. Sensory innervation for touch and pressure is limited to small regions of the external ear, including the ear canal and the external surface of the eardrum. Sensory fibers from these regions make an initial synapse in a ganglion outside the brainstem, within the skull, and enter the brainstem through the root of cranial nerve VII. These fibers terminate in the chief (also called principal) sensory nucleus of V (see Figure 6–22, right side). Taste fibers innervate the anterior two-thirds of the tongue, have an initial synapse in the same ganglion as the other sensory fibers and enter the brainstem with the root of cranial nerve VII, terminating in the nucleus solitarius.

The voluntary motor function of cranial nerve VII is of obvious importance to the speech-language pathologist. As one example, the motor component of cranial nerve VII controls the *orbicularis oris* muscles and the associated muscle complex (including muscles such as the *mentalis, levator anguli oris,* etc., see Chapter 5) that are critical to the production of vowel contrasts that depend on labial configuration, as well as labial motions and configurations for consonants such as /p/, /b/, /f/, and /v/. These muscles, as well as muscles of the cheeks, also have an important role in swallowing.

When a speech-language pathologist or neurologist tests the integrity of the voluntary motor component of cranial nerve VII, the face is evaluated at rest or when movement is requested from the person. For example, damage to cranial nerve VII on one side of the brainstem will result in paralysis of the muscles on the entire half of the same side (ipsilateral to the damage) of the face. With such damage the speech-language pathologist or neurologist usually observes a drooping lower corner of the mouth, a smoothed nasolabial fold, and a smooth (crease-free) forehead on the side of the lesion when the face is at rest. These at-rest observations are typical of, for example, observation of the face in Bell's palsy (see Duffy, 2005). For evaluation of movement, a patient can be asked to smile rapidly, blink several times, and lift her eyebrows. Unilateral damage resulting in paralysis of muscles innervated by cranial nerve VII causes a rapid smile to be produced with lateral movement of the corner of the mouth only on the undamaged side; blinks are possible only with the eyelid on the unaffected side; and only the eyebrow on the unaffected side can be raised.

Cranial Nerve VIII (Auditory-Vestibular Nerve)

The auditory-vestibular nerve is sensory. The nerve has a double name because it carries information to the brainstem from both the cochlea and the vestibular apparatus of the inner ear. The cochlea contains the end organ cells for hearing, and the vestibular apparatus the cells for balance and movement coordination of the eyes, head, and trunk.

The cochlea and vestibular apparatus are related structures, containing fluid-filled chambers embedded within the temporal bone of the skull. Within these fluid-filled chambers are hair cells whose position and shape are changed by displacement of the fluid. In the case of the cochlea the fluid displacement and resulting effect on the hair cells is typically due to sound energy entering the external ear canal, vibrating the ear drum and the three ossicles (bones) of the middle ear, causing the ossicle coupled to the cochlea (the *stapes*) to move in and out of one of the fluid-filled chambers. In the case of the vestibular apparatus, the hairs cells are displaced when the head turns. The hair cells of both structures are connected to sensory fibers that are depolarized or hyperpolarized when the hair cells are displaced by fluid motion. These sensory fibers make a first synapse in ganglia outside the brainstem (the spiral ganglion in the case of the cochlea; vestibular [Scarpa's] ganglion in the case of the vestibular apparatus). The sensory fibers exiting these ganglia run together as the two parts of cranial nerve VIII — the auditory (cochlear) nerve and the vestibular nerve — to their respective nuclei in the brainstem.

The two nerve bundles of cranial nerve VIII approach and enter the dorsolateral aspect of the brainstem close to the junction of the medulla and pons (the pontomedullary junction). Figure 6–27 shows a transverse section of the brainstem, slightly inferior to the pontomedullary junction and therefore technically in the medulla. Note the entry point of the auditory portion of cranial nerve VIII, and the close proximity of the cerebellum to the inferior, dorsolateral surfaces of the pons. The narrow space between the pons and cerebellum is referred to as the *cerebellopontine angle* (see Figure 6–27). Cerebellopontine angle tumors are a class of tumors in which a mass at or within the angle presses on the ventral and ventrolaterlal surface of the brainstem and (most commonly) affects the function of cranial nerves V, VII, and VIII.

Fibers of the cochlear (auditory) division of cranial nerve VIII synapse on cells in the cochlear nuclei (two on each side), located just below the dorsolateral surface of the pontomedullary junction, as shown in Figure 6–27. Fibers from the vestibular division of the nerve synapse on cells of the vestibular nuclei (four on each side), located dorsally, more or less facing the ventral surface of the cerebellum. In the inferior-superior dimension shown on the right side of Figure 6–22 (in purple), the vestibular nuclei are seen to extend well above and below the pontomedullary junction.

The *central auditory pathways* consist of fiber tracts and several intervening nuclei connecting the cochlear nuclei to auditory cortical regions. A signal moves along the auditory pathway from the cochlea to auditory nerve, from the auditory nerve to the cochlear nuclei, from the cochlear nuclei to several other nuclei in the brainstem, the last of which are the inferior col-

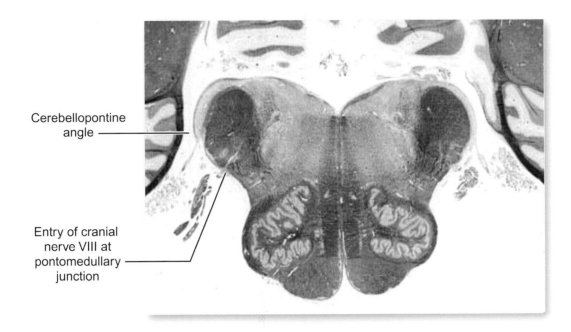

Cerebellopontine angle ——

Entry of cranial nerve VIII at pontomedullary —— junction

Figure 6–27. Horizontal section through a human brainstem, in the high medulla just below its junction with the pons. The section shows the brainstem tissue surrounded by cerebellar tissue (note the small white space at the midline, between the posterior edge of the brainstem tissue and the more posterior cerebellar tissue; that white space is part of the fourth ventricle). The section shows the entry point of cranial nerve VIII to the brainstem, as well as the small, lateral space between the lower pons and the surrounding cerebellar tissue; this space is the cerebellopontine angle. The "coiled" nuclei in the ventrolateral part of the brainstem section are the inferior olivary nuclei (also see Figure 6–28) whose lateral-most "bend" forms the inferior olive landmark on the ventral surface of the brainstem (see Figure 6–20).

liculi in the midbrain, then to the medial geniculate bodies of the thalamus and finally to the primary auditory cortex. Signals are processed from the auditory nerve through the brainstem very, very quickly, with about a 5- to 6-ms lag between the firing of auditory nerve fibers and firing of cells in the inferior colliculus. An audiometric test called the Auditory Brainstem Response (ABR), in which electrical signals generated by nervous system structures are measured with scalp electrodes and amplifiers, takes advantage of these very rapid but measurable transit times along the auditory nerve and brainstem pathways. One popular use of this test is in screening for the presence of possible hearing problems in newborns (see Picton, 2010).

The central pathways for the vestibular system are complex, consistent with the complex tasks of eye-head-trunk coordination. The vestibular nuclei send information received from the vestibular component of cranial nerve VIII up the brainstem to the oculomotor, trochlear, and abducens nuclei for coordination of head and eye movements; the nuclei also send informtion down the spinal cord and to the cerebellum for coordination of head and trunk movement.

There are batteries of tests for the integrity of both the cochlear and vestibular components of cranial nerve VIII. These are not described here, but may include pure tone, speech discrimination, and ABR evaluation for the cochlear component, and observation of eye movement and balance for the vestibular component.

Cranial Nerve IX (Glossopharyngeal)

The glossopharyngeal is a mixed nerve. As seen in Figure 6–20, the nerve is attached to the upper medulla in the groove just lateral to the swelling of the inferior olive on the ventral surface of the brainstem. Voluntary motor fibers of cranial nerve IX originate in the superior portion of the nucleus ambiguus (a long column of motor neuron cells located (in cross-section) about midway between the ventral and dorsal surfaces of the medulla, and somewhat lateral to the midline. Figure 6–28 shows a horizontal section of the medulla, taken roughly between the superior and inferior borders of the medulla, in which the nucleus ambiguus is seen just dorsal to the inferior olive. Figure 6–22, left side, shows the nucleus ambiguus extending throughout

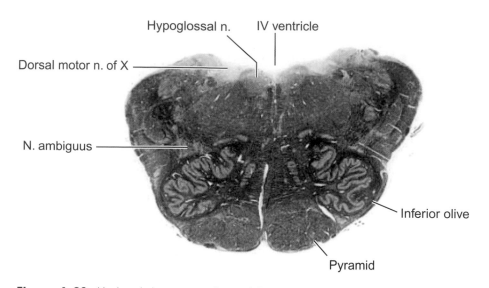

Figure 6–28. Horizontal cross-section of the medulla, roughly midway between the superior and inferior boundaries of the medulla. Note the positions of the nucleus ambiguus, the hypoglossal nucleus, and the ventral pyramids.

the entire superior-inferior length of the medulla. The motor component of cranial nerve IX, derived from the top of the nucleus ambiguus column, innervates a single pharyngeal muscle, the *stylopharyngeus*. As described in Chapter 4, contraction of the paired *stylopharyngeus* muscles may lift and widen the pharyngeal tube; the specific role of this muscle in speech production is unknown, but it almost certainly plays a role in swallowing by shortening the pharyngeal tube (Meng, Murakami, Suzuki, & Miyamoto, 2008; see also Chapter 13).

The glossopharyngeal nerve also has an autonomic motor component. The inferior salivatory nucleus (see Figure 6–22, see left side of brainstem, nucleus in upper medulla, close to the midline) gives off fibers that exit the brainstem along with the voluntary motor fibers derived from the nucleus ambiguus. The autonomic fibers then separate from the fibers en route to the *stylopharyngeus* muscle, the former innervating cells in the parotid gland. The parotid is the largest salivary gland of the head and neck, and is located—actually wrapped around—the ramus of the mandible. When stimulated by the autonomic fibers of cranial nerve IX the gland secretes saliva into the oral and pharyngeal cavities.

The sensory component of the glossopharyngeal nerve transmits information on touch, temperature, and pressure from the posterior one-third of the tongue, parts of the pharynx, and the external ear and surface of the eardrum facing the middle ear cavity. The various sensory fibers serving these regions make first synapses in a pair of related ganglia, then enter the brainstem together at the root of cranial nerve IX (see Figure 6–20) and terminate in the brainstem, within the spinal part of the sensory trigeminal nucleus (see Figure 6–22, right side of brainstem, lower part of light green nucleus). There is also an autonomic sensory component to cranial nerve IX, part of which carries taste information from the posterior one-third of the tongue to cells at the top of the columnlike solitary nucleus. The other autonomic sensory component of cranial nerve IX conveys information on blood gases and blood pressure from receptors near the split of the common carotid artery into the internal and external carotid arteries (carotid bodies; see Chapter 2). Fibers from these receptors go to cells at the bottom of the solitary nucleus column.

There are no clinical tests for the *independent* integrity of cranial nerve IX. Most of the clinical tests employed by neurologists and speech-language pathologists are designed to evaluate the *motor* function of the various cranial nerves. As noted above the role of the *stylopharyngeus* in speech is not clear, nor is it clear how this muscle can be tested separately from the many other muscles of the pharynx, which as explained below are innervated by cranial nerve X (vagus). Cranial nerves IX and X are sometimes evaluated together via the gag reflex, which depends for its sensory input on fibers from cranial nerve IX (stimulated when the posterior pharyngeal wall is touched) and for its motor response (contraction of the pharyngeal constrictor muscles, among other muscles) on fibers from cranial nerve X.

Cranial Nerve X (Vagus)

Cranial nerve X is a mixed nerve. The nerve is attached to the brainstem as a series of roots in the groove just lateral to the inferior olive, immediately inferior to the point of attachment of cranial nerve IX (see Figure 6–20). Also like cranial nerve IX, the voluntary motor fibers of the vagus nerve originate in cells of the nucleus ambiguus (see Figures 6–22 and 6–28). These cells and the fibers they give rise to innervate the pharyngeal constrictor muscles, the *palatal levator*, the *salpingopharyngeus*, the *palatopharyngeus* and *palatoglossus* muscles, and the intrinsic muscles of the larynx (*cricothyroid, thryoarytenoid, posterior cricoarytenoid, lateral cricoarytenoid*, and *arytenoid*) (see Chapters 3 through 5). The voluntary muscle component of cranial nerve X clearly plays an important role in speech and swallowing, given its control of muscles that adjust the dimensions of the velopharyngeal port, the pharyngeal lumen, aspects of tongue motion, and the tension and configuration of the vocal folds.

Cranial nerve X also has an autonomic motor component. Most of these fibers arise from the dorsal motor nucleus of X, which like the nucleus ambiguus forms a column throughout the medulla (though not quite as long as the nucleus ambiguus). The dorsal motor nucleus of X is medial to the nucleus ambiguus, more dorsal (hence its name), and close to the floor of the fourth ventricle (see Figure 6–28). Fibers arising from cells in the dorsal motor nucleus of X (and possibly from a small region of the nucleus ambiguus as well) stimulate mucous glands within the pharynx and larynx, and glands within the gut and other organs. Autonomic motor function, with fibers derived from the dorsal motor nucleus of X, is also supplied by cranial nerve X for control of the smooth (nonvoluntary) muscle of the heart and gut.

Information on touch, pressure, and temperature is carried by sensory fibers from the pharynx, larynx, parts of the external ear and eardrum and the meninges from the posterior part of the cerebral hemispheres. Like touch, pressure and temperature information traveling in any cranial nerve (see information above on cranial nerves V, VII, IX), these sensory fibers make initial synapses in ganglia outside the brainstem, enter the brainstem where the nerve roots for cranial nerve X are indicated in Figure 6–20 and travel to the lower part of the sensory nucleus of V (see Figure 6–22, right side of brainstem, light green column).

Cranial nerve X includes an autonomic sensory component that carries sensation from the gut. These sensations are not conscious, as in the case of touch or pressure, but may result in a sense of "feeling good" or "feeling bad" (Wilson-Pauwels et al., 2002). Autonomic fibers also arise from chemoreceptors, baroreceptors, and the mucosal surfaces of the larynx. This information makes a first synapse in one member of a pair of ganglia, which sends fibers into the brainstem at the point of attachment of the vagus roots and subsequently to the nucleus solitarius (see Figure 6–22, right side, dark green column).

Several clinical tests are used to evaluate the integrity of the voluntary motor function of cranial nerve X. One involves asking a patient to open her mouth and say the vowel "ah" as the clinician observes the velum. Typically, at the onset of phonation the velum is pulled up, symmetrically, by the paired *palatal levator* muscles. This is consistent with expected velopharyngeal closure for vowels. Upward movement of one side of the velum, but not the other, indicates a problem with cranial nerve X or the nucleus ambiguus (or both) on the side opposite to the observed movement (that is, damage is suspected on the side that does not lift). If both sides fail to lift when the vowel is phonated, bilateral damage to the nucleus ambiguus and/or cranial nerve X may be indicated, or there may be bilateral lesions in the cortical regions for velopharyngeal muscles (or to the tracts issuing from these cortical regions whose targets are the velopharyngeal motor neuron cells in the nuclei ambiguus).

Clinical evaluation of cranial nerve X can also be performed by listening to a person's voice quality, and/or requesting that the person execute voluntary laryngeal maneuvers. The vagus nerve provides innervation to the intrinsic muscles of the larynx, which acting together create a muscular tone somewhat like a background, postural setting for vibration of the vocal folds. When the contraction levels of the intrinsic muscles are set properly, each cycle of vocal fold vibration has a relatively quick closing phase, and a closed phase (see Chapter 8). These closing and closed phases of vocal fold vibration produce a glottal spectrum rich in harmonics, and a voice quality perceived as "good." Damage to one side of the vagus nerve, or particularly one of its branches called the *recurrent laryngeal nerve* which innervates the intrinsic laryngeal muscles that adduct the vocal folds, results in weakness or paralysis of the adductors and a compromised ability to create the proper postural setting described above. When this situation occurs, as in cases of unilateral vocal fold paralysis (for example, due to crushing injuries of the neck or upper thorax, where the recurrent laryngeal nerve runs before entering the larynx, or as a result of neck surgeries), typical voice quality is likely to be weak, breathy, hoarse, and/or raspy. Whereas such voice qualities may suggest a problem with the vagus nerve (or the laryngeal motor neurons in the nucleus ambiguus), they do not provide information on the precise location (side) of damage.

Voluntary laryngeal maneuvers can provide further information regarding the function of cranial nerve X. For example, a patient can be asked to produce a quick, strong cough, which requires rapid and forceful contraction of the adductor muscles innervated by the recurrent laryngeal nerve. Some clinicians use laryngeal diadochokinetic tasks consisting of rapid repetitions of a single vowel such as /i/, with a request of the patient to initiate each vowel with a "hard" glottal attack, to evaluate the integrity of the laryngeal adductors; each /i/ is assumed to require quick and forceful contraction of the adductor muscles. When the adductors are weakened or paralyzed by damage to one or both sides of the vagus nerve, the onset of the cough or repeated /i/'s is perceived as weak and ineffective. Another clinical test involves asking the person to increase the pitch of her voice; for example, "Say 'ah' using the highest pitch possible." Difficulty with this task may indicate impairment of the superior laryngeal nerve, a branch of cranial nerve X, which innervates the *cricothyroid* muscles that stretch and stiffen the vocal folds. As with listening to typical voice quality, these clinical tests may suggest damage to the vagus nerve, but no firm conclusion can be reached concerning the exact location of damage. Damage on either the left or right side can cause breathiness, a weak-sounding cough, or weak onsets for the vowels in a laryngeal diadochokinetic sequence.

These tests of vagus nerve integrity for phonatory function are described here because they are used fairly frequently in a speech-language pathologist's evaluation of the cranial nerves. The interpretation of voice abnormalities is complicated because many neural, structural, or functional disorders may produce similar perceptual results. The best way to test for the presence of vagus nerve dysfunction affecting the laryngeal muscles is to view the vocal folds directly, either by indirect laryngoscopy (via a laryngeal mirror) or through an endoscope (see Chapter 3).

As noted above in the discussion of cranial nerve IX, the gag reflex is mediated by a neural loop whose sensory branch travels in cranial nerve IX, and whose motor branch travels with cranial nerve X. When the posterior wall of the pharynx or the soft palate is touched, the sensory receptors in the pharyngeal mucosa are depolarized and send a signal via the sensory fibers of cranial nerve IX to the brainstem, via a sensory ganglion. These fibers travel to the lower part of the sensory nucleus of V, where they make synapses with cells whose axons project to the nucleus ambig-

uus. The nucleus ambiguus, as discussed in the present section, contains motor cells that control contraction of the pharyngeal constrictor muscles, *palatal levator* muscles, and laryngeal adductor muscles. Stimulation of these motor cells through the reflex arc causes rapid contraction of all these muscles, effectively protecting the airway from potentially dangerous material. The gag reflex is simple yet mysterious. Why don't we gag when, for example, eating or drinking? As food or liquid passes the soft palate and through the pharyngeal tube the sensory receptors in the mucous membranes and muscle tissues surely respond to the touch, pressure, and temperature of the food or liquid. Although the precise mechanism is unknown, some aspect of swallowing must inhibit the elicitation of the gag reflex. Another mystery concerning the gag reflex is its absence in at least 20–25% of the population with "normal" neurological mechanisms. The absence of a gag reflex, when elicited properly (such as touching the posterior pharyngeal wall with a cotton swab) does not necessarily imply a neurological problem. Because the gag reflex can be elicited from either side of the posterior pharyngeal wall (either to the right or left of the midline pharyngeal raphe: see Chapter 5), a positive reflex on one side but not on the other is generally taken to suggest something wrong in one of branches of the gag reflex loop, or perhaps in the brainstem nuclei (sensory nucleus of V and nucleus ambiguus) where the loop makes central synapses.

Cranial Nerve XI (Spinal Accessory Nerve)

Cranial nerve XI, which only has motor fibers, is called the spinal accessory nerve because its motor neurons are located in the ventral horn of upper segments of the cervical spinal cord, rather than in the brainstem. Figure 6–22 shows the approximate location of this column of spinal cells, called the spinal accessory nucleus, extending from the junction of the medulla and spinal cord four or five segments down into the cervical spinal cord. Note how the spinal accessory nucleus is in line with the columnar nucleus ambiguus.

Why is a nerve with cells of origin in the spinal cord considered a cranial nerve? First, the nerve supplies motor innervation to two muscles of the head and neck, the *sternocleidomastoid* muscle and the *trapezius* muscle. The former muscle turns the head and lifts the chin toward the side opposite the contraction (when the right *sternocleidomastoid* contracts with its sternum end fixed, the head is turned and lifted toward the left side, and vice versa), and the latter muscle produces rotation of the scapula and raises the arm above the shoulder. Second, many authors regard the accessory nucleus as a continuation of the nucleus ambiguus; both columns seem to be derived from the same embryological tissue. In fact, as reviewed in Chapter 3, some authors believe the spinal accessory nucleus may innervate muscles of the larynx along with branches of cranial nerve X. Third, and perhaps most importantly, the fibers issued from the accessory nucleus emerge from the spinal cord, and ascend into the skull to travel with fibers of cranial nerves IX and X. Note in Figure 6–20 how the several rootlets of the accessory nerve emerge lateral to the inferior olive, like the rootlets of cranial nerves IX and X, and travel superiorly along the edge of the spinal cord. In fact, cranial nerves IX, X, and XI exit (or, in the case of the sensory components of IX and X, *enter*) the skull through the same opening (the jugular foramen, a fairly large opening in the base of the skull through which nerves pass).

Cranial nerve IX is evaluated by testing the separate actions of the two muscles. Evaluation of the *sternocleidomastoid* muscle is performed by asking the patient to turn and raise her head to one or the other side against a clinician-imposed resistance. For example, the patient rotates and lifts the head to the right side while the clinician imposes pressure against the side of the head to which the turn is attempted. If the clinician detects weakness, innervation to the side opposite the turn (in the case of this example, innervation to the left *sternocleidomastoid* muscle) is suspected of damage. The *trapezius* muscle is evaluated by asking the patient to lift both shoulders or to raise each arm above the level of the shoulder while the clinician resists the raising motion with downward pressure on the arm. Asymmetric shoulder raises, or weakness detected during the attempt to raise the arm above the head, are both possible indications of damage to the accessory nucleus or the fibers of cranial nerve IX that innervate the *trapezius* muscle. These tests may be performed routinely by some speech-language pathologists as part of the cranial nerve exam, but at best the *sternocleidomastoid muscle* and *trapezius muscle* have no more than a supplementary role in speech production.

Cranial Nerve XII (Hypoglossal)

Cranial nerve XII is generally regarded as strictly a motor nerve, innervating all the intrinsic muscles and all but one of the extrinsic muscles of the tongue (the exception being the *palatoglossus* muscle, innervated by cranial nerve X). The fibers of cranial nerve XII originate in the hypoglossal nucleus, a column of motor cells near the midline of the medulla (see Figure 6–22). A horizontal section through the medulla, approximately halfway between its upper and lower borders, shows the hypoglossal nuclei in the floor of the fourth ventricle, on either side of the midline (see Figure 6–28). Axons from these cells run ventrally and laterally to emerge as cranial nerve XII on the ventral surface of the medulla, in the sulcus between the pyramid and the inferior olive (see Figure 6–20).

The control of both intrinsic and extrinsic tongue muscles by cranial nerve XII means that virtually any lingual behavior relevant to speech production is ultimately vested in the integrity of this nerve and its brainstem nuclei. This includes both fine adjustments to create the precision configurations required for the grooved tongue of fricatives such as /s/ and /sh/ as well as the presumably gross adjustments of tongue position associated with distinctions between (for example) front and back vowels. Although some older theories of lingual muscle function and speech production viewed the intrinsic muscles as mostly associated with consonant production and the extrinsic muscle with vowel production, both muscle groups almost certainly work together to produce tongue configurations and gestures for intelligible speech and all of its phonetic components.

Clinical tests for the integrity of cranial nerve XII involve visual examination of the tongue at rest, as well as an evaluation of tongue protrusion when the patient

---

The Final Common Pathway

What is this? The last path we will all travel? No, it is a term used when referring to a certain part of the motor system, the part containing nuclei of cell bodies whose axons go directly to muscles. The term "motor neuron" is typically reserved for the cells in these nuclei, which receive information primarily from descending fiber tracts coming from the cortex. They are the last stop before motor commands are sent via cranial and spinal nerves to muscles in the jaw, lips, rib cage wall, and other parts of the speech apparatus and body. The idea of a final common pathway recognizes that a particular motor nucleus in the brainstem or spinal cord may receive input from several different sources and be subject to a "net effect" of all those different inputs. The idea of a final common pathway in motor systems was originally formulated by the famous neurophysiologist Charles Sherrington, and described in his then revolutionary 1906 text, *The Integrative Action of the Nervous System.*

is asked to stick out her tongue in a straight line. Visual examination with the tongue inside the mouth, at rest with the jaw slightly open, is to assess the mass of the tongue tissue and/or the presence of small contractions that appear on the tongue surface as transient bumps, ripples, and shakes. The tongue protrusion test is performed to determine if the tongue deviates to either the left or right side when the patient is asked to do the protrusion in a straight line. The interpretation of these signs is explained in the section "Cortical Innervation Patterns" below, where the innervation patterns for the cranial nerve nuclei and the concept of upper versus lower motor neuron innervations and disease is discussed.

CORTICAL INNERVATION PATTERNS

This section describes the innervation of brainstem motor nuclei by cortical cells, and specifically of the motor nuclei associated with speech-related muscles of the head and neck. These nuclei include the motor nucleus of V (trigeminal), the facial motor nucleus, the nucleus ambiguus, the spinal accessory nucleus, and the hypoglossal nucleus. The cortical innervation of the oculomotor nuclei (oculomotor, trochlear, and abducens nuclei) is not discussed here, nor is the innervation of nuclei associated with outflow of the autonomic system (salivatory nuclei, dorsal motor nucleus of X).

Table 6–5 summarizes the innervation patterns for the five, paired brainstem motor nuclei that control speech musculature of the head and neck. When both members of a specific motor nucleus pair receive input from the left and right motor cortices (from the primary motor cells in both the left and right hemispheres), the nuclei are bilaterally innervated. Table 6–5 classifies the motor nucleus of V, part of the facial motor nucleus, the nucleus ambiguus, and the accessory nucleus as receiving bilateral innervation. For example, both motor nuclei of V—on the left and right sides of the pons—receive corticobulbar projections from both the left and right hemispheres. Stated in another way, the left motor nucleus of V receives an ipsilateral projection from the left hemisphere and a contralateral projection from the right hemisphere; the right motor nucleus of V receives an ipsilateral projection from the right hemisphere and a contralateral projection from the left hemisphere.

Table 6–5 shows the innervation of the facial motor nucleus to be both contralateral and bilateral. The facial motor nucleus contains cells specific to muscles of the upper face and cells specific to muscles of the lower face. Cells for control of the lower face receive only contralateral innervation from the cortex, whereas cells for control of the upper facial muscles receive bilateral innervation from the motor cortex. Raising your eyebrows in surprise, for example, involves commands from both sides of the motor cortex to both facial motor nuclei, whereas movement of the corner of your right lower lip is produced by commands from the left motor cortex to the right facial motor nucleus.

Like the facial motor nucleus, the accessory nucleus has both contralateral and bilateral innervation from the motor cortex. There is some dispute about the pathways from the motor cortex to the upper regions of the cervical spinal cord, where the accessory nucleus is located, but the most conservative view seems to be that the *sternocleidomastoid* muscle is innervated

Table 6–5. Cortical Innervation Patterns of the Brainstem Motor Nuclei for Speech Musculature

MOTOR NUCLEUS	INNERVATION
Motor Nucleus of V (V)	Bilateral
Facial Motor Nucleus (VII)	Bilateral (upper face)
	Contralateral (lower face)
Nucleus Ambiguus (IX, X, XI)	Bilateral
Accessory Nucleus (XI)	Bilateral (**sternocleidomastoid** muscle)
	Contralateral (**trapezius** muscle)
Hypoglossal Nucleus (XII)	Contralateral

Note: The cranial nerves associated with these motor nuclei are indicated in parentheses.

bilaterally, and the *trapezius* muscle contralaterally (DeToledo & David, 2001); however, some authors (Wilson-Pauwels et al., 2002) claim that the *sternocleidomastoid* muscle is innervated only ipsilaterally—that is, the left motor cortex only innervates the left accessory nucleus, the right motor cortex only innervates the right accessory nucleus. Because these muscles probably have relevance to speech performance only under high-effort conditions, further description of the innervation patterns of the accessory motor nucleus is not pursued here.

The hypoglossal nucleus, which controls muscles of the tongue, is the only motor nucleus of the brainstem with strictly contralateral innervation from the motor cortex. Tongue cells in the left motor cortex innervate cells in the right hypoglossal nucleus, and vice versa.

Why These Innervation Patterns Matter

These innervation patterns have significance for clinical signs of neurological disease. Because the brainstem motor nuclei innervate the *muscles* of the speech apparatus ipsilaterally—that is, motor nuclei on the left and right sides of the brainstem innervate muscles on the left and right sides of the head and neck, respectively—knowledge of the innervation of the brainstem nuclei by cortical structures can lead to important clues concerning lesion location based on the appearance of head and neck structures at rest, or their performance during voluntary maneuvers. For example, a unilateral, cortical lesion of cells that control muscles of the face should not result in a deficit of upper face control, but may result in a loss of lower face control on the side opposite the lesion. The unilateral cortical lesion will cause loss of input to the facial motor nucleus on the same side (ipsilateral to the lesion) and to the facial motor nucleus on the opposite side (contralateral to the lesion), but these facial motor nuclei still receive healthy input from the undamaged motor cortex on the other side of the brain, allowing for more or less normal appearance and functional muscle contraction for muscles of the upper face. The unilateral cortical damage does, however, result in a deficit in appearance and control of the lower face contralateral to the lesion. This is because the cells in the facial motor nucleus that control lower face muscles receive cortical input only from the contralateral hemisphere.

Consider several hypothetical clinical presentations. One person appears to have impairment of *all* facial muscles (upper and lower) on one side of the face, with normal-appearing muscles on the other side. With the face at rest, the impaired side might show, in varying degrees, a smoothed forehead (as opposed to the furrows created by normal tone in the muscles of the forehead), a reduced depth or complete absence of the nasolabial fold (the fold of skin forming a line between the side of the nose and the corner of the mouth), and/or a drooping lower lip. Based on the innervation patterns described above, the presence of both upper and lower facial paralysis on one side but normal-appearing facial characteristics on the other side, suggest a unilateral lesion in the facial motor nucleus in the pons, or in cranial nerve VII close to its exit from the brainstem and the skull, before it splits into various "local" nerves that supply individual muscles of the face (this is called a lower motor neuron lesion; see sidetrack on "Upper Versus Lower Motor Neuron Lesions"). Because the brainstem motor nuclei innervate head and neck muscles ipsilaterally, the lesion in the brainstem or the cranial nerve is on the same side as the observed paralysis.

Why is it relatively easy to rule out a *cortical* lesion in the case of this half-face pattern of weakness/paralysis? The explanation is the bilateral innervation of the facial motor nuclei for muscles of the upper face, which means that a unilateral cortical lesion does not produce noticeable impairment of the upper face at rest; only a unilateral, lower motor neuron lesion produces this set of signs. Bilateral cortical lesions result in paralysis on *both* sides of the face, as do bilateral lesions of the facial motor nucleus or cranial nerve VII close to its exit point from the brainstem. When both sides of the face are paralyzed, the distinction between bilateral cortical versus bilateral brainstem/cranial nerve lesions is not so difficult because a brainstem lesion large enough to affect both sides of the pons also produces marked effects on other behaviors, a description of which is beyond the scope of this chapter.

Similar reasoning applies to apparent paralysis of the velopharyngeal muscles or the larynx. The brainstem motor nucleus for the majority of velopharyngeal and laryngeal muscles is the nucleus ambiguus, which is innervated bilaterally from the motor cortex (see Table 6–5). If you ask a neurologically normal individual to open her mouth and observe the motion of the velum when she says "ah," the upward motion of the velar tissue flap is rapid and symmetrical as the velopharyngeal port is closed for the vowel production. A unilateral cortical lesion in cells associated with velopharyngeal muscles does not typically affect this rapid and symmetrical motion to a significant degree, because the nucleus ambiguus receives bilateral innervation from the cortex. A unilateral lesion in the nucleus ambiguus or in cranial nerve X, however, results in weakness on the same side of the lesion. When the patient says "ah," the upward movement of the velum is asymmetrical, with rapid elevation on the side of the healthy nucleus ambiguus and weak or no movement on the side of the brainstem/cranial nerve lesion. Similarly, a unilateral cortical lesion among laryngeal motor cells has little or no effect on normal vibration of the vocal folds, whereas a unilateral lesion in the nucleus ambiguus or cranial nerve X results in vocal fold paralysis on the same side as the lesion, which in many cases affects voice quality.

Unlike the cases of bilateral innervation reviewed above, in which a unilateral cortical lesion does not result in an observable appearance or movement deficit of the upper face, velum, and vocal folds, a unilateral lesion of tongue cells in the motor cortex should result in an observable deficit. The contralateral-only innervation of the hypoglossal nuclei suggests this expectation. For example, a unilateral lesion among tongue motor neurons in the right motor cortex affects the strength of muscles on the left side of the muscular complex of the tongue. The several muscles of the tongue are capable of very complex tongue motions and configurations, but a simple test of the integrity of tongue motion is to request an individual to protrude his tongue, in a straight line. In the neurologically healthy individual, the tongue is centered as it is protruded, balanced by the roughly equivalent strength of the paired musculature (primarily the genioglossus muscle) producing the protrusion. In a person with a unilateral cortical lesion in tongue cells, the tongue muscles on the side opposite the lesion are weak; therefore, when the tongue is protruded from the mouth the healthy side pushes the tongue "away from the lesion." For example, a lesion in the left motor cortex results in weakness of the genioglossus muscle on the right side of the tongue, which causes the tongue to deviate rightward when protruded from the mouth, away from the left-side, cortical lesion. The tongue deviates toward the weak side during a protrusion gesture because the "strong" genioglossus on the left side of the tongue is not balanced by an equally strong genioglossus on the right side of the tongue.

This scenario makes sense for a unilateral cortical lesion because of the exclusively contalateral innervation of the hypoglossal nuclei from the motor cortex. Deviation of the tongue on protrusion to one side or the other, however, is also symptomatic of a lesion to the hypoglossal nucleus or hypoglossal nerve on the *same side* as the lesion (and therefore, the same side of the weakness). Recall that the muscles of the head and neck are innervated *ipsilaterally* from the brainstem motor nuclei. A lesion in the right hypoglossal nucleus, or to the hypoglossal nerve exiting the right side of the

Upper Versus Lower Motor Neuron Lesions

There are motor neurons in the cortex, the brainstem, and the spinal cord. Cortical motor neurons send long axons to cells in both the brainstem and the spinal cord, which in turn send axons into the peripheral nervous system to end on muscles. Muscle control problems can result from damage anywhere along this path from cortex to muscle fiber. Neuroscientists and neurologists have a professional jargon to refer to sites of lesions along these motor pathways. "Upper motor neuron" lesions are those occurring in the cortical motor neurons or in the axons they issue, *before those axons make synapses with the motor neurons in the brainstem or spinal cord.* "Lower motor neuron" lesions are those occurring in the nuclei of the brainstem or motor cells of the spinal cord, or in the axons they issue and the peripheral nerves in which those axons travel. "Upper" motor neuron lesions result in muscles with excessive resting tone (stiff muscles) and hypersensitive reflexes. "Lower" motor neuron lesions result in loss of muscle mass (wasting, or atrophy), small muscle twitches visible to the naked eye (called fasciculations), and in some cases insufficient resting tone. In both upper and lower motor neuron lesions the involved muscles tend to be weak.

brainstem, produces weakness of the muscles on the right side of the tongue. In the case of such a lesion, the tongue deviates to the right (weak) side when protruded, just as it does when there is contralateral, cortical lesion.

In both cases described above, the tongue deviates to the side with weak muscles. In one case the weakness is the result of a contralateral, upper motor neuron lesion, in the other the result of an ipsilateral, lower motor neuron lesion (see sidetrack on Upper Versus Lower Motor Neuron Lesion). Because the clinical sign—deviation to the weak side—is the same for both lesion locations, is it possible to use other signs to identify the site of lesion? Lower motor neuron lesions typically produce fasciculations and muscle wasting (atrophy), so a combination of tongue deviation to one side on protrusion, with loss of muscle mass and fasciculations on the half of the tongue to which the deviation occurs, suggest that the lesion is in the hypoglossal nucleus and/or cranial nerve XII. Conversely, tongue deviation to one side with no loss of muscle mass and no fasciculations is suggestive of an upper motor lesion on the side opposite the deviation.

The Cranial Nerve Exam and Speech Production

Table 6–5 and the summary provided in the preceding section are guides to interpretation of lesion location when orofacial and laryngeal gestures deviate from expectations for the healthy brain. The various tests described here, and especially those to distinguish upper from lower motor neuron damage, are conducted primarily with nonspeech (e.g., lifting the eyebrows versus lateralizing the corner of the mouth; protrusion of the tongue) or speechlike (saying /a/ quickly, or phonating an extended vowel) tasks. The value in understanding these tasks is partly in appreciating the "wiring" of the craniofacial apparatus, in knowing what a speech-language pathologist is looking for when she asks a patient to protrude the tongue or examines the appearance of the face at rest, and in grasping an important part of the standard neurological examination. The results of these evaluations do not predict, with any degree of precision, actual speech production performance. A patient may have some deviation of the tongue and some obvious facial weakness yet still have intelligible speech; conversely, a patient whose cranial nerve exam appears to be within normal limits may have some obvious problems with conversational speech or when evaluated by more formal speech intelligibility tests. The cranial nerve exam yields valuable information, but this information is specific to the tasks used to evaluate the cranial nerves. Speech motor control, like general motor control, has been shown to be *task-specific*. A speech-language pathologist should not assume the results of the cranial nerve exam tells her all she needs to know about a patient's *speech* motor control abilities. Additional reasons for caution in interpreting these standard neurological tests in terms of speech motor control are discussed in the concluding section of the chapter.

SPINAL CORD AND SPINAL NERVES

Spinal Cord

The spinal cord includes gray and white matter, and extends as a long cord of tissue from the first cervical vertebrae (C1) to the first or second lumbar vertebrae (L1, L2). The superior edge of the spinal cord is continuous with the inferior edge of the medulla; the inferior edge of the spinal cord terminates at L1 or L2, but the protective coverings of the brain (including the dura and arachnoid mater, labeled in Figure 6–29; see section below, "Meninges, Ventricles, Blood Supply") continue to nearly the bottom of the sacral vertebrae and spinal nerves exit inferiorly to the inferior termination of spinal cord tissue.

A view of a vertical segment of spinal cord tissue, plus its protective coverings and nerves exiting and entering the cord, is shown in Figure 6–29. The view is from the front and slightly above and to the right of a horizontal (transverse) slice across the cord. The roughly H-shaped, darker part seen in this transverse slice are clusters of cell bodies of neurons (gray matter), and the whitish area surrounding these cells (white matter) are axons ascending and descending in the spinal cord, and entering and leaving the spinal cord. The specific form of the H-shaped cluster of cell bodies varies according to the level of the spinal cord at which a horizontal slice is made. Figure 6–29 shows a horizontal cut made at the lower end of the cervical cord, but the anatomical facts described in the next paragraph apply to any level of the cord.

The anterior (ventral) midline of the spinal cord is defined by a fissure, the *anterior median fissure*; the corresponding midline groove on the posterior (dorsal) aspect of the spinal cord is called the *posterior median septum* (see Figure 6–29). At any level of the spinal cord, the H-shaped cluster of cell bodies is more or less symmetrical with respect to these anterior and posterior median landmarks. In Figure 6–29, the spinal cord gray matter is labeled as having paired posterior horns and paired anterior horns. The "horns" are the clusters of cell bodies in the ventral (anterior) or dorsal (posterior) halves of a given transverse section. The notion of dorsal and ventral horns in the gray matter of the spinal cord goes past simple anatomical description; dorsal horn cells are typically sensory, receiving input from axons traveling from peripheral body structures to the spinal cord, and ventral horn cells issue axons that exit the spinal cord to provide motor innervation to muscles.

The white matter of the spinal cord is a dense composition of axons running in all different directions. In any transverse section, spinal cord white matter includes axons entering and leaving the cord, ascending and descending in the cord, and even traveling between cell bodies within the cord. The details of each of these fiber tracts are outside the scope of this text, but as in the cerebral hemispheres the fibers are arranged systematically and can be described by a general "geography" within any transverse section of the

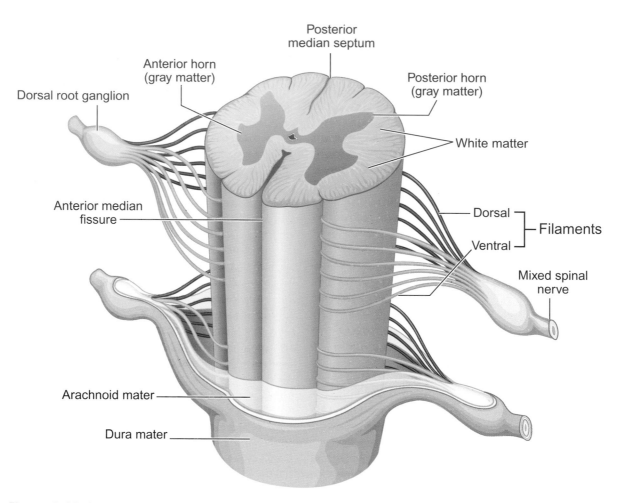

Figure 6–29. View of a section of the spinal cord from the front and slightly above a horizontal cut through the lower cervical cord. The horizontal cut shows the central gray matter in an H-shaped pattern, and the white matter surrounding it. The dorsal and ventral root filaments entering and leaving the spinal cord, respectively, are also shown, as are the meningeal coverings.

cord. For example, the corticospinal tract (which originates in the primary motor cortex and other parts of the frontal lobe, and continues through the internal capsule until most of the fibers decussate in the medulla) runs down the spinal cord as a fairly tight bundle in the lateral part of the spinal cord. At each level of the spinal cord, the lateral corticospinal tract issues axons to the anterior horn cells on the same side. These anterior horn cells issue axons that travel outside the spinal cord in peripheral nerves to innervate muscles. Recall that a small proportion (about 20%) of motor fibers originating in the motor cortex (both primary and premotor) and traveling through the internal capsule and upper brainstem do not decussate in the medulla, but rather continue into the spinal cord on the same side as their origination. These fibers form the anterior corticospinal tract, which runs in the anterior (ventral) part of

the spinal cord white matter, just lateral to the anterior median fissure. Other motor tracts in the spinal cord are not discussed here. Sensory fibers, primarily ascending in the spinal cord from posterior (dorsal) horn cells through the brainstem and thalamus and eventually to the cortex, run primarily in the posterior (dorsal) white matter columns lateral to the posterior median septum. These fibers carry information from peripheral body structures on touch, pain, and temperature.

Spinal Nerves

As shown in Figure 6–29, spinal nerves are attached to each segment of the spinal cord. The general organizational scheme for the spinal nerves is as follows. Motor and sensory fibers are attached to the spinal cord at different locations. Dorsal root filaments, which carry sensory information, enter the spinal cord close to the most posterior (dorsal) tip of the spinal gray matter. Ventral root filaments exit the spinal cord lateral to the anterior median fissure, close to the most anterior border of the anterior (ventral) horns. Note the use of the term "filaments": at each segment of the spinal cord, an entering or exiting nerve gives off several separate nerves. Figure 6–29 shows the sensory (dorsal) filaments as red fibers entering the the spinal cord, and the motor (ventral) filaments as blue fibers exiting the spinal cord.

At a very short distance from the entrance or exit of these nerves into or from the spinal cord, in the PNS, there is a gangion for each spinal nerve. They are called dorsal root ganglia (see Figure 6–29) because they contain the first synapses for sensory fibers from peripheral structures en route to the spinal cord. When sensory fibers enter the spinal cord, therefore, the synapse they make in a posterior horn cell is the *second* synapse in the sequence of information transfer from periphery to cortex. This is generally true for all sensory information in transit through the spinal cord, with the exception of sensory information derived from muscle spindles in voluntary muscle of the limbs and trunk. Just as in the case of the muscle spindles of the jaw for which the sensory fibers from the spindles go directly into the brainstem mesencephalic nucleus of V (described above in section on Jaw Jerk reflex), sensory fibers from muscle spindles embedded in limb and trunk muscles bypass a synapse in dorsal root ganglia and make direct connections with posterior (dorsal) horn cells within the spinal cord. This increases the speed of limb reflexes, just as the jaw jerk reflex is so fast due to the direct connection between spindles and the brainstem.

Although the dorsal root ganglia contain the cell bodies of first synapses for many sensory fibers, Figure 6–29 shows motor nerves derived from anterior (ventral) horn cells exiting the spinal cord and running through a ganglion. These motor filaments do not make synapses within the ganglia, but run through them "bundled" together with sensory fibers. Beyond the ganglia, toward the periphery, motor and sensory fibers associated with the spinal cord always run together; spinal nerves are therefore mixed (both sensory and motor) nerves. For example, the spinal nerves associated with the *internal intercostal* and *external intercostal* muscles are derived from from the first (T1) through eleventh (T11) thoracic segments (Chapter 2). Sensory fibers from receptors in these muscles carry information back to the spinal cord concerning touch, pressure, and stretch (the latter via muscle spindles). Motor fibers in these nerves control the contrac-

tion properties of the muscles. In general, the level at which a spinal nerve exits the spinal cord is consistent with the body level of the structures innervated by the nerves. Thus, arm and hand muscles are innervated by spinal nerves from cervical segments of the cord, rib cage wall muscles by spinal nerves from thoracic segments, and abdominal wall muscles from lumbar segments. Two well-known exceptions to this general rule are the diaphragm, which corresponds in position to the lower level of the thoracic cord but is innervated from the third through fifth cervical segments of the spinal cord, and the feet and legs, which are innervated from lumbar segments of the spinal cord.

NERVOUS SYSTEM CELLS

The CNS is composed of fluids, blood vessels, and several cell types. The cell types can be divided into the two major categories of *neurons* and *glia*. Imagine all the cells of the nervous system sitting in fluids—the *extracellular space*—with very precise, yet changeable, chemistry. This chemistry is regularly changed on a short-term basis—in fact, millions of times per second—and on a long-term basis as well. Interactions between neurons and glial cells contribute to both the precision and changeability of this chemical profile. The traditional understanding of the difference between the two major types of cells is that neurons are the signaling cells in the brain, whereas glia function as support and nourishment for the neurons and do not transmit signals. Signaling cells are those that send information to other cells and are also capable of receiving information from one or many cells; this idea is familiar to students who have studied synaptic transmission in the brain (discussed more fully below). According to recent research, some glial cells may also receive and send signals, but in this chapter the traditional distinction between neurons and glial cells is emphasized.

Depending on the source, the human brain is said to contain roughly 80–95 billion neurons and either the same number or many more glial cells. Whatever numbers one chooses to accept, the brain contains a lot of cells packed into the relatively small container of the skull. The signaling cells send and receive an enormous amount of information per unit time, and in doing so generate and expend a tremendous amount of energy. There is practical value in understanding the structure and physiology of nervous system cells, because many neurological diseases that have consequences for speech, language, and hearing behavior are explained partly or largely in terms of dysfunction of basic cellular anatomy and physiology. In addition, pharmacological and other treatments for these diseases often target aspects of basic cellular physiology. The following sections cover the structure and function of glial cells and neurons, the nature of the neuronal potentials (resting and action), synaptic transmission and neurotransmitters, and the neuromuscular junction.

Glial Cells

Figure 6–30 shows a neuron and some glial cells with which it shares brain space. The primary role of glial cells, according to present understanding, is to support the integrity of the signaling cells — the neurons — in a number of ways. Glial cells come in several forms, including *astrocytes, oligodendrocytes,* and others, as listed in Table 6–6.

The most numerous glial cells are *astrocytes,* shown in Figure 6–30 by a star-shaped cell with appendage-like projections from a central body (other subtypes of astrocyte may have different forms). Astrocytes used to be thought of as not much more than biological filler material between neurons, but recent research

suggests a much more important role for these cells in brain function. This role includes a contribution to the control of the chemical makeup of the extracellular (outside the cell) environment, including regulation of the molecules permitted to pass from the blood supply of the brain to the extracellular fluid. In addition, astrocytes form protective barriers around synapses (locations where information is transmitted from one neuron to another), apparently to ensure that neurotransmitters released at a particular synapse do not spread to other locations where they are not needed or where they might interfere with other transmissions. Similarly, astrocytes play a role in the removal of excess neurotransmitter after it has been released. Astrocytes also provide "anchors" for neurons, almost as if they were the skeletal framework on which neurons are hung.

Another type of glial cell lays down myelin on axons, the relatively narrow projections that carry electrical impulses from the cell body of a neuron to its terminus. In the CNS such glial cells are called *oligodendrocytes* (in the PNS the analogous glia are *Schwann* cells). In Figure 6–30 the simple-looking oligodendrocytes are shown extending short "arms" to the axon.

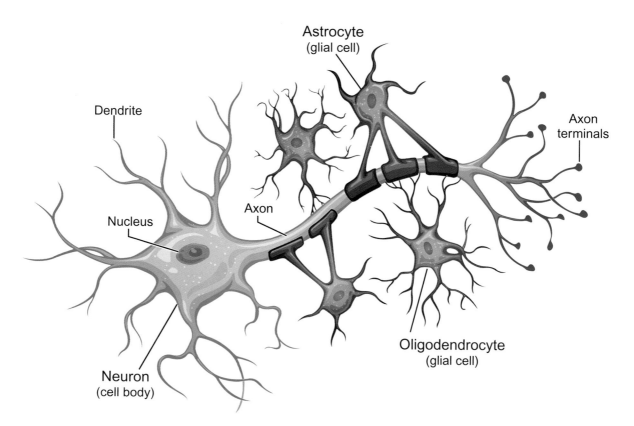

Figure 6–30. Neuron and glial cells.

Table 6–6. Types and General Functions of Neurons and Glial Cells

TYPE	FUNCTION
Glial	Nonsignaling
Astrocytes	"Anchor" neurons to blood supply
	Regulate neuron extracellular environment
Oligodendrocytes (Schwann cells in PNS)	Myelin-forming
Microglia	Clean up dead material
Ependymal	Produce cerebrospinal fluid
Neurons	Signaling
Many types	

These arms wrap the axon with the fatty substance myelin, described in greater detail below.

Other glial cells include those responsible for "cleaning up" dead material in the brain; these are called *microglia*. Finally, the fluid-filled ventricles of the brain contain ependymal cells along their walls. These cells generate the fluid (CSF) inside the ventricles. Ependymal cells are not technically glia because their embryological origin is different from the origins of astrocytes and oligodendrocytes.

Neurons

The structure of the neuron is critical to understanding its normal physiology, and how this physiology is affected by disease. Figure 6–31 is a schematic image of a neuron and several of its component structures. Neurons differ in size, shape, and complexity, dependent on their location and function within the brain. This is why Table 6–6 lists "many types" under the general heading of "neurons." All neurons, however, have a cell body (soma), dendrites, axon, and axon terminal, called a terminal button (also referred to as a terminal segment or terminal bouton). Neurons reside in a fluid medium, or *extracellular environment* (shaded blue area in Figure 6–31). The structures inside the neuron are its intracellular components. The intracellular components of a neuron are separated from the extracellular environment by a membrane with very special properties. The membrane is impermeable to a number of different molecule types, but can change its permeability to certain molecules by the action of substances manufactured within the cell body.

Cell Body (Soma)

The cell body or *soma* is typically a relatively large, spherical structure. To call the cell body "relatively large" is to describe the size of a tiny structure in a brain-world of other tiny structures; a typical soma is about 20 μm in diameter (0.000020 meters, perhaps 100 times smaller than the diameter of a poppyseed). Inside the cell body is the nucleus, as well as a number of critical structures called *organelles*. Among the organelles shown schematically in Figure 6–31 are mitochondria (Mi), endoplasmic reticula (ER: where reticulum is the singular), golgi apparatus (GA), and ribosomes (protein-synthesizing organelles, not labeled in the figure). These organelles serve the neuron's metabolic functions, generate proteins that affect the cell membrane's properties, and also manufacture and transport the neurotransmitters used to signal from one neuron to another.

The cell body and its contents are separated from the extracellular environment by a membrane composed of lipids (fatty and/or oily substances that are insoluable in water) in which numerous protein molecules are embedded. The membrane's permeability to various elements can be changed very rapidly by the action of these proteins. These changes in permeability are critical to understanding the neuron's basic function of conducting electrical impulses (see below, section on Action Potential).

The nucleus of a neuron, like the nucleus of almost any cell in the body, contains deoxyribonucleic acid (DNA). Information in the DNA is transported out of the nucleus by messenger ribonucleic acid (typically abbreviated mRNA) and into the main fluid of the cell

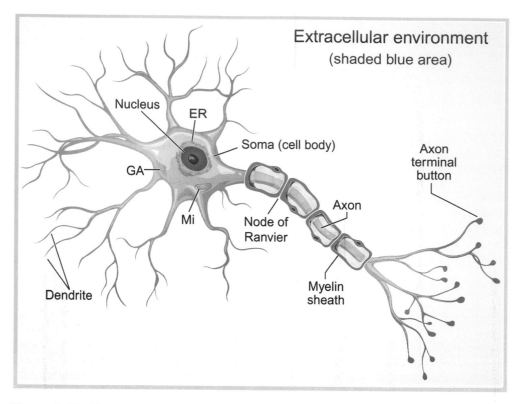

Figure 6–31. Neuron showing structures within the soma (ER = endoplasmic reticulum; Mi = mitochondria; GA = golgi apparatus) that manufacture proteins and neurotransmitters, and the myelin sheath of the axon. The myelin sheath is not continuous down the entire length of the axon; the small gaps between adjacent myelin wraps are called nodes of Ranvier. Note the many dendrites associated with the soma, and the many terminal buttons of the axon.

body where the organelles are located. The function of mRNA is to link up with organelles such as the endoplasmic reticula and ribosomes so that proteins can be synthesized. These newly synthesized proteins serve a number of critical functions, one of which is to allow the cell body membrane to make very brief changes in its permeability to specific molecules. Changes in the membrane's permeability allow molecules to pass from the extracellular environment into the cell body, or from the cell body to the extracellular environment. Additional details of the process of protein synthesis in neurons are outside the scope of this chapter; the interested reader is referred to one of several outstanding neuroscience and general biology textbooks in which this information is presented in a highly readable form (Bear et al., 2007; Kandel et al., 2000).

The cell body also contains microtubules which extend down the axon. These miniature tubes can be thought of as railway tracks extending from the cell body to the end of the axon. Proteins and other substances synthesized in the cell body are transported by means of these "tracks," down the axon to its terminal button.

Finally, as shown in Figure 6–31, many short projections from the cell body extend into the extracellular space. These projections are called *dendrites*, and the entire set of them extending from the cell body is called a *dendritic tree*. The membranes of the dendrites contain protein molecules, known in the neuroscience community as *receptors*; receptors detect specific neurotransmitters. The section below on Synaptic Transmission and Neurotransmitters provides information on how the terminal buttons of one neuron interact with the dendritic tree of a different, nearby neuron.

Axon and Terminal Button

As shown in Figure 6–31, the axon is a cablelike projection from the cell body. The location where the axon "arises" from the cell body is called the axon hillock. The axon ends at the terminal buttons. Axons can be very short in length (less than a millimeter) or very long (close to a meter). The axon is the means by which a neuron transmits an electrical impulse from the cell body to the terminal button(s).

The intracellular content of axons is distinct from that of the cell body of a neuron. As noted above, microtubules extend from the cell body to the terminal buttons, but the protein-synthesizing organelles—the ribosomes—are not found in axons. The proteins found in an axon are synthesized solely in the cell body, and transported, via microtubules, to the terminal buttons. The intracellular contents of the terminal button(s) of an axon, which may include just a few or many terminal buttons (Figure 6–31 shows about a dozen buttons), include numerous small "packets" called synaptic vesicles. These vesicles are tiny, membrane-encased packages of neurotransmitter. There are also many mitochondria in the terminal buttons, which indicate a high level of energy expenditure at the terminal buttons of axons.

The length of axon between the axon hillock and the terminal buttons has a wrapping-like covering called *myelin*, the fatty substance produced by oligodendrocytes. The oligodendrocytes wrap the axon with multiple, concentric rings of myelin. Figure 6–31 shows the myelin wrapping to be discontinuous from axon hillock to terminal buttons, so that intervals of myelin-covered axon are interrupted by very small breaks in the wrapping. These small breaks in the myelin wrapping are called *nodes of Ranvier*. As explained below, the myelin wrapping and nodes of Ranvier have great importance to the conduction of electrical impulses from cell body to terminal boutons. Most axons in the CNS and PNS are myelinated, but certain functional systems (such as the pathways responsible for pain perception) have a fair number of unmyelinated axons.

Synapse

Figure 6–32 illustrates the essential features of a synapse. The typical synapse is the terminal button-to-dendrite synapse, but other synapse types—such as terminal button-to-soma, or even terminal button-to-axon—are also found in the CNS; attention is focused here on the standard synapse. The inclusion of synapses under the general heading of "Neurons" may be slightly misleading, because a synapse involves a collection of structures, as well as part of the extracellular environment. The collection of structures comprising a synapse gains its anatomical status by virtue of its functional importance. The collection of structures comprising a synapse includes a neuron's *presynaptic membrane* (membrane of the terminal buttons), the *postsynaptic membrane* (most typically the membrane cover-

ing a branch of the dendritic tree arising from the soma of a second, nearby neuron), and the extracellular substance separating and even *joining* the two membranes, called the *synaptic cleft*.

Presynaptic Membrane. The presynaptic membrane is the cell wall at the end of the axon and encases the synaptic vesicles within the terminal buttons. Embedded within the presynaptic membrane are special proteins where synaptic vesicles can, under the right conditions, attach and subsequently "dump" their neurotransmitter contents into the synaptic cleft. A single terminal button may contain synaptic vesicles storing different kinds of neurotransmitters; individual neurons are not limited to a single neurotransmitter. The presynaptic membrane can be thought of as the component of a synapse from which neural signals are sent.

Postsynaptic Membrane. The postsynaptic membrane is the receiving part of a synapse. This is where signals sent from the presynaptic membrane of one neuron are "picked up" for processing by another neuron. Like the presynaptic membrane, the postsynaptic membrane is partly composed of protein molecules that serve the specialized purpose of receiving these signals. These molecules form receptors designed not only to pick up neuronal signals in general, but which are specialized for particular neurotransmitters. A postsynaptic membrane of a single neuron may contain receptors specialized for a variety of neurotransmitters, and even for subvarieties of one neurotransmitter.

Synaptic Cleft. The synaptic cleft is the "space" between the presynaptic and postsynaptic membranes. The scare quotes around the word "space" emphasize its miniature (between 20 and 50 millionths of a millimeter) width. This cleft consists of a meshwork of proteins which not only serves as the medium through which a neurotransmitter is conveyed from the presynaptic (sending) to postsynaptic (receiving) membranes, but also attaches the two membranes to each other. The presynaptic membrane, synaptic cleft, and postsynaptic membranes are bound together as an anatomical unit.

Resting Potential, Action Potential, and Neurotransmitters

Information is transmitted in the nervous system largely by the conversion of electrical energy into neurochemical energy, which is then transformed back into electrical energy. An important key to understanding how neurons send electrical signals from the soma to

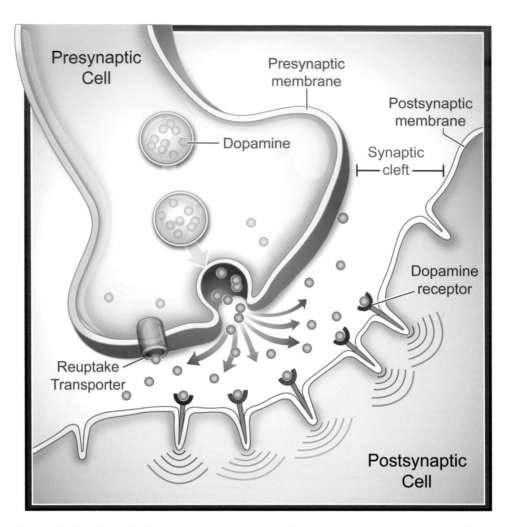

Figure 6–32. Essential features of a synapse. The drawing shows a terminal button, whose covering is called the presynaptic membrane. Inside the button are packets containing neurotransmitter molecules, illustrated in this drawing by dopamine molecules. The postsynaptic membrane, associated with a different neuron, is shown in light purple and separated from the presynaptic membrane by a small gap of extracellular fluid called the synaptic cleft. Embedded within the postsynaptic membrane are receptors specialized for a particular neurotransmitter; the receptors shown are dopamine receptors. The dopamine released from the presynaptic membrane "binds" to the receptors on the postsynaptic membrane. Usually excess neurotransmitter is released into the synaptic cleft, so a mechanism called the reuptake transporter brings the excess molecules back into the terminal button and repackages them for later use.

the terminal buttons is an appreciation of the changeable characteristics of cell membranes. The following paragraphs present a brief, simplified introduction to this signaling process.

Resting Potential

Figure 6–33 shows a schematic neuron with a focus on the chemical, ionic environment of the soma when the neuron is at "rest" (not stimulated). Some of these ions have a positive electrical charge, whereas others have a negative electrical charge. The two most important, positively charged ions in Figure 6–33 are potassium (K^+) and sodium (Na^+), shown in large concentrations outside the cell body, in the extracellular fluid. Within the cell body, in the intracellular fluid, a group of unspecified, negatively charged ions are shown. Keep in mind the schematic nature of this drawing: the

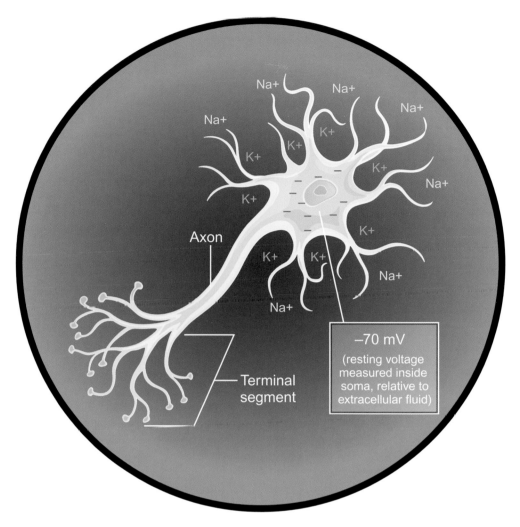

Figure 6–33. Drawing of a neuron showing the relative distribution of negative and positive ions inside the soma versus the extracellular fluid.

depiction of K^+ and Na^+ ions as restricted to outside the soma does not mean these ions are not also within the cell body, but rather that *after ionic equilibrium is established* they are much more highly concentrated in the extracellular fluid.

At rest, the membrane of a neuron cell body is relatively permeable—allows passage—to K^+ molecules. On the other hand, the membrane is not permeable to Na^+ molecules or the negatively charged ions concentrated inside the soma. The selective membrane permeability to K^+ is the result of openings within the membrane that are specially "tuned" to K^+ molecules; these special openings are a relatively constant characteristic of the cell membrane. The presence of these openings helps explain how "ionic equilibrium," the equal and opposite electrical forces across the cell membrane that define the rest state of the cell, is achieved. Before ionic equilibrium is established, K^+ molecules

are "naturally" concentrated *inside* the soma—their numbers inside the soma are much greater than in the extracellular fluids. Ions with unequal concentrations in two locations always seek to establish equilibrium of concentration between these locations, which in the present case are the intracellular and extracellular regions. Because of the unequal concentration of K^+ inside and outside the soma, the permanent openings to K^+ within the cell membrane result in more K^+ traffic outward to the extracellular fluid, as compared to traffic inward to the intracellular fluid. When more K^+ molecules pass out of the soma than move into it, the result is a more negative charge within the soma (intracellular fluid) relative to outside the soma (extracellular fluid). A critical phase in this process of net K^+ movement to the extracellular fluid is when the tendency of the positively charged ions to leave the soma is exactly balanced by the negative electrical charge inside the soma; when this occurs, equilibrium is reached and the movement of K⁺ ions stops. This can be likened to two forces pulling with identical magnitudes in opposite directions (K⁺ molecules exerting a force to "run down" its concentration gradient from inside to outside the cell to establish K⁺ equilibrium, versus the negative force created by loss of positive charges inside the cell due to K⁺ escape, trying to "pull back" the positively charged ions into the soma).

The balance of these two, oppositely directed forces establishes the resting potential of the undisturbed neuron; in this state the neuron membrane is said to be *polarized*. Potentials refer to voltage differences between two points, and the electrical potential difference between the inside and outside of the cell body is roughly 70 millivolts (mV) (0.070 volts). Because the voltage inside the soma is negative relative to outside the soma, the resting potential of a neuron is expressed with a negative sign, that is, −70 mV. In this electrical state, the neuron does not fire impulses down its axon.

Action Potential

An action potential is the change of the negative resting potential to a positive value, and the subsequent return of the potential to the negative resting value. These changes in membrane potential occur in response to stimulation of a sensory organ (induced by an external stimulus such as a change in shape of an end organ resulting from touch, or exposure of an organ to light, as in vision), or as a result of exposure of the neuron's membrane to neurotransmitters released by another, nearby neuron. The action potential occurs very rapidly (on the order of 1/1000th of a second, or 1 ms), and propagates down the entire length of the axon to its terminal button. The arrival of the action potential at the terminal button causes packets of neurotransmitter to be "dumped" into the synaptic cleft between the terminal button and the dendrites of an adjacent neuron (or neurons). The more detailed description of the action potential presented below is highly schematic; for greater detail on the molecular basis of the action potential, Kandel et al. (2000) is an excellent source.

Figure 6–34 shows a schematic action potential. The x-axis is time (units = ms), the y-axis is voltage (units = mV). The red trace shows the voltage measured inside the soma relative to the surrounding extracellular fluid (voltage is always measured as a difference in charge between two points) as a function of time. The narrow, blue-shaded rectangle extending across the time axis between (roughly) −60 mV and −80

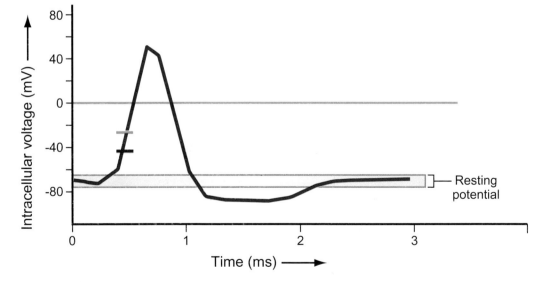

Figure 6–34. Graph of an action potential, showing intracellular voltage (in mV) on the y-axis and time (in ms) on the x-axis. The range of resting potential values is shown by the blue rectangle centered on an intracellular voltage around −70 mV. The dark purple, horizontal line shows the voltage change that must be reached to produce the "all-or-none" action potential, and the green horizontal line shows the cell potential at which the K⁺ channels are opened to re-establish the resting potential, as described in text. Both events are examples of voltage-gated membrane permeabilities to specific ion flows.

Faster Than the Speed Of . . .

Nerves conduct action potentials very, very quickly. A general rule is that myelinated nerves conduct impulses faster than unmyelinated nerves, and within the class of myelinated nerves those with larger axonal diameters conduct impulses faster than those with smaller axonal diameters. How quick is quick? The ulnar nerve, a mixed (motor and sensory) nerve that exits the spinal cord around the first thoracic (T1) segment of the spinal cord, carries motor impulses to muscles of the forearm and pinky finger at a speed of at least 60 m/sec. For those of you who do not like metric, that's about 134 miles per hour. Closer to home, the facial nerve conducts motor impulses at a speed of roughly 50 m/sec, and the motor part of the trigeminal nerve (to jaw muscles) conducts at a rate of about 55 m/sec. Some nerve fibers conduct at slower speeds, such as those that lack a myelin wrapping or have just a thin myelin sheath; these are primarily fibers that carry the sensations of pain and temperature, and their conduction speeds may be no more than 20 m/sec. Everyone has had the experience of touching something hot and realizing it only after what seems to be a long time; this is because thinly or unmyelinated temperature pathways conduct impulses relatively slowly, so the time between stimulation of the temperature receptors and recognition of the heat seems relatively long.

mV shows a range of membrane potentials consistent with the resting potential of about −70 mV, discussed above. Note that in this drawing, the action potential trace begins within this range. Less than half a ms after the beginning of the trace, the potential begins to move in the positive direction, toward zero, suggesting the neuron has been stimulated. The membrane potential begins to change in the positive direction because the stimulation causes the membrane to become permeable to Na^+ ions, which previously have been concentrated in the extracellular fluid relative to the inside of the soma. In theory, this imbalance in concentration of Na^+ ions across the membrane causes the ions to flow "down their gradient" (from areas of higher to areas of lower concentration), but the impermeability of the membrane to Na^+ in the resting state does not allow this flow. The stimulation of the neuron, by an external event or neurotransmitter, causes some Na^+ specific channels in the soma membrane to open, allowing a modest flow down the concentration gradient, into the cell body. This is why the membrane potential begins to change in a positive direction.

The real action in the action potential begins, however, when the changing membrane potential reaches a value of roughly −45 mV. At this voltage level, a "threshold effect" occurs and a huge number of Na^+ channels in the membrane are instantly opened, allowing a rush of Na^+ into the cell body; this threshold is indicated in Figure 6–34 by the short, horizontal, dark purple bar that crosses the rising action potential trace. The term "voltage-gated sodium channel" is used to refer to a special membrane pore that is switched on, like flipping a switch, when a certain membrane potential (voltage) is reached. Considering the thousands and thousands of voltage-gated channels on each neuron membrane, their simultaneous opening at the threshold voltage allows a great deal of Na^+ to rush in to the soma. As can be seen in Figure 6–34, this causes the potential to shoot up past zero and perhaps as high as +40 mV, *depolarizing* the membrane in less than 1 ms. A depolarized membrane is one in which the normal (resting) negative potential is "flipped" into the positive region for a very brief interval. A depolarized membrane initiates the conduction of electrical impulses down the axon, to the terminal button.

As shown in Figure 6–34, the action potential is not only defined by the rapid increase from a negative to positive membrane potential, but also by the reversal of this process and a return to a negative potential. The return to a negative potential is, for a brief time, to a value slightly *more negative* than the resting potential of −70 mV. Why does this happen? First, when the action potential approaches its peak positive value, the Na^+ channels are closed as suddenly as they were opened; this is another voltage-gated channel effect. The cessation of Na^+ ions rushing into the soma initiates the process of repolarizing the cell membrane. But another mechanism is equally if not more important in repolarizing the membrane potential, and this is the result of the large number of voltage-gated K^+ channels in the cell membrane. Very shortly after the threshold voltage has been reached and the Na^+ channels have been instantly opened (see Figure 6–34, purple bar), the depolarization triggers a relatively slow (relatively slow on a "neuron-time" scale, that is) opening of K^+ channels; the voltage at which this occurs is indicated by the green bar on the action potential trace. Keep in mind, when the membrane is strongly depolarized —when positive ions inside the membrane are far more concentrated than outside the membrane—there should be a strong gradient for K^+ to flow from the inside to outside of the membrane (the reverse of the gradient direction during the resting potential). When the voltage-gated K^+ channels are turned on shortly after depolarization, by the time the action potential has reached its maximum value the K^+ channels should be wide open and ready to allow these positive ions to rush out of the soma into the extracellular fluid and in so doing drive the membrane potential into the negative range, in fact below the resting potential value of around -70 mV for a short period of time (see in Figure 6–34 how the potential dips below the resting potential rectangle, between roughly 1 and 2 ms along the time scale, before returning to a typical resting potential value). This period of time is when the neuron is said to be *refractory*, or relatively unresponsive to stimulation. Some people refer to the neuron being *hyperpolarized* (the resting membrane potential more negative than usual) during this brief period.

When the cell membrane is depolarized, the change in electrical potential from negative to positive propagates down the axon, to the terminal buttons where neurotransmitter is stored in tiny packets. One way to think about the conduction of the action potential down the axon is like a fuse, that when lit at the end, continuously ignites along the extent of the burning material until reaching its destination where the effect produced is, say, an explosion. This analogy is a bit off the mark for two reasons. First, the end effect of the propagating action potential, when it reaches the terminal button, is not to initiate an explosion but rather a set of complicated processes designed to unload neurotransmitter into the synaptic cleft. Second, the fuse analogy is explicitly one of continuous depolarization down the axon, but for the great majority of neurons the propagation is not continuous, but rather "jumps" from section to section of the axon.

The explanation for the action potential jumping down the axon, rather than propagating continuously, is revealed by the anatomy of a typical neuron as shown in Figure 6–31. As described earlier, the axon is wrapped in myelin, which functions as an electrical insulator to current flowing down the axon, this current being the result of the voltage changes of the action potential. Myelin is wrapped around axons in sections, with small interruptions, called *nodes of Ranvier*, at regular intervals from the soma to the terminal buttons. Figure 6–31 shows these lengths of myelin as purple rectangles, with the axons visible inside the myelin wrapping by the artist's trick of making the wrapping transparent. The action potential appears to jump down the axon from one node of Ranvier to the next. The jumping action potential is referred to as *saltatory transmission* (the word "saltatory" having a Latin ori-

gin meaning leaping, or dancing). The net effect of the myelin wrapping and the jumping action potential is to make transmission of electrical impulses from soma to terminal button very, very fast. Healthy myelin wrapping is critical to an efficiently and effectively functioning nervous system; demyelinating diseases such as multiple sclerosis slow up neural transmission and may cause a large range of sensory and motor problems.

Synaptic Transmission and Neurotransmitters

The information presented above on the resting potential, depolarization, and hyperpolarization may seem like neural trivia, but a grasp of these concepts is important to understand how signaling is accomplished in the nervous system. The following discussion focuses on action potentials in the CNS, where the properties of neuron membranes and their ability to change polarity (electrical charge) are largely dictated by the chemicals to which they are exposed. Signaling in the nervous system — sending messages from one brain region to another — is largely a recurring process of conversion of energy forms. The most typical of these energy conversions is from an electrical to chemical form, and then back to an electrical form. When the action potential (electrical energy) reaches the terminal button of the axon, it initiates processes that cause neurotransmitter (chemical energy) to be released into the synaptic cleft. In the synaptic cleft these chemicals bathe the membrane of an adjacent neuron's dendrites, and in so doing affect the membrane properties. The effect on the membrane properties is to open or close ion channels, which may result in a change in the membrane's polarity, either depolarization or hyperpolarization. The electrical-chemical-electrical pattern of energy conversion in the brain recurs constantly over time and space (that is, in different brain regions at the same time). This constant demand for energy conversion and consumption in the brain explains why in humans the metabolic requirements of brain function are disproportionately large relative to the weight of the organ in comparison to the overall organism weight.

The terminal button of a neuron contains packets of neurotransmitter, shown in Figure 6–32 as blue dots that represent neurotransmitter molecules. The neurotransmitter and their packets are manufactured and packaged in the cell soma (or in certain cases in other parts of the neuron) and transported down the axon to the terminal button. When an action potential propagates down an axon and reaches the terminal button, a series of chemical reactions (not described here) cause some of these packets to dump their neurotransmitter contents into the synaptic cleft, represented in

Figure 6–32 as the very light blue "medium" between the terminal button and the curved, purplish surface depicted "across the way" from the end of the terminal button.

This curved surface represents the membrane of a dendrite extending from the soma of a postsynaptic neuron adjacent to the terminal button of the presynaptic neuron. This dendritic membrane is studded with special organs, shown here as small spikes with semicircular receptacles reaching into the synaptic cleft. These special organs are neurotransmitter receptors, typically "tuned" for specific neurotransmitter types. When the action potential propagated down the presynaptic axon reaches the terminal button, causing the neurotransmitter molecules to be dumped into the synaptic cleft, some of these molecules will "bind" to the dendritic receptors that are tuned for their chemical properties. The binding of neurotransmitter molecules to these receptor sites is shown by the blue dots sitting within the semicircular receptacles.

The effect of neurotransmitters on the dendritic membrane is to modify the permeability of the dendrite membrane. Some neurotransmitters make the membrane more permeable to Na^+, resulting in an inflow of positive ions to the cell body and an action potential. This neurochemical gating of ion channels is directly analogous to the voltage-dependent gating described above; the difference is simply in what causes the channels to open. A neurotransmitter effect that causes Na^+ channels to open and therefore flips the negative resting potential to a positive one is referred as an *excitatory* effect, because it causes the "next" neuron to fire. Other neurotransmitters actually close membrane channels that permit positive ions to flow into the cell body. This makes the membrane potential more negative (hyperpolarized) which inhibits the production of an action potential. The neurotransmitters that hyperpolarize membrane potentials are called *inhibitory*.

One of the many interesting aspects of brain neurochemistry is that the clinical effect (the effect on human behavior) of drugs that block or amplify a neurotransmitter depend on which part of the synapse the drug acts upon. Clinical effects are likely to be different for drugs that affect the presynaptic release of a given neurotransmitter than those that affect the postsynaptic uptake of the same neurotransmitter.

The discussion to this point has used a single neuron (see Figure 6–31), or a zoom view of parts of two neurons separated by a synaptic cleft (see Figure 6–32), to illustrate the action potential and the signaling capability of neurons by electrical-chemical-electrical conversion across synapses. In reality, each neuron in the CNS receives input from many neurons and delivers output to many neurons. In the schematic neuron drawing of Figure 6–31 the multiple dendrites extending from the cell soma, and the multiple terminal buttons (only one is labeled in Figure 6–31), make this many-to-one and one-to-many arrangement clear: the dendritic tree is extensive, as are the multiple terminal buttons projecting from the axon. The situation is even more complex because many neurons are not specialized for a particular neurotransmitter; they have receptors on dendrites for multiple neurotransmitters (even for subtypes of the same neurotransmitter), and may package more than one neurotransmitter in their terminal buttons. The receptors on the dendrites may be tuned to both excitatory and inhibitory neurotransmitters, and the terminal buttons may contain packages of both types. How does this work?

Think of the many inputs converging on the dendrites of a single neuron as summing their effects on the dendritic membrane, with the net effect determining the dendritic membrane potential. The dendrites of a given neuron may receive thousands of excitatory inputs (neurotransmitter baths from multiple neurons) that open Na^+ and K^+ channels, and thousands of inhibitory inputs that close these same channels and perhaps also allow negatively charged ions into the cell. If there are more excitatory inputs than inhibitory inputs, the net effect is excitatory and an action potential is generated in the neuron receiving the multiple inputs; the opposite situation silences the neuron, maintaining or exaggerating the negative membrane potential (that is, producing a hyperpolarized membrane). Summed over millions and millions of neurons, the state of brain activity at any given moment is very much a statistical process involving net inputs and outputs.

Neurochemically gated ion channels involve a relatively large range of neurotransmitter types. Some well-known (and well-studied) neurotransmitters are listed in Table 6–7, together with their primary function (excitatory or inhibitory) and primary role in behavior. It is very important to understand the use of the term "primary" function and role in this table. A neurotransmitter may have a primary excitatory function (such as acetylcholine) but still be able to produce inhibitory effects when binding to specialized, inhibitory receptors. Similarly, a particular neurotransmitter may play a primary role in motor control (such as dopamine or acetylcholine), yet also have major involvement in functions such as memory and attention. This summary table must therefore be understood as a simplification not only of the complex functions and roles of the selected entries, but also as omitting a good number of other neurochemicals known to affect signaling in the nervous system.

Table 6–7. Well-Studied Neurotransmitters in the Human Brain, Their Primary Function, and the Behaviors With Which They Have Been Linked

NEUROTRANSMITTER	PRIMARY FUNCTION	BEHAVIORS
Glutamate	Excitatory	Widespread (memory, learning)
GABA	Inhibitory	Widespread (muscle tone)
Dopamine	Excitatory	Motor, mood, reward
Norepinephrine	Excitatory	Mood, attention, sleep, pain
Epinephrine	Excitatory, inhibitory	Blood pressure, airway diameter
Serotonin	Excitatory, inhibitory	Mood, arousal
Acetylcholine	Excitatory	Muscle contraction (sk)
	Inhibitory	Muscle contraction (ht)

Notes: GABA = Gamma Aminobutyric Acid; sk = skeletal; ht = heart.

Neuromuscular Junction

The neuromuscular junction is a special type of synapse in the PNS. It is the location at which the terminal buttons of motor axons make contact with specialized receptors on the surface of muscle tissue. A schematic drawing of a neuromuscular junction is shown in Figure 6–35, where a terminal button of a motor axon is shown adjacent to muscle tissue and a motor endplate on that tissue. A motor endplate contains the specialized receptors sensitive to the neurotransmitter acetylcholine. As shown in Figure 6–35, packets of acetylcholine are stored in the terminal buttons of motor nerve axons. When an action potential travels down a motor nerve axon and reaches the terminal button, acetylcholine is released into the synaptic cleft separating the terminal button from the motor endplate. At a neuromuscular junction, therefore, the terminal button is the presynaptic membrane, and the motor endplate is the postsynaptic membrane; the membranes are separated by the synaptic cleft. The release of acetylcholine into the synaptic cleft results in binding of the neurotransmitter to the specialized acetylcholine receptors embedded in the motor endplate. This binding opens up Na^+ channels in the muscle tissue membrane, resulting in a postsynaptic potential that causes the underlying muscle fibers to slide across each other. This is the microview of what happens when a motor end plate is depolarized; the macroview is simply that the summed effect of the terminal buttons of many motor axons releasing acetylcholine onto many motor endplate receptors make a muscle contract and exert some force.

Voluntary (skeletal) muscles have many motor end plates, but as a general rule muscles involved in more precise movements (such as those of the fingers or larynx) have many more motor end plates per unit area of muscle tissue as compared to muscles that produce gross movements (such as muscles of the trunk). Motor endplate distributions have been studied a fair amount in limb and trunk muscles, but not so much in orofacial muscles. A disease called *mysasthenia gravis* (MG) is specifically associated with disease at the neuromuscular junction, and more specifically with disruption of the acetylcholine receptors on the motor endplates. In MG the immune system attacks the acetylcholine receptors (that is, MG is an autoimmune disease), rendering many of them nonfunctional. This results in muscle weakness and rapid fatigue among people with the disease. The weakness and fatigue may affect the speech apparatus and result in a speech motor control disorder. On the other side of the neuromuscular junction, the release of acetylcholine from storage packets in the terminal button can be inhibited by administration of botulinum toxin, more commonly known in medical settings as Botox. The drug works by preventing the packets from attaching to the presynaptic membrane, an important first step in the "dumping" of a neurotransmitter into the synaptic cleft. Botox is perhaps best known as a cosmetic drug, used to offset the effects of aging on muscles of the facial area (that is, to eliminate wrinkles). Botox is also used to treat

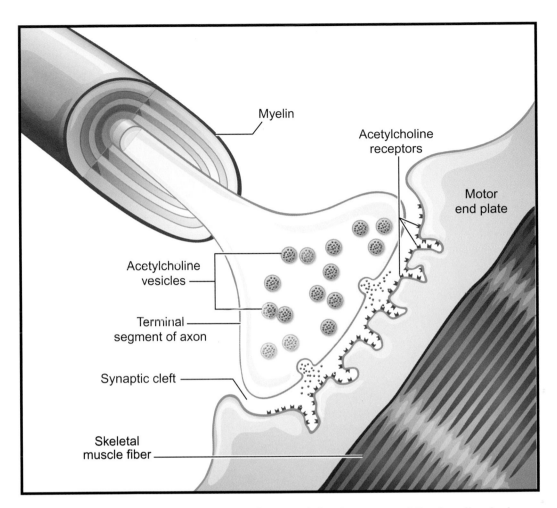

Figure 6–35. A neuromuscular junction, the specialized synapse at the junction between a peripheral motor nerve and muscle tissue. The terminal button containing packets of the neurotransmitter actelycholine is the presynaptic component of the synapse, and the motor endplate is the postsynaptic component. Embedded within the motor endplate are specialized receptors for acetylcholine. When acetylcholine released by the presynaptic membrane binds to receptors in the motor endplate, the muscle fibers are depolarized and contract.

certain neuromuscular disorders in which excessive amounts of muscle contraction cause disruption of movement. For example, Botox may be used to inhibit the excessive muscle contractions in the basal ganglia disorder called *dystonia*, in which the initation of a purposeful action (such as turning the head to look to the left or right) results in sustained and excessive muscle contractions. A specific type of voice and speech disorder called spasmodic dysphonia (SD) is thought to be a dystonia that is focused in the larynx and surrounding structures (Ludlow, 2011). Botox, injected directly into the vocal folds, can relieve the voice spasms and interruptions of phonation characteristic of this disorder. The presumed therapeutic mechanism, both in SD spe-

cifically and dystonia more generally, is the reduction of acetylcholine released at the neuromuscular junction and therefore less powerful muscle contractions.

MENINGES, VENTRICLES, BLOOD SUPPLY

In this section the coverings of the brain, the cavities within the CNS that produce, contain, and transport CSF, and the brain's blood supply are described. These three major areas of brain anatomy and physiology are considered together because they have interrelated functions.

Meninges

The cerebral hemispheres, the brainstem, and the spinal cord are masses of cells and fiber tracts encased by layers of nonneural tissue. These casings serve a protective function, as well as several other functions related to metabolic activities of neural tissue. The brain "floats" inside this protective housing. The layers of tissue pro-

viding this protective function are collectively called the meninges (the plural of the Greek word "meninx," meaning "membrane").

An artist's rendition of the relationship of the cortex and its underlying white matter to the meningeal covering layers is shown in Figure 6–36 (bottom image). Imagine this rectangular slab of multilayered tissue to be extracted from the top part of the head, a

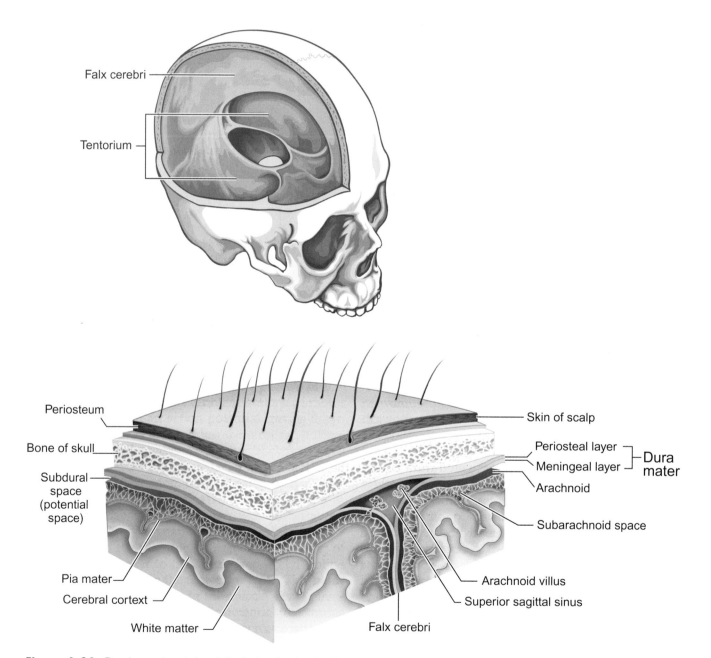

Figure 6–36. Rectangular slab of skull plus brain (*bottom image*), showing the meningeal layers and associated spaces relative to the underlying nervous system tissues. The various folds of the dura mater are shown (*top image*) with all brain tissue removed; note the falx cerebri and the tentlike covering—the tentorium cerebelli—of the brainstem and cerebellum created by the infoldings of the dura mater.

centimeter or two posterior to the top of the forehead and shown in the coronal plane. This view shows white matter toward the inferior edge of the slab, and the cortical layer of gray matter above it. The labels for white matter and cerebral cortex are shown in the sagittal plane view, on the left side of the slab.

Above the cortex and its underlying white matter are multiple layers of tissue, the top layer being the skin of the scalp (with hairs protruding from it), beneath which is a relatively thick, bony layer, commonly called the skull. Immediately beneath the skull is the most superficial layer of the meninges, the dura mater; deep to this layer is the arachnoid mater, followed by the pia mater, the deepest layer of the meninges. The dura, arachnoid, and pia mater layers form the meninges of the brain.

Dura Mater

The term "dura mater" means "tough mother," an appropriate term because the tissue has a leathery, hidelike texture. Figure 6–36 (bottom image) shows the dura mater as tissue in two layers, the more superficial of which is called the periosteal layer, the deeper one the meningeal layer. The periosteal layer of the dura mater adheres to the underside of the bony skull, whereas the meningeal layer is in contact with the arachnoid mater. These two layers of the dura mater are labeled toward the upper right edge of the coronal plane "wall" of our slab. Note that the dura mater also continues inferiorly to encircle the spinal cord.

The description of the dura mater as a two-layered meningeal structure is more than excessive anatomical detail. As shown on the coronal face of the slab (see Figure 6–36, bottom image), the meningeal layer separates from the periosteal layer toward the midline of the slab, to form a barrier between the left and right hemispheres. Note how as the bilayered dura mater approaches the midline, the meningeal layers on either side dip inferiorly and form a nearly vertical separation between the tissues of the two hemispheres. This partition is called the falx cerebri; it runs from the front to back of the hemispheres. When viewed in the sagittal plane, the falx cerebri forms a sheet having the shape of the letter C rotated 90 degrees clockwise. The anterior-to-posterior extent of the falx cerebri is roughly the same as the anterior-posterior extent of the corpus callosum, which sits immediately ventral to the inferior edge of the falx. The falx cerebri is shown in a separate image at the top of Figure 6–36, an image drawn with all brain tissue removed from the contents of the skull cavity. In this image the darker gray folds depict "infoldings" of the meningeal layer of the dura mater.

Another separation of the meningeal layer of the dura mater from the periosteal layer forms the tentorium cerebelli. This part of the dura mater is like a tent (hence, "tentorium") draped over the brainstem, separating it from the cerebral hemispheres. The tentorium cerebelli also forms a boundary between the cerebellum and the ventral surface of the occipital lobes. Although the configuration of the tentorium cerebelli is difficult to appreciate in a two-dimensional drawing, Figure 6–36, top image, shows the tentlike structure with an opening in the middle, formed by the infoldings of the meningeal layers of the dura. The cerebral hemispheres sit above this opening, the brainstem and cerebellum below it. The posterior edge of the opening is the midline of the dural covering separating the cerebellum from the ventral surfaces of the occipital lobes. When you hear the term "supratentorial," reference is being made to a structure or disease process (such as a stroke, or tumor) above the opening between the cerebral hemispheres and brainstem; "infratentorial" refers to structures or disease processes below this opening, in the brainstem and/or cerebellum. In clinical settings, the term "transtentorial herniation" refers to a pathological process in which parts of the cerebral hemispheres—most typically medial structures of the temporal lobes—are pushed through the tentorial opening shown in Figure 6–36, into the "compartment" normally occupied by the brainstem. This may happen when there is excessive pressure in the cerebral hemispheres (perhaps as a result of a stroke, or nonpenetrating brain injury resulting from a blow to head, or even a large tumor in one of the hemispheres), forcing the contents of the cerebral hemispheres inferiorly. Transtentorial herniation is an extremely serious event, typically causing death.

The dura mater serves an obvious protective function for the neural tissue of the CNS. The dura "holds in" the CSF in which the cerebral hemispheres and brainstem float. As discussed in the next section, the CSF circulates throughout the CNS. One prominent region within which the fluid circulates is immediately below the second layer of the meninges, the arachnoid mater.

Arachnoid Mater

The arachnoid mater is a thin membrane attached to the underside of the dura matter; below this membrane is a small space in which CSF circulates. As shown in the bottom image of Figure 6–36, the subarachnoid space appears as a honeycombed chamber. The typical thickness of this space, extending from the arachnoid membrane to the pia mater below, is roughly 5–6 mm but varies quite a bit depending on where the measurement is taken (for example, it is thicker if measured to the maximum height of a cortical gyrus, and thinner if measured to a fissure). The honeycombed appearance results from delicate membranes extending from the arachnoid layer adhered to the underside of the dura, down to the pia mater. These membranes, together with the CSF circulating in the subarachnoid space, create a spongy cushion that protects the neural tissue against damage.

Although not shown in Figure 6–36, arteries enter and veins exit brain tissue via the subarachnoid space. Arteries distribute blood to brain tissue via smaller vessels that penetrate the deepest layer of the meninges (the pia mater), and veins in the arachnoid space carry blood away from the brain by sending smaller veins into sinuses created by the separation of the two layers of the dura mater. The major venous return of blood to the heart is located in these sinuses; a cross-section of one such sinus, the superior sagittal sinus, is shown in Figure 6–36.

Pia Mater

The pia mater, the deepest layer of the meninges, is an extremely thin membrane that adheres closely to the surface of the cerebral hemispheres, following its curvatures and fissures. In a fixed brain prepared for dissection, in which the dura and arachnoid have been removed, the pia is often intact and appears as a filmy, milky-colored membrane that can be "pinched" away from the gyri and sulci. The pia mater is so closely adherent to the cortical surface it is sometimes not immediately apparent, on casual inspection by eye, that there is a membrane investing the surface of the hemispheres.

Meninges and Clinically Relevant Spaces

Clinically, the meninges are often referenced when a case involves bleeding in one of the spaces between the layers of these protective coverings. These are "potential spaces" in the sense of not having any measurable volume until something causes them to expand and create a "real" space. For example, the undersurface of the skull and the top surface of the dura are normally tightly bound to one another, but the potential space between them, called the epidural space, may be filled by blood when an artery bleeds. Similarly, the potential space between the dura and arachnoid layers can be filled by blood when an artery or vein bleeds. The term "subdural hematoma" refers to pooled blood in the space between the dura and arachnoid layers of the meninges. Any collection of blood within the menin-

geal spaces can exert pressure on the underlying brain tissue and cause loss of function, including loss of speech and/or language function.

Ventricles

The meningeal layers, as described above, include the honeycombed subarachnoid space filled with CSF. CSF is produced, circulated, and delivered back to the venous system (the drainage of blood from brain to heart) within a system of ventricles, chambers deep within the cerebral hemispheres and brainstem. CSF also flows through a central conduit in the spinal cord.

The ventricular system and associated conduits are shown in Figure 6–37. This sagittal view of the hemispheres and brainstem has been made transparent for better appreciation of the location and configuration of the ventricular system. The lateral ventricle is the complexly shaped, green structure, the third ventricle is shown in light blue, the cerebral aqueduct in purple, and the fourth ventricle in reddish orange. Below the fourth ventricle, in darker blue, is the foramen of Magendie and a downward projection that becomes the central canal of the spinal cord. Figure 6–38 shows these structures in a coronal view, looking from the front of the cerebral hemispheres toward the occipital lobes, and color-coded in the same way as in Figure 6–37. This view shows the lateral ventricles (green) to be paired, symmetrical structures in the two hemispheres, and the third ventricle and cerebral aqueduct to be midline (axial) structures. The fourth ventricle is a chamber between the brainstem and cerebellum, and is symmetrical with respect to both halves of the brainstem.

Lateral Ventricles

The sagittal view of Figure 6–37 shows the lateral ventricle to be a large, reversed C-shaped chamber occupying deep locations in all four lobes of the brain. The frontal horn of the lateral ventricle is in the frontal lobe, the body is in both the frontal and parietal lobes, and an occipital horn extends into the occipital lobe. The lower part of the reversed-C shape is the temporal horn of the lateral ventricle, which extends anterolaterally into the temporal lobe, from the junction of the body and occipital horn.

Some notable landmarks are associated with the complex shape of the lateral ventricle. For example, the corpus callosum, the massive fiber tract that connects cells in one hemisphere to cells in the other hemisphere, is located just superior to the upper edge of the frontal

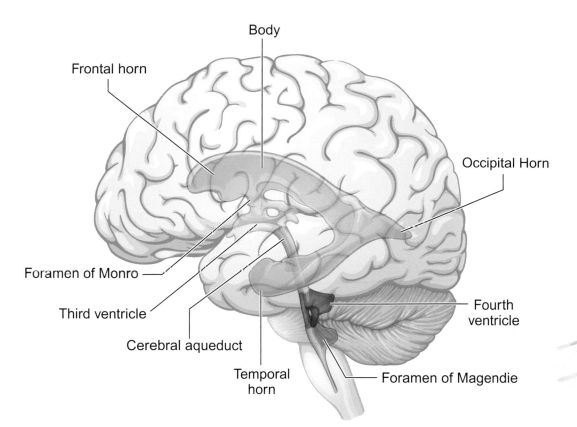

Figure 6–37. Sagittal view of the cerebral hemispheres, brainstem, and cerebellum, drawn to show the location and configuration of the ventricles. Lateral ventricles in green, third ventricle in light blue, cerebral aqueduct in purple, and fourth ventricle in reddish orange. The dark blue part of the ventricular system, seen inferior to the fourth ventricle, includes the beginning of the central canal of the spinal cord as well as other conduits through which CSF flows to the subarachnoid spaces in the cerebral hemispheres.

horn and body of the lateral ventricle (see Figure 6–5, upper right). The caudate nucleus, a component of the basal ganglia (see Figure 6–3), is the lateral boundary of the lateral ventricle and follows its inverted C shape (see Figure 6–16) from the frontal lobe to its curl into the temporal lobe. Immediately below the temporal horn of the lateral ventricle, in the temporal lobe, is the hippocampus.

Third Ventricle

In the sagittal view of Figure 6–37 the third ventricle is shown in blue as a flattened, complexly shaped cavity. The coronal view of Figure 6–38 shows the lateral ventricles connected to the third ventricle by narrow conduits which join in the midline and form a single channel, the *foramen of Monro*. The foramen of Monro drains CSF from the lateral ventricles into the third ventricle. In addition to its role in the transport of CSF

throughout the CNS, the third ventricle is an important anatomical landmark because it is the medial boundary of the two thalami (see the coronal view of Figure 6–3, in which the lateral ventricles are the two winglike cavities next to the caudate nuclei, and the third ventricle is the narrow "slit" between the thalami). There is often a connection between the left and right thalami, *through* the third ventricle; this is shown in Figure 6–37 as the circular opening in the third ventricle depicted in the same color as the brain tissue. This connection is called the interthalamic adhesion.

Cerebral Aqueduct, Fourth Ventricle, and Other Passageways for CSF

At the posterior, inferior end of the third ventricle, roughly at the top of the midbrain, the cavity narrows down and forms the cerebral aqueduct, shown in purple in Figures 6–37 and 6–38. This narrow channel

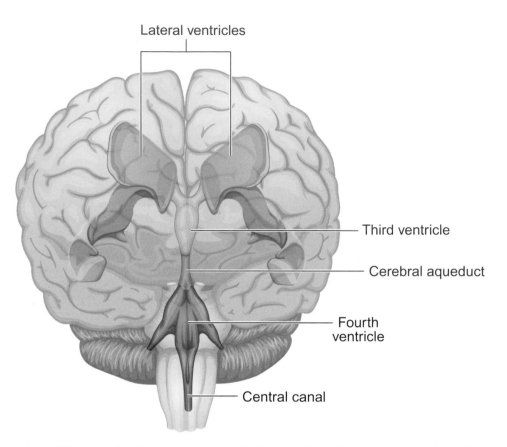

Lateral ventricles

Third ventricle

Cerebral aqueduct

Fourth ventricle

Central canal

Figure 6–38. Coronal view of the cerebral hemispheres, brainstem, and cerebellum, looking from the front of the hemispheres, drawn to show the configuration of the ventricles. Color coding of the ventricles is the same as in Figure 6–37.

courses through the midbrain and opens up in the pons and medulla as a complexly shaped cavity called the fourth ventricle. The fourth ventricle is just posterior to much of the pons and medulla, and anterior to the cerebellum; think of this fluid-filled cavity as a boundary between the cerebellum and the lower two divisions of the brainstem. In many textbooks the cerebellum is said to be the "roof" of the fourth ventricle, and the pons and medulla the "floor" of the fourth ventricle.

The fourth ventricle has several outlets that deliver CSF to the spinal cord and the subarachnoid space covering the cerebral hemispheres. In Figures 6–37 and 6–38 the thin blue passageway extending down from the fourth ventricle is the beginning of the central canal of the spinal cord. In horizontal cross-sections of the spinal cord (such as Figure 6–29) this canal is seen as the small circle in the center of the section, surrounded by gray matter. CSF flows through the canal and collects toward the bottom of the vertebral column in a small cavity below the inferior termination of spinal cord tissue, which is a few segments higher than the termination of the vertebral column. This inferior cav-

ity is the insertion point for a spinal tap, when a suspected medical condition requires the withdrawal of a small amount of CSF for laboratory analysis. Proper insertion of a needle to collect the sample, below the inferior termination of spinal cord tissue, produces the desirable result of accessing a quantity of CSF without damaging neural tissue.

Two additional conduits projecting from the fourth ventricle in posterolateral directions can be seen in Figure 6–38. These are passageways from the fourth ventricle into the subarachnoid space around the cerebral hemispheres.

Production, Composition, and Circulation of CSF

CSF is generated primarily by cells in the lateral ventricles. These cells, collectively called the choroid plexus, are derived from embryological ependymal cells (see Table 6–6). The choroid plexus cells are suspended from the roof of the lateral ventricles and generate roughly half a quart of CSF every 24 hours. CSF travels from the lateral ventricles via the foramen of Monro to the third ventricle and then via the cerebral aqueduct to the fourth ventricle. Some fluid from the fourth ventricle continues inferiorly into the central canal of the spinal cord, and some exits via the lateral passageways shown in Figure 6–38 to circulate in the subarachnoid space surrounding the cerebral hemispheres. Because the subarachnoid space can hold only about one-third of the volume of CSF produced by the choroid plexus, a mechanism exists to drain CSF from the brain into the bloodstream. Figure 6–36 (bottom image showing a slab of skull and underlying meningeal and neural tissue) includes a small structure labeled "arachnoid villus," also called arachnoid granulations. These structures (there are many arachnoid villi) extend from the subarachnoid space into the sinuses created by separation of the two layers of the dural mater. The arachnoid villi "dump" circulating CSF from the subarachnoid space into the venous system, effectively draining off excess CSF and maintaining a healthy pressure inside the ventricles and subarachnoid spaces. The draining of CSF into the venous system also serves the purpose of carrying neural waste products—the brain "trash" generated as neural and glial cells perform their metabolic tasks—out of the brain to be dissolved harmlessly in blood returning to the heart.

CSF is a clear fluid containing many different kinds of molecules, including proteins, chemical elements such as magnesium, chloride, potassium, and sodium, and other substances such as glucose, urea, and carbon dioxide. Normal values are available for each of these substances, and may be used as reference data when spinal tap fluid is analyzed as part of a diagnostic workup for diseases such as meningitis or certain cancers. However, the procedure is not performed routinely because of risk factors and the availability of other diagnostic tests for the same conditions.

Blood Supply of Brain

A frequently used organizing principle for the blood supply to the brain is to divide it into anterior versus posterior circulation. This very gross principle is illustrated in Figure 6–39, where the anterior circulatory components of the arterial supply to the brain are shown in brown and the posterior components in red. Both anterior and posterior circulations originate in major arteries emerging from the heart.

Anterior Circulation

For this part of the discussion, the reader should make frequent reference to the labeled arteries on the left side of Figure 6–39. The aorta, the largest artery in the body, emerges from the heart and ascends in the thorax before turning around and descending toward the abdomen. At the top of the aortic arch two major arteries arise and move blood toward the head. These are the common carotid arteries, one being the left common carotid artery (supplying the left side of the face and the left hemisphere of the brain) and other the right common carotid artery. For the sake of clarity, Figure 6–39 shows only the left common carotid artery and the left hemisphere; the anatomical facts on the right side are identical to the ones described in the next paragraph.

As the common carotid artery ascends in the neck it bifurcates (gives off two branches) roughly at the level of the mandible. One of these branches is the external carotid artery, which provides blood to structures such as the pharynx, tongue, face, and eyes. The other branch appears in Figure 6–39 as a continuation of the common carotid artery; this is the internal carotid artery, a main source of blood supply to the brain. Note how the internal carotid artery makes several sharp turns when it reaches the ventral surface of the temporal lobe. One of these is shown in Figure 6–39 as a hard right turn, along the line of the sylvian fissure. This branch of the internal carotid artery is called the middle cerebral artery (MCA). Another branch of the internal carotid artery is the anterior cerebral artery (ACA), shown in Figure 6–39 as a leftward turn off the main path of the internal carotid artery. The ACA supplies blood to medial portions of the frontal and parietal lobes, much of the corpus callosum, and small portions of basal ganglia structures. The importance of the MCA in speech, language, and hearing function is discussed below.

Posterior Circulation

This section focuses on the labeled arteries on the right side of Figure 6–39. Although the description that follows is for the left side of the brain only, the anatomy is identical for the right side of the brain.

The subclavian artery is a major branch of the aortic arch, supplying blood to the arm on the same side as the artery. The vertebral artery arises from the subclavian artery and ascends the neck within small openings in the ventral portions of the cervical vertebrae. When it reaches the base of the skull, the vertebral artery courses through the foramen magnum and continues to ascend on the ventral surface of the medulla until it joins with the vertebral artery from the other side, at the junction of the medulla and pons. When the two vertebral arteries join they form the basilar artery. Before the vertebral arteries join at the junction of medulla and pons, they deliver blood to one part of the cerebellum and the lateral part of the medulla via

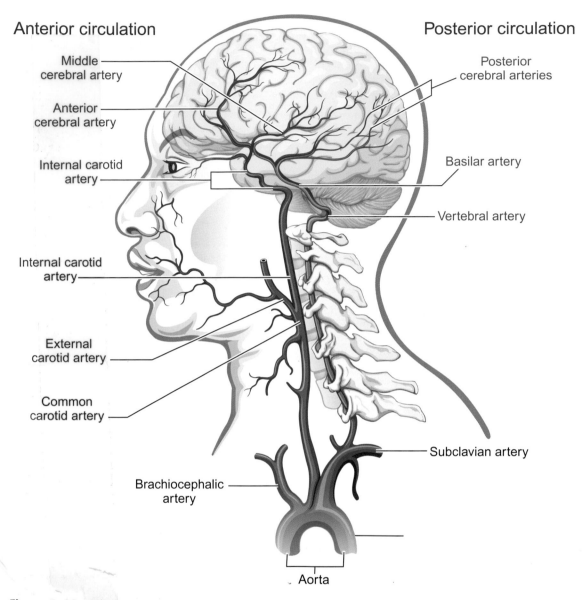

Figure 6–39. Arterial supply of the brain, shown originating at the heart. The anterior supply is shown as the brown arteries, the posterior supply as the red arteries.

the posterior inferior cerebellar artery (PICA). The PICA is shown in Figure 6–40, which presents a view of the ventral surface of the cerebral hemispheres, the cerebellum, and the medulla and pons, as well as an illustration of the joining of the two vertebral arteries to form the basilar artery. As the basilar artery ascends the pons it issues two more branches, the anterior inferior cerebellar artery (AICA) and the superior cerebellar artery (SCA). The AICA supplies blood to parts of the pons and the central part of the cerebellum, whereas the SCA serves the upper part of the cerebellum and some parts of the midbrain.

The basilar artery provides the posterior circulation for the cerebral hemispheres, by issuing the posterior cerebral artery (PCA; see Figures 6–39 and 6–40). The PCA provides blood to the posterior parts of the cerebral hemispheres, including the occipital lobes, and parts of the thalamus and corpus callosum.

Circle of Willis

A view of the arterial anatomy on the base of the brain shows the ACA and MCA, both major branches of the internal carotid artery, and the PCA, the main branch of

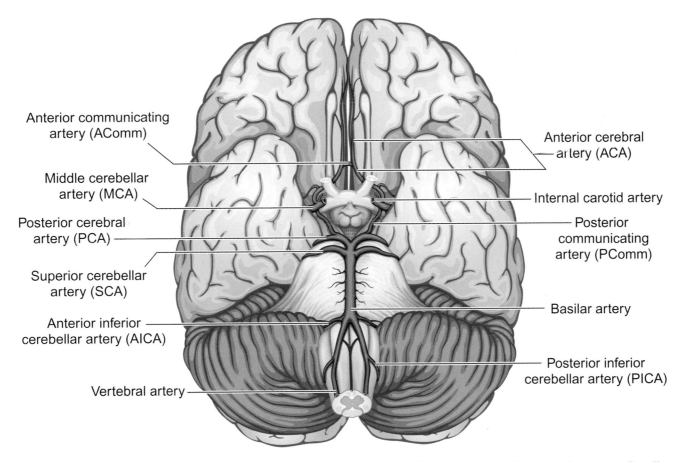

Figure 6–40. Ventral surface of the cerebral hemispheres, showing the paired vertebral arteries ascending the medulla, their junction to form the basilar artery at the base of the pons, and some of the important branches into the brainstem and cerebellum. The circle of Willis can also be seen in this drawing (see also Figure 6–41).

the basilar artery, forming a circular passageway. This circle, shown in Figure 6–41, is called the *circle of Willis* and is created by interposing linking arteries between the main arterial branches. Follow the basilar artery up the pons and note where the PCA branches off into the left and right hemispheres; both PCAs give off a branch called the posterior communicating artery (PComm), which links to the MCA. The MCA is labeled on the left side of Figure 6–41, and by comparing the left and right sides it is obvious that the MCA can be considered a continuation of the internal carotid artery (see below). The ACA's connect from the MCA to the anterior part of the brain, and the two ACA's are connected via the anterior communicating artery (AComm).

Blood at the base of the brain can flow in a circular pattern because the two main, paired branches of the carotid artery (ACA, MCA) and the one main, paired branch of the basilar artery (the PCA) are connected by communicating arteries. The circular blood flow pattern created by the circle of Willis has the capabil-

ity of compensating for loss of blood flow from one of the main blood supplies to the brain. For example, blockage of the internal carotid on one side of the circle of Willis could, in theory, be compensated for by increased flow from the basilar artery, because both main arteries can contribute to the circular blood flow pattern. This may be especially important in cases of temporary blockage. This classic description of circle of Willis anatomy must be taken with a grain of salt because there is a good deal of variation across individuals in the actual components of this circular arrangement. Some scientists believe this anatomical variation across individuals may help explain racial and ethnic differences in stroke risk (Eftekhar et al., 2006).

MCA and Blood Supply to the Dominant Hemisphere

The MCA is of particular interest to the speech-language pathologist and audiologist because it supplies blood to

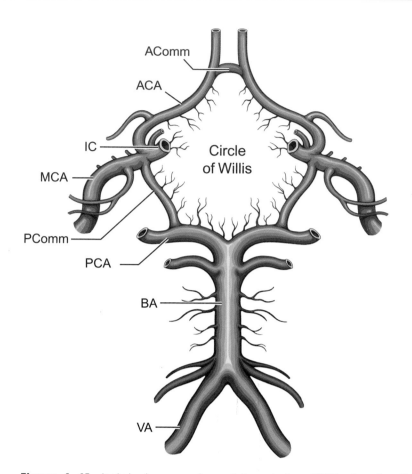

Figure 6–41. Isolated, zoom view of the circle of Willis showing its formation from the main blood supply sources to the brain: the basilar artery (*posterior supply; BA*) and middle cerebral arteries (*anterior supply; MCA*). The circle is completed by linking arteries (*posterior cerebral artery, PCA; posterior communicating artery, PComm; anterior cerebral artery, ACA; and anterior communicating artery, AComm*).

most of the lateral aspects of the cerebral hemispheres. More specifically, the MCA is the source of blood for the perisylvian speech, language, and hearing areas of the dominant hemisphere (the left hemisphere, in about 95% of the population). Blockage of the left MCA, or of one of its more local branches or associated small vessels deeper in the brain, has the potential to affect brain tissue critical to normal communication function. Many strokes associated with speech and language deficits are the result of loss of blood flow in the left MCA or its branches.

Figure 6–42 shows how the MCA distributes branches across the lateral surface of the left hemisphere; the same pattern can be assumed for the right hemisphere. Note how the MCA emerges on the surface of the hemisphere near the anterior tip of the temporal lobe and the lower surface of the frontal lobe. The MCA

courses along the sylvian fissure, posteriorly and superiorly, giving off an upper branch and a lower branch. The upper branch supplies blood primarily to frontal lobe tissue, whereas the lower branch distributes blood to parietal lobe tissue. In addition, note the offshoots from the main trunk of the MCA to the temporal lobe.

In theory, a blockage to blood flow can occur at any point along the course of the MCA and its branches. Blockages at the sharp turn from the internal carotid artery to the MCA (a more or less right-angle bend) are not uncommon, and affect the entire distribution of blood to the lateral surface of the hemisphere. Blockages can also occur in the turn to the upper or lower branches of the MCA, or in the offshoots into the temporal lobe. An overly simplified, but in many cases clinically useful, way to correlate these blockage possibilities with functional consequences is as follows.

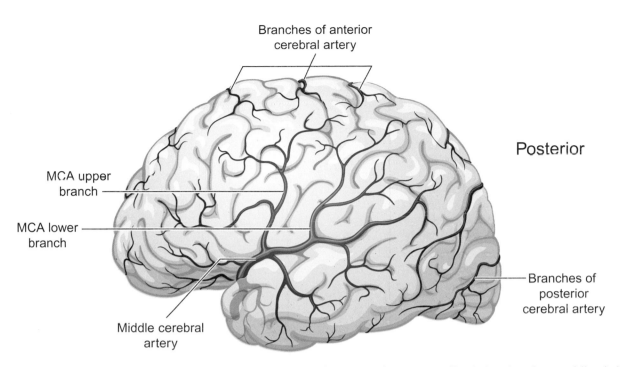

Figure 6–42. Distribution of middle cerebral artery (MCA) branches across the lateral surface of the left hemisphere. As the MCA emerges on the surface of the hemisphere between the anterior tip of the temporal lobe and lower, posterior lip of the frontal lobe, it gives off upper and lower branches as labeled in the figure. Branches of the anterior cerebral artery (ACA) and posterior cerebral artery (PCA) are also shown.

A blockage at the turn from the internal carotid artery to the MCA deprives the anterior and posterior parts of the left hemisphere of blood and therefore affects both expressive (anterior lesions) and receptive (posterior lesions) speech and language functions. Such a large area of damaged perisylvian tissue might lead to global aphasia — the massive disruption of both production and comprehension abilities. Blockage at the junction of the MCA and the offshoot labeled "MCA upper branch" (see Figure 6–42) might be expected to have a primary influence on production ability, whereas blockage at the junction of the MCA and the offshoot labeled "MCA lower branch" might be associated with a primary receptive problem. This is consistent with the idea of anterior and posterior lesions in the dominant hemisphere producing primarily production and comprehension problems, respectively. As noted above, this is an overly simplified view of speech and language functions of the brain, but it is a view consistent with certain diagnostic categories of communication function following stroke and left hemisphere damage. More is said about the issue of brain structures and specific speech and language functions in the section titled, "Speech and Language Functions of the Brain: Possible Sites and Mechanisms."

The MCA also is a significant source of blood for structures deep within the cerebral hemispheres. A general view of the distribution of MCA blood to the contents of the cerebral hemispheres is given in Figure 6–43, which is an artist's rendition of a coronal section roughly midway between the front and back of the hemispheres. The left side of the section shows labeled brain structures, and the right side shows the source of blood supply to these structures from the main components of the circle of Willis (MCA, ACA, PCA). The purple shaded regions indicate the areas of the hemispheres supplied by the upper and lower branches of the MCA, including the cortical regions on the lateral surface of the hemisphere and the underlying white matter of the coronal radiata. Deep branches of the MCA (light bluish gray) also provide blood to the caudate, putamen, parts of the globus pallidus, and parts of the internal capsule. Speech and language problems plus limb deficits on the right side of the body, a frequently seen combination in stroke clinics, are explained by interruptions of MCA blood flow which affect the perisylvian areas (speech and language) and the internal capsule (limbs). Figure 6–43 also shows regions of the internal capsule, caudate, and globus pallidus to be supplied by the anterior choroidal

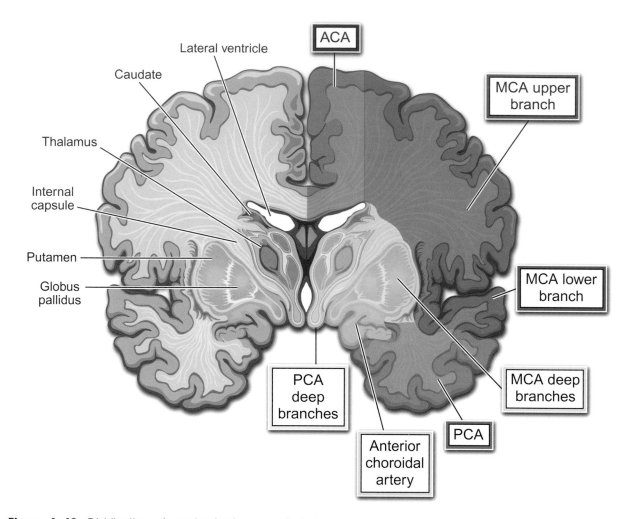

Figure 6–43. Distribution of cerebral artery supply to both surface and internal components of the cerebral hemispheres, shown in a coronal slice made roughly midway between the anterior and posterior ends of the hemispheres. The left side of the slice shows labels for subcortical structures; the right side of the slice identifies the arteries supplying different regions. MCA = middle cerebral artery; PCA = posterior cerebral artery; ACA = anterior cerebral artery.

artery, an offshoot of the internal carotid artery close to the branching of the MCA at the base of the brain. The PCA supplies the ventral part of the temporal lobe, with deeper branches of the PCA supplying the thalamus and hypothalamus. The most dorsal and medial aspects of the cerebral hemispheres are supplied by the ACA.

The advantage of knowing the detailed blood supply of the brain is the ability to understand the co-occurrence of symptoms and signs, such as the speech-language and limb problems mentioned above. Neurologists often use such co-occurrences to make educated estimates of where a stroke has occurred (that is, the location of blood flow interruption), estimates typically confirmed by imaging studies.

Not all strokes produce obvious problems at first. The very small vessels that penetrate to the deep struc-

tures of the hemispheres, such as the basal ganglia nuclei and internal capsule, may be blocked with a resulting loss of blood to very local regions of brain tissue. Eventually, a sufficient number of these small infarcts (loss of blood flow) can produce personality changes and dementia. Indeed, one category of dementia, broadly referred to as vascular dementia, seems to be the result of a large number of these very small regions of damage. On autopsy, the brain tissue sometimes has a "pin-cushion" appearance, with many small holes in the brain tissue.

Blood-Brain Barrier

In most parts of the body, substances flowing in the bloodstream can be transferred to tissue by passing through the walls of the vessels, directly into the tissue. The walls of vessels in the brain are different than walls of vessels in other parts of the body. Brain blood vessels have a structure that forms a protective barrier against chemicals or toxins that have the potential to destabilize the neurochemistry of the brain. This *blood-brain barrier* is especially relevant when certain drugs are administered to alleviate symptoms and signs of a CNS disease. For example, it is well known that Parkinson disease is at least partly a result of reduction of the neurotransmitter dopamine in the brain. Dopamine is manufactured by cells in the substantia nigra and plays an important role in the normal functioning of basal ganglia structures such as the striatum. To address the reduction of dopamine in the brain, why not administer a drug, orally, with the molecular composition of dopamine? As it turns out, dopamine molecules are blocked by the blood-brain barrier. In the 1960s, scientists figured out that a precursor of dopamine—a chemical compound that is one of the steps in the neuronal synthesis of dopamine—was able to cross the blood-brain barrier. Patients were given this precursor, called L-DOPA, which was able to cross the blood-brain barrier. Once in the brain, L-DOPA was converted into dopamine by "normal" neuronal processes. In this case knowledge of the blood-brain barrier and the chemical transformations in the synthesis of dopamine permitted an effective treatment for many of the problems associated with Parkinson disease.

SPEECH AND LANGUAGE FUNCTIONS OF THE BRAIN: POSSIBLE SITES AND MECHANISMS

Scientists have considered models of speech and language functions of the brain for well over a century (if not more). The models typically highlight sites (locations in the brain where certain functions are accomplished) and pathways connecting these sites. The models may also include mechanisms, which are accounts of how things happen. Early on, very simple models of speech and language sites and functions of the brain were offered by Broca and Wernicke, who attempted to interpret postmortem regions of brain damage in relation to speech and language performance of the patients prior to their death. According to these models, speech-language expression and comprehension were vested in tissue around Broca's and Wernicke's areas, respectively. A parallel, "site-based" development occurred in models of motor speech disorders, a group of speech disorders caused by neurological damage to a number of different locations

within the CNS and PNS. Motor *speech* disorders are typically separated from neurologically based *language* disorders (the type considered by Broca and Wernicke), because the former are assumed to reflect damage only to motor control systems, with language representations completely intact. The dominant model of motor speech disorders (Darley, Aronson, & Brown, 1975; Duffy, 2005) makes explicit associations between specific sites of damage (such as in the cerebellum, versus the corticobulbar tracts) and specific speech problems. Early models of aphasia and motor speech disorders were therefore very much concerned with sites, and somewhat less with mechanisms.

Over the last 20 years there has been an explosion of research on speech and language functions of the brain, especially due to the widespread use and increasing sophistication of brain imaging techniques. This research has brought us to a point where the strict idea of sites matching up with particular speech and language functions (and speech-language signs/symptoms in the case of brain lesions) does not seem reasonable. The *general* notion of a link between sites and function is probably still viable—posterior lesions in the dominant hemisphere are more likely to result in comprehension problems as compared to anterior lesions. Similarly, damage to the cerebellum is more likely to make a patient's speech sound slightly drunk as compared to the damage associated with Parkinson disease, which is likely to make a patient sound very soft, mumbly, and dysfluent. With the addition of imaging techniques designed to trace *connections* in the brain (see sidetrack on "DTI"), as well as accumulating evidence of certain neurological diseases having a major influence on these connections (in addition to, or rather than, major influence on the connected *sites*), clinicians and scientists are beginning to consider the brain as a network in which multiple sites and their connections are devoted to integrated functions. This is a *system*, as compared to site, view of speech-language functions of the brain. A system view might explain, for example, why different sites of brain damage can produce very similar motor speech signs/symptoms, or very similar comprehension problems.

One recent scientific approach to understanding brain systems is to combine imaging findings in healthy people and persons with brain diseases, with computer simulations of brain processes. The computer simulations are implemented by software written to mimic brain locations, their presumed functions, and the way in which information is transferred between specific cortical regions or subcortical nuclei. This kind of model can be used to run very elegant simulation experiments. The simulations can include hypothetical lesions in specific cortical regions or along the pathways connecting these regions. Selected speech and language forms may be "input" to the model to see how it "performs" under varied conditions of damage. This simulated performance can be compared to the performance of humans with documented lesions in the areas "damaged" in the simulation. If human performance matches the simulation peformance, a tentative conclusion is that the region of simulated damage is "responsible" for the speech and language performance matched between the patient and computer.

A well-known model of this sort is called DIVA (**D**irections **i**nto **V**elocities of **A**rticulators), developed originally by Dr. Frank Guenther of Boston University and under continuous development by Dr. Guenther and his coworkers (see Bohland et al., 2010; Guenther, 1995, 2006; Guenther, Ghosh, & Tourville, 2006; Peeva et al., 2010). DIVA is a neural network model of speech motor control that includes the programming of articulatory movements as well as the direct commands to guide the articulators after the programming has been done. To say that DIVA is a neural network model is to say it is a computer simulation of speech motor control. DIVA has been used to test the effects of simulated lesions in components of its speech motor control network, and the results have been compared to certain speech production signs reported in persons with documented lesions matching those tested in the simulations. A fitting way to end this chapter is to consider DIVA in a moderate amount of detail, and to ask how an understanding of such a model may be useful to speech-language pathologists who want to use their knowledge of brain function to diagnose and treat patients from an evidence-based, anatomicophysiological perspective.

A simplified adaptation of the DIVA model is shown in Figure 6–44. Three of the boxes represent cortical regions; arrows represent fiber tracts connecting these regions.

DIVA: Speech Sound Map (lvPMC)

The box titled "Speech Sound Map" represents an area of the frontal lobe, the *lateral ventral premotor cortex* (lvPMC), thought to "contain" basic units of speech production. More specifically, the lvPMC is a region of the premotor cortex just anterior to the face area of primary motor cortex; some scientists say it is adjacent to Broca's area, others may include portions of it *in* Broca's area. This region is thought to be very important in the planning of action—an area of the brain involved in the assembly and preparation of motor programs. The lvPMC is not necessarily a speech-specific region, but

plays a role in action production in general and may contain cells specialized for observing action ("mirror neurons") as well. The units of speech production contained within the lvPMC are thought to be syllables of the consonant-vowel (CV) type. It is possible that very frequently used syllables (in English syllables such as "the" and "neh" [as in the first syllable of the word "never"]) are tightly packaged there, almost like indivisible units, for easier access and assembly for production. Syllables having a lower frequency of occurrence (such as "wah" and "tih") may have to be assembled from individual sounds (that is, from phonemes) when producing a word containing the syllable.

The lvPMC plays an important role in the way DIVA accounts for certain "normal" speech phenomena, as well as for specific speech production deficits following strokes or other brain injuries that affect this area. For example, if lvPMC is the site for syllable selection and/or assembly, and more generally the programming of a speech task, the more complex the programming requirements the greater the expected activity in this brain region. Similarly, damage to lvPMC is expected to result in speech production behaviors that reflect programming problems.

How do scientists manipulate speech motor programming requirements, and what speech behaviors suggest a speech programming problem? Speech motor programming requirements are varied by manipulating the phonetic complexity of a speech task. These variations have taken two primary forms. One is to vary the number of syllables in a speech production task, by having conditions in which a speaker is required to produce single syllable, two-syllable, or three-syllable utterances. Two-syllable utterances are thought to require more programming resources than one-syllable utterances, three-syllable utterances more resources than two-syllable utterances. In fMRI studies the expected outcome for neurologically normal individuals is for greater lvPMC activity with increasing number of syllables to be produced (that is, with increasing programming demands). Various studies have supported this outcome, although the results are not uniformly consistent with this prediction (for a review see Peeva et al., 2010).

Another way to vary phonetic complexity is to change the structure of a syllable while holding constant the number of syllables in an utterance. For example, the syllables /sa/, /sta/, and /stra/ are thought to require increasingly complex speech motor programming as the utterance is changed from a consonant-vowel (CV) (/sa/), to CCV (/sta/), to CCCV (/stra/) form (see Wright et al., 2009). Part of this assumption may be related to the tendency for syllable frequency

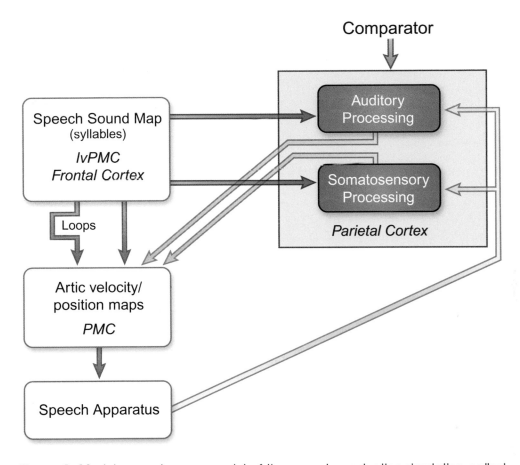

Figure 6–44. A box-and-arrows model of the speech production simulation called DIVA. The model shown here is adapted and modified from Guenther (2006), Peeva et al. (2010), and other publications from Professor Guenther's laboratory. Boxes represent cortical areas for speech motor control (and the speech apparatus), arrows represent tracts connecting these areas (or the apparatus to these areas). The speech sound map, where syllables are represented, is presumed to be in the lateral ventral premotor cortex (lvPMC), close to or including what is regarded as Broca's area. Articulatory velocity and position maps are located in the primary motor cortex (PMC). Auditory and somatosensory processing and comparisons are thought to take place in the parietal cortex.

to decrease as extra consonants are added to the syllable onset, part may simply reflect the added articulatory challenge of producing syllables with clustered consonants, as compared to singleton consonants (that is, CCCV vs. CV syllables). In experiments with neurologically normal speakers, participants are asked to say one of these syllable forms as quickly as possible when given a "go" signal (such as a brief tone). A frequently replicated finding is for the reaction time (RT: time from the onset of the "go" signal to the onset of the syllable) to increase as the syllable complexity increases (i.e., RT's for /stra/ are reliably longer than RT's for /sa/). The interpretation of the increasing RT across CV, CCV, and CCCV syllable forms is that it

takes more time to program a complex syllable such as /stra/ as compared to a simple syllable such as /sa/. In a sense, the longer RT for /stra/ as compared to /sa/ is the extra time required for processing in the lvPMC to "prepare" the utterance for production.

The linkage between these RT findings, DIVA, and the concerns of speech-language pathologists is the disorder called apraxia of speech (AOS: see sidetrack on "Apraxia of . . . Speech"). In adults, AOS is almost always associated with a known lesion, and is thought to be a speech motor programming disorder independent of weakness or paralysis of muscles in the speech apparatus (Darley et al., 1975; McNeil, Robin, & Schmidt, 2009). Many authors have noted the pres-

Apraxia of . . . Speech

The term "apraxia" was borrowed for application to speech from the general neurological literature. Following a stroke, some patients do not produce certain behaviors on command (e.g., "Show me how you use this pencil") but spontaneously produce the behavior (e.g., signing a document), demonstrating the ability to use the muscles to produce the action. This disorder —the inability to produce action on command— is called apraxia (meaning, "without action") to distinguish it from action disorders explained by obvious muscle weakness or sensory disturbance. Frederick Darley apparently was the first to graft the idea of apraxia onto poststroke, speech problems in adults; he used the term "apraxia of speech" in a 1969 paper presented at the annual convention of what was then called the American Speech and Hearing Association (see Ogar, Slama, Dronkers, Amici, & Gorno-Tempini, 2005). Fifteen years earlier, however, Morley, Court, and Miller (1954) had employed the term "articulatory dyspraxia" to mean precisely what Darley wanted to capture with the term "apraxia of speech." Morley et al. (1954, p. 9) said, when referring to their case studies of children with what seemed to be neurologically based, developmental speech disorders, "In the remaining six children . . . movements of the lips, tongue, and palate appeared normal on voluntary movements carried out at the examiner's request, but clumsy and awkward when the children attempted the more complex and rapid movements of articulation. We have regarded such cases as possible examples of 'dyspraxic dysarthria' or 'articulatory dyspraxia.'"

in lvPMC affects utterances having different numbers of syllables, or the different syllable shapes noted above. The model can be attached to an articulatory synthesizer, which permits an experimenter to determine how the model "produces" the utterances. Does the model hesitate longer before producing utterances with increased phonetic complexity, and is this hesitation exaggerated when the model contains a lesion in lvPMC? Does the model produce a greater number of errors when a lesion is mixed with greater phonetic complexity? These are examples of how a model such as DIVA can be manipulated and compared for performance matches to data from humans—in short, how the model can simulate human speech behavior.

Despite the value of DIVA in addressing the role of lvPMC in speech production, models such as these are limited in their ability to explain human speech and language behavior. For example, there is a disorder called childhood apraxia of speech (CAS) or developmental verbal dyspraxia in which the signs are described as very similar to those observed in adults, but the underlying cause is not. Whereas, in adults, AOS is almost always associated with a known brain lesion, in CAS it is almost always the case that brains scans *fail* to show the presence of a lesion. The presence of abnormal speech signs in CAS, with no known lesion, suggests other brain mechanisms, or deficits (or immaturities) in those mechanisms associated with programming behavior. Stated differently, if speech motor programming problems exist in children diagnosed with CAS but in whose brains no lesion can be found, other nervous system dysfunctions must be responsible for the behaviors. One view is that CAS is a problem with excessive "noise" (unwanted, random activity) in the speech motor programming mechanism. In fact, DIVA has been programmed with such noise and shown to produce instability (utterance-to-utterance variation greater than normal) in the simulated speech production of the model (Terband & Maassen, 2010). The instability may reflect immature or truly pathological brain function for speech motor control, but is not necessarily easy to relate to programming difficulties. In addition, brain lesions in locations other than the lvPMC, both cortical and subcortical, may produce signs consistent with a speech motor programming disorder (see Ogar et al., 2005; and Pramstaller & Marsden, 1996, for a general review of apraxia and subcortical lesions). This suggests that either multiple locations in the speech motor control network are capable of producing the same process—in this case programming—or that the network functions as a truly integrated system, in which the act of producing an utterance requires programming and execution by an integrated system, rather than a series of process-specific parts.

ence of a lesion in or around lvPMC when the signs of AOS are documented clinically (interested students are encouraged to read a classic paper by Mohr et al. [1978]).

Of greatest interest is the frequent claim that a diagnostic feature of AOS is an increase in articulatory errors with increasing phonetic complexity of utterances. Whether the phonetic complexity is in the form of multiple-syllable utterances, or single syllables with complex forms, adults with AOS are said to have a disproportionately difficult time producing words such as "statistical" and "Mississippi" as compared to "sat" and "miss" (Rosenbek, Kent, & LaPointe, 1984). DIVA can be programmed to evaluate how a simulated lesion

DIVA: Articulatory Velocity/ Position Maps (PMC)

The primary motor cortex (PMC) contains cells connected to brainstem and spinal motor neurons via the corticobulbar and corticospinal tracts, respectively. These PMC cells are the primary command cells for specification of muscle contraction characteristics —how forceful, how fast, how short or long, and so forth. In DIVA, the PMC cells of interest are the ones associated with head and neck (corticobulbar) and respiratory (corticospinal) muscles. These cells receive program instructions from the lvPMC via a fiber tract connecting the two areas; this is represented in Figure 6–44 by the unlabeled arrow from the "Speech Sound Map" to the PMC. Activity in PMC is presumed to be devoted strictly to execution. In fact, cells in the PMC are thought to be insensitive to phonetic complexity, unlike the complexity-sensitive lvPMC cells. For this reason damage to PMC cells presumably results in dysarthria, and there is good clinical evidence to support this expectation (Urban et al., 2003, 2006).

As Figure 6–44 shows, however, the input to the PMC is not restricted to the hypothesized programs constructed in the lvPMC. The arrow labeled "loops" in Figure 6–44 represents the potential modification of PMC cell activity by information circulating in the two cerebral sensorimotor loops described above: the cortico-striatal-cortical loop and the cortico-cerebellar-cortical loop. Both the basal ganglia and cerebellum have been identified as brain structures involved in aspects of motor programs, meaning that loops between these structures and the PMC must have something to do with "direct" motor activity in PMC cells. As stated eloquently by Terband and Maassen (2010), the dense interconnectedness of the many and widespread motor components of the brain makes it exceedingly difficult to use speech data of any single kind or from a single task to make clean distinctions between programming (i.e., apraxia) and execution (i.e., dysarthria) problems. The effect of these loops on the execution cells in the PMC also emphasizes the concept of sensorimotor control noted throughout this chapter. "Speech motor control" is more properly referred to as "speech sensorimotor control."

DIVA: Auditory and Somatosensory Processing: Parietal Cortex and Frontal-Parietal Association Tracts

Figure 6–44 shows projections from the lvPMC to the auditory and somatosensory parietal cortex (red arrows) and projections from the auditory and somato-sensory cortices to the PMC (blue arrows). The model also shows connections, indicated by green arrows, from the speech apparatus to somatosensory and auditory cortices. This group of connections within the CNS (red and blue arrows), and from the peripheral apparatus back to the CNS (green arrows), play a critical role in the uniqueness of DIVA as a model of speech sensorimotor control relevant to clinical issues in speech-language pathology.

Consider first the intrahemispheric association tracts, connecting cortical areas in the frontal and parietal lobes. The anatomical evidence for these connections is clear, and includes the arcuate fasciculus (to account at least for auditory information) as well as other fibers connecting the region near the lvPMC with the parietal lobe (to account at least for somatosensory information: see Martino et al. [2011]). Information in these association tracts flows in both directions—parietal to frontal lobe, and frontal to parietal lobe (Hickok & Poeppel, 2007).

Consider next the red arrows projecting from lvPMC to the parietal auditory and sensory association areas, a key feature of DIVA. For a syllable stored in lvPMC (or assembled from smaller, phonemic "parts" in the case of a low-frequency syllable), this projection tract carries a data-based model of the expected sensory consequences of the articulatory gestures required to produce that syllable. In the production of the word "sigh," for example, there are tactile and motion consequences of moving the front of the tongue from the tight, slightly leaking contact with the alveolar ridge required for the fricative /s/ to the constantly changing vocalic configurations required for the diphthong /aɪ/. Similarly, there are acoustic consequences of these movements—the frication noise for the voiceless /s/ to the rapid formant transitions (reflecting the rapid changes in vocal tract configuration) of /aɪ/. Over many repetitions of this syllable, from the time a child first starts to produce speech and throughout the thousands and perhaps millions of "sigh" syllables in many different words, a human speaker builds up a data-based model, or calibration, of how these particular movements should "feel" (tactile, motion sense, and so forth) and sound (acoustic) when the syllable is produced correctly. These calibrations are established by means of the connections between the speech apparatus and somatosensory and auditory association areas in parietal cortex. As the structures of the speech apparatus move during speech production, tactile receptors, baroreceptors (receptors sensitive to air pressure), and receptors sensitive to parameters of muscle contraction (such as muscle spindles) send information to somatosensory cortex, just like information that is sent to auditory cortex from sensory receptors in the cochlea. This information is encoded in the association cortex as a set of expectations for correct productions. It is as if the motor commands issued from the brain to the speech apparatus are linked, as a critical part of speech motor control, with the sensory movement consequences of those commands. The two-way pathways between the parietal and frontal lobes allow these expectations to be transferred to the lvPMC, where the programming of syllables is combined with the sensory consequences of their production. At the same time a syllable is being programmed and delivered to PMC, the set of sensory expectations is sent to the somatosensory and auditory association areas in the parietal lobe. These are additional reasons why the term "speech sensorimotor control" is preferable to "speech motor control."

Do the sensory expectations for a given syllable *match* the actual incoming somatosensory and acoustic data? This question is answered through the use of the Comparator, shown as the shaded box around the somatosensory and auditory processing boxes in Figure 6–44. If the incoming data match the sensory expectations, as they typically will in a person with a normal speech apparatus, the process of speech production continues without the need for any adjustments. But if the sensory input from the speech apparatus does not match the expected calibration signal delivered to the parietal association cortices, an error is detected by the comparator and corrections are sent, via the blue lines, to PMC for modification of the motor commands. Although not shown in Figure 6–44, comparisons that indicate a consistent error over many repetitions also send information back to the lvPMC where the calibration, or expectations, can be updated for future productions of the syllable. In other words, the model can learn from its mistakes.

Why is this process of developing and maintaining a calibration between speech movements and their sensory consequences, and the ability to detect errors and modify the calibrations, so important to the speech-language pathologist? The primary reason is that the integration of sensory consequences, and especially those related to the auditory channel, are critical to the concept of *speech* sensorimotor control. Note the avoidance of the term *tongue* motor control, or *jaw* motor control, but rather the focus on *speech* sensorimotor control. As suggested by DIVA, an important part of the speech sensorimotor control network is the comparison of expected and actual sensory consequences, and a major component of sensory consequences is the acoustic speech signal. Therefore, diagnostic or therapeutic efforts aimed at (for example) tongue or velar strength, jaw wags, and speed of lateral tongue motions are inappropriate. These oromotor, nonspeech

motions certainly have sensory consequences, but an acoustic signal generated by the vocal tract for purposes of communication is not among them. Nor are the tactile, aeromechanical, and motion sensory consequences of articulatory gestures the same as those associated with, say, maximum strength contractions of the tongue or jaw. The mounting evidence against the relevance of oromotor, nonverbal tasks for understanding speech sensorimotor control is consistent with DIVA's incorporation of the acoustic speech signal and somatosensory signals specific to speech gestures into the concept of speech sensorimotor control (relevant readings include Ballard, Robin, and Folkins [2003], Forrest [2002], Ruscello [2008], Weismer [2006b], and Ziegler [2003] among others).

DIVA: Where Is Aphasia, Where Are Dysarthria Types?

In the introduction to DIVA, it was noted that the model assumes the "correctness" of language representations in the brain. Also, in DIVA the primary command cells in PMC are not sensitive to the phonetic complexity issues that affect cells in lvPMC. PMC is strictly about the act of producing the sequences planned in lvPMC and adjusted by information circulating in the cortico-striatal-cortical and cortico-cerebellar-cortical loops. These aspects of the current version of DIVA can be generalized to say that the model does not, in its current form, handle language expression and comprehension issues seen in aphasia, where representations or access to them may be affected. In addition, the model cannot currently account for the fact that different locations of brain damage associated with dysarthria may result in different-sounding speech disorders (e.g., the dysarthria resulting from cerebellar damage may sound different from the dysarthria associated with damage to the corticobulbar tract). DIVA is a remarkable achievement and has already produced new and important insights to speech production and its disruption by brain lesions. Future developments are likely to include new simulations of aphasia, and new simulations of the execution functions of the model. The fact that a model cannot explain everything about a process as complicated as speech and language, and even makes mistakes or produces difficult-to-interpret results concerning the processes it is designed to explain, does not make it less valuable. It is, in effect, a highly structured guide to future theoretical (modeling) and clinical investigations of the nervous system basis of human communication.

REVIEW

The chapter is initiated with a summary of general concepts including central versus peripheral nervous system (CNS vs. PNS), anatomical planes and directions, white versus gray matter, tracts versus nuclei, nerves versus ganglia, afferent and efferent, and lateralization and specialization of function.

The cerebral hemispheres include cortical tissue (gray matter), fiber tracts (white matter), and subcortical nuclei (gray matter), and the surface of the cerebral hemispheres is defined by gyri (hills) and sulci (valleys).

Each cerebral hemisphere has four lobes, including the frontal, parietal, temporal, and occipital lobes, and regions within these lobes that have been proposed as serving specialized roles in speech, language, and hearing.

Two other areas of cortical tissue—the insula and components of the limbic system—may play important roles in speech, language, and hearing.

Cerebral white matter is composed of many types of tracts (association, striatal, commissural, descending, and ascending) that connect different parts of the CNS to each other, one of the most important of which for speech and language is the arcuate fasciculus.

Descending tracts from the cortex to the brainstem (corticobulbar tract) and spinal cord (corticospinal tract) innervate lower motor neurons that represent the final common pathway to muscles of the speech apparatus.

Ascending tracts are primarily associated with sensory pathways and carry information about touch, pain, temperature, hearing, vision, vibration, and proprioception.

The basal ganglia are subcortical nuclei (nuclei within the cerebral hemispheres and above the brainstem) that connect to the cortex via loops and are important in aspects of speech sensorimotor control such as the refinement and programming of motor behavior.

The thalamus is the major relay for all sensory information (except smell) ascending in the CNS to the cortex and is also an output target to the cortex, via the globus pallidus, for information processed in the basal ganglia.

The cerebellum is connected to the spinal cord, brainstem, and cerebral hemispheres by means of the cerebellar peduncles, and to the cortex (via loops, like the basal ganglia) and contributes to the coordination of complex motor behavior, and balance, and possibly plays a role in programming motor sequences such as successive articulatory gestures.

The brainstem, a stalk of tissue connecting the spinal cord to the cerebral hemispheres and cerebellum, has three levels, including (from superior to inferior) the midbrain (mesencephalon), pons, and medulla, each containing sensory and motor nuclei, as well as descending, ascending, and crossing fiber tracts.

Prominent features on the ventral and dorsal surfaces of the brainstem are entrance and exit locations of most of the cranial nerves, including those (cranial nerves V, VII, IX, X, XI, XII) associated with control of head and neck muscles.

The 12 cranial nerves have numbers and names (olfactory, optic, oculomotor, trochlear, trigeminal, abducens, facial, auditory-vestibular, glossopharyngeal, vagus, spinal accessory, and hypoglossal) and are composed of motor, sensory, or both motor and sensory fibers that transmit information between the CNS and the body.

A reflex called the jaw jerk is mediated by brainstem structures associated with cranial nerve V, and the mechanism of this reflex serves as a model of stretch reflexes throughout the body.

Standard tests administered by neurologists and speech-language pathologists are used to evaluate the integrity of the cranial nerves and determine potential site(s) of lesion (using knowledge of neural innervation patterns), but should not be used to make inferences about speech production skill.

The spinal cord, which is continuous with the inferior border of the medulla and extends from the first cervical vertebrae to the upper lumbar vertebrae, contains central gray matter consisting of neuron cell bodies (sensory cells in the back and motor cells in the front) and surrounding white matter consisting of axons that supply the muscles of the breathing apparatus as well as other voluntary musculature of the limbs and torso.

Cells in the nervous system include signaling cells (neurons) and glial cells (astrocytes, oligodendrocytes, Schwann cells) that provide metabolic and protective support to the neurons, and ependymal cells that secrete CSF.

Neurons, or signaling cells, are composed of a cell body (soma), dendrites, an axon, and a terminal button or buttons, and usually communicate with each other by conversion of electrical-to-neurochemical energy, which is then converted back to electrical energy.

An action potential is initiated at the dendrites, which depolarizes the soma, causing the electrical energy to be propagated down the axon to the terminal button (presynaptic membrane) where neurotransmitter is released into the cleft between the terminal button and the dendrites of an adjacent neuron (postsynaptic membrane), with the presynaptic/synaptic cleft/

postsynaptic structures and conversion of electrical-to-chemical-to-electrical energy being called a synapse.

The neuromuscular junction is where a motor nerve makes contact with a motor end plate attached to muscle fiber, and where acetycholine is released by the terminal button of the peripheral nerve to bind to special receptors embedded in the motor endplate, thereby causing an action potential to be generated in the muscle fiber and the muscle fiber to shorten (contract).

The meninges are protective coverings of the cerebral hemispheres, brainstem, and spinal cord and include the dura mater, arachnoid mater, and pia mater.

CSF flows throughout the ventricular system, which includes the lateral ventricles, third ventricle, fourth ventricle, and central canal of the spinal cord.

The blood supply of the brain includes an anterior and posterior supply, with one of the most important anterior arteries for speech, language, and hearing function being the middle cerebral artery.

The computer simulation model called DIVA is able to make certain predictions about damage to regions of the frontal lobe and speech output, as well as damage to parts of the parietal lobe and the effect on a speaker's ability to produce articulatory gestures with known acoustic results.

REFERENCES

Ackermann, H., & Riecker, A. (2010). The contributions(s) of the insula to speech production: A review of the clinical and functional imaging literature. *Brain Structure and Function, 214,* 419–433.

Alvarez, J. A., & Emory, E. (2006). Executive function and the frontal lobes: A meta-analytic review. *Neuropsychology Review, 16,* 17–42.

Ballard, K. J., Robin, D. A., & Folkins, J. W. (2003). An integrative model of speech motor control: A response to Ziegler. *Aphasiology, 17,* 37–48.

Bear, M. F., Connors, B. W., & Paradiso, M. A. (2007). *Neuroscience: Exploring the brain.* Baltimore, MD: Lippincott Williams & Wilkins.

Bernal, B., & Ardila, A. (2009). The role of the arcuate fasciculus in conduction aphasia. *Brain, 132,* 2309–2316.

Bohland, J. W., Bullock, D., & Guenther, F. H. (2010). Neural representations and mechanisms for the performance of simple speech sequences. *Journal of Cognitive Neuroscience, 22,* 1504–1529.

Blumenfeld, H. (2010). *Neuroanatomy through clinical cases* (2nd ed.). Sunderland, MA: Sinauer Associates.

Bostan, A. C., & Strick, P. L. (2010). The cerebellum and basal ganglia are interconnected. *Neuropsychology Review, 20,* 261–270.

Catani, M., & Mesulam, M. (2008). The arcuate fasciculus and the disconnection theme in language and aphasia: History and current state. *Cortex, 44,* 953–961.

Conturo, T. E., Lori, N. F., Cull, T. S., Akbudak, E., Snyder, A. Z., Shimony, J. S., . . . Raichle, M. E. (2008). Tracking neuronal fiber pathways in the living human brain. *Proceedings of the National Academy of Sciences USA, 96,* 10422–10427.

Culham, J. C., & Valyear, K. F. (2006). Human parietal cortex in action. *Current Opinion in Neurobiology, 16,* 205–212.

Darley, F. L., Aronson, A. E., & Brown, J. R. (1975). *Motor speech disorders.* Philadelphia, PA: W. B. Saunders.

Deacon, T. W. (1997). *The symbolic species: The co-evolution of language and the brain.* New York, NY: W. W. Norton.

DeToledo, J. C., & David, N. J. (2001). Innervation of the sternocleidomastoid aand trapezius muscles by the accessory nucleus. *Journal of Neuro-Ophthalmology, 21,* 214–216.

Doron, K. W., & Gazzaniga, M. S. (2008). Neuroimaging techniques offer new perspectives on callosal transfer and interhemispheric communication. *Cortex, 44,* 1023–1029.

Dronkers, N. F., Plaisant, O., Ibas-Zisen, M. T., & Cabanis, E. A. (2007). Paul Broca's historic cases: High-resolution MR imaging of the brains of LeBorgne and Lelong. *Brain, 129,* 1164–1176.

Duffy, J. D. (2005). *Motor speech disorders: Substrates, differential diagnosis, and management.* St. Louis, MO: Elsevier Mosby.

Eftekhar, B., Dadmehr, M., Ansari, S., Ghodsi, M., Nazparvar, B., & Ketabchi, E. (2006). Are the distributions of variations of circle of Willis different in different populations? Results of an anatomical study and review of literature. *BMC Neurology,* http://www.biomedcentral.com/1471-2377/6/22

Epelbaum, S., Pinel, P., Gaillard, R., Delmaire, C., Perrin, M., Dupont, S., . . . Cohen L. (2008). Pure alexia as a disconnection syndrome: New diffusion imaging evidence for an old concept. *Cortex, 44,* 962–974.

Fasano, A., Daniele, A., & Albanese, A. (2012). Treatment of motor and non-motor features of Parkinson's disease with deep brain stimulation. *Lancet Neurology, 11,* 429–442.

Forrest, K. (2002). Are oral-motor exercises useful in the treatment of phonological/articulatory disorders? *Seminars in Speech and Language, 23,* 15–26.

Galantucci, B., Fowler, C. A., & Turvey, M. T. (2006). The motor theory of speech perception reviewed. *Psychonomic Bulletin Review, 13,* 361–377.

Gazzaniga, M. (2000). Cerebral specialization and interhemispheric communication: Does the corpus callosum enable the human condition? *Brain, 123,* 1293–1326.

Geschwind, N. (1965). Disconnection syndromes in animals and man. *Brain, 88,* 237–294.

Grodzinsky, Y., & Santi, A. (2008). The battle for Broca's region. *Trends in Cognitive Sciences, 12,* 474–480.

Gunether, F. H. (1995). Speech sound acquisition, coarticulation, and rate effects in a neural network model of speech production. *Psychological Review, 102,* 594–621.

Guenther, F. H. (2006). Cortical interaction underlying the production of speech sounds. *Journal of Communication Disorders, 39,* 350–365.

Guenther, F. H., Ghosh, S. S., & Tourville, J. A. (2006). Neural modeling and imaging of the cortical interactions underlying syllable production. *Brain and Language, 96,* 280–301.

Heimer, L., & Van Hoesen, G. W. (2006). The limbic lobe and its output channels: Implications for emotional functions and adaptive behavior. *Neuroscience and Biobehavioral Reviews, 30,* 126–147.

Hickok, G. (2009). The functional neuroanatomy of language. *Physics of Life Reviews, 6,* 121–143.

Hickok, G., & Poeppel, D. (2007). The cortical organization of speech processing. *Nature Reviews: Neuroscience, 8,* 393–402.

Ito, T., & Gomi, H. (2007). Cutaneous mechanoreceptors contribute to the generation of a cortical reflex in speech. *NeuroReport, 18,* 907–910.

Kandel, E. R., Schwartz, J. H., & Jessel, T. M. (2000). *Principles of neural science* (4th ed.). New York, NY: McGraw-Hill.

Keller, S. S., Crow, T., Foundas, A., Amunts, K., & Roberts, N. (2009). Broca's area: Nomenclature, anatomy, typology, and asymmetry. *Brain and Language, 109,* 29–48.

Kent, R. D., Martin, R. E., & Sufit, R. L. (1990). Oral sensation: A review and clinical prospective. In H. Winitz (Ed.), *Human communication and its disorders* (vol. 3, pp. 135–191). Norwood, NJ: Ablex.

Knecht, S., Dräger, B., Deppe, M., Bobe, L., Lohmann, H., Flöell, A., . . . Henningsen, H. (2000). Handedness and hemispheric language dominance in healthy humans. *Brain, 123,* 2512–2518.

Kuehn, D. P., Templeton, P. J., & Maynard, J. A. (1990). Muscle spindles in the velopharyngeal musculature of humans. *Journal of Speech and Hearing Research, 33,* 488–493.

Langers, D. R. M., Backe, W. H., & van Dijk, P. (2007). Representation of lateralization and tonotopicity in primary versus secondary human auditory cortex. *NeuroImage, 34,* 264–273.

Lee, D., Swanson, S. J., Sabsevitz, D. S., Hammeke, T. A., Winstanley, F. S., Possing, E. T., & Binder, J. R. (2008). Functional MRI and Wada studies in patients with interhemispheric dissociation of language functions. *Epilepsy and Behavior, 13,* 350–356.

Lindenberg, R., Fangerau, H., & Seitz, R. J. (2007). "Broca's area" as a collective term? *Brain and Language, 102,* 22–29.

Ludlow, C. L. (2011). Spasmodic dysphonia: A laryngeal control disorder specific to speech. *Journal of Neuroscience, 19,* 793–797.

Martino, J., De Witt Hamer, P. C., Vergani, F., Brogna, C., de Lucas, E. M., Vázquez-Barquero, A., . . . Duffau, H. (2011). Cortex-sparing fiber dissection: An improved method for the study of white matter anatomy in the human brain. *Journal of Anatomy, 219,* 531–541.

McNeil, M. R., Robin, D. A., & Schmidt, R. A. (2009). Apraxia of speech. In M. R. McNeil (Ed.), *Clinical management of sensorimotor speech disorders* (2nd ed., pp. 249–268). New York, NY: Thieme.

Meng, H., Murakami, G., Suzuki, D., & Miyamoto, S. (2008). Anatomical variations in stylopharyngeus muscle insertions suggest interindividual and left/right differences in pharyngeal clearance function of elderly patients: A cadaveric study. *Dysphagia, 23,* 251–257.

Middleton, F. A., & Strick, P. L. (2000). Basal ganglia and cerebellar loops: Motor and cognitive circuits. *Brain Research Reviews, 31,* 236–250.

Mohr, J. P., Pessin, M. S., Finkelstein, S., Funkenstein, H. H., Duncan, G. W., & Davis, K. R. (1978). Broca aphasia: Pathologic and clinical. *Neurology, 28,* 311–324.

Morley, M., Court, D., & Miller, H. (1954). Developmental dysarthria. *British Medical Journal, 1,* 8–10.

Nambu, A. (2008). Several problems on the basal ganglia. *Current Opinion in Neurobiology, 18,* 595–604.

Obeso, J. A., & Lanciego, J. L. (2011). Past, present, and future of the pathophysiological model of the basal ganglia. *Frontiers in Neuroanatomy, 5,* 1–6.

Ogar, J., Slama, H., Dronkers, N., Amici, S., & Gorno-Tempini, M. L. (2005). Apraxia of speech: An overview. *Neurocase, 11,* 427–432.

Peeva, M. G., Guenther, F. H., Tourville, J. A., Nieto-Castanon, A., Anotn, J.-L., Nazarian, B., & Alario, F.-X. (2010). Distinct representation of phonemes, syllables, and suprasyllabic sequences in the speech production network. *NeuroImage, 50,* 626–638.

Picton, T. (2010). *Human auditory evoked potentials.* San Diego, CA: Plural.

Postuma, R. B., & Dagher, A. (2006). Basal ganglia functional connectivity based on a meta-analysis of 126 Positron Emission Tomography and functional magnetic resonance imaging publications. *Cerebral Cortex, 16,* 1508–1521.

Pramstaller, P. O., & Marsden, C. D. (1996). The basal ganglia and apraxia. *Brain, 119,* 319–340.

Price, C. J. (2010). The anatomy of language: A review of 100 fMRI studies published in 2009. *Annals of the New York Academy of Sciences, 1191,* 62–88.

Rasmussen, T., & Milner, B. (1977). The role of early left-brain injury in determining lateralization of cerebral speech functions. *Annals of the New York Academy of Sciences, 299,* 355–369.

Ridderinkhof, K. R., Ullsperger, M., Crone, E. A., & Nieuwenhuis, S. (2004). The role of the medial frontal cortex in cognitive control. *Science, 306,* 443–447.

Rosenbek, J. C., Kent, R. D., & LaPointe, L. L. (1984). Apraxia of speech: An overview and some perspectives. In J. C. Rosenbek, M. R. McNeil, & A. E. Aronson (Eds.), *Apraxia of speech* (pp. 1–72). San Diego, CA: College-Hill Press.

Ruscello, D. M. (2008). An examination of non-speech oromotor exercises in children with velopharyngeal inadequacy. *Seminars in Speech and Language, 29,* 294–303.

Said, C. P., Haxby, J. V., & Todorov, A. (2011). Brain systems for assessing the affective value of faces. *Philosophical Transactions of the Royal Society B, 366,* 1660–1670.

Saigusa, H., Yamashita, K., Tanuma, K., Saigusa, M., & Niimi, S. (2004). Morphological studies for retrusive movement of the human adult tongue. *Clinical Anatomy, 17,* 93–98.

Sanders, I., Han, Y., Wang, J., & Biller, H. (1998). Muscle spindles are concentrated in the superior vocalis subcompartment of the human thyroarytenoid muscle. *Journal of Voice, 12,* 7–16.

Sarikcioglu, L., Altun, U., Suzen, B., & Oguz, N. (2008). The evolution of the terminology of the basal ganglia, or are they nuclei? *Journal of the History of the Neurosciences: Basic and Clinical Perspectives, 17*, 226–229.

Saur, D., Kreher, B. W., Schnell, S., Kümmerer, D., Kellmeyer, P., Vry, M. S., . . . Weiller, C. (2008). Ventral and dorsal pathways for language. *Proceedings of the National Academy of Sciences of the United States, 18*, 18035–18040.

Schmahmann, J. D., Smith, E. E., Eichler, F. S., & Filley, C. M. (2008). Cerebral white matter: Neuroanatomy, clinical neurology, and neurobehavioral correlates. *Annals of the New York Academy of Sciences, 1142*, 266–309.

Springer, J. A., Binder, J. R., Hammeke, T. A., Swanson, S. J., Frost, J. A., Bellgowan, P. S. F., . . . Mueller, W. M. (1999). Language dominance in neurologically normal and epilepsy subjects: A functional MRI study. *Brain, 122*, 2033–2046.

Swanson, S. J., Sabsevitz, D. S., Hammeke, T. A., & Binder, J. R. (2007). Functional magnetic resonance imaging of language in epilepsy. *Neuropsychology Review, 17*, 491–504.

Takai, O., Brown, S., & Liotti, M. (2010). Representation of the speech effectors in the human motor cortex: Somatotopy or overlap? *Brain and Language, 113*, 39–44.

Terband, H., & Maassen, B. (2010). Speech motor development in childhood apraxia of speech: Generating testable hypotheses by neurocomputational modeling. *Folia Phoniatrica et Logopaedica, 62*, 134–142.

Tervaniemi, M., & Hugdahl, K. (2003). Lateralization of auditory-cortex functions. *Brain Research Reviews, 43*, 231–246.

Urban, P. P., Marx, J., Hunsche, S., Gawehn, J., Vucurevic, G., Wicht, S., . . . Hopf, H. C. (2003). Cerebellar speech representation: Lesion topography in dysarthria as derived from cerebellar ischemia and functional magnetic resonance imaging. *Archives of Neurology, 60*, 965–972.

Urban, P. P., Rolke, R., Wicht, S., Keilmann, A., Stoeter, P., Hopf, H. C., & Dieterich, M. (2006). Left hemispheric dominance for articulation: A prospective study on acute ischaemic dysarthria at different localizations. *Brain, 129*, 767–777.

Wahl, M., Lauterbach-Soon, B., Hattingen, E., Jung, P., Singer, O., Volz, S., . . . Ziemann, U. (2007). Human motor corpus callosum: Topography, somatotopy, and link between microstructure and function. *Journal of Neuroscience, 27*, 12132–12138.

Weismer, G. (2006a) (Ed.). *Motor speech disorders.* San Diego, CA: Plural.

Weismer, G. (2006b). Philosophy of research in motor speech disorders. *Clinical Linguistics and Phonetics, 20*, 315–349.

Willems, R. M., & Hagoort, P. (2009). Broca's region: Battles are not won by ignoring half of the facts. *Trends in Cognitive Sciences, 13*, 101.

Wilson-Pauwels, L., Akesson, E. J., Stewart, P. A., & Spacey, S. D. (2002). *Cranial nerves in health and disease.* Hamilton, Ontario: B.C. Decker.

Wright, D. L., Robin, D. A., Rhee J., Vaculin, A., Jacks, A., Guenther, F. H., & Fox, P. T. (2009). Using the self-select paradigm to delineate the nature of speech motor programming. *Journal of Speech, Language, and Hearing Research, 52*, 755–765.

Ziegler, W. (2003). Speech motor control is task-specific: Evidence from dysarthria and apraxia of speech. *Aphasiology, 17*, 3–36.

Zilles, K., Armstrong, E., Schleicher, A., & Kretschmann, H. J. (1988). The human pattern of gyrification in the cerebral cortex. *Anatomy and Embryology, 179*, 173–179.

Acoustics

INTRODUCTION

Physical acoustics encompasses a huge range of topics, many of which are not covered in this text. The information presented here is selected to serve as a foundation for the study of speech acoustics. Readers interested in a full, technical treatment of acoustics should consult the classic textbook of Beranek (1986). Entertaining histories of acoustics as a scientific discipline have been published by Hunt (1978) and Beyer (1999).

In this chapter, a series of questions are addressed. When these questions are answered, the foundation will be established for an understanding of the acoustic theory of speech production. The questions are as follows:

1. What are pressure (sound) waves, and how can they be measured?
2. What is sinusoidal motion, and which measurements are relevant to its description?
3. What are complex acoustic events, and how are they related to sinusoids?
4. What is the phenomenon of resonance, and how is resonant frequency determined in mechanical and acoustical systems?
5. What does it mean to say that a resonator "shapes" an input?

Secret Acoustical Society?

The leading acoustics organization in the world is the Acoustical Society of America (ASA), founded in 1929. Roughly 35 scientists attended the initial 1929 meeting of the Society (that's the number counted in a photograph taken of the attendees at the meeting). Today, ASA has over 7,000 members who study all aspects of acoustics. The Society encourages open exchange of ideas and education in acoustics. It wasn't always so. The science of acoustics goes way back to the Ionian philosopher Pythagoras (ca. 575–495 BC), the same fellow after whom a famous geometry theorem is named. Pythagoras enjoyed a sort of guru status, and his followers decided that their investigations should be kept secret to protect their intellectual sanctity. We know the Pythagoreans made numerous observations about acoustical events, but alas, we only learned about these through indirect sources—leaks in the system. So the first Acoustical Society was really a Secret Acoustical Society.

PRESSURE WAVES

This section considers the nature of pressure waves. It discusses the forces that govern such waves, how local changes in air pressure occur, how pressure waves propagate through space, and how such waves can be measured and represented.

The Motions of Vibrating Air Molecules Are Governed by Simple Forces

Sound can be defined as the propagation of a pressure wave—a *sound wave*—in space and time. Clarification of this definition requires a precise definition of exactly what is meant by the term *pressure wave*.

Sound is always propagated throughout some medium. The various media that may conduct sound waves (e.g., water, steel, air) are all composed of molecules that are more or less compressible. In other words, the molecules of these media may, under the influence of a force, be displaced away from their rest positions (where "rest positions" means the positions when no forces are applied to the medium) and moved closer to nearby molecules. The resulting "bunching up'"of molecules, relative to their distribution at rest, shows that the medium is compressible.

The molecules of all sound-conducting media share the characteristics of *elasticity* and *mass*. Elastic objects oppose displacement, and do so with greater magnitude as they are moved farther from their rest positions. A common example of this is a rubber band. When the rubber band is completely collapsed (unstretched), it is in its rest position. As the rubber band is stretched, it becomes stiffer and increasingly difficult to stretch. Massive objects oppose being accelerated and decelerated (that is, they have *inertia*: ("a body in motion tends to stay in motion"), and do so with greater magnitude as they become more massive. The effect of mass on motion is easily appreciated by the speeding automobile that does not stop instantly when the brakes are applied.

Opposition to displacement (elasticity) and acceleration/deceleration (mass) actually result in energy storage. This stored energy can be expressed as motion of the object even in the absence of an external force. This topic is taken up in greater detail below.

The sound-conducting medium of interest for speech is, at least in most cases, air. The number of molecules in a cubic inch of air, referred to as the density of air and symbolized with the Greek letter *rho* (ρ), is approximately 4×1023. The density of molecules in water is about four times greater than that in air, and in steel about eleven times greater than air.

With air as the medium, a schematic drawing[1] can be used to illustrate the concepts mentioned above and to clarify the nature of pressure waves. Imagine, as shown in Figure 7–1, four columns of air molecules (labeled1, 2, 3, 4) extending across some distance. Five rows, labeled A, B, C, D, E, show the state of these molecules at successive moments in time. Row A (hereafter, time A) shows the molecules at rest, with no external forces applied to them. This rest position is indicated across all times by the dashed lines extending downward throughout the four columns of molecules. Note the even spacing between the molecules across time A.

Molecules at rest are actually still in motion (this rest motion is referred to as *Brownian* motion), but the average spacing between any pair of molecules will be roughly equivalent, as shown in Figure 7–1, time A. Because the molecules at time A are not being displaced from their rest positions and thus not being accelerated, they store no elastic or inertial energy (other than the small stored energies due to Brownian motion). At time B, the molecule in column 1 is subjected to a *force* (indicated by the rightward directed arrow) that moves it rightward, away from its rest position and in the direction of the molecule at position 2. For present purposes, a *force* can be thought of as any push or pull applied to an object. As the moving molecule gets farther from its rest position, it opposes increasing displacement by generating an increasing *recoil force*, which is exerted in the direction of the rest position, or a direction opposite to its current motion. Stated in a different way, the original force of the rightward push is transferred to the air molecule, whose rightward displacement is increasingly opposed by the tendency of the molecule to recoil back to its rest position. The current motion continues away from the rest position because the original force of the push still exceeds the recoil force. The recoil force is the stored energy resulting from the molecule's displacement, and is a hallmark of all elastic objects that are displaced from their rest positions.

At position 2, time B, several interesting things happen. First, the spacing between molecules 1 and 2 is

---

[1]A *schematic* drawing is basically a graphical model that attempts to capture the important aspects of a phenomenon while reducing or eliminating other information. For example, a stick person is a schematic of the human form, and a road sign indicating a curve is a schematic of the actual layout of a curving roadway.

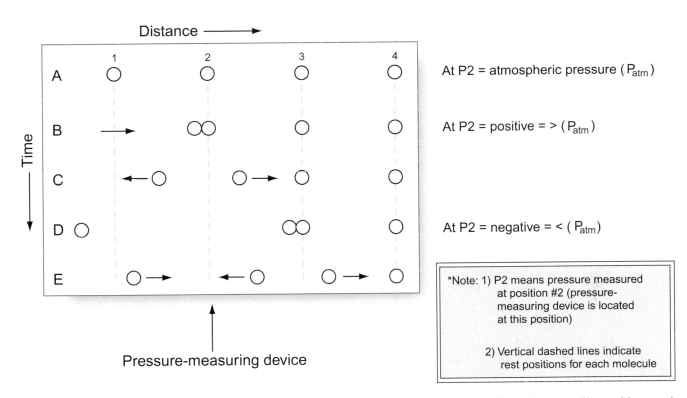

Figure 7–1. Schematic model of the vibration of air molecules around their rest positions. Rest positions of four molecules are shown at time "A" at positions 1, 2, 3, and 4. Time is indicated by the rows A, B, C, D, and E. A pressure-measuring device is located at the rest position of molecule 2. See text for details.

now minimal compared to their spacing at rest (time A). At position 2, time B, the molecules are bunched up, and molecule 1 bumps molecule 2, just as the push originally bumped molecule 1 to get this process underway. Second, the molecule that was originally pushed to start the process has, as described above, been displaced relatively far from its rest position and is generating a strong recoil force to return to its rest position. At some point, the recoil force will equal and then exceed the original force and thus cause the molecule to stop its rightward motion and begin to move leftward. Assume that the original molecule from position 1 is, at time B, not only just bumping the molecule at position 2 but also is about to reverse its direction. The reversal of direction is due to the recoil force overcoming the forces on the molecule due to the original push.

At time C, the molecule from position 1 is headed back toward the rest position (leftward-directed arrow). The molecule from position 2, having been bumped by the position 1 molecule, is now moving away from its rest position and in the direction of the molecule at position 3 (rightward-directed arrow). At time D, the molecule from position 2 is bumping into the molecule

at position 3, and is also about to reverse its direction—just like the situation discussed above for time B, position 2. The molecule from position 1, however, has gone *through* its rest position, and is displaced far to the left—note at time D the wide separation of the molecules from positions 1 and 2. Clearly, the elastic recoil forces caused the molecule from position 1 to move back toward the rest position at time E, but why doesn't the motion stop at the rest position—why has it passed the rest position at point 1? The answer is that inertial forces do not allow the molecule to "stop on a dime" at the rest position, but drive the molecule through rest and to the rightward extreme. The molecule, which has mass and opposes acceleration and deceleration, will not decelerate instantly to stop at the rest position, but rather will continue its motion through that point in space. As the molecule passes through the rest position and continues to move away from it, it is once again stretched and develops recoil force. The molecule continues this motion until the recoil forces again overcome the forces driving the molecule away from its rest position (primarily inertial). Once again, the motion is reversed, and the molecule heads back in the direction of the rest position. And once again, the motion does not stop at the rest position because of inertial forces; the molecule continues to move back and forth around the rest position.

It is important to understand that the forces maintaining the back and forth motion of the molecule around the rest position are a product of the motion itself: recoil and inertial forces result from the motion of the molecule. These forces are intrinsic to the motion of the molecule, rather than imposed from an outside source (as was the case with the bumping force that initiated the motion).

After the original application of the force at position 1, therefore, the back and forth motion is maintained by energy stored by the molecule itself. If the molecules were vibrating in a *frictionless* medium, where no energy was lost because of heat generation, the back and forth motion would continue indefinitely. Realistically, heat loss due to air molecules rubbing against each other and other surfaces eventually cause the back and forth motion to die out if external forces are not continuously reapplied to the air molecules. However, the principles of recoil and inertia forces still apply to a dying-out motion. The frictional forces compete with the recoil and inertial forces, and in the absence of external forces (such as another bump), eventually dominate the latter two and end the motion.

The Motions of Vibrating Air Molecules Change the Local Densities of Air

The motion of air molecules and the forces that control that motion have been described. How can this description lead to an understanding of pressure waves? Assume that a device for measuring air pressure is placed at position 2 in Figure 7–1. *Pressure* can be defined as the force exerted over a unit area ($P = F/A$) and is proportional to the density of air. When air molecules are more densely packed in some unit volume, they collide with each other more frequently and generate more force and more pressure within that volume. Conversely, when air molecules are less densely packed together, the collisions are less frequent and the pressures are relatively lower. At time A in Figure 7–1, there are no external forces applied to the air molecules and the density of air is that associated with air at rest (recall the 4×10^{23} figure given above). The pressure measured at time A, position 2 (or at any other position at time A, because the density of air at rest is the same

at any spatial location) is referred to as *atmospheric pressure*. The actual value of atmospheric pressure is not important to the current discussion,[2] but the *reference function* of this pressure is important. In the following discussion, atmospheric pressure (symbolized hereafter as P_{atm}) is considered as zero (0) pressure. At time B, the schematic drawing shows two molecules close together at position 2, indicating a relatively denser packing of air molecules at that position as compared to time A. The pressure measuring device at time B, position 2 should measure a higher pressure than at time A because the denser packing of molecules will involve more frequent collisions and higher forces. Any time a pressure is above the reference pressure P_{atm}, it is referred to as *positive pressure*. The more tightly packed the molecules, the more positive the pressure.

At time D, position 2, the first and second molecules are widely separated in space. This represents a case where the density of air is less than it is at P_{atm}. The pressure-measuring device records a value below P_{atm}, which is a *negative pressure*. The less tightly packed the molecules, the more negative the pressure.

These positive and negative pressures are not positive or negative in any absolute sense. They are only positive (above) or negative (below) with respect to the reference pressure P_{atm}. Figure 7–2 shows the result of the continuous bunching up and spreading apart of the air molecules schematized in Figure 7–1.

The three rows labeled A, B, D in Figure 7–2 correspond to the same rows in Figure 7–1 (rows C and E from Figure 7–1 have been omitted from Figure 7–2), indicating three different times in the evolving history of air molecule movement. At time A, each of the multiple dots represent an air molecule, and the collection of these molecules are shown evenly distributed across space, as expected if the medium is not being affected by an external force. The pressure at any point throughout the distribution, measured at any location in space from the left to right edge of the dot display, is P_{atm}.

At time B, this distribution has been changed to one in which regions of low and high density alternate across space. The heavily shaded areas represent high densities (as when two molecules are immediately adjacent, as in Figure 7–1, time B, position 2), and the lightly shaded areas represent low densities (as in Figure 7–1, time D, position 2). At time D, regions of high and low densities again alternate across space, but their locations have been reversed from those at time B. In other words, for a given point in space (such as position 2), what was a high density and high pressure area

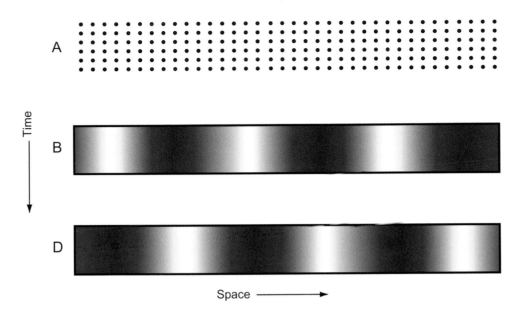

Figure 7–2. Schematic drawing of pressure waves, distributed in space and time. A, B, and D correspond to discrete times depicted in Figure 7–1. At a given point in space, pressure changes over time.

at time B, is a low density and low pressure area at time D. Areas of high density and high pressure are called areas of *compression* or *condensation*[3]; areas of low density and low pressures are called areas of *rarefaction*.

Pressure Waves, Not Individual Molecules, Propagate Through Space and Vary as a Function of Both Space and Time

Recall what was said earlier about the motion of individual air molecules. They moved around a rest position, the movement resulting from inherent elastic and inertial forces. The molecules themselves, however, do not *propagate* across space. What moves across space is the *pressure wave*, shown in Figure 7–2 from left to right as the sequence of high and low densities (pressures), or the sequence of compression (condensation) and rarefaction areas. Because these alternating regions of high and low pressures are the result of the back and forth movement of air molecules, which alternately bunches them up and spreads them apart, a given point in space will sometimes have high pressure (such as time B, position 2 in Figure 7–1), and sometimes have low pressure (time D, position 2 in Figure 7–1). Thus, a pressure

wave extends across space at a specific instant in time (examine Figure 7–2, across time B or D), and varies in time at a particular point in space (Figure 7–2, compare times B and D at any point in space).

When a pressure wave moves away from the *source* of the sound waves (the origin of the forces that initiated the displacement of air molecules), the alternating regions of high and low pressures often project in a straight line, as shown from left to right in Figure 7–2. These kinds of sound waves are called *plane waves*, because the sequence of high and low pressures can be thought of as a series of pressure "slices," or planes, extending away from the source. For the present discussion, only plane waves will be considered, but other kinds of pressures waves are possible (for example, those moving sideways from a source, rather than in a straight line away from the source: see comment on this in Chapter 10).

The Variation of a Pressure Wave in Time and Space Can Be Measured

There are specific measures of the temporal (time) and spatial (space) variation of pressure waves. A firm grasp of these measures is essential to understanding

---

[3]Condensation is the result of compression. For purposes of this text, compression and condensation are used interchangeably.

important aspects of the acoustic theory of speech production, covered in Chapter 8.

Temporal Measures

Figure 7–3A redraws a portion of the molecule motion shown in Figure 7–1. Of particular interest is the motion of the first molecule, shown in Figure 7–3A as a shaded circle. As in Figure 7–1, space (distance) is shown from left to right, and time from top to bottom (times A, B, C, D, E, occurring in succession). The numbers 1, 2, 3, 4, and 5 above the filled circles show the position of the first molecule at 5 discrete points in time, starting from the molecule at the rest position "1" and ending with the molecule back at the rest position "5." At time B, the molecule is immediately adjacent to the next molecule, which will create a region of compression, or high pressure, at the point in space indicated by the upward-pointing arrow. The pressure at this

point in space will become somewhat negative at time C (molecule labeled "3"), more negative yet at time D (molecule labeled "4"), and will return to P_{atm} at time E (molecule labeled "5").

The motion of the filled-circle molecule is shown as a function of time in Figure 7–3B. When any magnitude (such as displacement, pressure, speed, and so forth) is shown as a function of time, the plot is called a *waveform*. This waveform shows the position of the molecule from rest position (1), to the rightward extreme (2), the return through the rest position (3), at the leftward extreme (4), and finally back at the rest position (5). The discrete positions are connected to illustrate the continuous motion of the molecule throughout the vibratory cycle. This waveform shows one complete *cycle of motion* of the molecule. If the molecule continued to move after point 5, it would repeat the 1 through 5 sequence and produce another cycle with the same motion history.

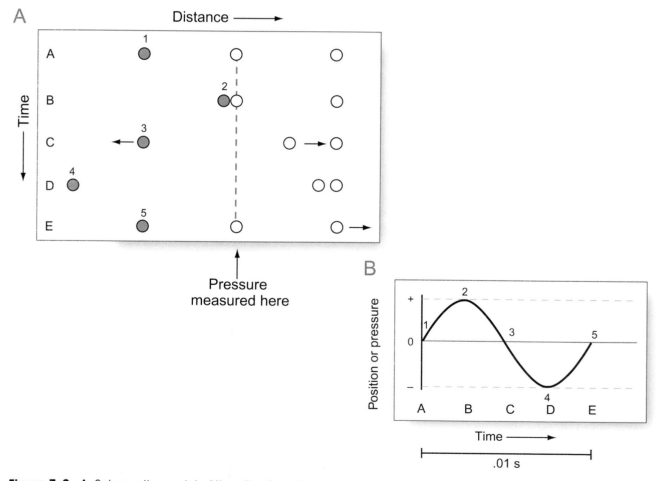

Figure 7–3. **A.** Schematic model of the vibration of an air molecule (*filled circles*) around its rest position. Numbers above the molecule indicate five successive points in time throughout its vibratory cycle. **B.** Plot of the position of the filled-circle molecule and the pressure measured at the location of the second molecule during one vibratory cycle.

The *y*-axis of the waveform in Figure 7–3B is also labeled pressure because it is easy to show that air pressure (measured at position 2) and position of the first molecule change in the same way over time. The right most extreme of molecule movement ("2" in Figure 7–3A) is also the time when air compression is maximum at the pressure measurement point, the leftmost extreme ("4") will occur at the same time as a rarefaction at the pressure measurement point, and the rest positions ("1" and "5") will be associated with P_{atm}. Positions between these discrete times will have pressures somewhere between compressions and P_{atm} or rarefactions and P_{atm}. Thus, the waveform in Figure 7–3B also shows the temporal variation of the pressure wave. The period (*T*) is the time taken to complete one full cycle of motion and is given by the formula: $T = 1/f$, where *f* = frequency. The filled-circle molecule is plotted as *a continuous function of time* as shown in Figure 7–3B. Figure 7–3A only indicates 5 discrete points in time, but Figure 7–3B shows every possible position of the molecule from time A through E, and how those positions change over time. Time is shown on the *x*-axis and molecule position (or air pressure) is shown on the *y*-axis. The horizontal line separating the upper and lower halves of the waveform indicates the rest position of the molecule, that is, when pressure = P_{atm}. The numbers 1, 2, 3, 4, and 5 given in Figure 7–3A are indicated on the time plot in their appropriate locations. The measurement of the temporal variation of a pressure wave that repeats over time, like the one shown in Figure 7–3B, is performed by computing the time taken to complete one full cycle. This is called the *period* of vibration and is denoted by the symbol *T*. For example, according to the time scale shown on the waveform in Figure 7–3B, it takes .01 second to complete one cycle of molecule motion. Thus for this waveform *T* = .01 second(s) or *T* = 10 milliseconds (ms).

In this example, .01 s and 10 ms are the same value, but expressed in different units. In speech and hearing applications, it is typical to express time units in ms. For reference purposes, 1 s = 1000 ms, 0.1 s = 100 ms, 0.01 s = 10 ms, and 0.001 s = 1 ms.

An alternate way to express the time variation of a repeating, cyclic motion, like the one shown in Figure 7–3B, is in terms of *frequency*, symbolized with an *f*. Frequency (*f*) is simply the inverse of period (*T*), and can be stated in the formula

$$f = 1/T \qquad \text{Formula (1)}$$

The units for frequency are *hertz*, abbreviated as Hz, which stands for "cycles per second." The number resulting from the formula indicates how many complete cycles of vibration occur in one second. For example, if Formula (1) is applied to the 10-ms period in Figure 7–3B, the result is $f = 1/10$ ms or $f = 1/.01 = 100$ Hz.

Because frequency (*f*) is the inverse of period (*T*), as one variable (e.g., *f*) increases, the other (e.g., *T*) decreases. Thus, longer periods are associated with lower frequencies, and shorter periods are associated with higher frequencies. Figure 7–4 shows the relationship between frequency and period ranging from 1.0 ms to 10.0 ms. For this graph, period is plotted on the *x*-axis, and is changed in steps of 0.5 ms (i.e., 1.0 ms, 1.5 ms, 2.0 ms, 2.5 ms . . . 10.0 ms). The corresponding frequency values, computed by $f = 1/T$, are plotted on the *y*-axis. The inverse relationship, where longer periods are associated with lower frequencies, is clearly seen in the way the plotted points descend on the *y*-axis as the value on the *x*-axis increases (moving to the right on the *x*-axis). Note also that the relationship between *T* and *f* is not *linear*. In a perfectly linear relationship between two variables, equal-sized change in one variable is accompanied by equal-sized change in the other variable. If the relationship between *T* and *f* were perfectly linear, each 0.5-ms step in *T* would be accompanied by a constant change in *f*. In Figure 7–4, however, the frequency changes (*y*-axis) accompanying the 0.5-ms steps in the region of 10 ms (*x*-axis) are clearly much smaller than the frequency changes accompanying 0.5-ms steps in the region of 1.0 ms. For example, the 0.5-ms change between 9.0 and 9.5 ms on the *x*-axis produces a change in *f* of approximately 6 Hz, but the same 0.5-ms change between 2.5 and 3.0 ms produces a change in *f* of more than 65 Hz. When the individual points in Figure 7–4 are connected by a continuous line, the relationship between the two variables is clearly curved. This kind of relationship, where equal steps along one variable do not produce equal steps on the second variable, is called a *nonlinear* relationship; in this case the relationship between the two variables is curvilinear.

Spatial Measures

In Figure 7–2, pressure waves were explained as "alternating regions of high and low pressures extending across space." Portions of two pressure waves are shown in Figure 7–5, one corresponding to a frequency of 100 Hz, and the other corresponding to a frequency of 1000 Hz. The *x*-axis is labeled as distance, and is scaled from 0 to 500 centimeters (cm) (equivalent to roughly 0 to 195 inches). The portions of the pressure waves for both frequencies shown in Figure 7–5 consist of sequences of high- and low-pressure regions. The high-pressure regions are shown as the more heavily

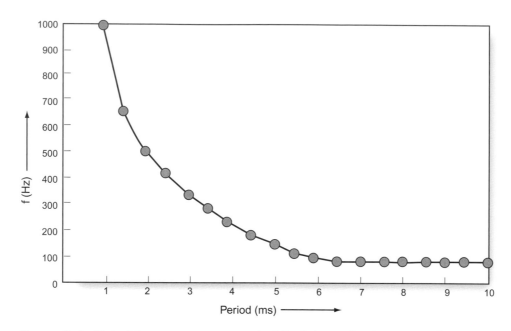

Figure 7-4. Plot of frequency versus period that shows the inverse and nonlinear relationship between the two variables.

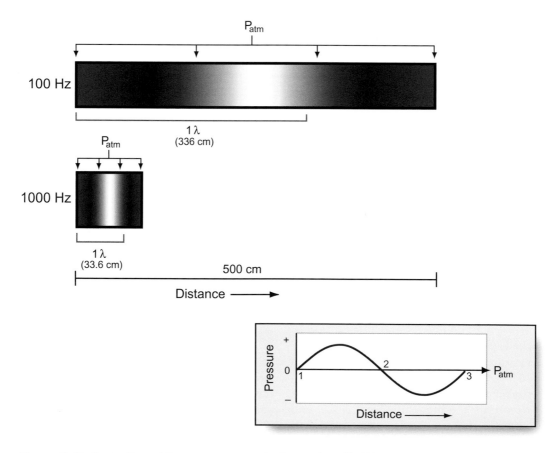

Figure 7-5. Illustration of the measurement of wavelength. Wavelength is the distance covered by a cycle of pressure variations. This distance is marked as 1λ on the 100-Hz and 1000-Hz signals. Wavelength is longer for the 100-Hz signal. The bottom right inset shows pressure variations plotted as a function of distance.

shaded areas indicating relatively dense packing of air molecules) and the low-pressure areas as the lightly shaded areas (indicating the relatively sparse packing of molecules). It is immediately apparent that one complete variation across space between high and low pressures associated with the 100-Hz sound covers a greater distance than the corresponding variation across space for the 1000-Hz sound. The formal measurement of the spatial variation of a pressure wave is called the *wavelength*, which is simply the distance covered by a high-pressure region and its succeeding low-pressure region (or, by a low-pressure region and its succeeding high-pressure region). Wavelength is symbolized by the Greek letter *lambda* (λ), and is shown for both pressure waves in Figure 7–5 as extending from the leading edge of the first high-pressure region to the leading edge of the next high-pressure region. In accord with the definition given immediately above, this includes the distance covered by the first high-pressure region and its succeeding low-pressure region.

Wavelength has an inverse relationship to frequency. The higher the frequency, the shorter the wavelength. This acoustic law is illustrated in Figure 7–5 where the 1000-Hz sound has a much shorter wavelength than the 100-Hz sound. The formula for wavelength is:

$$\lambda = c/f \text{ or } f = c/\lambda \qquad \text{Formula (2)}$$

where f = frequency and c = the speed of sound in air, which is a constant and has a value of approximately 33,600 cm/s (roughly 1100 ft/s). If the values of the frequencies shown in Figure 7–5 are plugged into the formula along with the value for the constant c, the wavelengths for 100 Hz and 1000 Hz are found to be approximately 336 cm (100 Hz) and 33.6 cm (1000 Hz).

Note also that the "boundaries" of the low and high pressure regions in Figure 7–5 are marked as P_{atm}. As described above, this indicates that as the pressure varies across space there are points where the pressure is equal to P_{atm}. The pressure varies across space by going above P_{atm}, below it, above it, and so on. The changes in pressure across space are gradual. When talking about high or low pressure regions, those regions are referred to as containing either the maximum positive or negative pressures. The graded nature of these pressure changes is illustrated in Figure 7–5 by the continuous changes in the shadings of the compression and rarefaction regions, with the heaviest shading occurring at the most positive pressure and the lightest shading at the most negative pressure.

The continuous changes in pressure across a single wavelength are also shown in the inset to Figure 7–5,

where pressure (y-axis) is shown as a function of distance (x-axis). The horizontal line in this inset is P_{atm}, the reference pressure. Pressure is seen to increase relative to P_{atm} ("1" in the inset) until it reaches a positive peak, then decreases and passes through P_{atm} ("2" in the inset) as it goes to the negative peak, then reverses again to return to P_{atm} ("3" in the inset). This is a different way to plot the pressure waves shown in the main part of the figure. As explained in the section of Chapter 8 dealing with articulatory configuration and the acoustic output of the vocal tract (the "tube" of air shaped by the articulators between the vocal folds and the lips), the concept of wavelength is critical to an understanding of why different articulations result in different vowel sounds.

Pressure Waves: A Summary and Introduction of Sinusoids

The motions of air molecules can produce pressure waves, which are the basis of sound. Pressure waves vary across space and time, and both variations can be described and measured using simple mathematics.

To this point, the examples and explanations of these events have been *schematic*, or simplified to some degree. For example, very little has been said about the causes, or *sources*, of these air molecule motions and resulting pressure waves. And the particular motions discussed are very simple, whereas many acoustic events—such as speech—involve very complex vibrations of air molecules, and very complex sources of those vibrations. It is the case, however, that even the most complex vibrations can be broken down into a set or group of the simple vibrations described above. It is also the case that a complex vibration can be generated by taking a set of these simple motions and adding them together. In other words, a complex acoustic event can be created by combining many individual simple acoustic events. The understanding of simple vibrations is the basis for understanding the more complex vibrations observed in most acoustic events.

The simple motions and resulting pressure waves discussed above are called *sinusoidal* motions and waves. Sinusoidal motions are the simplest form of vibration. More complex vibrations can be broken down into a set of individual sinusoids. Complex acoustic events occur when a group of sinusoids is combined together. A formal description of sinusoidal motion is presented next, along with the idea that complex sounds are the sum of their component sinusoids.

Sound Speed

Speed of sound in air varies as a function of air temperature, and to a lesser degree as a function of humidity and altitude. The higher the temperature, the faster the propagation of sound waves. Students will find slightly different values used in different texts. 33,600 cm/s is roughly the value that would be measured at 0 degrees Celsius (32 degrees F). Speed of sound also varies with the nature of the conducting medium. Sound propagation is about four times faster in water as compared to air, and about 11 times faster in steel, as compared to air (everyone knows the trick of putting an ear to a railroad track to "hear" an oncoming train that is at a great distance). The general rule is: the denser the medium, the faster the sound conduction.

SINUSOIDAL MOTION

In the foregoing discussion of pressure waves, the motion of air molecules was described as being governed by simple laws of elasticity and inertia. The effects of recoil and inertial forces produced the oscillation of the molecule around a rest position. This motion is a sinusoidal motion (also called *simple harmonic motion*), and it has a simple conceptual and mathematical basis.

Sinusoidal Motion (Simple Harmonic Motion) Is Derived from the Linear Projection of Uniform Circular Speed

Imagine, as shown in Figure 7–6A, a circle of some arbitrary radius with its four right angles AB, BC, CD, and DA. The filled dot at point A is meant to indicate an object that rotates continuously around the circumference of the circle, in a counterclockwise direction. In particular, this object rotates around the circle with

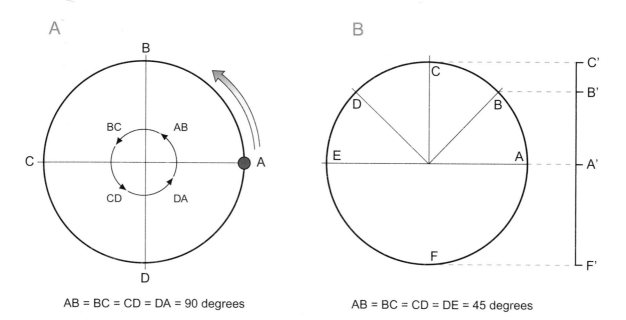

AB = BC = CD = DA = 90 degrees   AB = BC = CD = DE = 45 degrees

Figure 7–6. Derivation of sinusoidal motion from the linear projection of uniform circular speed. **A.** Filled circle moving around larger circle at uniform circular speed when it crosses equal angles in equal time intervals. **B.** Projection of points along the circumference of the larger circle to a line segment, showing how projection from equal angles does not result in equal linear segments. See text for details.

uniform circular speed (UCS). In UCS, the rotating object crosses equal angles in equal amounts of time. In the example shown in Figure 7–6A, this means that the time it takes the rotating point (*filled dot*) to travel from point A to B will equal the time it takes to travel from point B to C, or from point C to D, or from point D back to A. This is consistent with the definition of uniform circular motion given immediately above, because angles AB, BC, CD, and DA all equal 90 degrees and each 90-degree angle (or each 45-degree angle, or 30-degree angle, and so forth) is traversed in an equal amount of time.

Sinusoidal motion can now be defined as the *linear projection of uniform circular speed*. This is illustrated in Figure 7–6B, where one-half of the circle has been partitioned into four angles of 45 degrees each. Alongside the circle is a vertical line, the top and bottom of which have exactly the same location as the top and bottom of the circle (point C is located at the top of the circle). At each point along this half-circle motion, a horizontal dashed line has been drawn to intersect the vertical line. These horizontal lines *project* the labeled points (points A through E) along the circle over to the vertical line—hence the expression, linear projection of UCS. Remember that each of the 45-degree angles shown in Figure 7–6B is traversed by the rotating object in equal amounts of time.

The result of the linear projection of UCS can be best appreciated by comparing the points on the vertical line to the corresponding points on the circle. The projection of point A on the circle results in point A' on the line, which clearly divides the line into upper and lower segments of equal length. Point B on the circle projects to point B' on the line, and point C on the circle projects to point C' on the line. The interesting comparison here is the length of the linear segment A'-B' to B'-C'. Clearly the segment A'-B' is longer than the segment B'-C', yet these two segments result from the projection of points spanning *equivalent arcs*. In other words, when the circular motion involves equal distances (that is, motion covering equal angles), the linear projection of the points defining those angles does not yield equal linear distances.

As the point moves from point C to point E, its linear projection is superimposed on the same line segment (A'-C') originally covered when the point rotated from A to C. The movement of this projection is now from C' to A', which is the reverse of the original projection. As the rotating point moves from E to F, the linear projection would extend from A' to F', and the projection of the rotation from F to A would be superimposed on the A'-F' line segment, except in the opposite direction.

Discrete angles on the circle illustrate the linear projection of UCS, but obviously as the point rotates about the circle, the angles change continuously as they are projected along the line segment. The linear projection of a complete rotation around the circle looks very much like the motion of the air molecule in Figures 7–1 and 7–3. A' on the linear segment is the rest position, whereas C' and F' are the extremes of the linear displacement. One complete cycle involves motion from the rest position A' to the one extreme (C'), then back through the rest position to the other extreme (F') and then back to the rest position. In fact, if the line segment in Figure 7–6B is turned on its side with C' to the right and F' to the left, the motion described by the linear projection of the rotating point is the same as the motion of air molecules described above.

When the Linear Projection of Uniform Circular Speed Is Stretched Out in Time, the Result Is a Sine Wave

Imagine now that the rotating object in Figure 7–6A is a small ring through which a pencil is inserted, and that the motions described by UCS are marked on paper beneath the circle. If the circle could be moved from left to right across the paper at a constant speed and without disturbing the UCS of the rotating ring, the pencil line would draw the motion as a function of time. The resulting waveform would look like the one in Figure 7–7 (and the ones in Figures 7–3 and 7–5), and is called a *sine wave*. This is displacement shown as a function of time. If the timescale is known, the period (and its inverse, frequency) can be determined using the simple

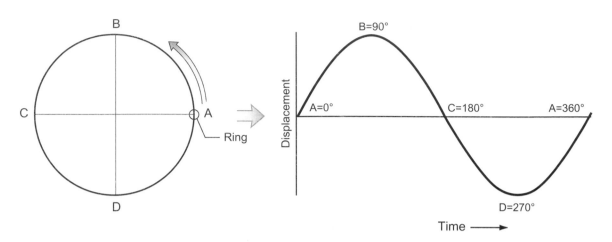

Figure 7–7. Linear projection of uniform circular speed, shown as a function of time. If a pencil is inserted through the ring at A on the large circle (*left side of figure*) during uniform circular speed, and the motion is traced as the pencil is moved from left to right, the sinusoidal waveform on the right side of the figure will result. Angular notation on the waveform at the right corresponds to angles crossed during motion around the circle on the left.

computation of Formula (1)—$f = 1/T$. Note also the corresponding positions on the circle and resulting waveform (given by A, B, C, D in Figure 7–7).

Sinusoidal Motion Can Be Described by a Simple Formula, and Has Three Important Characteristics: Frequency, Amplitude, and Phase

Sinusoidal motion can be described fully by three characteristics, or *parameters*. The first of these parameters is frequency, which has been defined above as the number of full cycles occurring in a 1-s interval. If one complete rotation about a circle is equivalent to one cycle of vibration, it is easy to see how a faster speed of rotation would result in a higher frequency. A faster speed of rotation would reduce the amount of time required to complete one full revolution around the circle, which is the same as saying that the period, T, would be reduced. As Formula (1), $f = 1/T$ and Figure 7–4 indicate, a reduction in T will be associated with an increase in f. The second parameter is amplitude, which will be symbolized as A. Amplitude can be thought of in terms of displacement of an air molecule from the rest position. The circle in Figure 7–6 can be used to provide a simple illustration of variations in A. The vertical line on to which points are projected from the circular motion is made to correspond in length to the size (diameter) of the circle. The extremes of the linearly projected motion are, therefore, defined by

the diameter of the circle. If the circle is made larger or smaller, the extremes of the linearly projected motion will be greater or smaller, respectively. Thus, the amplitude of the vibration, which in this case is considered to be the same as displacement, is related to the size of the circle.

The third parameter, phase, is symbolized by the Greek letter ϕ (*phi*) and describes the position of the sinusoidal motion relative to some arbitrary reference position. For example, in Figure 7–7, assume that position A is the reference point. Using the circular basis of sinusoidal motion, the location or *phase* of point B can be described as 90 degrees relative to point A, because the radii extending to points A and B form a 90-degree angle. Similarly, the phase of points C and D are 180 degrees and 270 degrees, respectively, relative to the reference point A. This phase angle description applies to the waveform in Figure 7–7 as well, because points along the waveform are simply points around the circle extended in time. With A as the waveform reference point, a time corresponding to a *lag* of 90 degrees is equivalent to a quarter of a complete cycle, 180 degrees would be a half cycle, and so forth. This example uses phase to compare points within a single waveform, but it can also be used to compare points across two waveforms of identical or different frequencies. Phase relations between two or more sinusoids of different frequencies are discussed below in the section dealing with complex waveforms.

A simple formula describes sinusoidal motion as a function of time. This *sinusoidal function* is used to determine the displacement of an object (i.e., an air molecule) at any instant in time, and is computed as follows:

$$D = A \sin(2\pi ft + \phi) \qquad \text{Formula (3)}$$

where D = the displacement of the object at a given instant, A = the maximum displacement of the object from the rest position, f = the frequency of the motion, t = the specific time at which the displacement D is being computed, and ϕ = the starting phase of the motion (like the reference point described above). 2π is a constant (equaling 360 degrees, or one full revolution around the circle) that reflects the circular origin of sinusoidal motion and when multiplied by "ft" converts the whole expression in parentheses to an angular notation. The *sin* is a trigonometric function, the sinusoid function that converts angles to real numbers.

Tables of sine values for angles between 0 and 360 degrees are available in any basic trigonometry text. Sine values vary between 0 and +1.00 for angles ranging from 0 to 90 degrees, and then fall from +1.00 back to 0 for angles ranging from 91 to 180 degrees. Between 180 and 360 degrees, these values have mirror-image negative values, ranging from 0 to –1.00 (270 degrees) and then back to 0 (360 degrees).

If the starting phase (ϕ) in Formula (3) is assumed to be zero (that is, if we are not concerned about the absolute starting phase of the waveform), the formula for sinusoidal motion can be simplified to:

$$D = A (\sin \phi) \qquad \text{Formula (4)}$$

where D = displacement, A = maximum displacement, as above, and ϕ = the angle formed between the reference radius (i.e., the radii projected to point A in Figures 7–6 and 7–7) and the radius projected to any other point along the circle. For the sequence of angles formed as an object rotates around the circle (that is, 0 to 360 degrees), application of this formula yields a sine wave.

Sinusoidal Motion: A Summary

A sine wave is a waveform that results from the linear projection of UCS. A sine wave can be said to be *periodic*, because multiple rotations around the circle will produce multiple waveforms having the same period. Because the period is the same for all cycles of the vibration, sinusoids by definition and derivation have only a single frequency. A sinusoidal waveform can be described by a simple formula in which period, amplitude, and phase are the parameters.

Because a sinusoid involves only a single frequency, it can be considered to be the simplest type of acoustic event. In fact, sinusoids can be considered as the basic "building blocks" of acoustic events containing many frequencies. Acoustic events that contain many frequencies have *complex waveforms*, which may or may not repeat over time. The next section describes complex acoustic events.

COMPLEX ACOUSTIC EVENTS

Two types of complex events are considered: (a) those in which the waveform pattern repeats over time, and (b) those in which no repeating pattern can be identified. When an acoustic event contains more than one frequency and has a waveform with a repeating pattern, it is called a *complex periodic* event. An acoustic event with more than one frequency and no repeating pattern is called a *complex aperiodic* event.

Complex Periodic Events Have Waveforms That Repeat Their Patterns Over Time, and Frequency Components That Are Harmonically Related

Figure 7–8 shows two different complex periodic waveforms and associated spectra. Both waveforms, shown above their respective spectra, share the property of repeating their pattern over time and, in fact, have the same period of roughly 8 ms and hence a *fundamental frequency* of around 125 Hz ($f = 1/8$ ms, $= 1/.008$ s $= 125$ Hz). The fundamental frequency is determined by the rate of repetition of the major waveform pattern, as indicated by the marked periods on the two waveforms. Note that, even though the fundamental frequency is nearly identical for the two wave forms, the appearance of the waveforms is clearly different. The frequencies in addition to the fundamental frequency, and their amplitudes and phase relations, give the waveforms their unique appearance.

Waveform displays are said to show an acoustic event in the *time domain*, because the event is shown as a function of time. This is a useful way to display an acoustic event, but if one is interested in the frequencies and their amplitudes that give waveforms their unique appearance, a different type of display is required. When an acoustic event is examined in the *frequency domain*, the individual frequencies and amplitudes that contribute to a complex acoustic event are displayed. The frequency domain of an acoustic event is shown by a

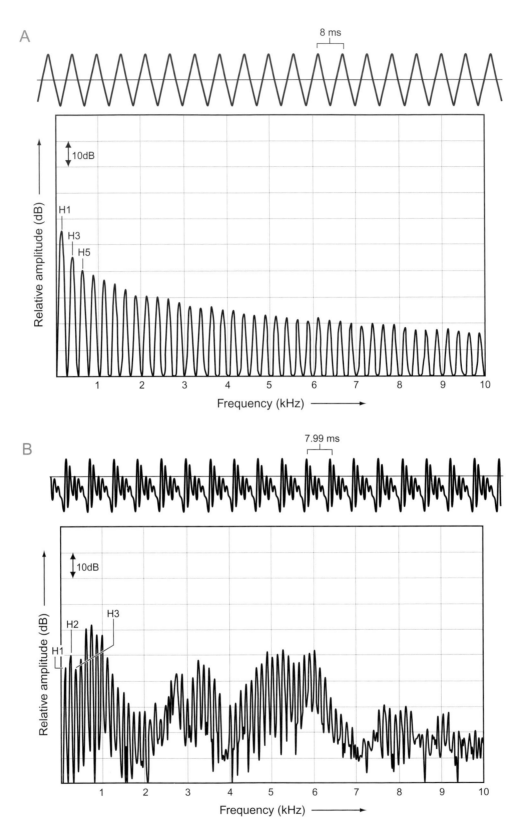

Figure 7-8. Two complex periodic waveforms and their spectra. **A.** Waveform and spectrum of a 125-Hz triangular wave. The period of one cycle (8 ms) is marked on the waveform, and the first (H1), third (H3), and fifth (H5) harmonics are marked on the spectrum. **B.** Waveform and spectrum of the vowel /a/ produced by an adult male. The period of one cycle (7.99 ms) is marked on the waveform, and the first (H1), second (H2), and third (H3) harmonics are marked on the spectrum.

spectrum, which can be defined as a plot of *relative amplitude* (y-axis) as a function of frequency (x-axis). Spectra are shown immediately below the two waveforms in Figure 7–8. These two spectra are quite different.

The spectrum of the waveform in Figure 7–8A shows frequency components at odd number multiples (1, 3, 5, 7, 9 . . . *n*) of the fundamental frequency (125 Hz). This spectrum, therefore, contains frequency components at 125 Hz (the fundamental frequency, or first harmonic (H1), 375 Hz (H3), 625 Hz (H5) . . . 125 × (2*n* − 1)Hz, where *n* is the number of frequency components in the spectrum. The relative amplitudes of the frequencies, as represented by the heights of the harmonic components (i.e., the magnitude on the y-axis), decrease consistently as frequency increases. In this spectrum, therefore, a higher frequency (e.g., 625 Hz, the fifth harmonic of 125 Hz) always has less energy than a lower frequency (e.g., 375 Hz, the third harmonic).[4] Waveform (A) is a common test signal used in electronics shops and laboratories, and is called a *triangular wave*. A triangular wave is said to have an odd-integer series of harmonics.

The waveform in Figure 7–8B is the time domain representation of the vowel /ɑ/ spoken by an adult male. The marked period of the waveform is 7.99 ms, almost identical to the 8-ms period of the triangular wave in Figure 7–8A. The periods of the two waveforms are not perfectly identical because it is very hard for a human, even one with some training in voice, to produce a vowel with a precise frequency (the triangular wave was produced with a computer program capable of synthesizing exactly a period of 8 ms). The frequency domain representation (i.e., the spectrum) shows why the /ɑ/ waveform is different from the triangular waveform in Figure 7–8A. First, the /ɑ/ spectrum contains harmonics at whole-number multiples of the fundamental frequency (that is, 1, 2, 3, 4, 5, 6, 7, 8, 9 . . . *n*), not just odd-number multiples. An easy way to verify this difference is to compare the two spectra for the number of harmonics between 0 and 1000 Hz. The triangular wave shows four harmonics from 0 to 1000 Hz, whereas the vowel /ɑ/ shows eight. The vowel spectrum is, therefore, harmonically denser than the triangular wave spectrum. A second difference between the two spectra is the pattern of amplitudes as a function of harmonic frequency. Unlike the spectrum of the triangular wave, the relative amplitudes of the frequency components do not decrease consistently with increases in frequency. Rather, the relative amplitudes fluctuate as frequency increases (moving rightward on the x-axis), sometimes increasing and sometimes decreasing. For example, note in the vowel spectrum the greater relative amplitude of the fifth and sixth harmonics (between roughly 600–750 Hz) as compared to the second harmonic (around 250 Hz). The different harmonic densities, the different variation of amplitude as a function of frequency, plus different phase relations among the frequencies (not discussed here) all contribute to the different appearance of triangular wave and vowel waveforms. Both, however, are clearly periodic and different in shape from a sinusoidal (single-frequency) waveform.

A Complex Periodic Waveform Can Be Considered as the Sum of the Individual Sinusoids at the Harmonic Frequencies

For each one of these complex periodic waveforms, there are multiple, harmonically related frequencies, which are shown clearly in the spectral representations of the sounds. The energy at these frequencies is *discrete*, which means that between the harmonic frequencies (e.g., at 250 Hz in Figure 7–8A, which is between the first and third harmonics of the triangular wave spectrum) there is little or no energy. The multiple harmonic frequencies are all occurring at the same time, and it is their combination that produces the complex waveforms seen in Figure 7–8. Earlier in this chapter, the idea was advanced that understanding sinusoidal vibration was important because even the most complex acoustic events can be broken down into their component sinusoids.

The spectral representations shown in Figure 7–8 provide a snapshot, for some interval of time, of the component sinusoids of a complex acoustic event. In a sense, the spectrum shows the acoustic event with the individual frequency components "pulled apart" and displayed with their individual, relative amplitudes. The formal analysis required to produce a spectrum of a waveform is called *Fourier analysis*, a mathematical tool that decomposes a complex time domain function (e.g., a complex periodic waveform) into the set of its simple functions (i.e., sinusoids). In this text, the mathematical details of Fourier analysis are not discussed, but the conceptual basis of the process, the ability to break down a complex acoustic event into its simple components, is very important. Fourier analysis is

---

[4]A formal discussion of sound intensity and sound pressure level (two ways to measure the energy in an acoustic event) is not provided here. For the present discussion, the term "relative amplitude" is used to describe the energy relations between two or more frequency components in a spectrum. These energy relations are expressed in decibels (dB).

implemented in almost every speech analysis computer program. For example, the spectra in Figure 7–8 were constructed using TF32 (Milenkovic, 2001), a computer program written by Professor Paul Milenkovic of the University of Wisconsin–Madison. Using mouse-controlled cursors, the user selects the portion of the waveform to be analyzed (in Figure 7–8, the waveform portions shown were the ones subjected to Fourier analysis) and selects a function that instructs the program to perform a Fourier analysis. The Fourier analysis function automatically displays spectra like those shown in Figure 7–8.

The conceptual basis of Fourier analysis can also be "stood on its head" to show that a group of simple functions can be added together to produce a complex acoustic event. For example, if a computer program were used to synthesize a sinusoid at 125 Hz, the result would be a sinusoidal waveform with a period of $T = 8$ ms. If the program were used to synthesize another sinusoid at 375 Hz, whose waveform was added to the 125 Hz waveform, the new waveform would clearly not be sinusoidal but would retain the original period of 8 ms. The new waveform would be a complex periodic event, with two frequency components. If this process were repeated for a large series of odd-integer harmonics, whose synthesized amplitudes decreased as a function of frequency, the waveform would eventually be triangular. The progression from sinusoidal to triangular waveform reflects the addition of all odd-integer harmonics whose amplitudes decrease across frequency in a specific way. The period of the triangular waveform, however, always equals the period of the lowest frequency component, which in this case is 8 ms (that is, the period of 125 Hz). This is the Fourier concept stood on its head. Instead of decomposing a complex acoustic event into its component sinusoids, a complex acoustic event is synthesized, or composed, from many different sinusoids.

When two or more sinusoids are related to each other by a whole number multiple, they are said to be in a harmonic relationship. Moreover, when the individual sinusoidal components of an acoustic event are harmonically related, the complex event will be periodic (see section below on complex aperiodic events). In the case of the spectrum shown in Figure 7–8A, the 375 Hz harmonic component is three times the fundamental frequency of 125 Hz and is, therefore, called the third harmonic of the fundamental frequency. In the triangular wave spectrum, there is no second harmonic (which would be 250 Hz for a 125-Hz fundamental frequency). The component at 625 Hz is the fifth harmonic (5 × 125 Hz), the component at 875 Hz the seventh harmonic (7 × 125 Hz), and so on. In the vowel spectrum, which has a consecutive integer series of harmonics, there is a second (250 Hz), third (375 Hz), and fourth (500 Hz) harmonic (and so on). In both cases, and more generally in any complex periodic event, the fundamental frequency, the lowest frequency component in the spectrum, is synonymous with the first harmonic. Later in this text, the spectrum associated with the acoustic result of vocal fold vibration will be discussed and the concept of harmonics will play an important role in understanding the acoustic theory of speech production.

Complex Aperiodic Events Have Waveforms in Which No Repetitive Pattern Can Be Discerned, and Frequency Components That Are Not Harmonically Related

As in Figure 7–8, Figure 7–9 shows two pairs of waveform-spectrum displays for two different complex aperiodic acoustic events. By definition, these waveforms are composed of multiple frequencies, but, in contrast to the waveforms in Figure 7–8, neither shows a repetitive pattern over time. The lack of a repetitive pattern reflects the lack of periodicity, hence the term complex *a*periodic acoustic event. Because there is no repetitive pattern, it is not possible to compute a period for these waveforms, which, therefore, do not have a fundamental frequency.

The frequency composition of complex aperiodic acoustic events cannot be inferred with much accuracy from their waveforms, but rather must be obtained from a direct examination of the spectrum (remember that in a complex periodic waveform, the ability to

---

Pending Further Notice

Ever wonder about the connection between words such as "pendant," "pending," "pendulous," "pendulum"? They all derive from a 17th century Latin word meaning "hanging down," which in turn probably derives from a 13th century Scandinavian word meaning "wag" or "fluctuate." In fact a pendulum does wag back and forth—it fluctuates in position as a function of time. It does so with simple harmonic motion, and obeys the same principles discussed here for the simple motions of air molecules.

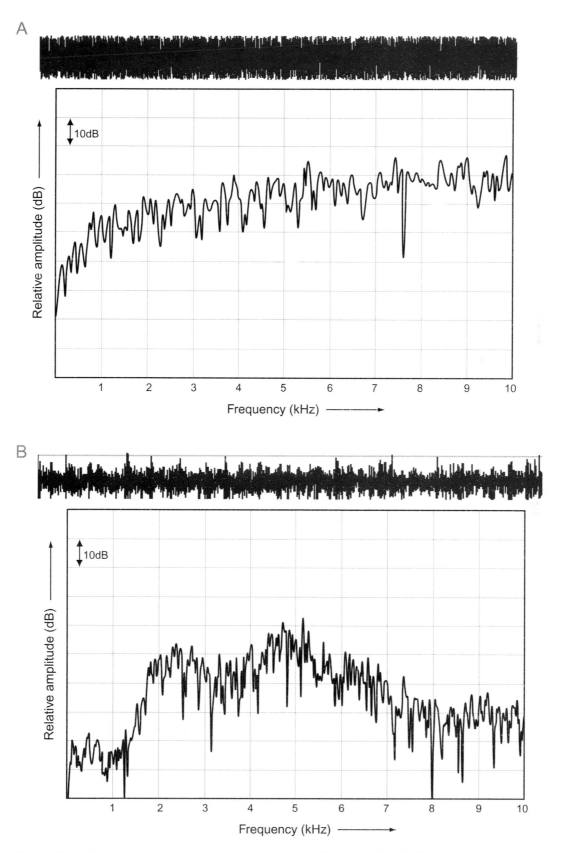

Figure 7-9. Two complex aperiodic waveforms and their spectra. **A.** Waveform and spectrum of a white noise produced by freeware on the Internet. **B.** Waveform and spectrum of a sustained /ʃ/ produced by an adult male. The two waveforms do not have periods, and discrete harmonics do not appear in their spectra.

compute the period and hence the fundamental frequency from a waveform allows at least a partial identification of other frequency components because of their harmonic relationship to the fundamental). The spectra shown in Figure 7–9 were obtained by Fourier analysis, just as they were for the complex periodic events shown in Figure 7–8. The decomposition of complex waveforms into their component sinusoids follows the same principles for both periodic and aperiodic events. Figure 7–9A shows the waveform and spectrum of a white noise sample. White noise is a type of complex aperiodic acoustic event that contains, in theory, all frequencies (from 1 Hz to infinity); the amplitudes of each of these frequencies vary randomly over time. In theory, white noise should have equal average energy at all frequencies. Stated otherwise, the spectrum of a "perfect" white noise should be flat.

The displayed white noise waveform in Figure 7–9A has a total duration of 150 ms, and the spectrum was computed for only this interval. The spectrum, which displays frequencies from 0 to 10.0 kHz, is not perfectly flat, but shows a more or less continuous and slow rise in energy from low to high frequencies. This white noise was obtained from free software on the Internet, so perhaps the algorithm for generating the noise was not accurate or something about the way the signal was processed resulted in the deviation from a perfectly flat spectrum. Nevertheless, as a result of the absence of harmonics in this spectrum it is much more difficult to identify discrete frequency components such as those seen in the spectra of Figure 7–8. Rather, the energy appears to be varying in a more or less continuous fashion.[5] The use of a truly flat-spectrum white noise as a test signal is important in the upcoming discussion of resonance and resonators (see later, Figure 7–18 and accompanying text). Figure 7–9B presents the waveform and spectrum of a sustained /ʃ/, a voiceless fricative produced by grooving the blade of the tongue against the hard palate. Like the white noise waveform there is no repeating pattern, and like the white noise spectrum it is difficult to identify discrete frequency components because of the absence of harmonics. This spectrum shows an increase of energy from very low frequencies to higher frequencies, but the peak energy in the /ʃ/ spectrum occurs around 5000 Hz. Above 5000 Hz, the energy declines gradually, giving the overall *spectral shape* an appearance of symmetry between 3000 and 7000 Hz. The characteristics of this spectrum

are consistent with /ʃ/ spectra reported in the literature and described in Chapters 10 and 12).

Complex Acoustic Events: Summary

Complex acoustic events are composed of more than one frequency, and may be periodic or aperiodic. Complex periodic events have a repetitive waveform pattern and, therefore, a fundamental frequency. The higher frequency components are harmonically related to this fundamental frequency. Complex aperiodic events do not have a fundamental frequency because the waveform pattern is nonrepetitive. The frequencies in the spectrum do not all stand in a harmonic relationship to one another.

Complex acoustic events can be displayed in either the time or frequency domain. When Fourier analysis is applied to a time domain representation (i.e., a waveform), a complex waveform is decomposed into its simple, sinusoidal functions. This process identifies the component frequencies and their amplitudes, which are displayed in the frequency domain as a spectrum. The time and frequency domains are merely two alternative representations of acoustic events. The two domains do not show different events, just different ways of look-

---

**Fourier Analysis Was
Hot in the 19th Century**

Sometimes the most important aspects of one scientific discipline have their origins in a different scientific area. Fourier analysis was "invented" by one Baron J. B. J. Fourier (1768–1830) who wrote a famous textbook whose French title can be translated as "Analytic Theory of Heat." This text had nothing to do with acoustics, but did take up the problem of periodic variations in heat. Fourier designed his analysis to decompose these complex variations into their simple harmonic components, and in the middle of the 19th century a German physicist named Georg Ohm (1789–1854) argued for the application of Fourier analysis to the decomposition of complex tones into simple ones.

---

[5]The actual shape of a computed spectrum depends in certain details on the way in which the acoustic signal has been processed (e.g., including such variables as the type of microphone and possibly tape recorder used, the specifications of the computer program used to perform the analysis, and so forth). In the spectra presented in this text, it is safe to assume that frequencies between 100 Hz and 9000 Hz are minimally affected by these variables. Some of these variables are considered further in Chapter 10.

ing at the same event. The simplest example of this was provided earlier, when the period and frequency of a sinusoid were defined as the inverse of each other ($f = 1/T$, or $T = 1/f$). The period is derived from the time domain representation, and the frequency, of course, is derived from the frequency domain. One of the major advances in acoustic phonetics occurred when an instrument was developed that combined the time and frequency domain representations into a single display. This instrument, the *sound spectrograph*, is discussed in Chapter 10.

To this point, the discussion of complex acoustic events has been restricted to cases where the sound can be related strictly to the vibration of one object. For example, when a tuning fork is struck, the vibrating tines of the fork displace the surrounding air molecules and are, therefore, the source of the pressure waves heard as sound. Similarly, the vibrating diaphragm (a woofer, or tweeter) in one of the loud speakers connected to a stereo system serves as the source of pressure waves heard as music. Many acoustic events, including the production of speech sounds and the sounds of most musical instruments, actually involve an interaction between a source of sound, like the ones discussed above, and a resonator (or resonators). A resonator is part of an acoustic system that emphasizes certain frequencies in a source vibration and rejects certain other frequencies. Attention is now turned to a detailed consideration of the phenomenon of resonance.

RESONANCE

Resonance is the phenomenon whereby an object vibrates with maximum energy at a particular frequency. Sometimes the term "natural frequency" is used synonymously with the term resonance. To say that an object has a natural frequency, or that it resonates at a particular frequency, does not mean that the object only vibrates at one frequency. It simply means that there is a frequency that "naturally" produces a vibration of greatest amplitude, even while other frequencies produce vibrations of lesser amplitude. The reasons why objects have "natural frequencies" are the main focus of this section.

Vibratory objects include almost anything in the world. The main vibratory object of concern in this book is, of course, air; but the phenomenon of resonance extends to other objects, sometimes with startling outcomes. For example, most people know about the ability of some vocalists to shatter a wine glass with a loudly sung note, or the comedic scene in films where

an opera singer hits a note of extremely high frequency and intensity, causing mirrors, windows, vases, eyeglasses, and other assorted objects to break apart. These are all examples of vibratory energy in air, emerging from a singer's vocal tract and being transferred to a mechanical object and causing it to vibrate. If a frequency produced by the singer coincides with the natural or resonant frequency of the solid object and the energy transfer from air to solid is sufficient, the solid may begin to vibrate. If the energy transfer from air to solid is very efficient at the natural frequency of the solid, the vibration of the solid may become violent enough to cause the solid to break apart. Perhaps one of the most startling examples of resonance is when a bridge set into vibration by the rhythmic marching of soldiers. If the synchronized marching frequency is the same as the resonant frequency of the bridge it is transferred very efficiently, and the bridge responds with large-amplitude swayings (vibrations) that can endanger its structural integrity.

The concept of resonance is introduced here by describing a simple mechanical model. Then, because energy can be transferred from vibrating objects to volumes of air, acoustic resonance is discussed in detail. This discussion shows how concepts from mechanical systems are directly applicable to acoustical systems.

Calm Yourself with Dissonance

Everyone is familiar with the peculiar sound evoked from a partially filled wine glass by rotating a finger around the lip of the glass. This party trick is rooted in the ancient practice of meditating with the assistance of Tibetan Singing Bowls. In ancient times, these bowls were constructed from a mixture of several different metals such as gold, copper, silver, and iron. The different proportions of metals used to craft the bowls determined their unique resonant properties, elicited by stroking the bowl's edge with a leather mallet. Here is what is interesting about these resonant characteristics: the peaks in the spectrum of a vibrating Tibetan Singing Bowl often produce a highly dissonant musical chord, unlike the nicely balanced chords we typically associate with soothing music. The multiple resonances of a Tibetan Singing Bowl sound vaguely like outer space sounds from a 1950s science fiction movie. Yet these sounds are considered well-matched to the calming practice of meditation.

Mechanical Resonance

Mechanical systems can be used to understand acoustical systems. This is illustrated using a spring-mass model to describe the phenomenon of resonance and how mass and elasticity determine resonant frequencies.

A Simple Spring-Mass Model Can Be Used to Explain the Concept of Resonance

Figure 7–10A shows a simple mechanism consisting of a mass (e.g., a small block of wood) labeled M, a spring labeled K, and a fixed surface to which the spring-mass assembly is attached. The spring-mass model in Figure 7–10A is not under the influence of any external forces (i.e., it is not being pushed or pulled) and is, therefore, at rest. Not surprisingly, if the mass is pulled away from the fixed surface (that is, the spring is stretched) and then released (Figure 7–10B), the result is a back-and-forth movement around the original rest position (rest position indicated by the vertical dashed line at the right of the figure). As the spring-mass assembly vibrates, the spring is sometimes stretched (Figure 7–10B) and sometimes compressed (Figure 7–10C) relative to its rest length (Figure 7–10A or 7–10D). Figure 7–10D

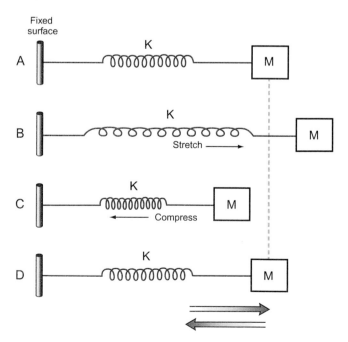

Figure 7–10. Spring-mass model that illustrates the concept of mechanical resonance. K = spring and M = mass. **A.** Model at rest. **B.** Model stretched from its rest position. **C.** Model compressed relative to its rest position. **D.** Model passing through its rest position during vibration.

shows the spring-mass model as it passes through the rest position, either in the direction of stretching (right-pointing arrow) or compression (left-pointing arrow). The difference between Figures 7–10A and 7–10D is that Figure 7–10A shows the model at rest (no forces applied), whereas 7–10D shows a single moment in time during vibration when the spring-mass model is at a length corresponding to the length at rest.

The period of this vibration is equal to the amount of time required to complete one full cycle of motion (from rest, to maximum stretch of the spring, back through rest to maximum compression of the spring, and then back to rest). Alternatively, one could measure the frequency simply by counting the number of complete vibrations occurring in some unit of time and then converting to Hz, the number of complete cycles in 1s. Notice that the motion being described—a back and forth movement around a rest position—is exactly like the one described above for the motion of air molecules (see Figures 7–1 and 7–3). The relevant question here is, "What determines the frequency of a spring-mass model after it has been set into motion by a manual stretch?"

The Relative Values of Mass (M) and Elasticity (K) Determine the Frequency of Vibration of the Simple Spring-Mass Model

As described earlier, the mass and elasticity properties of an air molecule play a critical role in maintaining the motion of the molecule. This idea is pursued here, but now with reference to the specific properties of M and K that determine vibratory frequency of the spring-mass model.

Mass. The mass of an object is defined as its weight divided by a constant, which is the value of acceleration due to gravity. Formally,

$$M = weight/g_o \qquad \text{Formula (5)}$$

where weight can be measured in pounds or grams and g_o is the symbol used to denote acceleration due to gravity, the value of which is 9.8 meters/s². Because g_o is a constant, mass can be considered to be directly proportional to weight for the remainder of this discussion.

Objects with mass have the property of inertia, meaning that they offer opposition to being accelerated and decelerated. This property explains why, when an air molecule recoils from a stretched or compressed position back toward the rest position, it does not stop at the rest position. The inertial forces inherent in the air molecule oppose deceleration as the molecule approaches rest position, and cause the motion to continue past rest and toward the other extreme position. Similarly, when recoil forces overcome inertial forces and reverse the direction of movement back toward the rest position, the molecule does not reach full speed immediately because the inertial forces oppose acceleration. These same inertial forces apply to the vibration of the spring-mass model. The foregoing explanation of mass and inertia provides the clues to how mass affects the frequency of vibration. Keep in mind, both recoil and inertial forces are acting at the same time during the vibration, with one or the other dominating depending on the position of the vibratory object.

Imagine that the mass in Figure 7–10 is replaced with a heavier one. Because the new mass is greater than the old one, it should demonstrate greater inertial forces. The new mass will, therefore, oppose being accelerated and decelerated to a greater degree than the old mass. How will this affect the motion of the spring-mass model? If the new spring-mass model opposes acceleration and deceleration more than the old one, it should take more time for the model to move through one complete cycle. This is the result of the greater time required to initiate movement at points in the cycle where the direction of motion is reversed (as at the end of a maximum displacement) or to slow down the movement as the spring-mass model goes through the rest position. Thus, the effect of adding mass to the spring-mass model is to increase the period of vibration, which of course is the same as decreasing the frequency. All other things being equal, an increase in mass will decrease the resonant frequency of a vibratory object.

Stiffness. The elasticity of an object is defined by the amount of force required to displace the object some distance. Elasticity is typically measured in terms of *stiffness*, which can be expressed formally as:

$$K = \text{Force/Meters} \qquad \text{Formula (6)}$$

where K is the symbol for the quantity *stiffness*, force is measured in units called *newtons*, and *meters* indicates a linear distance. Stiffness is typically schematized by a spring, as shown in Figure 7–10 and several upcoming figures. Force can be described in terms of an equivalent weight required to displace an object some distance. For example, 1 newton is roughly equivalent to the application of 0.224 pounds (or 98.7 grams; 1 pound = 439 grams) of force to an object. If there were a scale sensitive enough to register accurately fractions of a pound and enough force was applied manually to make the scale register 0.224 pounds, 1 newton of force would have been applied to the scale.

The elasticity formula shown above suggests that stiffer objects require greater force to displace them over some standard distance. This concept is illustrated in Figure 7–11, which shows two spring-mass models mounted on either side of a measuring rule marked off in centimeters. For this demonstration the two masses (M1 and M2) are assumed to be equal, but the springs, labeled K1 and K2, have some unknown difference in stiffness. The difference in the stiffness of K1 and K2 can be determined as follows. First, both spring-mass models are resting at "0" on the centimeter rule, so 1 cm can be designated as a standard displacement for both models. Next, a wire is attached to the mass of each model, and this wire is connected to a scale which registers the amount of weight applied to the spring-mass model when it is displaced 1 cm. The stiffer spring, according to formula (6), is the one requiring more weight (greater force) to produce a displacement of 1 cm. As shown in Figure 7–11, if K2 is greater than K1, then F2 (where F = force) will be greater than F1 to produce the standard displacement of 1 cm.

In the discussion of air molecule motion, it was noted that as a molecule is displaced from its rest position, a recoil force is developed and exerted in the direction of the rest position. When any spring is stretched or compressed away from its rest position, it stores these recoil forces, which become greater with increasing displacement from the rest position. When the two springs in Figure 7–11 are stretched 1 cm away from their rest positions, it follows that the stiffer spring—K2—will generate a greater recoil force to return to the rest position because it required a greater force to displace it from the rest position. If the two springs are suddenly let go after their extension to 1 cm, they will both spring back toward the rest position, but K2's movement will be faster because its recoil forces are greater than those of K1 at equivalent displacements. In other words, greater recoil forces are associated with greater rates of movement when the forces are permitted to produce motion (as in the case of "letting the spring go").

Now assume that the original spring in Figure 7–10 is replaced with one having greater stiffness. The greater recoil forces, and thus recoil speeds, of the new spring will decrease the time required for the model to complete a full cycle of vibration. Stated in another way, if the motion of the spring-mass model is faster because of a stiffer spring, it will take less time to move back and forth. Thus, the effect of increasing stiffness is to decrease the period, which is the same as increasing the frequency. All other things being equal, an increase in stiffness will increase the resonant frequency of a vibratory object.

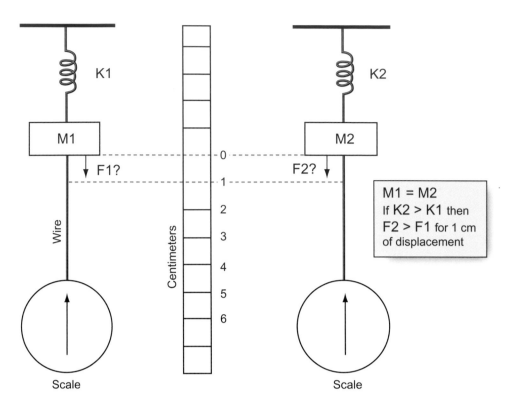

Figure 7–11. Measurement of stiffness. If the spring on the right (K2) is stiffer than the spring on the left (K1), all else being equal, it will take a greater force to displace the K2-M2 spring-mass model a 1-cm unit of length.

The Effects of Mass and Stiffness (Elasticity) on a Resonant System: A Summary

The foregoing discussion of the factors that determine the resonant frequency of a spring-mass model can be summarized by the following formula:

$$fr = 1/2\pi \times \sqrt{K/M} \qquad \text{Formula (7)}$$

where fr = resonant frequency, K = stiffness and M = mass; $1/2\pi$ is a constant related to the circular origin of sinusoidal motion. According to the formula, increases in the numerator K will increase the resonant frequency fr, whereas increases in the denominator M decrease fr. The formula and preceding discussion also show that a decrease in fr could be accomplished either by a decrease in stiffness or an increase in mass. Similarly, an increase in fr could be accomplished either by an increase in stiffness or a decrease in mass. In more complicated resonant systems, both stiffness and mass vary independently, and their combination determines the resonant, or natural frequency of the system.

Tacoma Narrows Bridge

A spectacular episode of apparent wind-induced resonance occurred in 1940, when the half-mile long Tacoma Narrows Bridge in Washington State responded to high winds with vibrations of increasingly large amplitude and eventually collapsed into the Puget Sound (see Petroski, 1992, for an interesting account of bridge structures and the potential dangers of resonance). There has been some con-troversy over the years about the exact cause of the bridge's collapse, but one factor seems to be that the wind "forced" the bridge to resonate and twist rhythmically until it broke apart and collapsed. If you enter "Tacoma Narrows Bridge" into a search engine on the Internet, you can see photographs and even a brief movie of the bridge as it responded to the winds.

Acoustic Resonance: Helmholtz Resonators

The concepts just developed in the discussion of mechanical resonance are directly applicable to a model of acoustic resonance called *Helmholtz resonance*. Helmholtz resonance is so named because Hermann von Helmholtz, a German scientist who lived in the late 19th century, constructed acoustic resonators and studied the laws governing their vibratory behaviors. A discussion of Helmholtz resonance will not only show how concepts of mechanical resonance are equally valid in an acoustical system, but is also directly applicable to certain aspects of vowel production, as discussed in Chapter 8.

Figure 7–12A shows a drawing of a Helmholtz resonator. The resonator consists of a neck having some length *l*, a circular opening with radius a, and a bowl having radius R. The air contained within this resonator can be separated into two functional components corresponding to the resonator neck and bowl, respectively.

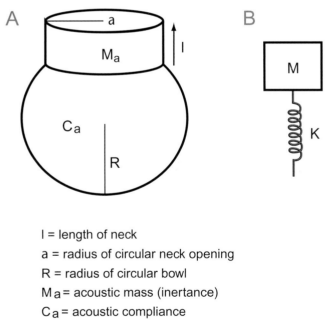

I = length of neck

a = radius of circular neck opening

R = radius of circular bowl

M_a = acoustic mass (inertance)

C_a = acoustic compliance

Figure 7–12. A. Helmholtz resonator and dimensions that determine its resonant frequency. **B.** Spring-mass model that is analogous to the Helmholtz resonator in A.

The Neck of the Helmholtz Resonator Contains a Column, or Plug of Air, That Behaves Like a Mass When a Force Is Applied to It

The air within the neck can be thought of as a plug of air having some mass. When a force is applied to this plug of air, or *acoustic mass*, it offers opposition to being accelerated and, once set in motion, offers opposition to being decelerated. This pluglike acoustic mass, which is symbolized as M_a and alternately called an *inertance* to highlight the analogy to inertial forces offered by mechanical masses, behaves just like the masses described above in the discussion of spring-mass models.[6]

To continue the analogy from mechanical resonators, an increase in M_a decreases the resonant frequency (*fr*) of a Helmholtz resonator. M_a can be increased in a Helmholtz resonator by one of two physical modifications to the neck section. First, the neck can be lengthened (greater *l* in Figure 7–12A). A longer neck will increase the number of air molecules within the plug, thus adding the mass of the newly included molecules to the ones in the original plug. This is a straightforward analogy to the mechanical case of increasing the weight of a solid mass. The second way to increase M_a is to decrease the size of the neck opening (decreasing a in Figure 7–12A), even with a constant neck length. At first glance, this seems counterintuitive, because a decrease in the size of the neck opening should decrease the number of molecules in the air plug (i.e., make it more narrow), and, therefore, make it less, rather than more, massive. Functionally, however, the effect of narrowing the neck size and hence the air plug is to cause the molecules within the plug to move at a greater speed during vibration, and hence require longer acceleration and deceleration times to and from this higher speed. When air molecules are flowing and encounter a constriction, they tend to speed up. The narrower the constriction, the greater the speed of the molecules. Thus, given two air plugs of the same length but differing degrees of narrowness, the narrower air plug will respond to an applied force in a more mass-like way because acceleration must be to higher speeds and deceleration must be from higher speeds. The narrower plug, therefore, offers greater functional opposition to acceleration and deceleration than the wider plug, because it takes longer to get up to, and come

---

[6]Technically, a "perfect" acoustic mass is a plug of air that can be accelerated, but not compressed. What this means is that when a force is applied to one end of a plug of air, the air molecules in the plug move (accelerate) as a unit without changes in air density (that is, pressure). In other words, the air molecules within the plug are not forced closer together as a result of the application of the force. The analogy to a mechanical mass is direct. When a force is applied to a solid mass, the laws of inertia dictate completely the movement of the mass provided there is no compression (e.g., bending, twisting, splitting) of the molecules making up the solid. See Footnote 7 for a similar explanation of a "perfect" acoustic compliance.

down from, the higher speed induced by the smaller constriction. These greater acceleration and deceleration effects will add to the period, and, therefore, decrease frequency. A narrower neck opening, therefore, reduces resonant frequency compared to a wider neck opening, because the narrower opening is associated with greater M_a.

The Bowl of a Resonator Contains a Volume of Air That Behaves Like a Spring When a Force Is Applied to It

The second functional component of the Helmholtz resonator is the bowl. When a force is applied to the air in the bowl, the molecules may be compressed or expanded, just like the spring in the spring-mass model. When the air is compressed, the molecules exert a recoil force to "spring out" to their rest position. When the air is expanded, the molecules exert a force to "'spring back" to their rest position. These recoil forces, summed over all the air molecules within the bowl, are expressed as pressures above or below P_{atm}. Compressions create positive pressures ($>P_{atm}$), and expansions create negative pressures ($<P_{atm}$). The term *acoustic compliance* (C_a) is used to denote the stiffness properties of the volume of air within the resonator bowl. Compliance is actually the inverse of stiffness, so a stiffer volume of air would be said to be *less* compliant, and vice versa.[7]

Following the analogy from mechanical resonators, an increase in C_a (i.e., a decrease in the stiffness) l decreases the f_r of a Helmholtz resonator. C_a can be changed in a Helmholtz resonator by simply changing the size of the bowl: larger bowls (those with larger internal radii, R in Figure 7–12) are more compliant, smaller bowls less compliant. For a given applied force to an acoustic compliance, molecules in a larger bowl have more room to be displaced from their rest positions and are therefore more compliant (i.e., less stiff). Molecules in a smaller bowl have less room to be displaced, and therefore are less compliant (i.e., more stiff). The analogy to a spring is straightforward. Imagine two springs of exactly the same material and

the same number of coils per unit length, but of different absolute lengths (say, 5 and 15 cm). If each of these springs is compressed the same distance (say, 1 cm), the shorter spring develops a greater recoil force than the longer spring. The small versus large air volume effect on acoustic compliance, where small bowls have low C_a (more stiff), and large bowls have high C_a (less stiff), can be explained in exactly the same way.

A mechanical model of a Helmholtz resonator looks just like a spring-mass model. The correspondence between the two systems is captured by the orientation of the spring-mass model to the right of the Helmholtz resonator in Figure 7–12B. In both systems, an increase in mass lowers the resonant frequency and an increase in stiffness (a decrease in compliance [C_a] in an acoustic system) raises the resonant frequency. An increase in mass lengthens the period (because of increased inertial effects) and an increase in stiffness shortens the period (because of increased recoil forces and, hence, recoil speeds).

Another way to demonstrate the analogies between the mechanical and acoustical resonant systems is to show what happens when the air in the Helmholtz resonator is made to vibrate. Figure 7–13 shows four "snapshots" of a Helmholtz resonator at different points in a vibratory cycle. In all four snapshots, the colored plug or cylinder in the vicinity of the neck represent M_a, and the "cloud" of dots within the bowl represents C_a. The movement of the air plug relative to the volume of air within the bowl can be likened to a piston moving in and out of a volume of air or, of course, to a mass alternately compressing and expanding a spring. In snapshot A, the plug (M_a) and volume (C_a) of air are essentially at their rest positions. The pressure measured inside the bowl would be "0" (P_{atm}), because the air molecules are not stretched or compressed relative to their rest positions and, therefore, no recoil forces are exerted. Snapshot B shows the air plug displaced into the bowl, which compresses the volume of air within the bowl and raises the pressure, as indicated by the denser cloud of dots. The compressed air molecules generate recoil forces in the outward direction, which eventually overcome the inertial force of the inward-

---

[7]In theory, a "perfect" compliance is a volume of air that can be compressed (or expanded), but not accelerated (this is the opposite of the definition of a perfect inertance, given in Footnote 6). This means that the molecules within the volume are all displaced from their rest positions by compression or expansion, but are not accelerated to new rest positions (for example, 3 cm away from their old rest positions). Under this definition, the compressing or expanding force is expressed equally throughout the air volume in the form of increased or decreased pressures. If some of the molecules were accelerated and thus moved from their original rest positions, the pressure changes would not be uniform throughout the volume. Another way to say this is that some of the applied compression or expansion force would be "lost" in the acceleration of air molecules. Imagine a mechanical spring to which a compression force is applied. If the spring does not move as a whole when the force is applied (i.e., if the spring as a whole does not change location, meaning it is not accelerated) as the force is applied to the other end, some of the applied force will be "lost" to the movement of the spring, and the recoil force will not equal the applied force.

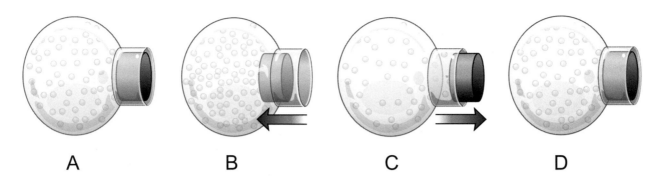

Figure 7–13. Four "snapshots" of the air in a Helmholtz resonator during vibration at resonance. The plug of air in the neck of the resonator is depicted by the shaded cylinder. The volume of air within the bowl of the resonator is depicted by the cluster of dots. Snapshots A, B, C, and D show four different moments in time during a vibratory cycle. **A.** Rest position. **B.** Plug of air displaced into the resonator bowl, causing the compression of air within the bowl. **C.** Plug of air extending out of the resonator bowl, causing expansion of air within the bowl. **D.** Plug of air passing through the rest position.

moving plug and drive it back toward the neck opening. The plug is driven outward, passes through its rest position because of its own inertial forces, and actually extends past the neck opening, as shown in snapshot C. At snapshot C, the molecules in the bowl are stretched relative to their rest positions and the pressure is negative, as indicated by the sparser cloud of dots. The stretched molecules generate an inward recoil force that ultimately overcomes the inertial force of the outward-going air plug and pulls it back through the rest position (snapshot D).

The analogy between mechanical and acoustical resonant systems can be summarized by means of the formula for the resonant frequency of a Helmholtz resonator. One version of the formula is exactly the same as that given for the spring-mass model, namely,

$$fr = 1/2\pi \times \sqrt{K/M} \qquad \text{Formula (7)}$$

but it is desirable for the expression to have direct relevance to the case of a Helmholtz resonator. Thus the resonant frequency of a Helmholtz resonator is given by:

$$fr = c/2\pi \times \sqrt{S/Vl} \qquad \text{Formula (8)}$$

In this formula, the constant "$c/2\pi$" differs from the mechanical case ($1/2\pi$) only by the inclusion of the constant c = speed of sound in air. S = the surface area of the opening of the neck. The inclusion of S in the numerator indicates that as the surface area increases (as the neck becomes wider) the resonant frequency will increase. This is consistent with the statement given above that wider necks are associated with smaller M_a. V = the volume of the resonator bowl, which when larger increases the Ca and thus lowers the resonant frequency (hence its placement in the denominator). And finally, l = length of the neck is in the denominator because longer resonator necks are associated with greater M_a and, therefore, a lower resonant frequency.

Acoustic Resonance: Tube Resonators

Not all acoustic resonators are shaped like a Helmholtz resonator, in which the neck and bowl are physically and functionally distinct. *Tubes* are a class of resonators which have substantial relevance to speech acoustics as well as other sonic events such as music. A critical concept in the understanding of tube resonance is that of *wavelength*, discussed earlier in this chapter (see Figure 7–5 and accompanying text). First consider what happens when a tube of *uniform cross-sectional area* (i.e., a tube having no constrictions), with both ends open to atmosphere, is exposed to sound energy.

Figure 7–14 pictures a tube open at both ends and a loudspeaker that produces sound energy at one end. If the loudspeaker is producing a complex acoustic event that has many different frequencies, the tube is exposed to pressure waves that have a wide variety of wavelengths (recall that frequency and wavelength, related by the formula $\lambda = c/f$, are inverse functions of one another). Many of the pressure fluctuations associated with these varying frequencies propagate through the tube only weakly, but a small group of frequencies produce very strong pressure fluctuations within the tube. These frequencies have wavelengths—distributions of sound pressure in space—that match the pressure conditions at the open ends of the tube.

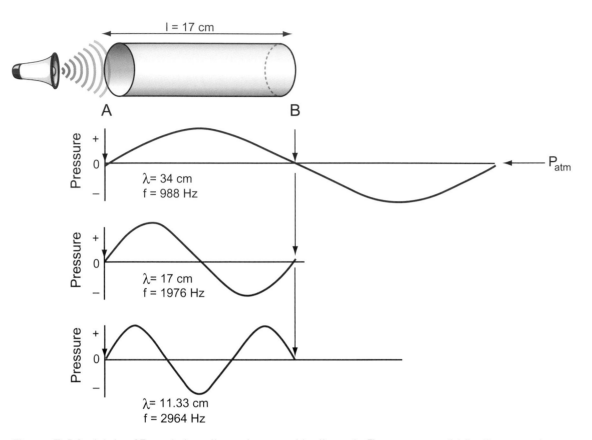

Figure 7–14. A tube 17 cm in length and open at both ends. The pressure distributions are shown for the first three resonant frequencies.

Three Shakers and Movers

The human body is subject to vibration and has an overall resonant frequency as well as different resonant frequencies for different parts. For example, the breathing apparatus has its own resonant frequency. One way to determine this resonant frequency is to seal the body inside a chamber below the shoulders. Powerful loudspeakers attached to the chamber are then used to create large sinusoidal pressure swings at the surface of the breathing apparatus (the torso), while airflow from the mouth is monitored. The frequency of pressure swings is changed up and down while the magnitude of the airflow is recorded. The greatest peak-to-peak airflow will occur at the resonant frequency of the breathing apparatus. Your authors have such resonant frequencies of about 4, 5, and 6 Hz. Thus, each of us has a breathing apparatus that shakes best at a different frequency. Maybe you can guess something about our body sizes from these numbers.

What are the pressure conditions at the two open ends of the tube in Figure 7–14? Under normal conditions, the pressure at the open ends is P_{atm}. Therefore, there must be frequencies whose wavelengths distribute pressure over space in such a way to have P_{atm} at the two ends of the tube. Immediately below the tube in Figure 7–14, a wavelength (pressure as a function of distance; review the inset of Figure 7–5) is shown along the same distance spanned by the tube. As described earlier, a wavelength is composed of the full range of pressure variations between the maximum positive and maximum negative pressures. In Figure 7–14, the complete wavelength immediately below the tube is shown beginning at P_{atm}, going to the maximum positive pressure, then passing through P_{atm} and going to maximum negative pressure, and then back again to P_{atm}. Note that the pressure at the beginning (point A) and at half of this wavelength (point B) matches the pressure at the open ends of the tube. The downward-pointing arrows in Figure 7–14 indicate the first two points along this wavelength where the pressure = P_{atm}. Those points correspond in space with the open ends of the tube. When this half-wavelength matches the pressure conditions at the open ends of the tube, the pressure fluctuation within the tube will be very strong and the tube will resonate at the frequency corresponding to the full wavelength.

The general concept of resonance, where an object vibrates with maximum amplitude at one frequency (or multiple frequencies, as in the case of a tube), can be shown to apply to tubes in the form of *standing waves*. Recall from the earlier discussion of sound waves that at a given point in space, the pressure varies over time from atmospheric, to maximally positive, to atmospheric, to maximally negative, and then back to atmospheric. In a continuing vibration, this pressure variation at one point in space repeats over and over. A standing wave occurs when the vibrating air molecules within a tube produce the same pressure variations at the *same location* within the tube, and these pressures reinforce each other and build up to their maximum value. These are called standing waves because even though the pressures at the one point within the tube do vary over time, the reinforcing of the pressures at the same locations within the tube produces what appears to be a "frozen" distribution of pressure within the tube. At some point along this "frozen" distribution of pressure, a pressure maximum will be located, and this maximum will represent a higher pressure than produced by other frequencies. The fact that it is the highest pressure for a group of frequencies indicates that the wavelength associated with this pressure distribution has a frequency that occurs at a resonance of the tube.

Standing waves occur at the resonant frequencies of the tube, and the pressure distributions shown in Figure 7–14 that "fit" the tube length are examples of such "frozen," maximum-amplitude pressure distributions. In the case of a tube open at both ends, this maximum pressure will always occur somewhere within the tube, but never at the ends where the pressure must always be P_{atm}.

This leads to a simple formula for the resonant frequencies of a tube open at both ends. The discussion above implies that if the length of the tube is known, one must double it to get the wavelength, and thus the frequency, that will produce the desired pressure match at the ends of the tube and the expected standing waves. Because it is half the wavelength that "fits" the pressure conditions at the ends of the tube for the lowest resonance, the formula is called the *half-wavelength rule* and is expressed as:

$$fr = n \times c/2l \qquad \text{Formula (9)}$$

where fr = resonant frequency, c = the constant, speed of sound in air, l = the length of the tube, and n = a multiplier that can be any integer from 1, 2, 3 . . . n. For

the 17 cm length tube in Figure 7–14, the computation of resonant frequency for $n = 1$ is $fr = 1 \times 33,600/2 \times 17 = 988$ Hz.

This is the lowest resonant frequency of this tube, but as implied by the multiplier n in the formula, not the only resonant frequency. An important difference between Helmholtz resonators and tube resonators is that tube resonators have multiple resonances, whereas Helmholtz resonators (and their mechanical counterparts, spring-mass models) have only a single resonance. Why do tube resonators have multiple resonances? It is easy to show that there are other frequencies whose wavelengths will meet the requirement of P_{atm} at both ends of the tube, and, therefore, produce standing waves within the tube. For example, a frequency of roughly 1976 Hz will have a wavelength of 17 cm ($\lambda = c/f$; $17 = 33,600/f$; $f = 33,600/17 = 1976$ Hz), exactly the same length as the tube. The spatial distribution of pressure for 1976 Hz will produce P_{atm} at both ends of the tube, as shown in Figure 7–14. Similarly, a frequency of 2964 Hz will have a wavelength of roughly 11.33 cm, with one-and-one-half of these wavelengths equaling 17 cm, the length of the tube. As shown in Figure 7–14, one-and-one-half wavelengths of the 2964-Hz component meets the pressure requirements at both ends. In theory, an infinite number of wavelengths will "fit" the tube according to the pressure requirements described here. A tube resonator, therefore, has an infinite number of resonant frequencies.

Another important class of tube resonators are those with one end closed, as seen in Figure 7–15 where the right-hand side of the tube is closed. As in the case of the tube open at both ends, a loudspeaker generates a wide variety of frequencies at one end of the tube, but the tube generates large-amplitude pressure fluctuations for only a selected few of these frequencies. These selected frequencies (i.e., the resonant frequencies) are determined by wavelengths whose pressure distributions match the pressures at the ends of the tube. The pressure condition at the open end of the tube in Figure 7–15 is already known—it is P_{atm}. But what is the pressure condition at the closed end of the tube? Recall from the earlier discussion of sound waves that pressures are proportional to the number of air molecule collisions per unit time. At the closed end of the tube, the number of these collisions is higher than at any other location within the tube, and certainly much higher than at the open end of the tube. This is because the closed end serves as a barrier to the motion of air molecules, so that as they move around they tend to be deflected into other molecules immediately adjacent to the barrier. This results in the largest number of air molecule collisions per unit time within the tube, and hence the highest pressure within the tube. Thus,

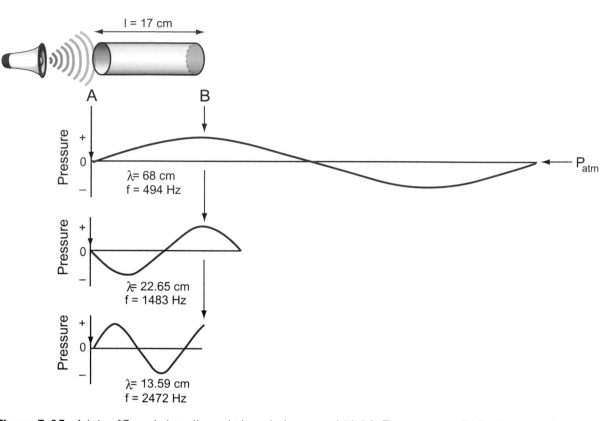

Figure 7–15. A tube 17 cm in length and closed at one end (*right*). The pressure distributions are shown for the first three resonant frequencies.

the correct "matching" pressure at the closed end of the tube is the greatest pressure along the wavelength. Pressure should be "0" at the open end (P_{atm}), and maximum at the closed end. When the pressures along a wavelength match these conditions, a standing wave will result where the "frozen" pattern will appear to have P_{atm} at the open end and maximum pressure at the closed end.

A complete wavelength contains two maximum pressures, one on the positive side of P_{atm} and one on the negative side (see Figure 7–5, inset). In Figure 7–15, the wavelength immediately below the tube is lined up in space with the tube so that 0 pressure is at the open end of the tube, and the first maximum pressure, which happens to be the positive maximum that occurs one-quarter of the way along the full wavelength, is at the closed end. Thus, one-quarter of a wavelength "fits" the pressure requirements for resonance of this tube. The resonance patterns of a tube closed at one end are summarized by the *quarter-wavelength rule*, which can be written as follows:

$$fr = (2n - 1) \times c/4l \qquad \text{Formula (10)}$$

where fr = resonant frequency, c = the constant, speed of sound in air, l = the length of the tube, and $2n - 1$ is a multiplier that specifies the pattern of higher resonances. For a tube 17 cm in length and $n = 1$ (the lowest resonant frequency), the computation is $fr = (2 \times 1 - 1) \times 33,600/68 = 494$ Hz.

Just as in the case of a tube open at both ends, other wavelengths meet the pressure requirements of a tube closed at one end. In Figure 7–15, the next shorter wavelength (i.e., the next higher frequency) that meets the pressure requirements is one that fits three-quarters of its length into the tube. If 0 pressure is located at the open end of the tube, at three-quarters of the wavelength, the pressure is at the positive maximum, which meets the pressure requirement of the closed end. The next shorter wavelength fits five-quarters (a full wavelength plus one-quarter) into the tube, the next one seven-quarters, and so forth. In each case, the next shorter wavelength—and thus the next highest frequency—has a pressure distribution that meets the requirements of the tube. Note that the series of wavelengths increases by odd integers, that is, 1/4, 3/4, 5/4, 7/4 . . . (2n − 1)/4. This explains the resonant frequency multiplier in the quarter-wavelength formula.

Resonance in Tubes: A Summary

An important aspect of a tube is that it resonates at multiple frequencies. This is because wavelengths of multiple frequencies—not just a single frequency—have pressure distributions that meet the pressure requirements at the ends of the tube. Examples of the multiple wavelengths that meet the pressure requirements of tubes open at both ends or closed at one end are shown in Figures 7–14 (*open at both ends*) and Figure 7–15 (*closed at one end*). It is very important to understand that when a tube resonates, the wavelengths of the multiple resonant frequencies are all producing their unique pressure distributions within the tube at the same time. If a snapshot could be taken of the pressure distribution within a tube closed at one end, the standing waves for *each* of the resonant frequencies would be visible. Figure 7–16 shows a hypothetical example of this for the first three resonant frequencies of a tube closed at one end. The snapshot shows the expected maximum pressure at the closed end for all three standing waves corresponding to the first three resonant frequencies, but also additional maximum pressures (e.g., see arrows) near the middle and toward the open end of the tube. These other maximum pressures are from the standing waves of the higher resonant frequencies, and all are present when the tube resonates. Stated differently, the pressure distributions are all superimposed on each other when the air in the tube is vibrating.

A fair amount of attention has been devoted to the resonant patterns of tubes because the physical principles are directly applicable to speech acoustics. In fact, a good model of the vocal tract as an acoustic resonator is a tube closed at one end. And, if the pressure distributions within a vibrating tube are understood, as described above, the relationship of the configuration of the vocal tract to the acoustic output of the vocal tract can be easily understood. Chapter 8 presents these ideas in specific detail.

Beer and Flutes

"Aeroacoustics" is the study of how air interacts with or influences mechanical structures. When you blow across the edge of that half-filled beer bottle in your hand, the air from your mouth is like a jet (a narrow "beam" of air) that exerts a force on the volume of air within the bottle; a resonant tone results. Typically, the less air in the bottle, the higher the tone. The air in the bottle and within the neck is like a Helmholtz resonator, and the air jet across the top like a displacing force. The interaction of these two factors produces the tone through a very complex set of resonance and air-jet phenomena. In a general sense, flutes produce tones by this kind of aeroacoustic interaction.

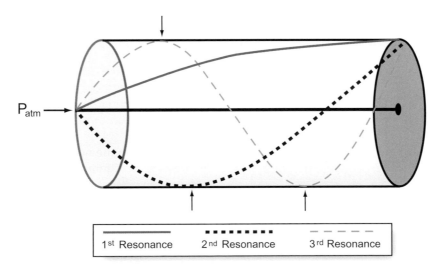

Figure 7–16. Simultaneous pressure distributions for the first three resonant frequencies within a tube closed at one end (*right*). Pressure distributions for all three resonant frequencies manifest at the same time in the vibrating tube. The thick horizontal line depicts atmospheric pressure as a reference point within the tube, in relation to the pressure distributions of the three resonances.

Resonance Curves, Damping, and Bandwidth

The examples of vibration discussed so far have not included considerations of energy loss, even though all natural vibratory phenomena are characterized by loss of energy over time. The effect of this loss of energy is to reduce the amplitude of vibration over time, and eventually to terminate the vibration. Thus, a spring-mass model, when set into sinusoidal motion, has increasingly smaller displacements over time as energy is lost, and ultimately ceases moving when the forces responsible for the loss of energy overcome recoil and inertial forces. This applies equally to acoustic systems such as Helmholtz resonators and tubes, where the displacement of air molecules responsible for propagation of a pressure wave gradually diminishes to zero if the source of sound (such as the loudspeaker in Figures 7–14 and 7–15) is removed from the vicinity of the resonator. A mechanical or acoustical resonator with no energy loss factors would, in theory, continue to vibrate forever after being set into vibration.

This introductory comment concerning the impact of energy loss in resonant systems refers exclusively to time domain phenomena. Energy loss is a typical characteristic of natural vibrations, and those vibrations, therefore, die out over time. Because time domain and frequency domain phenomena are in an inverse relationship to one another, it is not surprising that energy loss affects vibratory frequencies as well as times. After a brief review of factors responsible for energy loss in vibratory systems, the relationship between the time and frequency aspects of *lossy vibrations* (vibrations affected by the energy loss factors described below) is discussed. The term *damping* is used to describe energy loss in vibratory systems. *Lightly damped* systems have minimal energy loss and *heavily damped* systems have substantial energy loss.

Energy Loss (Damping) in Vibratory Systems Can Be Attributed to Four Factors

The factors causing energy loss in vibrating systems include friction, absorption, radiation, and gravity.

Friction is a substantial source of energy loss in vibratory systems and is produced when objects rub against each other or against other structures, thus producing heat. In a mechanical system such as a spring-mass model, the mechanical parts (the mass and spring) rub against air molecules as they move and generate heat. If the mass is mounted in a wooden track, additional heat is generated as the mass slides along the track. In acoustic systems, the rubbing of air molecules against each other and against the walls of the resonator (such as the soft tissues of the vocal tract) generates heat and thus expends energy. When frictional factors are present, some portion of the vibratory energy is dissipated (lost) in the form of heat. This dissipated energy cannot be recovered and, therefore, degrades the vibration.

Absorption of vibratory energy occurs when the vibrating object transfers (and thus loses) some of its energy to another structure. If a spring-mass model is mounted on a wall, some of the vibratory energy of the model may be taken up by the wall and lost. Air molecules vibrating within a human vocal tract can be absorbed by vocal tract tissues, causing the latter to vibrate. In this case, the transfer of vibratory energy may result in an effective vibration of (for example) the cheeks, but the energy is still lost from the vibrating air.

Radiation of sound is a form of energy loss typically associated with acoustic resonators. When air is vibrating within a resonator, some of the sound energy escapes, or radiates, from the tube and is lost. The obvious application of radiation loss in the vocal tract is the escape of sound energy from the lips and nose.

Gravity is the force that attracts any mass to the earth. Gravity can cause energy loss in any vibrating object by exerting a force on the object that opposes the forces inherent to the vibration (such as recoil and inertia). This is not a major consideration in energy loss in acoustic vibratory systems, but may become important in the simple vibration of a pendulum.

Time- and Frequency-Domain Representations of Damping in Acoustic Vibratory Systems

The top of Figure 7–17 shows a Helmholtz resonator of unknown resonant frequency. Obviously, the frequency could be determined with the proper formulas by making the appropriate physical measurements, such as the length and radius of the neck, and the volume of the bowl, but the resonator characteristics can also be determined by performing an experiment. The small outlet at the bottom right of the resonator bowl serves as an output through which acoustic energy is radiated and measured. Assume a microphone is mounted directly over this hole and attached to a computer that can record acoustic waveforms and compute spectra by Fourier analysis. The microphone-computer setup, therefore, permits acoustic measurements to be made at the output of the resonator.

A small-scale experiment performed with this resonator-computer setup demonstrates the effect of damping on the time- and frequency-domain representations of Helmholtz resonance. For this experiment, the

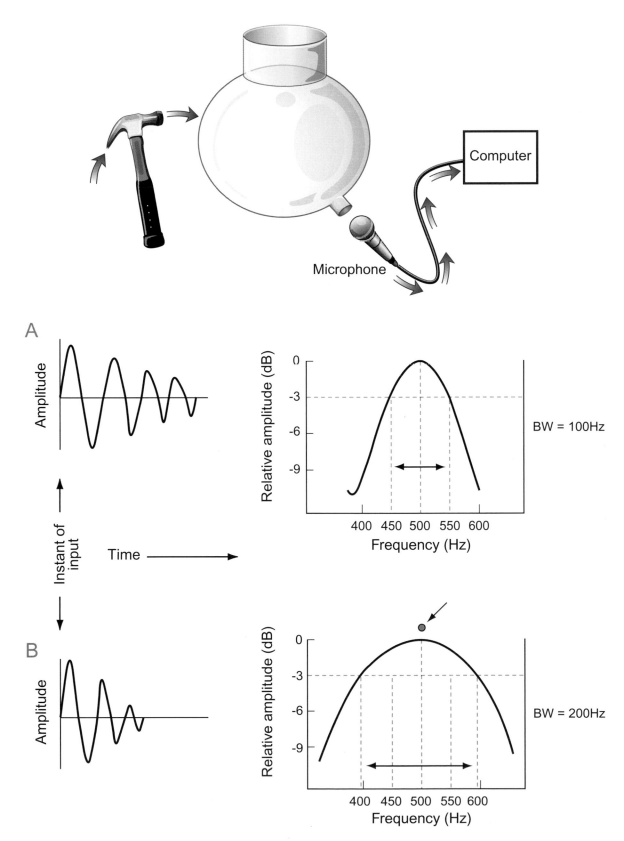

Figure 7-17. Excitation of a Helmholtz resonator (*top*) with a brief stimulus and the recording of its response (*bottom*). Time (*waveforms at left*) and frequency-domain (*spectra at right*) displays resulting from excitation are shown on the left and right, respectively, in both A and B. The resonator is more lightly damped in A than in B.

air within the resonator must be excited using a very brief *input* stimulus. For example, the air within the resonator could be excited by means of a single tap on the outside of the resonator, perhaps using a small hammer as shown in Figure 7–17. The tap is an *impulse-like* event, designed to have an extremely brief duration that will not interfere with the *response* (i.e., the vibration of the air within the resonator) of the resonator. This provides a source of vibration to the resonator—turning it on, so to speak—but the source is withdrawn immediately and the subsequent response is observed. Now imagine that the experiment is performed twice, once with the resonator having minimal energy loss factors (lightly damped) and the second time with increased energy loss factors (more heavily damped).

The damping factors could be increased for the second experiment by (for example) placing more of the resonator bowl in contact with some absorptive material or decreasing the ease with which air molecules move along the edges of the resonator by increasing the roughness of the interior surface (thus increasing friction). For both experiments, the brief input energy —the tap—must be identical so that differences in the acoustic measurements between the two resonator conditions can be attributed to the differences in damping, and not differences in the characteristics of the input.

Figure 7–17A shows a waveform (left) and a spectrum (right) of the acoustic energy associated with the resonator response in the condition of light damping. Two notable observations can be made about the waveform: (a) the amplitude is relatively large immediately following the input, and then decreases over time until it is zero; and (b) the waveform is periodic, but does not appear to be strictly sinusoidal, which suggests that the acoustic event is characterized by more than one frequency component.

The resonator response can also be seen in the spectrum to the right of the waveform, which shows frequency on the *x*-axis and relative amplitude on the *y*-axis. The relative amplitude scale has been arbitrarily marked 0 dB at the point of maximum energy in the resonator response, and the negative numbers simply indicate sound levels (in dB) less than this maximum energy point. The function shown in the spectrum is called a *resonance curve*, which displays the computer-generated measurements of sound levels at all frequencies of interest. Because resonance is defined as the frequency at which an object (in this case the air within the resonator) vibrates with maximum energy, this resonance curve shows the Helmholtz resonator to have a natural or resonant frequency of 500 Hz. The frequency at which peak sound energy occurs along the resonance curve defines the resonant frequency.

The other frequencies along the resonance curve —those not associated with peak energy, but clearly showing some vibratory energy— reflect energy loss factors affecting this vibration. If there were no energy loss factors in this Helmholtz resonator the spectrum would show a single line at 500 Hz, indicating vibratory energy at a single frequency. Such a resonator would be said to be *perfectly tuned*. Damping factors in a resonator change this tuning, and produce energy at frequencies other than the natural frequency. The frequency-domain index of this tuning, and thus of damping, is called the *bandwidth* of the resonator. Bandwidth is defined as the range of frequencies between the two *3-dB-down points* on either side of the peak energy. In Figure 7–17A, a horizontal dashed line has been extended from the −3-dB level on the *y*-axis to intersect the resonance curve on either side of the peak (500 Hz), and from each of these intersecting points a vertical line has been dropped to the *x*-axis (frequency). The vertical lines show the frequencies where the energy is 3 dB less than the energy at the resonant frequency of 500 Hz, namely, 450 Hz to the left and 550 Hz to the right. The bandwidth of this resonance, shown on the spectrum by the horizontal line terminated in arrows, is 100 Hz.

In Figure 7–17B, the time-and-frequency domain results are shown for the same resonator with greater damping. Here the waveform clearly decays faster and the bandwidth is wider than in Figure 7–17A. The spectrum in Figure 7–17B has been drawn to show an important feature of the effect of increased damping on the resonance curve: The single dot in the middle of the spectrum (arrow in Figure 7–17B) is the location of peak energy for the lightly damped resonator in 7–17A, and the peak of the more heavily damped resonance is shown at 0 dB, as in Figure 7–17A. The more heavily damped resonance of Figure 7–17B clearly does not produce the same amount of energy at the resonant frequency as the more lightly damped resonance of 7–17A, but the resonant frequency is the same for both resonators.

In other words, the peak energy in Figure 7–17B is still at 500 Hz, even though it is weaker than the peak energy in 7–17A. The most notable difference between parts A and B is the bandwidth, which is wider in B (200 Hz, indicated by horizontal line ending in arrows). Changes in damping do not affect the resonant frequency (ies) of an acoustic system.

Why is bandwidth defined in terms of the 3-dB-down points on the resonance curve? The energy in a sound wave is capable of doing some *work* (such as causing an effective displacement of the human eardrum, and thus having an important effect in the per-

Organic Music-Making: Hats Off to Tube Resonators

Everyone is familiar with pipe organs, the massive array of different-lengthed tubes rising above a keyboard, the heart-thumping sound a truly great instrument is capable of generating. Obviously, a pipe organ has the ability to generate tones of a wide range of pitches by having all those pipes of different length. But it also achieves pitch variation with *individual* pipes by providing the organist with controls for "capping" one end of the tube, or leaving both ends open. Really, pipe organs are simply tube resonators in disguise as ear candy.

ception of sound), and there is a range of sound levels below the peak that is still effective in doing this work. The term *power* is typically used by scientists to designate the work capability of energy, and it can be shown that half of the peak sound power is equivalent to 3 dB below the peak sound level. The concept of the *half-power points* designating the lower limit of effective sound energy is thus the origin of the use of 3-dB-down points to determine the bandwidth. The reader should understand that the half-power (3-dB-down) points are used by agreement of the community of individuals interested in sound, and do not necessarily reflect any inherent truths about the effective nature of sound energy. This kind of *operational definition* is very common in all sciences, and serves the purpose of allowing scientists to communicate with one another and share research experiences within a common measurement framework.

An Extension of the Resonance Curve Concept: The Shaping of a Source by the Acoustic Characteristics of a Resonator

In Figure 7–17 a brief input (the hammer tap) was used to show the relationship between the speed of decay of the resonant waveform and the bandwidth of the resulting spectrum (resonance curve). This impulse approach to the excitation of the resonator was useful in showing that damping can be defined in the time or frequency domains. Greater damping is indicated by faster speeds of waveform decay (time domain) and wider bandwidths (frequency domain). This idea is now extended by demonstrating how a resonator shapes the energy in an input signal.

Figure 7–18 shows an experimental arrangement similar to that in Figure 7–17, except now a continuous white noise is serving as the input signal to a Helmholtz resonator (Figure 7–18A), and a tube resonator (Figure 7–18B). A continuous, perfect white noise is an excellent input signal for evaluating the characteristics of a resonator, because the average sound level at any frequency is equivalent to the average sound level at any other frequency. This is shown in Figure 7–18 by the flatline spectrum for the input signals. Because the average sound level in the input signal is equivalent at all frequencies, any modification of the spectrum at the output of the resonator must be due to the characteristics of the resonator. Stated otherwise, any difference between the input and output spectra must be due to the resonator only, because the energy in the input spectrum is constant as a function of frequency.

Figure 7–18A shows how the Helmholtz resonator *shapes the input spectrum*. The air in the resonator vibrates with maximum energy at one frequency—the resonant frequency—and with less energy at other frequencies. The resonance curve is similar to the one shown in Figure 7–17, its shape being the result of both the physical dimensions of the resonator (which determine the resonant frequency) and the energy loss factors. The difference between the input and output spectra in Figure 7–18A is solely a result of the resonator characteristics.

Figure 7–18B shows the *input-output function* for a tube closed at one end. The tube shaped the flat input spectrum by resonating at multiple frequencies (only three are shown in Figure 7–18). Each peak in this output spectrum is a resonant frequency, and the bandwidth around each peak is determined by energy loss factors which may differ as a function of frequency (see Chapter 8).

The concept of resonators shaping an input to produce an output is a crucial one for understanding the acoustic theory of speech production. A flat input spectrum has been used to illustrate this concept, but the shaping idea applies to any situation where an input is applied to a resonator. Another way to think about the effect of a resonator on a sound source is to consider the former a *filter*. A filter is any device that passes certain inputs (i.e., allows those inputs to get through) and rejects others (i.e., stops them from getting through). Acoustic filters such as Helmholtz or tube resonators pass certain frequencies (especially the resonant frequencies) and reject others. In the case of speech production, the vocal tract can be considered as a filter that passes or rejects frequencies generated by different sources (such as the source energy generated by the vibrating vocal folds).

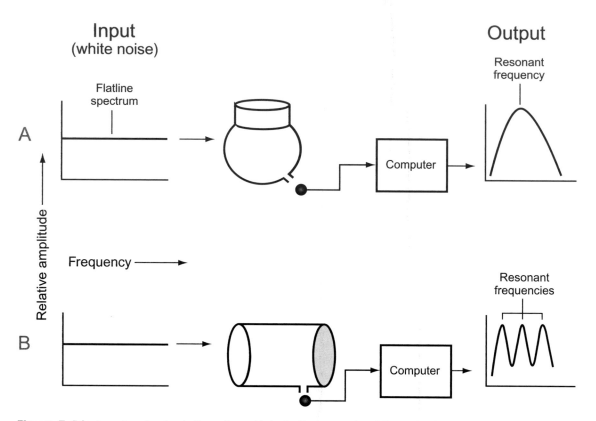

Figure 7–18. Input-output relations for a Helmholtz resonator (*A*) and a tube resonator (*B*), using white noise with a perfectly flat spectrum as the input signal. In both cases, the resonator "shapes" the input signal, as shown by the output spectra to the far right in the two panels.

Resonance, Damping, and Bandwidth: A Summary

The vibratory patterns of air in resonators are not only characterized by the resonant frequency (the frequency wth maximum vibratory energy), but by energy loss factors that determine the shape of the curve around the peak. The energy loss factors, or damping of a resonance, can be described in either the time or frequency domain. Greater energy loss is associated with more rapid decay of vibratory amplitude over time and with wider bandwidths. For a given resonator, variations in damping have no effect on the resonant frequencies (i.e., the locations of peaks in the spectrum). A simple way to determine the acoustic characteristics of a resonator is to perform an input-output experiment, wherein the input is a signal having the same energy at all frequencies. When this input signal is used to excite the resonator, any differences between the input and output spectra must reflect the characteristics of the resonator. Resonators are said to shape, or filter, inputs, and in so doing produce an output that reflects the combination of the input and resonator characteristics.

REVIEW

Pressure waves can be understood by examining the motions of air molecules during vibration.

These motions are governed by various forces, including those due to the elasticity and inertial properties of air molecules.

Factors that contribute to energy loss also determine how long the vibrations continue.

Sinusoids are the simplest type of acoustic vibration and can be considered as the elementary components of more complex vibrations.

A mathematical technique, Fourier analysis, allows a decomposition of a complex acoustic event into its component sinusoids.

When a computer program is used to construct a spectrum for a portion of a waveform, the program applies the Fourier technique to decompose the complexities in the time domain (the waveform) into the component sinusoids, and then displays the components in the frequency domain (a spectrum).

Fourier analysis is valid for acoustic events that repeat in time (complex periodic sounds) and for those that do not repeat in time (complex aperiodic sounds).

Resonance is the phenomenon where an object vibrates at a single frequency, or multiple frequencies, with maximal amplitude.

Two types of resonators—Helmholtz and tubes—were considered in detail.

The frequencies at which Helmholtz and tube resonators vibrate are governed by specific laws.

Resonators shape, or filter, the acoustic energy in a source of sound.

The shaping of a source by a resonator is critical to the understanding of the acoustic theory of speech production.

REFERENCES

Beranek, L. (1986). *Acoustics*. New York, NY: American Institute of Physics.

Beyer, R. (1999). *Sounds of our times*. New York, NY: Springer-Verlag.

Hunt, F. (1978). *Origins in acoustics*. New Haven, CT: Yale University Press.

Milenkovic, P. (2001). *TF32. User's manual*. Madison, WI: University of Wisconsin.

Petroski, R. (1992). *To engineer is human: The role of failure in successful design*. New York, NY: Vintage.

Acoustic Theory of Vowel Production

INTRODUCTION

Speech scientists and speech-language pathologists are indebted to Gunnar Fant, a Swedish speech scientist, for the development of the theoretical basis of speech acoustics. Fant performed much of the work on the theory in the 1940s and 1950s, and published his classic book, titled *Acoustic Theory of Speech Production*, in 1960. Previously, two Japanese scientists (Chiba & Kajiyama, 1941) had developed a similar mathematical theory of vocal tract acoustics, but this work was essentially unknown in western hemisphere countries until well after World War II. Fant, as well as a small group of scientists whose names are encountered throughout this text (Kenneth Stevens, Osamu Fujimura, Arthur House, James Flanagan), continued to develop and refine the theory in the 1950s, 1960s, and 1970s. Indeed, the theoretical development continues today. In particular, the texts of Flanagan (1972) and more recently Ste-

vens (1998) showcase developments in speech acoustic theory since the original work of Fant, and Chiba and Kajiyama (see also Story, 2005). Much of the information in this and the following chapter is drawn from these sources.

The acoustic theory of vowel production can be stated in very broad terms, as follows: for vowel production, the vocal tract resonates like a tube closed at one end, and shapes an input signal generated by the vibrating vocal folds. The two major concepts suggested in this broad statement of the theory—(a) the resonance patterns of a tube closed at one end, and (b) the shaping of an input by a resonator—are covered in Chapter 7. At this point, the broad statement of the theory refers only to vowel production. The theory is most precise for the case of vowels, primarily because its mathematical basis works best for the resonant frequencies of vowels (as compared to many consonants). The theory also addresses consonant acoustics, which is covered in Chapter 9. To explore the acoustic theory

Fathers of Speech Acoustics

Professor Gunnar Fant (1919–2009) was a famous speech acoustician and is widely regarded as one of the fathers of speech acoustics. Fant was born in Sweden in 1919 and spent most of his career in the Department of Speech, Hearing, and Music at the Royal Institute of Technology (KTH) in Stockholm. Fant founded this department in 1951 as the Speech Transmission Laboratory, after spending 1949 and 1950 at the Massachusetts Institute of Technology working with another giant in the field, Professor Kenneth Stevens (b. 1924). Over the years, Fant's department generated a wealth of valuable research

in the area of speech acoustics, all of which was reported in a famous, recurring publication called the *KTH Speech Transmission Laboratory Quarterly Progress Report*. Fant's 1960 book, *Acoustic Theory of Speech Production*, is one of a very few knowledge touchstones for the serious speech scientist. The student who reads and comprehends Fant's text, as well as Professor Stevens' (a second intellectual father) magnificent 1998 text *Acoustic Phonetics*, which can be considered a successor to, and enlarger of, Fant's classic book, can claim to be well-informed about the many aspects of speech acoustics.

of vowel production in greater depth, this chapter addresses the following set of questions:

1. What is the precise nature of the input signal generated by the vibrating vocal folds?
2. Why should the vocal tract be conceptualized as a tube *closed* at one end (as compared to open at both ends)?
3. How are the acoustic properties of the vocal tract determined?
4. How does the vocal tract shape the input signal?
5. What happens to the resonant frequencies of the vocal tract when the tube is constricted at a given location?
6. How is the acoustic theory of vowel production confirmed?

WHAT IS THE PRECISE NATURE OF THE INPUT SIGNAL GENERATED BY THE VIBRATING VOCAL FOLDS?

The periodic vibration of the vocal folds provides the input signal to the vocal tract resonator. This periodic vibration is referred to as the *source* for vowel acoustics. As discussed in Chapter 7, any signal can be studied in both the time and frequency domains. Much of what follows is a condensation of work done by Fant (1979, 1982, 1986) as refinement of the theory first published in 1960.

The Time Domain

The identification of the precise time-domain characteristics of the signal produced by vocal fold vibration is fairly complicated. The larynx, a structure of cartilage, membrane, ligament, and muscle, is not easily accessible for direct measurement of vocal fold behavior. If a microphone is placed directly in front of a speaker's lips while he or she phonates a vowel, the recorded acoustic event will reflect the *combination* of source (vocal fold) and resonator (vocal tract) acoustics. There is no simple way to look at the waveform (time domain) of a vowel recorded in this way (such as that shown in Figure 7–8B) and identify the components due only to vocal fold vibration. Some other approach must be found to "split" the waveform of a recorded vowel into the parts contributed by (a) the vibrating vocal folds and (b) the resonating vocal tract.

One of the earliest attempts to understand the details of vocal fold vibration was described by Farnsworth (1940), who took high-speed motion pictures of

the vibrating vocal folds by filming the image of the glottis as reflected in a laryngeal mirror. When played back in slow motion, these films allowed Farnsworth to view, on a frame-by-frame basis, movements of the vocal folds and the changing configuration of the glottis (the space between the vocal folds) throughout individual cycles of vocal fold vibration. A sequence of images of one vocal fold cycle, qualitatively similar to those examined by Farnsworth but collected with a contemporary device, is shown in Figure 8–1. The cycle begins with the vocal folds fully approximated (image 1). The folds separate gradually to a maximum width of the glottis (image 5), then begin to move back to the midline until they are once again fully approximated and there is no glottis (images 6–10). Scientists examined images such as these and for each one measured the width and length of the glottis, allowing them to derive the glottal area on an image-by-image basis. They then plotted *glottal area as a function of time* for a complete cycle of vocal fold vibration. A typical *glottal area function*, commonly symbolized as A_g, is shown for two cycles of vocal fold vibration in Figure 8–2A. The baseline in this plot represents full approximation of the vocal folds (i.e., $A_g = 0$), and upward movement of the function indicates increasingly larger separation of the vocal folds (i.e., increasing A_g). One cycle of vocal fold vibration is defined as the interval between successive separations of the vocal folds, as marked in Figure 8–2. Note that the vocal folds are fully approximated for a substantial portion of each cycle (nearly 40% of each cycle). The moment immediately before the vocal folds separate has been chosen arbitrarily as the initiation of each cycle. The duration of these cycles of vocal fold vibration may range from as little as 1 ms or less (for some opera or pop singers who can produce extremely high-pitched notes) to the more typical 5 ms (adult women, as shown in Figure 8–2) or 8 ms (adult men).

The A_g function shown in Figure 8–2 is not an acoustic signal, but rather reflects a pattern of vibration that produces an acoustic signal. How does one obtain the acoustic signal associated with vocal fold vibration—separate from the influence of the cavities in the vocal tract—and how is this signal related to the A_g function just described? Imagine that it was possible to suspend, immediately above the vocal folds, a device that measures the magnitude of airflow coming through the glottis as a function of time. When the vocal folds separate during a vibratory cycle (e.g., during phonation of a vowel) airflow through the glottis is expected because speech is produced with tracheal pressures greater than those in front of the lips (i.e., P_{atm}), and air always flows from regions of higher pres-

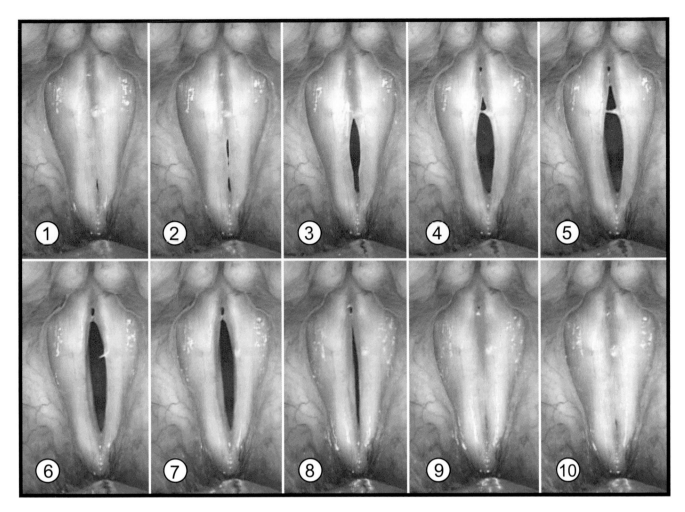

Figure 8–1. Successive images from one complete cycle of vocal fold vibration recorded via the Digital Strobe. The cycle begins in the upper left frame (*image 1*) with the vocal folds approximated. The folds begin to separate in image 2 and reach maximum separation in image 5. Closing of the vocal folds takes place in images 6 through 10. Images provided courtesy of KayPENTAX, Montvale, NJ. Reproduced with permission.

sure to regions of lower pressure. Intuitively, the magnitude of this airflow should be zero when the vocal folds are fully approximated (when there is no glottis to allow the passage of air), and maximum when the vocal folds are maximally apart (when A_g is the largest). In other words, the airflow coming through the glottis should increase as A_g increases, and decrease as A_g decreases. A plot of the magnitude of airflow coming through the glottis as a function of time should look a lot like the A_g function shown in Figure 8–2A. The time domain plot of airflow through the glottis is a *glottal flow* function, symbolized as $\dot{V}_g$. Because the $\dot{V}_g$ reflects movement of air molecules, this movement being responsible for the production of pressure waves (see Chapter 7), $\dot{V}_g$ is the proper signal to study as the source in vowel acoustics.

A $\dot{V}_g$ function is shown in Figure 8–2B. As expected, it looks very much like the A_g function (the detailed differences between the two types of waveforms will not be discussed in this text). Nevertheless, as noted above, actual measurement of the flow coming through the glottis in a phonating human is extremely difficult, if not impossible. Instead, scientists obtain $\dot{V}_g$ signals like the one shown in Figure 8–2B using an indirect approach.

Imagine a situation in which the input signal is the vibration of the vocal folds and the filter is a resonance curve associated with a specific shape of the vocal tract. From the discussion of tube resonators in Chapter 7 and introductory comments made above concerning the vocal tract resonating like a tube closed at one end, multiple peaks are expected in the resonance

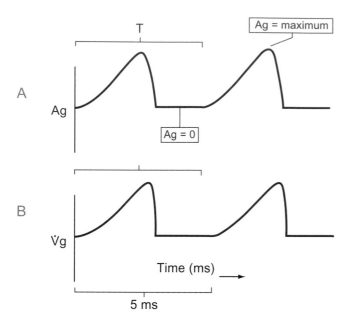

Figure 8–2. A. Glottal area function (A$_g$) for two cycles of vocal fold vibration. Upward displacements represent increasingly larger glottal areas, which are proportional to glottal widths measured from images like those in Figure 8–1. **B.** Glottal airflow function (V̇$_g$) obtained by inverse filtering (*see text*). Upward displacement indicates increasing magnitudes of airflow passing through the glottis.

curve. The input signal, plus a resonance curve (filter) for this hypothetical shape of the vocal tract, are shown in the upper part of Figure 8–3. When the input signal—here labeled "glottal source signal"—is applied to the vocal tract filter, the result is the output labeled "speech signal" (Figure 8–3, upper right panel). That speech signal represents the blending of the input and filter characteristics. Because of this blending, the output signal cannot reveal the exact characteristics of the input signal unless something is done to it. What is done to it, to "recover" the input signal, is a process called "inverse filtering" as demonstrated in the lower part of Figure 8–3. On the left is the speech signal, the same one as in the upper right-hand panel of the figure. This is the "blended" signal reflecting the influence of both the source and vocal tract filter. This blended signal serves as input to a resonance curve that is a "flipped" or mirror image of the one shown in the top of the figure. In this "flipped," or "inverse filter," there are valleys at the precise locations of the peaks in the upper filter function. If the inverse filter is constructed correctly, when the "blended" input signal is run through it, the resonances will be taken away from the signal and what remains at the output of the filter is

the glottal source signal. This is shown in the lower right panel as "recovered glottal source signal." In essence, the sequence of the bottom panel reverses that of the top panels, with the special adjustment of "flipping" or inverting the filter function. This is a time-honored approach to studying the glottal input signal independent of the filter function.

The technical details of inverse filtering are not important here, and the technique is more complicated (and often trickier) than implied by the straightforward logic of Figure 8–3. For current purposes, the ability to recover a glottal source signal—such as the V̇$_g$ signal— is the central issue. There are three important features of the V̇$_g$ signal shown in Figure 8–2B.

First, as noted above for the A$_g$ signal, the V̇$_g$ signal is periodic, meaning that its characteristic shape repeats over time. The rate at which it repeats over time is the fundamental frequency (F0) of vocal fold vibration, or how many times per second the vocal folds go through complete cycles of vibration. In adult women, a typical F0 is around 190 to 200 Hz, in men around 115 to 125 Hz, and in 5-year-old children around 250 to 300 Hz (Kent, 1997; Lee, Potamianos, & Narayanan, 1999). As shown in Figure 8–2 the period (T) of this time-domain signal can be measured easily, and the inverse of the period is the F0 (see Chapter 7 for a discussion of $f = 1/T$).

The second important feature of the V̇$_g$ signal for the kind of phonation used by most people in ordinary conversation is the shape of the opening and closing portions of each cycle. The slope of the opening phase is shallower than the slope of the closing phase, making each cycle appear as if it is "leaning to the right." This shape feature is seen clearly in the V̇$_g$ signal of Figure 8–2B. The steepness of the closing phase is important because it reflects how rapidly the vocal folds come together as each cycle ends. The more rapidly the vocal folds come together, the steeper the closing part of the V̇$_g$ signal. This has great importance to the frequency domain characteristics of the source, as discussed in the next section.

The third important feature is that the V̇$_g$ signal shows some portions where the vocal folds are apart (i.e., where airflow is coming through the glottis), and some portions where the vocal folds are approximated. The ratio of open time to closed time for each cycle, which in normal voices is typically around 1.2:2 (i.e., the vocal folds open approximately 60% of each cycle), may be an important determinant of how much of the source signal is periodic and how much is aperiodic. This is important when considering the physiological and acoustical basis of pathological voice quality.

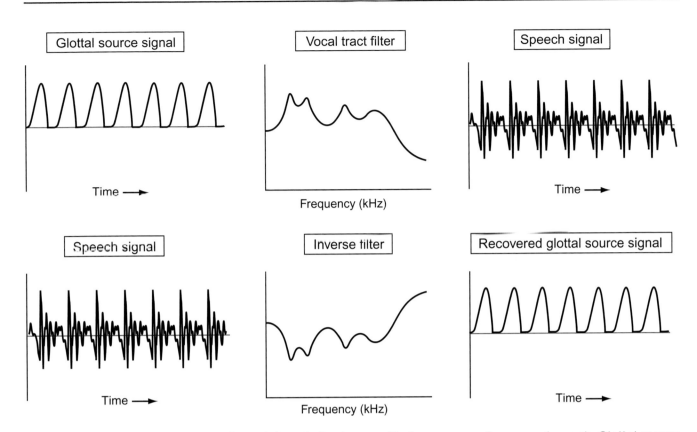

Figure 8–3. Schematic representation of steps in the inverse filtering process. *Top row of panels:* Glottal source signal serves as input to a multipeaked filter function associated with a vocal tract configuration and results in an output which is the speech signal recorded at the lips. The three-panel sequence summarizes the source-filter theory of vowel acoustics. *Bottom row of panels:* The output signal shown in the top right waveform now serves as the input to an "inverse filter," which is the "flipped" or mirror image of the filter function in the middle of the top row of panels. The inverse filter inverts the peaks shown in the top filter function and takes away the resonances from the input signal. The result of the process is the recovered glottal source signal shown in the bottom right panel. Figure provided courtesy of James Hillenbrand, Ph.D., Western Michigan University, Kalamazoo, Michigan. Reproduced with permission.

Figure 8–2 shows clearly that the $\dot{V}_g$ signal does not have a sinusoidal shape, but it is periodic. Material covered in Chapter 7 suggests, then, that the signal should be described as a complex periodic waveform. Determination of the frequency components of a complex periodic waveform requires analysis in the frequency domain, and, therefore, discussion of the spectral characteristics of the source waveform.

The Frequency Domain

Imagine that the $\dot{V}_g$ signal shown in Figure 8–4A was submitted to Fourier analysis to identify the frequency components contributing to this waveform. A typical spectrum resulting from this Fourier analysis would be like the one shown in Figure 8–4B. The important

features of this spectrum are: (a) there is a series of frequency components, at consecutive-integer multiples of the lowest-frequency component; and (b) the relative amplitudes of the frequency components decrease systematically as frequency increases. This is the *glottal source spectrum.*

The lowest frequency of the glottal source spectrum is the fundamental frequency (F0), which corresponds to the rate of vibration of the vocal folds. The F0 is also called the *first harmonic* (H1) of the source spectrum. The other frequency components in the glottal source spectrum are whole number multiples of the F0. There is a component at two times the F0 (the second harmonic, H2), three times the F0 (the third harmonic, H3), four times the F0 (the fourth harmonic, H4), and so on. In theory the number of harmonics in the glottal source spectrum is infinite, but the progressive

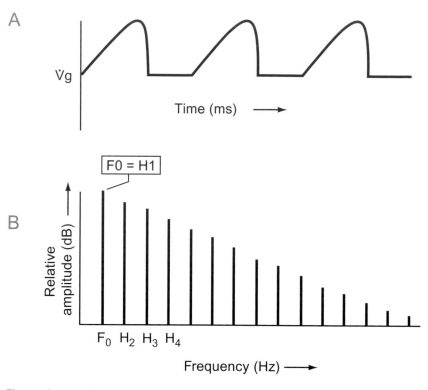

Figure 8–4. A. Time-domain and **B.** frequency-domain representations of vocal fold acoustics. The time domain is represented by the glottal airflow waveform ($\dot{V}_g$) and shows the acoustic result of vocal fold vibration. The frequency domain is represented by the glottal spectrum that results from vocal fold vibration and indicates F0, the fundamental frequency (first harmonic), and H2, H3, and H4 (the second, third, and fourth harmonics, respectively). The harmonics above H4 (arbitrarily chosen at the last-labeled harmonic on the graph) are whole-number multiples of the F0.

reduction in relative amplitude with increasing frequency greatly limits the significance of very high-frequency harmonics.

The reduction of energy (relative amplitude) in the harmonic components of the glottal source spectrum as frequency increases is clearly seen in Figure 8–4B. Moving from left (lower frequency) to right (higher frequency) on the *x*-axis, the vertical lines showing the amplitude of the components become progressively shorter. This energy reduction is systematic, with the relative amplitude decreasing approximately 12 dB for each octave increase in frequency. This gives the typical glottal spectrum a distinctly "tilted" appearance. As discussed below, changes in the nature of vocal fold vibration affect the extent to which the glottal spectrum is "tilted." In the summary of the time domain characteristics of the glottal source, three major characteristics were identified including: (a) the periodic nature of the waveform, (b) the shape of the waveform, and (c) the ratio of open to closed time. Discussion turns

now to how each of these features affects the glottal source spectrum.

The Periodic Nature of the Waveform

The $\dot{V}_g$ waveform repeats over time, is not sinusoidal, and is, therefore, a complex periodic event. The repetition of the $\dot{V}_g$ waveform is not perfectly periodic, but rather has very small variations in the periods of successive glottal cycles. This is why vocal fold vibration is referred to as *quasiperiodic*. Throughout this discussion, the term "period" refers to the average period—the small, period-to-period variations are not considered further here. The period of the glottal waveform depends on the rate of vibration of the vocal folds, which varies according to a number of factors including sex and age (see Chapter 3). Figure 8–5 shows two $\dot{V}_g$ waveforms (left part of figure) having different periods, and their associated glottal spectra (right part of figure). Note that both waveforms show the $\dot{V}_g$ over a

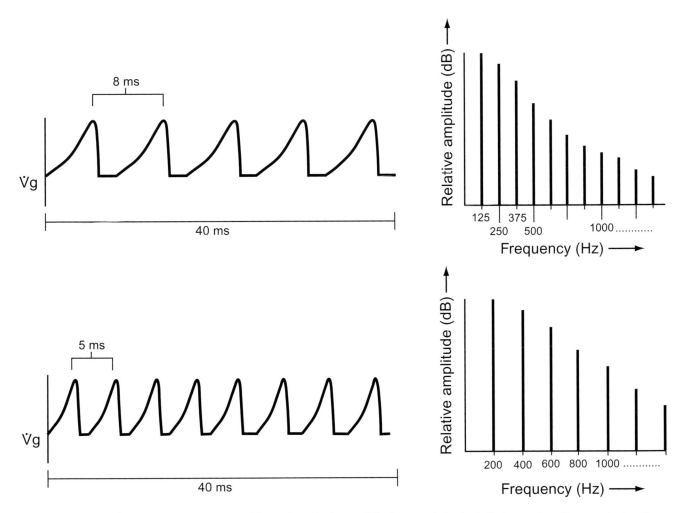

Figure 8–5. Two $\dot{V}_g$ waveforms having different periods, and their associated glottal spectra. *Top:* period = 8 ms, F0 = 125 Hz. *Bottom:* period = 5 ms, F0 = 200 Hz. Both waveforms show vibration of the vocal folds over a 40-ms interval. Note the greater number of cycles within this interval for the F0 = 200-Hz waveform (lower waveform), as compared to the F0 = 125-Hz waveform (*upper*). Note also in the glottal spectra the wider spacing of harmonics for F0 = 200 Hz (*bottom*), as compared to F0 = 125 Hz (*top*).

40-ms interval. The top waveform has a period of 8 ms (typical of many adult males), the inverse of which is an F0 of 125 Hz. This 125 Hz F0 is shown as the lowest-frequency component in the glottal spectrum to the right of the waveform. The bottom waveform has a period of 5 ms (typical of many adult females), the inverse of which is an F0 of 200 Hz. This F0 is shown as the lowest-frequency component in the corresponding glottal spectrum. The harmonics of the female glottal spectrum (bottom) are more widely separated than the harmonics of the male glottal spectrum (top). This follows from the fact that the glottal spectrum consists of a consecutive integer series of harmonics: Higher F0s will yield greater spacing between successive harmonics as compared to lower F0s. The glottal spectra of speakers with low F0s, therefore, are more densely packed with harmonics when compared to the glottal spectra of speakers with high F0s. This difference between the glottal spectra of low versus high F0s explains, in part, why spectrographic analysis of vowels produced by adult males tends to be easier than spectrographic analysis of vowels produced by adult females and children.

The Shape of the Waveform

The opening and closing parts of the $\dot{V}_g$ waveform create a shape that appears to be "leaning to the right," and the steepness of the closing slope reflects how rapidly the vocal folds return to the midline for each cycle.

There is a systematic relationship between this closing slope and the "tilt" of the glottal spectrum: the steeper the closing slope in the $\dot{V}_g$ waveform (the faster the vocal folds return to the midline on each cycle), the less tilted the glottal spectrum. This relationship is exemplified in Figure 8–6, where the $\dot{V}_g$ waveform on the left has a clearly steeper closing slope than the $\dot{V}_g$ waveform on the right (see arrows indicating slopes on the closing part of the waveforms). *CP* in Figure 8–6 is the closed phase of the glottal cycle, or the portion of each cycle when the vocal folds are fully approximated, whereas *OP* stands for open phase. Note the spectra associated with these two waveforms. The glottal spectrum for the waveform with the relatively steep closing slope shows reduction in relative amplitude with increasing frequency, but not nearly as dramatically as the glottal spectrum for the waveform with the shallower closing slope. The dashed line connecting the tops of the vertical lines in the two spectra shows the rapid reduction in

energy across frequency when the closing slope in the time-domain is shallow (right-hand part of figure), as compared to when it is steep (left-hand part of figure). The spectrum with the dramatic reduction in harmonic energy is said be more tilted than the spectrum with the more gradual reduction in energy. In theory, a glottal spectrum with "no tilt" would be one in which the relative amplitudes of all harmonic components were equal (the dashed line connecting the tops of the vertical lines would be strictly horizontal), and a glottal spectrum with "infinite tilt" would be one in which there was energy at the first harmonic (F0), but at no other frequencies.

Another way to express the concept of tilt of the glottal spectrum is to use the 12-dB-per-octave figure given above for the typical reduction in harmonic amplitude across frequency as a reference value. $\dot{V}_g$ waveforms with very steep closing slopes (e.g., Figure 8–6, left panel) should, therefore, have a smaller dB

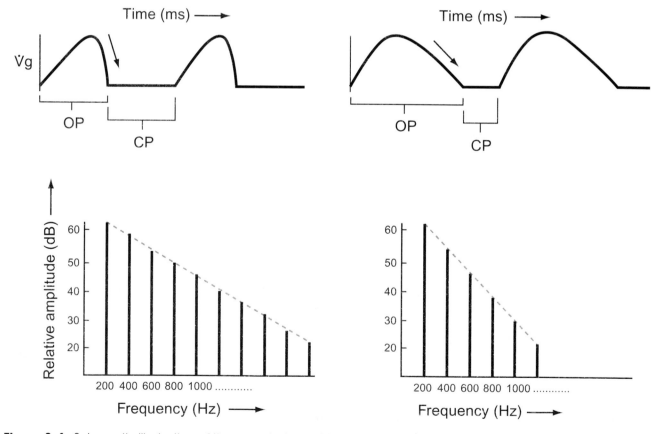

Figure 8–6. Schematic illustration of the speed of vocal fold closing and tilt of the glottal spectrum. The two upper panels show $\dot{V}_g$ waveforms, one with relatively rapid closure of the vocal folds (*left*), and one with relatively slow closure of the vocal folds (*right*). Relative speeds of closure are portrayed by the slope of the arrows alongside the closing phase of the functions. The glottal spectra immediately below the two waveforms demonstrate how speed of closure affects the tilt of the spectrum. OP = open phase (time). CP = closed phase (time).

Imperfect Perfection

The quasiperiodic nature of vocal fold vibration is largely a result of subtle aeromechanical imperfections. Vocal fold vibration is driven by aerodynamic forces and sustained by mechanical ones. These forces can hardly be expected to repeat themselves, across successive cycles, with perfect precision. If the forces do not repeat themselves exactly, the thing they are forcing—vibration of the vocal folds—will not either. In early versions of talking computers (speech synthesizers) scientists used a perfectly periodic, complex tone to simulate the source for vowels. Listeners didn't like it. It sounded mechanical, robotic, unfriendly. The solution was to take this complex periodic waveform and introduce into it a small amount of "jitter," or very minimal variation in the cycle-to-cycle period. Listeners found this much more pleasing. More human, you could say.

change per octave (<12 dB per octave), and those with very shallow closing slopes should have a larger dB change per octave (>12 dB per octave).

These concepts are important in understanding the physiological and acoustical bases of so-called *hyperfunctional* and *hypofunctional* voice disorders. In hyperfunctional voice disorders, the vocal folds move together too rapidly and forcefully on each closing phase of vocal fold vibration, resulting in a glottal spectrum with less-than-normal tilt, or too much energy in the higher-frequency harmonics. Listeners interpret this kind of voice quality as abnormal, sometimes using the term *pressed voice* to describe what they hear. A pressed voice sounds overly effortful or strained. In hypofunctional voice disorders, the vocal folds move together more slowly and less forcefully, the result being a highly tilted glottal spectrum because there is so little energy in the higher-frequency harmonics. This kind of voice is often heard by listeners as weak, breathy, and thin.

The Ratio of Open Time to Closed Time

For each cycle in a typical $\dot{V}_g$ waveform, the vocal folds are apart about 60% of the time, and approximated about 40% of the time. If the two waveforms in Figure 8–6 are examined, it is fairly obvious that a waveform with a shallower (slower) closing phase is also likely to have more open time throughout a complete

cycle. Similarly, a waveform with a steeper (faster) closing phase is likely to have a waveform with less open time and, therefore, a longer closed phase throughout a complete cycle. Because the speed of closing and the open time (and, therefore, the closed time) are in most cases correlated (greater speed, less open time; less speed, more open time), less open time will generally be associated with a less tilted glottal spectrum, and more open time with a more tilted glottal spectrum. The closing speed and ratio of open time to closed times (OP/CP) are, therefore, somewhat redundant descriptions of $\dot{V}_g$ waveforms (and spectral characteristics). However, in certain cases, they may provide independent information.

Nature of the Input Signal: A Summary

To answer the first question posed at the outset of this chapter, the precise nature of the input signal generated by the vibrating vocal folds is a complex periodic waveform whose spectrum consists of a consecutive-integer series of harmonics, at whole number multiples of the F0. The harmonics in the glottal spectrum systematically decrease in relative amplitude with increasing frequency. These harmonics serve as input to the vocal tract resonator, which shapes that input according to its resonant characteristics. Consideration turns now to the vocal tract resonator.

WHY SHOULD THE VOCAL TRACT BE CONCEPTUALIZED AS A TUBE CLOSED AT ONE END?

The vocal tract is an acoustic resonator. In Chapter 7, two general classes of acoustic resonators—Helmholtz and tube—are described. For the present discussion, accept on faith that the vocal tract is a tube resonator. It is easy to provide the proof of the tube-resonance characteristics of the vocal tract, as shown in a later section of this chapter.

If the vocal tract is regarded as a tube resonator, the question must be asked, "Does it resonate as a tube open at both ends, or closed at one end?" The answer to this question requires a brief reconsideration of the vibrating vocal folds, and how this vibration influences the acoustic output of the vocal tract.

Figure 8–7 shows two signals in the time domain, collected synchronously during phonation of a vowel. The upper signal is $\dot{V}_g$, discussed above at some length. Note the upward pointing arrows at the end of the

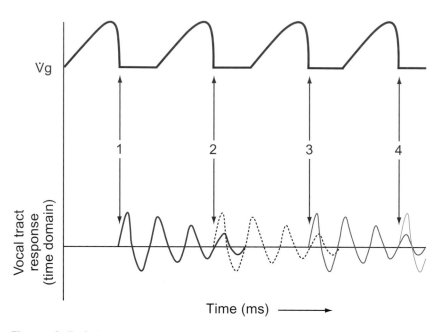

Figure 8–7. Schematic waveforms showing excitation of a vocal tract resonance (*bottom waveform*) by the vibrating vocal folds (*top waveform*). The top waveform, $\dot{V}_g$, shows four periods, with the instant of closing for each cycle marked by an upward-pointing arrow. The waveform of the vocal tract response shows a damped vibration at a resonant frequency of 500 Hz. This vibration is initiated each time the vocal folds snap shut, indicated by the downward-pointing arrows. The amplitude of the damped vocal tract resonance decays over time. Each new excitation of the resonance may overlap with the previous one, resulting in overlap (and summation) of the two damped response waveforms. All of the vocal tract resonances are excited by the closing of the vocal folds, but only a single resonance waveform (for 500 Hz) is shown for the sake of clarity.

cycles in the $\dot{V}_g$ signal. These arrows mark the instant in time at which the vocal folds snap together during each cycle of vibration. At these instants, when the airflow through the glottis is suddenly blocked by closure of the airway, the air immediately above the vocal folds becomes compressed and sends a pressure wave through the vocal tract. Now, consider the situation just described. At the glottal boundary of the vocal tract, there is, for an instant, no airflow and the air molecules become compressed, whereas at the open, oral boundary of the vocal tract air molecules move freely between the lips. This appears very much like the aeromechanical conditions found in a resonating tube closed at one end, where pressure is maximum at the closed end and flow is maximum at the open end (see Chapter 7). In fact, each time the vocal folds snap together, a pressure wave is set up in the vocal tract, and this wave obeys the rules of resonance in a tube closed at one end. Another way to say this is that the

vocal tract resonances are excited each time the vibrating vocal folds snap together. Because the excitation occurs when the folds approximate and the oral end of the vocal tract is open for vowel production, the vocal tract resonates like a tube closed at one end.

In Chapter 7, a model of resonance was described in which a hammer was used to tap a resonator, thus exciting the resonant frequency (Helmholtz resonator) or frequencies (tube resonator). Imagine the hammer being controlled by a periodic motor, rotating it toward the resonator and striking it, then pulling back away, rotating it back toward the resonator and striking it again, and so forth. The continuous motion of the hammer back and forth, toward and away from the resonator, is obviously important to producing the excitation of the resonator, but the actual *instant* of excitation of the resonator corresponds only to the point in time when the hammer strikes the resonator. The analogy to excitation of the vocal tract resonances is direct.

The motion of the vibrating vocal folds (the swing of the hammer) is important to the resonance of the vocal tract, but the actual excitation of the resonances occurs only at the instant in time of vocal fold approximation (the tap of the hammer on the resonator).

The Response of the Vocal Tract to Excitation

What does it mean to say that the vocal tract resonances are *excited* each time the vibrating vocal folds snap together? The answer is found in the bottom trace of Figure 8–7, where a waveform is initiated each time the vocal folds snap together. For purposes of simplification, a waveform for only a single resonant frequency is shown in the bottom signal of Figure 8–7, but waveforms are initiated for each resonant frequency of the tube. Think of the vocal tract response waveform shown in Figure 8–7 as corresponding to the first resonance of the tube, with a frequency of 500 Hz. The period of that waveform is 2 ms ($500 = 1/T$, $T = .002$ s or 2 ms). Note how the resonance waveform at the first excitation is initiated with relatively great amplitude, which then declines over each successive cycle until the vibration dies out completely (red waveform). In the example of Figure 8–7 note also that the resonance may be *re*-excited before the previous waveform has completely died out (compare the amplitude of the vocal tract response from excitation 1 (red waveform) and excitation 2 (black, dashed-line waveform). The large, 500-Hz vocal tract vibration at excitation 2 overlaps the small (decaying) vibration from excitation 1. Similar "re-excitations" are shown at excitations 3 (blue waveform) and 4 (green waveform). If Figure 8–7 showed the waveforms of all the excited and re-excited resonances, the vocal tract response signal would be visually too "busy" to illustrate the main point of this discussion. The main point is that the vocal tract responds to excitation with damped oscillations at each of its resonant frequencies. The oscillations are damped, meaning they die out over time because there is energy loss in the vocal tract due to the factors discussed in Chapter 7 (friction, absorption, and radiation).

To this point, emphasis has been placed on the time-domain characteristics of the source signal and the response of the vocal tract. The focus now turns to the question of how the vocal tract resonances shape the input signal to produce an acoustic output. Stated more simply: "What is the acoustic basis of the events known as vowel sounds?" The best approach to this problem is to consider the source signal and vocal tract resonances in frequency-domain terms.

Of Beer Bottles and Vocal Tracts

When the vocal tract is excited by the sudden "snapping shut" of the vocal folds, the excitation has the form of a glottal spectrum. A series of such excitations, such as the 190 or so per second expected for an adult female, gives the excitation spectrum its "nice" form of discrete harmonics. This harmonic spectrum is shaped by the vocal tract filter. A historical footnote in speech acoustics was the idea that the excitation of the vocal tract was like the edge tones described in the Chapter 7 sidetrack titled, "Beer and Flutes." In this view, the resonant chambers of the vocal tract are excited by the individual puffs of air coming through the vocal folds during each cycle of vibration. The air puffs "force" air in the vocal tract into resonance, much like blowing across a beer bottle opening forces the air inside the bottle to produce a tone. This footnote view was called the "inharmonic theory" of vocal tract acoustics; it is not correct. The correct view is called the "harmonic theory," for obvious reasons. The vocal tract shapes an acoustic spectrum according to its resonant properties, rather than having its resonant frequencies "forced" into vibration by an aerodynamic event such as the air puff.

HOW ARE THE ACOUSTIC PROPERTIES OF THE VOCAL TRACT DETERMINED?

As discussed in Chapter 7, acoustic resonators can be described in the frequency domain by a resonance curve (see Figure 7–18). The peak of the resonance curve defines the resonant frequency of the resonator, and the width of the curve between the 3-dB-down points — the bandwidth — provides an index of the amount of energy loss in the vibration. Assume, for this discussion, a vocal tract shape associated with the schwa (/ə/), a shape very much like a tube having uniform cross-sectional area from the glottis to the lips. This shape is like that of the straight tubes considered in Chapter 7, for which there are no constrictions, or narrowings, along the entire length of the tube. With such a tube, one should be able to simply apply the quarter-wavelength rule to obtain the multiple peaks of the resonance curve, provided the tube length is known. The shapes of the resonance curves (determined by the bandwidths) are also important, so some additional calculations would be necessary to arrive at a full resonance curve for the vocal tract tube.

If the mathematical tools were available to determine the bandwidths of the multiple resonances, the resonance curve for a vocal tract tube 15 cm in length and shaped for the vowel schwa would look something like the one shown in Figure 8–8. As expected, the lowest (first) resonant frequency is at $c/4l = 560$ Hz (where $c = 33,600$ cm/s and $l = 15$ cm), the second at 1680 Hz (3×560) and the third at 2800 Hz (5×560). Although the vocal tract tube has, like any other tube, an infinite number of resonances, only the first three are shown for the sake of clarity (as well as for other reasons that will become apparent as this discussion proceeds).

The bandwidths are indicated for each peak of the resonance curve by the range of frequencies between the 3-dB-down points. For the present discussion, the bandwidths for each of the three resonances have been set to 60 Hz.

The example in Figure 8–8 was generated using simple principles established in Chapter 6 (the quarter-wavelength rule), as well as an "on faith" assumption about bandwidths. Fant (1960) needed a more comprehensive theory, however, because for most vowels the vocal tract tube does not have a uniform cross-sectional area from the glottis to the lips. Rather, *vocal tract configurations* typically involve constrictions along the path from glottis to lips, some of which are extremely small (often referred to as "tight" constrictions). Fant

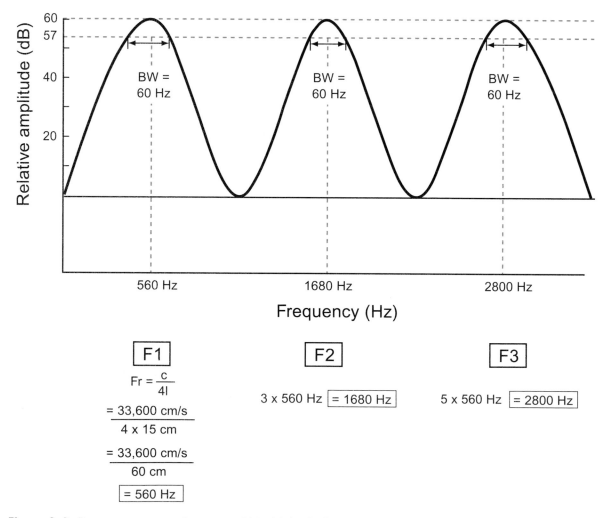

Figure 8-8. Resonance curve for a vocal tract tube in the shape of the schwa /ə/ and having a length of 15 cm. The resonant frequencies along the curve were computed by the quarter-wavelength rule, and the bandwidth of each resonance was assumed to be 60 Hz. Only the first three resonances of the tube are shown.

approached the problem of drawing the resonance curves for different vocal tract shapes in the following way. He took sagittal x-ray pictures of an adult male speaker's productions of a variety of Russian and Swedish vowels. The soft and hard tissues of the speaker's vocal tract (tongue, lips, hard palate, velum, part of the pharynx) were coated with barium paste, which allowed easier identification of the outlines of structures in the developed film. Figure 8–9 shows a magnetic resonance image (MRI) of a speaker producing a high back vowel, with the boundaries of the air tube outlined and the air tube itself slightly shaded. The outlined and shaded tube includes boundaries defined by the walls of the larynx superior to the vocal folds, the pharynx, hard palate, velum, tongue, lips, and other surfaces. Although Figure 8–9 is an image type much more advanced than the standard x-ray

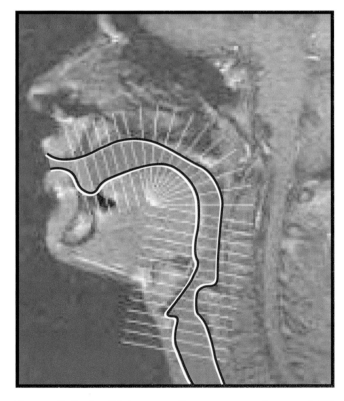

Figure 8–9. Sagittal magnetic resonance image (MRI) of a male speaker producing a vocal tract configuration for the vowel /u/. Boundaries of the vocal tract (tongue surface, hard and soft palates, pharynx, and so forth) are outlined to show the shape of the vocal tract tube and how its dimensions vary from glottis to lips. Background image obtained from Audiovisual-to-Articulatory Speech Inversion (ASPI). Retrieved September 2, 2012, from http://aspi.loria.fr. Reproduced with permission.

images used by Fant, his approach can be explained just as effectively using the MRI example. Fant used the x-rays he obtained of many different vowels to outline the varied vocal tract shapes. When the structures are outlined in this way, the column of air extending from the glottis to the lips can be conceptualized as a tube of varying cross-sectional area.

The vocal tract length of the speaker studied by Fant (1960) was approximately 17.5 cm. Fant plotted the varying cross-sectional area of the vocal tract by estimating the area of the air tube at 0.5-cm increments from glottis to lips. This kind of "sectioning off" of the vocal tract is shown in Figure 8–9 by the sequence of straight lines drawn through the vocal tract tube which is outlined in red. If a line is imagined running straight forward from the glottis to the lips, along the long axis of the vocal tract, each of the straight lines seen in Figure 8–9 can be thought of as intersecting this long axis line at a right angle. The part of the intersecting line within the vocal tract—between the red outline in Figure 8–9—defines the "size" of the vocal tract tube at that location. The distance between adjacent lines defines a small section, or "tubelette" within the vocal tract (Story, 2005), for which width measurements can be made. For example, the tubelettes are quite narrow toward the back of the oral cavity, where the tongue is raised toward the boundary of the hard and soft palates. However, the tubelettes are much wider toward the front of the vocal tract. Fant sectioned his vocal tract images into 35 "pieces" (2 measurements per cm of vocal tract, 2 × 17.5 = 35). The width of each one of these section lines was measured and entered into a simple formula used to compute the area for that slice of the vocal tract. What emerged from this exercise was an *area function of the vocal tract*.

Area Function of the Vocal Tract

An area function of the vocal tract is a plot of cross-sectional area as a function of distance along the vocal tract from glottis to lips. This distance is described by the succession of the measurement "slices" shown in Figure 8–9. Figure 8–10 shows an area function for the vowel /i/. Here area, in cm^2, is plotted on the y-axis and section (slice) number (i.e., distance) is plotted on the x-axis. The low section numbers are near the glottis (i.e., section 1 is immediately above the glottis), and the measurement moves toward the lips from left to right. Each section number has an area value, so the function is actually a string of discrete points. For illustration purposes, the discrete points have been connected and the area function is represented in Figure 8–10 as a

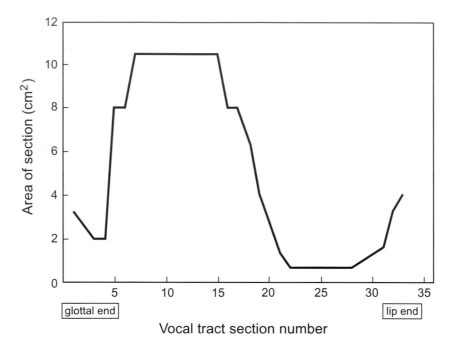

Figure 8-10. Area function for the vowel /i/ plotted from data reported by Fant (1960, p. 115). Vocal tract section number (from 1 to 35, with sections extending from the glottis to the lips) is plotted on the *x*-axis. Cross-sectional area (in cm²) is plotted on the *y*-axis. Even though the cross-sectional area is measured in discrete steps (for each section), individual points are connected by a straight line to give the impression of a continuous area function.

continuous line. This is justified because the measurements of successive slices were made sufficiently close together (in 0.5-cm increments) to minimize the likelihood of major changes in cross-sectional vocal tract area between the measurement steps along the vocal tract length.

The area function in Figure 8–10 shows relatively large cross-sectional areas in the lower and upper pharyngeal regions (the left side of the *x*-axis), with relatively smaller areas toward the front of the vocal tract. A very tight constriction — that is, small cross-sectional areas — is present between sections 22 and 27. This function is intuitively consistent with phonetic descriptions of the vowel /i/ as a high-front vowel, where the major constriction is in the front of the vocal tract.[1]

The area functions supplied the link between the configuration of the vocal tract tube, as shaped by the oral and pharyngeal structures, and the resonant frequencies of that tube. Fant (1960) developed a mathematical technique for estimating the tube resonances

from the area function. The specifics of the mathematical technique are not covered here, but the conceptual link between the area function and estimation of vocal tract resonant frequencies is straightforward, and makes use of information developed in Chapter 7. Chapter 7 described the role of mass and compliance in determining the resonant frequency of an acoustical resonator. Imagine that the air contained within the boundaries of any two adjacent measurement points (that is, within a tubelette corresponding to the small air column between two measurement lines) has certain mass and compliance properties. If these properties are specified for each of the 35 sections of air, all of the information relevant to the resonant frequencies of the vocal tract should be available. Fant's mathematical theory allowed him to estimate mass and compliance properties from the area measurement for each section, or tubelette. Based on the mass and compliance estimates from *all* 35 sections, the theory produced an estimate of the resonant pattern for the entire

---

[1]The relatively large areas in the back portion of the vocal tract may not be intuitive from a standard phonetic perspective, which typically classifies vowels according to: (a) the degree of tongue advancement and (b) the height of the tongue. Neither of these classificatory dimensions implies anything about the size of the pharyngeal airway, especially just above the glottis.

vocal tract. When mathematical information concerning energy loss factors was included, Fant was able to draw the complete resonance curve (resonant frequencies and bandwidths as in Figure 8–8) for a given vocal tract configuration.

The conceptual basis of Fant's (1960) theory is, therefore, fairly simple. If the mass and compliance characteristics of the vocal tract tube can be determined, the resonance curve for the tube can be constructed. Because the vocal tract resonates like a tube, there are multiple peaks (i.e., resonances) along the resonance curve, each with its own bandwidth.

At this point in the development of Fant's (1960) theory, it is important to recognize that the vocal tract resonance curve is computed from the measured area function. The resonant peaks are determined mathematically, rather than being measured by analyzing the spectrum of a produced vowel. For this reason the computed resonance curve is called a *theoretical spectrum*, or a *filter function*. This theoretical spectrum, or filter function, shows where the resonances for this particular vocal tract configuration should be. The term *filter function* is particularly interesting, because it implies that the vocal tract acts like a filter, allowing energy to pass through only at certain frequencies. The regions of the spectrum where energy passes through, of course, are those regions at and in the immediate vicinity of the resonant peaks. The next section discusses the way in which the source spectrum and filter function (theoretical spectrum) are combined to produce an output spectrum—a measured spectrum, as for a phonated vowel. This discussion will show why the theoretical spectrum (the filter function) is not always exactly the same as the output spectrum (the spectrum of a produced vowel).

HOW DOES THE VOCAL TRACT SHAPE THE INPUT SIGNAL? (HOW IS THE SOURCE SPECTRUM COMBINED WITH THE THEORETICAL VOCAL TRACT SPECTRUM TO PRODUCE A VOCAL TRACT OUTPUT?)

The two questions heading this section are merely variants of the same problem, which is to determine how the acoustic characteristics of the source and vocal tract combine to produce a vocal tract output, which in this case is a vowel sound. The frequency-domain representation of the vocal tract output is called an *output spectrum*. This is the spectrum measured, with appropriate instruments, from an actual vowel produced by a talker.

Figure 8–11 presents a simple graphic answer to the question posed above. The input (source) spectrum, as described in a preceding section, is shown at the left of the figure. The filter function is shown in the middle of the figure as a resonance curve with three peaks,

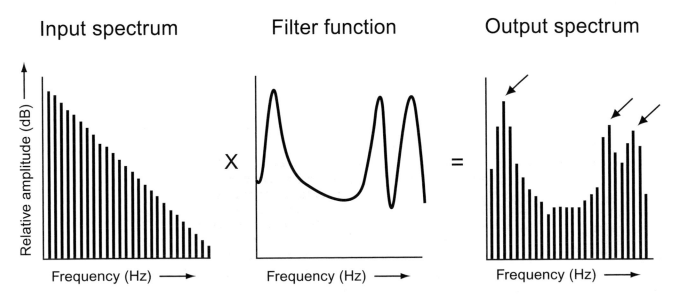

Figure 8–11. Schematic representation of how the source or input spectrum and filter function are combined to produce a vocal tract output. The left panel depicts the input spectrum, the middle panel the filter function for a vocal tract in an /i/ configuration, and the right panel the output spectrum. The output spectrum shows which harmonics are and are not emphasized by combining the input and filter functions. The peaks in the output spectrum are formants (F1, F2, F3) representing the first three resonant frequencies of the vocal tract.

corresponding to the first three resonances of a vocal tract tube in an /i/ shape. Note the multiplication sign between the input spectrum and filter function. To determine the output of the vocal tract (the right panel in Figure 8–11), the energy in the input spectrum is multiplied by the energy in the filter function.[2] To be a little more explicit about what this process of multiplication means, the axes of both the input (source) spectrum and the filter function are the same—frequency on the x-axis, relative amplitude on the y-axis (i.e., they are both spectra). The input spectrum shows the relative amplitude of discrete frequency components, and the filter function shows the frequencies at which energy applied to it will be "amplified" (the resonances) or "de-emphasized" (the valleys of the resonance curve, between the resonances). The multiplication described here is simply another way to understand the shaping of the input (source) spectrum by the filter function. The harmonics in the input (source) spectrum will be shaped by the form of the filter function. At resonant frequencies of the filter function, energy in the input (source) spectrum is multiplied strongly, and appears in the output spectrum as prominent energy components. At valleys in the filter function, energy in the input (source) spectrum is multiplied weakly or not at all, and does not appear (or appears only weakly) in the output spectrum.

The result of the multiplication of the input (source) spectrum by the filter function (equivalently, the shaping of the input [source] spectrum by the filter function) is indicated by the "=" sign and shown in the output spectrum of Figure 8–11. This spectrum shows the harmonics, now reshaped from their form in the input (source) spectrum. An important feature of the glottal source spectrum is the systematic decrease in harmonic amplitude as frequency increases, but in this output spectrum some of the higher frequency harmonics actually have greater relative amplitude than some of the lower frequency harmonics. This is because of the shaping of the input (source) spectrum by the filter function, which emphasizes some higher frequency harmonics while de-emphasizing some lower frequency harmonics. The rise and fall of the harmonic amplitudes in the output spectrum of Figure 8–11 follow pretty closely the locations of the resonances in the filter function. However, all of the peaks in the filter function were computed as having

roughly equal amplitudes, but in the output spectrum the higher-frequency "peaks" (see arrows) have less amplitude than the lower-frequency peaks (note the decline in peak amplitude across the three peaks in the output spectrum). This is because the energy available in the input (source) spectrum decreases with increasing frequency, meaning there is less energy to multiply by the roughly equivalent peaks in the filter function. So, an output spectrum may show a general decrease in harmonic energy with increasing frequency, but in some cases higher frequency harmonics have greater amplitude than lower-frequency harmonics.

The distinction between harmonics in the source (input) spectrum and peaks in the output spectrum can be confusing, so it is useful to pursue this description a little further. In the output spectrum of Figure 8–11, there is a series of harmonics whose amplitudes rise and fall according to peaks and valleys of the filter function. But there is no systematic relationship between the frequency locations of the harmonics in the source (input) spectrum and the frequencies of the peaks in the filter function. The frequencies in the source (input) spectrum are determined by the rate of vibration of the vocal folds (the F0), and the frequencies of the peaks in the filter function are determined by the configuration of the vocal tract. In the acoustic theory of vowel production the source and filter are independent.[3] Two simple examples of the independence of the source and filter in the theory are as follows: (a) for a given speaker, the same vowel (produced by a single filter function) can be produced with many different F0s and, therefore, many different source spectra; and (b) for a given speaker, many different vowels can be produced with the same F0. Thus, either the source or the filter can be adjusted without affecting characteristics of the other component.

A graphic example (Figure 8–12) illustrates the independence of the source and filter in the acoustic theory of vowel production. The example also highlights a distinction in the theory between *computed and measured* resonances. Figure 8–12 shows two graphs, both of which have a computed (theoretical) filter function with resonances at 300 Hz (.3 kHz), 2300 Hz (2.3 kHz), and 3000 Hz (3.0 kHz). This filter function would be a reasonable set of formant frequencies for an adult male's production of /i/. Because the source spectrum and filter function are shown as spectra,

---

[2]The idea of the source being multiplied by the energy in the filter function is somewhat of a simplification, but one that does not violate the essentials of the theory. In precise mathematical terms, the output of the vocal tract is determined by the convolution of source and filter energy. It is like a "blending" of the source and filter functions.

[3]This statement is true for the purposes of this textbook; it can be shown that there are some effects of the filter on the source under certain conditions, but these are beyond the scope of this text.

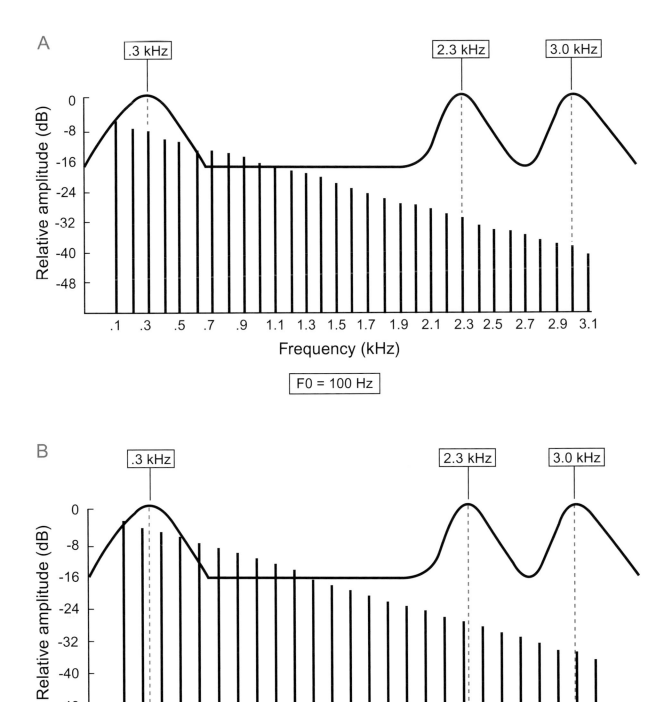

Figure 8-12. A single filter function (appropriate for the vowel /i/) superimposed on two source spectra having different fundamental frequencies and, therefore, different spacing between harmonics. In panels A and B, the filter function is superimposed on a source spectrum having an F0 = 100 Hz and 120 Hz, respectively. When F0 = 100 Hz, frequencies of the harmonics match the frequencies of the computed resonances of 300 Hz, 2300 Hz, and 3000 Hz. When F0 = 120 Hz, frequencies of the harmonics do not match the first and second resonances, but do match the third resonance (120 × 25 = 3000 Hz).

Hardheaded Speech Acoustics

First (Chapter 7) we used a hammer analogy for the excitation of resonators, then in the previous sidetrack we said that wasn't exactly the way the vocal tract was excited for speech, now we're going to say that the vocal tract *can* be excited "inharmonically," if you care to do so. Vowel-like vocal tract sounds can be produced by banging the skull (usually toward the front of the head, in the middle, with your knuckles) with the vocal tract open (flicking the neck with your fingers can produce roughly the same effect). Try this with your vocal tract in the shape of the vowel in "oh" and then "ee." You'll probably hear the difference, and most certainly a listener will. This is simply the case of the vocal tract being excited by a source different from the harmonic glottal spectrum. The vocal tract will respond with damped oscillation of the resonant frequencies, "ringing" in response to the skull bangs.

one can superimpose two different source spectra on these identical filter functions. Source spectra with F0s of 100 Hz and 120 Hz are shown in Figures 8–12A and 8–12B, respectively. Because the F0s of these two source spectra are slightly different (by 20 Hz), so are the frequencies of the consecutive-integer series of harmonics. For example, for the F0 of 100 Hz there is a 3rd harmonic at 300 Hz, a 23rd harmonic at 2300 Hz, and a 30th harmonic at 3000 Hz. In this case, there is harmonic energy *exactly* at the location of the computed resonances of the filter function, as well as harmonic energy 100 Hz above and below these frequencies. The harmonic energy around the peaks in this filter function, but especially exactly at the peaks, will contribute to emphasizing energy in the output spectrum in the immediate region of the computed peaks.

In fact, when the energy in this source spectrum is multiplied by the values along the filter functions, the peaks in the output spectrum are likely to coincide exactly with the computed (theoretical) peaks because there is harmonic energy precisely at the location of the computed peaks. This is the case for the superimposed source and filter characteristics in Figure 8–12A.

Now consider the case of the source spectrum and filter function in Figure 8–12B. Here the F0 of 120 Hz does *not* produce harmonics coinciding exactly with the computed peaks at 300 Hz and 2300 Hz, but the

25th harmonic matches the resonance at 3000 Hz. For example, the second and third harmonics in this source spectrum are located at 240 and 360 Hz, values only in the general neighborhood of the computed first resonance at 300 Hz. Similarly, the 19th and 20th harmonics of 120 Hz are located at 2280 and 2400 Hz, values that do not coincide exactly with the computed second resonance of 2300 Hz. When the energy at these harmonic frequencies is multiplied by the values along the filter function, the general region around the first and second computed resonances is emphasized in the output spectrum, but the location of these peaks in the output spectrum may not coincide exactly with the theoretical peaks in the filter function.

Harmonics in the source spectrum are not *purposely* matched up with the locations of the computed (theoretical) peaks of the filter function. They do not have to be matched up in this manner, because the general region of resonance given by a computed peak is emphasized in either case (i.e., whether or not a harmonic is exactly located at a peak in the filter function). But this discussion explains why the output peaks in the measured spectrum may not coincide exactly with the computed (theoretical) peaks in the filter function. A computed (filter function) and measured (output spectrum) peak are exactly the same only when a harmonic in the source spectrum has the same frequency as a *computed* resonance.

The general regions of resonance in the output spectrum have been emphasized in this discussion, rather than specific values of harmonics. In the output spectra—the kinds of spectra typically measured in the laboratory—these regions of high energy are called *formants*. Because the individual harmonics are not of great importance, output spectra are typically shown as smooth curves that can be described as tracing an *envelope* along the varying harmonic amplitudes resulting from the shaping of the source spectrum by the filter function. Figure 8–13 presents output spectra for the isolated vowels /i/ (top spectrum), /ɑ/ (middle spectrum), and /u/ (bottom spectrum), spoken by an adult male. These spectra show how a *spectral envelope* can be drawn by connecting the tops of the harmonic lines with a smooth curve. The harmonic spectra in Figure 8–13 were generated with Fourier analysis, whereas the smooth, spectral envelopes superimposed on the tops of the harmonics were generated by linear predictive code (LPC) analysis, a special computer algorithm for locating formant frequencies (discussed more fully in Chapter 10). Each spectral envelope shows three peaks, labeled *F1*, *F2*, and *F3* (F1 = first formant, F2 = second formant, F3 = third formant). The higher frequency

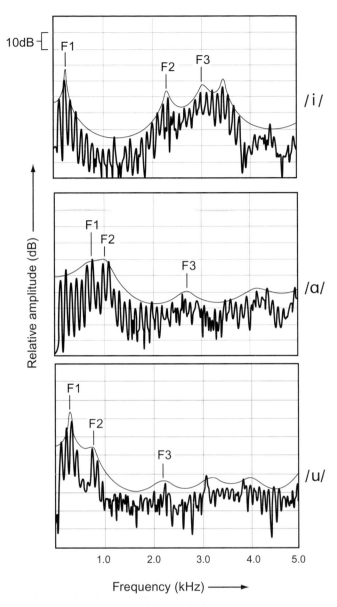

Figure 8-13. Output spectra for the vowels /i/ (*top panel*), /ɑ/ (*middle panel*), and /u/ (*bottom panel*), showing how the tops of the harmonics computed by Fourier analysis can be connected to draw a smooth curve, or spectral envelope, computed by linear predictive code (LPC) analysis. The peaks in the envelope are the formant frequencies, marked F1, F2, and F3 in each spectrum. Spectra are shown for the 0- to 5-kHz range. Each vertical division (*y*-axis, relative amplitude) is equal to 10 dB.

peaks in the output spectrum do not seem to be particularly important for either the acoustic or perceptual specification of vowels, so the frequency locations of the measured peaks—the formant frequencies—will dominate the discussion of vowels.

A great deal of research, some of which is reviewed in Chapter 11, has shown that the first three peaks in a vowel spectrum have great importance for the acoustic and perceptual specification of vowel identity. The frequency locations of these first three peaks is sometimes referred to as the *F-pattern* of a vowel, and this terminology will be used throughout this text. For example, the F patterns of the vowels shown in Figure 8–13 are F1 = 237, F2 = 2283, and F3 = 3058 Hz for /i/, F1 = 775, F2 = 1012, F3 = 2713 Hz for /ɑ/, and F1 = 280, F2 = 732, and F3 = 2218 Hz for /u/ (measurements made by author GW). Although the F-pattern of a vowel is always stated in terms of these three frequencies, the exact frequency value attached to each of the formants does not mean that other frequencies in the vowel spectrum are unimportant in the acoustic and perceptual specification of vowels. It is better to think of these numbers as *center frequencies* denoting a region of *spectral prominence*. In the region of spectral prominence for each formant, there is a small range of frequencies that reflects the resonance characteristics of the vocal tract (recall the discussion of bandwidth in Chapter 7). The F-pattern is always stated with respect to the frequencies measured at the highest peaks in the output spectrum.

All /i/'s and /u/'s Are Not Created Equal

As Fant proposed, formant frequencies completely specify vowels, but the more you look into the relationship between formant values and vowel identity, the more you realize this statement requires some qualification. One such qualification has emerged from the recent trend in speech acoustics research comparing acoustic phonetic data between different languages. Although many different languages "share" certain vowels, such as /i/ and /u/, the formant frequencies often differ across the languages. How is it that the same vowel—at least, one transcribed with the same phonetic symbol—has a different F-pattern in different languages? Think about it. We'll tell you more in Chapter 11.

---

peaks typically have somewhat lower amplitude than the lower frequency peaks, primarily because the energy in the source spectrum decreases with increasing frequency (see above). The relative amplitudes of

Formant Bandwidths

Chapter 7 presented a brief discussion of the factors responsible for energy loss in acoustic systems. These factors, which include friction, absorption, and radiation, are all operative in the vocal tract and contribute to the shape of the resonances (formants) in the output spectrum.

When air molecules vibrate within the vocal tract they rub against each other and also against soft and hard tissues. This friction generates heat, which dissipates a small amount of the vibratory energy. The vibration of the air molecules may also be taken up by nearby structures whose own resonant frequencies are close to the frequencies propagated through the vocal tract. For example, the cheeks and possibly the tongue appear to have resonant frequencies in the neighborhood of 200 Hz, close to the typical first formant frequencies of several vowels (Fujimura & Lindquist, 1971). When a formant frequency is close to the resonant frequency of a structure such as the cheek, the tissue will absorb some of the energy and transform it into its own vibratory event. This absorption of acoustic energy by vocal tract structures is another form of energy loss and contributes to the damping of vocal tract resonances. Under certain conditions, such as when the nasal cavities are connected to the oral cavity or the oral cavity is connected to the subglottal cavities (e.g., the trachea) because the vocal folds are abducted, the amount of energy loss may be greatly increased partly because there is more tissue to absorb sound energy. Thus, nasalized vowels tend to have greater formant bandwidths than nonnasalized vowels, and the bandwidth of the first formant is greater when a vowel is produced with breathy, as compared to regular, phonation. Finally, the radiation of sound from the mouth results in some loss of energy as the sound changes environment from an enclosed tube (the vocal tract) to the open atmosphere. Megaphones are effective in transmitting sound over a relatively great distance partly because their gradually flared design decreases the radiation loss from the vocal tract to the atmosphere. The flare of the megaphone provides a gradual transition from the vocal tract shape to the "shape" of the atmosphere, reducing the amount of energy loss in the propagation of sound from the vocal tract to the atmosphere.

Table 8–1 (data from Fujimura & Lindqvist, 1971) contains some estimates of formant bandwidths, and provides a rough range of the formant values associated with the bandwidths. The formant values are provided to support the statement that vowel resonances are relatively *sharply tuned*. In other words, the

Table 8–1. Approximate Bandwidths of the First (F1), Second (F2), and Third (F3) Formants of Vowels; Frequency Ranges for Those Formants Are Also Provided.

	F1	F2	F3
Bandwidth	45–90	40–90	40–150
Formant Frequency Ranges	250–800	500–2500	2400–3300

Source: These data were taken from graphs published by Fujimura and Lindqvist (1971). All values are in Hz, and include data for men and women.

resonances in the spectrum have rather narrow bandwidths compared to the actual frequencies of those resonances. For example, bandwidths of 45 to 90 Hz are relatively narrow compared to typical F1 values which range between 250 and 800 Hz, depending on the vowel. These bandwidths are very definitely narrow compared to the higher formant frequency values for F2 and F3.

How does bandwidth affect the acoustic categorization and perception of vowel sounds? Earlier it was noted that the F-pattern (the first three formant frequencies) seemed to be sufficient as an acoustic index of vowels. Information on formant amplitudes and bandwidths does not seem to be particularly useful for the acoustic categorization of vowels. When speech synthesizers are used to systematically increase the bandwidth of vowel formants while maintaining constant formant frequencies, listeners do not hear a change in vowel category. Rather, vowels are perceived as increasingly "muffled" as bandwidths are increased. This "muffling" effect is sometimes heard in the speech of children and adults with craniofacial deficits and associated velopharyngeal incompetence. The perception of muffled vowels in these speakers may be explained, in part, by the increased bandwidths resulting from the undesired coupling of the oral and nasal cavities. Even though the increased "muffling" of vowel quality may not have an effect on the perception of vowel categories, there may be an effect on general speech intelligibility and naturalness.

Acoustic Theory of Vowel Production: A Summary

Information presented to this point can be summarized as follows. First, the input, or source, for vowel production is the acoustic result of vocal fold vibration. This acoustic event can be described in the frequency domain as a series of consecutive integer harmonics whose energy systematically decreases with increasing frequency. The exact shape of this glottal spectrum depends on how fast the vocal folds snap together on each cycle of vibration. When the vocal folds snap together very quickly, the harmonic energy decreases relatively slowly with increasing frequency (less tilted spectrum). When the vocal folds move together slowly, the harmonic energy decreases relatively rapidly with frequency (more tilted spectrum).

The resonator in vowel acoustics is the vocal tract, which extends from the top margin of the vocal folds to the lips. The vocal tract resonates like a tube closed at one end, the closed end being the vocal folds, the open end being the lips. The vocal tract resonances are excited at the instant of closure for each cycle of vocal fold vibration. This excitation causes the vocal tract to respond with an infinite series of damped resonances.

A mathematical theory developed by Fant (1960) relates the area function of the vocal tract to the specific resonant frequencies of the tube. The area function is a plot of the cross-sectional area of the vocal tract from glottis to lips, and can be thought of as a description of the shape of the air column formed by the articulators and the more or less fixed structures of the vocal tract (such as the posterior pharyngeal wall and hard palate). By using this shape to estimate the mass and compliance of consecutive sections of the air column, Fant was able to calculate the resonant frequencies of differently shaped tubes (i.e., air columns). For current purposes, calculation of only the lowest three resonances is important. The resonance curve that results from these calculations shows the peaks at resonant frequencies, the bandwidths of those peaks, and the valleys between the peaks. This curve is called the filter function. At any frequency, the filter function shows how the energy at the corresponding frequency in the glottal spectrum will be transferred by the vocal tract. At frequencies where there are peaks in the filter function, energy transfer will be maximum, meaning that the energy will appear prominently in the output spectrum. At frequencies where there are valleys in the filter function, the energy at corresponding frequencies in the glottal spectrum will not appear prominently in the output spectrum.

The actual acoustic event that emerges from the lips—a vowel sound—is the product of the acoustic characteristics of the glottal spectrum (the amplitudes of the harmonic frequencies) and the varying amplitudes along the filter function. The output spectrum shows which frequencies are prominent, and which

are not. Peaks in the output spectrum, where energy transfer is maximal, are called formants. The first three formant frequencies of a vowel are referred to as the F-pattern of that vowel. The F-pattern is vitally important in the understanding of speech acoustics and perception.

The acoustic model of the vocal tract as a tube closed at one end is a central concept in the development of this theory. The tubes studied in Chapter 7, however, were all of uniform cross-sectional area, like a straight pipe having no constrictions along its length. As mentioned above, the articulation of the schwa may be performed with a vocal tract shape somewhat like a straight tube or pipe, but other vowels clearly require tube shapes of varying cross-sectional area from glottis to lips. Is there a straightforward way to understand how constrictions along the vocal tract tube cause changes in the resonant frequencies known to occur in a straight tube with one end closed? With no constrictions in a tube closed at one end, the quarter-wavelength rule accounts for the resonant frequencies, provided the length of the tube is known. What happens to these resonant frequencies when a constriction is introduced somewhere in the tube? Fortunately, the mathematical details of Fant's (1960) theory do not need to be studied to understand when and how the resonances change with constrictions in a tube. There is a simple conceptual basis for these changes, and the background for the concepts has already been established in Chapter 7. Discussion now turns to constrictions in the vocal tract tube, and their effect on formant frequencies.

WHAT HAPPENS TO THE RESONANT FREQUENCIES OF THE VOCAL TRACT WHEN THE TUBE IS CONSTRICTED AT A GIVEN LOCATION?

At the end of the discussion of tube resonances in Chapter 7, a graph (Figure 7–16) of the pressure distributions for the first three tube resonances was shown. This graph is reproduced in Figure 8–14A. The pressure distributions for the first three resonances correspond to one-quarter of the wavelength for the first resonance (solid blue curve), three-quarters for the second resonance (short-dashed red curve), and five-fourths for the third resonance (long-dashed green curve). (In these graphs "maximum pressure" can mean either maximum positive or maximum negative pressure. The sign of maximum pressure is not important for the discussion that follows.) As stated in Chapter 7, there

A

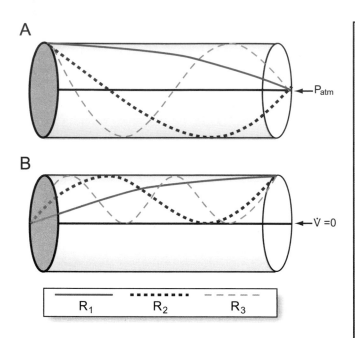

B

R₁   R₂   R₃

Figure 8–14. A. Reproduction of Figure 7–16 showing the pressure distributions corresponding to the first three resonances of a tube closed at one end. Pressure distributions follow the quarter-wavelength rule. **B.** Velocity distributions for the first three resonances of the tube shown in A. Velocities at any point in the tube are the exact mirror image of the pressure distributions. Thus, when pressure is maximum, velocity is zero, and vice versa. The center horizontal line in A represents P_{atm}, whereas the center horizontal line in B represents zero velocity. Maximum pressure in A means either maximum positive or maximum negative pressure.

are many other pressure distributions in this tube corresponding to the higher resonances. They are not shown here partly for reasons of clarity, but also because the first three resonances are the ones of chief concern in vowel acoustics.

As introduced in Chapter 7, Figure 8–14 shows the three pressure distributions superimposed on one another in the tube. The expected maximum pressures at the closed end of the tube can be seen for all three distributions, as well as other locations of maximum and zero (atmospheric) pressure that are specific to a particular wavelength. For example, the first resonance has maximum pressure at the closed end which falls to P_{atm} at the open end. The second resonance has maximum pressure at the closed end, which decreases to P_{atm} about one-third of the way toward the open end, decreases to maximum (negative) pressure about two-thirds of the way to the open end, and then returns to P_{atm} at the opening. Examination of the pressure pattern for the third resonance reveals two regions of maxi-

mum pressure in addition to the maximum pressure at the closed end. Thus, along the length of this tube there are a number of regions of maximum pressure associated with each of the three lowest resonances.

Regions of high pressure result when molecules are packed together and in a relatively motionless state (i.e., at one of the extremes of the simple harmonic motion). It follows that if a measurement were made of the velocity of air molecules at the regions of high pressure in the tube, the value would be zero (i.e., no displacement as a function of time = zero velocity). P_{atm} is indicated in Figure 8–14 by a horizontal, solid black line running through the center of the tube. When the wavelengths associated with the different resonances cross this line, meaning that their pressure value is equal to P_{atm}, the air molecules are minimally packed together and move at their maximum velocity. Note the inverse relationship between pressure and velocity in the tube. When pressure is maximum, velocity of air molecules is zero, and when pressure is zero (= P_{atm}), velocity is maximum. In fact, when the distributions for air molecule velocity are drawn for the first three resonances, they are exact mirror images of the distributions of pressure shown in Figure 8–14A.

Those velocity distributions are shown in Figure 8–14B. The velocity pattern for the first resonance is shown by the solid blue line, for the second resonance by the short-dashed red line, and by the third resonance by the long-dashed green line. The information in either the pressure or velocity distributions is redundant with respect to the other distribution. If the value of pressure at a given point within the tube is known, it implies the value of air molecule velocity at that same point (and vice versa). For current purposes, the important point is that, at regions of high pressure, the velocity is low and at regions of low pressure the velocity is high. This can be confirmed in Figure 8–14 by matching the regions of maximum pressure for a given resonance with regions of zero velocity. This relatively straightforward concept is critical to understanding why and how resonances of the tube change when a constriction occurs at a specific location.

Imagine a constriction placed in the tube, exactly at a location of maximum pressure (and, therefore, zero velocity of air molecule movement). This situation is schematized in Figure 8–15A, which shows the three-quarters-wavelength distribution of pressure associated with the second resonance. There is a maximum pressure at the closed end of the tube, and one about two-thirds of the way toward the open end (the maximum pressures are shown here on both the positive and negative sides, emphasizing the importance of the *absolute* maximum, rather than the sign of the pressure). The tube has been constricted at this latter pressure maximum (arrow, Figure 8–15A). What is the effect, if any, of this constriction on the air vibrating within the tube? The constriction in the region of maximum pressure compresses the air molecules even more, forcing them farther from their rest positions. As air molecules (or any elastic object) are displaced farther from their rest positions, they become stiffer. Thus, a constriction in a region of maximum pressure increases the stiffness of the air molecules. Increased stiffness in a vibratory system results in a higher resonant frequency, which is exactly what happens in this example. The second resonance of the tube in Figure 8–15A, with a constriction placed at a maximum pressure region along its wavelength, increases in frequency relative to the case when the tube has no constrictions. Stated otherwise, if the length of an unconstricted tube is known, the second resonance (symbolized here as fr_2) can be computed as $fr_2 = (3) \times c/4l$. When a constriction is placed at a region of maximum pressure, the second resonance increases relative to the value computed for the unconstricted

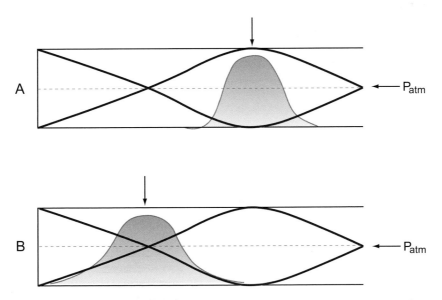

Figure 8–15. A. Tube closed at one end showing the three-quarter-wavelength distribution of pressure associated with the second resonance. A constriction is placed in the tube at the pressure maximum (*arrow*), about two-thirds of the way toward the open end. **B.** Same tube and pressure distribution as in A, but with the constriction positioned farther back in the tube, at a location where pressure = 0 and velocity, therefore, is maximum. Pressure distributions are shown as both positive and negative, emphasizing the maximum pressure locations regardless of sign.

tube. In this sense, the resonances of the unconstricted tube are reference frequencies, and the frequencies of constricted tubes can be regarded as deviations from these reference values.

What happens if the constriction is moved back in the tube to where the pressure is zero (P_{atm}) and velocity is maximum (Figure 8–15B)? In the region of the tube where velocity is maximum, the air molecules are moving at top speed. To attain that top speed, the molecules will have to undergo substantial acceleration. As described in Chapter 7, objects with mass (like air) demonstrate inertia, which is an opposition to acceleration and deceleration. When air molecules are flowing through a tube and encounter a constriction they speed up, increasing their effective mass at the point of constriction. The effective mass is increased because the maximum velocities are increased at the constriction, and the inertia of the molecules becomes greater with the requirement to accelerate to higher velocities. The narrower the constriction, the higher the velocities of the air molecules and hence the greater the inertial effects. This is the explanation for the increased acoustic mass of Helmholtz resonators with narrower necks. Logic would suggest, then, that when a constriction is placed at a location of maximum velocity (zero pressure) the tube resonance in question decreases relative to the case when the tube is unconstricted. This is because a constriction in the region of a velocity maximum has the effect of increasing the acoustic mass, which will lower the resonant frequency of a vibratory system. Thus, the second resonance of the tube in Figure 8–15B shows a decreased frequency, relative to an unconstricted tube, when the constriction is placed at a velocity maximum.

The examples given in Figure 8–15 make use of the pressure (or its mirror image, velocity) distribution only for the second resonance of a tube closed at one end, but the principles can be generalized to the pressure (or velocity) distributions of all tube resonances. The principles, and some subprinciples, are as follows:

1. A constriction located at a pressure maximum raises the frequency of the resonance whose wavelength "carries" the pressure maximum. This is because the constriction increases the stiffness of the air along that wavelength.
   - The greater the degree of the constriction at a pressure maximum, the stiffer the air molecules become and, therefore, the greater the increase in the resonant frequency (tighter constrictions at pressure maxima will result in greater increases in the resonant frequency).

2. A constriction located at a velocity maximum lowers the frequency of the resonance whose wavelength "carries" the velocity maximum. This is because the constriction increases the acoustic mass of the air along that wavelength.
   - The greater the degree of the constriction at a velocity maximum, the more inertive are the moving air molecules and, therefore, the greater the decrease in the resonant frequency (tighter constrictions at velocity maxima will result in greater decreases in the resonant frequency).

3. A constriction between a pressure or velocity maximum changes the frequency of the relevant resonance according to the relative magnitudes of the pressure and velocity at the point of constriction. Thus, a constriction at a point where the pressure is above P_{atm}, but not maximum, may increase or decrease the resonant frequency, depending on the actual magnitudes of the pressures and velocities at that point in the tube. In other words, the effects of constrictions on resonant frequencies are continuous (i.e., they do not apply only at pressure or velocity maxima).

In principles 1 and 2, the phrase "whose wavelength *carries* the pressure (velocity) maximum . . . " is important, because the constrictions shown in Figure 8–15 affect only the second resonance (because it is that resonance's pressure and/or velocity maxima that are being constricted). The effects of the constrictions are always specific to the pressure (or velocity) regions of a particular resonance. But the point has been made that the pressure (or velocity) distributions for *all* of the resonances are "superimposed" on each other as the tube vibrates. A reasonable question is: "What happens when a constriction occurs on these superimposed distributions?"

Figure 8–16 displays a mid-sagittal view of a vocal tract, below which are three tubes closed at one end. The vocal tract drawing is lined up with the tubes such that the glottal end matches the closed (right) end of the tubes, and the lip opening matches the open (left) end of the tubes. It is useful to think of the tubes as straightened out versions of the vocal tract, in which the right-angle bend of the pharyngeal-oral airway has been eliminated. The top tube shows the pressure distribution for the first resonance, the middle tube the pressure distribution for the second resonance, and the bottom tube the distribution for the third resonance. These pressure distributions are superimposed on each other in the vocal tract tube, but they are shown separately here for the sake of clarity. For this discussion, assume a tube length of 15 centimeters (like the length of an adult female vocal tract), which in the case of no constrictions would yield the first three resonances at

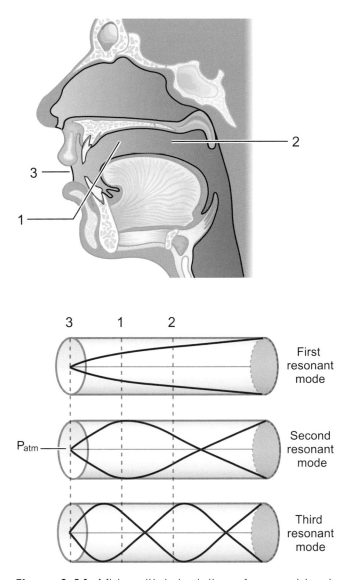

Figure 8–16. Mid-sagittal depiction of a vocal tract, below which are three tubes showing the pressure distributions for the first three resonances. The closed (*right*) end of the tube is analogous to the glottal end of the vocal tract, whereas the open (*left*) end of the tube is analogous to the lips. The numbers 1, 2, and 3 show locations of hypothetical constrictions within the vocal tract and their corresponding locations relative to the pressure distributions within the tube. High pressures within the tubes are indicated when the wavelength pressure distribution is against the edges of the tube. Sign of the pressure is not relevant. The thin horizontal line within each tube indicates atmospheric pressure.

$c/4 \times 15 = 560$ Hz, 1680 Hz (3×560), and 2800 Hz (5×560) (where $c = 33{,}600$ cm/s).

Imagine a constriction placed toward the front of the vocal tract, roughly at the location indicated by the number "1" in Figure 8–16. This is the constriction location expected for the high-front vowel /i/. The corresponding location of this constriction along the three pressure distributions is shown by the vertical, dotted line extending down from the number "1" above the top tube. The constriction falls at a region of relatively low pressure (i.e., relatively high velocity) for the first resonance, maximum pressure for the second resonance, and between zero and maximum pressure for the third resonance, perhaps closer to maximum than zero pressure. The effect of this constriction on the first resonance is to lower its frequency somewhat relative to the resonance when the tube is unconstricted (i.e., 560 Hz), because it occurs at a region of relatively high velocity, toward the front of the tube. The constriction, therefore, increases the acoustic mass, which produces a lower resonant frequency relative to the first resonance of the unconstricted tube. The same constriction, however, occurs at a maximum pressure region for the second resonance. The constriction will, therefore, increase the second resonant frequency relative to second resonance of the unconstricted tube, because the air along this wavelength becomes stiffer as the region of high pressure is compressed. Finally, the constriction occurs between zero and maximum pressure for the third resonance, but closer to the maximum pressure. The third resonance, therefore, has a slightly higher frequency when compared to the third resonance of the unconstricted tube. This is because the constriction slightly increases the acoustic stiffness for this resonance.

In this example, it is important to recognize that a single constriction causes different effects for the different resonances, depending on the location of the constriction and the distributions of pressure (velocity) along the tube. The effects of the constriction are all simultaneous, but may cause changes in resonant frequencies in different directions. Constriction "1," for example, causes a decrease in the first resonance, but a large increase in the second resonance and a somewhat smaller increase in the third resonance.

Example 2 in Figure 8–16 shows a more posterior constriction in the vocal tract, one that might be observed for the production of the high-back vowel /u/. The dotted line extending through the tubes from the number "2" shows a constriction at a mid-pressure (mid-velocity) location for the first resonance, close to a velocity maximum for the second resonance, and close to a pressure maximum for the third resonance. Compared to constriction "1," then, constriction "2" would produce a somewhat higher first resonant frequency, a much lower second resonant frequency (because constriction "2" occurs close to a velocity maximum for the second resonance, whereas constriction "1" occurs at a pressure maximum), and perhaps a higher third resonance.

Example 3 in Figure 8–16 is like a constriction at the lip opening of the vocal tract. This is an interesting case because the constriction occurs at a region of zero pressure (maximum velocity) for all three resonances. This constriction should, therefore, lower all three resonant frequencies, because the constriction increases the acoustic mass for all resonant modes. In fact lip rounding, which produces a constriction at the open end of the vocal tract tube, has the effect of lowering all resonant frequencies of the vocal tract. In addition, note that the tongue-constriction effects described above for constriction "2," as in the vowel /u/, may be changed if lip rounding (constriction "3") is combined with the tongue constriction. For example, the slight raising of the third resonance produced by the tongue constriction "2" (close to a pressure maximum— see Figure 8–16) may be offset by the lowering effect of lip constriction.

In summary, any constriction in the vocal tract affects all resonant frequencies of the tube. Because the pressure (or velocity) distributions for all resonances are superimposed on each other when the air in the tube vibrates, any constriction affects the pressure (or velocity) distributions for every resonance. The simple concepts of stiffness and mass explain why a constriction in the region of a pressure maximum raises a resonant frequency, and why a constriction in the region of a velocity maximum lowers a resonant frequency. A given resonance may be affected by two simultaneous constrictions, for example by the tongue and lips, but the stiffness and mass rules described here continue to explain what happens to the resonance when a previously straight tube is constricted.

Vowel articulation can be thought of as the creation of vocal tract tubes with different area functions. The area functions are modified by the kinds of constrictions described above, which result in different resonant frequencies for different vowels. Resonant frequencies in the vocal tract change according to the principles discussed here. There is a lawful connection between articulatory configuration and vocal tract resonant (formant) frequencies.

The theory of tube resonance presented above is referred to as *perturbation theory*. It is called perturbation theory because it explains how the resonances of a tube are changed when the cross-sectional dimensions of the tube are perturbed, or constricted. The theory explains why constrictions in a tube modify the resonant characteristics of the tube. Because the ultimate interest is in the relationship between articulatory

---

A Chance Encounter

Imagine being a professional speech acoustician, on vacation in the city of Odense, Denmark, and spending a July day in 2004 visiting several museums. At the end of the day you are tired, but you still have the Funen Art Museum on your list. On the second floor you discover the work of Martin Riches. Riches' art is the creation of what he calls "machines," two of which are arty speech synthesizers! Riches is not a speech acoustician, but he read Fant's book and then created a piece he calls "The Talking Machine." Riches studied Fant's area functions and carved vocal tract shapes out of wood blocks, for all sounds, then fitted them with a reed as a source and powered each reed/block with an air supply. The vocal tract blocks are mounted within a frame and the machine talks when the operator enters a word on a keyboard (visit http://www.youtube.com/watch?v=WClZcQo9l6Q). The synthesized speech is very intelligible. Not a bad demonstration of the "truth" of area functions, and pleasing art as well.

---

configurations and vocal tract resonances, it would be convenient to have a small set of articulatory rules that account for the changes in vocal tract resonant frequency with changes in vocal tract shape. This would be much simpler than asking exactly where a constriction was located relative to the pressure (velocity) distributions of the resonant modes. Stevens and House (1955) studied this problem intensively, and developed a *three-parameter model of vowel articulation* to account for the relationships between vowel articulations and vocal tract resonances. It is useful to describe this model in some detail because it illustrates one way in which the acoustic theory of vowel production was tested.

The Three-Parameter Model of Stevens and House

Fant (1960) worked on his theory by marking sagittal tracings of the vocal tract into 35 half-centimeter sections from glottis to lips. Based on the cross-sectional area of each of these sections, Fant estimated their effective acoustic mass and stiffness. If the acoustic mass and stiffness are known for each of the 35 vocal tract sections, then it is known for the entire vocal tract and the full set of vocal tract resonances can be computed.

Stevens and House (1955) created an analog model of Fant's theory by using their knowledge of electrical circuits and their resonant properties. The model can be explained by describing several simple characteristics of electrical circuits and components (prior knowledge of electrical circuit theory is not necessary to follow this discussion). The term *analog model* indicates that the electrical model is studied as an analogy of the acoustic properties of the vocal tract.

A simple electrical circuit is shown in the lower right-hand part of Figure 8–17. The circle labeled "S" represents a source of energy that supplies a flow of electrons to the circuit. This flow of electrons is called *current*, and the two long curved arrows around the bottom of the circuit show it flowing both from the negative side of the source to the positive side, and vice versa. This current source generates a sinusoidal signal, depicted in the upper left-hand part of Figure 8–17,

with the speed of electron movement varying between zero (e.g., at the peaks of the sinusoid, when the direction changes from upward to downward, or vice versa) and some maximum value (e.g., when the sinusoid is passing through the "rest" position as shown in the waveform in the upper left part of figure). The sinusoidal variation of the current also accounts for the alternating movement of the electrons (i.e., from negative to positive, and positive to negative) indicated by the two curved arrows around the bottom of the circuit.

The circuit in Figure 8–17 contains three components. The component labeled R is a *resistor*, whose primary characteristic is to create a certain amount of *frictional opposition* to the passage of electrons through the circuit. Friction, as discussed in Chapter 7, is a form of energy loss in which molecules rubbing against one another produce heat and, therefore, dissipate energy. Stevens and House (1955) used resistors in their model

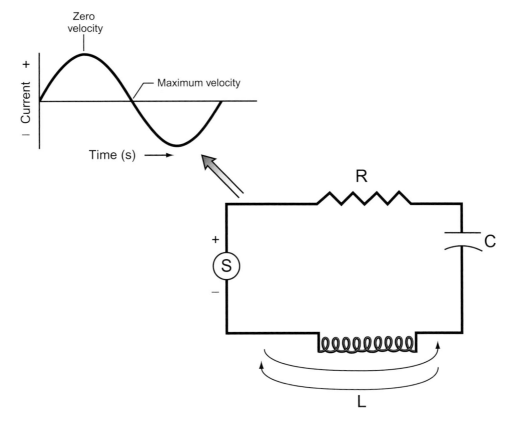

Figure 8–17. Schematic portrayal of a simple RLC electrical circuit (bottom right). S indicates a source of energy that produces current in the circuit. Current varies sinusoidally, as shown in the waveform inset (*top left*) of the figure. R = resistor. L = inductor. C = capacitor. When current flows through the circuit, R dissipates some of the energy in the form of heat, whereas L and C react to the current, as explained in the text. The waveform inset in the upper left part of the figure shows how current varies as a function of time.

to simulate energy loss in the vocal tract and thus the bandwidth characteristics of the formants.

The resonances (formants) of the vocal tract were simulated by Stevens and House (1955) with the components labeled L and C. L stands for an *inductor*, an electrical component that opposes the acceleration and deceleration of moving electrons. If electrons are moving around a circuit with changing velocities, the accelerations are sometimes very high, and other times very low and even zero. Acceleration is defined as the change in velocity over time, so at those times during sinusoidal motion when the velocity is approaching zero—when velocities have to change rapidly from very high to near zero—there will be very high accelerations. One example of a high acceleration is the part of the waveform in Figure 8–17 where velocity is changing rapidly over time to reduce to zero, just before the waveform changes directions from up to down. The inductor will oppose these high accelerations, which are greater for high, as compared to low, frequencies. Not only do the changes from high to low velocities (and, therefore, high accelerations) occur more rapidly for high, as compared to low frequencies, but there are more such changes per unit time for high frequencies. Note that the discussion of the role of acoustic mass in determining resonant frequencies depended on the concept of inertia, the tendency for objects to oppose being accelerated and decelerated. The inductor opposes acceleration of electrons in the way that objects having mass oppose acceleration and deceleration. The inductor can, therefore, be used in an electrical circuit to simulate an acoustic mass in the vocal tract.

The C in the circuit stands for a *capacitor*, an electrical component that stores electrons and offers opposition to the flow of current in proportion to how many electrons it has stored. The capacitor can be thought of as a closed container through which electrons try to flow. As electrons enter this container they sometimes get stuck inside, and the capacitor gradually "fills up" with more and more electrons. The fuller the capacitor, the harder it is to get more electrons inside, which results in a reduction of the current in the circuit. The current is reduced because the electron flow in the overall circuit is partially blocked by the nearly full capacitor, through which the electrons are trying to flow. Imagine a closed volume of air, such as you find in the bowl of a Helmholtz resonator (e.g., see Figure 7–13). If a plunger is placed in the neck of the resonator and moved into the bowl at an *intended* constant velocity, the air inside the bowl becomes increasingly stiff with increasing displacement of the plunger. Because the increasing stiffness develops a recoil force in proportion to the displacement of the air molecules

(i.e., the displacement of the plunger), the *intended*, constant velocity of the plunger is opposed by the increasingly stiff air molecules. Thus, even though the plunger velocity was intended to be constant, the developing and increasing recoil force slows down the plunger movement. This is a fancy way to explain the fact that, with any spring (i.e., any volume of air), the more it is displaced from its rest position, the more difficult it is to move. Note the direct analogy to the electrical capacitor. The fuller the capacitor gets (the more the air molecules are compressed), the more opposition it offers to current flowing into it (like a recoil force). The capacitor is, therefore, an electrical version of an acoustical compliance (the inverse of stiffness), and can be used in an electrical circuit to simulate an acoustical compliance in the vocal tract.

Inductors and capacitors come in different sizes, much like masses and springs come in different magnitudes. As Fant (1960) did, Stevens and House (1955) estimated the cross-sectional area, and hence the acoustic mass and compliance, of each one of 35 sections of the vocal tract. They then used rules (not discussed here) to select the proper inductor and capacitor to simulate the acoustic mass and compliance of each section. They ended up with a device having 35 connected "RLC circuits" (circuits with a resistor [R], inductor [L], and capacitor [C]). The selection of the LC components was a simulation of the vocal tract area function, which, of course, depends on articulatory configuration. The LC settings of the whole, 35-section device could, therefore, be interpreted in terms of articulatory configuration.

This last point, that the model could be interpreted in terms of articulatory configuration, is especially important. Ideally, it would be useful to know the precise acoustic output for every possible vocal tract configuration (assuming a constant source spectrum). For any number of reasons, it is impossible to command a human to produce all these different configurations. But, with an electrical simulation of vocal tract (articulatory) configuration, small and precise changes in the configuration can be made (i.e., simulated) and the ensuing output observed. This is exactly what Stevens and House (1955) did. They changed the model's L and C characteristics in small steps to generate a complete "map" of the relation of vocal tract configuration to vocal tract acoustic output. By using an appropriate, electronically generated wave to simulate the source waveform, and an instrument to measure peaks in the output spectrum of the 35-section model, they measured the "formants" of the model for all possible articulatory configurations.

Based on these manipulations of the model, Stevens and House (1955) offered the following conclusions. The mapping between vocal tract configuration and vocal tract output for the first three formants did not need to be specified for each possible articulatory configuration. Instead, this mapping could be described fairly accurately with just three parameters.[4] More importantly, the three parameters made sense in terms of traditional phonetic descriptions of vowel articulation. The parameters included (a) *tongue height*, (b) *tongue advancement*, and (c) *configuration of the lips*.

Tongue Height

In traditional phonetic descriptions, vowel tongue height describes the relative height of the tongue at the location of the major vocal tract constriction. For Amer-

ican English vowels made in the front of the vocal tract, the tongue height series from lowest (most open vocal tract) to highest (most closed vocal tract) is /æ,ɛ,e,ɪ,i/. The corresponding series for American English back vowels is /ɑ,ɔ,o,ʊ,u/. When Stevens and House (1955) simulated changes in tongue height (or equivalently, mouth opening) the main acoustic effect was on the first formant frequency (F1). Specifically, F1 decreased with increases in tongue height (as vowels went from low to high). This effect was more pronounced for the front vowel series as compared to the back vowel series (see section on perturbation theory on page 394). Figure 8–18 illustrates the tongue height-F1 relationship by plotting tongue height on the x-axis and F1 on the y-axis. High tongue heights (short distances between

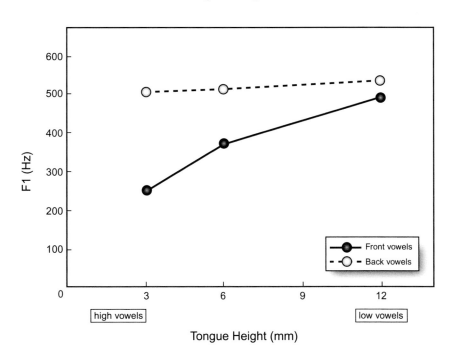

Tongue Height Rule

Figure 8-18. Graph illustrating the effect of changes in tongue height on the first formant frequency (F1). Tongue height is plotted on the x-axis as the distance between the highest point of the tongue and the palate. Higher numbers indicate lower tongue heights (that is, a more open vocal tract). Frequency of F1 is plotted on the y-axis. Filled circles, connected by solid lines, plot the effect for front vowels. Unfilled circles, connected by dashed lines, plot the effect for back vowels. Data extrapolated from Stevens and House (1955).

---

[4]Scientists typically deal with very complex phenomena, with many variables, but do not like to summarize their observations by describing each phenomenon and every variable. They are always looking to reduce the complexity of the real system to a few manageable parameters. If these few parameters capture the major performance characteristics of the system, this type of complexity reduction is deemed appropriate. Stevens and House's (1955) three-parameter model does not work perfectly, but it provides a good approximation to the relation of vocal tract configuration to vocal tract output.

the highest point on the tongue and the palate), as in vowels like /i/ and /u/, are indicated by low numbers on the x-axis ("0" represents complete closure of the vocal tract, as in a stop consonant). Moving from left to right on the x-axis, therefore, represents high to low tongue heights. The tongue height-F1 relationship is plotted separately for front (filled circles connected by a solid line) and back (unfilled circles connected by a dotted line) vowels. For front vowels, the graph shows clearly that F1 changes from about 250 Hz to slightly below 500 Hz as the tongue moves from a high to low position. For back vowels, there is only a small change with adjustments of tongue height, but it is in the same direction as the change for front vowels.

Tongue Advancement

Tongue advancement refers to the relative frontness or backness of the major constriction for vowels. In American English, the major constrictions for vowels such as /æ,ɛ,e,ɪ,i/ are toward the front of the vocal tract, whereas the major constrictions for /ɑ,ɔ,o,ʊ,u/ are toward the back of the vocal tract. There are also a few vowels in American English whose constrictions are in a relatively central location in the vocal tract (between front and back vowels). These would include /ɛ,ə,ɚ,ʌ/. When Stevens and House (1955) held all other factors constant as they simulated constrictions from the back to front of the vocal tract, two clear effects were observed. First, as the constriction moved from back to front, the frequency of F2 increased dramatically. This effect was more dramatic when the model was set for high tongue heights (as in moving from a /u/ to /i/ configuration) as compared to low tongue heights (as in moving from an /ɑ/ to /æ/).

Second, back-to-front movements also resulted in a decrease in the frequency of F1. A summary of these findings is that increases in tongue advancement result in an increasing F2 and a decreasing F1. The effect of tongue advancement on F2 is shown in Figure 8–19. Tongue advancement, plotted on the x-axis, is measured as the distance of the major vowel constriction from the glottis. Small distances (to the left of the x-axis) would represent relatively back constrictions, and large distances relatively front constrictions. To simplify the presentation, F2 values are plotted only for a constriction at 4 cm above the glottis (a back constriction) and at 13 cm above the glottis (a front constriction). Filled circles connected by solid lines plot F2 values for a relatively high tongue height (shown in Figure 8–19 by r = 0.4 mm indicating the radius of the constriction between the highest point on the tongue and the palate), and unfilled circles connected by dotted lines plot

F2 values for a relatively low tongue height (indicated by r = 0.8 mm). For high tongue positions (filled circles), moving the tongue from front to back results in an F2 change from about 1000 Hz to 2250 Hz. For low tongue positions (unfilled circles) the same increase in tongue advancement changes the F2 from roughly 1300 Hz to 1800 Hz. For the sake of simplicity, these effects are shown as linear changes (straight lines connecting the two measurement points) but articulatory-to-acoustic transformations are, in many cases, not linear. Readers interested in more details of the complex nature of articulatory-to-acoustic transformations are encouraged to consult Stevens and House (1955) and Stevens (1989).

Configuration of the Lips

Some vowels of American English are said to be produced with rounded lips. These vowels include /u,ʊ,o,ɔ/. American English does not have a vowel opposition that depends on rounded versus unrounded lips. For example, the high-back-rounded vowel /u/ does not have a high-back unrounded counterpart. Many languages of the world, however, do have vowels distinguished by lip rounding. For example, Swedish has a rounded and unrounded high-front vowel (/i/ versus /y/), and Japanese has a rounded and unrounded high-back vowel (/u/ versus /ɯ/). Stevens and House recognized the importance of lip rounding in languages of the world by systematically varying lip configuration in their model and observing the effects on formant frequencies. They conceptualized the lip section of the vocal tract as a separate "compartment," whose dimensions could be measured by calculating: (a) the area enclosed by the open lips, and (b) the length of the "compartment," measured as the distance between the front of the teeth and the most forward edge of the lips. Imagine a speaker's face when he or she is producing an exaggerated /u/, with lips rounded. If one were looking at the speaker from the front, the rounding of the lips would produce a very small mouth opening, or area. If one were looking from the side and knew roughly where the speaker's teeth were, the lips would extend well in front of the teeth and the lip "compartment" would be relatively long. When the lips were spread, as in /i/, the opposite would occur. Then, there would be a relatively large area between the spread lips, which would be pulled close to the teeth making the distance between the teeth and lips relatively small. Stevens and House used the ratio of the area of the opening enclosed by the lips (A) to the length of the lip compartment (l) as an index of lip rounding, with smaller values of the ratio A/l

Tongue Advancement Rule

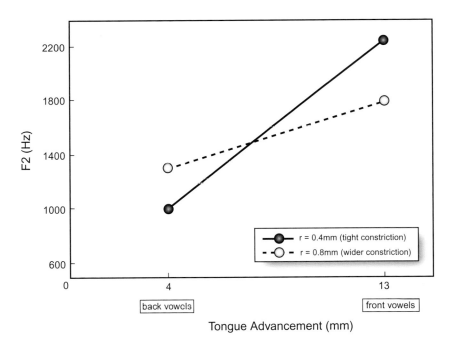

Figure 8-19. Graph illustrating the effect of changes in tongue advancement on the second formant frequency (F2). Tongue advancement is plotted on the *x*-axis as the distance of the major vocal tract constriction from the glottis. Higher numbers indicate constrictions made more forward (toward the front) of the vocal tract. Frequency of F2 is plotted on the *y*-axis. Filled circles, connected by a solid line, plot the effect for relatively small constriction radii (relatively high tongue heights). Unfilled circles, connected by a dashed line, plot the effect for relatively large constriction radii (relatively low tongue heights). Data extrapolated from Stevens and House (1955).

(smaller area, longer length) indicating more rounded lips. They applied the same principles of acoustic-to-electrical modeling used for tongue height and tongue advancement, and observed the effects of different degrees of lip rounding on formant frequencies. By varying lip rounding at different settings for tongue height and tongue advancement, Stevens and House were able to identify the entire range of acoustic effects due to lip rounding.

The general effect of lip rounding can be stated as follows: as the lips become more rounded, *all* formant frequencies decrease. Because rounding of the lips is like extending the length of the vocal tract, increased lip rounding should lower all formant frequencies of the vocal tract because a longer tube will have lower resonant frequencies than a shorter tube, all other things being equal. In addition, lip rounding decreases the area enclosed by the inside border of the lips, cre-

ating a narrower resonator neck which decreases the resonant frequencies of the vocal tract (see section in Chapter 7 on Helmholtz resonators). The vocal tract is typically not a tube with uniform cross-sectional area, however, so lip rounding does not affect all resonances equally. The greatest decreases in formant frequencies with lip rounding are seen in F2, with somewhat lesser (but roughly equal) effects on F1 and F3. Moreover, the influence of lip rounding on F2 depends substantially on tongue height: the higher the tongue, the more lip rounding will cause F2 to decrease. The general effects of lip rounding on F2 are illustrated in Figure 8–20. Two degrees of lip rounding are plotted on the *x*-axis. An *A/l* ratio of 0.4 represents a highly rounded condition and a ratio of 6.7 a highly spread (unrounded) condition. For each rounding condition, there are four plotted points. High-back vowels are shown by filled circles connected by a heavy solid line, low-back vowels

Lip Rounding Rule

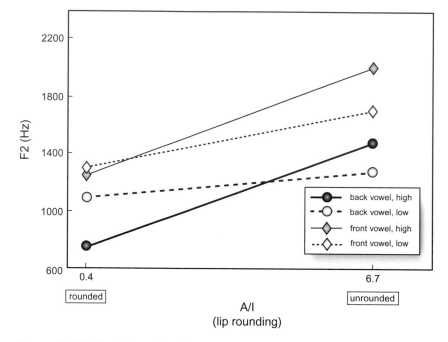

Figure 8–20. Data showing the effect of changes in lip rounding on the second formant frequency (F2). Lip rounding is plotted on the x-axis as the ratio of the area of the lip section to the length of the lip section (A/l). Higher numbers indicate more spread lips (less lip rounding). Frequency of F2 is plotted on the y-axis. Filled circles, connected by a thick solid line, show the effect for back, high vowels. Unfilled circles, connected by a thick dashed line, show the effect for back, low vowels. Filled diamonds, connected by a thin solid line, show the effect for front, high vowels. And, unfilled diamonds, connected by a thin dashed line, show the effect for front, low vowels. Data extrapolated from Stevens and House (1955).

by unfilled circles connected by a heavy dashed line, high-front vowels by lightly shaded diamonds connected by a thin solid line, and low-back vowels by unfilled diamonds connected by a thin dashed line. Consistent with Stevens and House's (1955) general findings concerning the effects of lip rounding on vowel formants, all of the points at the 0.4 A/l value have lower F2 values than corresponding points at the 6.7 value. If the amount of F2 change from the 0.4 to 6.7 value is studied for each vowel type, there are clearly greater effects of lip rounding on the F2s of high, as compared to low, vowels.

Dynamic Analogies

In the text, mechanical, aerodynamic, acoustic, and electrical systems have been introduced. In several cases, a single physical principle has been shown to be relevant to all systems. Take inertia, for example. Inertia is a property of things having mass, such as a block of wood. In an aerodynamic system, a plug of air has mass, called an inertance, which has relevance to acoustic resonance. Inertance, in turn, can be simu-lated with the electrical component called an inductor. The representation of a single physical concept in several different systems is referred to as a *dynamic analogy*. The term is used particularly for the representation of mechanical and acoustic concepts in an electrical circuit, like the Stevens and House model. Dynamic analogies have been exploited to create electrical models of the auditory system, as well.

Importance of the Stevens and House Rules: A Summary

The findings of Stevens and House (1955) are often stated in the form of simple rules for relating changes in articulatory configuration to changes in formant frequencies. A clear statement of these rules is a good way to summarize the preceding discussion.

Rule 1. F1 varies inversely with tongue height. The higher the tongue, the lower the F1. The rule applies more dramatically to front, as compared to back vowels.

Rule 2. F2 increases, and F1 decreases, with increasing tongue advancement. The rule applies dramatically for high vowels, and somewhat more weakly for low vowels.

Rule 3. All formant frequencies decrease with increased rounding of the lips, but the major effect is on F2. The rule applies more dramatically to high as compared to low vowels.

An additional aspect of Stevens and House's (1955) modeling experiment is worthy of mention. The behavior of the third formant was not as easily related to changes in articulatory dimensions (tongue height, tongue advancement, configuration of the lips) as were F1 and F2. The changes in F3 that were observed tended to be rather small, regardless of the articulatory change. The only rule relevant to F3, therefore, is the one concerning lip rounding.

The Connection Between the Stevens and House Rules and Perturbation Theory

The Stevens and House (1955) rules can be thought of as articulatory summaries of the resonance rules described in perturbation theory. In perturbation theory, constrictions in the region of high velocities produce a decrease in the resonant frequency. According to Rule 1, given immediately above, F1 varies inversely with tongue height. Figure 8–21A summarizes this articulatory rule within the framework of perturbation theory. There the pressure distribution is shown for the first tube resonance, and articulatory constriction locations are indicated for back and front vowels. The location for the front vowel constriction corresponds to a relatively low pressure, and, therefore, high velocity, along this wavelength. Constrictions at the front vowel location will decrease the frequency of the first resonance (i.e., the first formant), with greater constrictions producing greater frequency decreases. The same degrees of constriction for back vowels will not produce such dramatic decreases in the first resonant frequency

because the velocity is not as high at this location. This parallels the behavior of F1 with changes in tongue height. The effect on F1 of increasing the constriction is much greater for front, as compared to back, vowels.

Figure 8–21B shows how Rule 2 relates to perturbation theory. Rule 2 states that advancing the tongue from back to front vowel positions causes (a) an increase in F2 and (b) a decrease in F1. The effect of tongue advancement on F2 is illustrated by the lower tube, which contains the pressure distribution for the second resonance (i.e., a three-quarter-wavelength distribution of pressure). The location marked "back" is approximately at the constriction location for a vowel like /u/, where the pressure is near zero and the velocity is, therefore, near maximum. As the constriction is moved forward, the pressure increases to a maximum in the region of the vocal tract where an /i/ constriction would be made ("front" in Figure 8–21B). If tongue advancement from an /u/ constriction to an /i/ moves from a region of low to high pressure (high to low velocity), it is easy to see why the F2 increases. In addition, because the effect of constrictions on resonant frequencies is greatest for very tight constrictions, the effect on F2 will be greater for higher, as compared to lower, vowels. The upper tube in Figure 8–21B reproduces the distribution of pressure for the first resonance, and shows why tongue advancement results in a lowering of F1. As the tongue moves forward, the pressure for the first resonance is increasingly lower and the velocities increasingly greater. A more frontal constriction will, therefore, be located at higher velocities, and result in lower resonant frequencies.

Finally, Figure 8–21C illustrates the relationship between perturbation theory and Rule 3, which states that rounding the lips reduces the frequencies of all the formants. The downward-pointing arrow indicates a constriction at the open end of the tube, which shows the pressure distributions for the first three resonances. For each of these pressure distributions, the pressure is zero at the open end, and the velocity is maximum. A constriction at the open end of the tube, therefore, lowers all formant frequencies.

Importantly, Stevens and House's (1955) complete mapping of the relation of vocal tract configuration (articulatory configuration) to formant frequencies resulted in the interesting discovery that more than one vocal tract configuration could produce the same formant frequencies. This finding introduced a special consideration in the articulatory interpretation of formant frequency measures. If each set of formant frequencies had been associated with a unique vocal tract configuration, an acoustic analysis of formant frequencies would allow one to infer, exactly, the vocal tract configuration that produced the formant frequencies.

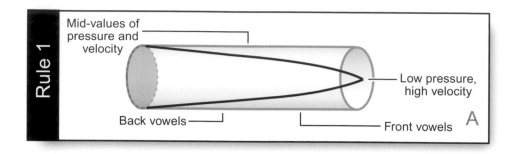

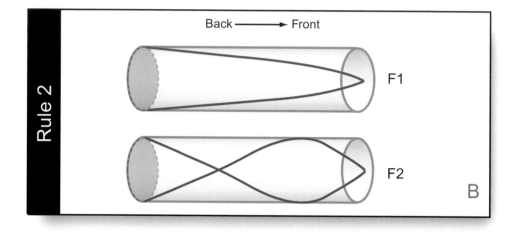

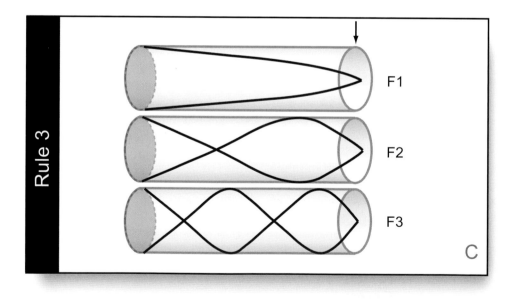

Figure 8–21. Schematic tube models illustrating the connection between the Stevens and House (1955) rules and perturbation theory. **A.** Pressure distribution for F1, showing perturbation relationship of front and back constrictions to the tongue height rule. **B.** Pressure distributions for F1 and F2, showing perturbation relationships of moving a constriction from back to front, to the tongue advancement rule. **C.** Pressure distributions of F1, F2, and F3, showing perturbation relationships of a constriction at the opening of the tube to the lip configuration rule.

As Stevens and House showed, however, this was not the case. The inference of vocal tract configuration from the F-pattern is, therefore, ambiguous in certain cases. The inability to specify a precise articulatory configuration from formant frequencies is referred to as the *nonuniqueness problem*, because there is not a unique (i.e., a single) vocal tract configuration that might produce a given F-pattern. In many cases, though, the F-pattern does provide enough information to make fairly accurate guesses about vocal tract configurations. This leads us to a consideration of the importance of the Stevens and House findings.

Why Are the Stevens and House Rules Important?

The systematic study of articulatory behavior in speech production has a relatively brief history. Certainly, interest in phonetics has a solid historical basis, but concentrated study of the physiological and acoustic behavior of the vocal tract did not occur until well after the beginning of the 20th century. The relative youth of the science of speech production can be explained on the basis of technical limitations. Before the 20th century, instruments for direct visualization of some of the "hidden" articulators (such as the tongue, velum, and larynx) were not available, nor was it possible to make acoustic recordings and spectral analyses of vocal tract output.

The seeds for the explosive growth in communication sciences as a vibrant academic discipline were sown in the 1950s and 1960s, a period during which Fant developed and elaborated his acoustic theory. This period also saw the first systematic collection and analysis of data concerning tongue behavior during speech. X-ray motion pictures, a technology originally developed for medical diagnoses of gastrointestinal function (upper and lower GI studies), were adapted to the study of speech production. A participant's tongue and other articulators were coated with barium paste to make the soft tissue more visible in the developed films. These films were analyzed by hand tracing the outlines of articulatory structures on a frame-by-frame basis. In later variations on this technique, small pellets were fixed to the tongue, lips, and velum and the movements of these points were measured by hand from the x-ray films. This approach eliminated the need to trace whole, sometimes poorly imaged vocal tract structures, but still required a fairly intensive effort on the part of an investigator or clinician. The latest development of this technology involves computerized tracking of the movements of pellets placed on the tongue and other articulators, using either x-rays or electromagnetic fields. The automated collection and storage of the moving pellets greatly reduces the amount of time spent in learning something about what an articulator is doing during an utterance.

This small digression on techniques of visualizing hidden articulators highlights the difficulty of obtaining information on the articulatory function of structures such as the tongue. Most of these techniques involve a substantial amount of subject preparation (e.g., fixing the pellets, or magnetic coils, to the tongue), and the instruments are not readily available to practitioners (see below). Moreover, any x-ray technique carries with it some health hazard (there are no currently known health hazards associated with electromagnetic techniques), and the cost of any of these techniques, plus the expertise needed to use them, limit their broad application.

This is where the importance of the Stevens and House rules enters the picture. The Stevens and House (1955) rules allow a practitioner to examine an acoustic record of an utterance, locate the formant frequencies from this record, and *infer* the likely vocal tract configuration(s) that produced those formants. Because of the nonuniqueness problem there may be some ambiguity in these inferences, but for the most part, the formant frequencies provide good information on articulatory positions and time histories (changes in position over time). All this can be done by making recordings of a person's speech, and then submitting the recordings to the proper analyses.

Who are the practitioners referred to above? These include researchers and clinicians, both of whom are interested in having access to techniques that allow them to draw objective, cost-effective, and *noninvasive* conclusions about a speaker's articulatory behavior. A noninvasive technique is one in which instruments do not have to be introduced into the body to obtain diagnostic and or prognostic information, or one that does not create a potential health risk to the participant or client. Obviously, x-ray procedures must be considered invasive, and the electromagnetic technologies mentioned above are not cost-effective. The use of acoustic analysis to draw reasonable inferences about articulatory behavior should be viewed as the most likely technique to upgrade the ability of speech-language clinicians to account for their diagnostic and management observations concerning speech production abnormalities. There is a high level of skill required to make these inferences, but it is the purpose of texts such as this one, and appropriate university-level coursework, to supply the framework for these skills.

Another Take on The Relationship Between Vocal Tract Configuration and Vocal Tract Resonances

The formant frequencies of the vocal tract tube can be understood using the rules for calculating the resonant frequencies of tubes with uniform cross-sectional area acoustics, and knowing how and why those resonances are modified when a constriction is placed somewhere in the tube. The shape of the vocal tract tube yields the area function, which is really another way to express the articulatory configuration for a given vowel. The continuous area function from glottis to lips, and its effect on formant frequencies, can be reduced to three variables whose changes affect formant frequencies in systematic ways. This is what Stevens and House (1955) accomplished, the expression of tube acoustics in terms of variables relevant to a phonetician—tongue height, tongue advancement, and lip rounding.

Another approach to understanding the effects of articulatory configuration on vowel acoustics is based on a simple resonator model. This approach deserves mention because it has been used in educational settings in which students are taught vocal tract acoustics, even at very young ages. The *Connected Tube Model* (Arai, 2012) represents the vocal tract as a sequence of connected but discrete tubes, as represented in Figure 8–22. Tubes models are shown for the vowels /i/, /e/, /a/, /o/, and /u/, with the glottal end of the vocal tract at the left end and the lip end on the right. In the tube model for /i/, the large-diameter, back tube is seen separated from the equally large-diameter but much shorter front cavity, by a long tube of very narrow diameter. The large back tube represents the cavity behind the front constriction for /i/, and the large front tube represents the short, open cavity in front of

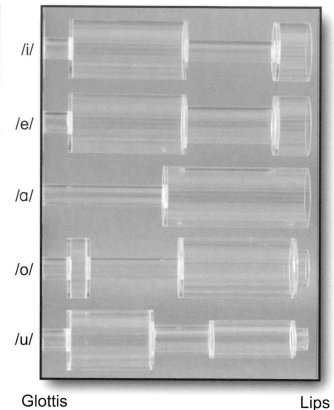

/i/

/e/

/a/

/o/

/u/

Glottis   Lips

Figure 8–22. Connected tube models of vocal tract configurations for the vowels /i/, /e/, /a/, /o/, and /u/, from top to bottom. The glottis end of the vocal tract is to the left, and the mouth end to the right. Photograph from Arai (2012), reproduced with modifications by permission.

the /i/ constriction. The /i/ constriction is represented by the narrow-diameter, connecting tube between the two larger tubes. What is interesting about this model is that the simple, mathematical rules discussed in Chapter 7 for determining the resonant frequencies of tubes and Helmholtz resonators can be applied to this rather crude model to determine the first three formant frequencies of a modeled vowel. For example, in the case of the three-tube model for /i/ at the top of Figure 8–22, the back cavity can be regarded as a tube open at both ends, the front cavity as a tube closed at one end (where the closed end is where the narrow constriction begins, and the open end is at the mouth), and the back cavity attached to the narrow passageway formed by the constriction as a Helmholtz resonator (the neck is formed by the narrow-diameter constriction, the bowl by the large-diameter back cavity). If the appropriate tube lengths and bowl radius (in the case of the back cavity when functioning as a Helmholtz resonator) are measured and the values plugged into the formulas given in Chapter 7 for tubes either open at both ends (half-wavelength rule) or closed at one end (quarter-wavelength rule), or for a Helmholtz resonator, an interesting result emerges from the computations. The Helmholtz formula produces a resonant frequency very similar to the F1 for /i/, the half-wavelength formula a resonant frequency very similar to F2 for /i/, and the quarter-wavelength formula a resonant frequency similar to F3 for /i/ (Arai, 2012, see his Figure 7 and 8). Resonator computations on the crude tube models shown in the Figure 8–22 for /e/, /ɑ/, /o/, and /u/ also produce F1, F2, and F3 values similar to those observed for the natural adult productions of these vowels. Note in Figure 8–22 the differences among the connected tube models for the five vowels.

On the one hand, this may seem like a trivial demonstration. After all, a brief examination of the five connected tube models in Figure 8–22 shows precisely the sort of vocal tract configuration differences expected in a comparison between any two of these vowels. For example, the primary difference between the tube models for /i/ and /e/ is the larger-diameter "constriction tube" for /e/, as compared to /i/, which in phonetic terms is the same as saying the tongue forms a constriction for both /i/ and /e/ in the front part of the vocal tract, but the constriction is not quite as tight for /e/. Another comparison example is that the tube model for /ɑ/ is distinguished from the other tube models by the long, large-diameter tube in the front of the model and the long, narrow-diameter tube in the back of the model. This is expected for a vowel typically described as having a substantial constriction between the tongue and the pharynx and a wide-open front cavity (that is, a low-back vowel). What is surprising, perhaps, is how well the simple-resonator model computations of formant frequencies match with actual formant frequencies measured from persons producing these vowels. Keep in mind that these good matches occur even though real area functions change *continuously* from glottis to lips (that is, smoothly). In contrast, in the resonator models of Figure 8–22 the connecting points between adjacent resonators often involve large, sudden changes in resonator diameter, as in the case of the sudden change in the /i/-tube model from the narrow tube to either the large back resonator or front tube. This suggests a certain degree of inexactness in the transformation from vocal tract configuration to formant frequencies; stated more simply, in certain cases it appears "precise" articulation is not required to achieve a target vowel output.

There are limitations to the connected tube model. It works best for vowels that separate the vocal tract into fairly easily recognizable cavities in front of and behind well-defined constrictions. The tube models shown in Figure 8–22 are for vowels in which there is a well-defined constriction somewhere in the vocal tract, with easily recognized cavities on either side of the constriction. For vowels with "straighter" tubes but some constriction, such as /æ/ and /ɛ/, a connected tube model may not be effective for predicting actual formant frequencies. As it turns out, however, the vowels for which the connected tube model is effective—the ones shown in Figure 8–22—are among the most frequently occurring vowels in languages of the world.

CONFIRMATION OF THE ACOUSTIC THEORY OF VOWEL PRODUCTION

Theories are proposed explanations of how something happens. Fant's (1960) theory is designed to explain how vowel sounds happen, but like all theories it may be false, either completely or, perhaps, just in parts. The confirmation of the acoustic theory of vowel production has taken several forms including analog experiments and human experiments.

Analog Experiments

As discussed earlier, the experiments of Stevens and House (1955) were based on an electrical model of the acoustic characteristics of the vocal tract. Stevens and House were able to get their model to sound like human vowels (albeit crudely) when they selected electrical components to simulate the area functions of the vocal tract. For example, because the model sounded like an /i/ when the components were mimicking an /i/ area function, this was fairly compelling evidence in favor of the theory. If the vocal tract did not resonate like a tube closed at one end and respond acoustically to constrictions according to the principles of perturbation theory, it is hard to see why the electrical model would have worked so well. Many scientists believed that the electrical analog experiments served as strong confirmation of Fant's (1960) theory.

Human Experiments

A powerful way to test the correctness of Fant's (1960) theory is to compare formant patterns predicted from the area functions to those actually measured when people produce vowels. The formant patterns predicted from area functions depend on the "goodness" of various aspects of the theory. If the calculated (theoretical) formants match the measured formants, the theory can be broadly confirmed. A comparison of theoretical and human formant frequencies is shown in Figure 8–23, in the form of F1-F2 (left) and F2-F3 (right) plots. These are very popular plots, where the values of two formant frequencies are plotted as coordinates in a simple scatterplot (in theory, a plot could be made of three or more simultaneous formant frequencies, as a set of coordinate points in three-space, or *n*-space for more than three formants). In the left plot, F1 is on the *x*-axis, and F2 is on the *y*-axis. In the right plot F2 is on the *x*-axis and F3 is on the *y*-axis.

In both plots, the filled circles (labeled "electrical analog") show theoretical locations of F1-F2 or F2-F3 coordinates as generated by an electrical analog of the vocal tract constructed by Fant, based on the area functions obtained from his x-rays of the vocal tract. Fant's analog was very much like the one studied by Stevens and House (1955), described above. These points are theoretical in the sense that they are based on an ability to use the area function to estimate the inertances (acoustic masses) and compliances of small sections of the vocal tract and to represent those with inductors and capacitors in an electrical model that can generate sound. The unfilled circles (labeled "human") are actual formant frequencies measured by Fant (1960, p. 109), from the sustained vowels produced by the speaker whose vocal tract was being x-rayed for the study. Data are shown for three vowels, /i/, /ɑ/, and /u/.

One test of the goodness of the theory is the extent to which the theoretical (electrical analog) points agree with the human points. Examination of the two plots in Figure 8–23 suggests that the agreement is fairly impressive, especially for F2. Even in cases where there are differences between the theoretical and human measurements (as in F1 for /u/ and /ɑ/, and in F3 for all three vowels), the differences are relatively small. These data suggest that Fant's (1960) theory predicts human formant frequency data with a fairly high degree of accuracy.

It should also be noted that the electrical analog generates formant measures from the area functions for /i/, /u/, and /ɑ/ that are consistent with the Stevens and House (1955) rules listed and explained above. For example, /i/ is the highest and most front vowel in the phonetic working space and, therefore, has a very high F2 and very low F1. The opposite case is seen for the back and low vowel /ɑ/, which has a very low F2 and very high F1. This is yet another piece of evidence in favor of the theory's goodness.

Why don't the human and electrical analog formant frequencies match exactly? There are several ways to answer this question, but the general answer is, "The lack of exact matches between the theoretical and human formant frequency coordinates does not invalidate the theory." First, it is very rare for a theory

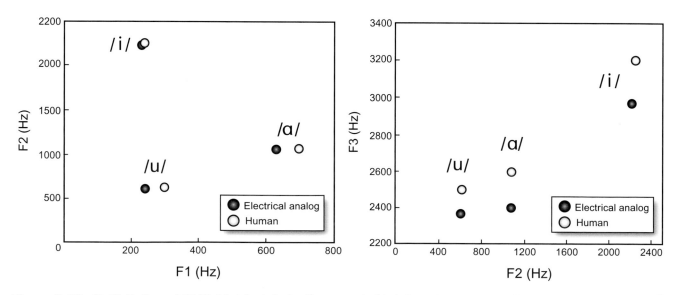

Figure 8–23. F1-F2 (*left*) and F2-F3 (*right*) plots for the vowels /i/, /u/, and /ɑ/ produced by an electrical analog based on Fant's (1960) theory (*filled circles*) and by a human producing the vowels during an x-ray filming procedure (*unfilled circles*). Agreement between the theoretical and human data suggests that the acoustic theory of vowel production is generally correct. Data plotted from Fant's Table 2.31-1 on p. 109 (1960).

to be confirmed by exact, quantitative matches to theoretical predictions. Scientists always expect some error between their predicted (theoretical) and obtained measurements. There may have been some error in estimating the area functions, perhaps deriving from certain inexact measures of the x-ray images. Alternatively, the actual measures of the formant frequencies, whether done by hand or by computer, may be subject to error. Second, and perhaps most importantly, a theory can be correct in many ways but subject to refinement in its details. This is certainly the case for the acoustic theory of speech production. It is correct, for example, to claim that the area function predicts the locations of formant frequencies, but the precision of those predictions—how close the theoretical values come to actual values—may depend on details that have yet to be discovered, or ultimately, may be unknowable.

Alternatively, the rules can be stated in articulatory terms as described by Stevens and House (1955), which include: (a) tongue height, (b) tongue advancement, and (c) configuration of the lips.

Such terms are consistent with traditional descriptions of vowel articulation.

Increases in tongue height (higher tongue heights) result in decreases in F1, increases in tongue advancement (moving the tongue from back to front) result in increases in F2 and decreases in F1, and increased lip rounding decreases all formant frequencies but most notably F2.

The lawfulness of the relations between articulatory configuration for vowels and the formant frequencies of the vocal tract acoustic output make it possible to infer articulatory behavior from just the acoustic analysis, without need for direct examination of articulators such as the tongue.

REVIEW

The acoustic theory of vowel production includes a source, or input (the vibrating vocal folds which produce a glottal spectrum) and a filter (the vocal tract resonator), which combine to produce an acoustic output measured directly in front of the lips.

The source produces a complex periodic waveform whose spectrum consists of a consecutive-integer series of harmonics.

The vocal tract filter, or resonator, can be modeled as a tube closed at one end.

When the source and filter combine to produce an output spectrum, the peaks in this spectrum are referred to as formants.

The formants are essentially the resonances of the vocal tract, which change according to changes in the shape of the vocal tract tube.

The vocal tract configuration for a schwa is most like the case of a tube closed at one end and having uniform cross-sectional area (i.e., no constrictions) from one end to the other; this tube has a set of formant frequencies predicted from the quarter-wavelength rule.

When constrictions are introduced into the tube—when articulatory configuration changes from schwa to other vowels—the formant frequencies change according to certain rules.

These rules can be stated in terms of the location of a constriction relative to pressure and flow distributions within the tube so that constrictions near a pressure maximum will increase the formant frequency whereas constrictions near a flow maximum will decrease the formant frequency.

REFERENCES

Arai, T. (2012). Education in acoustics and speech science using vocal-tract models. *Journal of the Acoustical Society of America, 131,* 2444–2454.

Carré, R. (2004). From an acoustic tube to speech production. *Speech Communication, 42,* 227–240.

Chiba, T., & Kajiyama, M. (1941). *The vowel: Its nature and structure.* Tokyo, Japan: Tokyo-Kaiseikan.

Fant, G. (1960). *Acoustic theory of speech production.* Hague, Netherlands: Mouton.

Fant, G. (1979). Glottal source and excitation analysis. *Speech Transmission Laboratory—Quarterly Progress and Status Report, 1,* 85–107.

Fant, G. (1982). Preliminaries to the analysis of the human voice source. *Speech Transmission Laboratory—Quarterly Progress and Status Report, 4,* 1–27.

Fant, G. (1986). Glottal flow: Models and interactions. *Journal of Phonetics, 14,* 393–399.

Farnsworth, D. (1940). High speed motion pictures of the human vocal cords. *Bell Laboratories Record, 18,* 203–208.

Flanagan, J. (1972). *Speech analysis, synthesis, and perception.* Berlin, Germany: Springer-Verlag.

Fujimura, O., & Lindqvist, J. (1971). Sweep-tone measurements of vocal tract characteristics. *Journal of the Acoustical Society of America, 49,* 541–558.

Kent, R. (1997). *The speech sciences.* San Diego, CA: Singular.

Lee, S., Potamianos, A., & Narayanan, S. (1999). Acoustics of children's speech: Developmental changes of temporal and spectral parameters. *Journal of the Acoustical Society of America, 105,* 1455–1468.

Stevens, K. (1989). On the quantal nature of speech. *Journal of Phonetics, 17,* 3–46.

Stevens, K. (1998). *Acoustic phonetics.* Cambridge, MA: MIT Press.

Stevens, K., & House, A. (1955). Development of a quantitative description of vowel articulation. *Journal of the Acoustical Society of America, 27,* 484–493.

Story, B. (2005). A parametric model of the vocal tract area function for vowel and consonant simulation. *Journal of the Acoustical Society of America, 117,* 3231–3254.

9

Theory of Consonant Acoustics

INTRODUCTION

Chapter 8 showed how fairly simple concepts from basic acoustics (Chapter 7) are put together to construct a theory of vowel acoustics. Essentially, the theory can be viewed as a combination of the following concepts: (a) input signals, (b) resonance and resonators, and (c) output signals. As stated in Chapter 8, the basic theory was presented for the case of vowels because the theory is most precise and accurate for this class of sounds. There is, however, an acoustic theory of *speech* production, not just vowel production. The purpose of this chapter is to establish the theoretical basis for the vocal tract acoustics of nonvowel sounds. Many of the concepts developed for the vowel theory are applicable in this chapter, but some new concepts, specific to the acoustics of consonants, are introduced. The following questions are addressed:

1. Why is the acoustic theory of speech production more accurate for vowels, as compared to consonants?
2. What are the acoustics of coupled resonators, and how do they apply to consonant acoustics?
3. What is the theory of fricative acoustics?
4. What is the theory of stop acoustics?
5. What is the theory of affricate acoustics?
6. What kinds of acoustic distinctions are associated with the voicing contrast for obstruents?

WHY IS THE ACOUSTIC THEORY OF SPEECH PRODUCTION MOST ACCURATE AND STRAIGHTFORWARD FOR VOWELS?

Table 9–1 lists several reasons why the acoustics of sound classes such as obstruents, nasals, and at least one semivowel require some theoretical elaboration over and above that provided for vowels. First, the theory of vowel acoustics is relatively simple because the resonators can be described as contained within a single tube which extends away from a source. The single tube, in this case, is the vocal tract, and the source is the vibrating vocal folds. There are sound classes, however, for which the single tube model is not adequate. For example, production of the nasal sounds /m/, /n/, and /ŋ/ involves two major tubes—the pharyngeal-oral and nasal—which communicate with each other.[1] This arrangement, wherein a "shunt" or "sidebranch" resonator is attached to a main resonating tube, produces certain acoustic effects different from those associated with vowel acoustics.

Second, the important frequencies for vowels, which are below about 4000 Hz, have wavelengths considerably longer than the cross-sectional dimensions of the vocal tract. To make this statement more concrete, consider the cross-sectional areas of the vowel /i/ along the length of the vocal tract. In measurements reported by Fant (1960, p. 115), the cross-sectional areas of the vocal tract for /i/ ranged between 0.65 cm^2 (at

---

[1]Chapter 4 contains detailed discussion of the double-barreled nature of the nasal cavities and its functional significance. Nevertheless, because the double-barreled nature is relatively inconsequential to the acoustic product, it is treated as a single tube in the present context.

Table 9–1. Reasons Why the Acoustics of Obstruents, Nasals, and Some Semivowels Are Not Completely Covered by the Theory of Vowel Production Presented in Chapter 8

1. The production of nasals, laterals, and obstruents involves *coupled* resonator tubes, rather than the single-tube resonators of vowels. The acoustics of coupled, or *shunt* resonators, are somewhat different from the acoustics of single-tube resonators.

2. The important acoustic energy in vowels is located at frequencies below 4000 Hz, for which the wavelengths exceed the cross-sectional dimensions of the vocal tract. In this case, only plane waves propagate in the vocal tract and the acoustics are easily related to the area function. Obstruents sounds have important energy at frequencies above 4000 Hz, where wavelengths are less than the cross-sectional dimensions of the vocal tract. In this case, the sound waves are more complex than planar and the area function does not completely describe the tube acoustics.

3. Vowels have a complex periodic source produced by vocal fold vibration, this source being located at one end of the single-tube resonator. Obstruents have aperiodic sources produced by air flowing through and against vocal tract structures. These sources may be located between resonant cavities of the vocal tract.

the site of the front constriction) and 10.5 cm² (in the region of the relatively open pharynx). The F-pattern for /i/ reported by Fant (1960, p. 109) for a representative speaker is F1 = 240 Hz, F2 = 2250 Hz, and F3 = 3200 Hz. By applying the wavelength formula ($\lambda = c/f$) to these frequencies and assuming the speed of sound in air (c) to be 33,600 cm/s, $\lambda1$ (wavelength for F1) = 140 cm, $\lambda2 = 14.9$ cm, and $\lambda3 = 10.3$ cm. Because the range of cross-sectional areas given above will be far greater than the simple distances (i.e., radii) used to compute the areas, the wavelengths computed for the first three formants are clearly greater than the cross-sectional dimensions of the vocal tract for the vowel /i/. The importance of this fact is that, in the case of vowels, *sound waves will travel through the vocal tract only as plane waves.* In other words, when the wavelengths of frequencies are greater than the cross-sectional dimensions of a tube such as the vocal tract, the pressure waves propagate along the long axis of the tube (from one end to the other), but not in other dimensions (such as from the center to the sides of the tube). When pressure waves are propagated mostly as plane waves, the area function of the tube can be used with great accuracy to predict the resonant frequencies of the tube, as discussed in Chapter 8.

At frequencies above 4000 Hz, many wavelengths are shorter than the cross-sectional dimensions of the vocal tract and pressure wave propagation in the vocal tract is more complex. The mathematics underlying the theory for cases in which wavelengths are smaller than the cross-sectional dimensions of the vocal tract are more complex, and more prone to error. Many consonants—especially obstruents, which include stops, fricatives, and affricates—have substantial amounts of

energy above 4000 Hz, so the theory is not as accurate for this class of sounds as compared to vowels.

Finally, the theory of vowel acoustics includes a complex periodic source, described in Chapter 8. The spectrum of the voicing source is related in a straightforward way to the complex, periodic motions of the vocal folds. In obstruent consonants, however, many sources are aperiodic and depend on complex interactions between airflow and structures within the vocal tract. In addition, some sources for obstruents may be located *between* resonant chambers of the vocal tract, rather than at one end of the vocal tract as in the case of vowels.

In this chapter the theoretical concepts required to understand coupled or "shunt" resonators are discussed. Then, vocal tract aeromechanics in obstruent production are described and related to previously discussed concepts from vowel acoustics. Subsequent sections cover points 2 and 3 in Table 9–1, and show how the acoustics of stops, fricatives, and affricates are logical consequences of aeromechanical events associated with the articulatory positions, configurations, and movements in obstruent production.

WHAT ARE THE ACOUSTICS OF COUPLED (SHUNT) RESONATORS, AND HOW DO THEY APPLY TO CONSONANT ACOUSTICS?

The English nasals /m/, /n/, and /ŋ/ are produced with oral airway closure and an open velopharyngeal port. Because the oral closure involves a complete obstruction to airflow through the vocal tract, /m/, /n/, and /ŋ/ are sometimes called "nasal stop consonants." In fact, the place of complete closure for the three nasals is essentially the same as the place of closure for the stops /b/, /d/, and /g/ (and cognates /p/, /t/, and /k/). Nasals are, therefore, like stop consonants produced with an open, rather than closed, velopharyngeal port. The interval during which the oral closure coincides with an open velopharyngeal port is referred to as the *nasal murmur*. This term is used to distinguish the acoustics of nasals produced with complete oral closure from the acoustics of vowels produced with a somewhat open velopharyngeal port—that is, nasalized vowels. The theory of nasal murmurs is discussed first, followed by the more complex case of *nasalization*, the term used to describe the acoustic effect of coupled resonators with an open oral tract.

Nasal Murmurs

Figure 9–1 shows a schematic tube model of the vocal and nasal tracts during production of an /m/. The nasal tract part of this model is highly simplified and schematic for the purposes of this discussion; for beautiful, computerized tomography (CT) and MRI-based images of a human nasal tract, see Serrurier and Badin, 2008, Figure 6. Several features of the model in Figure 9–1 are different from the vowel tube model discussed in Chapter 8. First, the lip end of the pharyngeal-oral tube is closed, consistent with labial closure for

/m/. The rest of the pharyngeal-oral tube has been constricted roughly in the shape appropriate for the vowel /i/ (tight constriction in the front of the vocal tract, more open tube in the back). Second, the velopharyngeal port is open, also consistent with the production of /m/ or any other nasal sound. As shown in Figure 9–1, the open velopharyngeal port couples the pharyngeal-oral and nasal tracts. Tubes coupled in this way are referred to as *shunt resonators*, one of the resonators being a shunt, or diverging tube, relative to the other resonator. Third, additional shunt resonators are coupled to the nasal tract, shown as tubelettes communicating with the nasal cavities. These tubelettes represent the sinuses, which contribute in important ways to the acoustics of nasal sounds (Dang & Honda, 1996; Dang, Honda, & Suzuki, 1994). The source is located at the glottal end of the tube and has a harmonic spectrum produced by the vibrating vocal folds, just as in the production of vowels. All English nasals are produced as voiced sounds.

As in the case of vowels, the resonators shown in Figure 9–1 shape the spectrum of the source. When shaping the source spectrum for vowels, there are frequency regions at which sound transmission through the vocal tract is maximum. Those regions appear in both the theoretical (i.e., computed from the mathematical theory) and measured spectra as peaks, otherwise known as resonances or formants. The frequency regions between these spectral peaks, or spectral valleys, have substantially less energy than the resonances because the vocal tract shape does not emphasize

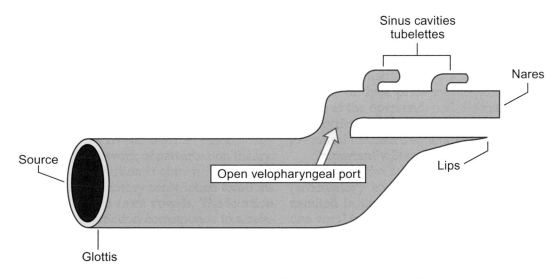

Figure 9–1. Tube model of the vocal tract with coupled resonators. The open velopharyngeal port couples the nasal and pharyngeal-oral cavities, and the sinus cavities are coupled to the nasal cavities. The front end of the tube, where the lips are located, is closed.

energy in these regions. Although the reasoning in this last statement may sound circular, it serves to highlight the primary difference between theoretical and measured spectra of vowels and nasals. In the case of the coupled (shunt) resonators shown in Figure 9–1, there are actually frequency regions where sound energy is "trapped," thus producing *antiresonances*. For example, the closed oral tube shown in Figure 9–1 will shape a frequency region of the source spectrum, but that energy will be "trapped" in the closed resonator.

Of Mufflers, Heating Systems, and Nasals

The concept of shunt resonators is well known to engineers interested in noise reduction in cars, motorcycles, and heating systems. A shunt resonator traps energy at certain frequencies and reduces the amount of energy radiating (coming out) from an acoustic system. This is why car mufflers are constructed with multiple side branches off the main pipe, and heating ducts often have small, dead-end chambers off their main path. Although nasals don't "require" sound reduction, listeners seem to take advantage of it and use it as one cue that a nasal has been produced.

Energy may also be trapped in the smaller sinus resonators shown in Figure 9–1, because the sinus cavities are closed resonators. These regions of antiresonance, where energy is trapped because two or more tubes are coupled together and one or more of the tubes has a dead end, can be calculated based on resonator type and size, just as in the vowel theory. An antiresonance affects a measured spectrum in several ways, most notably by eliminating or reducing energy in its vicinity.

Because the nose is an acoustic tube open to the atmosphere at the nares, nasal murmurs have resonances (formants) related to the shape and size of the nasal passages. Antiresonances originate in the sinus cavities, the closed oral cavity, and as a result of the asymmetrical left and right conduits through the nasal cavities, from just behind the nasal septum to the outlet of the nasal cavities at the nares (Pruthi, Espy-Wilson, & Story, 2007). Nasal sounds, therefore, have spectra consisting of a mix of resonances and antiresonances. The concept of an antiresonance is illustrated in Figure 9–2, which shows theoretical speech-sound spectra from Fant (1960) for a vowel (/ɑ/) and two nasals (/m/ and /n/). The theoretical spectrum for the vowel /ɑ/ was computed, as discussed in Chapter 8, based on the estimated area function derived from a midsagittal x-ray tracing of a single speaker producing the sustained vowel. The theoretical spectra for the nasals were also estimated from area functions of the nasal cavities, but the process was somewhat more complex than the case for vowels. Sagittal x-rays could not

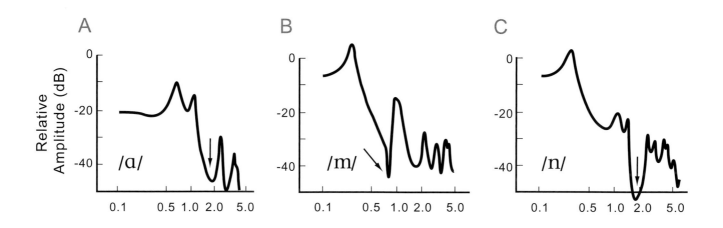

Figure 9–2. Computed spectra based on area functions, showing resonances for /ɑ/ (*panel A*) and resonances and antiresonances for two nasal murmur spectra /m/ (*panel B*) and /n/ (*panel C*). From *Acoustic Theory of Speech Production* (pp. 144, 153), by G. Fant, 1960, The Hague: Mouton. Copyright 1960 by Mouton de Gruyter. Modified and reproduced with permission.

produce a satisfactory image for the computation of nasal area functions, so Fant used a plastic model of the nasal cavities obtained from a cadaver, and adjusted this model to fit the dimensions of the single speaker. The nasal area functions derived from this model were then submitted to the mathematical theory that generated the nasal resonances and antiresonances resulting from the coupling of the nasal and pharyngeal-oral cavities. It should be noted that modern imaging techniques allow very accurate reconstructions of nasal and sinus cavity dimensions and, therefore, estimates of nasal cavity area functions (Dang & Honda, 1996; Dang et al., 1994).

The first three peaks in the theoretical vowel spectrum are shown clearly in Figure 9–2A. These peaks correspond to the first three formants of the vowel /ɑ/. Note how the peaks in this spectrum are *sharply tuned*, with relatively narrow bandwidths. Of special interest are the valleys of the computed resonance curve. The arrow on the vowel spectrum indicates a valley around 1800 Hz where the energy is nearly 40 dB less than the energy of the first peak. This is a substantial energy difference between the highest peak in the spectrum and the valley, but note that the valley develops between

---

The Sinuses Are Helmholtz Resonators, Part I

In a beautifully done experiment, Dang and Honda (1996) used Magnetic Resonance Imaging (MRI) to measure the structural characteristics of the sphenoid, maxillary, and frontal sinuses in three participants. These characteristics included the volume of each sinus, as well as the dimensions of the small anatomical "tube" connecting the sinus cavity to the main nasal pathways. For each sinus volume Dang and Honda computed a value for compliance, and for each connecting tube a value for inertance. They entered these values into the formula for Helmholtz resonators (see Chapter 7) and obtained the theoretical location of antiresonance frequencies for each sinus (remember: the sinuses are closed cavities). Then, they compared the calculated antiresonance frequencies to actual measurements of antiresonances during the participants' production of nasals. The calculated and measured antiresonance frequencies matched within 10% of each other!

---

the second and third peaks in a relatively gradual way. Stated otherwise, the vowel spectrum does not show anything resembling a sharply tuned, "upside down" peak along its resonance curve. The valley in the vowel spectrum is partly the result of the decreasing energy in the source spectrum with increasing frequency (see Chapter 8), and partly the result of the close spacing of F1 and F2 for this vowel (see Fant, 1973, Chapter 1, for information on formant frequency spacing and formant intensity).

The theoretical spectrum for /m/ shows peaks, much like the vowel spectrum, but it also shows a reverse, or upside down peak. This sharply tuned, reverse peak, which is indicated in Figure 9–2B by an arrow and occurs around 800 Hz, is the antiresonance which results from trapped acoustic energy in the closed pharyngeal-oral cavity. The antiresonance peak shows relatively sharp tuning, which distinguishes it from the broader valleys seen in vowel spectra. Fant (1960) showed that the frequency of this antiresonance is related to the size of the pharyngeal-oral cavity in which the acoustic energy is trapped. That is, the frequency location of these reverse (negative) peaks is based on the same resonator rules as the frequency location of the positive peaks typically referred to as formants. Larger cavities yield antiresonances with lower frequencies, smaller cavities yield antiresonances with higher frequencies.

This latter point is made clear by examination of the theoretical spectrum for /n/ shown in Figure 9–2C. The reverse peak in this spectrum—the antiresonance—is located just below 2000 Hz (see arrow) which is substantially higher than the 800-Hz antiresonance for /m/. Based on the relation of resonator size to frequency, these different locations for the antiresonance of /m/ versus /n/ make sense. The cavity in which acoustic energy is trapped for /m/ is substantially larger than the cavity in which energy is trapped for /n/. The antiresonance for /n/ should be located at a higher frequency than the antiresonance for /m/, just as shown in the comparison of spectra B and C of Figure 9–2. In the case of the velar nasal /ŋ/, the point of constriction may result in an extremely small cavity behind the constriction that is coupled to the nasal cavities, or even the absence of a small coupled cavity. When the coupled cavity is extremely small, the antiresonance is located at a relatively high frequency, probably well above 3000 Hz. The absence of a coupled cavity, and hence a cavity in which acoustic energy can be trapped, occurs if the point of constriction for the velar nasal is sufficiently posterior in the vocal tract so that the pharyngeal and nasal cavities appear as a single tube with no side branches. In this case, there may be no major antiresonance, but simply a pattern of resonances determined by the configuration of the continuous pharyngeal-nasal tube.[2] Midsagittal tracings of vocal tract configurations for /m/, /n/, and relatively anterior and posterior constrictions for /ŋ/, adapted from Fant (1960) and shown in Figure 9–3, summarize these concepts of side-branch resonance and coupled cavity size. Dashed outlines show the size of the closed pharyngeal-oral cavity in which energy is trapped.

Although this discussion has focused on the antiresonance feature of the nasal murmur spectra shown in Figure 9–2, there are also important resonance characteristics of nasal murmurs. In Figures 9–2B and 9–2C, the first peak in the nasal murmur spectra for both /m/ and /n/ occurs roughly between 250 Hz and 300 Hz and has a relatively high amplitude. According to Fant (1960), the first resonance of the velar nasal /ŋ/ also occurs in this frequency region. This relatively high-amplitude, low-frequency (between 250–300 Hz) formant can be considered a constant feature of all nasals.

The constancy of the formant frequency across all nasals suggests that it must be produced by a relatively constant area function, regardless of which nasal is produced. This relatively constant area function almost certainly reflects the combined pharyngeal and nasal cavities. In the speech production of a person with a structurally intact speech production apparatus, there are typically no time-varying constrictions of the nasal cavities—the nasal tract does not typically change shape during speech production, as does the oral tract. Similarly, the shape of the pharyngeal section of the vocal tract is fairly constant across the different places of articulation (bilabial, lingua-alveolar, dorsal) for nasal murmurs. The effect of this constant tube shape, extending from the pharynx through the nasal cavities, is the production of a low- frequency formant that is a kind of acoustic "signature" of a nasal murmur. In addition to this low frequency resonance—the nasal F1— nasal murmurs typically have a series of higher formants occurring roughly at 1000 Hz (nasal F2), 2000 Hz (nasal F3), 3000 Hz (nasal F4), and so on. These

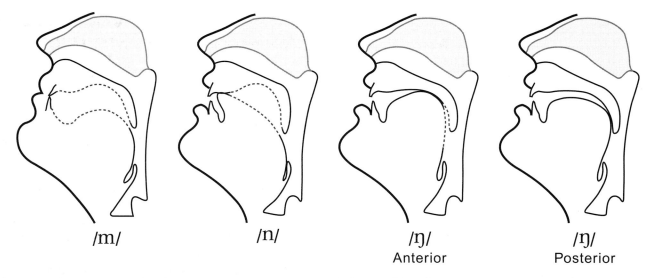

/m/   /n/   /ŋ/
Anterior
/ŋ/
Posterior

Figure 9-3. Midsagittal tracings of the vocal tract for /m/, /n/, and /ŋ/. The two right-hand vocal tracts show a relatively anterior and a relatively posterior constriction for /ŋ/, respectively. The size of the coupled oral cavity in the first three vocal tracts is indicated by dashed lines along the tracings. The size of this cavity is largest for /m/, somewhat smaller for /n/, and very small for /ŋ/ when the constriction is anterior. There is no dashed line tracing in the right-most vocal tract because the relatively posterior point of constriction does not permit any coupling between the oral and nasal cavities. In this case, the pharynx and nasal cavities act as a continuous, single-tube resonator. From *Acoustic Theory of Speech Production* (p. 140), by G. Fant, 1960, The Hague: Mouton. Copyright 1960 by Mouton de Gruyter. Modified and reproduced with permission.

---

[2]Even with an /ŋ/ constriction that is sufficiently posterior to eliminate any coupling between the oral and nasal cavities, there may still be antiresonances in the spectrum because of the sinuses, which function like resonators coupled to the nasal cavities (i.e., side-branch resonators to the nasal cavities). Dang and Honda (1996), have made direct measurements of the frequency locations of the sinus antiresonances. Their results suggest that the sinuses contribute antiresonances within the 500 to 1000 Hz region.

upper formants of the nasal murmur, however, tend to be quite sensitive to surrounding phonetic context and are very variable across speakers (Fujimura, 1962).

Energy Loss in the Nasal Cavities, Antiresonances, and the Relative Amplitude of Nasal Murmurs

The resonances generated by the nasal tract tend to have greater bandwidths than the resonances of a typical vowel spectrum. In Chapter 8, the factors of absorption, friction, radiation, and gravity were identified as sources of energy loss in the transmission of sound through the vocal tract and into the atmosphere. The wider bandwidths of nasal resonances are largely accounted for by high absorption factors in the nasal cavities. These high absorption factors are related to the extensive surface area within the nasal cavities, which contain many complicated folds and recesses. There is more tissue to absorb sound in the nasal cavities than there is in the vocal tract. The damping of nasal resonances, as revealed in the bandwidths of the nasal formants, tends to be greater than the damping of oral (vowel) resonances.

The combined effects of an antiresonance and the relatively greater damping of nasal resonances tend to make nasal murmurs weak in relative amplitude when compared to vowels (Pruthi & Espy-Wilson, 2004). Antiresonances not only eliminate energy at the exact frequency location of their "reversed peaks," but also reduce energy at surrounding frequencies. Increased damping results in less intense resonant peaks. Because the overall amplitude of a sound can be thought of as the sum of all energy along the resonance curve (i.e., the sum of all amplitudes at all frequencies in a spectrum), speech sounds with antiresonances and increased damping, such as nasals, naturally have less overall amplitude than sounds such as vowels that do not have antiresonances and have minimal damping.

Nasal Murmurs: A Summary

A *nasal murmur* is defined as the sound produced when the velopharyngeal port is open and there is a complete obstruction to the oral airstream. This description encompasses the sound class of English nasal consonants transcribed as /m/, /n/, and /ŋ/. In the production of nasal murmurs, two major tubes are coupled, the nasal tube which is open to atmosphere and the oral tube, which is completely sealed from the atmosphere by articulatory closure. The sealed, oral tube will shape the source spectrum according to its resonator size, but the energy shaped by that tube will be trapped there because its outlet to the atmosphere is closed.

This results in an antiresonance, or a reverse peak in the spectrum. The sinus cavities coupled to the nasal tract also function as closed resonators and contribute antiresonances to the spectrum of a nasal murmur. Antiresonances affect a measured spectrum by reducing or eliminating energy at and around the frequency of the reversed peak. The energy in the spectrum of a nasal murmur is also reduced because of the relatively high damping of the nasal formants that results from absorption of sound by the extensive tissue surface area in the nasal cavities. Whereas antiresonances are an important characteristic of nasal murmurs, there are also resonances of the nasal cavities, the most important of which is a low frequency formant between 250 to 300 Hz. This formant frequency is relatively constant for the three nasals of English, because the pharyngeal and nasal cavities responsible for the formant do not change shape for the different places of articulation. Higher formants for the nasal murmurs can be measured as well, roughly at 1000-Hz intervals beginning at 1000 Hz. These formants reflect resonances of the nasal cavities. The specific frequencies of these upper formants vary with context and across speakers.

Nasalization

The acoustic theory of nasalization has many similarities to the theory of nasal murmurs, but is somewhat more complicated. As in nasal murmurs, the pharyngeal-oral and nasal airways are coupled, but in the case of nasalization both tracts are open to atmosphere. The overall output of the vocal tract for nasalized vowels therefore represents a mixture of the resonant characteristics of the nasal and pharyngeal-oral cavities, as well as the effects of their coupling.

When the nasal and pharyngeal-oral airways are coupled, with both open to atmosphere, sound waves propagate through both airways and radiate from the mouth and nares. Each of these tracts has resonant characteristics dependent on the size of the cavities (and, hence, the inertance and compliance of the air in those cavities). The oral resonances should be roughly, but not exactly (see below) the same as when the nasal cavities are not coupled to the pharyngeal-oral cavities. Thus one major effect of coupling the nasal to the pharyngeal-oral cavity during a vowel should be the addition of resonances from the nasal cavities. To a large degree, this is exactly what happens. In effect, the spectra of nasalized vowels have extra formants due to the addition of a second resonant tube.

There is another effect of coupling the oral and nasal cavities. Recall from the discussion of nasal murmurs that sound is trapped in the closed oral cavity, introducing an antiresonance into the spectrum. In nasalized vowels, antiresonances are also introduced to the spectrum as a result of energy trapped in the paranasal sinuses (Dang et al., 1994; Stevens, Fant, & Hawkins, 1987). The main antiresonance in nasalized vowels appears to occur at a relatively low frequency, between about 300 Hz and 1000 Hz. Interestingly, the primary *resonance* of the nasal cavities also occurs in this frequency region, as does the first formant (F1) of most non-nasal vowels. Nasalized vowels, therefore, contain a low-frequency spectrum (between about 300–1000 Hz) having a nasal resonance, an antiresonance, and a pharyngeal-oral resonance (the F1 of the oral vowel). For several writers (Hawkins & Stevens, 1985; Stevens et al., 1987), this resonance-antiresonance-resonance pattern in the region around F1 of the oral vowel is the defining acoustic feature of nasalization.

The low-frequency spectra of four nasalized and nonnasalized vowels are shown in the four panels of Figure 9–4. Each panel shows the energy level, in relative amplitude (dB), across the frequency range from 0 to 1300 Hz. The "zero" point on the dB scale is arbitrary. The blue curve in each panel shows the spectrum for the nonnasalized vowel and the red curve shows the spectrum for the nasalized version of the vowel. The articulatory difference between the nonnasalized and nasalized vowels is found at the velopharyngeal port. For nonnasalized vowels, the port is closed, whereas for nasalized vowels, the port is open. Note for the vowel /ɑ/ the peaks in the non-nasalized spectrum (blue curve) at roughly 680 Hz and 1100 Hz, and the absence of any sharply tuned, reversed peaks (antiresonances). The frequency location of the peaks is consistent with the typical F1 and F2 values observed in the /ɑ/ spectra of adult males. The label $F1_0$ indicates the first oral resonance (i.e., the first formant) of the nonnasalized vowel. The spectrum for the nasalized /ɑ/ (that is, /ɑ̃/: red curve) shows peaks in roughly the same location as the $F1_0$ and F2 peaks of the nonnasalized spectrum, but the nasalized peaks are at somewhat higher frequencies than the nonnasalized peaks; this is especially the case for $\tilde{F}1$ compared to $F1_0$. Note the label $\tilde{F}1$ indicating the location of the first oral resonance for /ɑ̃/.

The /ɑ̃/ spectrum is different from the /ɑ/ (nonnasalized) spectrum in several important ways. First, $\tilde{F}1$ clearly has a lower amplitude than $F1_0$. There is a corresponding amplitude difference for the F2 peaks (around 1100 Hz), but not of the same magnitude. Second, there is a clear antiresonance, labeled AR on the graph, just above 500 Hz in the /ɑ̃/ spectrum. This antiresonance is a result of the coupling of the sinus cavities to the pharyngeal-oral and nasal cavities for the production of /ɑ̃/. The antiresonance also accounts for the relatively low amplitude of $\tilde{F}1$) as compared to $F1_0$. Recall that antiresonances tend to reduce energy at and around their frequency locations. The location of the antiresonance, just above 500 Hz is close enough to the F1 of /ɑ/ to have a major effect on its amplitude in the nasalized version of the vowel. Third, there is a low-amplitude peak in the nasalized spectrum, around 400 Hz, that is not present in the nonnasalized spectrum. This is the primary resonance of the nasal tract, labeled *NR*, which mixes with the oral resonances and is seen in the output spectrum of a nasalized vowel.

The Sinuses Are Helmholtz Resonators, Part II

Yes, the locations and shapes of the sinus cavities are fixed inside your head and, yes, they are relatively far from the action where articulatory changes modify the area function of the vocal tract; the sinuses are even relatively far from the ever-changing area of the velopharyngeal port. It might be assumed, then, that for a given person the resonant frequencies of these sinus Helmholtz resonators, and therefore the frequencies of the antiresonances they contribute to the spectrum of a nasalized vowel, are fairly constant: their acoustic consequences would seem to be above the fray of the acoustic consequences of moving the tongue, jaw, velum, and so forth to spew out yet another whining complaint. Not so, according to Pruthi, Espy-Wilson, and Story (2007), who combined MRI measurements of the vocal and nasal tracts with electrical modeling analysis to show that for nasalized vowels, the precise frequencies of antiresonances originating in the sinus cavities change with changes in the vocal tract area function, as well with the degree of openness at the velopharyngeal port! Interestingly, sinus resonant frequencies are not affected by different places of articulation for the nasal murmur—they are constant. But the hypernasality of dissatisfaction is basically a vowel thing, so the next time you are asked to stop complaining, nod knowingly and state that whining is acoustically complex, as are you.

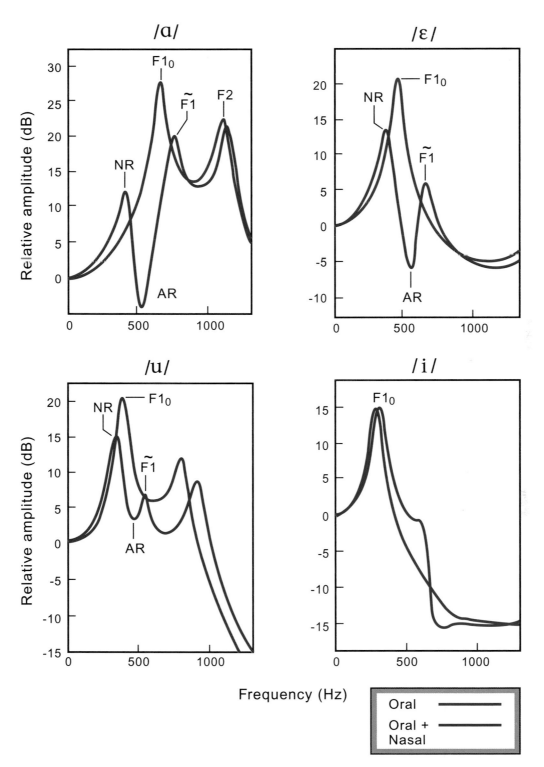

Figure 9–4. Spectra for the vowels /ɑ/, /ɛ/, /u/, and /i/ for nonnasalized (*blue curves*) and nasalized (*red curves*) conditions. Frequency, between 0 and 1300 Hz, is plotted on the abscissa and relative amplitude, in dB, is plotted on the ordinate. NR = nasal resonance. AR = antiresonance. $F1_o$ = F1 of nonnasalized vowel. $\tilde{F}1$ = F1 of nasalized vowel (combined oral and nasal outputs). For each vowel except /i/, note the nasal resonance-antiresonance-F1 pattern in the nasalized spectra. For /i/, the nasal resonance is canceled by the antiresonance because of the small coupling (small velopharyngeal port opening) between the oral and nasal cavities. From "Some acoustical and perceptual correlates of nasal vowels," by K. Stevens, G. Fant, and S. Hawkins in *In Honor of Ilse Lehiste* (p. 246), Edited by R. Channon and L. Shockey, 1987, Dordrecht, Netherlands: Foris. Copyright 1987 by Foris. Modified and reproduced with permission.

The resonance-antiresonance-resonance pattern in /ã/, therefore, consists of the nasal tract resonance (*NR*) around 400 Hz, the antiresonance (*AR*) just above 500 Hz, and the F1 in the vicinity of 700 Hz. This general pattern is seen for other nasalized vowels, with variations that depend on vowel identity. Note for the vowels /ã/, /ɛ̃/, and /ũ/ how $\tilde{F}1$ is shifted up in frequency relative to $F1_0$, as well as the lower amplitude of $\tilde{F}1$ as compared to $F1_0$. In each of these cases, the antiresonance resulting from the coupling of sinus cavities to the pharyngeal-oral and nasal cavities reduces the amplitude of the first oral resonance. Also noteworthy is the fairly consistent frequency of the nasal resonance (*NR*) for the vowels /ã/, /ɛ̃/, and /ũ/. This consistency has the same explanation as the consistent nasal resonance in nasal murmurs. The area function of the nasal tract does not change substantially during speech production and, therefore, neither do its resonances.

The nonnasalized and nasalized spectra shown for the vowel /i/ (see Figure 9–4) seem to violate these acoustic principles of nasalization. No antiresonance (*AR*) is indicated, nor is there a nasal resonance (*NR*). The absence of the resonance-antiresonance-resonance pattern in the /i/ spectrum can be attributed to the small amount of coupling between the pharyngeal-oral and nasal cavities for this vowel. It is well known that the size of the velopharyngeal port in nasalized vowels is greater for low and mid-vowels (such as /ɑ/ and /ɛ/) than it is for the high vowel /i/ (see Bell-Berti, 1993). Stated in acoustic terms, the coupling between the pharyngeal-oral and nasal cavities is greater for low and midvowels than it is for high vowels such as /i/. When the coupling between the pharyngeal-oral and nasal cavities is small, the nasal resonance (*NR*) and the antiresonance (*AR*) have essentially the same frequency. When a resonance and antiresonance associated with the same cavity have the same frequency, they cancel each other and their effects are not seen in the output spectrum. The absence of a nasal resonance and antiresonance in the /ĩ/ spectrum is a result of this cancellation. The lack of effect of an antiresonance on F1 for /ĩ/ is readily apparent in its amplitude, which is essentially the same as the amplitude of $F1_0$.

The specific acoustic characteristics of nasalized vowels depend very much on precisely which vowel is nasalized. In a study employing a computer-implemented, electrical model of the vocal and nasal tracts plus the sinuses, "equivalent" nasalization of high and low vowels (that is, the same area of opening of the velopharyngeal port) produced very different changes in the low-frequency spectrum of the respective vowels (Rong & Kuehn, 2010). An appropriate response to the question, How does an open velopharyngeal port change the formant and antireso-

nance characteristics of the nasalized vowel spectrum? requires a question in return: Which vowel are you asking about (a similar result was reported by Pruthi, Espy-Wilson, & Story, 2007)?

Nasalization: A Summary

Nasalization is the term used to describe the production of vowels with an open velopharyngeal port. The acoustic theory of nasalization differs from the theory of nasal murmurs because in the former the oral airway is open, whereas in the latter the oral airway is closed. The primary acoustic effects of nasalization are seen in the frequency range between 0 and 1000 Hz and include: (a) the introduction of an "extra" resonance from the nasal tract, usually in the 300- to 500-Hz region; (b) an antiresonance located at a slightly higher frequency than the nasal tract resonance, probably due to trapping of energy in the paranasal sinus cavities which act as side-branch resonators to the main nasal cavities; and (c) a first oral resonance ($\tilde{F}1$) which may be slightly higher in frequency than the non-nasalized F1 ($F1_0$) and is usually of lesser amplitude than the non-nasalized F1. The reduction of F1 amplitude is due to the nearby antiresonance. Because of the reduction in $\tilde{F}1$ amplitude, nasalized vowels typically have less overall amplitude than corresponding nonnasalized vowels.

The Importance of Understanding Nasalization

Why is nasalization important (see Stevens et al., 1987)? First, when English vowels are articulated either before

---

More to Vowels Than Meets the Ear

How are vowels distinguished in a language? Well, according to tongue height, tongue advancement, and lip configuration, right? Actually, a more precise answer is yes, but not absolutely. In their 1996 book, *The Sounds of the World's Languages*, the great phoneticians Peter Ladefoged (1925–2006) and Ian Maddieson described and discussed "minor features of vowel quality," meaning vowel differences involving contrasts of (for example) voice quality and nasalization. Among the several "minor" contrasts in vowel quality discussed by Ladefoged and Maddieson, the opposition between an oral vowel and its nasalized counterpart (/i/ vs. /ĩ/ for example, as in French or Portuguese) is said to be the most common among languages of the world.

or after nasals, some portion of the vowel is produced with an open velopharyngeal port. Even though the vowels of English are described as non-nasal, and, therefore, produced with a closed velopharyngeal port, the open velopharyngeal port required for the nasal consonant will "spread" an acoustic effect to adjacent vowels. This spreading of articulatory (and, therefore, acoustic) characteristics from one segment to another is called *coarticulation*, as discussed in Chapter 5. The open velopharyngeal port for the nasal murmur cannot be closed instantaneously for the articulation of a following vowel. Thus, a vowel following a nasal consonant is nasalized for a brief time, during which the output of the vocal tract will reflect the effects of combined oral and nasal acoustics. Similarly, a vowel preceding a nasal consonant is nasalized for a certain interval when the velopharyngeal port is opened prior to the oral articulation of the nasal murmur. This opening of the velopharyngeal port during the vowel is often thought to reflect anticipation of the articulatory requirements of the nasal murmur. These coarticulatory effects of nasalization may serve as important cues to phonetic perception (that is, the presence of an upcoming nasal), even though there is no contrast in English between nasalized and nonnasalized vowels.

The second reason for understanding nasalization is suggested by the closing statement of the preceding paragraph. Whereas English does not have a *phonemic* opposition for nasalized and non-nasalized vowels, such contrasts are phonemic in languages such as French and Hindi (a language spoken in northern India). A comprehensive theory of speech acoustics should be able to explain the acoustic basis of sound systems for many (if not all) languages of the world, not just English.

A third reason for considering an acoustic theory of nasalization is the more practical one of children and adults with structural or neurological disorders that prevent the decoupling of the pharyngeal-oral and nasal cavities in speech production. Craniofacial anomalies, seen in many different syndromes, often involve structural deficits of the velopharyngeal port area which make velopharyngeal closure impossible or inadequate. Many different neurological diseases cause *dysarthria*, which affects the ability of muscles of the speech apparatus to function properly. A typical sign in many cases of dysarthria is chronic or intermittent hypernasality, sometimes similar to that seen in craniofacial anomalies. Regardless of the cause of inadequate or absent velopharyngeal closure, the effect is the same:

the chronic or intermittent nasalization of vowels (as well as additional effects on consonant production and acoustics). Speech-language pathologists should know the theory of nasalization as part of their basic scientific knowledge and as a foundation for diagnostic, prognostic, and management plans and statements. A speech-language pathologist who understands the acoustics of nasalization will be able to provide a coherent account to other health care professionals, such as physicians, as to why the speech of a child with a repaired cleft palate, but lingering velopharyngeal inadequacy, produces "muffled" and soft speech. As a further example of how speech acoustics theory can inform clinical practice, recent theoretical work of Rong and Kuehn (2010) has shown how the acoustic results of nasalizing a vowel may actually be compensated for by adjustments of the oral cavity. Rong and Kuehn (2010) use modeling techniques—very similar to the techniques used by Stevens and House, described in Chapter 8, except with the electrical circuits implemented by computer software—to show that nasal formants and antiresonances may be minimized or even eliminated by proper adjustments of the oral articulators. It is the case, then, that the extra absorption of sound energy in the nasal cavities and the presence of antiresonances from the sinus cavities may result in the muffled, soft speech quality associated with velopharyngeal incompetence, but Rong and Kuehn's work suggests the possibility of speech-language pathologists teaching a child to modify oral postures to offset these nasalization effects.

Coupled (Shunt) Resonators in the Production of Lateral Sounds

Figure 9–5A shows a tracing from a midsagittal x-ray of a speaker producing an /l/. Note the contact of the tongue apex at the alveolar ridge (arrow). In back of this contact, MRI data have shown the tongue to be somewhat grooved, giving the tongue a convex shape with two parallel air passageways, one on either side of the midline of the vocal tract (Narayanan, Alwan, & Haker, 1997). This type of /l/ production is referred to as a *lateral* manner of articulation, to denote the articulatory configuration just described and hence the propagation of sound waves through the lateral passageways.[3] The cavity immediately behind the apical closure, however, traps sound energy at frequencies determined by the size of the closed resonator and therefore introduces an antiresonance into the /l/ spectrum. The cavity behind

---

[3]The articulatory configurations for /l/ may not always conform to the lateral description given here. For example, word-final /l/ (as in the words *bowl* and *heel*) is often produced with a retracted tongue and no contact with the alveolar ridge (the so-called "dark /l/" discussed in many phonetics textbooks). Some dialects use the lateralized version of /l/ more often than other dialects.

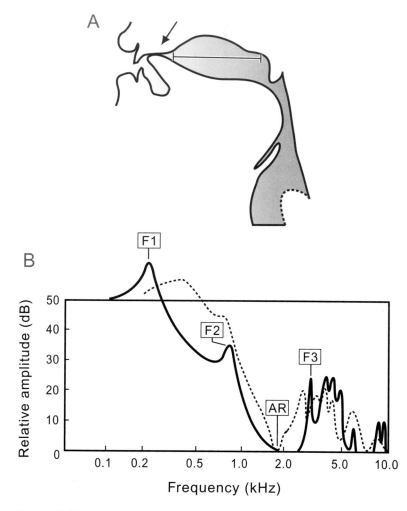

Figure 9–5. A. Midsagittal x-ray tracing of a lateral /l/ production. The contact of the tongue apex to the alveolar ridge is indicated by an arrow. The cavity where energy is trapped, thus introducing an antiresonance into the /l/ spectrum, is indicated by the horizontal line ending in short vertical bars. **B.** Theoretical (*solid line*) and measured (*dotted line*) spectra for lateralized /l/. Note the antiresonance (AR) in both the theoretical and measured spectra around 1800 to 2000 Hz. F1, F2, and F3 are indicated on the theoretical spectrum. From *Acoustic Theory of Speech Production* (pp. 163, 165), by G. Fant, The Hague: Mouton. Copyright 1960 by Mouton de Gruyter. Modified and reproduced with permission.

the apical closure can be considered a shunt resonator, in much the same way as described above for nasals.

The antiresonance in lateralized /l/ spectra derives from the cavity extending from the apical closure to the uvula, as indicated in the x-ray tracing of Figure 9–5A by the horizontal line ending in short vertical bars. Figure 9–5B shows the computed (theoretical) and measured spectra for an articulatory configuration like that shown in Figure 9–5A. If the spectra shown by the solid (theoretical) and dashed (measured) lines are compared, both show roughly the same frequency location of the antiresonance (*AR*), or reverse peak. This antiresonance occurs around 1800 to 2000 Hz and produces a substantial "dip" in the spectrum between the second and third formants. The antiresonance probably has the greatest effect on the amplitude of F3, which is quite low in both the theoretical and measured /l/ spectra in Figure 9–5B.

Coupled (Shunt) Resonators in the Production of Obstruent Sounds

Shunt resonators also occur in obstruent production. For all sounds considered so far (vowels, nasals, laterals), the theory involves a voicing source located at the back end of the vocal tract tube. The production of obstruents, however, involves a source of sound located *between* two resonating cavities. For example, in the production of /ʃ/ there is a noise (aperiodic) source generated in the vicinity of the supraglottal constriction. A magnetic resonance image (MRI) of a speaker producing an /ʃ/ is shown in Figure 9–6. The lips are to the right of the image and the air-filled cavities are shown as illuminated passageways. The /ʃ/ constriction is indicated by an arrow, and in and near this constriction a source of frication energy is generated (see

below for more details on frication sources). Just as the vibrating vocal folds produce a spectrum shaped by the vocal tract resonators, the /ʃ/ noise source has its spectrum shaped by the vocal tract. Even though the /ʃ/ noise source sits roughly between two resonators—the cavity in front of the constriction (Figure 9–6, "front cavity"), and the cavity in back of the constriction (Figure 9–6, "back cavity")—both cavities contribute to the vocal tract output because sound waves propagate away from the source in both directions (forward and backward). Because the back cavity is effectively closed, it traps energy at frequencies determined by its size and, therefore, generates an antiresonance. In this sense, the back cavity acts as a coupled or shunt resonator in the production of /ʃ/, and the antiresonance has an influence on the shape of the output spectrum. These kinds of coupled or shunt resonators are seen in the production of fricatives, stops, and affricates, as discussed more fully in the next section.

WHAT IS THE THEORY OF FRICATIVE ACOUSTICS?

Special features of fricatives make the theory of fricative acoustics different from those of the other sounds discussed thus far. These features can be understood by considering the general nature of fluid flow in pipes, and how different conditions within a pipe may change the nature of the flow and its acoustic results.

Fluid Flow in Pipes and Source Types

As mentioned above, obstruents are typically produced with a noise source, usually located in the vicinity of the major constriction or at the point where an obstacle (e.g., the teeth) interrupts airflow within the vocal tract. These noise sources are aperiodic (unlike the periodic voicing source), and can be related to patterns of airflow in the vicinity of the major constrictions or obstacles. In cases where the obstruent is voiced (such as a /b/, /z/, or /dʒ/), the voicing source may be superimposed on the vocal tract noise source. This case of *mixed sources* is discussed more fully in a later section of this chapter.

An understanding of aperiodic noise sources requires some background information on how patterns of airflow in tubes are modified at constrictions along the path of flow. Figure 9–7 shows a tube in which air molecules are flowing, as indicated by the parallel arrows. The arrowheads show the direction

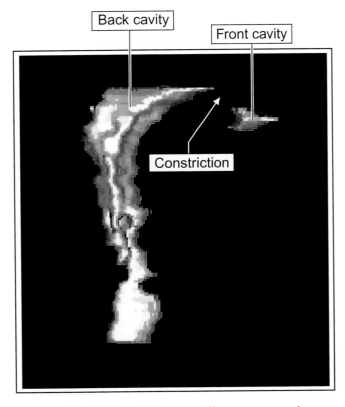

Figure 9–6. Midsagittal magnetic resonance image (MRI) of a speaker's vocal tract in the articulatory configuration for /ʃ/. The arrow indicates the /ʃ/ constriction, which is one location of the noise source whose spectrum is shaped by the front and back cavities. The back cavity is effectively a closed resonator and can be considered as a coupled, or shunt, resonator, contributing an antiresonance to the /ʃ/ spectrum. Image provided courtesy of Brad Story, Ph.D., University of Arizona, Tucson, Arizona. Reproduced with permission.

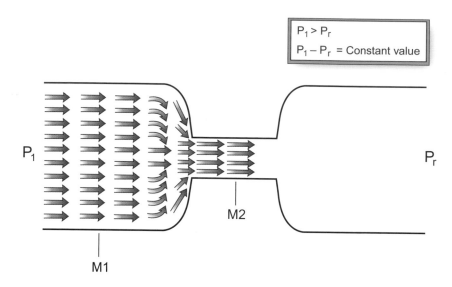

$P_1 > P_r$

$P_1 - P_r$ = Constant value

P_1

P_r

M2

M1

Figure 9-7. Laminar airflow within a tube. Laminar airflow is indicated by the parallel lines ending in arrowheads. Because pressure at the left of the tube (P_1) is greater than pressure at the right of the tube (P_r), air flows from left to right, toward the lower pressure. M1 indicates a measuring device placed at a relatively wide part of the tube and M2 indicates a measuring device placed at a relatively constricted part of the tube.

of the flow. Air is flowing through this tube because there is a *pressure differential* between the two ends of the tube. Air flows from regions of higher pressure to regions of lower pressure, so the movement of air molecules from left to right implies that P_1 is greater than P_r (where r means "reference"). The pressure differential $P_1 - P_r$ is assumed to be constant for the remainder of this discussion.

When air molecules flow through a tube in parallel streams, as shown in Figure 9–7, the flow is referred to as *laminar*. If the air flowing within the tube is not compressed as it moves from one end of the tube to the other, the air volume flowing past any one point in the tube per unit of time must be equivalent to the air volume flowing past any other point in the tube in the same unit of time. "Volume" can be interpreted as an amount, such as one might place in a container. It is typically measured in liters (L) (like milk, soda, or any other fluid, air being a fluid) or milliliters (mL).

Consider the tube shown in Figure 9–7 and imagine two volume-measuring instruments, one placed at a wide section of the tube (M1) and the other at a narrow section (M2). According to the law stated above, the volume of air moving past M1 in 1 s must equal the volume moving past M2 in the same time interval. The only way to get the same volume per unit time through a narrow section of the tube (at M2) as through a wide

section of the tube (at M1) is for the speed of the air molecules to be greater through M2, as compared to M1. Thus, air molecules flowing through a tube speed up as they go through a constriction.

Figure 9–8 reproduces the essential features of Figure 9–7 and adds two new conditions that have direct relevance to obstruent production, including the immediate case of fricatives. First, the flowing air molecules are shown both entering and exiting the constriction. Second, the flowing air molecules are shown striking a small rectangular obstacle, near the right-hand end of the tube.

As discussed above, as the air molecules enter the constriction they increase their speed. These fast-moving molecules then "shoot out" of the constriction exit in the form of a narrow stream or *jet* which expands as it moves downstream, toward the end of the tube. This jet of air is shown emerging from the constriction exit as a group of narrowly focused parallel lines. Note also in Figure 9–8 the circular motions of air molecules indicated along the edges of the jet. This circular flow pattern, which is clearly different from the parallel streaming of laminar flow, is called *turbulent flow*, or *turbulence*. When a constriction is narrow enough and the flow through it is sufficiently rapid, turbulent flow is produced in the manner shown in Figure 9–8. Because the temporal and spatial char-

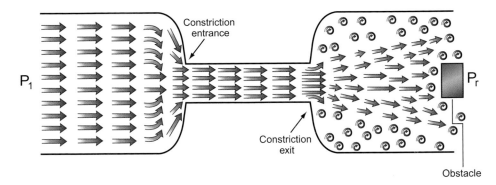

Figure 9–8. Air flowing in a tube, as in Figure 9–7, except that this tube has a very narrow constriction through which air is forced by a pressure differential across the two ends of the tube. Parallel lines indicate laminar airflow. Laminar airflow emerges from the constriction as a narrow jet, at the edges of which are rotating, erratically moving air molecules called turbulent flow. An obstacle is in front of the constriction and in the path of the airflow. When the laminar jet strikes the obstacle, air molecules move erratically and create additional turbulent airflow.

acteristics of these rotating air molecules are random (i.e., they are not periodic), their acoustic correlate is an aperiodic sound. The complex aperiodic acoustic event resulting from turbulent flow provides a sound source for fricatives, which have the narrow constrictions and high flows discussed in conjunction with Figure 9–8. Just as in the tube shown in Figure 9–8, air molecules speed up as they move through fricative constrictions and emerge from the constrictions as jets surrounded by regions of rotating, erratically moving air molecules, or turbulent flow. In fricative production, the turbulence generated at the exit of the supralaryngeal (above the larynx, that is, within the vocal tract) constrictions results in a *frication source*. This frication source is shaped by the resonant characteristics of the vocal tract, just as the vocal tract shapes the glottal source spectrum in vowel production.

The obstacle shown in Figure 9–8 produces a similar effect on the moving air molecules. When molecules strike the obstacle, they rotate and move erratically if certain conditions are met,[4] producing a significant amount of turbulent flow. The turbulence in the region of the obstacle functions as a frication source, just like the turbulence in the region of the constriction exit. When there is a sufficiently narrow constriction and a flow of sufficient magnitude (the conditions necessary for turbulence to be produced), plus an obstacle in the path of the expanding air jet "shooting out" from the constriction, multiple frication sound sources may

exist. For example, one source might be located near the constriction exit with the other at the "downstream" obstacle. In addition, air molecules moving along the walls of the vocal tract may also generate rotational patterns of airflow that result in aperiodic acoustic energy, and function as sound sources for fricatives. These "wall sources" are typically of weak intensity and associated with fricative articulations toward the back of the vocal tract (as in the velar fricative /x/ or pharyngeal fricative /ħ/.

What is the difference in the acoustic characteristics of a frication sound source with and without an obstacle like the one shown in Figure 9–8? Imagine an experiment in which the frication source characteristics generated by air rushing through a constriction is first measured without the obstacle in place, followed by an experiment in which the obstacle is placed in the path of the air jet. The primary difference in the source spectrum is a greater amount of overall energy in the "constriction + obstacle" case as compared to the "constriction only" case. The presence of the obstacle results in an acoustic event of greater amplitude (see below). In fact, if the linear distance between a constriction and a downstream obstacle is not too great, the frication source at the obstacle is powerful enough to dominate the amplitude of the acoustic event.

The tube model shown in Figure 9–8 is a fairly good representation of the aeromechanic and acoustic conditions generated in actual fricative productions.

---

[4]The conditions include the speed of the flow, the sharpness of the obstacle's edges, and the angle at which the flow strikes the obstacle.

Fricatives are associated with narrow constrictions and relatively high airflows, as mentioned above, and some fricatives (certainly /s/, /z/, /ʃ/, /ʒ/) have obstacles, in the form of teeth, located downstream from the constriction, in the path of the air jet.

An estimate of the source spectrum for fricatives is presented in Figure 9–9. Just as in the case of the voicing source for vowels, the spectral characteristics of frication sources are nearly impossible to measure directly, but must be inferred from the study of mechanical models and acoustical theory (Shadle, 1985, 1990). The spectrum shown in Figure 9–9 is not exactly correct, but is likely to be a very close approximation to the aperiodic source spectrum for fricatives. Stevens (1998), based on his own work and that of Shadle (1985, 1990), has argued that a source spectrum such as the one shown in Figure 9–9 is generally applicable to *all* fricatives. This "prototype" fricative source spectrum has slowly declining energy over the 0- to 10-kHz frequency range, with a roughly 20-dB difference between the highest-amplitude, low-frequency energy and the lowest-amplitude, high-frequency energy. In the 0- to 5-kHz range, the spectral energy changes only a little, and across this frequency range the spectrum can be described as more or less flat. There are fricative-specific modifications of this general spectrum, the most prominent one being the relative amplitude of the whole spectrum. As suggested by Stevens (1998), fricatives with greater source energy—those with obstacles (teeth) relatively close to the constriction—move the spectrum up the relative amplitude scale but leave the basic spectral shape unchanged. Those fricatives with lesser source energy—the ones made in the front of the vocal tract, near its exit to the atmosphere—have the source spectrum moved down on the relative amplitude scale. These fricative-specific changes in the overall level of the "prototype" source spectrum are indicated in Figure 8–9 by the arrows pointing up for /sʃzʒ/ and down for /fθvð/. In addition, because voiceless fricatives have greater oral pressure (P_o, see below) and hence greater airflow through the constriction as compared to their voiced cognates, the "prototype" fricative source spectrum is of greater amplitude for voiceless as compared to voiced fricatives.

Actual fricative source spectra may deviate from the prototype shown in Figure 9–9 for several reasons. As demonstrated by Shadle (1985, 1990), the shape and degree of the fricative constriction, the magnitude of

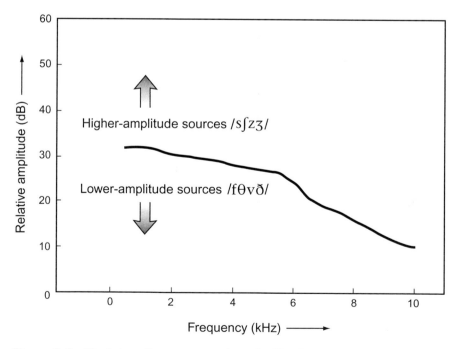

Figure 9–9. "Prototype" source spectrum for fricatives, modeled after data described by Stevens (2000) and work of Shadle (1985, 1990). The entire prototype spectrum is moved up the relative amplitude scale for fricatives in which an obstacle in the path of airflow contributes heavily to the source of energy (/sʃzʒ/) and down the scale for fricatives in which obstacles play only a minor role or no role at all (/fθvð/).

Good Dental Health = Nice Fricatives

Even before Shadle's (1985) experiments on how obstacles influence the aperiodic source for fricatives such as /s/ and /ʃ/, the University of Michigan phonetician J. C. Catford had described a relevant little experiment in his 1977 text, *Fundamental Problems in Phonetics*. He located two people with full dentures and asked them to produce /s/ and /ʃ/ with their dentures in, and with them out. Catford compared the teeth-in to teeth-out fricative spectra and found a dramatic difference in spectral intensity. The more intense fricative spectra occurred for the teeth-in productions, of course.

airflow through the constriction, the angle at which air flow strikes an obstacle, and the distance of the constriction from an obstacle are all factors that adjust details of the fricative source spectrum shape. These modifications, however, do not change the general description of an aperiodic source spectrum that gradually declines in energy from low to high frequency, and is more or less flat from 0 to 5 kHz.

Aeromechanic/Acoustic Effects in Fricatives: A Summary

The source of sound in fricatives represents a transformation of aeromechanical energy (in the form of turbulent flows) to acoustic energy (in the form of aperiodic waveforms and their spectra). The tube model of Figure 9–8 shows how air flowing through a constriction leads to the formation of a jet, around which turbulent flow is generated. This air jet may strike obstacles in its path and generate additional sound sources, which in some cases are the primary (dominant) source of acoustic energy. Air flows through a constriction because there is a pressure differential across it. In fricative production, pressure is higher in back of the constriction than in front of it. If the size of the constriction stays constant and the pressure differential across the constriction varies, what happens to the source spectrum? This is a very reasonable and relevant question, because

the same fricative may be produced with very different pressures depending on factors such as the stress, speaking style, and position of the fricative in a word. For example, fricatives occurring in the word-initial position (e.g., the /s/ in *sake* (/seɪk/) are produced with greater pressure than fricatives in word-final position (e.g., the /s/ in *case* (/keɪs/). If the pressure differential is greater in the word-initial position, the magnitude of flow through the constriction is greater as well. With all other factors constant, an increase in the pressure differential results in increased airflow through and out of the constriction.

Fortunately, the answer to the question concerning the source spectrum is not complicated. When the pressure differential and, therefore, airflow through a fricative constriction increases, the major effect appears to be an overall increase in the sound amplitude of the source. There do not appear to be major effects of increased airflow on the *shape* of the spectrum. So, if the probable source spectrum shown in Figure 9–9 is adjusted for changes in the magnitude of airflow through the constrictions, the significant adjustment involves moving the whole curve up or down the relative amplitude axis, but does not require changing the shape of the curve.

A Typical Fricative Waveform and Its Aeromechanical Correlates

An acoustic waveform for the sequence /æsæ/ is shown in Figure 9–10. Note the contrast between the periodic glottal pulsing of the surrounding vowels with the aperiodic amplitude variations in the fricative waveform. The fricative waveform may be called a *noise waveform* to indicate its lack of periodicity.

Immediately below the acoustic waveform are two additional waveforms, one showing the time history[5] of the air pressure in the vocal tract, the other the time history of air flowing through the vocal tract. For this example, assume that the pressure was measured *behind* the point of constriction (e.g., for /s/, in back of the point where the apex and anterior blade of the tongue form a groove in the vicinity of the alveolar ridge and anterior palate), and that airflow was measured as it emerged from the mouth. The air pressure and airflow histories are synchronized with the acoustic waveform, meaning that all three signals share a common and syn-

[5]"Time history" is a term used to describe the variation of a signal over time. In the case of an acoustic waveform, the time history is of variations in amplitude. Time histories may be shown for any number of other signals, including pressures, flows, movements of the articulators, voltages associated with muscle contraction (electromyograms, or EMG), and formant frequencies, to name a few measurable phenomena relevant to speech production.

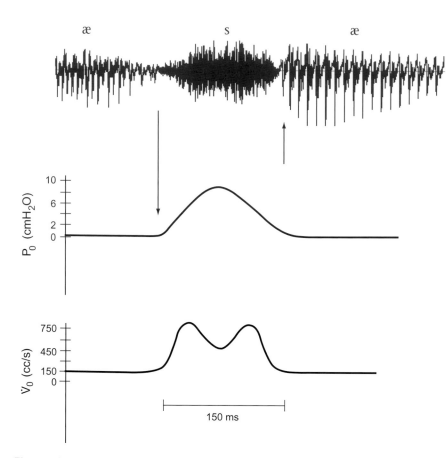

Figure 9–10. Acoustic waveform for /æsæ/ (*top panel*), shown with a synchronized oral pressure (*middle panel*), and oral airflow (*bottom panel*) records. Oral pressure, P_o, is near zero during the first vowel and begins to rise at the onset of aperiodic energy in the acoustic waveform. Pressure returns to near zero for the second vowel. Oral airflow, $\dot{V}_o$, is 150 cc/s for the first vowel, increases during the /s/ and shows two peaks during the fricative, before returning to 150 cc/s for the second vowel.

chronized time base. The air pressure measured within the vocal tract, called *oral air pressure* (P_o), is nearly zero during the first vowel and begins to increase (become positive) roughly at the instant when the acoustic signal changes from periodic to aperiodic (downward arrow pointing to P_o trace). The P_o reaches a maximum value of about 8 cm H_2O in the middle of the aperiodic /s/ waveform and then begins to fall back toward zero as the end of the fricative and onset of glottal pulsing

for the second vowel approaches (see upward arrow pointing to the acoustic waveform, Figure 9–10). P_o is nearly zero during the vowels because the vocal tract is open to atmosphere for production of these sounds (pressure inside and outside the vocal tract is nearly the same).[6] The airflow during the fricative is fairly high, roughly five times the magnitude of flow during the vowels, and has a "double-peaked" appearance very common for fricative production (Klatt, Stevens, &

---

[6]A reader attempting to put the information in this chapter together with material from Chapter 8 may detect what appears to be a contradiction. Here the text states that the pressure inside the vocal tract is zero during vowels because there are no substantial supralaryngeal constrictions, yet the discussion of perturbation theory in Chapter 8 included description of pressure variations along the wavelengths associated with vocal tract resonances. At the maximum pressure peaks of these wavelengths the pressure was clearly above P_{atm}. How can the statements made in this chapter about P_o being nearly zero during vowel production be resolved with the clearly positive pressures at certain points along the wavelengths of the resonant (formant) frequencies of vowels? In the case of the positive pressures along the wavelengths, these are at local points only (at a given cross-sectional slice of the vocal tract), and reflect relatively high-frequency pressure fluctuations (typically above 500 Hz). These are *acoustic* pressures in the sense that they are a characteristic of sound waves, as described in Chapter 7. P_o, an aeromechanic phenomenon, is a measure of the low-frequency (slow) compressibility of the *entire air volume in the vocal tract*, rather

Mead, 1968). The double peaks during fricative production probably reflect the time-varying tightness of the fricative constriction throughout the fricative duration. For present purposes, the relatively high airflow is of primary interest because of its capacity to produce turbulence.

Mixed Sources in Fricative Production

The production of the English fricatives /v/, /ð/, /z/, and /ʒ/ involves the turbulent airflow events discussed above, but may also be accompanied by vibration of the vocal folds. These voiced fricatives are, therefore, produced with two types of sources—one associated with the aperiodic, turbulent flow generated in the vocal tract and the other with the periodic vibration of the vocal folds. Fant (1960) used the term, "mixed source" to describe the case in which two sources were active in the production of a sound. In the case of a mixed source, both source spectra are shaped by the resonant characteristics of the vocal tract. It is as if the two sources are superimposed on each other, and the vocal tract resonators act on them (i.e., shape their spectra) simultaneously.

Shaping of Fricative Sources by Vocal Tract Resonators

The foundation for the understanding of resonances in fricative production has been prepared by: (a) the discussion of resonator size and resonant frequency (Chapter 7), and (b) the discussion of antiresonances in cases where sources are located between two resonant cavities.

The narrow vocal tract constriction required for fricatives can be thought of as dividing the vocal tract into a front and back cavity. The source is located in the vicinity of the constriction, or in front of the constriction (e.g., at the teeth), and its energy is propagated in both directions along the long axis of the vocal tract and possibly in other directions as well. Both the front and back cavities shape the source spectrum. However, the back cavity behaves as if it is "closed" and traps energy at frequencies determined by its size (i.e., just as open cavities—cavities that radiate sound to the atmosphere—amplify energy at frequencies determined

by their size). Thus, the back cavity shapes the source spectrum by introducing antiresonances into the fricative output spectrum. The front cavity, being open to the atmosphere, shapes the source spectrum by emphasizing a region of the spectrum. These emphasized frequencies appear in the output spectrum as high-amplitude regions, or peaks, at particular frequencies. A general, simplified rule for the way in which these cavities shape fricative spectra is as follows. As the cavity in front of the constriction gets smaller, the resonances of the frication spectra move to higher frequencies, consistent with the idea that air volumes in smaller resonating cavities are stiffer than air volumes in larger cavities. As the cavity behind the constriction gets smaller, the frequency of the antiresonances increases for the same reason.

Fricative spectra contain peaks, but they are not nearly as easy to identify as they are in vowel spectra. The peaks in fricative spectra are often broad, extending over a fairly large frequency region (perhaps 300–700 Hz). This is unlike vowel spectra in which the peaks are relatively narrow, with bandwidths in the 40- to 70-Hz range. Figure 9–11 presents examples of fricative spectra for /f/, /θ/, /s/, and /ʃ/. The fricatives were spoken in an /æCæ/ frame, where C = fricative, and the spectra were computed from the middle 50 ms

---

Sound Change

Speech sounds are subject to evolutionary selection pressures. One selection pressure is for a sound to be sufficiently distinct from other sounds so that it can function phonemically. When two phonemes in a language have very similar acoustic characteristics, their effectiveness as separate phonemes may be compromised. The two sounds may begin to merge into a single sound class and function more or less as allophones of one phoneme. Some believe this is happening to /f/ and /θ/ in African-American English, where the two sounds appear to be interchangeable in certain word positions. The weak, very similar spectra for these two fricatives make them ideal candidates for this kind of sound change—well known in the history of many languages.

---

than at a single cross-sectional slice of the tube. It is low frequency because the rise and fall of the pressure occurs over a period of roughly 0.06 to 0.12 s (60–120 ms), which is roughly the duration of the closure interval of stops and fricatives (see Figure 9–10 and Figure 9–16). The aeromechanical pressure symbolized by P_o is, therefore, a whole-volume, slowly varying event, whereas the acoustic pressures along the resonant wavelengths within the vocal tract tube are local (single-slice), rapidly varying events. This explains why the apparent contradiction is, happily, only apparent, and illustrates the difference between the acoustic and aeromechanic levels of observation introduced in Chapter 7.

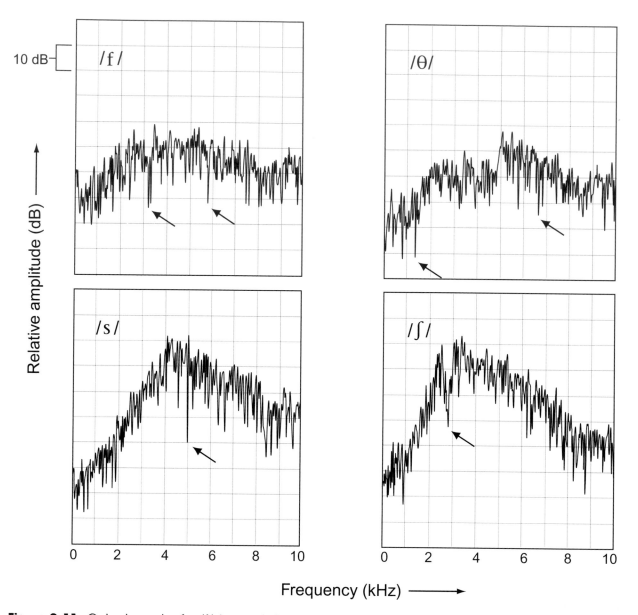

Figure 9–11. Output spectra for /f/ (*upper left*), /θ/ (*upper right*), /s/ (*lower left*), and /ʃ/ (*lower right*), produced by a 57-year-old adult male with complete dentition. The fricative spectra were computed from 50-ms intervals extracted from the middle of the frication noises in an /æCæ/ frame, where C = fricative. Arrows indicate probable antiresonances.

of the frication noises. These spectra have a frequency range of 0 to 10 kHz on the *x*-axis and relative amplitude, in 10-dB steps, on the *y*-axis. The fricatives were all recorded under exactly the same conditions, so relative amplitudes can be compared directly across the four spectra.

Both the /f/ and /θ/ spectra are relatively weak compared to the /s/ and /ʃ/ spectra. The peak amplitudes in the latter spectra are roughly 20 dB greater than the peak amplitudes of the former spectra. The /f/ spectrum is relatively flat, whereas the /θ/ spectrum has increasing amplitude up to 5.0 kHz and has relatively flat or slightly decreasing energy above 5.0 kHz. There is either a very small or nonexistent cavity in front of the constrictions for /f/ and /θ/, so the spectra of these fricatives might be expected to have an extremely high resonance frequency, or perhaps no clear region of resonance. In the case of an extremely small resonating cavity, the resonant frequency may be above the frequency limit of the spectra in Figure 9–11

(10 kHz) and, therefore, not visible in these plots. If the constriction is sufficiently anterior in the vocal tract and there is no effective front resonating cavity, the spectra may look like unfiltered versions of the source spectrum. Compare, for example, the shape of the prototype fricative source spectrum shown in Figure 9–9 to the /f/ output spectrum shown in Figure 9–11. With the exception of the low frequencies, the two spectra are quite similar. The /f/ and /θ/ spectra of Figure 9–11 also reflect the influence of antiresonances, as indicated by the upward-pointing arrows aimed at sharp "dips" in the spectra. As noted above, these result from energy trapping in the large back cavity.

A comparison of the /s/ and /ʃ/ spectra in Figure 9–11 illustrates nicely the principle of cavity size and resonant frequency. The constriction location for /s/ is more forward in the vocal tract than it is for /ʃ/, resulting in a smaller front cavity for /s/. Higher frequency peaks should, therefore, be observed for /s/, as compared to /ʃ/. Examination of the /s/ and /ʃ/ spectra in Figure 9–11 confirms this, showing a prominent, broad peak between 4.0 and 5.0 kHz for /s/ as compared to the peak in the /ʃ/ spectrum located between 2.5 and 3.5 kHz. The probable locations of antiresonances in the /s/ and /ʃ/ spectra have been indicated by upward-pointing arrows.

Figure 9–12 summarizes the relation of constriction location to the frequency location of major resonances by showing a sequence of spectra from a vocal tract maneuver in which one of the authors moved his tongue continuously from an /x/ to an /s/ position, sliding it forward from the back position while generating frication noise. The /x/ sound is a fricative heard in languages such as German and Yiddish (as in German "ach" /ɑx/ and Yiddish "chutzpah" /xʊtspɑ/). The three spectra shown are "slices" in time from the beginning (top spectrum), middle (middle spectrum), and end (bottom spectrum) of the back-to-front gesture. Note how the major concentration of spectral energy moves from a lower to a higher frequency region as the constriction is moved forward. The peak energy in the /x/, /ʃ/, and /s/-like positions of the tongue are indicated by arrows, and are located roughly at 1.5, 2.4, and 5.3 kHz, respectively. This is consistent with the increasingly small front cavity as the constriction is moved from back-to-front in the vocal tract.

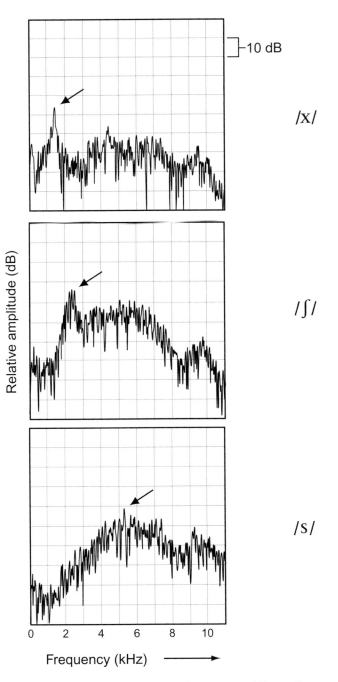

Figure 9-12. Sequence of spectra as one of the authors moved his tongue continuously forward from an /x/ to /s/ position while generating frication noise. Each spectrum is a "slice in time" from the continuous back-to-front gesture. The change in frequency emphasis as the tongue moves forward is related to the increasingly smaller front cavity. Arrows indicate peaks in the spectra.

Measurement of Fricative Acoustics

Both spectral and temporal measures are important in the description of fricative acoustics. The measures reviewed below are used frequently in scientific and clinical applications, but do not exhaust the possible measures that could be used to describe fricative acoustics.

Spectral Measurements

In the acoustic theory of vowel production, the measurement of formant frequencies is highlighted as an important way to capture the essential acoustic characteristics of vowels. The F-pattern (the frequencies of the first three formants) is an accepted way to represent the acoustic characteristics of vowels. Unfortunately, there is no standard way to measure and summarize fricative spectra. The goal of a measurement strategy for fricative spectra is to obtain a number, or small set of numbers, that reliably distinguishes between fricatives having different places of articulation, and possibly even between fricatives having the same place of articulation but different voicing characteristics.

Figure 9–13 shows two different approaches to the measurement of fricative spectra, using /f/ (top) and /s/ (bottom) spectra as examples. These fricative spectra are smoothed versions of the ones shown in Figure 9–11. "Smoothed" means that the general shape of the spectrum is shown as a curve connecting the peaks of the Fourier spectrum. The smoothing technique is discussed further in Chapter 10, but for present discussion the spectra are shown in this simplified way to facilitate the explanation of fricative spectral measurement. The arrows in each spectrum point to the primary peak, or the frequency associated with the greatest amplitude. This measurement is called the *peak frequency* of a fricative spectrum. This simple and straightforward approach to the measurement of fricative spectra is conceptually similar to the measurement of peaks (formants) in vowel spectra. In particular, because the primary resonance of fricatives depends on the size of the front cavity (the cavity in front of the constriction) the peak frequency is, in many cases, correlated with the place of articulation. Higher peak frequencies are expected for fricatives with smaller front cavities (such as /s/), and lower peak frequencies for fricatives with larger front cavities (such as /x/ or /ʃ/). In Figure 9–13 the /f/ peak frequency of 3.5 kHz is clearly different from the /s/ peak at 4.6 kHz.

Although there has been some success classifying fricative place of articulation with peak frequency measurements (Jongman, Wayland, & Wong, 2000), the measures are not as reliable in separating fricatives as formant frequency measures are for separating vowels. Many fricative spectra have multiple peaks of relatively similar amplitude, making the use of a single peak frequency relatively unreliable in distinguishing among different places of fricative articulation. This is illustrated in Figure 9–13 by the /f/ spectrum which has three peaks— at 2.6, 3.5 (highest peak), and 5.2 kHz—

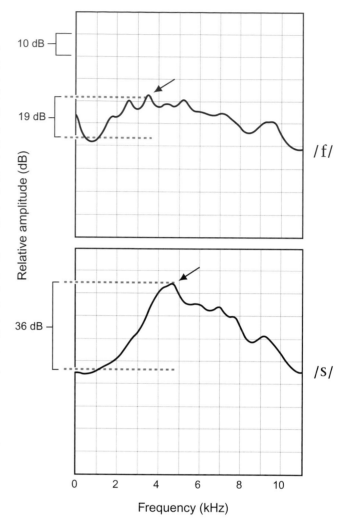

Figure 9–13. An /f/ (upper panel) and /s/ (lower panel) spectrum, showing two different ways to quantify spectral characteristics. Peak frequencies in both spectra are shown by downward-pointing arrows. Dynamic range of each spectrum is indicated by the distance between the upper and lower dashed lines in each panel.

of very similar relative amplitude. What if measurements were made of the frequencies of the two or three highest peaks in a fricative spectrum? This increases the *dimensionality* of the measurement (as in vowels, where three peaks are used) and may lead to better acoustic discrimination of fricative place of articulation. Unfortunately, the peaks in fricative spectra are often not as well defined (sharply tuned) as in vowel spectra and can be difficult to identify. It would seem as if other types of measurements should be explored, possibly in combination with the measurement of peak frequency(ies).

One such measurement is the *dynamic range* of a fricative spectrum. Figure 9–13 shows, for the two spectra, the range of amplitudes between the highest and lowest energies along the smoothed curves. This range is indicated on each spectrum by the two horizontal, dashed lines, and the range value in decibels is shown to the left of each spectrum. In this example, the dynamic range measurement has been limited to the frequency range 1.0 to 10.0 kHz to avoid low energies at the extremes of the spectrum. This approach is taken because the energy at the extremes of the fricative spectra are likely to be influenced as much by the way the fricatives were recorded and analyzed as by the articulatory characteristics of the fricatives. The substantially larger dynamic range of 36 dB for /s/ as compared to 19 dB for /f/ is a quantitative approach to capture the subjective visual impression of the relative flatness of the /f/ spectrum as compared to the /s/ spectrum. Although dynamic range measurements have not been explored in great detail for fricative spectra (see Shadle, 1985), the combination of such a measure with peak frequencies could result in better ability to distinguish between the acoustic characteristics of fricatives like /s/ and /ʃ/, or /f/ and /θ/ (or their voiced cognates).

Finally, fricative spectra can be quantified by treating the spectrum as a distribution of numbers and computing parameters that describe the central tendency, dispersion, tilt, and "peakiness" of the set of numbers. One of the first lessons of basic statistics concerns the existence and characteristics of a *normal distribution*. Using the normal distribution as a reference, any distribution can be described by: (a) an average, or *mean* of all the numbers (i.e., the central tendency); (b) a *variance*, which is the tendency of the numbers to spread more or less around the mean (dispersion); (c) a *skewness*, an index of how much the distribution curve deviates from strict symmetricality and leans left or right (tilt); and (d) a *kurtosis*, an index of how much the distribution deviates from "normal" peakiness (either more "peaky" or more flat). These four measures are called the first four *moments* of a distribution, and when applied to acoustic spectra they are called *spectral moments*. It is easy to see how the spectra in Figures 9–11, 9–12, and 9–13 look like distributions of numbers that deviate from the typical "bell-shape" of the normal distribution. Computer programs are available to compute spectral moments. These programs provide a four-number index (mean, variance, skewness, and kurtosis) of a fricative spectrum, or of any speech sound spectrum for that matter. These measures can be obtained automatically and rapidly, and certain fricatives can be distinguished from each other quite

---

Parsing Parsimony

The term "reducing the dimensionality" of a measurement problem is well known in all branches of science, including speech acoustics. How many numbers does it take to represent the fricative /ʃ/ so that it is completely distinguishable from other fricatives? Is the peak frequency measured at the halfway point of a fricative waveform sufficient, or do you need additional numbers (such as secondary and tertiary peak frequencies, fricative amplitude, and so forth). Scientists typically prefer the simplest measurement possible, so they spend a lot of time trying to determine the smallest set of numbers required to capture the essence of a physical phenomenon. The concept of *parsimony*—achieving adequate description or explanation using the simplest devices—is deeply entrenched in the souls of scientists.

---

well using this approach (Forrest, Weismer, Milenkovic, & Dougall, 1988). The articulatory interpretation of spectral moments, however, is sometimes not straightforward, which may limit their application in clinical settings. Spectral moments are discussed in greater detail in Chapter 11.

Temporal Measurements

The waveform in Figure 9–10 illustrates clearly the different appearance of vowel (periodic) and fricative (aperiodic) energy. Even in the case of voiced fricatives, for which the acoustic result of vocal fold vibration may be mixed with frication noise, vowels and fricatives look quite different in a waveform display. The different appearance of vowels and fricatives permits *segmentation* of the waveform into pieces that correspond to vowels, and pieces that correspond to fricatives. The "pieces" will correspond to *segment durations*, where "segment" refers to a sound category (vowel or fricative). The "pieces" are equivalent to durations, because they are defined along the *x*-axis of the waveform, which is time. Specific rules for the temporal segmentation of speech waveforms and *spectrograms* are given in Chapter 10. There is an extensive literature on segment durations (see Chapter 11), which have been used more than any other measure to describe and sometimes classify different types of speech disorders.

The Acoustic Theory of Fricatives: A Summary

The acoustic theory of fricatives shares with the acoustic theory of vowels the concepts of source and filter. In fricative production there is a source generated supralaryngeally, as a result of turbulent airflow: (a) in the vicinity of the constriction, (b) at an obstacle in the path of airflow, or (c) along the walls of the vocal tract. A particular fricative may have turbulent noise sources at any combination of these three sites. This turbulent source is aperiodic and produces a spectrum that is nearly flat, or in some cases slightly falling, as a function of frequency. When airflow strikes an obstacle directly, as in the case of /s/ and /ʃ/ where flow hits the teeth, the frication source has relatively great amplitude. When airflow strikes other surfaces in a more indirect manner, as in the case of /f/ and /θ/ where airflow may glance off the teeth and/or lips, or when the airflow moves along the vocal tract walls or encounters no obstacles in its pathway, the frication source is relatively weak. These differences in source amplitude are largely responsible for the pronounced, overall amplitude differences between English fricatives with constrictions in the vocal tract (/s/, /ʃ/, /z/, /ʒ/) vs. those with constrictions at the outlet of the vocal tract (/f/, /θ/, /v/, /ð/).

The filter in fricative production is the vocal tract, as it is for vowels. Because the source propagates in both directions along the long axis of the vocal tract and even from side to side of the tube, all cavities contribute to the shaping of the source spectrum, even though the source location may be well in front of the cavity behind the constriction. The primary resonances in fricative spectra originate in the cavity in front of the constriction. As this cavity decreases in size, as when a fricative constriction is moved from the back to front of the vocal tract, the primary resonances will increase in frequency. Fricative spectra also contain antiresonances, which are due primarily to the back cavity and its behavior as a closed resonator that traps acoustic energy.

There is no standard approach to the measurement of fricative spectra, as there is in the case of vowels. However, three candidate measurements — peak frequencies, dynamic range, and spectral moments — appear to be useful. Future research should show which of these (or other) measures does the best job of distinguishing between the fricatives, and which can be most easily interpreted in articulatory terms.

WHAT IS THE THEORY OF STOP ACOUSTICS?

Figure 9–14 shows a tube model similar to the one shown for fricative aeromechanics (see Figure 9–8). Unlike the tube in Figure 9–8, which contains a narrow constriction through which air flows, the tube in Figure 9–14 has a complete constriction (at the downward-pointing arrow) that can be conceptualized as a closed valve blocking the flow of air. When a pressure differential exists between the two ends of the tube, with P_1 greater than P_r, air flows from the left end of the tube to the right end, as shown by the arrows in Figure 9–14. The airflow is blocked by the complete constriction, causing compression of the air molecules behind the constriction. Compression of air molecules results in increasing pressure that continues to rise until the constriction is broken or the air volume becomes maximally stiff and cannot be compressed further.

During speech production, completely closed tubes such as the one shown in Figure 9–14 occur

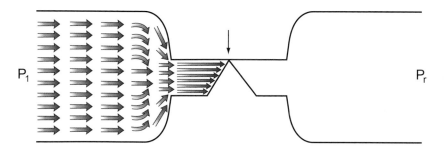

Figure 9–14. Airflow in a tube like that in Figures 9–7 and 9–8, except that a complete constriction in the tube (arrow) prevents air from passing through to the right side. Pressure builds up behind the constriction, as is the case for stop consonants. P_1 is the pressure behind the constriction and P_r is the reference pressure (atmospheric pressure).

for the articulation of stop consonants. The complete blockage of airflow for stops may be formed at several places throughout the vocal tract (at the lips, between the tongue and various locations along the hard and soft palates, and at the glottis), and generally lasts no longer than about 100 ms (1/10 of a second). When air flowing through the vocal tract is blocked by a stop constriction, the molecules within the volume behind the constriction are compressed simultaneously and uniformly. For example, in the production of a voiceless stop consonant, the vocal folds are separated and the volume in back of a vocal tract constriction includes the air spaces of the trachea and lungs (as well as those of the vocal tract). The nasal cavities are excluded from this volume because the velopharyngeal port is closed for the production of stops (as it is for all obstruents in English). The complete blockage of airflow at the stop constriction results in compression of air molecules throughout the volume behind the constriction. This compression is uniform and occurs nearly instantaneously throughout the enclosed volume, so the pressure should be the same—especially when it reaches its peak value—at all points in back of the constriction.

This condition is illustrated in the schematic speech production apparatus of Figure 9–15A, where a complete lingua-alveolar constriction is shown for the voiceless stop /t/, and the volume in back of the constriction is indicated by the shaded area. Three pressures are indicated within this volume. *Oral air pressure* is symbolized by P_o, which as reviewed above in the section on fricatives is the pressure measured within the vocal tract. P_t is *tracheal air pressure*, measured immediately below the vocal folds. P_{alv} is *alveolar air pressure*, or the pressure inside the lungs. When air is compressed behind a complete vocal tract constriction for a voiceless stop, the peak (highest) value of P_o is roughly equivalent to the peak values of P_t and P_{alv} because the vocal folds are separated during the stop closure, creating a continuous volume of air from the vocal tract constriction through to the trachea and lungs. In an utterance such as /ɑtɑ/, P_o is nearly zero (P_{atm}) during the first vowel, begins to rise when the

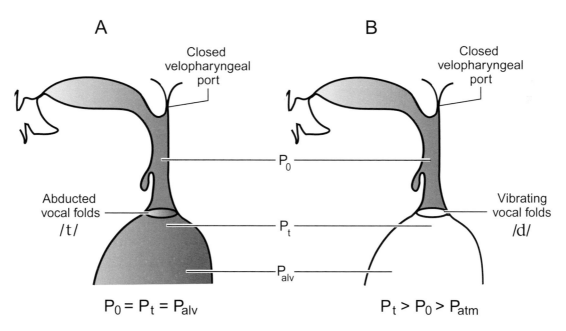

Figure 9–15. **A.** Schematic drawing of the speech production apparatus, showing a complete constriction at the alveolar ridge for the voiceless stop /t/. The volume of air that is compressed during the stop closure interval is indicated by the shaded parts of the drawing and includes the vocal tract spaces behind the constriction as well as the spaces within the trachea and lungs. Oral, tracheal, and alveolar air pressures are all equal during the stop closure interval. **B.** Schematic drawing of the speech production apparatus, showing a complete constriction at the lingua-alveolar ridge for the voiced stop /d/. The volume of air that is compressed during the stop closure interval is indicated by the shaded parts of the drawing and includes only the spaces between the constriction and the larynx. Tracheal air pressure is greater than oral air pressure and both are greater than atmospheric air pressure. The unshaded oval at the level of the glottis indicates laryngeal closure during the closed phase of the vibratory cycle.

complete constriction is made for the /t/ until a magnitude of 5 to 10 cm H_2O is reached, and drops rapidly back to nearly zero when the constriction is released into the following vowel. During vowel production, of course, P_t and P_{alv} will be above zero (around 5–10 cm H_2O) so that air can flow from the trachea and through the vocal folds, setting the latter into vibration. As mentioned above, the complete constriction for voiceless stops is generally maintained for no longer than 100 ms. It is during this closure interval that air is compressed and P_o rises above zero.

In the case of voiced stop consonants, the aeromechanical situation is somewhat different because the vibrating vocal folds separate the tracheal and pulmonary air volumes from the vocal tract air volume. In this case, the peak value of P_o typically does not equal P_t and P_{alv} because as air flows through the vibrating vocal folds there is some loss of pressure, resulting in P_o values that are generally lower than the pressures in the trachea and lungs. In Figure 9–15B the shaded area behind the lingua-alveolar constriction shows the compressible volume associated with P_o for voiced stops. This volume extends only between the constriction and the vocal folds, the latter shown as an unshaded oval to indicate the closed phases during each vibratory cycle. As long as P_t is greater than P_o by a critical amount (usually about 2 cm H_2O) the vocal folds continue to vibrate during the voiced stop closure interval, because air flows from the higher (tracheal) to lower (vocal tract) pressure region.[7]

Values of P_o for voiced stops, ranging between about 3.5 to 8.0 cm H_2O, are typically about 1.5 cm H_2O less than values for voiceless stops. The duration of the closure interval for voiced stops is about the same as that for voiceless stops, usually not exceeding 100 ms.

Both voiceless and voiced stops, therefore, have a buildup of P_o during their closure intervals. The vocal tract is "sealed" by the stop articulation (e.g., between the lips, or between the tongue and palate) as well as by closure of the velopharyngeal port. The seal briefly prevents air from escaping the vocal tract to the atmosphere and results in the P_o buildup. The next step is to link these aeromechanical events with the acoustic characteristics of stop consonants.

Intervals of Stop Consonant Articulation: Aeromechanics and Acoustics

Stop consonant articulation is often said to have several successive components. These include the closure, release (burst), frication, and aspiration intervals (the latter only occurring for voiceless stops). Voice-onset time (VOT) includes the burst, frication, and aspiration intervals in the case of voiceless stops, and the burst and frication intervals for voiced stops.

Closure (Silent) Interval

In an articulatory sequence such as /atɑ/ the vocal tract is open for the first vowel and then closed for the /t/ by contact of the tongue tip with the alveolar ridge. The closure interval of the stop is also called the *silent interval*, because during this interval the vocal tract generates little or no acoustic energy. In other words, if the vocal tract is completely sealed, there is no orifice from which acoustic energy can be radiated. The closure intervals of voiceless stops are typically completely silent, but the closure intervals of voiced stops may show evidence of weak periodic energy from vibration of the vocal folds. This weak periodic energy during the closure interval is not the result of a pressure wave emerging from the mouth or nose, because the vocal tract is completely sealed. Rather, vocal fold vibration during a closure interval causes the walls of the vocal tract to vibrate, these vibrations transferring to the air surrounding the head and neck in the form of low-energy pressure waves which may be sensed by the ear or by a microphone.

Figure 9–16 shows two speech waveforms to illustrate the closure interval for /atɑ/ (left) and /adɑ/ (right). P_o and $\dot{V}_o$ (oral air pressure and airflow) traces

---

[7]There are cases in which P_o rises to the same magnitude as P_t during the closure interval of a voiced stop. When this occurs, there is no pressure differential across the glottis, and hence no airflow and vocal fold vibration. This set of conditions might even be more common if it were not for an articulatory gesture that seems to be specific to voiced stops. In several studies (Bell-Berti, 1975; Kent & Moll, 1969), it has been shown that the volume of the cavity behind the vocal tract constriction and above the glottis actually *enlarges* during the closure interval of voiced stops (the same pharyngeal enlargement occurs for voiced English *fricatives*, suggesting the enlargement is associated with obstruent voicing in general, and not just stop voicing: see Proctor, Shadle, & Iskarous, 2010). The enlargement is accomplished by muscular mechanisms that widen the pharynx, lower the larynx, and raise the velum. In a closed volume, the product of pressure and volume is a constant; this aeromechanical characteristic of closed volumes is known as *Boyle's law*. Thus, if the volume behind the constriction and above the vocal folds is enlarged during the closure interval, the pressure within that volume should be reduced to meet the constancy described by Boyle's law. The reduced pressure tends to keep P_o below P_t, and allows vocal fold vibration to be maintained throughout much or all of the closure interval. This enlargement of the vocal tract volume behind the constriction does not occur for voiceless stops because there is no need to maintain a pressure difference across the glottis (i.e., there is no need to maintain vocal fold vibration, which requires a pressure difference across the glottis).

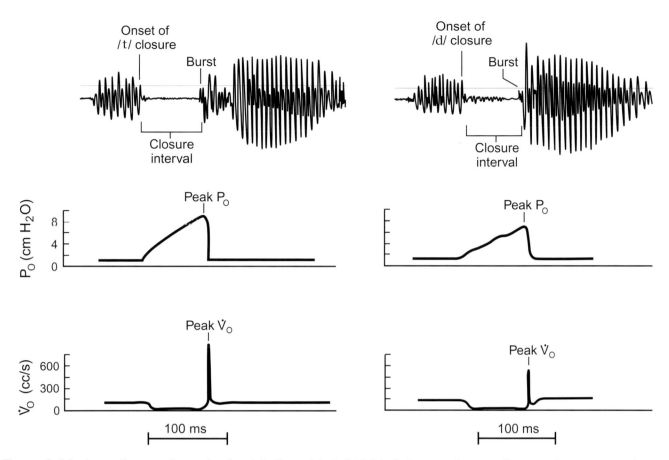

Figure 9–16. Acoustic waveforms for /ata/ (*left*) and /ada/ (*right*). Below each acoustic waveform are synchronized oral pressure (P_o) and oral airflow ($\dot{V}_o$) signals. See text for details.

are shown below and synchronized in time with each acoustic waveform. The vowels surrounding the closure intervals are easily identified by their large amplitude, periodic energy. For the /ata/ traces, a pointer marked "onset of /t/ closure" indicates the final glottal pulse of the first vowel, after which there is minimal or no acoustic energy for a period of about 70 ms. This is the closure interval of the voiceless stop consonant. The onset of the /d/ closure is also indicated by a pointer, but in this case the following closure interval contains some weak, periodic energy, as shown by the low-amplitude glottal pulses that terminate shortly before the burst. This is the energy from vocal fold vibration, transmitted to the microphone via vibration of orofacial tissue such as the neck and cheeks.

The airflow coming through the mouth ($\dot{V}_o$) is approximately 130 cc per s during the first vowel, and decreases rapidly to zero at the onset of the closure interval. For both voiceless and voiced stops, P_o is nearly zero (P_{atm}) during the vowels and begins to rise at the onset of the closure interval. The P_o continues

to rise until it is released at the point on the acoustic waveforms marked "burst" (see next section). Note the very brief, high airflow (peak $\dot{V}_o$) at the instant of release of the stop. This results when the stop constriction is opened suddenly and the high P_o developed during the closure interval decreases to nearly P_{atm} over an interval of just a few milliseconds or less. The relationship between the aeromechanical and acoustical events shown in Figure 9–16 for /ata/ and /ada/ is elaborated in the following descriptions of the burst, frication, and aspiration intervals.

Release (Burst) Interval

The sudden drop of P_o at the instant of stop closure release creates an acoustic source of energy, originally referred to by Fant (1960) as *shock excitation*. Shock excitation sources typically have very brief durations (perhaps no longer than 2 ms) and relatively flat spectra. As in the case of turbulent noise sources for fricatives, shock excitation sources for stops are located in the vicinity of the constriction and their spectra are shaped mainly by the cavity in front of the constriction. In Figure 9–16, the acoustic result of the sudden release of P_o is shown as the sudden "spike" at the end of the closure interval, labeled as the *burst*. Bursts are distinctive acoustic characteristics of both voiceless and voiced stops, although they are not always present for stop production (see Byrd, 1993, and Chapter 11). The typically greater P_o for voiceless, as compared to voiced stops (compare peak P_o for voiceless and voiced stops in Figure 9–16) generally results in greater amplitude for voiceless stop bursts (Stevens, 1998).

Frication and Aspiration Intervals

When the constriction is released, the pressure differential between the cavity behind the constriction (P_o) and the cavity in front of the constriction (P_{atm}) generates an airflow of relatively great magnitude. This event is shown in Figure 9–16 by the sudden "spikes" of airflow — the peak $\dot{V}_o$ — marking the end of the closure intervals during which airflow is zero. The passage of this flow through narrow constrictions in the vocal tract and at the glottis explains the final two phases of stop consonant acoustics.

In the discussion of the aeromechanical basis of the acoustic characteristics of fricatives (see Figure 9–8), turbulence was said to occur when a flow of sufficient magnitude passed through a sufficiently narrow constriction. Turbulent airflow produces the aperiodic acoustic energy of fricatives, as shown in the waveform of Figure 9–10. In the production of stop consonants there is a brief interval during which the conditions are met for the generation of turbulent airflow, and hence fricative-like aperiodic energy. In /ɑtɑ/, for example, as the tongue breaks the stop constriction and moves toward an open vocal tract configuration for the following vowel there is a brief interval when a very narrow constriction is formed between the tongue and alveolar ridge. The airflow "spike" shown in Figure 9–16 moves through this narrow constriction and, as in the case of fricatives, generates turbulence at the outlet of the constriction and perhaps at the teeth as well.

The acoustic time-domain result of the turbulent flow is illustrated in the waveform shown in Figure 9–17. This waveform is like a zoom-lens view of the intervals from the burst to the following vowel. The burst in Figure 9–17 is clearly followed by an interval of aperiodic energy, labeled the *frication interval*. This acoustic interval, which typically lasts for roughly 30 to 50 ms, reflects the period of time during which the conditions for turbulent flow are met at the stop constriction as it expands into the configuration for the following vowel. The frication interval of stops lasts only a brief time because as the tongue continues to move away from the alveolar ridge, the size of the constriction increases and eventually becomes too large to sustain turbulent flow. In addition, the flow decreases rapidly from its peak and quickly becomes too low to generate turbulence.

Figure 9–17 also shows a brief *aspiration interval* following the frication interval. Like the frication interval, the aspiration interval is the acoustic product of turbulent airflow. In this case, however, turbulence is produced at the glottis rather than at or around a constriction formed by the upper articulators. In the case of voiceless stops between two vowels, the vocal folds vibrate for the first vowel but then must be separated to prevent vocal fold vibration during the closure interval. The separation of the vocal folds is followed by their return to midline for the phonation requirements of the following vowel. As the vocal folds are moving together, there is a brief interval, immediately before complete approximation, during which there is a very narrow glottal constriction. The airflow through this narrow constriction produces turbulent airflow, the acoustic result of which is the aspiration interval shown in Figure 9–17. A typical aspiration interval has a duration of 10 to 30 ms. In stop consonant production, the aspiration interval is only found for voiceless cognates. This is because the vocal folds are not separated from the midline in voiced stops and, therefore,

---

Good Things Come in Small Packages

Stop bursts have extremely short life spans — typically less than 0.002 s in duration — and often have rather low amplitudes, at least when compared to vowels. Yet despite their seemingly small physical attributes, they have played a large role in theories of speech production and perception. A small experiment using speech analysis software can demonstrate the power of this little acoustic event: On the hard disk of the computer, record a speaker saying /pɑ/, /tɑ/, and /kɑ/, and then use any speech analysis program to isolate a 4- to 5-ms "piece" of each stop, beginning from the onset of the burst. Play each of the three very brief "pieces" to listeners and ask them if they hear a /p/, /t/, or /k/. From these tiny bits of information, most listeners will hear the "correct" stop!

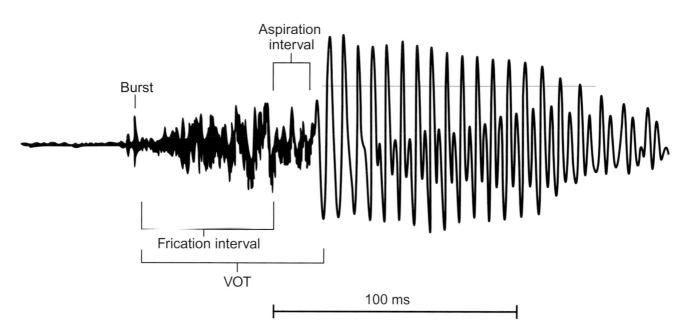

Figure 9–17. A "zoom" picture of a speech waveform showing the burst, frication, and aspiration intervals of a voiceless stop consonant. The sum of the time intervals for the burst, frication, and aspiration intervals is the voice-onset time (VOT).

do not have to be brought back together for voicing of the following vowel.

Both the frication and aspiration intervals are the result of turbulent airflow. Fant (1960) proposed the terms *frication noise* and *aspiration noise* to designate the location of the turbulent flow. Frication noise is the term for the acoustic result of turbulence generated in the vocal tract (at or around a constriction formed by the upper articulators) and aspiration noise is the term for turbulence generated at the glottis. The use of the word "noise" in these terms indicates the aperiodic nature of acoustic energy in the frication and aspiration intervals. Note in Figure 9–17 the much lower amplitude of the aperiodic energy during the aspiration, as compared to the frication, interval. Aspiration noise is typically quite weak, but the fairly clear amplitude distinction seen in Figure 9–17 between the frication and aspiration noise is not always so obvious.

Voice-Onset Time

The interval from the stop burst to the first glottal pulse of the following vowel is called the *voice-onset time* (VOT). The VOT of voiceless stops includes the burst, frication, and aspiration intervals, as marked in Figure 9–17. The VOT for voiceless stops is usually somewhere between 40 to 80 ms, but may vary according to a number of factors which are discussed more

fully in Chapter 11. VOT for voiced stops is generally less than 20 ms, and voicing may precede the stop burst (see Chapter 11).

Shaping of Stop Sources by Vocal Tract Resonators

As in vowels and fricatives, the acoustic output of the vocal tract for stops is the result of source spectra shaped by vocal tract resonators. Stop sources are considered first, followed by a discussion of how those sources are shaped by the resonators.

The Nature of Stop Sources

In the preceding discussion, the silent, burst, frication, and aspiration intervals of stop consonant production are described. Each of these intervals is produced with a different source, so it appears that stops are produced with a *succession* of changing sources. In the silent interval there is no source, followed by the shock excitation source of the burst, which gives way to two turbulent noise sources in the case of voiceless stops (frication and aspiration) or a single turbulent noise source in voiced stops (frication).

Earlier it was noted that it is very difficult to state the precise spectral characteristics of fricative noise sources. This comment also applies to sources associated with stop consonant production. Reasonable estimates of stop source spectra are available in the acoustic phonetics literature, however, and can be offered here. No description is required for the silent interval, of course, because there is no source.

The shock excitation source of the burst is a very brief event, lasting only as long as the time required for the peak P_o developed during the closure interval to decline to near P_{atm}, following release of the stop (see Figure 9–16). This interval lasts only a few milliseconds, and may be as brief as 0.5 ms (Stevens, 1998). Shock excitation qualifies as an *impulse-like event*, or one that is characterized by a large change in amplitude (in this case, pressure) over a very brief interval. Impulse-like events are known to "spread acoustic energy" across a wide range of frequencies, producing a spectrum having roughly equal energy at all frequencies. The source spectrum of shock excitation is roughly consistent with that of an impulse-like event; like the frication source spectrum, the shock excitation spectrum decreases in energy as frequency increases. For the purposes of this text it can be assumed that the source spectrum of shock excitation is roughly like that shown for fricatives in Figure 9–9. The different places of articulation for stop consonants have only a slight effect on the shock excitation source spectrum. Fant (1960) suggested that the source spectrum for /t/ shock excitation is flatter (shows a shallower decrease in energy across frequency) than the source spectra for /p/ and /k/. This description of shock excitation source spectra also applies to the voiced cognates (/b,d,g/).

The source spectra for the stop frication interval are also essentially the same as the source spectra for fricatives shown in Figure 9–9. The aeromechanical phenomena that produce sources for fricatives, and sources for the stop frication intervals, are identical. Figure 9–9 showed some place-of-articulation differences in the source spectra for fricatives, and these apply to the frication intervals of /p,b/ versus /t,d/ and /k,g/. The frication source for bilabials typically has weaker energy than the frication sources for lingua-alveolar and dorsal stop consonants, consistent with the place-related differences in frication source energy shown in Figure 9–9.

The source spectrum for the aspiration interval of voiceless stops has energy concentrated in the mid-frequencies (1.0–4.0 kHz), with less energy in the lower and higher frequencies. A single aspiration source spectrum applies to all three places of articulation of stops, because variation in place of articulation should not affect the acoustic result of turbulence at the glottis. This source spectrum is, therefore, somewhat different from the relatively flat source spectra of the shock excitation and frication intervals.

The Shaping of Stop Sources

The acoustic shaping of the shock excitation and frication sources in stop articulation is consistent with the shaping of fricative sources, described above. Shock excitation and frication sources are typically located within the vocal tract, between two resonators. As in the case of fricatives, the cavity in front of the source provides the primary emphasis of energy (resonance) in the output spectrum and the cavity behind the source contributes one or more antiresonances to the output spectrum.

Figure 9–18 presents fairly typical spectra for the three stop places-of-articulation, measured over a 10-ms interval beginning at the burst. The spectra have been smoothed in the same way as the fricative spectra in Figure 9–13. These spectra were derived from the voiceless stops, but the description provided here can be applied to the voiced cognates, as well. The shapes of these three burst spectra are consistent with the ideas developed above in the section on fricative spectra. For example, for the bilabial stop /p/ there is no vocal tract cavity in front of the constriction. A relatively flat output spectrum for the /p/ burst might be expected because there is no front cavity to emphasize a particular region of the shock excitation source spectrum. The /p/ burst spectrum shown in Figure 9–18 (left spec-

---

Counteracting Pop

Rock vocalists are famous for appearing to chew the microphones they are singing into. This is one way to control variations in voice intensity that result from changing the distance between the mouth and the microphone. If the singer is always lip-to-foam, the only variations in voice intensity heard by the adoring crowd will be those with artistic intent—that is, changed by the singer as she or he delivers the song. The "foam" to which the singer's lips are applied is called a wind or pop screen. Pop screens are designed specifically to disperse the bursts produced for /p/s and /b/s. When the intraoral pressure is released for bilabial stops, the sudden spike of airflow has the potential to overdrive the microphone, producing acoustic distortion. Pop screens scatter bilabial airflow spikes and prevent them from creating aural unpleasantries.

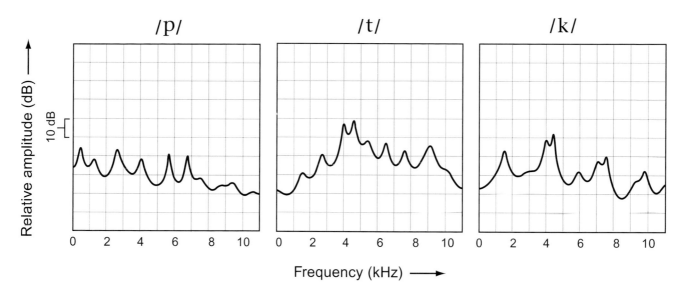

Figure 9–18. Sample output spectra (smoothed) for the burst interval of voiceless stop consonants. Each spectrum is computed from a 10-ms interval starting at the burst. The spectra for voiced stop consonants are similar to these, but may show somewhat less overall energy and some additional low-frequency energy.

trum) is, in fact, relatively flat between roughly 0 Hz and 7000 Hz (compare this to the description of the /f/ output spectrum, and Figure 9–11). Note the slight, rightward tilt of the /p/ burst spectrum, indicating a relatively gradual decrease in energy with increasing frequency. This flat or gradually declining spectrum is considered a classic characteristic of bilabial stops. As in fricatives, the cavity behind the shock excitation source contributes antiresonances to the spectrum.

The effect of the size of the cavity in front of the constriction is illustrated by comparing the burst spectra for /t/ (Figure 9–18, middle spectrum) to that for /k/ (Figure 9–18, right spectrum). The energy in the /t/ burst spectrum rises sharply from 0 Hz to roughly 4.5 kHz, with a clear spectral emphasis (the location of greatest energy) between 4.0 and 5.0 kHz. The /k/ burst spectrum, on the other hand, shows a prominent peak at 1.5 kHz, in addition to peaks in the vicinity of 4.0 kHz. The emphasis at higher frequencies in the /t/ burst spectrum makes sense because the cavity in front of the constriction is smaller than in the case of /k/ (or, stated otherwise, the large peak at 1.5 kHz in the /k/ burst spectrum, in contrast to the weak energy at this frequency in the /t/ spectrum, makes sense because the cavity in front of the /k/ constriction is larger than in the case of /t/). As the cavity in front of the stop constriction becomes smaller, the emphasis in the spectrum moves to higher frequencies. In this sense, the general *spectral shapes* of stop bursts are related to articulatory configurations in the same way as discussed above for

fricatives. Chapter 11 contains a detailed discussion of spectral shapes for stop bursts.

Stop burst spectra contain antiresonances. The same rules relating cavity-size to location of frequency peaks (or reverse peaks) apply to the locations of antiresonances as well as to resonances: Large cavities yield low-frequency resonances or antiresonances, and small cavities yield high-frequency resonances or antiresonances. The spectra in Figure 9–18 do not show antiresonances because the smoothing of the spectra ignores the locations where large "dips" occur.

Measurement of Stop Acoustics

Both spectral and temporal measurements have been used to quantify the acoustic characteristics of stops. As in the case outlined earlier for fricatives, the discussion below is not exhaustive but rather describes frequently made measurements.

Spectral Measurements

Surprisingly, even though stop burst spectra have played a prominent role in theories of speech production and perception, there has not been much agreement concerning their measurement. Earlier in this chapter it was pointed out that there is much discussion (and not much agreement) concerning the proper way to measure fricative spectra. The issues are similar for the measurement of stop burst spectra, with one important difference as reviewed below.

As in the case of fricative spectra, the goal of a measurement strategy for stop burst spectra is to obtain a small set of numbers that distinguishes among the three places of articulation. Stop burst spectra have numerous peaks and valleys, as is evident in the three spectra shown in Figure 9–18. In fact, these spectra are quite similar to fricative spectra (compare spectra in Figure 9–18 to those in Figure 9–11). Thus, peak frequencies can be measured for stop burst spectra but have the same problems as those discussed for fricatives. Similarly, dynamic range could be measured for burst spectra, but laboratory experience suggests that this would not provide a useful way to distinguish stop place of articulation.

Many researchers have focused their attention on the shape of the stop burst spectrum. Earlier, spectral moments were described as one means to obtain a numerical index of the shape of fricative spectra. When spectral moments are applied to stop burst spectra, they do a very good job of distinguishing place of articulation (Forrest et al., 1988; see additional discussion in Chapter 11). A nonnumerical, *prototype* approach to the classification of place of articulation for stop consonants involves the use of *spectral shape templates*. These templates, developed originally by Blumstein and Stevens (1979), provide a prototype burst spectrum for each place of articulation and an allowable range of variability for a particular stop burst spectrum to fit one of the prototypes. For example, if a stop burst spectrum fits within an allowable range of variability for the bilabial template, or prototype, it is classified as a bilabial stop.

Blumstein and Stevens (1979) constructed the templates based on their careful examination of many burst spectra computed over the 0–5000 Hz frequency range, and quantified the number of spectra from naturally spoken stops that were correctly classified using the templates. They had relatively good success in this exercise, classifying the place of articulation correctly about 85% of the time. This success makes the template approach attractive because it offers a relatively simple procedure for classifying acoustic events (burst spectra) according to phoneme category (i.e., place contrasts). For example, a computer could store the templates developed by Blumstein and Stevens (1979) and measure real burst spectra (for example, produced by clients with speech disorders) for comparison to the templates. In a clinical setting, this may serve as a simple approach to an objective evaluation of a client's articulatory capabilities for stop consonants. The procedure has certain limitations, however, which would have to be worked out prior to widespread clinical or research use. The classification accuracy of the original templates was evaluated by Blumstein and Stevens using a small number of speakers (3) who articulated simple syllables in a very careful way. It is not known if the same template approach would work for child speakers, older speakers, or any speaker using a more casual form of articulation. Also, it is not clear how to interpret an "unclassifiable" burst spectrum. In Blumstein and Stevens' study, some spectra did not fit *any* of the templates; how should these be classified? Persons with speech disorders often produce stops that sound as if they are "in between" the normal places of articulation. The template system would have to be expanded to capture these important articulatory events. These are areas in need of careful research if these objective measures are to have an impact in the clinic (see Chapter 11 for more material on spectral templates for stop consonant place of articulation).

Spectral measures can also be made of the frication and aspiration intervals following the stop release. The measurement issues for these spectra are the same as discussed above for the burst. The details of frication interval spectra for the different places of articulation are very similar to the details of burst spectra. In other words, the shape of the burst spectrum for an apical stop is very much like the shape of the frication interval spectrum for that stop. Spectra of aspiration intervals of voiceless stops have not been studied extensively, but generally show a pattern similar to the formant pattern of the following vowel. This is because the aspiration source, located at the glottis, excites the resonances of the vocal tract as it is opening following the stop release to the position for the following vowel. Unlike burst and frication interval spectra, spectra of aspiration intervals do not show significant variation across stop place of articulation.

Temporal Measurements

As in the case of fricatives, temporal segmentation of stop consonant waveforms is relatively straightforward. The waveforms in Figures 9–16 and 9–17 show the closure interval and VOT segments quite clearly. In real speech waveforms, it is often more difficult to find the dividing lines between the burst, frication, and aspiration intervals. Many measurements of closure intervals and VOTs have been reported in the literature and applied to clinical populations.

Stop Consonants: A Summary

Stops are produced when there is a constriction in the vocal tract that completely blocks the airstream for a brief interval. During this closure interval the pressure behind the constriction (P_o) builds up and is suddenly released when the articulators break the constriction. The sudden drop in pressure serves as an acoustic source called shock excitation, the spectrum of which is shaped by the vocal tract cavities. Typically, the cavity in front of the stop constriction provides the major resonance that shapes the shock excitation source, whereas the cavity in back of the constriction contributes antiresonances to the output spectrum.

Following the closure interval, there is a sequence of acoustic events associated with stops. For voiceless stops, the sequence is the burst, frication interval, and aspiration interval. The burst is associated with the release of P_o, the frication interval with high airflow rushing past the narrow vocal tract constriction immediately following the release, and aspiration interval with high airflow rushing past the vocal folds as they move together. The aeromechanical basis of the frication and aspiration intervals is turbulent airflow, the acoustic counterpart of which is aperiodic energy (i.e., noise). Voiced stops have burst and frication intervals, but lack an aspiration interval because the vocal folds are not separated from the midline during the closure interval, as they are for voiceless stops.

The spectra of the burst and frication intervals are unique for each of the three stop places of articulation. The uniqueness of these spectra can be traced largely to the size of the cavity in front of the constriction. In bilabial stops, the cavity is infinitely large (i.e., there is no vocal tract cavity), so the output spectrum tends to be flat. In lingua-alveolar stops, the cavity is very small, which results in a high-frequency emphasis in the output spectrum. In dorsal stops, the cavity is relatively large, resulting in a concentration of energy in the mid-frequencies of the output spectrum.

The output spectra of voiced and voiceless stops at the same place of articulation are essentially the same, with greater overall amplitude for the voiceless stop spectra. Voiced and voiceless stops may be distinguished from each other by: (a) the appearance of glottal pulses during the closure interval of voiced, but not voiceless stops; and (b) longer VOTs for voiceless, as compared to voiced stops.

WHAT IS THE THEORY OF AFFRICATE ACOUSTICS?

Affricates combine features of stop consonants and fricatives. Like stops, affricates have a closure interval during which P_o rises and is released when the articulatory constriction is broken. When the constriction is broken, there is a fairly long interval of frication energy generated by turbulent airflow in the vicinity of the expanding constriction. What seems to distinguish affricates from stops is the fairly long interval of this frication noise. In stops, the frication may last for about 30 to 50 ms, whereas in affricates this interval may be as long as 60 to 80 ms. As described above, frication noise results when the conditions for turbulent airflow exist, these conditions being: (a) a flow of sufficient magnitude (i.e., "high enough" flow) and (b) a sufficiently narrow constriction. The longer frication interval in affricates, as compared to stops, suggests that following the release of an affricate, the conditions for turbulence exist for a greater amount of time than they do following the release of a stop. This is why affricates are sometimes referred to as "slowly released stops." The affricates of American English, which include /tʃ/ and /dʒ/, may also have a place of articulation that is different (slightly posterior) from the lingua-alveolar place of /t/ and /d/. Affricates are discussed more fully in Chapter 11.

WHAT KINDS OF ACOUSTIC CONTRASTS ARE ASSOCIATED WITH THE VOICING DISTINCTION IN OBSTRUENTS?

Four intervals for stop consonants have been defined and discussed above. The first three of these (closure interval, burst, and frication interval) apply to both voiceless and voiced stops, whereas the aspiration interval is only found for voiceless stops. VOTs of voiceless stops are typically longer than those of voiced stops, partly because of the aspiration interval in the former case. Typical VOTs for voiced stops are between 0 and 20 ms, whereas VOTs for voiceless stops are typically between 40 to 80 ms. A VOT of zero means that glottal pulsing begins at the same time as the release of the stop (i.e., the burst). The difference in VOTs for voiceless and voiced stops is illustrated by comparing the left and right waveforms in Figure 9–16.

The relatively short VOTs of voiced stops are not only due to the absence of the aspiration interval, but also reflect burst and frication intervals that are somewhat shorter than those found in voiceless stops. The shorter burst and frication intervals are probably the result of the lower P_o in voiced, as compared to voiceless, stops. In addition, the vocal folds begin vibrating almost immediately after release of the vocal tract closure for voiced stops. This follows because, during the stop closure, the vocal folds are held near or at the midline, and may actually vibrate to produce voicing, as shown in the closure interval of Figure 9–16 (right). At

Slowly Released Slops

Affricates combine stop (closure and burst) and fricative features (a relatively long period of frication noise). This phonetic double-identity is represented in the transcription symbols for English affricates, /tʃ/ and /dʒ/. But are affricates really two sound classes—stops and fricatives—in rapid succession, or should they be accorded their own unique sound class? The famous linguist/phonetician Leigh Lisker (1918–2006) called affricates "slowly released stops," by which he meant to say they were neither stops nor fricatives, but something different. Another form of evidence for the unique status of affricates is what happens when the sound class is involved in a spoonerism. "Flipping the channel" becomes "chipping the flannel"; the /tʃ/ in "channel" does not separate into a stop and fricative component, with either one moving independently (nor does the /fl/ cluster separate for this switch— that's another story). Here is another one that makes the same point for /dʒ/, spoken by the actor Peter Sellers in the Pink Panther classic, *A Shot in the Dark* (1964): "killed him in a rit of fealous jage."

the release of a voiced stop, the vocal folds are immediately (or nearly so) ready to begin vibration for the following vowel.

The activity at the level of the larynx for voiceless stops (and for any voiceless obstruent), however, is substantially different than in the case of voiced stops. This activity receives detailed consideration in Chapter 11, where acoustic data and physiological interpretations are presented on the voicing distinction for stops, fricatives, and affricates.

REVIEW

In this chapter, the theory of consonant acoustics was presented, with special emphasis on the acoustic basis of antiresonances and the aeromechanical basis of noise sources.

Antiresonances occur when two resonators are coupled, as in the case of nasals and laterals, or when a source sits in between two vocal tract resonators, as in the case of stops, fricatives, and affricates.

Turbulent airflow is generated when a great enough airflow is forced through a sufficiently narrow constriction.

The acoustic correlate of turbulence is noise, which accounts for frication and aspiration sources in the speech production apparatus.

Stop consonants have a shock excitation source, which is the acoustic result of sudden release of the positive oral pressure developed during the silent interval.

The measurement of consonant spectra is fairly complicated, but several alternative approaches are discussed.

Data from several studies in which stop, fricative, and nasal spectra have been measured are presented in Chapter 11.

REFERENCES

Bell-Berti, F. (1975). Control of pharyngeal cavity size for voiced and voiceless stops. *Journal of the Acoustical Society of America, 57*, 456–461.

Bell-Berti, F. (1993). Understanding velic motor control: Studies of segmental context. In M. Huffman & R. Krakow (Eds.), *Phonetics and phonology: Nasals, nasalization, and the velum* (pp. 63–85). New York, NY: Academic Press.

Blumstein, S., & Steven, K. (1979). Acoustic invariance in speech production: Evidence from measurements of the spectral characteristics of stop consonants. *Journal of the Acoustical Society of America, 66*, 1001–1017.

Byrd, D. (1993). American stops. *UCLA Working Papers in Phonetics, 83*, 97–116.

Catford, J. (1977). *Fundamental problems in phonetics.* Bloomington, IN: Indiana University Press.

Dang, J., & Honda, K. (1996). Acoustic characteristics of the paranasal sinuses derived from transmission characteristic measurement and morphological observation. *Journal of the Acoustical Society of America, 100*, 3374–3383.

Dang, J., Honda, K., & Suzuki, H. (1994). Morphological and acoustical analysis of the nasal and paranasal cavities. *Journal of the Acoustical Society of America, 96*, 2088–2100.

Fant, G. (1960). *Acoustic theory of speech production.* The Hague, Netherlands: Mouton.

Fant, G. (1973). *Speech sounds and features.* Cambridge, MA: MIT Press.

Forrest, K., Weismer, G., Milenkovic, P., & Dougall, R. (1988). Statistical analysis of word-initial voiceless obstruents: Preliminary data. *Journal of the Acoustical Society of America, 84*, 115–124.

Fujimura, O. (1962). Analysis of nasal consonants. *Journal of the Acoustical Society of America, 34*, 1865–1875.

Hawkins, S., & Stevens, K. (1985). Acoustic and perceptual correlates of the non-nasal-nasal distinction for vowels. *Journal of the Acoustical Society of America, 77*, 1560–1575.

Jongman, A., Wayland, R., & Wong, S. (2000). Acoustic characteristics of English fricatives. *Journal of the Acoustical Society of America, 108*, 1252–1263.

Kent, R., & Moll, K. (1969). Vocal tract characteristics of the stop cognates. *Journal of the Acoustical Society of America, 46*, 1555–1559.

Klatt, D., Stevens, K., & Mead, J. (1968). Studies of articulatory activity and airflow during speech. *Annals of the New York Academy of Sciences, 155*, 42–55.

Ladefoged, P., & Maddieson, I. (1996). *The sounds of the world's languages.* Oxford, UK: Blackwell.

Narayanan, S. S., Alwan, A. A., & Haker, K. (1997). Toward articulatory-acoustic models for liquid approximants based on MRI and EPG data. Part I. The laterals. *Journal of the Acoustical Society of America, 101*, 1064–1077.

Proctor, M. I., Shadle, C. H., & Iskarous, K. (2010). Pharyngeal articulation in the production of voiced and voiceless fricatives. *Journal of the Acoustical Society of America, 127*, 1507–1518.

Pruthi, T., & Espy-Wilson, C. (2004). Acoustic parameters for automatic detection of nasal manner. *Speech Communication, 43*, 225–239.

Pruthi, T., Espy-Wilson, C. Y., & Story, B. H. (2007). Simulation and analysis of nasalized vowels based on magnetic resonance imaging data. *Journal of the Acoustical Society of America, 121*, 3858–3873.

Rong, P., & Kuehn, D. P. (2010). The effect of oral articulation on the acoustic characteristics of nasalized vowels. *Journal of the Acoustical Society of America, 127*, 2543–2553.

Sellers, P. (1964). *A shot in the dark* [Motion picture]. B. Edwards (Director). United States: MGM Entertainment.

Serrurier, A., & Badin, P. (2008). A three-dimensional articulatory model of the velum and nasopharyngeal wall based on MRI and CT data. *Journal of the Acoustical Society of America, 123*, 2335–2355.

Shadle, C. (1985). *The acoustics of fricative consonants.* Doctoral dissertation, Massachusetts Institute of Technology, Cambridge.

Shadle, C. (1990). Articulatory-acoustic relationships in fricative consonants. In W. Hardcastle & A. Marchal (Eds.), *Speech production and speech modeling* (pp. 187–209). Dordrecht, Netherlands: Kluwer Academic.

Stevens, K. (1998). *Acoustic phonetics.* Cambridge, MA: MIT Press.

Stevens, K., Fant, G., & Hawkins, S. (1987). Some acoustical and perceptual correlates of nasal vowels. In R. Channon & L. Shockey (Eds.), *In honor of Ilse Lehiste* (pp. 241–254). Dordrecht, Netherlands: Foris.

10

Speech Acoustic Analysis

INTRODUCTION

Chapters 8 and 9 are devoted to the theoretical bases of speech acoustics, with acoustic patterns of various speech sounds presented to illustrate the theory. There are a variety of techniques for generating the speech acoustic displays shown in Chapters 8 and 9, and for using the displays to obtain speech acoustic measurements. These displays and measurements are the subject matter of the current chapter.

The current use of the term "techniques" goes beyond consideration of the instruments used to store, analyze, and *represent* (i.e., graph) the speech acoustic signal. In this chapter, the term includes the *conceptual* tools that have been developed to make sense of vocal tract output. When a speech signal—the acoustic output of the vocal tract—is displayed in the several ways discussed below, a large amount of information is available, not all of which is relevant to each of the many reasons for studying speech acoustics. For example, some individuals study the speech signal to make inferences about the articulatory behavior that produced the signal (as discussed in Chapters 8 and 9). Others may be interested in the characteristics of the signal used by listeners to understand speech. Still others may be interested in which parts of the speech signal are the best candidates for computer recognition of speech (i.e., machines that understand speech). And, of course, many scientists have studied the speech acoustic signal to develop computer programs for high-quality speech synthesis. Sometimes, what is important about the speech signal is relevant to all four of these areas of interest, but this is not always the case. Thus, the conceptual tools that make sense of the speech signal may be specific to a particular purpose.

Computers Are Not Smarter Than Humans

Speech recognizers are computer programs that analyze a speech signal to figure out what was said. The programs use acoustic analysis and other data (such as stored information on the probability of one sound following another) to produce a set of words that represents a best "guess" about the true nature of the input signal. These programs typically learn the patterns of a single talker 's speech, and in doing so improve their recognition performance over time for that talker. Unfortunately, the improved performance does not typically transfer to a new talker, whose acoustic-phonetic patterns are just different enough from the original talker's to confuse the speech recognition program. Humans, it should be noted, typically have no trouble transferring their speech recognition skills from one talker to another.

A BRIEF HISTORICAL PRELUDE

A brief history of the technology of speech acoustics research illustrates how much progress has been made in a relatively short time. A good starting point is the multitalented German scientist Herman von Helmholtz (1821–1894), who in the 1850s was very much interested in explaining the acoustical basis of vowel quality. Like most phoneticians who puzzled over the relationship between "mouth positions" and different vowel qualities, Helmholtz used an ancient piece of equipment—the ear—as a spectral analyzer to determine the rules linking vocal tract shape and vocal tract output. Helmholtz's innovation in the study of vowels was to insert between the mouth of the speaker and his own ear a kind of spectral analysis tool—in some cases a series of tuning forks, in others a series of Helmholtz resonators (Figure 10–1). When he used tuning forks

(see Figure 10–1, top), Helmholtz asked a laboratory assistant to set his vocal tract in the position of a particular vowel, and then struck the tuning fork and held it close to the assistant's lips. If the tuning fork produced a very loud tone, Helmholtz assumed that the cavity inside the vocal tract was excited by the sound waves and, therefore, "tuned" to the frequency of the fork. If the sound was weak, the natural frequency of the mouth cavity was assumed to be far from the frequency of the fork. Helmholtz was using the resonance principle discussed in Chapter 7, with the tuning fork serving as input, the vocal tract as resonator, and his ear as the detector of the output (see Figure 7–18 for a model of an input-resonator-output system). When a tuning fork produced a tone that was resonated by the assistant's vocal tract held in a particular vowel configuration, Helmholtz assumed that the frequency of the fork was a "natural" frequency of that vowel. By using a whole series of tuning forks, ranging from very low

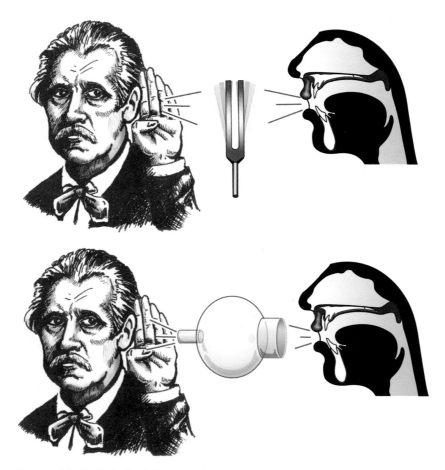

Figure 10-1. Helmholtz's experimental arrangements for determining the important frequencies of vowels. *Top panel* shows the tuning fork approach. *Bottom panel* shows the resonator approach.

frequencies to very high frequencies, Helmholtz was able to draw a diagram of the important frequencies for different vowels, or stated differently, the frequencies that distinguish the vowels from one another. In another series of experiments, Helmholtz's assistants phonated different vowels into the neck of a resonator while he listened at the other end (see Figure 10–1, bottom). By changing resonator size to sample a wide range of frequencies Helmholtz was able to identify which resonators, and hence which frequencies, seemed to produce the loudest sound at his ear. These frequencies were taken as the "natural" frequencies of the vowels. Both types of experiments show how the principle of resonance was applied to the problem of frequency analysis for vowels.

Helmholtz tried to circumvent a strictly *subjective* ear analysis by *objectifying* his judgments through the medium of physical instruments (i.e., tuning forks and Helmholtz resonators) with known frequency characteristics. After all, if there were a sufficient number of tuning forks, or resonators, the end result would be like a low-tech Fourier analysis. In Helmholtz's case, however, the *perceptual* magnitudes (i.e., the loudnesses), rather than the physical amplitudes, were identified for each frequency component in the spectrum. This was quite innovative and creative for the middle of the 19th century, long before electronic instruments were available to analyze and quantify the energy at different signal frequencies.

There were other attempts, prior to the electronics age, to objectify the speech signal. For example, in the latter part of the 19th century W. König knew that the acoustic output of the vocal tract was in the form of pressure waves, which had alternating regions of high and low pressures as described in Chapter 7 (see Figure 7–2). These rapidly varying regions of high and low pressures, König reasoned, could be studied by looking at the *effect* they produced on some easily observed event. König found such an event in the form of a gas-fed flame similar to that used in chemistry labs. Figure 10–2 shows a schematic diagram of the König apparatus. Gas was fed to a chamber beneath the burner ("inflow of gas" in Figure 10–2), and if the volume of the chamber was constant the flame had a constant height. If one side of the chamber had a flexible wall, in the form of a distensible membrane, movements of the membrane into the chamber compressed the gas and raised the height of the flame, whereas outward movements of the membrane expanded the volume of the chamber, which rarefied the gas and lowered the height of the flame. König had speakers phonate vowels into a pipe terminated by this distensible membrane, and the compressions and rarefactions of the speech wave within the pipe caused rapid inward and outward movements of the membrane, making the flame dance up and down as the gas volume was alternately compressed and expanded. By filming the movements of the dancing flame during

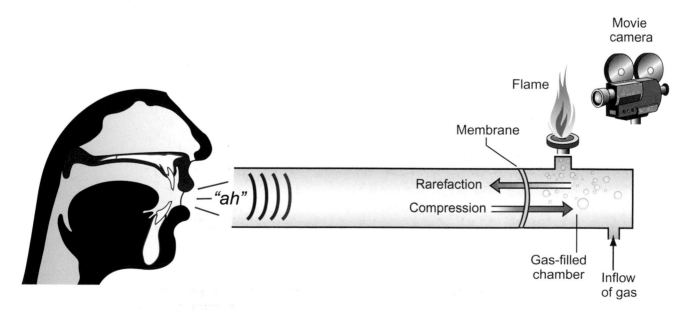

Figure 10–2. The König device for visualizing and recording pressure fluctuations in the speech wave. Compressions and expansions of the gas volume produced rises and falls in the flame height, which were filmed to obtain primitive speech waveforms.

these speech events, König was able to record *speech waves*. The conceptual basis of König's technique, of having sound waves create movement in a structure that is then *transformed* into an observable event, is the basis of modern electronic recording of speech signals. For example, many microphones transform acoustic to electrical energy by means of a very thin membrane whose vibratory movement creates varying voltages in response to air pressure fluctuations. These varying voltages are recorded on magnetic or digital tape, or directly onto computer disks, where they provide an electronic replica of the speech wave.

Devices for the transformation of mechanical to electrical energy, such as the transformation of the vibratory variations of a delicate membrane to voltage variations, did not become readily available until the early part of the 20th century. The great advantage of electronic devices was the ability to record and analyze a wider range of frequencies than was possible with strictly mechanical devices, and the related ability to capture very accurate details of sound waves, which other nonelectronic devices (such as König's) could not.

It is worth considering why electronic devices were able to extend the range of frequency analysis past that of a device like König's. As described in Chapter 7, there is an inverse relationship between frequency and period. When sound waves contain energy at higher frequencies the motion of the air particles is very rapid (i.e., they have relatively short periods). In a device like König's, the ideal situation would be for these very rapid motions of air particles to strike the membrane and set it into vibration at exactly the same high frequencies. The high-frequency motions of the membrane would be reflected in high-frequency fluctuations in flame height, and the flame would provide a precise representation of the energy in the sound wave.

Unfortunately, this is not always the case with a mechanical vibrator such as the membrane in König's device. Because the membrane has mass and therefore demonstrates inertia, it resists being accelerated by certain forces—especially those that last only a short time. The rapidly vibrating air molecules associated with high-frequency energy result in very short-lasting compressions and rarefactions. Because the membrane demonstrates inertia it is likely to move in response to these high-frequency vibrations only a little bit, or perhaps not at all, because high-frequency forces are not applied over a long enough time interval to overcome the opposition to acceleration. Think of it this way: A short-lasting compression applied to the membrane should push it inward, toward the gas chamber, but the membrane does not respond immediately to the applied force because it has mass and opposes being accelerated. By the time the membrane begins

to respond with inward motion, the rapidly varying pressure applied to the membrane has changed to an area of rarefaction, which tends to pull the membrane outward, away from the gas-containing chamber. In a sense, the membrane never gets a chance to respond accurately to the applied forces because of its inertial properties. The membrane acts like a filter, responding with motion to the lower frequency signals whose energy can be applied to it over a long enough time interval, but being insensitive to, and hence filtering out, the energy associated with higher frequency vibration. Therefore, the vibration of the membrane will not represent precisely all details of the actual pressure wave applied to it. The vibration of the membrane is said to *distort* the details of the pressure wave, and this distortion will be passed on to the variation in flame height. The fluctuation in flame height over time is not an entirely accurate representation of the acoustic event.

In the case of the König device, the relatively massive membrane *transduced* the pressure waves via compression or rarefaction of the gas in the chamber. König's membrane had to be relatively massive to produce effective compressions and rarefactions of the gas molecules. When electronic recording and storage of acoustical signals became available, this problem with relatively massive transducers, and hence distortion of acoustic signals, was more or less eliminated. Electronic transducers, which form the heart of a microphone, are still membranelike but are extremely delicate and have minimal mass. The vibrations of these transducers do not have to produce compressions and rarefactions of gas volumes, but rather produce changes in the motion of *electrons* in electrical circuits. The ease of electron acceleration and deceleration (due to negligible mass) allows the use of these thin, minimal-mass membranes to respond *faithfully* to very high frequencies in sound waves. The original devices used to display and analyze electronically recorded waveforms also made use of electron flow, which meant that there was very little distortion of the acoustic signal throughout the process of recording, displaying, and analyzing an acoustic signal.

Early electronic recordings and analyses of vocal tract output resulted in waveforms such as those shown in Figure 10–3. A (roughly) 70-ms waveform "piece" is shown for each of the four corner vowels of American English (/ɑ/, /i/, /æ/, /u/, clockwise from upper left-hand panel). These vowels were produced as sustained phonations by an adult male, and the 70-ms pieces shown in the figure were extracted from the sustained sounds using computer-editing techniques. These waveforms *are* faithful representations of the pressure waves associated with the vocal

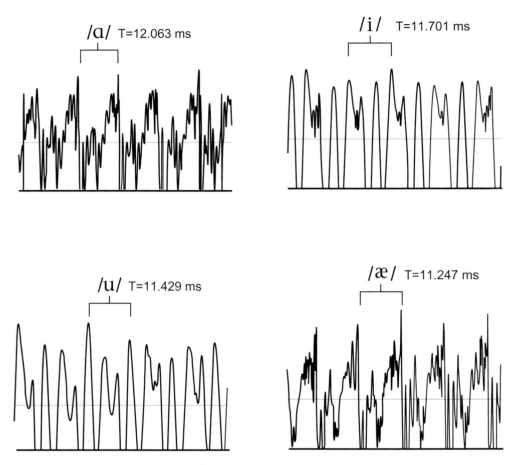

Figure 10–3. 70-ms waveform pieces from each of the four corner vowels of English. Pieces were extracted from sustained vowels. Note the individual glottal pulses, and the period (T) marked on each vowel waveform. Note also the different waveform appearance depending on which vowel was produced.

tract outputs for the corner vowels, and there are certain obvious similarities across the four waveforms. First, each of the waveforms has a repeating period, one of which is marked in each panel. The repeating period is to be expected because all vowels in English are produced with successive vibrations of the vocal folds (i.e., vowels usually are voiced). Second, each of the waveforms shows a number of smaller amplitude vibrations between the largest amplitude peaks. The largest amplitude peaks reflect the energy produced at the instant of vocal fold closure (see Chapter 8), and the smaller energy peaks are produced by resonances in the vocal tract. From the vowel theory presented in Chapter 8, it is known that the vocal tract resonances will be different for the four corner vowels; these different resonances explain the different appearance of the four waveforms in Figure 10–3. For example, the /ɑ/ and /æ/ waveforms seem to have more complex energy patterns within a given period as compared to the /i/ and /u/ waveforms. Note the many amplitude

fluctuations within the periods of the first two vowels, as compared to the smaller number of amplitude peaks within periods of /i/ and /u/.

Shouting at Early Microphones

The earliest microphone was developed in 1876 or 1877. It used a membrane that was displaced by sound waves, and the motion of the membrane was transmitted to a metal pin sitting in an acid solution. The motion of the membrane moved the pin to various depths of the acid solution, which changed the electrical characteristics of the system. Happily, this "liquid transmitter" system didn't catch on, because Alexander Graham Bell found he had to shout at the membrane to produce even a barely audible sound at the other end of the device (3 miles away!).

Although the resonance patterns are reflected in the different waveform patterns displayed in Figure 10–3, the differing resonant frequencies of the vowels cannot be determined merely by looking at the waveforms. The resonant frequencies can be determined using the technique of Fourier analysis, where a complex waveform is decomposed into the frequencies and amplitudes of the component sinusoids (see Chapter 7). Originally, this may have been done with paper and pencil, or with a mechanical device called a Henrici analyzer, but in either case the process was fairly tedious. As electronic devices became more sophisticated, specialized instruments were developed for automatic computation of a Fourier spectrum. These devices, called *spectrum analyzers*, took a waveform as input and stored some part of it in an electronic memory. The stored part might be a 70-ms piece such as the ones shown in Figure 10–3. The spectrum analyzer performed a Fourier analysis on that piece and showed the computed spectrum on a display screen. These analyses were quite accurate, but required a fair amount of computation time. Moreover, the spectrum results were more accurate when the stored piece was longer, rather than shorter.

The duration of the waveform undergoing analysis was of great concern for speech scientists, who had a good idea even at the dawn of the electronic age that the articulators, and hence the shape of the vocal tract, were in nearly constant motion. In Chapter 8, the relationship of vocal tract resonances to the shape of the vocal tract was discussed. When the shape of the vocal tract changes, so do the resonant frequencies. During speech production, many phonetically relevant changes in vocal tract configuration are quite rapid, in some cases occurring within intervals as brief as 40 to 50 ms. For example, when a lingual stop consonant such as /d/ is released into a low vowel such as /æ/, the vocal tract changes from the consonant to vowel configuration in about 40 ms. This large change in the shape of the vocal tract results in rapidly changing vocal tract resonances which are called *formant transitions*.

Imagine a situation in which a clinician or researcher was interested in analyzing the frequency range covered by one of these formant transitions, or the rate at which the frequency changes as a function of time (that is, the slope of the frequency change). A schematic of a second formant (F2) transition for the syllable /bæ/, produced by an adult male speaker, is shown in Figure 10–4. The upward-pointing arrow at 0 ms indicates the beginning of the formant transition, which occurs roughly at the first glottal pulse following release of the /b/. The downward-pointing arrow at 50 ms marks the end of the formant transition, or the point at which the frequency ceases changing as a function of time (note the relatively constant F2 value after the

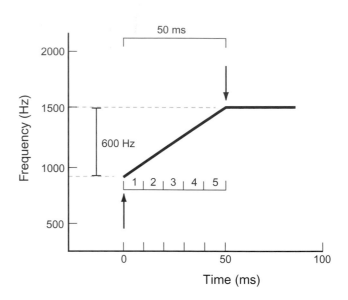

Figure 10–4. Schematic drawing showing an F2 transition for /bæ/. Upward-pointing arrow at 0 ms shows beginning of the transition. The end of the transition is shown by the downward-pointing arrow at 50 ms along the time axis. The pieces spanning the duration of the transition, labeled 1 through 5, show individual 10-ms intervals that could be extracted from the transition for analysis. See text for details.

downward-pointing arrow, indicating a steady vocal tract shape for the vowel /æ/ "target"). This F2 transition, which has a duration of 50 ms and covers a frequency range of 600 Hz (see Figure 10–4, vertical line between horizontal, dashed lines showing frequency range between the beginning and end of the transition) might present some obvious problems for the "static" spectrum analyzer described above. If the entire 50-ms piece of the waveform corresponding to the schematic transition in Figure 10–4 were submitted for spectral analysis, the resulting spectrum would be an average of all the changing frequencies along the transition. This analysis would clearly misrepresent the true vocal tract output. The "smeared" spectrum resulting from this kind of analysis would be virtually useless, at least with respect to an interpretation of the articulatory behavior that produced the acoustic event. The analysis could better match the true frequency event, however, by picking very small pieces along the transition, analyzing each piece, and combining the successive spectra to reconstruct the transition. This is shown by the successive, short-time pieces, along the bottom edge of the transition, each having a duration of 10 ms. As shown in Figure 10–4, a complete analysis of the transition using these 10-ms pieces would require five consecutive spectral analyses (5 pieces × 10 ms per piece = 50 ms, or the duration of the entire transition).

This approach would minimize the obvious spectral smear that occurs when the 50-ms piece is analyzed as a single interval, but it is not particularly attractive because (a) the amount of work involved in separately isolating and analyzing each 10-ms piece is substantial; (b) the short time pieces, as noted above, require a loss of accuracy in the analysis of the frequency components; and (c) the spectral smear problem is not entirely eliminated, because each 10-ms piece covers roughly a 120-Hz change (120 Hz for each of five 10-ms pieces = 120 × 5 = 600 Hz), this being a significant frequency change in vocal tract output.

The static, electronically based spectrum analyzers available to early speech researchers, therefore, had notable limitations. The analyzers allowed a previously unknown precision of frequency analysis, but the requirements of the analysis were not well matched to many of the important features of vocal tract output, which involve rapidly changing frequencies over relatively brief time intervals. It is true that these spectral analyses could be used quite effectively for waveforms extracted from sustained vowels (see Figure 10–3), or the occasional target intervals for a vowel in connected speech. In these cases, the vocal tract shape remains constant over a long time (sustained vowels) or a long enough time (targets in connected speech) to permit a reasonable, fast spectral analysis. But constancy of resonant frequencies over time is not typical of speech production. Rather, rapid frequency change over time is the rule in speech acoustics for both vowels and consonants, and almost certainly plays an important role in speech perception as well.

In summary, electronics allowed the recording and analysis of acoustic waveforms associated with vocal tract output. These electronic waveforms represented the actual fluctuations in the pressure waves with a high degree of accuracy, but did not provide immediate (i.e., visible) access to the formants, the information critical to an understanding of vocal tract shape (see Chapter 8). Inspection of the waveform revealed the *presence* of formants, which was reflected in the complex vibratory features within each waveform period (see Figure 10–3), but not the actual *frequencies* of those resonances. Spectral analyzers were able to take pieces of waveforms and perform very accurate determinations of resonant frequencies (peaks in the spectrum), but only for some relatively long time interval. Because speech production involves rapidly changing vocal tract shapes over relatively short time intervals, these were not ideal analyses. Clearly, what was needed was an analyzer that *could display formants as a function of time*. Such an analyzer would perform a spectral analysis as a (nearly) continuous function of time and display the spectral peaks (formants) in such a way that a

changing shape of the vocal tract could be inferred from a mere glance at the physical record. The development of the instrument capable of doing this kind of analysis was, in part, an ironic by-product of the human race's oldest failure of communication—war.

THE ORIGINAL SOUND SPECTROGRAPH: HISTORY AND TECHNIQUE

Throughout the course of World War II (1939–1945), there was an increasing use of encoded messages sent between different command posts, or from central locations to troop locations on the battlefield. This encoding, sometimes called *encryption*, was necessary because the warring parties were constantly monitoring each others' communications. One side employed the talents of many different people to develop the codes for effective encryption of a message, and the other side employed an equal number of people to figure out how to break these codes. The code breakers typically worked with paper and pencil, laboring over an encoded message and working through possible decoding solutions. At some point during the war, the allies (United States, the Soviet Union, Great Britain, and France) assembled a team of linguists, puzzle and code experts, mathematicians, engineers, psychologists, and other specialists to develop an automated decoding device. The theory behind such a device was relatively simple. An encoded message, such as a radio voice transmission, would be fed into a machine that performed various types of analysis to decode the message. The project failed to solve the problem of automated decoding of encoded messages, but one of its products was a device called the *sound spectrograph*.

The ideal spectrum analyzer for speech, as suggested above, would display formants as a continuous function of time. This is precisely what was produced when the sound spectrograph was used to analyze speech. Scientists in the Soviet Union—*prisoner* scientists, forced to work on projects ordered by the state—developed a sound spectrograph in the late 1940s, as related by the renowned writer A. I. Solzhenitsyn (1969) in his documentary novel, *The First Circle*. In the novel, Solzhenitsyn's character Major Adam Roitman explains how the spectrograph displays the speech signal in what he calls a *voice print*:

> In these voice prints speech is measured three ways at once: frequency, across the tape;—time, along the tape; and amplitude—by the density of the picture. Therefore, each sound is depicted so uniquely that it can be recognized easily, and everything that has been said can be read on the tape. (p. 217)

A sample spectrogram, with a time-synchronized waveform immediately above, is shown in Figure 10–5. When Major Roitman described frequency *across the tape*, he was referring to the *y*-axis of the spectrogram which extends in this example from 0 Hz (the baseline of the spectrogram) to just below 8.0 kHz. The *x*-axis in this spectrogram is time, corresponding to Roitman's *along the tape* dimension. In the present case, this time axis is marked off in 100-ms increments. The spectrogram shows a number of dark bands, all of which seem to vary in height (i.e., along the *y*-axis) across time. When Major Roitman described amplitude in terms of the density of the picture, he was referring to the varying darkness of different locations on the spectrogram. The darker the spectrogram at any given point in time and frequency, the greater the energy at that point. In Chapter 8, the formants of vowels were described as peaks in the spectrum, that is, as the locations in the spectrum where energy is at a maximum. Because the dark bands in the spectrogram shown in Figure 10–5 indicate locations of very high energy, they are the formants of the vowels. These dark bands vary in height (along the *y*-axis) across time, showing that the formant frequencies change substantially throughout an utterance.

Today, a spectrum analyzer is available that is well matched to the needs of speech analysis—one that displays the formants as a function of time. Figure 10–6 illustrates how the early versions of the spectrograph (the instrument) generated spectrograms (the pictures produced by the spectrograph). The operator of the spectrograph flipped a switch that caused rotation of the turntable platter shown in Figure 10–6. Wrapped around the edge of the platter was a magnetic strip that served as an electronic recording medium. A speech signal[1] was recorded onto the rotating magnetic band, which functioned as a closed tape loop permitting storage of no more than about 2.5 seconds of continuous speech. The frequency and amplitude information in the speech signal, as a function of time, was stored as magnetic patterns on this loop. With the recorded signal in place on the magnetic loop, the turntable was then rotated much faster than the recording speed[2] and the magnetic patterns served as the input to a spectrum analyzer.

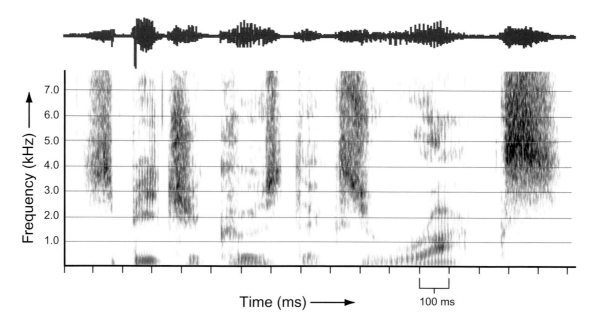

Figure 10–5. A sample spectrogram, showing time along the *x*-axis, frequency on the *y*-axis, and intensity as the darkness of the trace. The interval between each vertical tick on the time axis is equal to 100 ms, and horizontal lines running across the spectrogram from bottom to top (*y*-axis) mark 1000-Hz increments. The darkness of the tracing at any location indicates the relative intensity at that time-frequency coordinate. The speech waveform is above the spectrogram.

---

[1]This book is about speech, so it focuses on the use of the spectrograph to analyze speech signals. The spectrograph has been used to analyze signals produced by dolphins, birds, the act of swallowing, blood flowing through the carotid arteries, and stomachs in the process of digesting food (both efficiently and not so well!).

[2]We do not go into the details of why the turntable speed during analysis was so much faster than the turntable speed during recording; the speed difference was required for efficient analysis of the speech signal and production of the spectrogram.

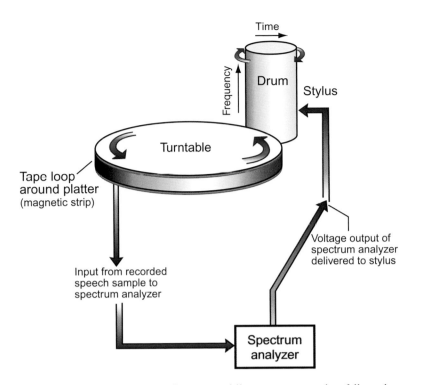

Figure 10-6. Schematic diagram of the components of the classic sound spectrograph. Speech is recorded onto the continuous magnetic tape around the turntable platter, and the magnetic fluctuations corresponding to the speech signal are passed to a spectrum analyzer. The voltage output of the spectrum analyzer is sent to a heated stylus that burns patterns onto special paper mounted on the rotating drum. See text for details.

Writing from Experience

When the world-famous writer Alexander Solzhenitsyn (1918–2008) wrote *The First Circle*, he had firsthand experience of the *Sharashka*, the Russian word for a prison camp for scientists. In the Soviet Union, many writers, artists, and politically active people were imprisoned simply for their beliefs. Most were sent to forced-labor camps, described in Solzhenitsyn's monumental work *The Gulag Archipeligo*.

A very few, like Solzhenitsyn, were more fortunate and were sent to a *Sharashka* to work on a scientific project. Solzhenitsyn's role in the development of the spectrograph was as a linguist. Life at a *Sharashka* was infinitely better than in the regular prison camps, but Solzhenitsyn's title reveals his feelings about his time there. It is taken from the "first circle of hell" in Dante's *The Divine Comedy*.

The spectrum analyzer performed its analysis by moving a fixed-width *analysis band*, or *filter*, across the entire frequency range. This is illustrated in Figure 10–7, which shows the hypothetical results of a Fourier analysis of the vowel /i/. In this figure, frequency is shown on the vertical *y*-axis, increasing from bottom to top, and amplitude is shown on the *x*-axis. Each of the lines in this Fourier spectrum is a harmonic

(the first three are indicated on the spectrum), and the length of each line extending to the right from the frequency baseline indicates the relative amplitude of the harmonic (e.g., the third harmonic has greater amplitude than the second harmonic). At the bottom of the frequency scale is a small bracket that extends over a frequency range of 300 Hz. This bracket is the fixed-width (width = 300 Hz) analysis band mentioned at the

/ i / Fourier Spectrum

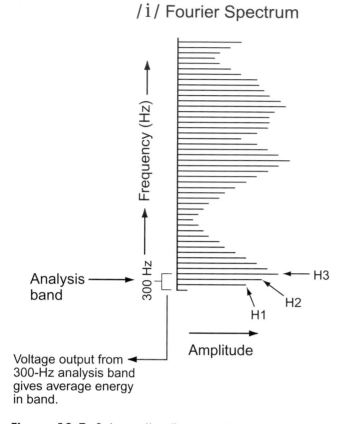

Figure 10–7. Schematic diagram showing how the spectrograph performs spectral analysis by sweeping an analysis band of fixed width (e.g., 300 Hz) across the frequency range of interest, and recording the average voltages from the analysis band as a continuous function of time and frequency. In this display, frequency is on the y-axis, intensity on the x-axis. Each harmonic of a vowel is shown as a line extending to the right; the length of the line indicates the relative intensity of that particular harmonic (H1 = first harmonic (F0), H2 = second harmonic, H3 = third harmonic, and so forth).

beginning of this paragraph. The arrow pointing down and to the left from this analysis band is labeled *voltage output*, and this output is the key to the spectrum analysis performed by the spectrograph. The analysis band senses the overall energy on the magnetic tape, which it transforms into a voltage. Higher voltages are associated with greater energy, lower voltages with lesser energy. Because the analysis band covers a range of only 300 Hz, the voltage output is only for the frequencies within the band and can be thought of as an average of all energy within the band. If the analysis band is swept continuously across the entire frequency range *it will provide overall voltage outputs as a continuous function of frequency.* In Figure 10–7, the arrow pointing

up from the 300-Hz analysis band indicates the direction in which the band is moved continuously across the frequency range. The band started at the lowest frequencies, where the output voltage reflected the overall energy from 0 to 300 Hz. As it moved continuously upward in frequency, the analysis band produced output voltages from the 5- to 305-Hz interval, the 10- to 310-Hz interval, and so forth. The band was always 300-Hz wide, but as it moved across the frequency scale it sampled and output the average energy for successive 300-Hz bands at progressively higher frequencies.

Recall that the magnetic patterns on the tape were fed into (i.e., served as input to) the spectrum analyzer while the turntable was rotating. The rotation of the turntable means that the spectrum analysis is conducted as a function of time because different "pieces" of the utterance pass the analysis band at different points in time. Thus, at any instant in time, the 300-Hz analysis band provides a voltage output for the frequencies it is covering. When the analysis band is swept across the frequency range continuously, and the turntable rotates enough times to allow the analyzer to sample every instant of an utterance, the result is a set of voltages at all frequencies (i.e., within some predetermined frequency range) and at every instant in time around the tape loop. Thus, the example of Figure 10–7 is for a single instant in time—a spectral "slice in time"—and the sum of all such slice analyses results in a spectrogram of the type presented in Figure 10–5.

How did the voltages from the analysis band end up as marks of varying darkness on the spectrogram? The schematic drawing of the spectrograph (see Figure 10–6) shows a drum attached to the turntable, and a stylus marking the drum. When the turntable rotated for the spectral analysis of the recorded speech signal, the attached drum rotated at the same speed. A piece of special heat-sensitive paper was wrapped around the drum, and the stylus was applied to this paper and heated in proportion to the voltage output from the analysis. As the analysis band was swept slowly across the frequency range, the stylus was synchronously transported up the vertical dimension of the spectrogram (see frequency dimension along the drum in Figure 10–6). The varying voltages from the analysis band were burned onto the special paper, with darker regions representing areas of relatively greater acoustic energy, and lighter regions representing areas of relatively lower acoustic energy. The entire process of recording a speech signal onto the tape loop, mounting the paper around the drum and burning a complete frequency-by-time pattern onto the paper, took about 100 seconds to complete. All this to obtain acoustic knowledge of no more than 2.5 seconds of speech!

The Original Sound Spectrograph: Summary

There are several reasons why a fair amount of discussion has been devoted to the origins and function of the sound spectrograph. Most importantly, the invention of this instrument initiated a scientific revolution in the study of speech production, because for the first time, and with relative ease, the *time-varying* characteristics of articulatory processes could be studied by inference from acoustic records. These time-varying characteristics were revealed most prominently by the always changing formant frequencies. The discovery of these changes led to new ideas and insights about the behavior of the articulators in speech production.

The discussion of the spectrograph should demystify, at least in part, the general engineering concepts of speech acoustic analysis. An engineering degree is not necessary to understand the conceptual basis of spectrographic analysis. The amplitude and frequency characteristics of a speech signal are stored as a function of time on magnetic tape. The time-varying patterns of electromagnetic strength are submitted to a spectrum analyzer in the form of time-varying voltages (corresponding to the time-varying intensity of the magnetic fields on the tape), where voltage is proportional to sound intensity (greater voltage = greater intensity) and the speed with which the voltage changes is proportional to frequency (faster voltage changes [shorter periods] = higher frequencies). The energy in the spectrum is sampled using an analysis band, or filter, that covers a 300-Hz range and is swept continuously across the entire frequency range of interest. Because the voltage output from the analysis band is available for all frequencies and at every point in time, it can be used to create a total picture of the speech spectrum as a function of time. This picture is created by burning the energy patterns onto a piece of heat-sensitive paper, which results in a spectrogram. This process is summarized in Figure 10–6, by following the arrow from the turntable (the magnetic tape) all the way around to the stylus at the spectrograph drum.

Today, when scientists or clinicians make spectrograms to study speech they do so digitally, using a desktop or laptop computer. These *digital spectrograms* are displayed on computer monitors and look very much like the one shown in Figure 10–5, but can be produced almost instantaneously after an utterance has been recorded onto the computer (some instruments actually display the spectrogram in *real time*, as the utterance is being produced). The computer allows a spectrogram to be generated in just a fraction of the time required to produce the burned records described

---

Speech Acoustics as a Health Hazard?

Those of us of a certain age, who were making spectrograms before digital spectrograms became a reality, may read the title of this sidetrack and find themselves smiling and sniffing nostalgically. As the pattern was burned onto the special paper, carbon smoke would float away from the spinning drum and fill the room with the smell of speech acoustics. That smell was something like the exhaust of a car with a corroded, burned-out muffler. The wearing of light-colored clothes to the lab was discouraged—one would find fine black specks on a nice white sweater after a few hours of spectrogram-making. Some people—especially graduate students assigned to prepare spectrograms—took to wearing surgical masks in the lab.

---

above, but the analysis technique is essentially the same as that used in the original spectrograph. The rapid development of computer-based analysis of speech has also resulted in a host of new analyses for speech acoustics, but the spectrogram remains the gold standard because it is such an immediate and rich source of information about speech production and perception. Especially in clinical settings, the spectrogram has great, but unfortunately unrealized, potential for providing both qualitative and quantitative data concerning a client's speech production deficit.

A detailed presentation of spectrograms and their interpretation is now provided. Selected information on the application of spectrographic analysis to the understanding of speech disorders is presented in Chapter 11.

Interpretation of Spectrograms: Specific Features

Figure 10–8 shows a spectrogram of the utterance, *Peter shouldn't speak about the mugs*. A broad phonetic transcription of the sounds in the utterance is provided at the bottom of the display. Immediately above the spectrogram, on the same time scale, is the waveform of the utterance. The utterance was produced by an adult male aged 52 years, at a normal rate of speech and without any special emphasis on a particular word. The utterance was chosen for its ability to showcase

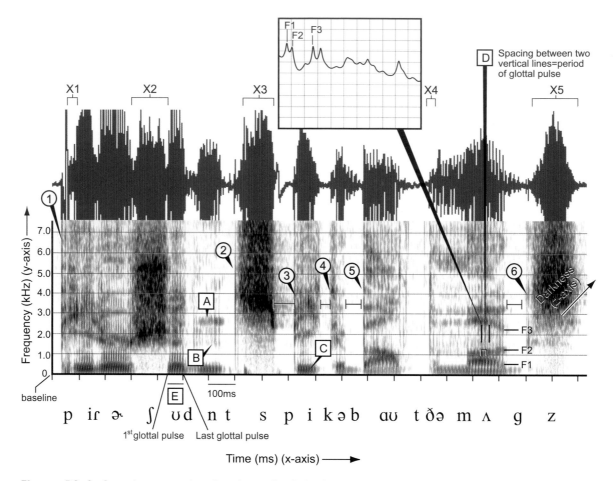

Figure 10–8. Spectrogram showing important features of a spectrographic display. Follow text description for information on axes, glottal pulses, formant frequencies, silent intervals, stop bursts, and aperiodic intervals.

certain spectrographic patterns, not because it has special meaning (as far as we know, Peter does not plan on ruining a surprise birthday present of really nice coffee mugs by telling the intended gift-receiver about them before the package is opened). This spectrogram was produced with the computer program *TF32*, written by Professor Paul Milenkovic of the Department of Electrical and Computer Engineering at the University of Wisconsin–Madison. *TF32* is a complete speech analysis program that includes algorithms for recording, editing, and analyzing speech waveforms, as well as displaying the speech signal as a spectrogram. Most of the speech analysis displays shown in this text were produced with *TF32* (see http://userpages.chorus.net/cspeech/).

The important features of the spectrographic display in Figure 10–8 include the *x*-, *y*-, and *z*-axes; *glottal pulses; formant frequencies; silent intervals; stop bursts;* and *aperiodic intervals.* Each of these features is dis-

cussed below, but it is important to point out here that a casual glance at the spectrogram suggests a series of chunks, or *segments*, as the pattern is inspected from left to right. If an individual with no training in speech acoustics was shown this spectrogram and asked to find natural "breaks" in the pattern along the time axis, he or she could probably do this quite easily (try it!). The chunks, or segments, are important because they often correspond roughly to speech sounds. Chapter 11 presents detailed information on the specific acoustic characteristics of the sound segments of English, and in some cases of other languages as well.

Axes

A general orientation to the axes of a spectrographic display has been given above (see Major Roitman's explanation of what he called a *voice print*). The *x*-axis is time, and is marked off in successive 100-ms intervals by the short vertical lines occurring at regular intervals along the baseline of the spectrogram. These 100-ms *calibration intervals* are similar in length to many of the segments in this spectrogram, suggesting a relatively short time span for important events of speech production. Using these calibration intervals, it is possible to estimate the entire duration of the utterance at just under 2000 ms, or a little less than 2 s. This does not seem like a particularly long time, but it is fairly typical for utterance durations, and even such a relatively brief interval contains many distinct segments.

The y-axis is frequency, which in the current spectrogram extends from 0 kHz to about 7.5 kHz. Calibration of the frequency axis is shown as the series of horizontal lines marked off in 1.0-kHz increments. The 0- to 8.0-kHz range is often considered as a standard for spectrographic displays because most of the important acoustic energy for understanding articulatory events, as well as how the speech signal provides phonetic information in the perception of speech, is thought to be contained within this range. This is true for the most part, but spectrograms can be generated for any frequency range. In the current text, a variety of spectrographic frequency ranges is used, depending on the purpose of the illustration. It is always important to check the frequency calibration along the y-axis of a particular spectrogram.

The z-axis (indicated on the right side of the spectrogram in red print), or third dimension of the spectrogram, is intensity. Unlike time (x-axis) and frequency (y-axis), in this type of spectrographic display intensity cannot be measured directly. Rather, intensity is coded by the darkness of the pattern at any time-frequency coordinate (that is, at any point on the spectrographic display). The darkness at any time-frequency coordinate can be compared to the darkness at any other time-frequency coordinate *only in relative terms*. This kind of coding is called a *gray scale*, which allows only *ordinal* comparisons between event magnitudes. For example, the intensity of the formant indicated by arrow A, roughly at the time-frequency coordinate of 600 ms (x-axis) and 2.7 kHz (y-axis) where the segment is marked phonetically as [n], is clearly greater (i.e., darker) than the formant above arrow B at the same segment (time-frequency coordinate of roughly 600 ms and 1.5 kHz). Similarly, the formant marked by arrow C, which occurs at a time-frequency coordinate of roughly 950 ms and 0.3 kHz where the segment is marked as [i], is slightly darker (more intense) than A. These comparisons are not stated in terms of numbers, but only as "greater than" or "less than" relations. This is what is meant by the gray scale allowing only ordinal comparisons. Time and frequency, on the other hand, can be

measured directly from the spectrogram and numerical differences between points can be determined. There are other ways to determine numerical intensity differences (e.g., difference in decibels) between two different regions of a spectrogram, but not in the type of display shown in Figure 10–8.

Glottal Pulses

Certain segments in Figure 10–8 have a characteristic appearance of a series of dark, vertical lines. These segments are the ones containing the dark bands identified above as the vowel formants. In fact, the vertical lines appear to be running throughout the segments containing the most obvious formants, such as the /i/ in /pi/ and the /ʊ/ in /ʃʊd/. The vertical lines are the acoustic result of vocal fold vibration, with each individual line reflecting a single glottal pulse. More precisely, in Chapter 8 the vocal tract resonances are said to be excited each time the vocal folds snap shut during a series of glottal cycles. Each of the vertical lines in the spectrogram represents this point of excitation, when the vocal folds close quickly at the end of a glottal cycle and create a pressure wave whose spectrum is shaped by the vocal tract filter. The shaping of the source spectrum by the vocal tract filter is shown on the spectrogram as darkened areas—that is, the dark bands—at the frequencies of the vocal tract resonances. Thus, the vertical lines and formants are not really different characteristics of the spectrogram. Rather, the formants are darkened areas along the vertical lines, showing where energy in the glottal source spectrum is emphasized (i.e., resonated) by the vocal tract filter.

Within any segment having the series of glottal pulses represented by vertical lines, the spacing of the lines appears to be very consistent. As described in Chapter 8, vocal fold vibration is quasiperiodic, with consecutive periods of nearly the same duration. The consistent spacing of the vertical lines along the time dimension (x-axis) of the spectrogram reflects the quasiperiodic nature of vocal fold vibration, and the spacing between any two vertical lines is equal to the period of the glottal cycle (see example D, incomplete red box in Figure 10–8 showing the distance between two glottal pulses). Although this kind of spectrogram does not provide a direct display of the F0 of vocal fold vibration, segments can be compared visually for the relative spacing of the glottal pulses and, thus, their relative F0s. For example, compare the spacing of the glottal pulses in the two segments marked as /i/ (in /spik/) and /ʌ/ (in /mʌgz/). The vertical lines, or glottal pulses, are closer together in /i/, as compared to /ʌ/. Another way to make this comparison is to say that the number of vertical lines *per unit time* is greater for /i/ than for /ʌ/. A greater number of glottal pulses per unit time implies a shorter period and a higher F0. Thus, a quick glance at this spectrogram tells us that /i/ has a higher F0 than /ʌ/.

Formant Frequencies

The dark bands seen in the patterns with regularly spaced glottal pulses have already been identified as formants. This pattern is seen for any speech sound produced with a relatively open vocal tract and voicing, including vowels, diphthongs, and semivowels (/l/, /w/, /ɹ/, /j/). In addition, nasals are voiced and radiate sound through the open nares, thus producing a similar kind of pattern. The spectrographic patterns seen above the phonetic symbols for these kinds of segments (in Figure 10–8, /i/, /ɚ/, /ʊ/, /n/, /i/, /ə/, /aʊ/, /ə/, /m/, /ʌ/, from left to right) confirm this distinctive appearance.

In most cases, it is relatively easy to look at a spectrogram and determine which dark band is F1, which is F2, and so forth. The general rule is to start at the baseline (where frequency = 0 Hz) and move up the frequency scale, or *y*-axis, until the first dark band is encountered. This is the first formant, or F1. Continue up the frequency axis until the next dark band is found, which is F2. The next dark band above F2 will be F3, and so forth. In Figure 10–8, the first three formants for the terminal part of the vowel /ʌ/ in the word /mʌgz/ have been identified in this way. This is exactly the same approach used to identify formants in the spectrum plots presented in Chapter 8 (e.g., Figure 8–13), where frequency is on the *x*-axis and relative amplitude is on the *y*-axis. Starting from zero frequency on these plots, the first peak is labeled as F1, the next peak as F2, and the next as F3 (see spectrum inset, Figure 10–8, where the formant peaks are shown from the middle of the vowel). When the formants are labeled as F1, F2, F3 . . . Fn in a spectrographic display, the peaks in the spectrum are identified exactly as in the spectrum plots, except that the spectrogram displays frequency on the *y*-axis and the spectral peaks are shown as the darkened bands.

There is another important difference between a spectrum plot and a spectrographic display of speech. The advantage of the spectrogram is that it shows the formants *over time*, whereas a spectrum plot is constructed for some slice in time, or *time window*. The spectrum inset shown for the vowel /ʌ/ in /mʌgz/ was constructed for a carefully selected piece of the /ʌ/ waveform. A closer look at the formants throughout the duration of this vowel shows why the selection of

a *part* of a vowel waveform is an important step in the determination of formant frequencies. All the formants, but especially F3, have changing frequency values as a function of time. At the first glottal pulse of /ʌ/, F3 seems to be approximately 200 Hz below the 3.0-kHz calibration line, but the formant falls steadily after the temporal middle of the vowel and appears to finish, at the final glottal pulse, about 300 Hz above the 2.0-kHz line. If the question is asked, "What are the formant frequencies of the vowel /ʌ/ in the word /mʌgz/?" the answer is very much dependent on where, during the course of the vowel, the measurements are taken. When scientists or clinicians talk about vowel formant frequencies in connected speech, they are usually referring to a set of measurements taken at or near the *temporal middle of the vowel*. In Figure 10–8, this point is indicated for the vowel /ʌ/ by the vertical line labeled "D" extending through the formant pattern. In practice, a time window of relatively brief duration (20–30 ms) is centered around this temporal midpoint and the spectral analysis is performed on the signal within this window. The interval corresponding to this brief window is shown by the two short vertical lines crossing the 2.0-kHz line, and a line from this window extends to the inset spectrum at the top of the spectrogram. That inset spectrum shows the formant frequencies averaged across this brief window. The formants will not change much over such a brief window, so the average is not a "smear" of rapidly changing frequencies (recall the discussion of Figure 10–4).

Formant frequencies are indicated by the dark bands, but where along their *vertical extent* should the measurement be taken? At the temporal middle of the vowel /ʌ/ in /mʌgz/, the lower edge of the F2 band is slightly below 1.0 kHz, but the upper edge is clearly above 1.0 kHz. Formant frequencies are identified by the peaks in the spectrum — that is, by single frequency values associated with energy maxima — but the formant bands cover a *range* of frequencies, so how is the single formant frequency determined? The answer is simple. At any given point in time, such as the temporal middle of /ʌ/, *the center of the formant band, halfway between the bottom and top of the band, is taken as the formant frequency*.

The great majority of the formant frequencies shown in Figure 10–8 are changing as a function of time. When connected speech is examined, this movement is the rule, rather than the exception. The constant movement of the formants during speech production reflects the constant change in the configuration of the vocal tract. One of the earliest revelations to emerge from studies of speech movements was the continuous motion of the articulators, and the absence of many "held," or static, vocal tract postures. This fact has made it difficult to identify *targets* for speech sounds, and indeed has led some scientists to *deny* the existence of such targets. Nevertheless, formant frequencies measured at the temporal middle of a vowel, as in the /ʌ/ example of Figure 10–8, have often been regarded as acoustic targets for vowels.

Silent Intervals and Stop Bursts

The aeromechanical characteristics of stop consonants were presented in Chapter 9. Recall that the vocal tract is completely sealed for a brief interval, during which time a positive pressure (oral pressure, or P_o) is developed within the closed cavity. When the articulators separate, the seal is broken, pressure is released suddenly, and airflow rushes from the vocal tract (see Figure 9–16). The acoustic result of this interval of complete vocal tract closure is called a *closure interval*, *silent interval*, or *stop gap*. The sudden release of pressure is called, appropriately, a *stop burst*.

Closure intervals are usually easy to identify in spectrograms. Because the vocal tract is, in theory, completely sealed during the vocal tract closure, acoustic energy should not be radiated from the vocal tract and the interval should appear as a brief blank spot, or *gap* on the spectrogram. If intensity is scaled on a spectrogram as the darkness of the trace (see above), then a white or nearly white "chunk" on the spectrogram should indicate an interval of no acoustic energy — a "silent" vocal tract. In Figure 10–8, the spectrographic appearance above the /p/ and /k/ in /spik/, the /b/ in /əbaʊt/, and the /g/ in /mʌgz/ confirms this expectation in varying degrees. The closure intervals for these stops are indicated by the red horizontal bars terminated by vertical tick marks between 3.0 and 4.0 kHz (placed in this frequency region for convenience of display only). The closure interval for the /p/ in /spik/ shows some energy between about 2.5 and 7.5 kHz, which is not uncommon when stops follow /s/ in /s/ + stop clusters. A small amount of energy is also seen in the closure interval for /k/ in /spik/. The energy in these intervals suggests an incomplete vocal tract seal during the closure interval. Some acoustic energy "leaks" through the mouth and is sensed by the microphone, appearing on the spectrogram as relatively weak-to-moderate aperiodic energy.

The gap for /b/ also shows a small amount of energy on the baseline, which appears to be periodic as indicated by a series of three or four small, regularly spaced pulses. The same kind of periodic energy is seen along the baseline during the /g/ closure interval. The presence of the periodic pulses during the /b/ and /g/ closure intervals makes sense because these are *voiced* stops, produced with vocal fold vibration during the vocal tract closure.

The periodic acoustic energy recorded on the baseline for these voiced stops cannot be radiated through either the mouth or nares openings, because these are sealed during the closure intervals. Rather, the pressure wave resulting from vibration of the vocal folds during a closure interval causes vibration of the *walls* of the vocal tract (i.e., the neck walls, the cheeks), which transmit their vibratory energy to the surrounding air. A pressure wave is propagated from the external surface of the vocal tract walls to the microphone used to record the acoustic event. This energy is seen only in the very lowest frequencies of the spectrogram because the walls of the vocal tract vibrate only at the lowest frequencies of vocal fold vibration, filtering out the higher source harmonics and preventing their energy from being sensed by the microphone.

As reviewed above, the termination of a closure interval is defined acoustically as a stop burst. Stop bursts are, at least in carefully articulated speech (like that elicited in laboratory experiments), very easy to identify in spectrograms. Figure 10–8 shows six of them, numbered 1 through 6. The distinctive spectrographic characteristic of a stop burst is a spikelike event — a dark, single vertical line — following a closure interval. The spectrographic feature of a dark vertical line signifying a stop burst seems to be similar to the description of glottal pulses, but there are several ways to distinguish the two acoustic events. First, as noted above, stop bursts are typically seen following a well-defined closure interval, so if one stop characteristic (i.e., the closure interval) is present, the occurrence of a second characteristic (i.e., the burst) may be expected. Bursts 2, 5, and 6 in Figure 10–8 conform to the pattern of a burst following an obvious closure interval. Second, stop bursts often have a much broader frequency representation than nearby glottal pulses. Stop bursts typically (but not always) contain energy at frequencies where the adjacent vowel does *not* have formant energy. Note how the energy of stop bursts 1, 2, 3, and 5 extends throughout most of the vertical scale of the spectrogram. Third, bursts are not often associated with the *clear* formant structure associated with glottal pulses. This is especially exemplified by burst 2. And fourth, when a stop burst occurs in succession with a series of glottal pulses, it typically is separated from the immediately adjacent pulse by an interval that is different from the separation between consecutive glottal pulses within the vocalic event. In other words, the interval between the burst and the immediately adjacent glottal pulse is not consistent with the period of vocal fold vibration as reflected by the intervals between the regularly spaced glottal pulses within the vocalic nucleus. For example, the interval between burst 3 and the first glottal pulse of /i/ in /spik/ is somewhat greater than the intervals between the following glottal pulses. If a vertical line on the spectrogram were actually a glottal pulse, and not a stop burst, it would be expected to fit in with the repetitive pattern of the following or preceding glottal pulses.

In practice, none of the individual criteria for identifying stop bursts should be relied on by themselves. Some or all of these criteria can be applied simultaneously to make the best decision about the identity of a spectrographic event. The choice of which criteria to apply may depend on the specific case under study. The /b/ burst in /əbaʊt/ (burst 5 in the spectrogram) is a good example of how some of the criteria described above may or may not apply to a given case. First, there is a clear closure interval preceding the burstlike feature, suggesting the articulation of a stop consonant. Second, this spike has substantial energy at frequencies other than those associated with the formants of the adjacent vowel. Note, for example, the spike energy from 1.5 to 2.0 kHz, 3.5 to 4.0 kHz, and 7.0 to 7.5 kHz. The following vowel does not contain formant peaks at these frequencies. However, the next two criteria for identifying stop bursts are more ambiguous. This burst does seem to have a formant structure, with darker marks in the vicinity of F1, F2, and F3 of the adjacent vowel. And the interval between the burst and the following glottal pulse is not so different from the intervals between any of the glottal pulses in the /aʊ/ diphthong. Does the failure to meet clearly the third and fourth criteria for distinguishing a stop burst from a glottal pulse cast doubt on the identification of this acoustic event as a stop burst? Probably not, in this case, because the evidence for the closure interval is very clear, as is the evidence for voicing (glottal pulses) during the closure interval. This reasoning is consistent, of course, with knowledge that a /b/ was intended by the speaker. Thus, a voiced closure interval would be expected, and it would follow that a /b/ burst would be superimposed on the continuous series of glottal pulses extending through the closure interval and into the diphthong.

There are many cases, however, in which this kind of simple reasoning—which includes expectations about what has been spoken, who has spoken it, and how it has been spoken—cannot be applied. For example, acoustic analysis of disordered speech must often proceed with very imperfect knowledge of what has been spoken. In this case, the *who has spoken the utterance* (for example, a client with a neurologically based speech disorder) and the *what has been spoken* are very much intertwined. If the client has reduced speech intelligibility and the examiner has difficulty generating a reliable gloss of the utterance, a decision about the spikelike event labeled as #5 in Figure 10–8 (is it, or is it not a burst?) becomes more problematic. This may even be a problem in the speech of persons with no speech disorder, depending on *how* an utterance is produced. The utterance displayed in Figure 10–8 was spoken by one of the authors in a somewhat formal way, very unlike his speech patterns in more casual speech. In casual speaking styles, speakers often produce much blurrier acoustic landmarks than those seen in Figure 10–8, and in the case of stop consonants may even omit bursts all together. This goes against textbook descriptions of stop consonant production. Crystal and House (1988) and Byrd (1993) concluded from their acoustic analyses of connected speech that as many as 50% of stop consonants have no identifiable burst!

How does one distinguish between a pause and a closure interval for a voiceless stop consonant? As described above, voiceless stop closures are identifiable on a spectrogram by an interval of no energy—a silent interval—but isn't the same spectrographic display expected for a pause, for which no energy is being generated by the vocal tract?[3] Obviously, if an interval of no energy is terminated by a burst, there is a good chance it is the acoustic result of a voiceless stop closure. Not all stops, however, have bursts (see above) and in some speech disorders bursts may be present but extremely weak. The potential for confusion between pauses and voiceless stop closures, therefore, must be recognized. In the speech of individuals who are free from speech disorders, there is a general criterion for distinguishing voiceless stop closure intervals from pauses, based on the duration of the silent interval. Actual pauses in speech are typically no less than about 150 ms in duration, whereas voiceless stop closure intervals are typically no more than about 120 ms. To be on the conservative side, many scientists have adopted a criterion of 200 ms for the minimal duration to consider a silent spectrographic interval as a pause. Silent intervals 200 ms or greater are identified as pauses, those less than 200 ms are subject to further evaluation (using information such as the presence of a burst). This criterion is somewhat less reliable in certain speech disorders, for which very long stop closure intervals may be one

---

[3]Reference is made here only to the kind of pause that is silent, typically called an *unfilled* pause. Obviously, in the case of *filled* pauses, such as the many "um's" found in everyday spoken discourse, there would be no confusion with a voiceless stop consonant.

result of a very slow speaking rate, quite common in many cases of motor speech disorders. Clearly, in these cases, the 200-ms criterion may not be effective, and the potential for confusion between stops and pauses is increased.

Aperiodic Intervals

As described in Chapter 9, aperiodic energy is produced within the vocal tract in several different ways and is an important component of the acoustic characteristics of fricatives, stops, and affricates. Aperiodic energy is shown in a spectrogram as an interval of energy having no repeating pattern. These aperiodic intervals are most commonly associated with fricatives and the release phase of stops and affricates. Aperiodic energy may also be mixed with periodic energy for certain sound segments (such as voiced fricatives) or phonation types (such as breathy voice).

In Figure 10–8, five intervals of aperiodic energy, labeled X1, X2, X3, X4, and X5, are marked at the top of the spectrogram by horizontal bars terminated by short, downward vertical lines. These five intervals vary in their duration (i.e., their extent along the x-axis), the range of frequencies over which energy is distributed, and the intensity of the energy. The duration of each interval can be estimated by comparing the length of each horizontal bar to the length of the time calibration ticks (at 100-ms increments) at the base of the spectrogram. The short, vertical lines extending downward from the ends of each horizontal bar show the location of the operationally defined onset and offset of each interval. The range of frequencies is indicated by the locations along the y-axis where there are light, medium, or dark tracings, and the relative intensity of that energy is indicated by the darkness of those tracings. Based on these characteristics, intervals X2, X3, and X5 appear fairly similar to one another, each having relatively long duration and fairly intense energy distributed across a wide range of frequencies. In general, aperiodic intervals of relatively long duration and intense energy are the result of voiceless fricative articulations, especially those produced with a lingua-alveolar or linguapalatal constriction (i.e., /s/ and /ʃ/, see Chapter 9). There are subtle, but important differences in the distribution and intensity of energy for intervals X2, X3, and X5. For example, very dark tracings indicating relatively intense energy extend down to about 1 kHz for segment X2, but not much lower than 2.5 kHz for segments X3 and X5. These differences are discussed in Chapter 9, where the relations of place of articulation to fricative frequency and intensity characteristics are considered.

Segments X1 and X4 differ from X2, X3, and X5 by virtue of their extremely brief durations. At its outset, segment X1 shows aperiodic energy in the form of a very brief "spike," the darkness of which is fairly constant between 0 and 7.0 kHz. This is, of course, a stop burst, and its distribution of energy across frequency is related to the place of articulation of the stop, as discussed in Chapter 9. Immediately following the burst is an interval of roughly 40 ms during which aperiodic energy is distributed broadly across frequency, but is relatively more intense in the 2.0- to 5.0-kHz range. This is the frication interval of the stop (see Chapter 9), and its distribution of energy is also related to the place of articulation. Segment X4 is very brief, showing a spikelike event that, in this case, is not associated with a stop articulation, but rather with the voiced fricative /ð/. Some fricatives, especially those produced at the front of the vocal tract (e.g., /θ,ð,f,v/), may show little, if any, energy on a spectrogram, and in some cases the energy that is visible will be very brief as in segment X4.

Segmentation of Spectrograms

The process of segmenting a spectrogram involves the identification of pieces of the display that correspond roughly to phonemic or phonetic units. The distinction between "phonemic" and "phonetic" is important, because typically there are more phonetic than phonemic units per spectrographic interval (see example below).

Glottal pulses play an important role in the measurement of various attributes of the spectrogram. The term *segment* has been introduced above as a temporal chunk or piece of the spectrogram that is somehow distinguishable from an adjacent chunk. These chunks also have some rough correspondence with sound categories, as indicated by the phonetic symbols at the bottom of the spectrogram. When scientists and clinicians want to know something about these chunks, however, they want to go past the very coarse observation of matching a given chunk with a sound type. Specifically, they are interested in making measurements to provide *quantitative information* about a segment. For example, a clinician might be interested in measuring the duration of the vowel /ʊ/ in the word /ʃʊd/, but cannot do so unless there are some rules for defining the onset and offset of the vowel. The rules for the boundaries, or onsets and offsets of many segments, often depend on the first and last glottal pulses of voiced segments. The glottal pulses shown as vertical lines in the spectrogram, therefore, play an important role in segmentation of spectrograms. Segmentation of the vowel /ʊ/ in

/ʃʊd/ is shown in Figure 10–8 as example E, where the upward-pointing lines indicate the first and last glottal pulses of the vocalic segment. The first glottal pulse is considered to be the onset, or beginning of the vowel, and the last glottal pulse the offset or end of the vowel. The distance between the first and last glottal pulses along the x-, or time axis—the interval "E"—can be converted to time to determine the duration of /ʊ/.

The use of glottal pulses to identify onsets and offsets of segments in a spectrogram is a well-accepted practice, but must be recognized as a form of *operational definition,* and not as the *truth.* Investigators, whether they are in the laboratory or clinic, use such definitions to describe measurements precisely and to allow other investigators to make exactly the same measurements using the same criteria. When an investigator identifies the first glottal pulse of a vowel as the onset of the vocalic event, it does not necessarily imply a belief that this point in time is where the brain initiates a vowel, or even that the brain represents onsets and offsets of speech segments.

Segmentation of vowels is relatively straightforward when vowels are located between two obstruents. The beginning of the vowel is taken as the first "full" glottal pulse, and the end of the vowel is the last full glottal pulse. A full glottal pulse is one that extends from the baseline at least through F2 of the display. The requirement that the glottal pulse go at least as high in frequency as F2 distinguishes it from the glottal pulses seen in voiced stops, affricates, and fricatives, as well as some low-intensity pulses that extend only through F1. According to this reasoning, a glottal pulse that extends through at least F2 is only visible because the vocal tract is open. If the vocal tract were closed, the sound energy generated within the vocal tract would not be visible at such high frequencies because these frequencies are filtered out by the vocal tract walls. Clearly, when trying to find the acoustic boundaries of a vowel, a clinician or scientist would like to identify the first and last instants in time when the vocal tract is open. When vowels are located before or after nasals, the "full glottal pulse" criterion cannot be used to segment a vowel from a nasal, but the change from an oral to nasal filter function, discussed in Chapter 9, can be used to find a vowel-nasal or nasal-vowel boundary. A sudden change in intensity at the boundary between a nasal and a vowel, and the sudden appearance of the low-frequency F1 characteristic of nasal cavity resonance, are good criteria for this segmentation problem. When vowels are located before or after semivowels (/ɹ,l,w,j/) or diphthongs (/aɪ, ɔɪ, aʊ, eɪ, oʊ/) the segmentation problem is very difficult because there are no natural boundaries. In general, the conservative approach in sequences such as "yellow" (/jɛloʊ/ or "I honor" (/aɪjɑnɚ/) is not to attempt a phonetic or phonemic segmentation. The duration of semivowels is often combined with the duration of surrounding vowels.

Segmentation of obstruents is, in many cases, fairly simple. When an obstruent follows a vocalic segment (vowels, diphthongs, semivowels), the last full glottal pulse of the preceding vocalic is taken as the instant before closure of the vocal tract, and, thus, as the beginning of the closure or constriction interval. The same criterion can often be applied to nasal + obstruent sequences because nasals are voiced and have an obvious formant pattern. In the case of stops, the offset (or end) of the closure interval is taken as the burst (same for the closure offset of affricates). In the case of fricatives, the offset is taken as the end of the frication noise, or the first full glottal pulse of the following vowel. Even though this latter measurement point (the glottal pulse following the frication noise) results in a fricative interval that may be slightly longer than the actual frication, it is more reliable than trying to locate the precise ending of the frication noise. When fricatives and stops are abutted, as in an /s/ + stop sequence, separation of the frication from the closure interval must rely on the termination of frication noise and the onset of silence (i.e., no energy in the closure interval). When two fricatives follow each other, the changing spectrum must be used to identify the end of one and beginning of the other. When two stops follow each other, the only way to distinguish the closure intervals is if the first stop is released, and produces a burst.

Returning briefly to the issue of phonemic versus phonetic segmentation, the case of voiceless stops provides a good example of this problem because the stop includes a closure interval, a burst, a frication interval, and an aspiration interval. These intervals can all be identified as segments on the spectrogram, but they are all associated with a single stop. If these intervals were identified by segmentation, the segmentation is labeled "phonetic" because the different segments all relate to the same phoneme (i.e., the stop). If the closure, burst, frication, and aspiration are combined and regarded as one interval this would be a "phonemic" segment. This is not a problem with segments such as vowels, where "subsegments" are not likely to be identified. However, when dealing with spectrograms produced by speakers with speech disorders this can be a problem, and it is wise to keep in mind that segmentation may result in two or more pieces that actually relate to the same phoneme. The opposite case is also true, that two or more consecutive phonemes may not be segmentable as two separate "pieces," as described above for vowel-vowel,

vowel-semivowel, and other sequences for which clear boundaries cannot be identified.[4]

Spectrographic segmentation of the utterance, "The blue spot is a normal dot," spoken by a 53-year-old male, is shown in Figure 10–9. A broad phonetic transcription is provided below the spectrogram, with the phonetic symbols located along the time axis

roughly in the middle of the acoustically identified segments. The vertical lines immediately below the baseline mark the segmentation boundaries, determined according to the rules outlined above. The pieces of the acoustic signal identified with these rules—the segments—are numbered in sequence from left to right. Seventeen segments are identified.

Can Unlabeled Spectrograms Be Segmented and Labeled?

The answer to this question is yes, and no. Speech acousticians have always been interested in their ability to examine an unlabeled spectrogram of an utterance, and determine the phonetic segments and ultimately the words displayed as acoustic patterns. This is a really, really difficult task, and even highly experienced speech scientists are reduced to babbling confusion when asked to "read" an unlabeled spectrogram. Many years ago, a speech scientist named Dr. Victor Zue, of the Massachusetts Institute of Technology, got so good at this that a colleague made a film of him reading an unlabeled spectrogram with what seemed to be unworldly quickness. Zue trained himself for this task, however, spending many hours learning the subtle phonetic variants of speech sounds that trip up seasoned speech scientists. Zue and a colleague also showed that students could be trained to read unlabeled spectrograms fairly well (Zue & Cole, 1979), although not with his remarkable speed and accuracy.

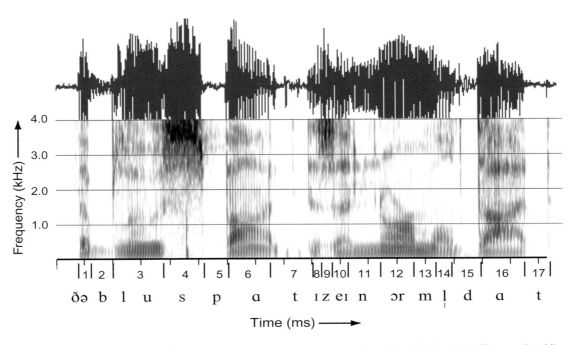

Figure 10-9. Spectrogram segmented according to the rules described in the text. The vertical lines immediately below the baseline of the spectrogram show the onsets and offsets of the segments, and the sound class corresponding to a segment is shown between the segment boundaries.

---

[4]Segmentation of a spectrogram does not have to be guided by sound classes (the approach described here), although that is certainly the most typical strategy. Segmentation could be guided by the underlying vocal tract gestures, an example of which is the vocalic articulatory gesture for the /uɪ/ sequence in the utterance, "The stew is good" (/ðəstuɪzgʊd/). Here the interest is in the relatively rapid and smoothly executed transition from a high-back (/u/) to a high-front (/ɪ/) configuration. These sorts of articulatory sequences, for which the "units" (segments) are defined on the basis of gestures rather than sound classes, have not been explored much in the clinical literature but are potentially of great diagnostic and theoretical value in understanding speech disorders.

Some of the segments shown in Figure 10–9 result from straightforward application of rules. For example, segments 1, 6, 8, 10, and 16 are vowels or diphthongs, for which the identification of first and last glottal pulses is fairly obvious. Segments 3 and 12, however, have obvious glottal-pulse boundaries but include two phonemes because there is no reliable way to separate the /l/ from the /u/ in segment 3 or the /ɔ/ from the /r/ in segment 12. It appears to be relatively easy to segment the nasals (segments 11 and 13), the stops[5] (segments 2, 5, 7, 15 and 17), and the fricatives (segments 4 and 9), although the intervocalic /z/ in /ɪzeɪ/ and the /t/ in segment 7 present certain segmentation challenges.[6]

Of course, the ease of segmenting any spectrogram depends on a number of factors, including the speaker, the speaking style (e.g., casual vs. formal), the context in which a given sound is spoken, and so forth.

Why segment a spectrogram? This question can be answered in several different ways, but the general response is this: to mark off a piece of the signal for the purpose of discovering the typical acoustic characteristics associated with that piece, and similar pieces. Similar pieces would be, for example, the same phoneme produced by different speakers, or by the same speaker under different speaking conditions (e.g., stressed or unstressed, fast or slow rate, etc.). If one knows the acoustic characteristics of well-defined pieces of the speech signal, one is in a position to write computer code for high-quality speech synthesizers and speech recognizers; to provide a quantitative description of the articulatory problem in a speech disorder; to identify the acoustic properties that should be processed optimally by a hearing instrument, be it a hearing aid, cochlear implant, or classroom-based assistive hearing device; and to incorporate the specifics of these characteristics into theories that attempt to explain the origin of, for example, disorders such as stuttering, apraxia of speech, and specific language impairment. When conversing with an individual who, because of some disease process, cannot produce oral speech and instead uses a speech synthesizer to produce intelligible responses and engage in what we humans love to do—talk, talk, talk—keep in mind that it is the study of the acoustic characteristics of speech sounds—acoustic phonetics—that created the possibility of the enjoyable experience of communicating with this particular person.

SPEECH ACOUSTICS IS NOT ALL ABOUT SEGMENTS: SUPRASEGMENTALS

A discussion of the techniques of speech acoustic analysis would not be complete without mention of phonetic events whose characteristics extend beyond the duration of the kinds of segments shown in Figure 10–9. These events are often called "suprasegmentals"—that is, bigger (i.e., longer) than segment-sized. Some authors refer to suprasegmental variables as *prosodic* variables.

A well-known example of a suprasegmental is the *fundamental frequency (F0) contour*, the variation in F0 over several segments. To obtain an F0 contour, one must have a way to measure the periods of many successive vibrations of the vocal folds—however, many glottal vibrations occur across an utterance. Take the segmented utterance of Figure 10–9 as an example. There are approximately 90 glottal pulses in this utterance. One way to obtain the F0 contour is to measure each of the periods, convert each to F0 by $F0 = 1/T$, and graph the resulting values as a function of time. With a proper display of a speech waveform, this is an easy but incredibly tedious thing to do. (One of the authors, who used to do this kind of hand analysis before the computer age, performed a period-by-period measurement of the utterance in Figure 10–9 and completed it in about 40 minutes.)

It would be desirable to have an automated procedure to measure F0. Most computer programs designed for speech acoustic analysis, like *TF32*, include algorithms for the measurement and display of F0 contours. Scientists typically refer to these algorithms as *pitch trackers*, even though the name is a technical misnomer because pitch is a perceptual phenomenon and F0 is the physical event being measured. There are many different algorithms for the measurement of F0, each using somewhat different strategies and computations, but in the end they perform the analysis essentially by

---

[5]In this text, when the term "stop duration" or "stop segment," is used, it refers to the closure interval. This is the conventional usage in the acoustic phonetics literature (Klatt, 1976; Umeda, 1977). The burst and VOT are sometimes allied with the stop, sometimes with the vowel.

[6]In English, word-final /t/ is often produced as a glottal stop (/ʔ/), and the /t/ in /spɑt/ may have been produced in this way. The weak "spike" seen a little more than halfway through interval 7 of Figure 10–9 could be an example of a momentary "leak" in glottal closure (not unusual for glottal stops), and the release at the end of the stop interval has energy concentrated at the formant frequencies of the following vowel /i/, also fairly common for glottal stop releases.

measuring the period of each glottal cycle. Above the spectrogram in Figure 10–10 is the F0 contour for "The blue spot is a normal dot," spoken with a small degree of emphasis on the word "normal." The F0 contour was computed automatically by *TF32* ("automatically" means, selecting a command such as, "perform pitch analysis") and is shown exactly as it was computed on a frequency scale of 75 to 200 Hz. Values are computed for each glottal pulse, and typically are *not* computed where there are no glottal pulses, although there are exceptions to both of these statements. For example, there are no values computed for the voiceless /s/ in *spot* (except for two at the end of the frication energy), which makes sense because of the absence of a periodic waveform for the voiceless fricative. However, a couple values were computed during the /t/ closure interval of the utterance-final word *dot*. More surprising, perhaps, is: (a) the uncertain performance of this analysis throughout the /ɪzeɪ/ sequence, for which the F0 contour appears to be discontinuous, as if there are missing values; and (b) the strange behavior of the analysis for the /n/, where the F0 values seem to jump between roughly 175 and 135 Hz, giving the contour an "up and down" staircase appearance that most certainly reflects

errors in computation rather than rapidly changing rates of vocal fold vibration. The sequence of F0 values starting with /ɪ/ in *is* and going through the word-initial /n/ of *normal* (segments 8 through 11 in Figure 10–9) is continuously voiced, and in theory should yield good F0 values for each of the glottal pulses.

These examples of F0 contour errors illustrate certain weaknesses of most "pitch tracker" analysis programs. Specifically, the programs make errors when the glottal period being estimated from the waveform is not "clear." What makes a glottal cycle unclear? The answer is, a lot of things, many of which are found in normal speech production and certainly are present in many speech disorders. For example, glottal cycles associated with breathy voice quality typically have both periodic and aperiodic energy and, therefore, present problems for F0 analysis programs. The aperiodic energy makes it difficult for the measurement algorithm to detect the beginnings and endings of individual glottal cycles. In general, F0 measurement algorithms will have increasing difficulty with accurate identification of glottal periods as the level of aperiodic energy increases. In the case of the /z/ in /ɪzeɪ/, periodic energy can be seen mixed with the

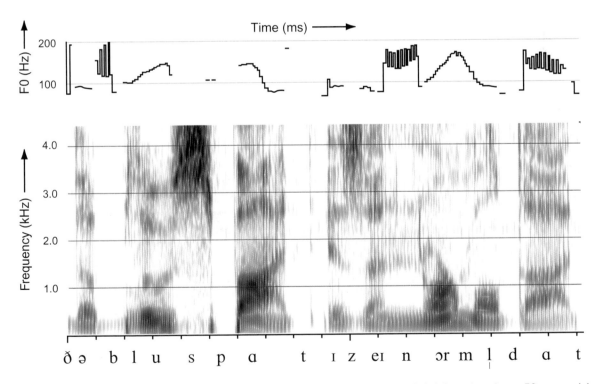

Figure 10–10. F0 contour (*top of display*) for "The blue spot is a normal dot," spoken by a 53-year-old male. The F0 data are displayed on a scale from 75 to 200 Hz. The spectrogram is shown below the F0 contour. See text for additional details.

frication energy above 3.0 kHz, but the program "lost" the periodicity and failed to compute F0 values during the middle of the fricative. The errors during the nasal /n/ may be attributed to one or both of two factors. First, the segment has relatively low energy (compare the darkness of the formants with that of the /ɑ/s in *spot* or *dot*), which often confuses F0 analysis programs because consecutive glottal cycles may not be clearly distinct from one another. Second, some F0 analyses, like the one in Figure 10–10, generate values by first computing the formant frequencies and then subtracting them from the overall spectral analysis, leaving the part of the signal associated with vocal fold vibration. This residual part of the signal is then used to generate the F0 value (see the discussion of inverse filtering in Chapter 8, especially Figure 8–3 and the associated text). Recall from Chapter 9 that nasals have antiresonances, as well as resonances. The antiresonances can make the separation of resonances from glottal vibrations problematic, and may result in analysis errors of the type indicated for /n/ in Figure 10–10.

The purpose of the foregoing discussion is not to dwell on the intricacies and delicate nature of F0 analysis programs. There is a larger point to be made, that automated analyses of speech acoustics are very, very fast—the F0 contour in Figure 10–10 was generated with a single point-and-click maneuver and appeared on the screen in less than a second—but are prone to error, even when the speaker is "normal." The F0 analysis in Figure 10–10 is not unique in this respect. All "pitch trackers" suffer from the kinds of errors shown in Figure 10–10. A good F0 analysis program performs the computations rapidly, provides a display such as the one in Figure 10–10, and allows the user to examine the display for errors and *correct them* interactively. There are, therefore, two caveat emptor lessons to take away from this discussion: (a) programs make errors; and (b) programs should allow the user to make corrections rapidly and easily. Corrections for the F0 contour shown in Figure 10–10 (not shown here) required about 5 min of time from one of your authors, well under the 40-some min required for the complete hand-analysis described above.

Despite errors in the F0 contour of Figure 10–10, its general shape is consistent with theories of prosody and previous laboratory observations. Generally, declarative utterances are expected to show an increasing F0 at the start of the utterance which quickly reaches a maximum value. For the remainder of the utterance, F0 falls gradually, reaching a lowest value at the end of the utterance. In the utterance shown in Figure 10–10, there is an F0 peak soon after the utterance begins, toward the end of the word "blue," with a value of roughly 145 Hz. Later in the utterance, there is another peak F0

of roughly 170 Hz, on the emphasized word "normal." This later peak F0, due to a stressed word, is assumed in many analyses to be superimposed on the gradual F0 fall following the early peak referred to above. The gradual fall of F0 from the high to low point in a declarative utterance is referred to as "declination." F0 details along the contour in Figure 10–10 are not discussed here, but a general shape description of F0 contours is amenable to a kind of contrast analysis similar to that used for segments. The general declination pattern for declarative utterances, for example, can be contrasted with the fall-rise pattern of F0 common for question utterances (e.g., "Are you going to help out?"). The shape of an F0 contour carries contrastive information concerning the grammatical function of the utterance.

In *tone languages* such as Thai, Igala (a language spoken in Nigeria), and the Mandarin and Cantonese dialects of Chinese, shape of the F0 contour across a vocalic segment has exactly the same contrastive function as, say, the difference in formant frequencies between two vowels. In these languages, the different F0 contours function as phonemes. For example, in Mandarin the sequence /bɑ/ produced with a flat F0 contour means "eight," but /bɑ/ spoken with a rapid fall-rise contour means "to hold" (Catford, 2000). The specific shape of the segment-sized F0 contour changes the meaning of the sequence, even as the articulatory characteristics of the segments (that is, the /b/ and the /ɑ/) stay the same. This is analogous to the case of English where the change of a vowel from "bat" to "bit" changes the meaning of the sequence. Both the Mandarin and English cases are examples of minimal pairs, but implemented using different phonetic strategies.

F0 analysis is clearly important, then, especially because tone languages are very widespread among peoples of the world (more people speak Mandarin than any other language in the world) and at the utterance level the contour shape has important grammatical functions. In addition, F0 variation during conversation plays an important role in conveying a speaker's emotional state, in providing signals concerning the rules of turn-taking, and in marking some very important aspects of an individual's personality. Some of these issues, as well as a broader consideration of the acoustics of prosody, are discussed in Chapter 11.

DIGITAL TECHNIQUES FOR SPEECH ANALYSIS

This chapter is not a technical manual of hardware and algorithmic details for speech analysis, but some discussion is provided below concerning the basics of computer analysis of speech. Digital analysis of speech has the same general goal as spectrographic analysis of speech: to produce an accurate spectral analysis as a function of time. As in the case of the F0 analysis outlined above, there are many different algorithms and hardware solutions to obtaining a quality analysis of speech waveforms. Here, the focus is on the main components and procedures for speech acoustic analysis by computer.

Spectrographic analysis using the original spectrograph from the 1950s (see Figure 10–7) or any of its several modernized models through the late 1980s required a recording of speech on some permanent medium and, of course, the instrument itself. Typically, a speech sample was recorded on a tape recorder (the tape being the permanent medium) and at some later time "fed into" the spectrograph for production of a spectrogram. All processing of the signal—the frequency analysis, the type of display, and so forth—was done by the fixed electronic circuitry of the instrument. That circuitry processed and displayed the *continuous* fluctuations of the magnetic field's strength recorded on the tape and stored temporarily on the tape loop of the spectrograph. These continuous fluctuations in the strength of the magnetic field were converted to continuous fluctuations in the voltage applied to the marking stylus, which then burned patterns of relative darkness onto the paper in proportion to the strength of the voltage. The word *continuous* is important to this

discussion: everything in this process was based on original recordings and transformations of the signal (i.e., from voltage to magnetic field, and then back to voltage, and ultimately to the darkness of the burned pattern) that did not change the continuous nature of the speech signal. A process such as this, in which the transforms and representations (magnetic, voltage, darkness of the trace, and so forth) are in the same form as the input signal—in this case the speech signal—is called an *analog process*. Computer analysis of speech requires a conversion of this analog representation to digital form.

Speech Analysis by Computer: From Recording to Analysis to Output

Figure 10–11 presents a simple block diagram of the important steps in speech analysis by computer. A microphone is used to transduce the continuously varying pressure waveform of speech into a continuously varying electrical signal. High-quality microphones achieve this transduction in a number of different ways, producing an electrical replica of the pressure wave in all respects, including frequency, amplitude, and time. The microphone signal can be used as input to a tape recorder, or to the hard disk of the computer. The left side of Figure 10–11 shows these two different input paths for the microphone signal.

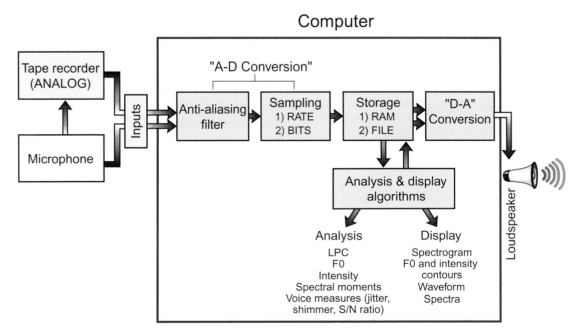

Figure 10–11. Block diagram of speech analysis by computer. See text for details.

Digital Speech Samples and the Aural Flip Book

When speech is synthesized by computer, or when a natural speech signal is digitized, the computerized form of the signal is a series of discrete time points—samples—each of which contains a spectrum. When these time points are output from a computer—when they undergo digital-to-analog conversion—the human ear will connect the discrete samples and hear them as a smoothly flowing speech signal. It is just like the flip books you enjoyed, and perhaps created, as a child (and maybe even as an adult). Each individual picture in the flip book is like a digital sample. When the stack of individual pictures is flipped, the human visual system connects the sequence of images and voilà! We have animation! Think of the process of digital-to-analog conversion as aural animation.

When a tape recorder (assumed to be an analog device for this discussion) is the destination for the microphone signal, at some point the tape-recorded signal must be delivered to the computer.

Computers (or digital tape recorders, essentially simple computing devices dedicated to sampling and storing analog signals) perform *digital* transformations of input signals, in which the analog signals are converted to a series of discrete numbers, each of which has the form of sequences of zeros (0s) and ones (1s). How that transformation is done is all important in computer-based speech analysis. The important factors in this transformation are: (a) sampling rate, (b) filtering, and (c) quantization.

Sampling Rate

Because the computer stores an acoustic waveform as a series of discrete numbers, a decision must be made concerning how frequently the computer "picks" and stores values from the continuously varying waveform. The conversion of analog to digital representation—A-to-D conversion, as indicated in Figure 10–11—is done by a piece of hardware called a sound card. The *sampling rate* determines how frequently numbers are picked off the analog event. Most computer programs and sound cards allow the sampling rate to be adjusted according the user's needs. These needs can be summed up pretty easily: What is the highest frequency in the analog waveform that is of interest for analysis, or perhaps playback to a listener?

Figure 10–12 illustrates the concept of sampling rate and how it is tied to the highest frequency of interest in a speech signal. For simplicity, a sinusoidal signal is used for this illustration, but the concept applies to complex waveforms. Panels A, B, and C of Figure 10–12 show one complete cycle of the same 1000-Hz sinusoidal signal, in its analog form, sampled by a computer at three different rates. Locations along the waveforms where samples are taken by the computer are shown by the red circles for sampling rates of 500 Hz (500 samples per second; panel A), 2000 Hz (panel B), and 5000 Hz (panel C). In panel A, the 500 Hz sampling rate extracts only a single sample from the cycle. The location of this sample, indicated by the red circle slightly before the completion of the first half-cycle, is arbitrary. However, for this 1000-Hz sinusoid, a 500-Hz sampling rate will result in only one sample extracted per cycle, regardless of where the sample is located. This is because a 500-Hz sampling rate picks samples from the analog waveform every 2 ms (that is, the period of 500 Hz), which is *twice the duration of a 1000-Hz cycle.* In other words, the 500-Hz sampling is much too slow (i.e., selects samples too infrequently) to produce a correct digital estimate of the frequency of this 1000-Hz signal. This sampling rate could never produce two samples *within* a single cycle of this 1000-Hz waveform, regardless of where a first sample is taken during any single cycle. The next (or previous) sample would always be taken in the next (or previous) cycle.

The example in panel A reveals an important axiom of computer sampling of analog waveforms. The axiom is directly related to the discussion in Chapter 7 of the relationship between frequency and period. A period (T) is a time interval along a repeating waveform whose inverse is frequency. The measurement of such a time *interval* requires at least two points: one to identify the start of the interval, the second to identify the end of the interval. With this in mind, the sampling axiom is as follows: *An accurate determination of a given frequency (not necessarily of the waveform details; see below) requires a sampling rate that extracts at least **two** samples from each individual cycle of the waveform.* The two samples allow estimation of the period of the cycle, and thus its frequency. The way to ensure that two samples are obtained per cycle is to use a sampling rate that is twice the frequency one wishes to measure. Panel B shows how a sampling rate of 2000 Hz, with samples extracted from the analog waveform every 0.5 ms (half the time it takes to complete a single 1000-Hz cycle), results in the two samples-per-cycle required for an accurate estimate of the period. As in panel A, the placement of the first sample is arbitrary, but with a 2000-Hz sampling rate the next sample must fall within this particular cycle.

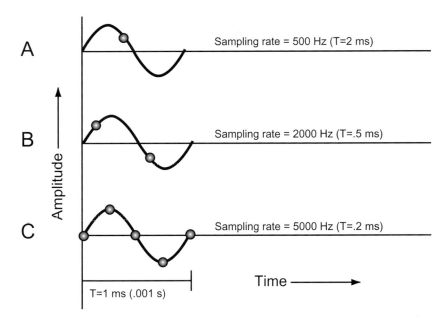

Figure 10–12. The concept of sampling rate, and its relation to the frequencies being sampled. Panels A, B, and C show how progressively higher sampling rates (computer samples of analog signal indicated by red circles on the waveforms) extract samples from a 1000-Hz sinusoid. "T" refers to the period of successive computer samples (the inverse of sampling rate). The "T" of 1 ms, shown under the sinusoidal waveforms, is the period of the signal being sampled. See text for explanation.

A general lesson from this discussion is that the sampling rate should always be at least twice the highest frequency that needs to be measured. According to information on vowels and consonants presented in Chapters 8 and 9, across *all* speech sounds there is phonetically relevant frequency information at least in the 0- to 8.0-kHz range, and for a limited number of sounds definitely up to 10.0 kHz. If one takes 10.0 kHz as the highest frequency of interest for most speech analysis applications, a sampling rate of no less than 20.0 kHz is required. Many speech analysis programs use 22.05 or 44.10 kHz as the default sampling rate (44.10 kHz is the standard sampling rate for digital audio equipment). Obviously, the more times per second a waveform is sampled, the more accurate the match between the analog waveform and its digital representation. In the absence of any other considerations, a high sampling rate is always desirable to increase the match between the analog and digital versions of the signal.

Sampling Rate Sidebar: Anti-Aliasing Filters

Figure 10–11 shows the input to the computer, whether from tape recorder or microphone, going through an *anti-aliasing filter* before the sampling phase of A-to-D conversion. The anti-aliasing filter is necessary to eliminate mistakes arising from the digital sampling process when no filter is used. These mistakes take the form of frequencies derived from the sampled signal, estimated from an *apparent* period between two sample points, that are not really in the signal but are natural results of a very specific (undesired) condition of sampling. That condition is in effect *when the sampling rate is not at least twice the highest frequency in the signal being sampled.* This may seem like a restatement of the sampling rate rule given above, but there is an important difference. To restate that rule: The sampling rate must be at least twice the highest frequency of *interest* to estimate it correctly. The aliasing rule says that if there are frequencies in the signal greater than *half* the sampling rate, the sampling process will estimate these frequencies erroneously — that is, the process will produce alias frequencies, which are not truly in the signal.

Why does this occur? A reconsideration of panel A of Figure 10–12 helps to answer the question. In this example, the frequency being sampled (1000 Hz) is, in fact, greater than half the sampling rate of 500 Hz. As stated above, with this sampling rate only one sample is picked from the 1000-Hz waveform and the signal frequency is not be estimated correctly. However, because there are samples occurring every 2 ms, *something* is estimated because the process produces successions of points and, therefore, time intervals that masquerade as real periods in the signal, even though the true signal does not contain those periods.

In a spectral analysis of the 1000-Hz sinusoid shown in Figure 10–12, the aliased frequency is easily recognized, but in a complex signal, such as speech, aliasing can present a major problem if not addressed correctly. And even though 10.0 kHz was identified as the highest frequency of interest for *phonetic relevance*, the speech signal contains frequencies well above 10.0 kHz, especially for certain consonants. These very high frequencies are prevalent for some fricatives (Tabain, 1998), as well as when speakers have very short vocal tracts (e.g., when analyzing infant speech; see Bauer & Kent, 1987). This is where the anti-aliasing filter comes into play. To prevent frequencies greater than half the sampling rate from creating an aliasing problem, the signal is *filtered* before it is submitted to the A-to-D process. An effective anti-aliasing filter has a low-pass configuration (i.e., passing frequencies from 0 Hz to some high frequency cutoff), with the cutoff frequency at half, or slightly less than half, the sampling rate. The object is to remove all frequencies more than half the sampling rate and so prevent aliasing—hence the name *anti-aliasing filter*.

Speech analysis systems with sampling rates of 22.05 kHz usually set the cutoff frequency of the anti-aliasing filter somewhere between 8.0 and 10.0 kHz. The actual filters may be built into the sound card as a hardware solution, or may be implemented with software. The exact details of cutoff frequencies are beyond the scope of this discussion; ask your instructor if you have a sudden, burning interest in the intricacies of anti-aliasing filters.

There is a familiar example of aliasing, familiar not from speech analysis but rather from the movies. Everyone has seen a movie scene in which a vehicle accelerates and the wheels initially appear to spin in the right direction (forward). As the vehicle continues to pick up speed, however, the wheels appear to freeze, as if they have stopped spinning, or may seem to spin in *reverse* even as the vehicle continues moving forward. The perception of frozen or reverse wheel motion is a case of aliasing. The illusion of no motion, or reverse motion, is produced by a sampling process like the one described above. Think of the motion of a rotating wheel on a car or stagecoach as an analog event, and the process of filming the motion as a sampling problem. Motion pictures are constructed from a series of individual frames, photographed at a fairly high rate—typically 24 frames per second (fps). Each frame is a sample picked from the analog motion, just like a sample taken by a sound card from an acoustic waveform. When the discrete motion picture frames are played back for viewing, the visual system connects the discrete frames and interprets them as continuous motion (because of a phenomenon called "persistence of vision"). As long as the sampling rate, 24 fps, is twice as great as the frequency of wheel rotation, there will be two sampling points per rotation to allow a correct visual estimation of the relative speed and direction of the wheel's motion. When the wheel rotation frequency (~12 rotations per second) reaches half the sampling frequency (24 fps), however, the wheel rotation is illuminated over and over at exactly the same point in the rotation cycle and the wheel motion appears to stop. As the frequency of the wheel rotation increases past the one-half sampling frequency point, the sampling points occur across several cycles of the wheel motion and the direction of that motion seems to reverse. These alias motions (clearly the wheel is not frozen in time, nor spinning in reverse as the car speeds toward some spectacular encounter with a wall, the Hulk, or garden-variety James Bond villain) are a byproduct of the sampling process. In film, it is no big deal, but in the analysis of speech it could lead to the "finding" of signal frequencies not truly there.

Quantization (Bits)

The preceding discussion describes how a computer implements A-to-D conversion along the time scale, but not the amplitude scale. Information concerning waveform amplitude must also be coded in digital form, a process called quantization. The number of *bits* used in A-to-D conversion determines how accurately the amplitude of an analog waveform is represented in digital form. Quantization is illustrated by the schematic diagrams in Figure 10–13. A 1000-Hz sinusoid having an arbitrary peak-to-peak amplitude is shown in both the upper and lower panels. In both panels, the sinusoid is shown with a series of equidistant, horizontal lines spanning the entire amplitude scale. In the upper panel these horizontal lines are less closely spaced than in the lower panel. Think of these horizontal lines as amplitude levels that can be digitized by the sound card. These are called quantization levels. At points along the sinusoid where a horizontal line—a quantization level—crosses the waveform, the amplitude stored by the computer is faithful to the amplitude in the analog waveform. But what happens for points sampled along the time domain for which the analog waveform amplitude is between two quantization levels? For example, if the 1000-Hz sinusoid is sampled at a high rate (e.g., 22.05 kHz; individual sample times in Figure 10–13 marked by the short ver-

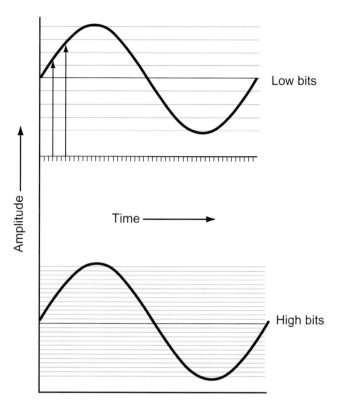

Figure 10-13. Quantization of analog waveform during the A-to-D process. Quantization levels are shown by the series of horizontal lines extending from the top to bottom of the amplitude scale. Time samples for conversion of the analog signal to digital form are shown on the x-axis of the upper graph. *Upper panel* = few quantization levels, low bit rate. *Lower panel* = many quantization levels, high bit rate. On the upper, low-bit chart, arrows pointing upward from the third and sixth samples show samples for which an exact quantization level is not available.

tical lines along the x-axis) with the quantization levels shown in the upper panel in Figure 10–13, there are a number of time samples along the waveform for which a quantization level is not available. These are shown in Figure 10–13, upper panel, by the time samples falling in between two of the adjacent amplitude levels available for digital storage (arrows extending upward from the third and sixth time samples). The value stored by the computer for an amplitude of an analog waveform that is "between" quantization levels is the one corresponding to the closest quantization level. This means that, during the digitization process, some real (analog) amplitudes "jump up," and some "jump down," to the nearest quantization level. The absence of a quantization level at a given point along the amplitude variation of a waveform, therefore, does not pre-

vent storage of that sample, which seems like a good thing. The amplitude represented for such a sample, however, is not the correct one and, in fact, produces a digital representation that distorts the shape of the analog waveform. This is not desirable, although in some cases it may be unavoidable. The ideal solution to the problem is to have the quantization levels spaced as closely as possible along the amplitude scale, as simulated in the lower panel of Figure 10–13. In this case, the quantization offered produces a digital representation of the sinusoid amplitudes much more like the analog waveform, because more analog amplitude variations can be stored directly, at the available quantization levels, and the "jumps" for in-between time samples are smaller than the ones required in the upper panel of Figure 10–13.

The number of quantization levels available in A-to-D conversion is generally described by the number of bits (bits = binary digits) used to store amplitudes in digital form. The greater the number of bits, the greater the number of quantization levels available for storing waveform amplitudes. It follows that a greater number of bits produces a better match between the amplitudes of the analog and digital versions of the waveform. The A-to-D conversion illustrated in the lower panel of Figure 10–13 has a greater number of bits compared to the upper panel because it allows more amplitudes to be represented during the conversion process. Speech waveforms have been digitized (that is, undergone the process of A-to-D conversion) at 8, 12, 16, and 32 bits. Sixteen bits provide very good representation of the amplitude fluctuations in a speech waveform. Speech digitized with 8 bits of amplitude resolution is fairly intelligible, but the overall quality of the signal is noticeably improved when a 16-bit conversion is used.

Analysis and Display

Most speech analysis programs have algorithms for display, editing, and analysis of speech waveforms. The basic display of a speech analysis program is the speech waveform, shown above the spectrograms in Figures 10–8 and 10–9. A waveform of the utterance *To feed the cat one must shoo the dog* is shown in Figure 10–14. This utterance was produced by one of the authors as a direct-to-disk recording (microphone input directly into the computer; see Figure 10–11), with a sampling rate of 22.05 kHz and 16 bits of amplitude resolution. The utterance waveform was displayed in near-real time as it was spoken, and immediately stored as a file. The waveform display at the top of Figure 10–14 is essentially identical to the one that appeared on the screen as it was being recorded.

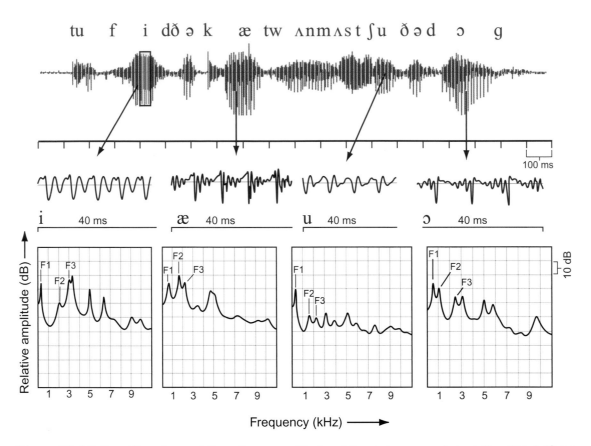

Figure 10-14. Top: Waveform of the utterance, "To feed the cat one must shoo the dog." 40-ms pieces are extracted from each of the four corner vowels, by centering an analysis window at the temporal middle of the vowel. One such window is shown by the shaded box over the /i/ waveform. Each waveform piece is shown in the middle row of the display, and the bottom row of panels shows the LPC spectra for each of these pieces.

Speech analysis programs allow the user to manipulate and process waveforms in many different ways, and to display the results of those processes. As listed in Figure 10–11, the typical speech analysis program allows linear predictive code analysis of formant frequencies (see below), different types of F0 and intensity measurement, computation of spectral moments (see Chapters 9 and 11), as well as other analyses beyond the scope of this book. Programs can generate a digital spectrogram, F0 contours, intensity contours, spectra for different "chunks" of a waveform, measures of voice production (jitter, shimmer, signal-to-noise ratio), and so forth. As a case study of computer analysis of speech and as a teaser for information on vowels presented in Chapter 11, consider Figure 10–14 from top to bottom as a demonstration of computer analysis of vowel formant frequencies.

The utterance whose speech waveform is shown in Figure 10–14 contains an example of each of the corner vowels of English (the phonetic symbol for the vowel

in *dog* is given as /ɔ/, but the low-back corner vowel is usually thought to be /ɔ/'s near neighbor /ɑ/. In the dialect of the individual who produced the display shown in Figure 10–14, a weird farrago of Philadelphia origin and Cheesehead spirit, the vowel in *dog* sounds to most listeners as something between /ɔ/ and /ɑ/). Formant frequencies are often measured for the corner vowels as a way to map out, in acoustic terms, the limits of vowel articulation for a given speaker. The conventional way to make formant frequency measures is to locate and segment the vowel of interest, select for analysis a relatively brief piece ("window") from the overall vowel waveform, and calculate for this piece the values of F1, F2, and F3.

The waveform editing function of *TF32* was used to isolate brief pieces of the /i/ in *feed*, the /æ/ in *cat*, the /u/ in the *shoo*, and /ɔ/ in *dog*. A shaded rectangle indicates the small time window of the waveform selected for analysis from the vowel /i/. In practice, these windows are not taken from a random part of the

[kɔrnɚ] or [karnɚ] Vowels?

"Corner" vowels play a major role in speech acoustics research and in clinical applications of speech acoustic analysis. These sounds define the limits—high-front, high-back, low-front, low-back—of vowel articulation. /ɑ/ is almost always identified as the low-back corner vowel, but in some dialects /ɑ/ may be realized as [ɔ], or /ɔ/ may be realized as [ɑ]. /ɔ/ may even involve a more extreme articulatory position as compared to /ɑ/. If so, *it* should be the low-back corner vowel, not /ɑ/. English /u/, the high-back corner vowel, is even more slippery than /ɑ/ and /ɔ/, as it seems to be losing its lip-rounding characteristic over the last 10 or 15 years. Perhaps /i/ will be like that perfect older brother, always doing the right thing, always stable, never changing. /æ/? Let's not even talk about that vowel . . .

vowel waveform, but in fact are 20 to 50 ms in duration and centered around the temporal middle of the vowel. Traditionally, "targets" for vowels have been located at their temporal midpoint and the use of a time window of 20 to 50 ms around this midpoint ensures a more stable spectral analysis than a shorter window (say, 5 ms). The 40-ms piece of the full /i/ waveform in Figure 10–14 is shown in detail immediately below the arrow pointing away from the /i/ in the full utterance. The 40-ms piece shows individual cycles of vocal fold vibration—about four cycles—expanded from their more compressed appearance in the full waveform. Most waveform editing functions of speech analysis programs allow a user to zoom in and zoom out on specific parts of the waveform, using cursor control and simple point-and-click maneuvers. Similar 40-ms windows around the vowel midpoints were extracted and "zoomed in" for the three other vowels. Their 40-ms pieces are shown below the arrows issuing from each of the vowels.

For these time windows, a type of analysis specific to speech analysis by computer was used to generate a spectrum from which formant frequencies are estimated. The analysis is called *linear predictive coding*, or *LPC* analysis. LPC analysis of speech spectra was first described in 1971 by two scientists from Bell Telephone Laboratories (Atal & Hanauer, 1971) and has become, with various refinements over the years, the standard approach to measuring formant frequencies. Figure 8–13 showed spectra for three vowels with two superim-

posed analyses, one a Fourier spectrum containing all the details of the harmonics and their amplitudes, the other a smooth curve showing the location of the peaks minus the distracting details of the Fourier spectrum. The simplified, smoothed spectra in Figure 8–13 were, in fact, LPC spectra. LPC spectra for the 40-ms windows extracted from the four corner vowels in *To feed the cat one must shoo the dog* are shown in the bottom four panels of Figure 10–14. The x-axis of each spectrum has a frequency range of 0 to 11.0 kHz, marked off by the grid lines in 1.0-kHz steps. The y-axis is marked off by grid lines in 10-dB steps. The spectra show peaks labeled F1, F2, and F3, the locations of which for the different vowels are very much consistent with expectations from the acoustic theory of vowel production. The mathematical mysteries of the software that make the analysis happen are beyond the scope of the present discussion. Rather, our emphasis is on the happy outcome of LPC analysis, which is to show the locations of the prominent frequency components (i.e., the formants) without the individual harmonic content of a Fourier spectrum. The spectra along the bottom of Figure 10–14 illustrate just how obvious the peaks are in these displays, and how easy it is to "pick" them as F1, F2, and F3.

It is a welcome outcome to have the well-defined and easily pickable peaks provided by LPC analysis, but as in any automatic procedure—like the F0 analysis described above—errors are made and have to be recognized as such. For example, the likelihood of erroneous formant estimates from LPC analysis increases as the speech signal becomes noiser (that is, contains more aperiodic energy) and is affected by acoustic transmission through the nasal cavities. In more direct clinical terms, speakers with breathy voices or with a moderate or substantial degree of hypernasality are not the best candidates for LPC analysis. Of course, these kinds of speech characteristics are common in many different speech disorders, so the use of LPC analysis to estimate formant frequencies in clinical populations has to be undertaken with a great deal of care. As in the case of F0 errors made by automatic pitch trackers, speech analysis programs that allow correction of miscalculated formant frequencies are best suited to clinical applications.

REVIEW

A brief history of speech analysis shows how the transduction of pressure waves produced during speech moved from mechanical to electronic transduction; the electronics age allowed recording and measurement devices to be more faithful to the details of the speech waveform.

Speech waveforms provide information on amplitude fluctuations as a function of time, allow computation of fundamental frequency (F0) for voiced sounds but do not provide direct access to formant frequencies.

The spectrogram, a display that shows formant frequencies as a function of time, allows a user to infer changes in vocal tract configuration resulting from movement of the articulators.

Strategies are presented for how to identify from spectrograms different segment types, how to perform segmentation, and how certain conventional measurements are performed.

Much of what is known about speech acoustics has been derived from spectrographic-type analyses, especially in the area of articulatory characteristics of speech.

Computer software such as *TF32*, allows a user to generate a spectrogram, measure segmental durations, vowel formant frequencies, obstruent spectral characteristics, as well as suprasegmental characteristics such as F0 contours.

The fundamentals of computer-based analysis of speech are presented, including discussions of sampling rate and quantization.

Computer-based techniques for analysis of formant frequencies, as one important example, are fast, reliable, automatic (do not require many user decisions) and for the most part accurate except in cases where a speaker has a breathy voice quality and/or excessive nasality.

An important caution about the use of digital speech analysis techniques is the possibility of computational errors, due to a noisy source or excessive nasality, and the need to employ a computer program that allows expert analysis of the automatic results and corrections of errors when needed.

REFERENCES

Atal, B., & Hanauer, S. (1971). Speech analysis and synthesis by linear prediction. *Journal of the Acoustical Society of America, 50,* 637–655.

Bauer, H., & Kent, R. (1987). Acoustic analyses of infant fricative and trill vocalizations. *Journal of the Acoustical Society of America, 81,* 505–511.

Byrd, D. (1993). 54,000 American stops. *UCLA Working Papers in Phonetics, 83,* 97–116.

Catford, J. C. (2000). *A practical introduction to phonetics* (2nd ed.). Oxford, UK: Oxford University Press.

Crystal, T., & House, A. (1988). The duration of American-English stop consonants: An overview. *Journal of Phonetics, 16,* 285–294.

Klatt, D. (1976). Linguistic uses of segmental duration in English: Acoustic and perceptual evidence. *Journal of the Acoustical Society of America, 59,* 1208–1221.

Solzhenitsyn, A. (1969). *The first circle.* New York, NY: Bantam Books.

Tabain, M. (1998). Non-sibilant fricatives in English. Spectral information above 10 kHz. *Phonetica, 55,* 107–130.

Umeda, N. (1977). Consonant duration in American English. *Journal of the Acoustical Society of America, 61,* 846–858.

Zue, V., & Cole, R. (1979). Experiments on spectrogram reading. *Acoustics, Speech, and Signal Processing, IEEE International Conference on ICASSP '79, 4,* 116–119.

11

Acoustic Phonetics Data

INTRODUCTION

This chapter provides a selective summary of acoustic phonetics data. The presentation must be selective because the research literature is voluminous. The large quantity of data available reflects the many uses of acoustic phonetics research—the discipline of acoustic phonetics serves many masters. For example, acoustic phonetics data are used by linguists who wish to enhance their phonetic description of a language; by speech communication specialists who are interested in developing high-quality speech synthesis and recognition systems; by scientists who wish to test theories of speech production, and prefer to use the speech acoustic approach to the interpretation of articulatory patterns rather than data obtained using one of the more invasive and time-consuming physiological approaches (such as x-ray tracking of articulatory motions); by speech perception scientists who want to understand the acoustic cues used in the identification of vowels and consonants by normal hearers and persons with hearing loss and prosthetic hearing devices; and by speech-language pathologists who want information concerning a client's speech production behaviors—information that can be documented quantitatively and, in some cases may be too subtle or transient to be captured by auditory analysis.

The majority of this chapter is concerned with the acoustic characteristics of *speech sound segments*—the vowel and consonant segments of a language. A brief discussion of the acoustic characteristics of prosody concludes the chapter.

VOWELS

The upper part of Figure 11–1 shows a spectrogram of two vowels, /æ/ and /i/, spoken by a 57-year-old healthy male in the disyllable frames /ə'hæd/ and /ə'hid/. The /ə'hVd/ frame (where V = vowel) is a famous one in speech science, originally used by Peterson and Barney (1952) in their landmark study of vowel formant frequencies produced by men, women, and children. Peterson and Barney (1952) wanted to measure formant frequencies in vowels under minimal influence from the surrounding phonetic context—that is, with little or no coarticulatory effects. The obvious way to get this kind of "pure" information on vowel articulation, and the resulting formant frequencies, is to have speakers produce isolated, sustained vowels. However, when participants are asked to do this, they have a tendency to sing, rather than speak, the vowels. Peterson and Barney designed a more natural speech task in which the unstressed schwa preceded a stressed syllable initiated by the glottal fricative /h/. The reasoning was that a segment whose articulation required primarily laryngeal gestures would minimally influence the vocal tract gestures required for a following vowel. The /d/ at the end of the syllable was necessary to provide a "natural" ending to the syllable, and also accommodated the production of lax vowels such as /ɪ/, /ɛ/, and /ʊ/, which in English do not occur in open syllables.

Clearly, the /d/ at the end of the syllable might have some influence on the vowel articulation. But Peterson and Barney (1952) made their formant frequency measurements at a location where the formants were "steady" (not changing in frequency), which they believed minimized any influence from the final /d/. Conveniently, this measurement point also seemed likely to capture the "target" location of the vowel. In other words, the point at which formant frequencies were stable was likely to coincide with the articulatory configuration aimed at by the speaker when trying to produce the best possible version of the vowel. Also, the inclusion of the schwa as the first syllable provided some control over the prosodic pattern of the disyllable, placing stress on the /hVd/ syllable.

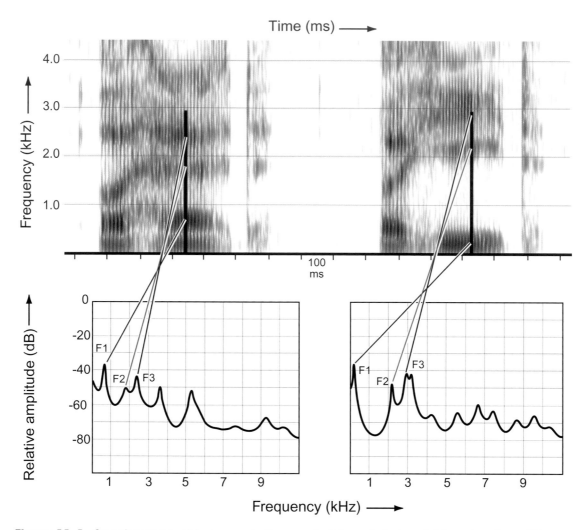

Figure 11–1. Spectrograms of two vowels (*top part of figure*), /æ/ and /i/, spoken by a 57-year-old healthy male in the disyllable frames /əˈhæd/and /əˈhid/. Bottom part of the figure shows LPC spectra for the two vowels, measured at the temporal middle of the vowels. The colored lines connect the middle of the formant bands on the spectrograms to the peaks in the LPC spectra.

Forty-three years following the publication of Peterson and Barney's (1952) classic work, Hillenbrand, Getty, Clark, and Wheeler (1995) published a replication of the study using updated analysis methods. Like Peterson and Barney, Hillenbrand et al. studied men (*n* = 45), women (*n* = 48), and children aged 10 to 12 years (*n* = 46, both girls and boys) producing the 12 monophthong vowels of English (/i,ɪ,e,ɛ,æ,ɑ,ɔ,o,ʊ,u,ʌ,ɝ/ in an /hVd/ frame.[1] Hillenbrand et al. measured the first four formants (F1-F4) at their most stable point, in

much the same way as shown in Figure 11–1 (in the figure, measurement of the fourth formant is omitted). The heavy vertical line through the spectrogram shows the point in time at which the formant frequencies were measured (in these cases, roughly in the middle of the vowel duration). Formant frequencies were estimated using linear predictive code (LPC) analysis, discussed in Chapter 10. The LPC spectra for the measurement point shown on the spectrograms are provided in the lower half of Figure 11–1. Lines point from the middle

---

[1]The vowel inventory of English is not always described as having 12 monophthongs. In particular, /e/ and /o/ are diphthongized in many dialects, but less often in the upper Midwest dialects included in the Hillenbrand et al. (1995) study. /ɝ/ is sometimes also not included as an English monophthong, but may be considered a rhotacized (/ɪ/-colored) vowel. Also note that Hillenbrand et al. did not use the schwa preceding the /hVd/syllable, as in Peterson and Barney (1952).

of the formant bands to the corresponding peaks in the LPC spectra. For these vowels, values of the first three formant frequencies for /æ/ are approximately 700, 1750, and 2450 Hz, and for /i/ are roughly 290, 2200, and 2950 Hz.

Figure 11–2 shows some of Hillenbrand et al.'s (1995, p. 3104) data in the form of an F1-F2 plot. Each phonetic symbol represents an F1-F2 coordinate for a given speaker's production of that vowel. Two of the vowels (/e/ and /o/) are not plotted to reduce crowding of the data points. The ellipses drawn around each vowel category enclose roughly 95% of all the observable points for that vowel.

These data show clearly how a single vowel can be represented by a wide range of F1-F2 values. For example, the vowel /i/ shows points ranging between (approximately) 300 to 500 Hz on the F1 axis and 2100 to 3400 Hz on the F2 axis. The ellipse enclosing the /i/ points is oriented upward and leaning slightly to the

right. Points in the lower part of the ellipse are almost certainly from men, points in the middle from women, and points at the upper part and to the right from children. This follows from the material presented in Chapters 7 and 8 on resonance patterns of tubes of different lengths, and age and sex-related differences in vocal tract length. The same general summary can be given for almost any vowel in this plot, even though the degree of variation and orientation of the ellipses vary from vowel to vowel. Despite the wide variation across speakers in formant frequencies for a given vowel, Hillenbrand et al. (1995) replicated Peterson and Barney's (1952) finding that the vowel intended by a speaker was almost always perceived correctly—consistent with the speaker's intention—by listeners. Somehow listeners heard the same vowel category even when confronted with a wide variety of formant patterns.

Figure 11–2 also shows that the formant frequency patterns of one vowel often overlap with those

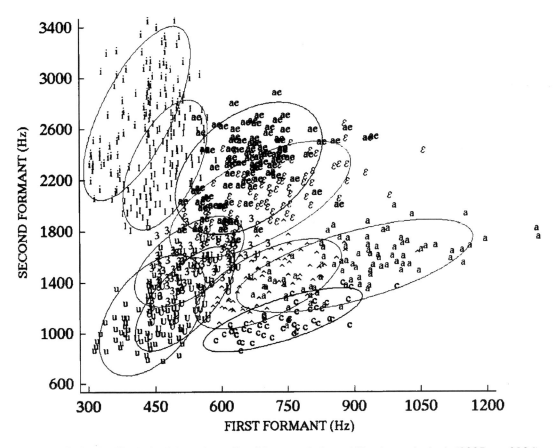

Figure 11–2. F1-F2 plot of American English vowels from Hillenbrand et al. (1995, p. 3104). Each phonetic symbol represents an F1-F2 coordinate for a given speaker's production of that vowel. Two vowels (/e/ and /o/) are not plotted to reduce crowding of the data points. The ellipses drawn around each vowel category enclose roughly 95% of all the observable points for that vowel. Reproduced with permission.

of another vowel. There is a small region of overlap between the ellipses of /i/ and /ɪ/, and a larger region of overlap between /æ/ and /ɛ/. In the lower left-hand part of the plot, roughly around F1 = 525 Hz and F2 = 1400 Hz, there is a three-way overlap of the vowels /u/, /ʊ/, and /ɝ/. In many cases, these areas of overlap are for vowels produced by speakers with vocal tracts of different lengths. For example, a good portion of the overlap between /æ/ and /ɛ/ seems to come from adult male /æ/ values with adult female, or child /ɛ/ values. But there are many cases where the overlap is not so clearly explained by differing vocal tract lengths. Still, the question remains, how do we hear the *same* formant frequencies produced by different speakers as *different* vowels? For the time being, Hillenbrand et al.'s (1995) data, like those of Peterson and Barney (1952), demonstrate that knowing a pattern of formant frequencies does not necessarily provide sufficient information to identify the intended (spoken) vowel category. At the

least, the identity of the speaker, including age, sex, and almost certainly dialect, must be known to link a specific formant pattern to a vowel category.

Figure 11–3 plots a summary of a subset of the data reported by Hillenbrand et al. (1995). The subset includes averaged F1-F2 data from men, women, and children, for American English corner vowels that were "well-identified" by a panel of listeners. Corner vowels define the limits of vowel articulation, with /i/ the highest and most front vowel, /æ/ the lowest and most front, /ɑ/ the lowest and most back, and /u/ the highest and most back. If these are the most extreme articulatory configurations for vowels in English, the formant frequencies should also be at the most extreme coordinates in F1-F2 space. By including only data from "well-identified" vowels, the plotted data can be regarded as excellent exemplars of these vowel categories. When the average F1-F2 coordinates for each of the four corner vowels are connected by a line for each

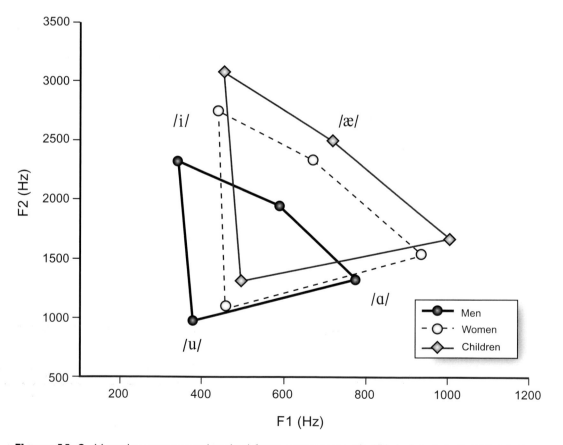

Figure 11–3. Vowel spaces constructed from corner vowels (/i/, /æ/, /ɑ/, /u/) of American English for men (*filled circles connected by solid lines*), women (*unfilled circles connected by dashed lines*), and children aged 10 to 12 years (*lightly shaded diamonds connected by solid lines*). These data are replotted from Hillenbrand et al. (1995, Table V., p. 3103) and are averages of vowels that were well identified by a crew of listeners.

Things Are Never That Simple, Even When They Are Complex to Begin With

Students sometimes have difficulty embracing the gray areas in science, because black and white answers are more comfortable. The overlap of vowel formant frequencies shown in Figure 11–2, coupled with listeners' apparent ease in identifying vowels in the overlapped areas, seems to be one of those hard-to-embrace gray areas: how do listeners do it? One possible answer is that the relationship of vowel acoustics to vowel identification is both more complex and more simple than suggested by the scatterplots in Figure 11–2. Both Peterson and Barney (1952) and Hillenbrand et al. (1995) constructed scatterplots based on F1 and F2 measured at a single point in time during vowel productions; in identification experiments, however, listeners heard the *whole* vowel. What if changes in formant frequency throughout the vowel duration are important for vowel identification? If this is the case, plots such as Figure 11–2 underrepresent the mapping between vowel acoustics and vowel identification (see Jacewicz & Fox, 2012, p. 1414, for just this argument!). The scientific problem is more complex because there is more to the acoustics of vowels than formant frequencies measured at a single point in time, and less complex because plots such as those in Figure 11–2 may miss the point. Think gray: it's so much more fun than thinking black and white.

of the three speaker groups, three vowel quadrilaterals are formed. In an F1-F2 plot, the area enclosed by such a quadrilateral is called the acoustic vowel space.

Three general characteristics of these F1-F2 plots are noteworthy. First, the vowel quadrilaterals for men, women, and children move from the lower left to upper right part of the graph, respectively. This is because the vocal tract becomes progressively shorter across these three speaker groups, and shorter vocal tracts produce higher resonant frequencies. Second, the area of the vowel quadrilaterals—the acoustic vowel space—appears to be larger for children, as compared to women, and larger for women as compared to men. This probably has little to do with articulatory differences between the groups (although there there may be some sex-specific articulatory effects), but rather is another consequence of the different-sized vocal tracts. Exactly the same articulatory configurations for

the corner vowels in a shorter, as compared to longer vocal tract, not only generate higher formant frequencies in the shorter vocal tract but also greater distances between F1-F2 points for the different vowels. The larger vowel space for the children, as compared to the men, therefore, does not mean the children use more extreme articulatory configurations for vowels. Third, the acoustic vowel quadrilateral for one group of speakers cannot be perfectly fit to the quadrilateral for a different group by moving it to the new location and uniformly expanding or shrinking it to achieve an exact match. Imagine the quadrilateral for men in Figure 11–3 moved into the position of the quadrilateral for women, followed by a uniform expansion of the male space to "fit" the female space. This attempt to scale the male quadrilateral to the female quadrilateral fails because the magnitudes of the sex-related vowel differences are not the same for each vowel. For example, note the relative closeness in F1-F2 space of the male and female /u/, as compared to the other three vowels. A similar inability to scale the vowels of one group to another is seen in Figure 11–4, which is an F1-F2 plot for the lax vowels (/i/, /ʊ/, /ɛ/), based on data reported by Hillenbrand et al. (1995). The group differences in these vowel triangles are very much like the ones shown for the corner vowel quadrilaterals (Figure 11–3), including vowel-specific differences across groups. Note especially the small difference between males and females for /ʊ/, as compared to the much larger male-female differences for /ɪ/ and /ɛ/. The lax-vowel triangle for men clearly cannot be scaled in a simple way to obtain the triangle for women.

The acoustic vowel space for corner vowels has a potential clinical application as an index of speech motor integrity. Evidence from several studies of speakers with dysarthria (speech disorders resulting from neurological disease (see Liu, Tsao, & Kuhl, 2005; Turner, Tjaden, & Weismer, 1995; Weismer, Jeng, Laures, Kent, & Kent, 2001), glossectomy (removal of tongue tissue, usually because of a cancerous tumor; see Whitehill, Ciocca, Chan, & Samman, 2006), cochlear implants (Chuang, Yang, Chi, Weismer, & Wang, 2012), and even neurologically normal speakers (Bradlow, Torretta, & Pisoni, 1996) suggests that the size of the acoustic vowel space is modestly correlated with independent measurements of speech intelligibility. There are at least two ways to interpret this correlation. First, because the acoustic vowel space for corner vowels is constructed from the most extreme articulatory positions for vowels (i.e., most high and front vowel /i/, most high and back vowel /u/, and so forth), the size (area) of the space may be an index of articulatory mobility. Those speakers who can position their

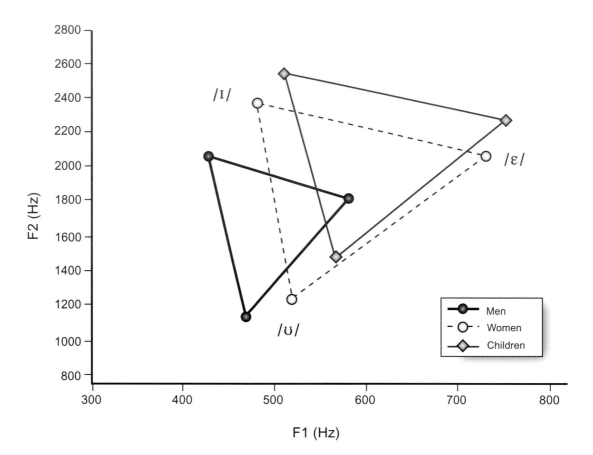

Figure 11–4. Vowel spaces constructed from three American English lax vowels (/i/, /ʊ/, /ɛ/) for men (*filled circles connected by solid lines*), women (*unfilled circles connected by dashed lines*), and children aged 10 to 12 (*lightly shaded diamonds connected by solid lines*). These data are replotted from Hillenbrand et al. (1995, Table V., p. 3103) and are averages of vowels that were well identified by a crew of listeners.

articulators most differently for the four corner vowels may have the greatest articulatory flexibility. Greater articulatory flexibility should produce greater acoustic distinctiveness for speech sounds and, therefore, better speech intelligibility. This interpretation of the vowel space measure considers the size of the acoustic vowel space as a global index of articulatory integrity. The interpretation seems most obviously appropriate for speakers with dysarthria and glossectomy, where it is easy to imagine speakers with reduced articulatory flexibility being those who do not make good acoustic distinctions and, therefore, experience deficits in speech intelligibility.

A second interpretation of the correlation between the size of the acoustic vowel space and speech intelligibility is that more poorly articulated vowels have a direct impact on speech intelligibility. In this view, the smaller vowel space is not simply a sign of overall speech motor control problems (as in the first interpre-

tation) but is an important, independent component of a speech intelligibility deficit. This is the view of Liu, Tsao, and Kuhl (2005) and may also explain why children with cochlear implants, whose auditory input is not as rich as children with normal hearing, produce smaller vowel spaces than normal-hearing children (Chuang et al., 2012).

There is a critical distinction between the first and second interpretations of the size of the vowel space. The second interpretation predicts an improvement in speech intelligibility for a client who, as part of a management program, learns to produce corner vowels with more extreme positions and, therefore, expands the acoustic vowel space. If the vowels are really an independent component of speech intelligibility, the larger vowel space resulting from management should result in improved speech intelligibility (Liu et al., 2005). The first interpretation, that a smaller vowel space merely reflects some limitation on articulatory

Speech Acoustics and Your Smile

In a 1980 paper delivered to the 100th meeting of the Acoustical Society of America, held in Los Angeles, the famous phonetician/phonologist John Ohala (now Professor Emeritus of Linguistics at UC Berkeley) proposed an acoustic explanation for smiling. By pulling the corners of the mouth back and against the teeth, Ohala argued, the vocal tract is effectively shortened. Shorter vocal tracts mean higher formant frequencies, and higher formant frequencies are typically associated with smaller people. Smaller people, such as children, are generally not viewed as a physical threat. Speaking while smiling — think game-show host — sends a signal that says, "I'm small, I'm not a threat, I'm friendly, like me and don't hurt me." In evolutionary terms, vocalizations while smiling eventually were dispensed with, and the soundless smile was enough to send a signal of friendliness.

flexibility, does not necessarily require that the smaller vowel space be associated with reduced intelligibility. In fact, a given speaker produces vowel spaces of very different size depending on their speaking style (formal versus casual) and even the kind of speech material they produce (e.g., vowels in isolated words versus vowels in an extended reading passage) without any significant loss of speech intelligibility (Kuo, 2011; Picheny, Durlach, & Braida, 1986).

It is not clear which of these interpretations is correct, or even if they should be considered opposing viewpoints. Both views may be correct to some degree. In any case, the measurement of vowel formant frequencies has potential as a noninvasive, clinical index of the integrity of speech motor control and its effect on speech intelligibility.

Vowel Acoustics, Dialect, and a Multicultural View of Acoustic Phonetics

In recent years there has been enormous interest in *comparative acoustic phonetics*. Comparative acoustic phonetics has two main, interrelated branches. One concerns the acoustic characteristics of similar speech sounds in two or more different languages or in two or more dialects of the same language. The other branch deals with the effect of native language (or dialect) phonetics (usually abbreviated as L1) on the acoustic characteristics of speech sounds in a second language (or dialect) (L2).[2] The relationship between these two branches is simple in concept, but complex in practice. How does the speech sound system of an L1, and its acoustic characteristics, affect the ability to produce sounds in an L2? Both branches are relevant to preclinical speech science because of the presence in the United States of many people who speak English as an L2, as well as the variation of American dialects across the country. A significant proportion of these individuals are currently or will be seeking the services of speech-language pathologists for communication concerns. These concerns could involve the influence of disease on speech production, or a desire among healthy speakers for accent modification or reduction.

Acoustic characteristics of vowels have been a major focal point of interest for both branches of inquiry. Figure 11–5 shows the interesting case of F1-F2 patterns for "shared" vowels, measured roughly at the temporal midpoint (where the formants are changing minimally), produced by adult male speakers in four languages — Madrid Spanish; American English as spoken in Ithaca, New York (presumably corresponding to the "Inland North" dialect: see Labov, 1991); modern Greek (primarily from Athens); and modern Hebrew as spoken in Israel. These four languages share the vowels /i/, /e/, /o/, and /u/. A fifth vowel, /a/, is shared by Spanish, Greek, and Hebrew. A "shared" vowel means that, when a phonetician uses transcription to assemble vowel inventories of several languages, the same phonetic symbol is used to represent a vowel sound produced in different languages. In Figure 11–5, the F1-F2 values for shared vowels are enclosed by visually fit ellipses. Clearly, the same vowels in Hebrew and English (for example) have different F1-F2 values, and the magnitude of these differences varies across vowels. The Hebrew-English differences for the high front vowels /i/ and /e/ are more dramatic as compared to /u/ and /o/. Similar comparisons for different language pairs suggest the same conclusion: The use of the same phonetic symbol does not mean the sound is actually the "same." Data such as these may explain

---

[2]The "L1-L2" terminology is typically used to designate speakers of two different languages, but the usage could be generalized to two different dialects of the same language (perhaps the designation should be "D1-D2"). At least one linguist (McWhorter, 2001) argues that the differences between languages and dialects are not so clear cut, with dialects and languages (including their phonetics) blending into each other as if they are on a continuum, rather than being categorically different.

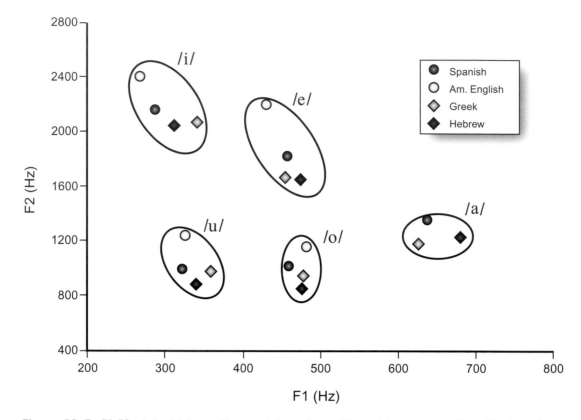

Figure 11–5. F1-F2 plot of "shared" vowels from four different languages. Spanish, American English, modern Greek, and Hebrew all have the vowels /i/, /e/, /o/, and /u/ in their phonetic inventories. In addition, Spanish, modern Greek, and Hebrew share the vowel /a/. Spanish data are shown by filled circles, American English data by unfilled circles, Greek data by lightly shaded diamonds, and Hebrew data by filled diamonds. The sources for the data are Bradlow (1995; Spanish and English), Jongman, Fourakis, and Sereno (1989; Greek), and Most, Amir, and Tobin (2000; Hebrew). All data are for adult male speakers.

why an L2 speaker's production of a vowel shared by L1 and L2 (e.g., an Israeli speaker's production of the vowel /i/ when speaking American English) can still be detected as accented by a native speaker of the L2 (Bradlow, 1995).

The cross-language comparison of shared vowels presented in Figure 11–5 is a simplistic one, even though it makes a valid point. The comparison is simplistic because "shared" vowels across different languages may vary in more ways than the F1-F2 values measured at a single point in time. The vowels may also differ (or be similar) by the higher (F3, F4) formant frequencies, the formant transitions going into and out of the so-called vowel "steady-states," the overall vowel duration, the relation of the vowel duration to the duration of adjacent syllables, and other potential factors. The acoustic comparison of shared vowel sounds in different languages is potentially very complex.

Despite this complexity, a simple F1-F2 comparison of L2 vowels (e.g., Korean speakers producing American English) and the L2 native vowels (e.g., Americans producing English) can reveal a good deal about the influence of an L1 on an L2 vowel system. Chen, Robb, Gilbert, and Lerman (2001) studied the formant frequencies of American English vowels produced by native speakers of Mandarin, the primary language of Taiwan and many parts of mainland China. The Mandarin vowel system includes six vowels, /i/, /e/, /u/, /o/, /a/, and /y/ (similar to a lip rounded /i/), the first five of which are also found in American English. American English is usually said to include 11 or 12 monophthong vowels, including the lax vowels /ɪ/, /ʊ/, and /ʌ/ which are "new" vowels for the Mandarin speaker learning English (just as /y/ would be a new vowel for the American speaker learning to produce Mandarin). Figure 11–6 shows F1-F2 data from

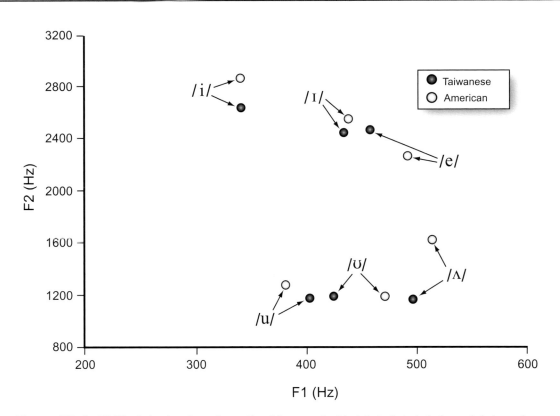

Figure 11-6. F1-F2 data for American English vowels /i/, /ɪ/, /e/, /u/, /ʊ/, and /ʌ/, spoken by adult female speakers from Taiwan whose native language is Mandarin (*filled circles*) and adult female speakers whose native language is American English (*unfilled circles*). Arrows project from each phonetic symbol to the points representing a specific, average F1-F2 coordinate for vowels produced by both groups of speakers. Data replotted from Chen et al., (2001).

the Chen et al. study, specifically for the American English vowels /i/, /e/, /ɪ/, /u/, /ʊ/, and /ʌ/ produced by Taiwanese adult females whose native language is Mandarin (filled circles) and by native female speakers of American English (unfilled circles). Each plotted point is labeled with the phonetic symbol matching the American English vowel that was intended by the Mandarin speakers.

These data suggest several important conclusions concerning the way in which the vowel pairs [ɪ]-[e] and [u]-[ʊ] were produced by the two groups of speakers. Native speakers of English produced these vowel pairs (unfilled circles) with a fair degree of separation in F1-F2 space, as expected for vowels with categorical (that is, phonemic) status. English [ɪ] and [e] differ both in the F1 and F2 dimensions, the differences implying a somewhat more open (higher F1) and slightly more posterior tongue position for [e]. English [u] and [ʊ] were separated only minimally along the F2 dimension, but differed by close to 100 Hz on the F1 dimen-

sion, suggesting a more open vocal tract for the latter vowel. In contrast, the F1-F2 points for the [ɪ]-[e] and [u]-[ʊ] English vowel pairs produced by Taiwanese speakers were very close together, differing only by small amounts along the F1 dimension. These vowel pairs in Mandarin-accented English were, therefore, closer together than any other vowel pair in the graph. It is as if the Mandarin speakers were treating the two English vowels of both pairs as members of a single vowel class.

There are competing theories of why the patterns in Figure 11–6 occur. Without pursuing in too much depth these very complex explanations of L2 phonetic performance, in both cases described above the Mandarin speakers produced a "new" vowel ([ɪ] in one case, [ʊ] in the other) almost as if it were a member of one of the "shared" vowels ([e] and [u]). Because the formant frequencies for the "shared" vowels are not identical across the two languages (see above), perhaps it may be more accurate to say the Mandarin speakers took the "shared"-"new" vowel pairs, and treated them as one category by producing F1-F2 values for both the "shared" and "new" vowels at an intermediate location between the American's well-separated F1-F2 points for the two vowels. Think of it as a phonetic compromise when the skill of producing two nearby, but separate, vowels is not yet available to a speaker.

Within-Speaker Variability in Formant Frequencies

The formant frequencies plotted in Figures 11–3 to 11–6 are averages across speakers. Figure 11–2, from Hillenbrand et al. (1995), presents a more realistic picture of variability in formant frequencies for a given vowel, but even this presentation shows only *across*-speaker variability. Within a speaker, vowel formant frequencies vary with a number of factors. These factors include—but may not be limited to—speaking rate, syllable stress, speaking style, and phonetic context.

Traditionally, the effects of these different factors on vowel formant frequencies have been referenced to a speaking condition in which the vowel is produced in a more or less pure form. Presumably, the best way to obtain a "pure" vowel production is for a speaker to produce it in isolation, perhaps much like the sustained vowel often used in a clinical evaluation of the speech mechanism. A problem with this is the tendency for speakers to sing, rather than speak the vowel. As mentioned above, in their original study of vowel formant frequencies, Peterson and Barney (1952) designed the /ə'hVd/ frame as a speech production event similar to real speech but largely free of many of the influencing factors noted above. Stevens and House (1963), in their classic paper on phonetic context effects on vowel formant frequencies, demonstrated for three phonetically sophisticated speakers (i.e., speech scientists) the lack of any difference in F1 and F2 for isolated vowels and vowels spoken in the /hVd/ frame. This result, as well as some other data reviewed by Stevens and House, suggested that formant frequencies measured at the midpoint of a vowel in the /hVd/ frame are representative of vowels articulated under minimal influence from factors such as context, rate, and so forth. Because of this, vowels measured in the /hVd/ frame are often referred to as *null context vowels*.

When null context vowels are plotted in F1-F2 space together with the same vowels produced in varied phonetic contexts, at different rates, and in different

speaking styles, an interesting pattern emerges. Figure 11–7 shows such a plot for the corner vowels (/i/, /æ/, /ɑ/, /u/) whose formant frequencies were derived for male speakers from several different sources in the literature. Two sets of "null context" data are plotted, one from Peterson and Barney (1952; filled circles connected by solid lines), the other from Hillenbrand et al. (1995; open circles connected by dashed lines). The decision to include F1-F2 data for null context vowels from two different data sets underscores the potential variability in these kinds of measurements. The two sets of null context data are most different for the low vowels /æ/ and especially /ɑ/. The speakers in the two studies were from the same geographical region (Michigan, with a few speakers from other areas), but their recordings are separated in time by close to 50 years. A likely explanation for the difference in the low vowel formant frequencies is changing patterns of vowel pronunciation over the period from about 1950 to 1990.

How do formant frequencies deviate from null context values when they are produced under different speaking conditions? The data shown in Figure 11–7 include F1-F2 data for the corner vowels for vowels spoken at a fast rate, but with syllable stress (Fourakis, 1991; filled triangles), in conversational-style production of sentences (Picheny et al., 1986; unfilled triangles), in a "clear-speech" production style of sentences (Picheny et al., 1986; filled diamonds), and in a /bVb/ context (Hillenbrand, Clark, & Nearey, 2001; lightly shaded diamonds).

With certain exceptions,[3] and especially when the Hillenbrand et al. (1995) null context vowel space is used as a reference, vowels spoken in any of the other conditions tend to have F1-F2 points that move "inside" of the vowel space created by the null context quadrilateral. Somewhat more specifically, the F1-F2 points for the different conditions seem to move away from the null context points for any of the corner vowels in the direction of a point roughly in the center of the quadrilaterals, indicated by the red circle. This point plots F1 = 500 Hz, F2 = 1500 Hz, the first two formant frequencies associated with the "neutral vowel" configuration, or a vocal tract with uniform cross-sectional area from the glottis to the lips. As discussed in Chapter 8, this is the vocal tract configuration most closely associated with schwa (/ə/). The F1 = 500 Hz, F2 = 1500 Hz pattern is appropriate for an adult male.

One way to interpret the overall pattern seen in Figure 11–7 is to regard the null context formant frequencies (and underlying vocal tract configuration)

---

[3]The most notable exceptions are the points from Fourakis (1991) for /ɑ/ and /i/.

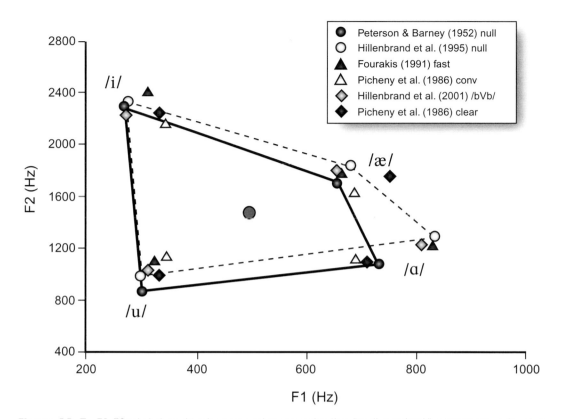

Figure 11–7. F1-F2 plot showing two vowel spaces for the "null context" corner vowels, plus corner-vowel data from studies in which the vowels were produced in other speaking conditions. Null context data are from tabled means published by Peterson and Barney (1952) and from careful pencil-and-ruler estimates of figures shown in Hillenbrand et al. (1995). Data from Fourakis (1991) are from tabled formant frequencies for fast-speech, stressed vowels pooled across various phonetic contexts. Values plotted from Picheny, Durlach, and Braida (1986) are for vowels extracted from sentence productions in conversational and clear-style speech and were estimated by the pencil-and-ruler technique from their published figures. The same estimation technique was used to obtain the /bVb/ data from Hillenbrand et al. (2001). The red circle in the middle of the plot is the F1-F2 pattern expected from a male vocal tract with uniform cross-sectional area from glottis to lips (the expected vocal tract shape for schwa). All plotted data points are from male speakers.

for a given vowel as an idealized target. In this view, described most explicitly by Bjorn Lindblom (1963, 1990), the speaker always aims for the idealized target, but misses it in connected speech by varying degrees because the articulators do not have sufficient time to reach the target before transitioning to the target for the next sound. For example, the target vocal tract shape (the area function) for the vowel /i/ would have a relatively tight constriction in the front of the vocal tract, and a wide opening in the pharyngeal region. This vocal tract shape is a significant deviation from the straight-tube configuration of schwa, and, of course, fits the description of /i/ as a high-front vowel. In Lindblom's view, when a vowel such as /i/ is produced in a condition other than the null context,

the idealized target will be missed in a specific way, namely, by producing a vocal tract configuration (and resulting formant frequencies) that reflects a slightly lesser deviation from the schwa configuration. It is as if all vowels are viewed as deviated vocal tract shapes (and formant frequencies) from the straight-tube configuration of schwa. Under optimal conditions, these deviations are maximal. In connected speech, however, the deviations from the schwa configuration are not as dramatic. By not producing the most extreme configuration associated with the sound, the speech mechanism has more time to produce a sequence of sounds in an acceptable manner. An /i/ in connected speech is still a high-front vowel, but not quite as high and front as in the null context.

Lindblom (1963) called this phenomenon "articulatory undershoot." Undershoot, in his opinion, occurred as a result of phonetic context, increased speaking rate, reduced stress, and casual speaking style, but all these different causes could be explained by a single mechanism. Simply put, the shorter the vowel duration, the greater the undershoot. In the language of phonetics, vowels experience greater reduction as vowel duration decreases, regardless of the condition in which the shorter vowel duration is elicited. Although this is not a universally accepted interpretation of undershoot, it often explains a good deal of variation in formant frequencies for a given vowel produced by a specific speaker. Most likely, factors other than vowel duration may, in some cases, have an independent effect on formant frequencies. For example, in Figure 11–7, the vowels /ɑ/ and /i/ from Fourakis (1991) do not fit the duration explanation of undershoot because they fall outside the null context quadrilaterals, even though the "fast condition" vowel durations were relatively short (as reported by Fourakis, 1991, Table III, p. 1821). Because these vowels were stressed, an independent effect of stress on vowel formant frequencies must be considered a possibility.

In a carefully controlled experiment, Kuo (2011) varied speech materials so that American English vowels occurred in simple, single-syllable utterances, words in sentences, and words in long reading passages. The Lindblom-inspired logic of this manipulation was that as speech material changed from formal, simple syllables (close to the "null" vowel) to more "connected" and conversational utterances (more casual), vowel durations would shorten, resulting in an increasing amount of undershoot of formant frequencies. Kuo reported data from ten adults males producing American English vowels embedded in the varied speech materials, and demonstrated that undershoot of "target" vowel formant frequencies increased as the speech material became more "casual." The degree and patterns of undershoot, however, depended on speaker and vowel. Some speakers were dramatic undershooters, some less so. In addition, the extent of undershoot across the speech materials was not the same for all vowels, and the vowel-specific patterns varied across speakers! An important lesson from Kuo's experiment, as well as several other experiments (e.g., Johnson, Ladefoged, & Lindau, 1993), is that almost any "pattern" in acoustic or articulatory phonetics, for any sound segment, is likely to have a broad range of variability when a sufficient number of speakers is studied. The across-speaker variability may be so dramatic that the identification of a well-defined acoustic and/or articulatory pattern for given sound segment is challenging. The reader is encouraged to keep this in mind as the acoustic characteristics of speech sounds are reviewed in this chapter.

Summary of Vowel Formant Frequencies

The take-home messages from this discussion of vowel formant frequencies and their variability across and within speakers are as follows. First, sex and age have a dramatic effect on the formant frequencies for a given vowel because these variables are closely associated with differences in vocal tract size and length. In general, the longer and larger the human vocal tract, the lower the formant frequencies for all vowels. This explains why, for a given vowel, there is such a large range of formant frequencies across the population (see Figure 11–2). The issue of how humans recognize a wide range of F-patterns as the same vowel is taken up in Chapter 12. Second, even when vocal tract length/size factors are held roughly constant, "target" formant frequencies for a given vowel may vary for several reasons. One of these reasons may reflect the inherent constraints on a phonetic symbol system. Even though a vowel may be transcribed as /u/ in several different languages, the F-pattern associated with productions of this vowel "category" may be substantially different (see Figure 11–5). The same conclusion can almost certainly be made about the same vowel produced by speakers of different dialects of the same language (Clopper, Pisoni, & de Jong, 2005). Additional reasons for variation with constant vocal tract length include the effects of phonetic context, syllable stress, speaking rate, and speaking style.

The implication of the variation in "target" formant frequencies for a particular vowel is that if one is asked the question, "What are the formant frequencies for the vowel ___?" an answer cannot be supplied without additional information on the speaker, the nature of the speech material, the language being spoken, the style of the speech (formal versus casual), and so forth. Even with all these questions answered, a definitive, precise answer is probably not feasible. It is more likely that a definitive, precise answer is not necessary because vowels may be perceived by focusing on relations among the formant frequencies, rather then absolute values of individual formants. In addition, it is likely that the formant frequencies measured near the temporal middle of vowels—the so-called "target" values—are only part of the information critical in distinguishing among the vowels of a language (see next section). These and other issues concerning vowel perception are discussed in Chapter 12.

A Brief Note on Vowel Formant Frequencies Versus Formant Trajectories

The discussion above presented what can be called a "slice-in-time" view of vowel formant frequencies. In this view, formant frequencies measured *at a given point in time* during the vowel nucleus provide a good representation of the vowel articulation—and presumably, the contribution of the vowel to speech intelligibility—if the time point for measurement is chosen wisely. Typically, speech scientists have tried to select the time point for formant frequency measurement by estimating the location of the vowel "target." These target locations have sometimes been estimated at the temporal middle of the vowel, where the formants seem to remain steady (the steady state of the vowel) after the initial transition from the consonant preceding the vowel, or perhaps one-third of the distance from the beginning to the end of the vowel. Each of these measurement points, when used alone, is likely to separate vowels with a high degree of success. This has been demonstrated in experiments in which single-slice measurements have been used to obtain either human classification of vowels or classification by statistical routines (Hillenbrand & Nearey, 1999). However, when single-slice formant frequencies are supplemented with information on formant frequency change throughout the vowel nucleus, identification/classification accuracy increases, sometimes substantially (Assman, Nearey, & Hogan, 1982; Hillenbrand & Nearey, 1999; Jacewicz & Fox, 2012). Simply put, both single-slice formant frequencies *and* formant movement throughout a vowel nucleus make important contributions to vowel identity.

The complexity of the mapping from articulatory to acoustic phonetics comes as no surprise to anyone who has studied tongue, lip, and jaw motions during speech for even the simplest CVC syllable. Figure 11–8 shows these motions for the vowel [ɪ] in the word [sɪp] produced by a young adult female. These data were collected with the x-ray microbeam instrument which tracked the motions of very small gold pellets attached to the tongue, jaw, and lips. In Figure 11–8 the lips are to the right and the outline of the hard palate is seen in the upper part of the x-y coordinate system. The motions of two lip pellets (UL = upper lip; LL = lower lip), two mandible (jaw) pellets (MM = mandible at molars; MI = mandible at incisors), and four tongue pellets (T1-T4 arranged front to back roughly from tip [T1] to dorsum [T4]) are shown for the vowel [ɪ]. The shaded portion on the waveform in the lower part of the figure corresponds to the time period of the motions shown in the upper part of the figure (arrows pointing up to the waveform indicate the onset and offset of the vowel, hence the beginning and end of the displayed motions of the various pellets). This interval lasts approximately 115 ms. The direction of the pellet motions throughout the vowel is shown by arrows with dashed lines. The final position of each pellet, at the last glottal pulse of the vowel before lip closure for [p], is marked by a small circle at the end of the motion track. All tongue pellets move down throughout the vowel, with the exception of the small upward motions in T2 and T3 at the beginning of the vowel. Throughout the syllable, the mandible moves up very slightly and the lips come together, as would be expected when a vowel is followed by a labial consonant. Although this display does not show the motions as a function of

---

Articulatory and Acoustic Phonetics

When speech scientists use the term "articulatory phonetics," they have in mind the positions and movements of the articulators, as well as the resulting configuration of the vocal tract, as they relate to speech sound production. The term "acoustic phonetics" describes the relations between the acoustic signal (resulting from those positions, movements, and configurations) and speech sounds. Many scientists have studied the relations between articulatory and acoustic phonetics, and found them to be fantastically complex. Why is this so? There are many reasons, but here are two prominent ones: First, exactly the same acoustic phonetic effect can be produced by very different articulatory maneuvers. For example, the low F2 of /u/ can be produced by rounding the lips, backing the tongue, or lowering the larynx. And second, certain parts of the vocal tract—the pharynx, for instance—are exceedingly difficult to monitor during speech production, yet play a very important role in the speech acoustic signal. Scientists who study the relations between articulatory and acoustic data often use very advanced mathematical and experimental techniques to determine just how an articulatory phonetic event "maps on" to an acoustic phonetic event.

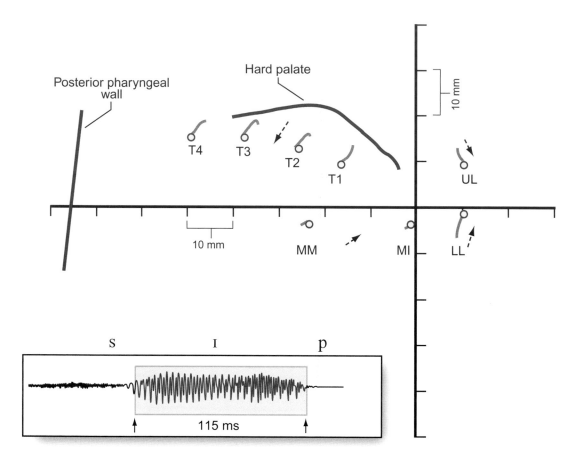

Figure 11–8. Tongue, jaw, and lip pellet motions for the vowel [ɪ] in the word [sɪp], produced by a young adult female. The directions of the pellet motions throughout the vowel are shown by dashed arrows, and the final pellet positions are marked by circles at the end of the motion tracks. Data are shown in the x-ray-microbeam coordinate system (Westbury, 1994), with the x-axis defined by a plate held between the teeth and the y-axis by a line perpendicular to the x-axis and running through the maxillary incisors. The portion of the speech waveform for which the motions are shown is highlighted by the shaded box on the waveform in the lower part of the figure.

time, they are more or less continuous throughout the vowel nucleus and do not have obvious steady-state portions where the motion "freezes." This is especially so for the tongue pellets, for which the downward motion is smooth and continuous from the beginning to end of the vowel.

The continuous motions of the articulators for the simple, relatively short-duration vowel [ɪ] are consistent with changing formant frequencies throughout the vowel nucleus. Based on these motions and the resulting formant transitions, it is not surprising that portions of the vowel in addition to the "slice-in-time" target measurement contribute to vowel identification. One future area of research is to generate better descriptions of these simple vowel motions, and to understand the role of such motions in vowel identification. This is an important area of research because of the significant contribution of vowel articulation to speech intelligibility deficits in the speech of individuals who are hearing impaired (Metz, Samar, Schiavetti, Sitler, & Whitehead, 1985) and who have dysarthria (Weismer & Martin, 1992), among other disorders.

Vowel Durations

Vowel durations have been studied extensively because of the potential for application of the data to speech synthesis, machine recognition of speech, and description and possibly diagnosis of speech disorders in which timing disturbances are present. What follows is a brief discussion of the major variables known to affect vowel durations.

Intrinsic Vowel Durations

An "intrinsic" vowel duration is one deriving from the articulation of the vowel segment itself, as opposed to an external influence on its duration (as described more fully below). The easiest way to understand this is to imagine a fixed syllable such as a consonant-vowel-consonant (CVC) frame, with vowel durations measured for all vowels inserted into the "V" slot of the frame. Figure 11–9 shows three sets of vowel duration values from a /CVC/ frame, as reported by Hillenbrand et al. (2001). In this experiment the Cs included /p,t,k,b,d,g,h,w,r,l/, in all combinations (consonants such as /h/ and /w/ were restricted to initial posi-

tion). In Figure 11–9 vowel duration in ms (*y*-axis) is presented for each vowel (*x*-axis), averaged across all consonant contexts (filled circles, solid lines), across vowels surrounded only by voiceless Cs (unfilled circles, dotted lines), and only by voiced Cs (lightly filled diamonds, solid lines). The pattern of durations across vowels is essentially the same for these three contexts. Because the contexts stay constant for any one of the three curves, any differences in vowel duration must be a property of the vowels themselves—precisely what is meant by an "intrinsic" property. Clearly, for each of the curves, low vowels such as /æ/ and /ɑ/ have greater durations than high vowels such as /i/, /ɪ/, /ʊ/, and /u/. The differences between low and high vowel durations typically are on the order of 50 to 60 ms, a very large effect in the world of speech timing. The explanation for the intrinsic difference in the duration of low versus high vowels has sometimes been based

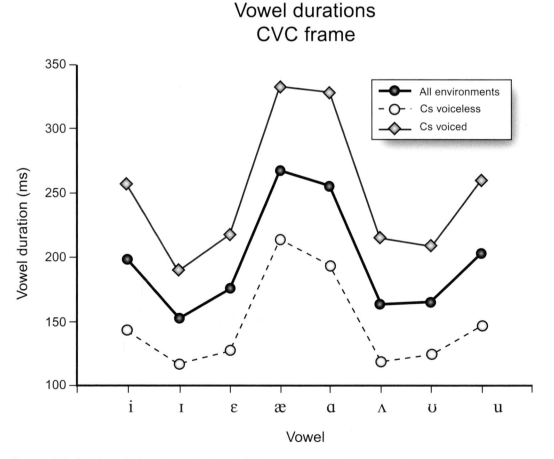

Figure 11-9. Vowel durations in fixed CVC frames for eight vowels in American English. Data are shown for environments in which C = voiceless (*unfilled circles*), C = voiced (*lightly shaded diamonds*), and for all C environments combined (*filled circles*). Data replotted from Hillenbrand et al. (2001).

on the greater articulatory distance required for the consonant-to-vowel-to-consonant path when the vowel is low, as compared to high. According to this idea, if one syllable requires articulators to travel greater distances than another syllable, it will take more time. This may explain part of the high-low intrinsic duration difference, but doesn't seem to account for all of the 50- to 60-ms difference.

The data in Figure 11–9 also show one other well-known intrinsic vowel duration difference, between tense and lax vowels. In any one of the three consonant contexts, tense vowels are longer than their lax vowel "partners" (compare the durations of the /i/-/ɪ/ and /u/-/ʊ/ pairs for any of the three curves). The difference in the duration of tense and lax vowels has a wide range (from about 22 to 65 ms in the data shown in Figure 11–9, depending on the consonant context), but always favors tense vowels when the consonant environment is held constant. This very consistent difference between tense and lax vowel durations is not easy to explain, and may be related to the spectral similarity of tense-lax pairs and the resulting need to distinguish them by duration.[4]

Listeners are sensitive to the high-low and tense-lax intrinsic differences in vowel duration. When high-quality speech synthesizers are programmed, for example, the differences just described are built into the algorithms to generate natural-sounding speech.

Extrinsic Factors Affecting Vowel Durations

Many factors influence vowel duration, certainly many more than can be covered in this chapter. What follows is a brief discussion of a few of the often-studied influences on vowel duration. Readers interested in comprehensive surveys of how and why vowel duration varies in speech production can consult House (1961), Klatt (1976), Umeda (1975), the series of papers by Crystal and House (1982, 1988a, 1988b, 1988c), and Van Santen (1992).

Consonant Voicing

Vowels are typically longer when surrounded by voiced, as compared to voiceless consonants. This effect is seen clearly in Figure 11–9 by comparing the "Cs voiceless" curve (unfilled circles, dashed lines) to the "Cs voiced" curve (lightly shaded diamonds, solid lines). The effect varies from vowel to vowel, but a reasonable general-

ization from the Hillenbrand et al. (2001) data is that vowels surrounded by voiced consonants are about 100 ms longer than vowels surrounded by voiceless consonants. The voicing of both the initial and final C in the CVC frame contributes to changes in vowel duration, but the largest influence is the voicing status of the final consonant of the syllable. If the syllable frame is marked as C_1VC_2, a voiced C_1 will lengthen a vowel by somewhere between 25 to 50 ms as compared to a voiceless C_1, whereas a voiced C_2 will lengthen a vowel by 50 to 90 ms relative to a voiceless C_2. The magnitude of these effects is lessened, perhaps greatly so, in more natural speaking conditions (Crystal & House, 1988a, 1988b).

Stress

Lexical stress is a characteristic of multisyllabic words in many languages, the best known examples in English being noun-verb contrasts such as "rebel-rebel" (/ˈrɛbl̩/-/rəˈbɛl/), and "contract-contract" (/ˈkɑntrækt/-/kənˈtræːkt/). Of course, many other multisyllabic words have alternating patterns of stressed and unstressed syllables as in "California" /kæləˈfɔrnjə/), where the first and third syllables have greater stress than the second and fourth syllables. When single syllables are stressed for emphasis or contrast ("Bob stopped by earlier"; "Did you say *Barb* stopped by?" "No, *Bob* stopped by"), the vowel in the emphasized syllable has greater duration than the original, lexically stressed production. All other things being equal, vowels in lexically or emphatically stressed syllables have greater duration than vowels in unstressed or normally stressed syllables (Fourakis, 1991). The magnitude of the duration difference between stressed and unstressed syllables, or between contrastively stressed and "normally stressed" syllables, is quite variable across speakers (Howell, 1993; Weismer & Ingrisano, 1979).

Speaking Rate

Vowel duration varies over a large range when speakers change their speaking rate. Slow rates result in longer vowel durations, fast rates in shorter vowel durations. Speaking rate also varies widely *across* speakers. Some speakers have naturally slow rates, some fast. Speakers who have habitually slow speaking rates have longer vowel durations than speakers with habitually fast rates (Tsao & Weismer, 1997). Perhaps these speaker-specific vowel durations should be considered intrinsic, rather than extrinsic influences on vowel duration.

---

[4]The thinking is that /i/ and /ɪ/, and /u/ and /ʊ/ have formant frequencies that are only subtly different, so vowel duration may have evolved in phonological systems to create an additional cue to the tense-lax vowel distinction.

Utterance Position Effects

The same vowel has variable duration depending on its location within an utterance. If the duration of /i/ in the word "beets" is measured in the sentence, "The beets are in the garden" versus "The garden contains no beets," the vowel is about 30 to 40 ms longer in the second sentence. This effect is referred to as phrase-final or utterance-final lengthening (see Klatt, 1975). The degree of lengthening depends on the depth of the grammatical boundary. A major syntactic boundary yields more vowel lengthening as compared to a "shallower" boundary; an extreme example is the greater lengthening at a truly end-of-utterance boundary (when the speaker is finished talking)—as compared to a syntactic boundary between two consecutive phrases.

Speaking Style

Over the past quarter-century, since Picheny, Durlach, and Braida (1985, 1986) introduced the notion of "clear speech" as a phenomenon worthy of experimental attention, research on the acoustics and perception of speaking style has been popular (for recent reviews see Calandruccio, Van Engen, Dhar, & Bradlow, 2010 and Smiljanić & Bradlow, 2011). Clear versus casual speech styles are potentially relevant to such diverse considerations as speaking to someone with a hearing impairment, someone whose native language is different from the language being spoken, someone who is listening to a native language but may not be a fully effective processor of spoken language input (such as infants or toddlers, or persons with intellectual challenges, or to a computer programmed to recognize speech). A clear speech style is thought to enhance acoustic contrasts that may be useful to a listener or machine trying to decode and identify segmental components of the incoming signal.

When speakers are asked to produce "clear speech," as if they are speaking to someone with a hearing loss or in a noisy environment, they typically slow their speaking rate and produce longer vowel durations. Whether clear speech exaggerates duration contrasts between vowels is, however, unclear. For example, in American English vowel duration is not a critical contrastive characteristic—phoneme categories are not contrasted strictly by vowel duration—which may explain why clear speech does not clearly exaggerate the duration distinction of vowel pairs such as /ʌ/-/ɑ/ and /ɪ/-/i/, which vary in duration (the first member of each pair is typically shorter than the second member: see DeMerit, 1997) but also in spectrum (formant frequencies). On the other hand, there is evidence of greater lengthening of tense, as compared to lax vowels in clear English speech (Picheny et al., 1986), even though tense and lax vowels also have different formant frequencies. Croatian, a language in which each of the five vowels may be either long or short, appears to have some tendency for clear speech to emphasize the duration difference (and thus the contrast between the long and short versions of the vowel; see Smiljanić & Bradlow, 2008). However, clear speech in Finnish, another language in which there are short and long vowels, does not seem to exaggerate the long-short vowel duration difference relative to its conversational speech difference (Granlund, Hazan, & Baker, 2012). A careful reading of the clear speech literature, at least to date, suggests a lot of speaker-to-speaker variability in the acoustics of speaking clearly. The question remains open of whether or not clear speech exaggerates contrasts consistently and in a uniform way across the phonetic contrasts of a given language.

Are We Wired for Rate?

Imagine a large sample of talkers—say, 100 people—each of whom reads a passage from which speaking rates (in syllables per second) are measured acoustically. If the talkers were chosen randomly, you would find a huge range of "typical" speaking rates, from very slow talkers, to talkers of average rate, to very fast talkers. These experimental measurements would confirm the everyday observation that some people speak very slowly, some very rapidly. Now imagine that you chose the slowest and fastest talkers in this sample, and asked them to produce the passage as fast as possible. If all talkers were able to produce the passage at the same, maximally fast speaking rate, regardless of their "typical" rate, that would indicate that the very slow or fast "typical" rates were a kind of conscious choice on the part of individual talkers. However, if the slow talkers couldn't speak as fast as the fast talkers, that would suggest that speaking rates reflect some basic neurological "wiring" that determines the "typical" rate. This experiment was performed by Tsao and Weismer (1997), who found that the maximal speaking rates of slow talkers were, in fact, significantly less than the maximal rates of fast talkers. It seems we are not all wired the same for typical speaking rate, and probably a bunch of other stuff, as well.

Why present such a complicated summary of clear versus conversational speech? Speech-language pathologists often ask persons receiving articulatory therapy to hyperarticulate, that is to say, to produce a clear form of speech as a strategy to master a particular sound or distinguish among a group of sounds (see Lam, Tjaden, & Wilding, 2012). The object may not be to have someone producing clear speech as an everyday form of speech, but in many cases it is a starting point for therapy.

DIPHTHONGS

American English has five or six diphthongs, depending on the dialect of the speaker and which authority is describing the sounds. The standard group of six includes /ɑɪ/ ("guys"), /ɔɪ/ ("boys"), /aʊ/ ("doubt"), /eɪ/ ("bays"), /oʊ/ ("goes"), and /ju/ ("beauty"). Spectrograms of the first five of these are shown in Figures 11–10 and 11–11. Diphthongs, somewhat surprisingly,

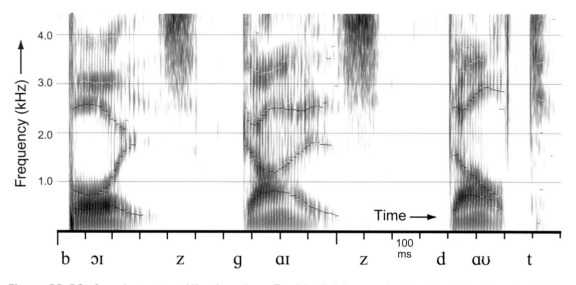

Figure 11–10. Spectrograms of the American English diphthongs /ɔɪ/, /ɑɪ/, and /aʊ/, spoken in the words "boys," "guys," and "doubt," respectively. LPC tracks are shown in red for F1, F2, and F3. Speaker is a 57-year-old, healthy male.

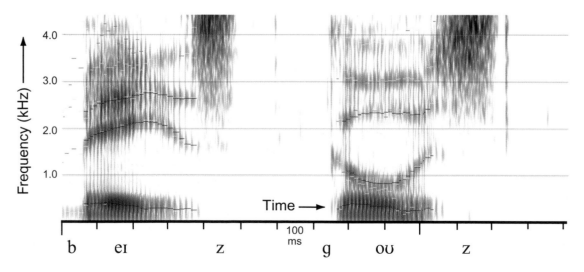

Figure 11–11. Spectrograms of the American English diphthongs /eɪ/ and /oʊ/, spoken in the words "bays" and "goes." LPC tracks are shown in red for F1, F2, and F3. Speaker is a 57-year-old, healthy male.

have not been studied nearly as extensively as vowels, possibly because the former have sometimes been considered as sequences of the latter. The symbols used to represent diphthongs, after all, are combinations of two vowels. Is the diphthong /ɔɪ/, for example, an /ɔ/ connected to an /ɪ/ by a relatively rapid change in vocal tract configuration? In Figure 11–10, at least for /ɔɪ/ and /aɪ/, the spectrographic data can be studied to address this question.

LPC tracks for F1-F3 are shown as red dashed lines throughout the vocalic nuclei. An LPC track is a sequence, over time, of estimated formant frequencies based on LPC analysis; in the case of the LPC tracks in Figure 11–10 a formant frequency is estimated at each glottal pulse throughout the diphthong. For /ɔɪ/ there is a large, rising F2 transition preceded and followed by intervals of unchanging formant frequencies—these are the so-called steady states mentioned earlier. Clearly, for this /ɔɪ/, the steady state preceding the large F2 transition is of greater duration than the steady state following it, the latter being very brief and perhaps only visible in F2. For the /aɪ/ in Figure 11–10, there is also a large F2 transition preceded and followed by steady states. The formant tracks for /aɪ/ are somewhat more complicated than the ones for /ɔɪ/ because of the influence of the initial /g/ which causes the initial falling (decreasing frequency) transition in F2. The steady state is the brief interval following this initial downward transition, immediately before the sharp rising transition in F2. The steady state following the transition is, as in the case of /ɔɪ/, most evident in F2.

The spectrographic data relevant to the question of whether diphthongs are two vowels connected by a rapid change in vocal tract configuration can now be addressed. The research logic is simple. Measure the formant frequencies at the steady states, and the hypothesis of two connected vowels is confirmed if they are similar to the formant frequencies of the vowels indicated by the transcription. For example, are the formant frequencies for the first steady state in /ɔɪ/ like those measured for the vowel /ɔ/, and the formant frequencies for the second steady state like those for the vowel /ɪ/?

The answer seems to be "no." Studies by Holbrook and Fairbanks (1962) and Gay (1968) do not support the idea of diphthongs as sequences of two vowels, for several reasons worth considering in more detail. Holbrook and Fairbanks had 20 male speakers produce each of the diphthongs in an /hVd/ frame at the end of a short sentence. They located spectrographic measurement points at the first and last glottal pulses of the diphthongs, as well as three additional points roughly equidistant between the initial and final points. The

formant frequencies of each diphthong were, therefore, represented by five measurement points throughout the duration of the vocalic nucleus. The data of Holbrook and Fairbanks are summarized in Figure 11–12, which shows averages of the five measured F1-F2 points throughout each diphthong. The direction of the arrow next to each phonetic symbol indicates the direction of the five plotted points from beginning to end of that diphthong. For example, the points for /ɔɪ/ (filled triangles) are indicated by a bent arrow pointing up. The first measurement point, at the first glottal pulse, is located roughly at F1 = 550 Hz and F2 = 800 Hz, and the final measurement point, at the last glottal pulse, is roughly at F1 = 500 Hz and F2 = 1900 Hz. The four other diphthong paths in F1-F2 space can be interpreted in the same way. Also plotted in Figure 11–12 are the F1-F2 values for the vowels /ɪ/, /ʊ/, /ɔ/, and /a/ reported for adult males by Hillenbrand et al. (1995) for the same /hVd/ frame used by Holbrook and Fairbanks for diphthong production. The phonetic symbol for each vowel identifies its location in F1-F2 space. The oval enclosing the symbol has no meaning other than to set off the vowel locations from the diphthong points. These vowel points were chosen either because the diphthong symbols include them as an end point (/ɪ/ being the end symbol for /ɔɪ/, /aɪ/, and /eɪ/; /ʊ/ the end symbol for /oʊ/ and /aʊ/) or as a starting point (/a/ the start for /aʊ/ and /aɪ/; /ɔ/ the start for /ɔɪ/).

Compare the F1-F2 points for the vowel /ɪ/ to the end points for the diphthongs /ɔɪ/, /aɪ/, and /eɪ/. It is no exaggeration to describe the endpoints for /ɔɪ/ and /aɪ/ as very distant from /ɪ/. Although the endpoint for /eɪ/ is relatively closer to /ɪ/, it is still substantially different in the F2 dimension. A similar analysis seems to apply to the comparison of /oʊ/ and /aʊ/ end points to the plotted point for /ʊ/. For the start points of /aɪ/ and /aʊ/, F1-F2 points for /a/ are a good match for /aʊ/ (filled boxes), somewhat less so for /aɪ/, and the plotted point for /ɔ/ is very far from the start point for /ɔɪ/.

Holbrook and Fairbanks (1962) concluded that the trajectory of diphthongs in F1-F2 space did not typically begin and end in well-defined vowel areas. They noted, however, that a careful examination of the diphthong paths would suggest virtually no overlap between the five diphthongs shown in Figure 11–12. When the starting and ending frequencies plus the direction of the F1-F2 change are considered, these five diphthongs separate nicely. Based on this apparent acoustic distinctiveness, characterized not only by formant frequencies at the beginning and end of diphthongs but also on their direction of formant frequency change over time,

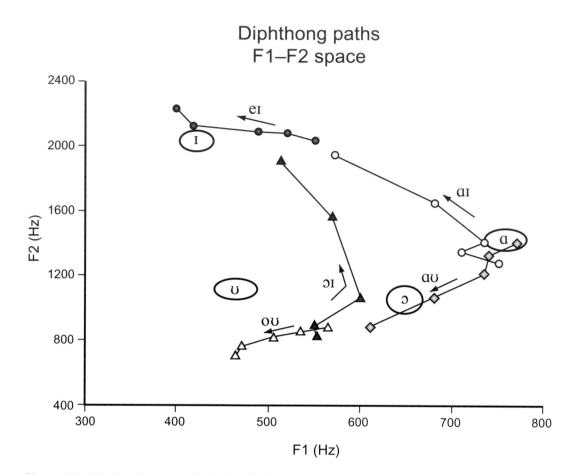

Figure 11–12. Diphthong paths in the F1-F2 plane, and F1-F2 points for four monophthongs. Each diphthong path is represented by five, equally spaced measurement points throughout the diphthong duration; the first point (at the beginning of the diphthong) for each diphthong path is the one preceding the arrowhead, and the last point is the one terminating the path, in the direction indicated by the arrow (see text for a worked example). Diphthong path symbols, clockwise from /aʊ/, lightly shaded diamonds; /ɔɪ/, filled triangles; /oʊ/, unfilled triangles; /eɪ/, filled circles; and /aɪ/, unfilled circles. Diphthong data from Holbrook and Fairbanks (1962), vowel data from Hillenbrand et al. (1995).

it might be predicted that diphthongs are relatively easy to classify with a statistical procedure. This is exactly what was found by Gottfried, Miller, and Meyer (1993) in an automatic (statistical) classification analysis of a large number of diphthongs produced by four Midwestern speakers. Over 90% of the diphthongs produced in this study were classified correctly, based on only a small number of measurements per diphthong.

Perhaps the difficulty of representing diphthongs as two sequenced vowels should have been obvious simply by examining spectrograms of natural productions of the sounds. As noted earlier, initial and final steady states can be identified for /ɔɪ/ and /aɪ/ (see Figure 11–10), but in the case of /aʊ/ F1 and F2 are changing at the beginning and end of the diphthong, where steady states might be expected. A similar

absence of initial and final steady states can be seen for /eɪ/ and /oʊ/ (see Figure 11–11). The absence of steady states in many cases of diphthong production has been noted by previous scientists (Lehiste & Peterson, 1961), and cited as a potential complication in classifying diphthongs as a sequence of two vowels.

If steady states are not a reliable characteristic of diphthongs, what is? A close look at Figures 11–10 and 11–11 suggests that each of the diphthongs has an identifiable, and in some cases substantial, transitional segment. The transitional segments, usually most pronounced in F2 but also seen in F1 and F3, reflect the rapid change in vocal tract shape between the initial and final parts of the diphthong.

Gay (1968) performed a simple experiment to determine which aspects of diphthong production varied, and which remained more or less constant over changes in speaking rate. Gay asked speakers to produce diphthongs at slow, conversational, and fast speaking rates, and measured F1 and F2 steady states at the beginning and end of the diphthongs as well as the slopes of F2 transitions. Across the speaking rate conditions, which resulted in substantial changes in the duration of the diphthongs (see below), Gay found the F1 and F2 onset measurement (like the initial steady-state measures described above) to remain fairly stable across rate. In contrast, the F1 and F2 offset measures (like the final steady-state measures) varied substantially. Of special interest, however, was the finding that the slope of the F2 transition was essentially constant across the rate changes: "the second formant rate of change [that is, the slope] for each diphthong remains relatively constant across changes in duration and *distinct from the rates of change of the other diphthongs*" (Gay, 1968, p. 1571, emphasis added). For Gay, the slope

of the F2 transition was a constant and distinguishing characteristic of diphthongs. His findings argued against the notion of diphthongs as merely sequences of two vowels connected by a transition. The transitional component of diphthongs was, in a sense, their defining feature and showed them to be a different sound class than vowels (see Watson & Harrington, 1999, for similar comments on the difference between vowels and diphthongs in Australian English).

The duration characteristics of diphthongs have not been well studied, but if asked, most speech scientists would probably expect diphthongs to be somewhat longer than monophthong vowels in equivalent environments and speaking conditions. Data published by Umeda (1975) for a single speaker suggest that /ɑɪ/, /ɑʊ/, and possibly /eɪ/ have greater duration than monophthongs. Comparisons between studies, such as the diphthong duration data published by Gay (1968) and the vowel duration data published by Hillenbrand et al. (1995, 2001) are complicated by nonequivalent phonetic contexts and speaking rates.

What's a Diphthong, What's a Vowel?

Figure 11–12 makes the case that direction of movement in F1-F2 space, when included with starting and ending frequencies, separates the American English diphthongs nicely. It is as if inherent vocal tract movement characteristics must be taken into account to make sense of diphthong differences. This conceptual strategy for distinguishing among diphthongs apparently applies to some vowels as well. Like diphthongs, vowels such as /ɪ/, /ɛ/, and /ʊ/ seem to have inherent movement (and therefore acoustic) characteristics (Nearey & Assman, 1986) important for their identification. These particular vowels—the lax vowels, mostly—are also quite variable across dialects, and their inherent movement characteristics may be specific to particular dialects. Recently, Jacewicz and Fox (2012, see their Figures 1 and 2) plotted data for lax vowels produced by speakers from southern Wisconsin and western North Carolina, in a way similar to the diphthong data in Figure 11–12. The plot shows that, when *movement* is taken into consideration for these apparently monophthongal vowels—at least that is what the textbooks call them—much of the confusion among these vowels, both in terms of their formant frequencies and their identification, disappears. So, are /ɪ/, /ɛ/, and /ʊ/ vowels or diphthongs?

NASALS

Data on the acoustic characteristics of nasals are more limited than those on vowels. There are no large-scale studies on formant and zero (antiresonance; see Chapter 9) frequencies in nasals, or their variation across speakers due to age and sex. The relatively small body of work on nasals has been concerned with the acoustic characteristics associated with nasal manner and place of production.

As discussed in Chapter 9, nasal articulations are described acoustically in two broad categories. One, the nasal murmur, concerns acoustic characteristics during the interval of complete oral cavity closure with an open velopharyngeal port. For example, the nasal murmur for /m/ occurs during the interval when the lips are sealed and sound waves travel through the open velopharyngeal port and radiate from the nostrils. During the nasal murmur, the speech spectrum includes resonances of the combined pharyngeal and nasal cavities, as well as antiresonances originating in the closed oral cavity and the sinus cavities. The second category of nasal articulation is nasalization, or the articulation of vowels (that is, with an open oral cavity) with a velopharyngeal port sufficiently open to "add" nasal resonances and antiresonances into the oral vowel resonances. The spectrum of nasalization is complex, consisting of both vocal tract and nasal tract resonances as well as antiresonances from the sinus cavities.

Nasal Murmurs

Figure 11–13 shows spectrographic characteristics of the nasal murmur interval for /m/ in stressed CVC syllables surrounding an /i/ (left side of upper panel) and /ɑ/ (right side of upper panel). The boundaries of the prestressed (first /m/) murmur intervals are marked below the spectrogram baseline by short, ver- tical bars. These murmur intervals are slightly greater than 100 ms (left spectrogram) and just under 100 ms (right spectrogram) in duration. These measurements are slightly longer than the 86 ms duration of /m/ in prestressed position reported by Umeda (1977) for a single speaker.

The nasal murmur intervals of both utterances shown in the upper panel of Figure 11–13 are clearly

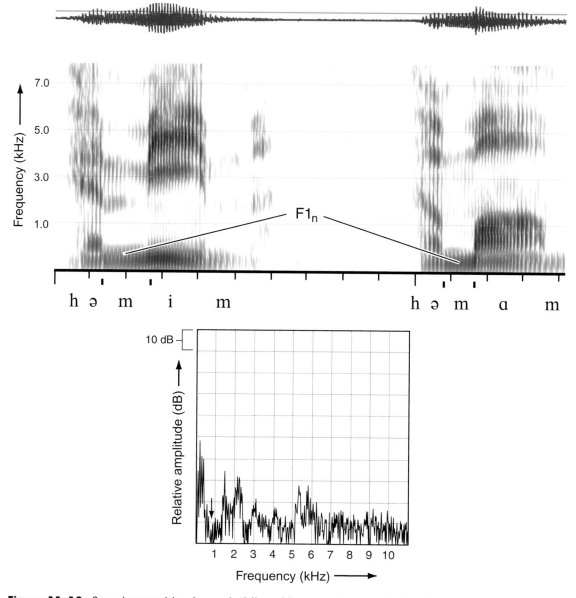

Figure 11-13. Spectrographic characteristics of the nasal murmur interval for /m/ in stressed CVC syllables surrounding an /i/ (*left side of top panel*) and /ɑ/ (*right side of top panel*). Short, vertical bars immediately below the baseline of the spectrogram mark the onsets and offsets of the nasal murmur intervals. An FFT spectrum from the middle 50 ms of the /m/ preceding the /i/ is shown in the lower part of the figure; the downward-pointing arrow indicates the approximate location of an antiresonance.

much less intense as compared to the surrounding vowels. Using the marked boundaries of the intervals as reference points, note the dramatic change in intensity from vowel to murmur or murmur to vowel. The intensity difference is reflected in the relative darkness of the vowel and nasal murmur traces. As discussed in Chapter 9, nasals tend to be less intense than vowels and other sonorant sounds (such as liquids, glides, rhotics) for two reasons. One is the presence of antiresonances (zeros) in the spectrum, which not only result in a substantial absence of energy at the exact frequency of the zero, but also reductions in energy at frequencies in the immediate vicinity of the zero. An antiresonance from the middle 50 ms of the first nasal murmur of /həmim/ is indicated at 750 Hz by a downward-pointing arrow in the FFT spectrum shown below the spectrogram. Note the general depression of spectral energy around 1000 Hz, as well as the "white space" from 500 to 1100 Hz in the spectrogram, reflecting the broad influence of the antiresonance. Because a speech sound's total energy is the sum of all energies at all frequencies, the presence of antiresonances in nasal murmur spectra makes their overall intensity relatively low, as compared to vowels. The second reason for the relatively weak intensities of nasal murmurs is the greater absorption, and, therefore, loss, of sound energy when acoustic waves propagate through the nasal cavities (see Chapter 9). The greater absorption of sound results in wider formant bandwidths and lower peak amplitudes of resonances.

The first formant of the nasal murmur is marked in both spectrograms as $F1_n$. The subscript "n" indicates that the resonance is from the combined pharyngeal and nasal cavities (hereafter, nasal cavities). This lowest resonance of the nasal cavities is a very constant characteristic of nasal murmurs, having relatively great intensity and a frequency of about 300 Hz (Fujimura, 1962). The rest of the nasal murmur spectrum usually contains a fair number of resonances and antiresonances. The spectrograms in Figure 11–13 illustrate this well, with the prestressed murmur of /həmim/ showing an $F2_n$ around 1500 Hz (at least for the first part of the murmur), a possible pair of formants ($F3_n$, $F4_n$) around 2000 Hz, and another around 3000 Hz. In the prestressed murmur of /həmɑm/ (Figure 11–13, upper right panel), there is a similar pattern of resonances above $F1_n$ but of much weaker intensity when compared to /həmim/. Fujimura described how variable

the patterns of nasal resonances and antiresonances were, both across and within speakers. Presumably, the within-speaker variation is primarily a result of changing phonetic contexts. The differences in the nasal resonances for the /i/ and /ɑ/ contexts is plain to see in Figure 11–13, and a consideration of the different frequency ranges occupied by the white spaces in the two spectrograms suggests differences in the antiresonance locations as well.

It may seem odd to see spectral evidence of different vowels during a nasal murmur, for which sound transmission is fully (or almost nearly so) through the nasal cavities because of the completely open velopharyngeal port. Such vowel-context effects on nasal murmur spectra have, in fact, been demonstrated in modeling studies based on human vocal tract and nasal tract cavity measurements. In such studies the vocal tract is represented with different vowel shapes while the velopharyngeal port is set to "wide open" to see what happens to nasal spectra as the vocal tract configuration is varied. Serrurier and Badin (2008, Figure 23) present a beautiful plot showing how their model reveals subtle vowel effects on nasal murmur spectra. Such model data are consistent with the spectrographic differences for /mim/ versus /mam/, described above.

Perhaps one explanation for the absence of an acoustic data base for nasals comparable to vowels is the difficulty of identifying formants and antiresonances during the nasal murmur. Many nasal formants above $F1_n$ are challenging to locate because of their weak intensity, and antiresonances are often inferred from the absence of energy, rather than by something definitive in the spectrogram or spectrum.[5] An alternative approach to identifying important acoustic characteristics of nasal murmurs (or any speech sound) is to make several measures of the murmur spectrum and use those measures in an automatic classification analysis. This is the kind of work done by scientists interested in computer recognition of speech. They want to know which acoustic features allow the most rapid and accurate identification of individual speech sounds.

A good example of this work is found in Pruthi and Espy-Wilson (2004). These investigators were interested in machine recognition of segments having a nasal *manner* of articulation. Pruthi and Espy-Wilson (2004) noted that nasals are often confused with liquids (/l/, /r/) and glides (/w/, /j/) when computers classify speech sounds on the basis of automatically

---

[5]Sharp dips in an FFT spectrum (downward-pointing arrow around 750 Hz in the spectrum shown in the lower panel of Figure 11–13) or white spaces in a spectrogram can occur in the absence of an antiresonance. A definitive identification of an antiresonance depends, in part, on knowing that an antiresonance *should* be found in a spectrum—that the spectrum is derived from a speech sound whose underlying articulation involves a parallel resonator (see Chapter 9).

extracted acoustic measures (that is, a computer algorithm that identifies segments through temporal and spectral measures). They designed four acoustic measures, based on consideration of the acoustic characteristics of nasal murmurs relative to those associated with the constriction interval of liquids and glides, as classification parameters for nasal manner of articulation. In a sense, the selection of the four measures was a hypothesis concerning the acoustic characteristics required to identify the nasal manner of production. These measures, with a brief explanation of why they were chosen, are listed in Table 11–1.

The point of this discussion is not to consider in detail the four measures selected by Pruthi and Espy-Wilson (2004), but to demonstrate the value of their experiment for understanding critical acoustic features of speech sounds. Pruthi and Espy-Wilson, using a combination of these four measures, correctly classified nasal manner of production for 94% of the more than 1000 nasal murmurs in a large database of sentences spoken by many different speakers. These measures were chosen carefully, to reflect certain aspects of nasal murmur acoustics that had been described in the literature. Moreover, the measures made sense in terms of the theory of vocal and nasal tract acoustics. The very successful classification performance suggests that these measures are strong candidates for further acoustic studies of nasal production and perception.[6]

Nasal Place

There is a long history of documenting the acoustic correlates of place of articulation for consonants, including nasals. Much of this history is concerned with the acoustic cues used by *listeners* to identify place of articulation. Although speech perception is considered in greater depth in the next chapter, the case of nasal place of articulation provides a good introduction to the interplay between studies of acoustic characteristics of speech sounds and their role as cues in speech perception.

Consider the following thought experiment. Imagine a CV syllable, where C = /m/ or /n/ and V = /i/,

Table 11–1. Four Acoustic Measures Used by Pruthi and Espy-Wilson (2004) for Automatic Classification of Nasal Manner of Articulation

MEASURE	EXPLANATION
Energy onset/offset at vowel-nasal (liquid/glide) boundaries	Energy change from vowel to nasal or nasal to vowel is greater than from vowel to liquid or liquid/glide to vowel
First spectral peak	Nasal murmurs have lower F1 as compared to F1s of liquids and glides
$dB_{0-320Hz}/dB_{320-5360Hz}$	Nasal murmurs have most energy concentrated below 320 Hz (at the $F1_n$), little energy above, so energy ratio would be high; liquids and glides have more energy in the 320- to 5360-Hz band, so ratio would be lower
Energy fluctuation	Level (in dB) of energy throughout a nasal murmur is more stable than throughout the constriction interval of a liquid or glide

Note: The measures were chosen as most likely to separate nasal manner from liquid and glide manner, because nasals are often mistaken as liquids or glides by speech recognition devices. Descriptions and explanations of the measures have been modified slightly from the original presentation.

---

[6]Simply because an acoustic measure can be used in a statistical or machine recognition procedure to obtain correct classifications of the manner (or any other feature) of articulation of a speech sound does not mean that humans use the same kind of information to make the same decisions. But the statistical/machine data do suggest testable hypotheses for perception experiments.

/ɛ/, /æ/, /ɑ/, /o/, or /u/. The consonants are chosen to represent the two nasals that occur in syllable-initial position of English words. The vowels are chosen to sample different locations around the vowel quadrilateral, to maximize potential coarticulatory influences on murmur acoustics—that is, to create variability in murmur acoustics due to phonetic context. The complete set of 12 syllables (2 nasal consonants × 6 vowels) is spoken by several speakers and saved as computer wave files. Speech analysis programs are used to make certain measurements as well as to "pull out" from each syllable wave file selected pieces for presentation to listeners. The waveform pieces are chosen to have one representative from the murmur, one from the vowel close to the murmur-vowel boundary (therefore containing formant transitions from murmur to vowel)

and one straddling the murmur-vowel boundary. Figure 11–14 illustrates these waveform pieces with a spectrogram of the utterance /əˈmɛ/. The boundaries of the nasal murmur are indicated by the short, upward-pointing arrows at the baseline. The three waveform pieces are shown by narrow rectangles ("windows") superimposed on the spectrogram. Each window is approximately 25 ms in duration. The left-most window is the murmur piece, the middle window the piece straddling the boundary between murmur offset and vowel onset (murmur + transition piece), and the right-hand window the transition piece—the piece of the vowel containing transitions from the consonant to the vowel.

These waveform pieces can be used to address the question, "Which piece(s) of the waveform, or which

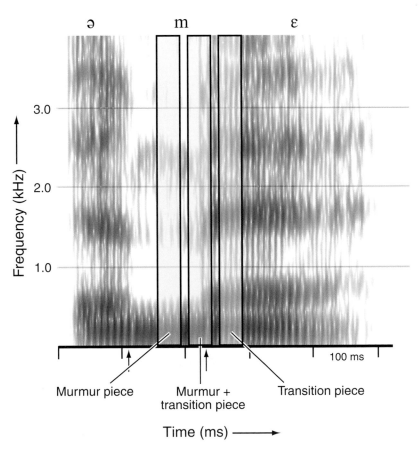

Figure 11-14. Spectrogram of the utterance /əˈmɛ/, shown with three 25-ms "windows" centered at different times. The left-most window (light green shading, "murmur piece") is within the nasal murmur, the center window (light blue shading, "murmur + transition piece") straddles the murmur-vowel boundary, and the right-most window (light yellow shading, "transition piece") is completely within the vowel, during the formant transitions from the murmur to the vowel.

acoustic characteristics within each piece, allow a classification of place of articulation (bilabial vs. lingua-alveolar) for the nasal consonant?" The classification can be performed by a statistical procedure (see below), or by human listeners. Stated in a different way: "Do the three pieces allow equivalent accuracy in classifying place of articulation for nasals, or is one piece 'better' than another?" For example, if the nasal murmur piece (the left-most box) is presented to listeners, can they use just this acoustic information to assign place of articulation accurately? Alternatively, if certain acoustic characteristics are extracted from the murmur window for /m/ and /n/, can these measures be used by an automatic classification algorithm to separate the two places of articulation? These types of experiments appear several times in the speech acoustics literature (e.g., Harrington, 1994; Kurowski & Blumstein, 1984, 1987; Repp, 1986). The results of the various experiments, although not always precisely consistent, suggest that *any* of these three pieces, when presented to human listeners or classified statistically, allow fairly accurate identification of place of articulation for syllable-initial nasals. Moreover, when two or more of the pieces are presented (or classified) together, the accuracy of place identification improves.

First consider the results for isolated murmurs. If nasal place of articulation can be identified (classified) accurately from just the murmur, something about its acoustic characteristics must be systematically different for labials versus lingua-alveolars. The duration of the

murmur can be ruled out as a measure that separates /m/ from /n/, but there are almost certainly spectral differences between these two nasal murmurs. The spectral differences are a result of different resonances and antiresonances of the coupled pharyneal and oral tracts. In Chapter 9, the frequency locations of the anti-resonances for /m/ versus /n/ were discussed, the former having a lower region (according to Fujimura [1962], roughly 750–1250 Hz), the latter a higher region (1450–2200 Hz). The unique resonances for /m/ in Fujimura's study included a two-formant cluster in the vicinity of 1000 Hz, and for /n/ a similar cluster above 2000 Hz. Qi and Fox (1992), in an analysis of the first two resonances of nasal murmurs for /m/ and /n/ produced by six speakers, reported average second resonances for /m/ and /n/ of 1742 and 2062 Hz, respectively. A careful examination of the /m/ and /n/ murmurs in Figure 11–15 shows formant patterns, and inferred antiresonance locations, generally consistent with the observations of Fujimura, and Qi and Fox. Both /m/ and /n/ have the expected first formant around 300 Hz, but in the frequency range above this formant, the spectra are different. Between the F1 and the next evidence of a higher resonance, both murmurs have an obvious "white space." For /m/, the white space extends roughly from 500 to 1150 Hz, and for /n/ it is located between 500 and 1600 Hz. Under the assumption that the exact antiresonance frequencies are approximately in the middle of these white space ranges, their center frequencies are 850 Hz for /m/ and

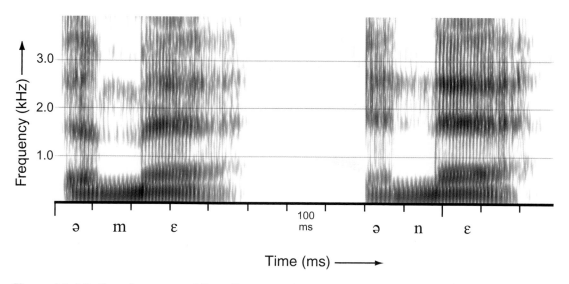

Figure 11–15. Spectrograms of the utterances /əˈmɛ/ and /əˈnɛ/, produced by a 57-year-old, healthy male. Note between-place differences in the murmur spectra and the pattern of formant transitions as the nasal is released into the vowel.

1050 Hz for /n/. Immediately above the antiresonance, the /m/ murmur has a second and perhaps third resonance around 1500 Hz, and above that a resonance around 2300 Hz. In comparison, the /n/ murmur has a second resonance around 1800 Hz, and what appears to be a cluster of two resonances around 2500 Hz. Clearly, the two murmurs have different spectral characteristics. It is reasonable to expect that listeners can use these differences to identify place of articulation.[7] In Repp (1986), listeners made accurate place judgments for /m/ and /n/ when given only the murmur piece of CV syllables, and Harrington (1994) obtained excellent statistical classification for these two nasals when using acoustic information from single spectrum "slices" taken from the murmur.

The spectrograms in Figure 11–15 also show different patterns of formant transitions as the murmur is released into the following /ɛ/. There is a long history of considering formant transitions at CV boundaries as strong cues to consonant place of articulation. This history originated in the late 1940s and early 1950s, at the Haskins Laboratories, where experiments showed that synthesized formant transitions cued place of articulation in the absence of consonant spectra (Liberman, Delattre, Cooper, & Gerstman, 1954). Figure 11–16 shows a spectrogram of the utterance /ənɛ/ to contrast its transitions with those of /əmɛ/ and /ənɛ/ in Figure 11–15. The pattern of F2 and F3 transitions over the first 40 or 50 ms following release of the murmur are unique to the different places of nasal articulation. For the transitions coming out of the /m/ murmur both F2 and F3 are rising, from /n/ they are more or less flat, and from /ŋ/ F2 is falling and F3 rising. This latter pattern (see Figure 11–16) seems to show F2 and F3 starting at nearly the same frequency and separating throughout the transition. The details of these F2-F3 transition patterns depend on the identity of the vowel following the murmur, but in most cases the patterns are uniquely different for the three places of articulation. Of course, in English the velar nasal /ŋ/ does not appear in the prestressed position shown in Figure 11–16, but this is not a physiological limitation—there are languages in which

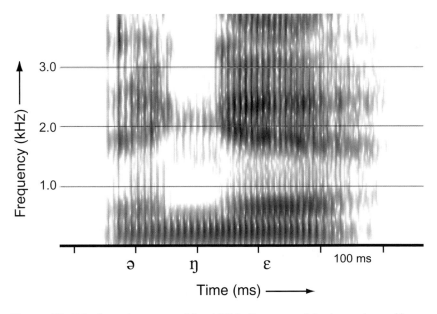

Figure 11–16. Spectrogram of the VCV utterance /əˈŋɛ/, produced by a 57-year-old male. Note the F2-F3 transition pattern immediately following release of the nasal murmur.

---

[7]The antiresonance and upper resonance locations for the murmurs in Figure 11–15 are different from those reported by Fujimura (1962) based on his theoretical calculations and data from two subjects, but the spectral relations (e.g., higher antiresonance for /n/ as compared to /m/, different patterns of resonances above the constant F1 at 300 Hz) are consistent with Fujimura's general description. The resonances and antiresonances for /m/ and /n/ shown in Figure 11–15 are also somewhat different from the modeling results reported by Rong and Kuehn (2010). Fujimura, and many other authors, have pointed to the wide range of variability expected across speakers for nasal murmur spectra as a result of variations in nasal tract and sinus cavity morphology (Dang & Honda, 1995).

the sound can appear in this position—so the point concerning place-specific transition patterns is a valid one.

Place of articulation information is present in these unique transition patterns, as demonstrated for listeners (Repp, 1986) and statistical classification (Harrington, 1994). The accuracy of place identification from the transitions (i.e., from the "transition piece" of the spectrogram shown in Figure 11–14) is essentially similar to the accuracy from the "murmur piece," as described above. Place information for nasals, therefore, seems to have acoustic correlates in at least two different locations throughout a CV syllable, and these correlates are both sufficiently stable to be reliable for listener and statistical classification of nasals.

Finally, in Figure 11–14 the middle "piece" straddles the boundary where the murmur ends and the transition begins. This interval has a very rapid change from the low-energy, unique resonance patterns associated with murmurs to the high-energy formant patterns for vowels. Several scientists (Kurowski & Blumstein, 1984, 1987; Seitz, McCormick, Watson, & Bladon, 1990) have argued that each place of articulation is associated with a unique frequency pattern for this rapid change. Whether or not this particular "piece" is more important in the classification of nasal place of articulation, as compared to the murmur or transitions alone, is a matter of considerable debate.

Nasalization

Nasalization, as reviewed in Chapter 9, is a concept with broad application in general and clinical phonetics. Nasalization of vowels, which is of concern here, involves complex acoustics as a result of the mix of oral and nasal tract formants with antiresonances originating in the sinus cavities.[8] Because measurement and interpretation of the spectrum of nasalized vowels is challenging, only a few studies have reported data on nasalization acoustics. Interesting theoretical treatments of vowel nasalization can be found in Stevens, Fant, and Hawkins (1987), Feng and Castelli (1996), Rong and Kuehn (2010), Pruthi, Espy-Wilson, and Story (2007), and Serrurier and Badin (2008). Chen (1995, 1997) developed two acoustic measures of nasalization, one of which is described here.

Recall that a Fourier spectrum of a vowel shows the amplitude of the consecutive harmonics (where the first harmonic = F0) produced by the vibrating vocal folds. Furthermore, the amplitude of variation of these harmonics reflects, in part, the resonance characteristics of the vocal tract when the speech signal is recorded by a microphone in front of the lips. When a vowel is produced with an open velopharyngeal port and is nasalized, some glottal harmonics in the region of the nasal resonances have increased amplitude (relative to the amplitudes when the vowel is not nasalized), and some harmonics in the region of oral formants have reduced amplitudes, as a result of nearby antiresonances and the extra damping due to increased absorption of sound energy in the nasal cavities (see Chapter 9). Chen (1995) took advantage of these facts and constructed a spectral measure of nasalization in which the amplitude of the harmonic closest to the first formant is compared to the amplitude of a harmonic close to the location of the second nasal resonance. The technique is illustrated in Figure 11–17.

Figure 11–17 shows two FFT spectra, both for the middle 30 ms of the vowel /i/ in the CVC [bib] (left spectrum) and [min] (right spectrum). In both spectra, two harmonics are of interest. One, labeled "A1," is the harmonic in the immediate vicinity of the low-frequency F1 of the vowel /i/. As expected, the A1 harmonic in the two spectra has relatively high amplitude as compared to the other harmonics. This makes sense because the amplitude of this harmonic is "boosted" by the typical first resonant frequency (that is, F1) of /i/. The other harmonic of interest is the one labeled "P1." Chen (1995) identified this harmonic as one "boosted" when the oral and nasal cavities are coupled via opening of the velopharyngeal port. The P1 harmonic is in the vicinity of the second resonance associated with the nasal cavity. In theory, the amplitude of the P1 harmonic should be quite small when the velopharyngeal port is closed and relatively greater when the port is open. Based on theoretical and experimental work, Chen recommended identifying the P1 harmonic by locating the FFT peak closest to 950 Hz.

Chen's (1995) index of nasalization requires measurement of the A1-P1 amplitude difference within a vowel spectrum. In Figure 11–17, the A1 and P1 *relative* amplitudes for [i] surrounded by [b] are roughly

---

[8]Recall that nasalization occurs when the velopharyngeal port is open at the same time the oral tract opens for vowel production. This combination of events is characteristic of "normal" speech production in at least two ways. First, vowels are typically not produced with perfect velopharyngeal port closure, but have variable amounts of small opening that depend on tongue height (higher the vowel, tighter the closure). Second, the coarticulatory patterns of nasal-vowel and vowel-nasal sequences almost always involve some velopharyngeal port opening during the vowel that reflects the previous (in nasal-vowel sequences) or upcoming (in vowel-nasal sequences) open port requirement of the nasal consonant.

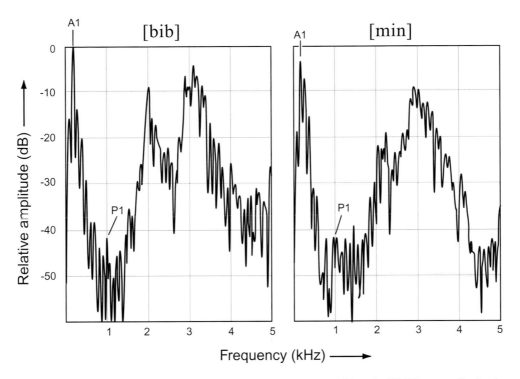

Figure 11-17. Two /i/ spectra showing the application of Chen's (1995) acoustic technique for quantifying the degree of vowel nasalization. The left spectrum is for /i/ in a nonnasal context, the right spectrum for /i/ in a nasal context. "A1" is the highest-amplitude harmonic in the vicinity of the F1 for /i/, "P1" a harmonic around 950 Hz, associated with the second resonance of the nasal tract. The acoustic measure is the amplitude difference, in dB, between A1 and P1.

0 and −42 dB, respectively, yielding an A1-P1 index of 42 dB. When [i] is surrounded by nasal consonants (right spectrum), and therefore likely to be partially nasalized due to coarticulatory influences, A1 = −4 dB, P1 = −42 dB, giving an A1-P1 index of 38 dB. As expected, the A1-P1 index for the vowel in a nasal environment is smaller than the index when the vowel is between nonnasal consonants.

The 4-dB difference between the A1-P1 amplitudes in oral and nasal consonant environments is small, and probably at the low end of the distribution for normal speakers. This oral versus nasal difference can be referred to as the (A1-P1$_{oral}$)–(A1-P1$_{nasal}$) index. For the vowel /i/, Chen (1997) reported the (A1-P1$_{oral}$)–(A1-P1$_{nasal}$) index to range between 4.2 and 22.3 dB across 10 normal speakers producing CVCs like the ones used for the example in Figure 11–17. The magnitude of this index also depends on which vowel is measured. Chen reported the greatest average index

for /i/ (15 dB), with average indices for /u/, /ɛ/, and /ʌ/ of 11, 10, and 12 dB, respectively.

Why would the measure vary across vowels? The amplitudes of A1 and P1 depend on the proximity of a formant to the FFT peaks of interest. For example, if P1 is always located as the harmonic peak closest to 950 Hz, it follows that its amplitude is affected by its distance from an oral formant. In a vowel such as /i/, the relatively low F1 (around 300 Hz) and high F2 (above 2000 Hz) are distant from the target region of 950 Hz, and so have only small influence, if any, on the P1 amplitude. But a vowel such as /u/, for which F2 is likely to be somewhere in the 1000- to 1200-Hz range, may have a greater effect on P1 amplitude. Low-back vowels such as /a/, which have a relatively high F1 and low F2, virtually surrounding the 950-Hz target region for the P1 amplitude measure, are even more problematic. Chen (1997) found the average [A1-P1$_{oral}$]–[A1-P1$_{nasal}$] index to be only 5.2 dB for /a/).[9] A clinician

[9]Chen (1997) described an approach to correcting for these vowel influences. Interested readers are encouraged to consult her paper for details.

interested in establishing a normative data base of the $(A1\text{-}P1_{oral})\text{--}(A1\text{-}P1_{nasal})$ index for comparison to clients with suspected or known velopharyngeal incompetence would do well to use speech materials in which low vowels are avoided.

Although a large-scale, normative database does not exist for A1-P1 amplitude differences in nonnasal environments, there is preliminary evidence for the clinical potential of this measure. Chen (1995) measured A1-P1 amplitude differences for vowels produced in nonnasal environments by children with impaired and normal hearing. She chose children with impaired hearing for this comparison because an important component of their reduced speech intelligibility is thought to be excessive nasalization of vowels. The children with normal hearing had A1-P1 differences for these vowels ranging from about 10 to 30 dB, with an average around 20 dB. In contrast, children with impaired hearing had A1-P1 amplitude differences ranging from about 1 to 15 dB, with the mean of these values clearly below 10 dB (values estimated from Chen, 1995, Figure 3, p. 2448). Of particular interest is Chen's finding of a relatively strong, negative correlation between A1-P1 differences and perceptual ratings of nasality for the children with hearing impairment. As the

A1-P1 amplitude difference decreased, children were perceived as increasingly nasal.

Because nasalization is a pervasive problem in a wide range of speech disorders, measures such as the Chen index (1995) should be pursued as supplements to other forms of nasality assessment. As presented in Figure 11–17, the measure is fairly simple, but identification of the A1 and P1 peaks is not always easy, especially when voice quality is poor and the glottal harmonics are not well defined. The technique may, therefore, have limited utility in clients with co-occurring velopharyngeal and laryngeal (voice) dysfunction.

SEMIVOWELS

In this chapter, /w/, /ɹ/, /l/, and /j/ are considered semivowels. /w/ and /j/ are also referred to as glides, /ɹ/ and /l/ as liquids, and the latter two sounds are also called rhotic and lateral, respectively. The term "semivowel" is a convenient way to group all four sounds because it captures a shared aspect of their production. All four sounds require movement to and away from a vocal tract constriction tighter than that for vowels, but not nearly so tight as required for obstruents (fricatives, stops, and affricates).

Figure 11–18 shows spectrograms of the four semivowels in VCV frames where V = /ɛ/. A quick glance at these spectrograms suggests a few prominent acoustic features of all semivowels. All have an interval during which F1, F2, and F3 are more or less constant, and relatively large transitions in at least one of the first three formants going into and out of these steady formant frequencies. The interval of relatively "flat" formants is called the *constriction interval*, and it is assumed to correspond to the articulatory phase of semivowel articulation when the vocal tract is *most* constricted. The length of the constriction interval for each semivowel is marked in Figure 11–18 by a horizontal bar between the 1.0- and 2.0-kHz calibration lines (the precise location of the horizontal bar along the frequency scale is not important; the position is different from semivowel to semivowel to avoid obscuring formants within the constriction interval). The duration of the each of the constriction intervals in Figure 11–18 is less than 100 ms, and in less carefully articulated speech is probably about 40 to 50 ms, on average (Dalston, 1975).

The constriction interval has a formant pattern in much the same sense as a vowel. The relative stability of these formant frequencies allows target values to be measured for the different semivowels. Do these formant frequencies distinguish the semivowels from

---

Spectrographic Challenges

Experienced acoustic phoneticians know that some spectrograms are easy to analyze, others are much more difficult. The "goodness" of a spectrographic display is usually easy to predict, based on characteristics of the person whose speech is being analyzed. Talkers with very high F0s and/or breathy voices are notoriously difficult to analyze, as are persons with a lot of nasal resonance. The low-amplitude, broad bandwidth formants in hypernasal speech complicate the precise identification of formant frequencies. Moreover, the most popular computer technique for formant frequency identification — linear predictive code (LPC) analysis — is based on a mathematical model that neglects the antiresonance "dips" described in Chapter 9. LPC formant estimates for a nasalized vowel are, therefore, often incorrect, and must be checked carefully on a spectrogram-by-spectrogram basis. This obviously complicates the use of LPC analysis in many speech disorders associated with velopharyngeal incompetence.

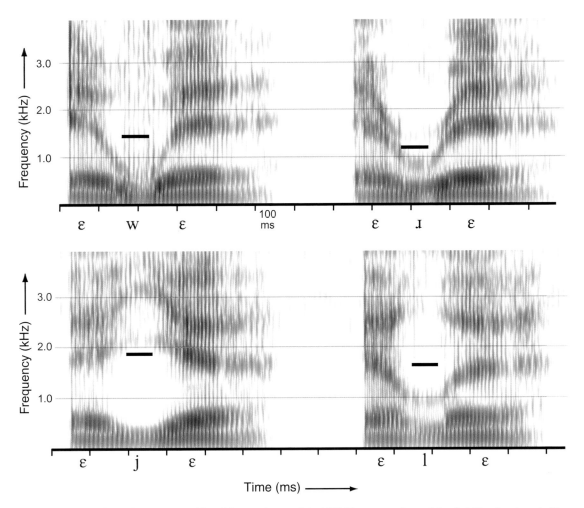

Figure 11-18. Spectrograms of English semivowels in VCV frames where V = /ɛ/. The horizontal bar located between 1.0 and 2.0 kHz in each spectrogram shows the approximate time interval corresponding to the constriction interval of each semivowel. See text for further explanation.

each other? F1 is quite similar across the semivowels, but unique F2-F3 patterns seem to characterize each of the sounds. Figure 11–19 shows how the semivowels in Figure 11–18 are separated in F2-F3 space. These formant frequencies, estimated by eye at the temporal midpoint of the horizontal bars in Figure 11–18, are plotted in Figure 11–19 (filled circles) together with values reported for young adult speakers by Dalston (1975; unfilled triangles = males, filled triangles = females) and Espy-Wilson (1992; unfilled squares). The values for a given semivowel are fairly consistent across the three different data sources, even though there are differences in speaker sex, age, and phonetic context of the semivowels (see Figure 11–19 caption). The ellipses are included to show the separation of the points for the four semivowels. Most obvious in this plot is the low F3 associated with /ɹ/, clearly different

from the F3s of the other semivowels. A distinguishing acoustic characteristic of rhotic articulation is the low F3, usually below 2000 Hz and very close to F2. Figure 11–19 shows just such a pattern: a horizontal line at roughly 2100 Hz can be drawn across the graph to separate /ɹ/ data from the other three semivowels. /w/ and /l/ both have a wide frequency separation between F2 and F3, as indicated by their general location in the upper left quadrant of the plot. /w/ and /l/ are distinguished from each other, however, by the generally lower F2 and F3 of /w/ as compared to /l/. Overall, this typically results in a greater F2-F3 separation between /l/ as compared to /w/. Finally, /j/ has a much higher F2 than the other semivowels. F3 of /j/ is also higher than the F3 of /w/, /ɹ/, and /l/. /j/ appears to occupy its own corner of the F2-F3 plot, clearly separated from the other semivowels.

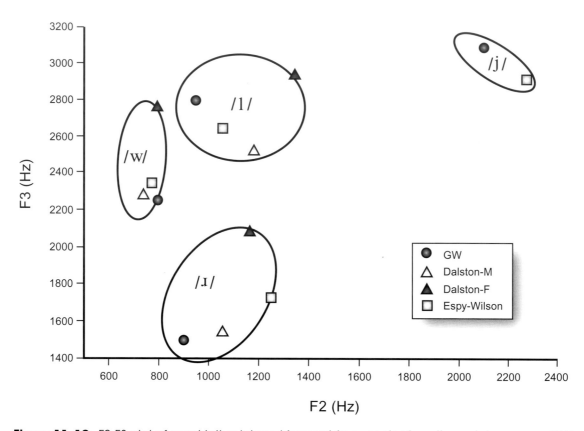

Figure 11–19. F2-F3 plot of constriction interval formant frequencies from three data sources. GW points (*filled circles*) are estimated formant frequencies (by eye) from the semivowels shown in Figure 11–18. Dalston-M and Dalston-F points (*unfilled and filled triangles, respectively*) are averages from Dalston (1975) for semivowels spoken as word-initial consonants in isolated words by three adult males and two adult females. Espy-Wilson (1992) points (*unfilled boxes*) are averages for intervocalic semivowels produced by two adult males and two adult females.

The pattern of formant transitions into and out of the constriction intervals also distinguishes among the semivowels. In very general terms, the important characteristics of these patterns are: (a) the specific formants that have large transitions into and out of the constriction interval, and (b) the direction (rising versus falling) of the transitions. For the purposes of this discussion, the direction of transitions is always referenced to the constriction interval. For example, in Figure 11–18, the VC (V = /ɛ/, C = semivowel) F1 transitions for all semivowels are falling into the constriction interval, and are rising for the CV part. With a special-case exception described below, the F1 transitions do not seem to distinguish among the four semivowels.

The direction of the F2 transitions into and out of the constriction interval easily separates /j/ from the other three semivowels. For /j/ the transition is rising into the constriction, and falling out of it. For /w/, /ɹ/, and /l/, there are fairly large, falling transitions into

the constriction interval, and rising transitions out of it. The magnitude of these transitions—the frequency range covered from the onset of the transition to its end—and the transition rate (transition magnitude/transition duration) are affected by the vowel context in which the semivowel is articulated. These context effects are very detailed and numerous. Interested readers should consult Espy-Wilson (1992, 1994) for relevant information.

The F3 transitions allow further distinction of /w/, /ɹ/, and /l/. /ɹ/ has a large falling (VC) and rising (CV) transition. This F3 transition is often immediately above (of greater frequency than) the F2 transition. The F3 transition seems to follow the F2 transition closely, especially just prior to and after the constriction interval. An F3 transition is often absent for /w/, or possibly has only very slight movement. The large F3 transition for /ɹ/ effectively separates its acoustic characteristics from those of /w/. The F3 transition for /l/, as shown in Figure 11–18, is rising slightly into the constriction interval and falling slightly out of it.

CV transition characteristics when C = semivowel are summarized in Table 11–2. When semivowels are in a symmetric VCV frame as in Figure 11–18, the VC and CV transitions are mirror images of each other. Table 11–2 uses a simple classification approach to transition type, much like that published by Espy-Wilson (1994). In this classification scheme, no two semivowels have exactly the same pattern of transitions to or from the following or preceding vowel. To be sure, the F1 and F2 transitions in this classification system are identical for /w/, /ɹ/, and /l/, but the F3 transition distinguishes among them. Note, however, the qualifications in Table 11–2 concerning the F3 transition of /w/ and the F1 and F3 transitions of /l/. These transitions may be especially sensitive to the identity of the following or preceding vowels. The F1 transition for /l/ + vowel sequences often appears to "jump" from the constriction interval to the following vowel, which may be the result of a sudden change in area function from a lateral articulatory configuration to the configuration for a following vowel (Narayana, Alwan, & Haker, 1997). Figure 11–18 shows this F1 "jump" in the CV part of /ɛlɛ/.

When the constriction interval and transition acoustics of semivowels are taken together, there is ample reason to believe the acoustic information is rich enough to distinguish among these sounds. Much like the case of nasals, discussed above, if the acoustic information is sufficient to distinguish among the

Table 11–2. Classification of CV Transition Type for the CV Sequence of a VCV Frame Where V = /ɛ/ and C = Semivowel

SEMIVOWEL	F1	F2	F3
/w/	rising	rising	flat[a]
/ɹ/	rising	rising	rising
/l/	rising[b]	rising	falling[c]
/j/	rising	falling	falling

[a]Some may rise, some may fall depending on context.
[b]Rise may look like a "jump"; see text.
[c]Very context-sensitive; some may be flat, some may rise.

semivowels, an automatic classification based on these acoustic characteristics should be successful in getting the sounds "right." As reported by Espy-Wilson (1994), however, there are frequent classification confusions between /w/ and /l/. These confusions occur because /w/ and /l/ are so similar acoustically (note the proximity of /w/ and /l/ data in Figure 11–19), and different phonetic contexts blur the subtle acoustic distinctions between them.[10]

The speech-language pathologist should know about semivowel acoustics because semivowel errors are frequent during phonological development. In both typical and delayed phonological development, /w/ for /ɹ/, /w/ for /l/, and /j/ for /l/ errors are not unusual. Perhaps the unique gesture characteristics of semivowels, of fairly rapid articulatory movement to and away from a constriction greater than required for vowels, but not so great as fricatives, make the sounds highly confusable. A somewhat different perspective is that the difficulty of mastering these sounds is not due to the similarity of their articulatory gestures, but rather to the similarity of the acoustic models of semivowels heard by the child as she is trying to connect perceptual representations of speech sounds with their production requirements. In this latter view, the child could produce the semivowels correctly if she were able to distinguish between them on a consistent basis.

This issue has been given some attention in the literature, by asking a simple question. When, for example, a child produces what appears to be a [w] for /ɹ/ error (as when a child is heard to say [waɪt] for the word "right"), is the error [w] acoustically similar or identical to a correctly produced [w] (when a child says [waɪt] for the word "white")? The question has been asked in two ways, when both the error and correct versions of the sound are obtained from the same child, or when the error sound is obtained from a single child and is compared to acoustic characteristics of the correctly produced sound collected from a group of children with normal articulation. Either approach seems to yield the same result: The acoustics of a [w] in a [w] for /ɹ/ error (or any other substitution error) are often *not* like the acoustics of normally articulated [w] (Chaney, 1988; Dalston, 1972; Hoffman, Stager, & Daniloff, 1983). In these analyses, the error [w] is different from correct [w] by having acoustic characteristics more or less between the error sound and the correct

---

[10]Speech-language pathologists are familiar with the distinction between light and dark /l/ ([l] vs.[ɫ]). Dark /l/ usually involves an articulatory configuration with a tighter constriction in the velar region or more posterior tongue position, as compared to light /l/. The dark /l/ constriction interval, therefore, has a higher F1 and lower F2 as compared to light /l/ (Narayanan, Alwan, & Haker, 1997). The higher F1 and lower F2 of dark /l/ may make it more confusable than the light /l/ with /w/, especially because of the lowered F2 in dark /l/ (see Figure 11–19, and notice how a lowering of F2 for /l/ would move it toward the /w/ region).

sound. A distinction is made by the child, but may be too subtle for human listeners to hear it, or even if they do hear a subtle distinction they may have a tendency to place it in a "comfortable" phoneme category—that is, to consider the distinction as a phonetic variant of a single phoneme category.

This finding seems to be consistent with the child's ability to hear the differences between the semivowels, but to have a limited ability to reproduce those distinctions. Acoustic characteristics that distinguish error [w] from correct [w] provide evidence for the child's knowledge of the required distinction between [w] and other semivowels. This knowledge is presumably obtained from the distinctions heard by the child, as produced by normally articulating adults and children. The acoustic analyses described above provide a level of understanding of a child's articulation behavior that appears to be unavailable when perceptual analyses alone are used to understand speech sound errors.[11]

Semivowel Durations

Specific data on semivowel durations are difficult to provide because it is challenging to segment semivowels from adjacent vowels (see Chapter 10). When constriction intervals can be segmented from the surrounding transitions—essentially a *phonetic* segmentation, as described in Chapter 10—they will have durations of 30 to 70 ms, with the majority of values toward the lower end of this range (Dalston, 1975). The duration of transitions into and out of the constriction interval are also in the 30- to 70-ms range. The combined time for the transitions and constriction intervals of semivowels may, therefore, be very brief (as short as 100 ms). This suggests a conclusion of very rapid, complex articulatory gestures occurring in a short amount of time, perhaps explaining, in part, why children master these sounds relatively late in the overall scheme of phonological development.

FRICATIVES

Fricatives are characterized by an interval of aperiodic energy whose spectrum and overall amplitude depend on place of articulation and, in some cases, voicing status. In English, fricatives are categorized as sibilants

(/s,z,ʃ,ʒ/) and nonsibilants (/f,v,θ,ð/) (the glottal fricative /h/ is discussed toward the end of this section). The sibilant-nonsibilant distinction is acoustically and perceptually meaningful because sibilants are more intense and have better-defined spectra than nonsibilants. "Better defined spectra" implies the presence of more easily identified spectral peaks and concentrations of spectral energy.

A general illustration of the acoustic bases of the sibilant-nonsibilant distinction is shown in Figure 11–20. Spectrograms are shown of the fricatives /s/ and /f/ in a VCV frame where V = /ɛ/. Superimposed LPC spectra for /s/ and /f/, computed over a 50-ms time interval centered at the midpoint of the frication noise, are shown immediately below the spectrogram. Along the baseline of the spectrogram, upward-pointing arrows show the frication onsets and offsets, based on the last glottal pulse preceding, and the first glottal pulse following the frication noise, respectively. The /s/ and /f/ durations are 174 ms and 154 ms, respectively.

The intensity difference between the sibilant /s/ and nonsibilant /f/ is seen easily in the spectrogram by the much darker frication noise for /s/. Note in the superimposed spectra the overall higher level of /s/ as compared to /f/. This kind of intensity difference is consistent for any sibilant-nonsibilant comparison, such as the /ʃ/ versus /θ/ comparison.

Behrens and Blumstein (1988) reported a typical intensity difference of 14 dB between voiceless sibilant and nonsibilant frication noises. Data reported by Jongman, Wayland, and Wong (2000) suggest a slightly smaller difference of about 9 to 10 dB. The sibilant-nonsibilant intensity difference applies to voiced fricatives (e.g., /z/ vs. /v/, or /ʒ/ vs. /ð/) as well, but the difference is probably not as great as in the case of voiceless fricatives (see Jongman et al., 2000, Table V, p. 1259). The higher intensity for sibilants is largely due to the presence of an obstacle, the teeth, in the path of the airstream emerging from the fricative constriction for /s,ʃ,z,ʒ/. As discussed in Chapter 9, the airstream striking the teeth creates a second turbulent flow source and boosts the overall energy of the source spectrum for these fricatives. The nonsibilants /f,θ,v,ð/ are produced with little or no obstacle in front of the constriction, and, therefore, have a weaker source spectrum than sibilants.

The difference in sibilant versus nonsibilant spectra is further appreciated by studying the superimposed spectra of the two sounds. The /f/ and /s/ spectra in

---

[11]The [w] for /ɹ/ examples presented here were chosen because of their clarity and frequency as errors in normal and delayed phonology. Many other examples could have been described; interested readers should consult Weismer, Dinnsen, and Elbert (1981), Weismer (1984), and Forrest, Weismer, Hodge, Dinnsen, and Elbert (1990) for additional examples.

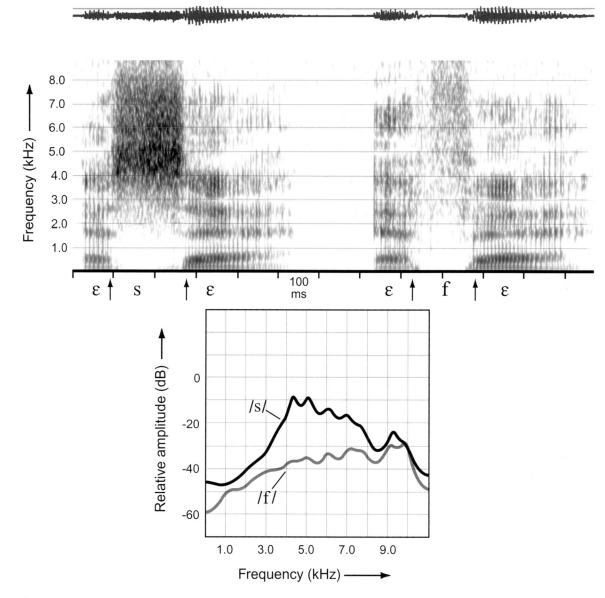

Figure 11-20. Spectrograms of the fricatives /s/ and /f/ in VCV frames where V = /ɛ/. Note the 0- to 8.4-kHz frequency range in these displays, to demonstrate the characteristic higher-frequency energy of frication noise. The upward-pointing arrows indicate the onsets and offsets of the fricatives, indicated by the last glottal pulse preceding the frication noise (onset) and the first glottal pulse following the frication noise (offset), respectively. Below the spectrograms LPC spectra ranging from 0 to 11.0 kHz are shown for the middle 50 ms of the frication noise; lighter line = /f/ spectrum, darker line = /s/ spectrum.

Figure 11–20 differ by the prominence (that is, the definition) of their peaks. The /s/ spectrum has two distinct, intense peaks, one around 4.3 kHz and the other just above 5.0 kHz. Both peaks are roughly 35 dB more intense than the lowest amplitude in the spectrum. In contrast, the /f/ spectrum has its greatest peaks just above 9.0 kHz and just below 10.0 kHz, roughly 30 dB more intense than the lowest energy in its spectrum (close to 0 kHz). Basically, the /f/ spectrum can be described as flatter than the /s/ spectrum (or the /s/ spectrum can be described as "peakier" than the /f/ spectrum). Sibilants typically have peakier spectra than nonsibilants, as shown in Figure 11–21 for the /ʃ/-/θ/ (left) and /z/-/v/ (right) contrasts.

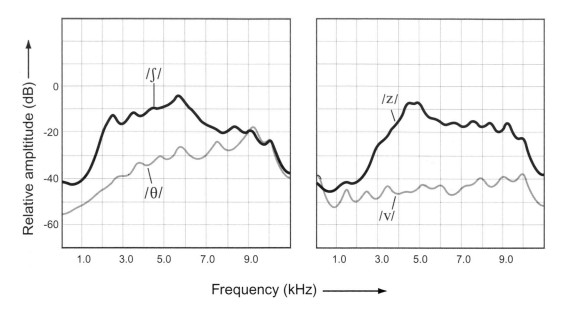

Figure 11–21. *Left panel:* LPC spectra for /θ/ (*light trace*) and /ʃ/ (*dark trace*). *Right panel:* LPC spectra for /v/ (*light trace*) and /z/ (*dark trace*). All fricatives were produced in a VCV frame where V = /ɛ/. Spectra were computed from the middle 50 ms of the frication noise.

As discussed in Chapter 9, quantification of the frequency characteristics of fricative spectra is not straightforward. Fricative spectra have sometimes been characterized with a single number, the peak frequency, defined as the frequency in the spectrum with maximum amplitude. For example, in Figure 11–21 the peak frequency for /ʃ/ is roughly 5.8 kHz, for /θ/ 9.2 kHz, for /z/ 4.5 to 5.0 kHz (there is a broad peak spanning this frequency range), and for /v/ 10.0 kHz. Jongman et al. (2000) reported that the simple measurement of peak frequency *statistically* distinguished fricative place of articulation when data were averaged across 20 speakers. The average, peak frequencies obtained by Jongman et al. for the four places of English fricative articulation are shown in Table 11–3. These peaks decrease in frequency as place of articulation moves backward in the vocal tract. As discussed in Chapter 9, this makes theoretical sense because the primary resonance of the vocal tract in fricative production derives from the cavity in front of the constriction, whose size increases as the place of articulation becomes more posterior. Larger resonators mean lower resonant frequencies.

The match between Jongman et al.'s (2000) peak frequency data and speech acoustic theory, however, should be approached with a certain degree of caution. The data, averaged across speakers (including sex) and vowel contexts, hide the substantial variation

Table 11–3. Average Peak Frequencies for Four Fricative Places of Articulation Reported by Jongman et al. (2000) for 20 Speakers Producing CVC Words in a Carrier Phrase

PLACE		PEAK FREQUENCY (Hz)
Labiodental	/f,v/	7733
Dental	/θ,ð/	7470
Alveolar	/s,z/	6839
Palatoalveolar	/ʃ,ʒ/	3820

Note: Data are for the first C in the CVC word. Peak frequencies were derived from spectra computed from the center 40 ms of the frication noise. Measurements were made from inspection of both FFT and LPC spectra.

in spectral details occurring from repetition to repetition for a given speaker, and across different speakers. One of these spectral details is the location of the peak frequency. In Figure 11–21, for example, the peak frequency of one of the author's /ʃ/ spectra (left panel) is approximately 1000 Hz higher than that of his /z/ spectrum (right panel). Not only are these numbers inconsistent with the *direction* of the effect reported by Jongman et al., in which alveolar fricatives have higher peak frequencies as compared to palatoalveolar fricatives,[12] but the actual values of the peak frequencies shown in Figure 11–21 are quite different from those listed in Table 11–3. For example, the peak frequency in Figure 11–21 for /ʃ/ is 5800 Hz, as compared to an average for /ʃ/ and /ʒ/ of 3820 Hz reported by Jongman et al. (2000). Substantial intra- and interspeaker variation in fricative spectrum details has been described by Narayanan (1995). Peak frequency as a descriptor of fricative spectra may separate fricative place of articulation with statistical reliability, but there is a great deal of error variation (unexplained data noise) in the statistical findings, and as Figure 11–21 shows it is easy to find exceptions to the trends reported in Table 11–3.

The measure "peak frequency" does not take advantage of a good deal of additional information in the fricative spectrum. For example, the fricative spectra in Figures 11–20 and 11–21 have varying shapes. Some seem to have energy "bunched up" in the middle (e.g., /ʃ/ and /z/), some have energy "tilted" to the right half of the spectrum, (e.g., /f/ and /θ/), and some seem nearly "flat" (e.g., /v/). These descriptions are based on the pattern of energy across all frequencies of the spectrum and, therefore, go substantially past the limited information of a single frequency at which maximum energy occurs. As discussed in Chapter 9, there is a way to represent the shape characteristics of an acoustic spectrum using the language of statistical distributions. The amplitude-by-frequency information in the *entire* spectrum is used to generate four numbers that represent the spectral shape. These numbers are called *spectral moments*.

Spectral moments are nothing more complex than basic statistical properties of a distribution of numbers. A distribution has a mean, a variance, a skewness, and a kurtosis. The mean is the average of all the numbers in the distribution, the variance is the degree to which those numbers are dispersed about the mean, the skewness is the degree of tilt of the distribution to the right or left of center, and the kurtosis is the extent to which the distribution is peaked or flat. In the language of acoustic phonetics, mean = the first spectral moment (M1), variance = the second spectral moment (M2), skewness = the third spectral moment (M3), and kurtosis = the fourth spectral moment (M4). The relationship of different distribution shapes—in the current case, spectral shapes—to number values is illustrated

in Figure 11–22. At the top of the figure is the symmetrical, normal distribution, typically described as having a mean of zero and variance of one. For present purposes, the normal distribution serves as a reference shape for other distribution shapes. This reference shape not only has a mean of zero and variance of one, but skewness and kurtosis values of zero. The two distribution shapes immediately below the normal shape show positive (left shape) and negative (right shape) skewness. When the majority of numbers in a distribution are bunched to the left-hand side and the right-hand tail is relatively long, the value of skewness is positive. The opposite case, where numbers are bunched to the right-hand side and the left-hand tail is long, is associated with a negative value of skewness. From an acoustic phonetics perspective, the concentration of vowel energy in the low frequencies should produce positive skewness values for vowel spectra. However, a sound such as /s/ has the majority of its energy in the higher frequencies (see the /s/ spectrum in Figure 11–20, and the discussion below of the pitfalls of spectral moments analysis) and, therefore, should have a negative value of skewness.

Variations in the "peakiness" of a distribution are illustrated in the bottom panel of Figure 11–22, with the normal distribution reproduced in blue. A distribution with a more pronounced peak than normal, shown by the green curve, has positive values of kurtosis. A shallower peak than normal, shown in red in Figure 11–22, has negative values of kurtosis. A comparison of the /v/ and /z/ spectra in the right-hand side of Figure 11–21 provides a good contrast in kurtosis values for two speech sounds. The /v/ spectrum is clearly flat and has a negative kurtosis, whereas the /z/ spectrum has distinct peaks and, therefore, a substantially more positive kurtosis.

The second spectral moment, variance, can be explained by considering the kurtosis shapes in the bottom panel of Figure 11–22. The very peaky distribution shown in green has its values "bunched up" near the center. This distribution has a low value of variance. In contrast, the relatively flat distribution in red has values spread across a wider range, which is associated with a higher value of variance. The /z/-/v/ spectrum comparison in Figure 11–21 shows the difference between a distribution having many values "bunched" toward the center (/z/) versus values spread across a

---

[12]The reversal of the direction expected from Jongman et al.'s (2000) data, and from speech acoustic theory, still holds even when the Figure 11–21 comparison is adjusted for mixing of place and voicing. Jongman et al. reported that voiced fricatives had somewhat lower peak frequencies than voiceless fricatives—about 300 Hz on average—but even when this is applied to the Figure 11–21 spectra the peak frequency difference is still around 700 Hz, and in the wrong direction.

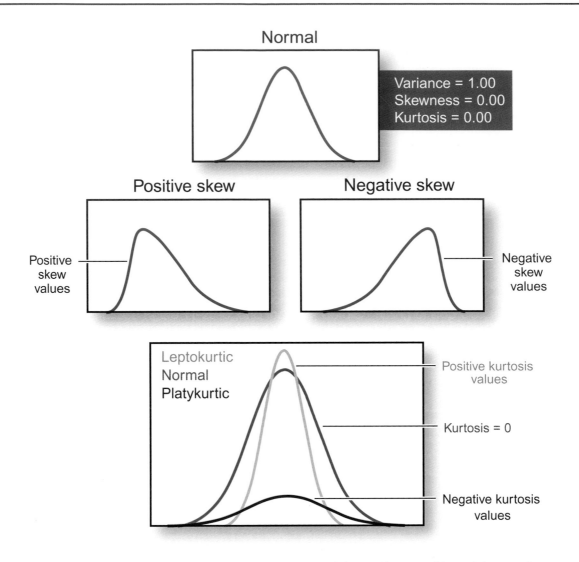

Figure 11–22. Distribution shapes illustrating a normal shape (*top graph*), and shapes showing skewness (*middle two graphs*), and kurtosis (*bottom graph*). Distributions with different variances are also illustrated in the bottom graph; see text for additional detail.

wider range (/v/). The /v/ spectrum is expected to have a larger variance than the /z/ spectrum.

Scientists have been interested in spectral moments for fricatives because the peak frequency approach to quantifying the spectra, as described above, focuses on only a single piece of information. This single piece of information presumably reflects the primary resonant frequency of the fricative (and, perhaps, not completely) and ignores other spectral variation that could be specific to different fricatives. In addition, early publications presenting qualitative analyses of fricative spectra (Hughes & Halle, 1956) suggested spectral shape as one possible distinguishing characteristic of fricative place of articulation. Forrest, Weismer, Milenkovic, and Dougall (1988) performed a spectral

moments analysis of the four English voiceless fricatives (/f,θ,s,ʃ/) and used these data to classify place of articulation in much the same way as the classification experiments discussed above for nasals. This classification experiment was performed not only to determine if the moments were useful in separating the four fricatives from each other (therefore demonstrating that spectral shape was an important characteristic of fricative acoustics), but to identify which moment(s) played the primary role in successful classification. In some sense, the results of Forrest et al. were disappointing, because the four voiceless fricatives were classified correctly only about 50% of the time. However, when sibilants were classified separately from nonsibilants, the latter were implicated as the reason for the poor classification results. Roughly 90% of the /s/-/ʃ/ classifications based on moments were correct, with skewness providing most of the classification accuracy. The classification of /f/ and /θ/, however, was near chance, suggesting that the moments did not distinguish them at all.

The confusions between /f/ and /θ/ in the Forrest et al. (1988) experiment are not surprising, given the weak intensity and often flat spectral characteristics of these sounds. Many classification errors, however, involved /s/ and /ʃ/ productions classified as /f/ or /θ/. Forrest et al. noted that the use of the four moments to classify fricatives neglects an important difference between sibilants and nonsibilants, namely, intensity of the frication noise. Many of the classification errors in Forrest et al., where sibilants were classified as nonsibilants, could have been avoided if frication intensity was included as a fifth classification variable.

Jongman et al. (2000), in a more extensive study of fricative acoustics, obtained spectral moments for all English fricatives produced by men and women in a variety of vowel contexts. Their moments data, averaged across speakers and vowels, are reproduced in Table 11–4. The data for the first moment (M1), which are given in units of Hz, are consistent with the theoretical discussion of fricative acoustics presented in Chapter 9.[13] M1 is nearly 2000 Hz higher for /s,z/ as compared to /ʃ,ʒ/, reflecting the difference in size of

Table 11–4. Spectral Moments Data for Fricatives

	M1	M2	M3	M4
/f,v/	5108	6.37	0.007	2.11
/θ,ð/	5137	6.19	−0.083	1.27
/s,z/	6133	2.92	−0.229	2.36
/ʃ,ʒ/	4229	3.38	0.693	0.42

Source: Data from Jongman et al. (2000, Table I, p. 1257).

Note: M1 = mean, M2 = variance, M3 = skewness, M4 = kurtosis. M1 values are in Hz, M2 values in MHz, and M3 and M4 values have no units (they are dimensionless, having been normalized). See Forrest et al. (1988) for computational details.

the resonator in front of the fricative constriction. The nearly identical M1 values for /f,v/ and /θ,ð/ are consistent with the absence of a resonating cavity in front of the constrictions for these nonsibilants. The M1s for /f,v,θ,ð/ are located roughly in the center of the analyzed frequency band (approximately 1–11,000 Hz). In the absence of a resonating cavity to shape the source spectrum, nonsibilant output (source × filter) spectra tend to resemble the aperiodic source spectra (see Chapter 9), which are relatively flat. This is why the M1s are so close to 5000 Hz, close to the center frequency of the analysis band.[14]

The M2 values listed in Table 11–4 also contrast the nonsibilants with the sibilants. Sibilant spectra have much smaller variances than nonsibilant spectra, which follows from the tendency of sibilant spectra to be peaky (that is, to have energy concentrated in peaks) and nonsibilant spectra to be flat (to have energy spread out across the entire spectrum).

The M3 data show a dramatic contrast between /s,z/ and /ʃ,ʒ/, the former having negative skewness, the latter positive skewness. This skewness contrast can be seen by comparing the /z/-/ʃ/ spectra displayed in Figure 11–21. The peaks for the palatoalveolar /ʃ/ are pushed to the lower-frequency, left-hand side of the spectrum, as compared to the higher-frequency peaks of the alveolar /z/. If the two spectra are thought of as distributions, the /z/ spectrum is tilted much more to the right than the /ʃ/, hence the negative skew value for /z/ and positive skew value for /ʃ/. The M3 values for /f,v,θ,ð/ are very close to zero, consistent with the essential flatness of their spectra.

In contrast to the values of the first three moments, values for M4 (kurtosis) reported by Jongman et al. (2000) are less easy to connect with known or expected characteristics of fricative spectra. The M4 values in Table 11–4 suggest that /f,v/ spectra are peakier than /ʃ,ʒ/ spectra, but this seems at odds with the large resonance peaks observed around 2000 to 4000 Hz for /ʃ,ʒ/ as compared to the typically flattened spectrum of /f,v/.

Some time has been spent explaining spectral moments and reviewing the relationship of values reported by Jongman et al. (2000) to spectral character-

---

[13]Although the mean of a normal distribution is zero, computation of the first spectral moment is based on frequency (Hz) and is not normalized like the zero mean of the normal distribution. M1 is computed by taking each frequency in the analysis band and weighting it by its amplitude. Thus, frequencies with greater amplitude are given more weight than frequencies with lesser amplitude in determining the M1 value of the spectrum. M1 can be interpreted as the primary energy concentration within the spectrum.

[14]Spectral moments are calculated within fixed frequency bands; the end frequencies of the moments reported in Table 11–4 are 1 Hz on the low end, and 11,000 Hz on the high end. The width of the band can be varied in whatever way an investigator desires, but it is typically dictated by the sampling rate and the low-pass filter cutoff frequency used when digitizing speech waveforms. For example, the moments reported in Table 11–4 (Jongman et al., 2000) were derived from waveforms sampled at 22,000 Hz and filtered with a cutoff frequency of 11,000 Hz.

istics of exemplar fricatives presented in Figures 11–20 and 11–21, or to characteristics expected from theoretical considerations. Spectral moments have become quite popular as a way to characterize fricative and stop-burst spectra. Most speech analysis programs, such as the one used to generate the spectrograms and spectra shown in this chapter, include algorithms to compute moments. One keystroke and four moments are reported. There are, however, three main problems with spectral moments that should be kept in mind when these measures are used as acoustic indices of fricative (or stop) production. First, the actual value of the moments is quite variable across different studies, and highly variable across speakers within a study. The reader is encouraged to compare fricative moments data published by Jongman et al., Fox and Nissan (2005), Tjaden and Turner (1997), Newman, Clouse, and Burnham (2001), and Tabain (2001) to gain a sense of the cross-study variation in these measures. Second, although moments quantify a lot of information in fricative spectra, they have not been successful in classifying fricative place of articulation. Forrest et al. (1988), Jongman et al., and Fox and Nissan all obtained the same results when classifying fricatives with moments (and some other variables). Typically, correct classification rates are about 90% for sibilants but only 60 to 70% for nonsibilants.[15] If spectral moments were the most inclusive and best way to represent the fricative spectrum, higher classification rates would be obtained.

The third problem with spectral moments consists of two interrelated subproblems. One of these subproblems is the tendency for high correlations between the moments, suggesting a lack of independence of the different measures. For example, because spectral moments are computed from a fixed analysis band, an M1 (spectral mean) of higher frequency is likely to have a more negative M3 (skewness). Stated otherwise, as the concentration of energy is "pushed" to the right of the analysis band (higher M1, as in /s/) the spectrum is tilted more to the right (more negative M3). Similarly, a more positive M4 (kurtosis), reflecting a spectrum in which there are very prominent peaks, likely has a smaller M2 (variance) because the energy is concentrated in a small frequency range (see bottom graph of Figure 11–22). The extent to which the moments are intercorrelated has not been reported in the literature

in a formal, large-scale analysis, but speech scientists who have used the analysis are aware of the lack of independence among the four measures.

The other subproblem is a lack of uniqueness between the numbers obtained in a moments analysis, and the actual shape of the observed spectrum. To understand this issue, consider the following thought experiment. A speech scientist is shown a list of formant frequencies in which each row consists of F1, F2, and F3 values. Based on these three formant frequencies, the speech scientist is asked to identify a vowel category. For example, the values F1 = 310, F2 = 2000, and F3 = 2800 would most likely be assigned the vowel category /i/. This would be a fairly easy task for a person with experience in acoustic phonetics. Even when the wrong vowel category was chosen it would almost certainly be adjacent in the vowel diagram to the correct category. Now, assume a similar experiment with the four spectral moments, the speech scientist's task being to select the most likely fricative category, or to draw the approximate spectral shape based on the numbers. This would be a daunting task for even the most seasoned expert. The difficulty of the task derives from the lack of independence of the moment values, as described above, and because a particular moment value can be associated with very different spectral shapes. This latter issue is especially relevant to the M2, M3, and M4 values.

These cautionary comments are not meant to negate the use of moments in describing fricative spectra. Spectral moments probably capture more information about a fricative spectrum than a peak frequency measure, and for certain distinctions, such as /s/-/ʃ/, seem to function quite well and are useful in revealing aspects of articulatory dysfunction in motor speech disorders and their response to clinical manipulations (Tjaden & Wilding, 2004). It may be the case that M1, in particular, is an excellent estimate of the peak frequency of *some* fricative spectra, particularly those of the lingual fricatives /s,z,ʃ,ʒ/ that tend to be relatively peaky. A claim has been made for /s/ spectra that M1 and the measurement of a single peak frequency produce essentially the same result (Iskarous, Shadle, & Proctor, 2011), but the underlying data are not shown and, even if true, the claim may not be applicable to analysis of other fricatives. Spectral moments are excel-

---

[15]The frequent confusions in classification experiments between /f/ and /θ/ and /v/ and /ð/ are almost certainly due to the similarity of their spectra and their weak intensity. Sounds that are not easily distinguished, or in the language of phoneticians, that do not meet a reasonable criterion of acoustic contrast, are often merged over time and lose their contrastive value. In English, for example, there are many dialects where the /ɪ/-/ɛ/ distinction is not made (in southern Indiana, for example, one both writes with a [pɪn] "pen" and wears a [pɪn] "pin"). A similar merger seems to be occurring between the labiodental and dental fricatives in African-American English, where forms such as [bof] "both" and [bɚfdeɪ] "birthday" are commonly heard (Craig, Thompson, Washington, & Potter, 2003). It is reasonable to assume the merger is being "provoked," in part, by the lack of discriminability between these sounds.

The Ultimate Social Consequence

The literature on speech sound development makes frequent reference to the negative social consequences faced by children who have speech sound errors. These are, of course, important, but none results in such extreme punishment as was meted out for an /s/-/ʃ/ confusion to the Ephramites of Biblical fame. As told in the Book of Judges in the Old Testament, a battle between the Gileadites and Ephramites resulted in the passages of Jordan being held by the Gileadites. Ephramites who desired safe passage were required to pass a verbal screening test that revealed whether or not they were friend or foe. Chapter 12, verse 6 says "Then said they unto him, Say now Shibboleth: and he said Sibboleth: for he could not frame to pronounce it right. Then they took him, and slew him at the passages of Jordan." Verse 6 goes on to say that 42,000 fell at the time. There is no record of how many went because their speech revealed them to be foe. The concept of a specific utterance that marks a person's geographical home was borrowed from this biblical story for the TIMIT (Texas Instruments/MIT) speech database, a huge collection of utterances from many different speakers, carefully transcribed and recorded for research use by speech scientists. The dialect group of the speakers in this database is revealed by two "shibboleth sentences," designed to be phonetically sensitive to dialect variation around the United States.

reliable marker of place of articulation for fricatives has often been driven by concerns with the lack of a consistent distinction in fricative *spectra* between /f,v/ and /θ,ð/. The fricative spectra of /s,z/ and /ʃ,ʒ/ are sufficiently distinctive from each other, and from /f,v/ and /θ,ð/, to cue place of articulation for listeners, but some other part (or parts) of the acoustic signal must contain the information to distinguish labiodentals from dental nonsibilants.[16] In an early experiment on fricative perception, Harris (1958) showed that the primary cue for the labiodental-dental distinction was the pattern of formant transitions at the release of the fricative. This idea has been accepted in the speech science community for many years, even in the absence of supporting data from acoustic measurements of actual speaker productions. As reviewed by Jongman et al. (2000), the evidence for the importance of formant transitions in distinguishing place of articulation for nonsibilant fricatives is mixed. Indeed, Jongman et al. failed to identify formant transition patterns that consistently separated the four places of fricative articulation, including the critical labiodental-dental distinction. Perhaps these sounds are inherently confusable and will disappear, over time, as a useful contrast in English (see footnote 14).

Fricative Duration

The literature on fricative duration has produced a fair amount of agreement on some basic facts. First, voiceless fricatives are longer than voiced fricatives, all other things being equal. The "all other things being equal" qualifier is important, because such factors as position-in-word (e.g., /ʃæk/ "shack" versus /kæʃ/ "cash"), stress level of the syllable in which the fricative occurs, speaking rate, immediate phonetic context (e.g., /sæk/ "sack" versus /stæk/ "stack"), among other variables, modify the duration of a particular segment. Second, among the voiceless fricatives and possibly also voiced fricatives, sibilants have slightly greater duration than nonsibilants.

Figure 11–23 is a spectrogram of the syntactically well-formed but semantically curious utterance, "Two scenes at the zoo failed to verify the shame." This utterance was constructed solely to illustrate fricative duration measures. Precise measures of fricative duration were made using a speech analysis program

lent measures, but care should be taken in their use and interpretation, and their relations to other measures of fricative spectra.

Formant Transitions and Fricative Distinctions

In the earlier section on nasal acoustics, the role of formant transitions at the release (CV) or onset (VC) of the nasal murmur was discussed as an acoustic correlate of place of articulation. Interest in formant transitions as a

---

[16]Most spectral analyses of frication noises have been confined to a highest frequency of 10.0 to 11.0 kHz, so there is always the possibility that /f,v/ could be distinguished from /θ,ð/ noise on the basis of spectral features above 10 kHz. Tabain (1998) examined just this hypothesis for speakers of Australian English and found no evidence for consistent spectral distinctions between the labiodental and dental fricatives in the frequency region above 10.0 kHz.

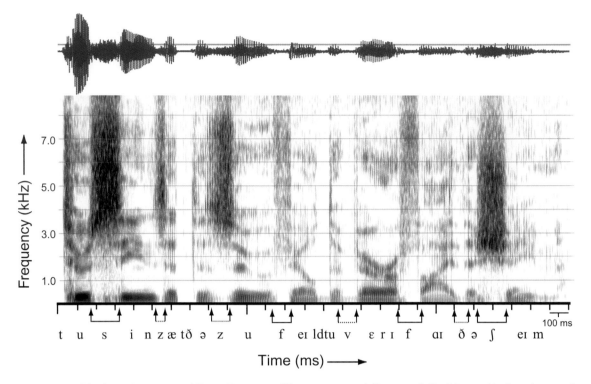

Figure 11-23. Spectrogram of the utterance "Two scenes at the zoo failed to verify the shame," constructed to show aspects of fricative duration. Eight fricatives in the utterance have been marked for duration; from left to right the fricative durations (all in milliseconds) are /s/ = 165; /z/ = 59; /z/ = 127; /f/ = 114; /v/ = 88; /f/ = 130; /ð/ = 71; and /ʃ/ = 162 (the /ð/ in /ætðə/ was not measured because the preceding stop makes it impossible to locate the /ð/ onset). Solid horizontal bars connecting the onset and offset arrows are for voiceless fricatives, dotted bars for voiced fricatives.

(TF32: Milenkovic, 2001) and the segmentation rules presented in Chapter 10. The actual durations for the eight fricatives marked in Figure 11–23 are provided in the legend. Fricative onsets and offsets are marked by arrows at the spectrogram baseline, and a horizontal bar connecting the base of the arrows shows the duration (solid lines = voiceless fricatives; dotted lines = voiced fricatives). The two voiceless sibilant durations (/s/ = 165 ms, /ʃ/ = 162 ms) are clearly a good deal longer than the voiceless nonsibilants (/f/ = 114 ms; /f/ = 130 ms). And, although one /z/ (in "zoo") has a duration of 127 ms, each of the other three voiced fricatives have durations less than 100 ms. Even these single examples of fricatives, in a connected-speech utterance (as compared to citation forms: see below) with variation in phonetic context and stress level, show patterns of duration largely consistent with the generalizations noted above. Voiceless fricatives are longer than voiced fricatives, sibilants are longer than nonsibilants.

A summary of published fricative duration data is provided in Table 11–5. Consideration of these data does not contradict the general outline of the two gen-

eralizations about fricative duration, but it does show that the magnitude of the voiceless/ voiced and sibilant/nonsibilant difference varies a good deal across studies. For example, among the three studies in which both /s/ and /ʃ/ were compared to /f/ and /θ/ durations (Behrens & Blumstein, 1988; Jongman et al., 2000; Umeda, 1977), only one (Behrens & Blumstein, 1988) reported findings supporting a decisive difference between sibilant and nonsibilant durations. The difference is slightly more convincing for the voiced sibilant-nonsibilant difference. Similarly, the difference in fricative duration for voiceless versus voiced stops is quite large in some studies (Jongman et al., 2000) and more subtle in others (Baum & Blumstein, 1987).

Two reasonable questions arise from this review of fricative duration. First, are there good explanations for the two general effects identified above? Is there a straightforward reason why sibilants would be longer than nonsibilants, and voiceless fricatives longer than voiced fricatives? Second, why do fricative duration values, and the magnitude of the sibilant-nonsibilant and voicing effects vary so much across studies?

Table 11-5. Selected Fricative Durations from Sources in the Literature

	/f/	/v/	/θ/	/ð/	/s/	/z/	/ʃ/	/ʒ/
Umeda[a]	122	78	119		129	85	118	85*
Baum & Blumstein[b]	149	116	134	107	174	152		
Behrens & Blumstein[c]	149		134		174		175	
Crystal & House[d]			72	41				
Jongman et al.[e]	166	80	163	88	178	118	178	123

Note: All data are for prestressed (fricatives preceding stressed vowels) fricatives, and are reported in milliseconds.

[a]Umeda (1977); *N* = 1 speaker, connected speech (reading).
[b]Baum & Blumstein (1987); *N* = 3 speakers, citation form syllables.
[c]Behrens & Blumstein (1988); *N* = 3 speakers, citation form syllables.
[d]Crystal & House (1988d); *N* = 6 speakers, connected speech (reading).
[e]Jongman et al. (2000); *N* = 20 speakers, citation form syllables.

Explanations for the effects are tentative, but may reveal something about the relationship of fricative duration measures to underlying speech physiology. More specifically, the process of making the measurements from acoustic records may explain part or all of the effects. For example, the longer duration of sibilants, as compared to nonsibilants, could reflect the generation of longer-duration, turbulent noise sources for sibilants. As presented in Chapter 9 and above, sibilants have more intense frication noise than nonsibilants largely because of the obstacle (teeth) effect. Perhaps the turbulent source is not only stronger, but also active over a longer period of time for /s,z,ʃ,ʒ/ as compared to /f,v,θ,ð/. This may be a reasonable explanation when scientists use the onset and offset of *frication noise* as the criterion for marking the boundaries of a fricative duration. Many scientists use this approach to measure fricative durations (e.g., Baum & Blumstein, 1987; Behrens & Blumstein, 1988; Jongman et al., 2000). The possible impact of this approach is illustrated by the subtle case shown in Figure 11–24, which shows two VCVs spoken by one of the authors with V = /ɑ/ and C = /θ/ (left) and /ʃ/ (right). Every attempt was made to produce these VCVs at the same rate and with stress on the second syllable. The vertical lines mark off the frication interval, defined by the onset (left line) and offset (right line) of the visible frication noise. When the measurements were made with maximal time expansion of the spectrographic display (to provide the best

temporal resolution), the frication intervals of /θ/ and /ʃ/ were 114 and 124 ms, respectively. This difference is fairly consistent with the sibilant-nonsibilant duration difference reported by Umeda (1977) and Jongman et al. If the duration of the frication noise is taken to reflect directly the duration of the fricative articulatory configuration, data shown in Table 11–5 and Figure 11–24 suggest that sibilants are indeed longer than nonsibilants.

As suggested above, however, fricative durations measured from a spectrographic or waveform display may not capture the entire duration over which a fricative configuration is maintained. Turbulent airflow, the source of aperiodic energy seen in acoustic displays of fricatives, occurs when airflow of sufficient magnitude is driven through a sufficiently narrow constriction or strikes an edge of a sharp object. It is easy to imagine a situation in which a fricative configuration is maintained but aperiodic energy is either not generated or is of such weak intensity as to be undetected in a spectrographic or waveform display. For example, the lingual nonsibilants /θ/ and /ð/ have a very broad, loose constriction (Tabain, 2001) which may not always be tight enough to generate turbulence, even though the fricative configuration is produced. Moreover, the conditions under which such loose constrictions occur may be more likely at the onset and offset of the fricative, when the constriction is being formed and released, respectively.

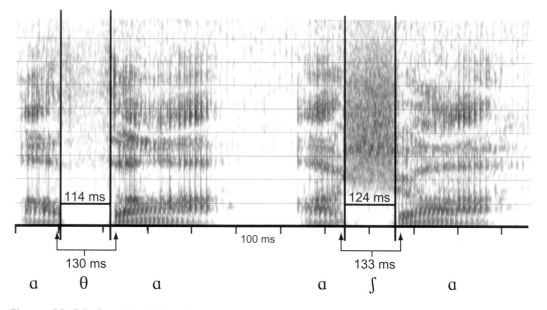

Figure 11–24. Spectrograms of the utterances /aθa/ (*left*) and /aʃa/ (*right*), illustrating the measurement of fricative duration under two criteria, one where the onsets and offsets of frication noise define the segment boundaries (*vertical lines running the length of the spectrogram*), the other where the preceding and following glottal pulses define the segment boundaries (*upward-pointing arrows*).

One way to address the possible mismatch of onset and offset of frication noise versus onset and offset of fricative *configuration* is to measure fricative durations from the last glottal pulse preceding the frication noise to the first glottal pulse following the noise. From an articulatory point of view, this makes sense because the last glottal pulse preceding frication is often timed to coincide with the onset of the supraglottal constriction (see review in Weismer, 2006, and below). In Figure 11–24, /θ/ and /ʃ/ durations measured with the glottal pulse criterion (boundaries marked by upward-pointing arrows) are 130 and 133 ms, respectively. Weismer (1980), using the glottal pulse criterion to measure fricative durations for nine speakers, reported mean, citation-form durations for /f/, /s/, and /ʃ/ of 180, 189, and 182 ms, respectively. These means were statistically indistinguishable from each other.

These considerations are offered to the reader in the spirit of an interesting scientific problem, rather than an endorsement of one measurement approach relative to another. The scientific problem shows how a measurement decision may affect conclusions about underlying articulatory processes. In particular, this issue shows how interpretation of acoustic data may require a good working knowledge of speech physiology. In the current case, the relevant physiology concerns the aeromechanics associated with fricative production.[17]

The second general effect for fricative durations, of consistently longer voiceless as compared to voiced fricatives, also requires a working knowledge of speech physiology. Data in Table 11–5 from Umeda (1977) and Jongman et al. (2000) suggest that voiceless fricatives in the prestressed position (in a CV or VCV frame where the vowel following the fricative is stressed) are nearly twice the duration of voiced fricatives. Why should there be such a large difference between the durations of cognate fricatives? The answer is most likely found in the different laryngeal behavior for voiceless versus voiced fricatives. Voiceless fricatives require the laryngeal devoicing gesture (LDG), an opening-closing movement of the vocal folds observed in many

---

[17]There is, at least in theory, a simple answer to the problem posed here. When fricative configurations are evaluated *directly* (by electropalatography techniques, or perhaps x-ray or electromagnetic techniques), are sibilant configurations longer than nonsibilant configurations, all other things being equal? This seems to be a straightforward question that might have been answered over the last 50 years of speech research, but, in fact, an answer requires very precise technical tools and measurement decisions. This is a fancy way to say that the relevant experiment has not been done.

languages for virtually all voiceless obstruents (e.g., Hirose, 1977; Löfqvist, 1980). The LDG differs from the opening-closing motions of the vocal folds during phonation in two important ways. First, the opening and closing movements of the LDG are produced under muscular control—the *posterior cricoarytenoid* muscle producing the opening, the *interarytenoid* (perhaps assisted by the *lateral cricoarytenoid*) the closing, with some assistance from the *cricothyroid* muscle to stiffen the folds and contribute to the cessation of phonation (Hirose, 1976; Löfqvist, Baer, McGarr, & Story, 1989). In contrast, the opening and closing movements during phonation are the result of aerodynamic and mechanical forces acting against the background forces exerted by laryngeal muscles (see Chapter 3). Second, the opening and closing motion of the LDG results in a very long event compared to the short-duration, opening and closing motion of a single cycle of vocal fold vibration. The LDG typically lasts roughly 120 to 150 ms, whereas a "long" period for one phonatory cycle would be roughly 10 ms in duration (for an F0 = 100 Hz, a rather low, average speaking fundamental frequency). The long duration of the LDG is critical to understanding the relatively long duration of voiceless, as compared to voiced, fricatives.

The laryngeal and supralaryngeal events shown schematically in Figure 11–25 for a VCV where C = /f/, /θ/, /s/, or /ʃ/, explain the relatively long duration of voiceless fricatives. Laryngeal events are shown as a function of time on the line labeled A_g, or "area of the glottis." These data are collected through an endoscope positioned directly above the vocal folds and connected to a recording device. The opening and closing motions of the vocal folds produce closely related variations in the area of the glottis (i.e., the area of the opening between the vocal folds). Upward deflections of the trace reflect opening of the vocal folds, downward deflections reflect closing of the vocal folds. The baseline represents full vocal fold approximation, such as occurs at the end of every phonatory cycle. The short duration cycles of opening-closing movements are the phonatory cycles associated with the vowels and the long-duration, larger opening-closing movement is the LDG. The time course of the LDG can be compared to events on the line labeled "Timing of fricative configuration." This is a schematic representation of the onset, duration, and offset of the grooved fricative configuration made by the tongue in contact with parts of the palate, or between the lower lip and upper teeth. This contact is shown as a raised box meant to represent the timing of the fricative configuration relative to the laryngeal events depicted on the top line. When the joint timing of laryngeal and supralaryngeal events is considered, the following conclusions can be drawn. First, the onset of the fricative configuration is synchronous with the onset of the LDG. Second, the

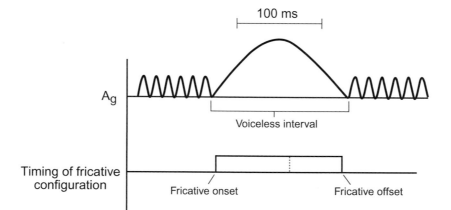

Figure 11-25. Schematic representation of laryngeal and supralaryngeal events for a VCV utterance in which C = a voiceless fricative. A_g = area of the glottis; upward movement on this trace indicates opening motions of the vocal folds, downward movement closing motions of the folds. The short-duration cycles are phonatory motions of the folds, the long-duration motion is the LDG. Voiceless interval = the duration of the laryngeal devoicing gesture. "Timing of fricative configuration" indicates the onset, duration, and offset of the supralaryngeal configuration required for fricative production. See text for additional details.

offset of the fricative configuration, presumably when the fricative is released into the following vowel, occurs approximately at the same time as the return of the vocal folds to the phonation-ready position (the closed position that permits aerodynamic and mechanical forces to create repeated oscillations of the vocal folds for phonation). Third, the LDG is in excess of 100 ms, as indicated by comparison of the LDG duration to the timescale indicated above the trace. In Figure 11–25 the duration of the LDG is labeled as the voiceless interval because it is the time during which the vocal folds are prevented from vibrating for phonatory purposes.

The LDG appears to "run off" as a preprogrammed gesture for production of a voiceless obstruent. "Preprogrammed," as used in this context, means that once the gesture is initiated it follows a more or less fixed amplitude and time course. The gesture does not seem to be subject to precise voluntary control (Löfqvist, Baer, & Yoshioka, 1981), supporting the idea that its amplitude and duration are relatively fixed, at least for a given stress condition and speaking rate. If the LDG is implemented for production of a voiceless fricative (as it should be for correct production of the sound class), and if its "programmed" duration is a fair amount in excess of 100 ms as shown in Figure 11–25, the duration over which the fricative configuration is maintained also must be in excess of 100 ms and, in fact, must nearly match the duration of the LDG. This is because an earlier release of the fricative, such as the point in time shown in Figure 11–25 by the dotted, vertical line, slightly past the most open phase of the LDG, would result in a substantial period of aspiration noise. The aspiration noise would extend from the time of fricative release until the LDG brought the vocal folds back to midline in preparation for phonation. This is clearly not desirable because aspiration noise following release of an English obstruent is a hallmark of voiceless stops, as well as the single voiceless affricate. An extended interval of aspiration noise following a fricative could result in misidentifications of fricatives as stops or affricates, and ultimately affect speech intelligibility.

The explanation for the relatively long duration of voiceless fricatives is, therefore, the need to "match" the duration of the supralaryngeal fricative configuration to the duration of the LDG—that is, to the voiceless interval duration. This duration is almost always in excess of 100 ms, and is likely to be somewhere within the 120- to 150-ms range, on average. Because voiced fricatives are not produced with an LDG, their duration is not required to be so long. The duration of most voiced fricatives is in the neighborhood of 100 ms, and often 15–20 ms less.

/h/ Acoustics

/h/ is often described as a glottal fricative because an aperiodic, continuant-type source is generated in and around the glottis. The glottis is partially or largely open during the production of /h/, and the aperiodic source is produced when the air jet emerging from the constriction between the vocal folds strikes the edges of the ventricular folds and epiglottis, generating turbulent airflow (Stevens, 1998, pp. 428–436). This is like the teeth-obstacle model presented above for fricatives /s/, /z/, /ʃ/, and /ʒ/, except in the case of /h/ the obstacles are structures immediately above the vocal folds.

The source-filter acoustics for /h/ are quite complex (Stevens, 1998). Here, /h/ acoustics are summarized in a few major points with reference to spectrograms of the utterances "Ohio" (/ohɑɪjo/) and /əˈhe/ (Figure 11–26). In both utterances, /h/ is in the intervocalic position, and the approximate onsets and offsets of the /h/-intervals are indicated by upward-pointing arrows at the spectrographic baseline. The /h/-interval clearly contains aperiodic energy, as expected when the

---

Survival of the Phonetic Fittest

Speech and language are constantly changing, always evolving. This is certainly the case in phonetics, where "strong" phonetic segments maintain their contrastive identity, weak phonetic segments do not. In Chapter 9 the ongoing merger of the /f/-/θ/ contrast in African-American English was cited as one such case. /h/ qualifies as phonetically "weak" for the same reason as /f/ and /θ/—it has very low amplitude. The sound is, therefore, subject to possible disappearance from sound inventories or deletion in connected speech. The weak energy of /h/ gives it poor survival potential in, say, noisy or difficult communication settings. Mielke (2003) reported an experiment in which Turkish speakers deleted /h/ at fast speaking rates, but only in phonetic environments where the /h/ energy was most likely to be extremely weak and, therefore, hard to perceive. It is almost as if speakers recognized the phonetic conditions in which /h/ was likely not to be heard, and took advantage of this knowledge by deleting the sound production from their utterances. /h/ deletion is common in other languages as well, the best known example being Cockney English (Norman, 1973).

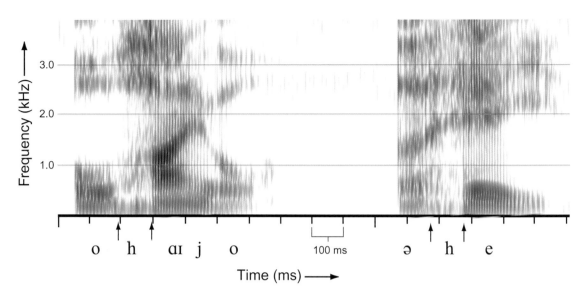

Figure 11-26. Spectrograms of the utterances /ohaɪjo/ (*left*) and /əˈhe/ (*right*), illustrating the acoustics of /h/. The onsets and offsets of the /h/ interval are indicated by upward-pointing arrows.

sound source is the result of turbulent airflow. Careful examination of the /h/-intervals indicates evidence of relatively weak glottal pulses—compared to the pulses in the surrounding vowels—mixed in with the noise. Intervocalic /h/ often has a combination of aperiodic and weak, periodic energy, suggesting that the abducted vocal folds are still vibrating loosely, with minimal or absent closed phases (Ladefoged, 2005).

Formants can be detected during the /h/-intervals. These regions of dark, aperiodic-plus-voicing energy seem to line up with the formants of the following (and to some extent, preceding) vowel. This makes sense under the assumption that /h/ is produced with the vocal tract shape of the surrounding vowel(s), except with a largely aperiodic source. Perhaps this is why Ladefoged (2005, p. 58) described /h/ as a "noisy vowel." The most complete treatment of the formant structure of /h/-intervals is found in Lehiste (1964, pp. 141–180). A recent study by Robb and Chen (2009) provides evidence that formants during the /h/ noise are basically the same as formants of following vowels. The consideration of /h/ as "phonetically neutral"—such as in the studies of vowel acoustics in /hVd/ frames—seems to be justified.

A dramatic feature of this noisy, formant-bearing interval is the relative weakness of energy around F1 as compared to the much more intense energy of the upper formants. This intensity difference is shown clearly in both /h/s in Figure 11–26. The weak energy in the F1 region of the /h/ noise is the result of sound absorption in the trachea. Interestingly, this fact explains why

a person with a breathy voice may also suffer intelligibility problems as a result of indistinct vowels. The loss of F1 energy due to vocal fold vibration characterized by poor closure, a physiological correlate of breathy voice, may result in a loss of vowel distinctiveness. The effect of a breathy voice on communication may, therefore, be more than just a voice problem. The effect may extend to segmental (acoustic) integrity and, therefore, speech intelligibility.

STOPS

Stop consonants enjoy a special status in speech acoustics. Their acoustic characteristics have been the subject of much study and debate, and their role in the perception of speech has a very long and contentious history. Stops are also attractive for acoustic-phonetic study because they are the only consonant type to occur in *all* languages of the world (Ladefoged & Maddieson, 1996). Within languages, stops are among the most frequently occurring consonant segments (Maddieson, 1997). Study of the acoustic phonetic characteristics of stops can, therefore, be considered as a "high-yield" effort in understanding both speech production and perception.

Spectrograms illustrating the basic properties of stop consonants are shown in Figure 11–27. The stops /t/ and /d/ are shown in VCV frames, where V = /ɑ/. The upper spectrograms show the stops produced with

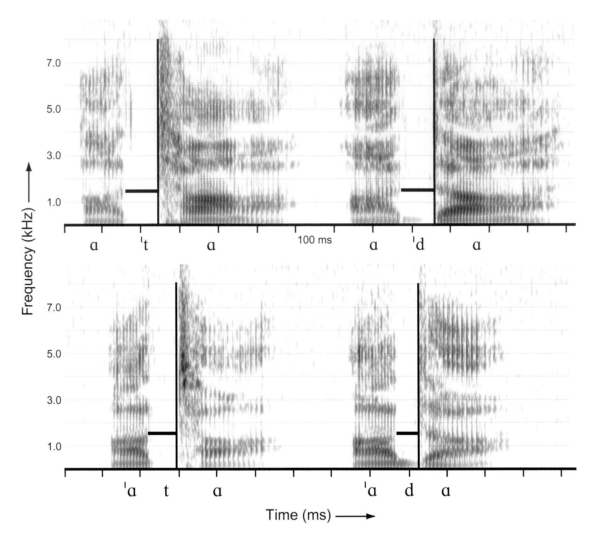

Figure 11-27. Spectrograms of the utterances /a'ta/ and /a'da/ (*top*) and /'ata/ and /'ada/ (*bottom*). Each stop has a closure interval consisting of no energy (voiceless stops) or a small amount of periodic energy on the baseline (voiced stops). The duration of each closure interval is shown by the length of the heavy, horizontal bar between 1.0 and 2.0 kHz. The vertical line at the end of each closure interval shows the location of the burst.

stress on the second syllable (/a'ta/, /a'da/), whereas the lower spectrograms show stops with stress on the first syllable (/'ata/, /'ada/). The frequency range for these spectrograms is roughly 0 to 8.5 kHz.

Closure Interval and Burst

As discussed in Chapter 9, the familiar acoustic markers—the manner cues—of a stop consonant are a closure interval followed by a burst. The closure interval corresponds to the period of time during which the vocal tract is completely sealed by the closed velopharyngeal port and the contact between the lips (for

/p/ and /b/) or between the tongue and points along the palate (for /t/, /d/, /k/, and /g/). Closure interval durations are indicated in Figure 11–27 by the heavy horizontal bars placed around 1.5 kHz. Spectrographically, closure intervals for voiceless stops appear as the white (no energy) intervals seen in Figure 11–27 for the two /t/s. For voiced stops, the closure interval is white with periodic energy along the baseline indicating vibration of the vocal folds (see /d/ closures in Figure 11–27). In connected speech, including sentences and extended reading passages, closure intervals for any of the stop consonants are rarely greater than 70 ms, the majority having durations of around 60 ms (Byrd, 1993; Crystal & House, 1988b). When closure duration measures are made for more formal utterances, such as CVCs or other simple syllabic frames, sometimes called "citation forms" (and sometimes produced in carrier phrases such as "Say ____ again"), the values are often longer than 70 ms but rarely exceed 100 msec (Luce & Charles-Luce, 1985; Stathopoulos & Weismer, 1983).

A fair amount has been written about variation in closure durations due to stop voicing and place of articulation. Various sources in the literature claim that stop closure durations are longer for voiceless, as compared to voiced stops, and become increasingly shorter as place of articulation moves back in the vocal tract (that is, /p/ closures are longer than /t/, which, in turn, are longer than /k/). The claims for the voicing effect are most interesting, because they clearly have their origin in a famous perceptual experiment performed and reported by Lisker (1957). Lisker measured for a single speaker the closure durations of a small number of /p/s and /b/s in words such as "rapid-rabid," "staple-stable," and "rupee-ruby." For this intervocalic, poststressed environment, Lisker measured average /p/ and /b/ closure durations of 120 and 75 ms, respectively. He then showed, using tape-splicing techniques, that an original "ruby" utterance (with glottal pulses eliminated in the closure interval) having a stop closure duration of 65 ms could be made to sound like "rupee" by lengthening the closure interval, leaving all other aspects of the signal unchanged. Lisker showed the same effect by systematically shortening an original 130-ms closure interval for /p/ in "rupee," which produced "ruby" responses at relatively short durations even though the closure interval contained no glottal pulses. Lisker concluded from these and other experiments that "closure durational differences play a major role in the voiced-voiceless stop distinction *in the type of context studied*" (1957, p. 48, emphasis added).

Lisker's (1957) carefully conducted experiment was overgeneralized by subsequent scientists who studied the link between stop voicing and closure duration. First and foremost, Lisker was careful to restrict his conclusion to the specific context of intervocalic, poststressed stop consonants. Selected closure duration data from the literature are summarized in Table 11–6, where values are included both for individual places of articulation (first six columns of data) as well as averaged across place but within voicing category (last two columns). The phonetic context and conditions under which stop closure durations were measured are described in the notes at the bottom of the table. These data support only a very subtle version of Lisker's proposed voicing effect on stop closure durations, especially when data are taken from connected speech. For example, Umeda (1977) reported only a

6-ms difference between the closure durations of voiceless and voiced stops for the 'VCV environment (see the two right-hand columns in Table 11–6 for Umeda, note b). Luce and Charles-Luce (1985) reported larger differences in the 'VCV environment (27 ms when the stop was followed by a vowel, 18 ms when the stop was followed by an /s/; see Table 11–6, notes e and f). The four speakers studied by Luce and Charles-Luce produced CVC citation forms in carrier phrases. Similar findings were reported by Stathopoulos and Weismer (1985; Table 11–6, note d). Even so, the effects reported by Luce and Charles-Luce and Stathopoulos and Weismer are of substantially lesser magnitude than the closure duration difference (~60 ms) used by Lisker as a starting point for typical voiceless and voiced stops. What is clear, however, is that the voiceless-voiced difference for closure durations does not extend to stops generally, across different contexts. Crystal and House (1988b), and Byrd (1993) reported voiceless stop closure durations to be between 2 and 6 ms longer than voiced stops in connected speech (Table 11–6, notes g and h), certainly not a difference of sufficient magnitude to serve as a useful perceptual cue to the voicing status of a stop.

The preceding discussion of closure duration as a potential marker of the voicing status of a stop consonant says nothing about the role of periodic energy during the closure interval. Lisker (1957) was careful to qualify his perceptual findings with the same concern, as he had eliminated glottal pulsing during the closure interval as a potential cue to the voicing status of the labial stop in the "rupee-ruby" pair he studied. Voiceless stops as produced by speakers who are free from speech disorders typically have no glottal pulsing during the closure interval. Occasionally, one or two glottal pulses extend from a preceding vowel into the beginning of a voiceless closure interval, as can be seen along the baseline of /ɑtɑ/ in Figure 11–27. This represents a small mistiming between the onsets of the LDG and the vocal tract closure for the stop. In the case of voiced stops, however, voicing of the closure interval is often incomplete. The typical pattern, illustrated nicely by /ɑdɑ/ in Figure 11–27, is for voicing to be present at the start of the closure interval but to terminate some milliseconds prior to the burst (voicing terminates roughly 30 ms prior to the burst in this example). As discussed in Chapter 9, this may occur when the oral air pressure developed in the vocal tract approximates the magnitude of the tracheal pressure. If there is an insufficient pressure difference across the vocal folds, they will not vibrate; it makes sense for the pressure difference to become insufficient later, rather than earlier in the closure interval.

Table 11–6. Selected Stop Closure Durations from Sources in the Literature. All data are reported in milliseconds.

	p	b	t	d	k	g	Voiceless	Voiced
Umeda[a]	89	90	77	83	69	69	78	81
Umeda[b]	67	57	25	26	61	53	51	45
Stathopoulous & Weismer[c]	96	92	82	76	72	68	83	79
Stathopoulous & Weismer[d]	87	66	44	41	71	56	67	54
Luce & Charles-Luce[e]	93	61	68	51	84	52	82	55
Luce & Charles-Luce[f]	89	77	89	62	75	60	84	66
Crystal & House[g]	66	55	—	—	61	60	54	52
Byrd[h]	69	64	53	52	60	54	59	56

[a]Umeda (1977); *N* = 1 speaker, connected speech (long reading passage), V'CV environment.

[b]Umeda (1977); *N* = 1 speaker, connected speech (long reading passage), 'VCV environment.

[c]Stathopoulos & Weismer (1983); *N* = 6 speakers, CVCVC citation forms in carrier phrase, V'CV environment.

[d]Stathopoulos & Weismer (1983); *N* = 6 speakers, CVCVC citation forms in carrier phrase, 'VCV environment.

[e]Luce & Charles-Luce (1985); *N* = 4 speakers, CVC citation forms in long carrier phrases, closure for second C measured preceding vowel /ɪ/, stops, therefore, in 'VCV environment, with C = word final.

[f]Luce & Charles-Luce (1985); *N* = 4 speakers, CVC citation forms in long carrier phrases, closure for second C measured preceding fricative /s/, stops, therefore, in 'VC/s/ environment, with C = word final.

[g]Crystal & House (1988b); *N* = 6 speakers, connected speech (two reading passages), data for /p,b,k,g/ are for stops in prevocalic, word-initial stops; voiced/voiceless data are for stops in all positions.

[h]Byrd (1993); *N* = 630 speakers, connected speech (sentences), all phonetic contexts pooled.

Flap Closures

The case of /t/ and /d/ in the intervocalic, poststressed position of words is particularly interesting, and serves to illustrate how the style of speech—formal versus less formal—can influence speech segment durations. The single speaker studied by Umeda (1977) produced /t/ and /d/ closure durations of 25 and 26 ms in the 'VCV context, respectively (Table 11–6, note b). For the same kind of context, Luce and Charles-Luce (1985) reported /t/ and /d/ closure durations of 68 and 51 ms (see Table 11–6, note e). At first glance, Umeda's (1977) values seem very short compared to other closure durations in Table 11–6, but, in fact, they are almost

identical to intervocalic, poststressed flap durations (/t/ = 26 ms; /d/ = 27 ms) reported by Zue and LaFerriere (1979) for six speakers producing words such as "rater" (/reiɾɚ/) and "matter" (/mæɾɚ/). Luce and Charles-Luce's much longer intervocalic, poststressed closure durations for /t/ and /d/ almost certainly reflect, in part, the more formal speech style associated with citation form. Luce and Charles-Luce's lingua-alveolar closure durations also reflect the word-final position from which their stop closure durations were measured (see Table 11–6, notes e and f). As Byrd (1993) has reported, flaps occur in this word-final position when they are intervocalic and poststressed, but are less likely to occur than when the lingua-alveolar stop is located *within* a word (e.g., flaps would be expected in the words "rooter" and "ruder," but perhaps not so frequently in "root a lot," where the lingua-alveolar stop occurs in word-final position).

Closure Duration and Place of Articulation

Data in Table 11–6 can be used to evaluate the effect of place of articulation on stop closure duration. When closure duration values in the two columns for labial stops are compared to the lingua-alveolars and dorsals, there is clearly a tendency for labials to have the longest durations. Differences between lingua-alveolar and dorsal closure durations are less convincing.

Stop Voicing: Some Further Considerations

The acoustics of stop consonant voicing are complex. A famous article by Lisker (1986) listed *16* potential acoustic measures that could differentiate the /p/ and /b/ in minimal pairs such as "rapid" versus "rabid." It seems, therefore, as if there are multiple "candidate" acoustic cues to the voicing distinction for stop consonants. According to Lisker, the notion of "candidate" cues for stop voicing means that they *may* signal the difference between voiced and voiceless stops, but are not *all* necessary to make the distinction a good one. In fact, the particular cues that may signal the voicing status of a stop are context dependent. This context dependency includes not only where the stop is located relative to other sounds and the prevailing prosodic conditions (e.g., word medially versus word-initially? pre- or poststressed?), but also the relational status of the candidate cues to the voicing distinction. Lisker provides an excellent example of the latter dependency, noting that even though the duration of the closure interval can signal the difference between "rabid" and "rapid," it will not do so if the [b] closure interval is fully voiced. In this case, the word will be heard as "rabid" no matter how long or short the closure interval.

In fact, the simplest acoustic cue to the voicing of stop consonants would seem to be this most straightforward one, namely, whether or not the closure interval contains glottal pulses. It seems logical to expect voiced stops to be produced with closure intervals containing glottal pulses, and voiceless stops to have no voicing during the closure. Whereas the absence of glottal pulses during a voiceless closure interval is almost always the case, the presence of glottal pulses during the closure interval of a voiced stop is a more complicated phenomenon. First, as discussed earlier in the chapter, glottal pulses do not always fill the entire closure interval of a voiced stop closure. The pulses may begin at the onset of the closure interval but terminate well before the stop is released. Depending on how much of the closure interval is actually voiced (i.e., contains periodic energy generated by the vibrating vocal folds) as well as the intensity of the pulses that are present, the closure may have a voiced or voiceless quality when judged by a listener. In the absence of consideration of other potential cues to the stop voicing distinction, the voiced stops could, therefore, be considered more vulnerable to perceptual errors (i.e., voiceless-for-voiced stop errors) than voiceless stops (voiced-for-voiceless errors). Interestingly, literature on stop voicing errors in dysarthria and apraxia of speech is consistent with this asymmetry, that speakers are more often heard to produce voiceless-for-voiced than voiced-for-voiceless errors (Marquardt, Reinhart, & Peterson, 1979; Platt, Andrews, & Howie, 1980). The extent to which this asymmetry reflects true substitution errors, as compared to phonetic errors in which voiced closure intervals are only partially voiced and, therefore, perceptually ambiguous and judged by listeners as voiceless stops, is unknown.

The potential ambiguity of a partially voiced closure interval may be reduced or eliminated as a result of the value(s) of one or more of the other cues to stop voicing. The best-studied cue to stop voicing is voice-onset time (VOT), defined as the time interval between the burst and the first glottal pulse of a following vowel. Because the value of VOT is grossly correlated with the presence or absence of glottal pulses within the closure interval, VOT may remove any ambiguity concerning the voicing status of a stop. This is true in English (at least) and for stops preceding stressed vowels (at least). Why should the value of VOT be associated with the presence versus absence of glottal pulses within the closure interval?

The answer has to do with the laryngeal devoicing gesture, discussed above with reference to the voicing distinction for fricatives (see Figure 11–25). Figure 11–28 repeats the schematic presentation of Figure 11–25, but with the vocal tract timing (labeled as "Timing of stop closure") now appropriate for a voiceless stop closure (rather than a voiceless fricative constriction). The LDG is identical to the one shown in Figure 11–25 for a voiceless fricative. In particular, note how the onsets of the LDG and supralaryngeal closure for the stop are synchronized, as well as the LDG duration of well over 100 ms. All this is the same as in Figure 11–25. The striking difference in Figure 11–28, as compared to Figure 11–25, is the release of the stop consonant closure interval roughly 60 to 70 ms after its onset (as

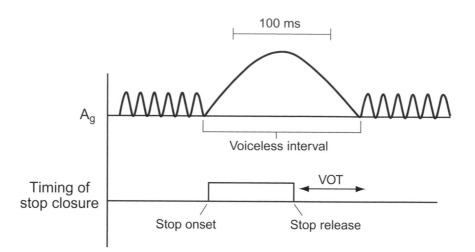

Figure 11-28. Schematic representation of laryngeal and supralaryngeal events for a VCV utterance in which C = a voiceless stop. A_g = area of the glottis. See Figure 11–25 legend for other details. "Timing of stop closure" indicates the onset, duration, and offset of the supralaryngeal configuration required for stop consonant production.

compared to the maintenance of the fricative constriction for the entire duration of the LDG in Figure 11–25). This earlier release, shortly after the widest separation of the vocal folds during the LDG, means that a significant interval of time will elapse between the stop release and the time when the vocal folds are brought together to resume vibratory activity. This interval is the VOT, and its relatively long duration results because the stop is released well before the LDG has completed its opening-closing movement. Voiced stops do not have an LDG. During the closure interval, the vocal folds remain more or less in the midline, close to, or in, the phonation-ready position. The vocal folds vibrate and cause glottal pulses to appear within the closure interval as long as there is a sufficient pressure differential (tracheal pressure minus oral pressure) across the vocal folds. But even if vocal fold vibration ceases halfway through the closure interval, when the supralaryngeal stop closure is released, the vocal folds are near or in the midline position and ready to resume vibrating almost immediately. This is the reason why the value of VOT is grossly correlated with the presence versus absence of glottal pulses within a stop closure interval. The absence of glottal pulses throughout the closure interval implies the presence of the LDG, which in turn results in a relatively long VOT. Glottal pulses within the closure interval, even if ceasing well before the stop release, imply the absence of the LDG and, therefore, the readiness of the vocal folds to resume vibrating very soon after the stop release.

VOT values have been reported many times since the classic study of Lisker and Abramson (1964) defined the measure and showed how it varied in different languages and speaking conditions. Extensive reviews of VOT data are available in Cho and Ladefoged (1999), Auzou et al. (2000), and Weismer (2006). Figure 11–29 summarizes VOT data for English by showing typical values along with selected factors known to modify the measured values. The VOT continuum shown in Figure 11–29 ranges between −30 and 50 ms and is marked off in 10-ms steps. Immediately above the horizontal time line phonetic symbols indicate typical VOT values for stops in sentences, as reported by Lisker and Abramson for four speakers. For example, Lisker and Abramson (their Table 17) reported average VOTs for /p/, /t/, and /k/ of 28, 39, and 43 ms, respectively. Each of the voiced stops has two entries along the VOT time line. One set is in the positive part of the continuum (7, 9, and 17 ms for /b/, /d/, and /g/, respectively), the other shows the three sounds grouped together with an arrow pointing to values more negative than −30 ms. Lisker and Abramson (1964) noted that some voiced stops are produced with voicing beginning *before* their release, and designated these as *prevoiced* with negative VOT values. Just as positive VOT values represent the delay between the burst and first glottal pulse of the following vowel, negative VOT values represent the time by which glottal pulses within the closure interval *precede* the burst. Both positive and negative VOT values are common in voiced stop production. The pre-

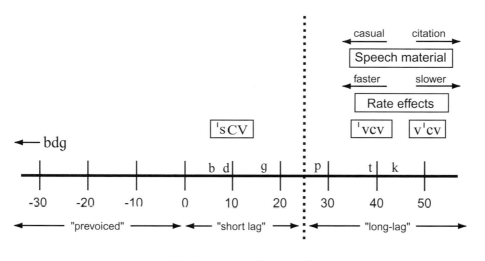

Voice-onset time (ms)

Figure 11-29. Graphic summary of VOT data from English speakers. A VOT continuum ranging from −30 ms to +50 ms is shown, and effects are indicated by the phonetic symbols and boxes above the continuum line. See text for additional detail.

voiced, voiced stops reported by Lisker and Abramson all had VOTs more negative than −30 ms, the last negative value on the continuum shown in Figure 11–29.

Figure 11–29 shows a vertical dotted line at 25 ms along the VOT continuum. This line designates a boundary between typical positive VOTs for voiced and voiceless stops. Voiceless stops can be expected to have VOTs exceeding 25 ms (*long-lag* VOTs), whereas voiced stops have VOT's less than 25 ms (*short-lag* VOTs) (Weismer, 2006).

The boxes above the VOT continuum and to the right of the 25-ms boundary identify factors that cause VOT to vary in systematic ways. These boxes are in the long-lag range of the VOT continuum because the effects are typically most prominent for voiceless stops, with much smaller effects on the short-lag VOTs of voiced stops. VOT is affected by the position of a voiceless stop relative to a stressed vowel. Longer VOTs are measured when the stop precedes, as compared to follows, a stressed vowel. The box containing the V'CV frame has been placed to the right (longer VOTs) of the 'VCV box to indicate this effect. In fact, VOTs for voiceless stops in 'VCV frames may be so short as to place them in the short-lag range (Umeda, 1977). The effect of speaking rate on VOT, indicated in Figure 11–29 by the box and arrows immediately above the stress effects, are predictable from the direction of rate change. Slower rates produce longer VOTs for voiceless stops (shown by the arrow pointing to the right), and faster rates produce shorter VOTs (left-pointing arrow) (Kess-

inger & Blumstein, 1997). The reduction (shortening) of long-lag VOTs at very fast speaking rates, however, is rarely so dramatic as to encroach on the short-lag range (Kessinger & Blumstein, 1997; Summerfield, 1975). Finally, the topmost box indicates that speaking style affects the value of long-lag VOTs. Longer VOTs for voiceless stops are produced in more formal speaking styles, sometimes referred to as citation form or "clear" speech (Krause & Braida, 2004; Smiljanic & Bradlow, 2005). Casual speech styles yield shorter VOTs. The difference between formal and casual speaking styles is likely to involve a difference in speaking rate. Formal speaking styles typically have slower rates than casual styles (Picheny et al., 1986).

A special case of VOT modification for voiceless stops is indicated by the "sCV" box above the short-lag range. "sCV" stands for prestressed s + stop clusters, in words such as "stop," "skate," "speech," "astounding," and so forth. Voiceless stops in s + stop clusters have short-lag VOTs (Umeda, 1977), as illustrated by the spectrograms in Figure 11–30. The first two words in this spectrogram are "peach" and "speech," with the VOT measurement for the two /p/s shown along the baseline. These intervals have a left-hand boundary at the /p/ burst and a right-hand boundary at the first glottal pulse of the following vowel. The 55-ms VOT for the /p/ in /pitʃ/ clearly fits the long-lag expectation for voiceless stops, whereas the 10-ms VOT for /p/ in /spitʃ/ illustrates the short-lag outcome of producing a voiceless stop in an s + stop cluster. This shortening

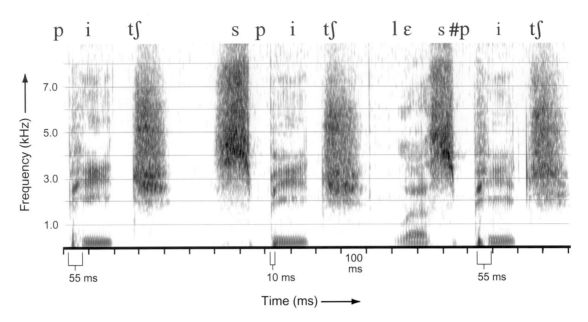

Figure 11–30. Spectrograms of the utterances /pitʃ/, /spitʃ/, and /lɛs#pitʃ/, showing how VOT varies when preceded by an /s/ in the same syllable (/spitʃ/) and across a word boundary (/lɛs#pitʃ/). VOT intervals are shown on the baseline.

effect seems to require that the s + stop cluster be part of one syllable, however (Davidsen-Nielsen, 1974). In Figure 11–30, the right-most spectrographic pattern is for the sequence /lɛs#pitʃ/, where the s + stop cluster crosses a word boundary (symbolized by "#"). In this case, the VOT for /p/ is in the long lag range, essentially the same as the /p/ VOT in "peach."

In summary, the value of VOT can be used in many cases as a correlate of the voicing status of a stop consonant. Long-lag stops are typically voiceless, and short-lag stops are typically voiced. The "mismatches" between VOT values and the voicing status for stops usually occur only for voiceless stops whose VOT values are measured in the short-lag range. This can occur when voiceless stops are in the poststressed position of a word, and should occur with near certainty when a voiceless stop is part of an s + stop cluster within a single syllable.

Finally, something must be said about VOT values in other languages. Many languages have stop voicing distinctions, but "cut up" the VOT range in different ways as compared to English. For example,

Korean has a three-way voicing distinction for each place of articulation, with the VOT range of roughly +20 to 120 ms "cut up" in three ways for the contrast (Cho, Jun, & Ladefoged, 2002). In contrast, French has a two-way voicing contrast in which the VOT continuum is "cut up" differently than in English. The voiced stops of French all have negative VOTs (i.e., they are prevoiced), and *short-lag*, positive VOTs for voiceless stops (Kessinger & Blumstein, 1997). This is why the voiceless stops of French are said to be unaspirated. Cho and Ladefoged (1999) provide an excellent analysis and interpretation of how very many different languages exploit the VOT continuum to "implement" their unique voicing contrasts.[18]

Bursts

Material presented in Chapter 9 describes the burst as the acoustic result of the sudden and rapid loss of oral air pressure at the release of a stop constriction. In practice, the isolation of a burst from the following fri-

[18]Voicing contrasts may be implemented in several different ways, including manipulation of the VOT continuum. This is not to say that VOT is the only way to effect a voicing contrast, just one of the more popular, at least among speech scientists who enjoy measuring it and perhaps among speakers of different languages, too (Kingston & Diehl, 1994). The popularity of VOT as a measurement object in languages of the world can be gauged by the results of a citation search one of your authors did on October 4, 2012. He used "VOT" as the keyword in the *Linguistics and Language Behavior Abstracts* (LLBA) database and received 558 "hits" (articles with "VOT" in the title), extending back to the 1970's. That's a lot of research on VOT!

cation interval (see Chapter 9) is exceedingly difficult. Theoretical analyses (Stevens, 1998; and see Johnson, 2003) suggest a duration of less than 5 ms for the true burst interval of a stop. In the acoustic phonetics literature, the term "burst" is often used in a somewhat broader sense to include the burst plus the following 10 to 20 ms into the frication interval. This broader use of the term "burst" is justified by the following summary of material from Chapter 9. Although the aeromechanical bases of the burst source and frication source are different, their spectra are quite similar. Because both source spectra are shaped significantly by the resonator in front of the source, the output spectra for the "true" burst and the following frication interval tend to be very similar. The use of the term "burst" to include the burst plus a brief part of the frication interval is, therefore, not a case of mixing apples and oranges. For the discussion that follows, the term "burst" is used in this broader sense of the 20–30 ms interval following the burst "spike" seen on waveforms and spectrograms.

Bursts are considered one of the hallmarks of the stop manner of production. In laboratory experiments involving citation-form speech, stops are almost always produced with a clear burst. Interestingly, in more connected forms of speech such as reading, a significant number of stop consonants have no identifiable burst even when perception suggests a "good" stop has been produced (Byrd, 1993; Crystal & House, 1988c). This is yet another example of how speech style can modify acoustic phonetic phenomena.

Stop bursts have been the focus of a great deal of research. In particular, the spectrum of stop bursts has been studied in an attempt to demonstrate that each of the three places of stop articulation in English is associated with a unique spectral shape. This problem was framed early in the history of speech acoustics research by Halle, Hughes, and Radley (1957) who measured spectra for stop bursts in simple CV syllables, where C = each of the English stops and V = /i/, /ɪ/, /ʌ/, /ɑ/, and /u/. Their analyses were similar to ones shown in Figure 11–31, where speech waveforms are shown for /pʌ/, /tʌ/, and /kʌ/ and a 20-ms increment beginning at the burst is marked off for spectral analysis. This interval is shown below each waveform in Figure 11–31 by the horizontal line whose endpoints are indicated by upward pointing arrows. Halle et al. isolated these 20-ms intervals and for each one computed a Fourier spectrum for the frequency range 250 to 10,000 Hz (the Fourier spectra shown in Figure 11–31 have a slightly wider frequency range, namely 0 to 11,000 Hz).

Halle et al.'s (1957) observations concerning the spectra of these burst intervals have been replicated

(with some minor differences) in several studies. Halle et al.'s observations were stated in terms of spectral shapes, that is, the relative distribution of energy across frequency. They described labial bursts as having primary concentration of energy in the lower frequencies, lingua-alveolar bursts with flat spectra or an emphasis of energy in the high frequencies (by which they meant, above 4.0 kHz), and dorsal stops as having prominent energy peaks in the midfrequency regions, meaning roughly between 1.5 and 4.0 kHz. In Figure 11–31, the /p/ burst has a relatively flat spectrum between 0 and 5.0 kHz and decreasing energy between 5.0 and 11.0 kHz; the /t/ burst has clearly increasing energy from 0 to 5.0 kHz and decreasing energy at the higher frequencies; and the dorsal burst has two large, midfrequency peaks of energy, one around 1.8 kHz and the other at 4.2 kHz. Despite the difference in speakers and (probably more importantly) the different frequency analysis bands, the spectral shapes in Figure 11–31 are very consistent with the major summaries offered by Halle et al. in their study of stop burst spectra. Based on these observations, it seems reasonable to claim that place of articulation is differentiated by the spectrum of the stop burst. If this is true, listeners presumably can use this information to identify place of articulation for stop consonants.

Perhaps it seems obvious that the burst has unique spectral characteristics for the three different places of articulation. After all, the acoustic theory of speech production predicts different resonant frequencies depending on the location of a constriction in the vocal tract. Clearly, the different constriction locations for the three places of articulation are accompanied by differences in vocal tract shape over the first few milliseconds following the release of a stop. Reliable differences in stop burst spectra as a function of place of articulation should, therefore, be expected. Speech scientists use the term *acoustic invariance* to refer to the stable, place-specific acoustic characteristics discussed here. An acoustically invariant characteristic of a particular speech sound is one that is always found in the waveform, regardless of who is producing the utterance or under what conditions the utterance is spoken.

This view, although attractive and apparently logical, neglects the well-known phenomenon of coarticulation. There are different ways to define coarticulation, but a more or less conventional definition makes the point: Coarticulation is the influence of one segment on another. Stated otherwise, the articulatory (and hence acoustic) characteristics of a particular segment depend on the articulatory (acoustic) characteristics of adjacent, and in some cases nonadjacent, segments. In the case of

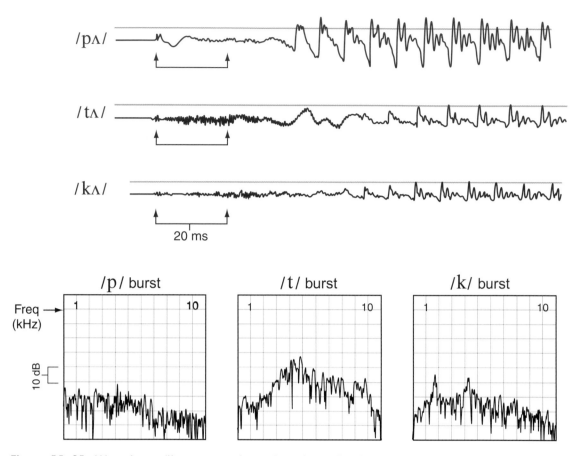

Figure 11–31. Waveforms (three upper traces) and spectra (lower three panels) for the stop consonants and initial part of vowels in /pʌ/, /tʌ/, and /kʌ/. A 20-ms interval, beginning at the stop burst, is indicated in the upper three traces by the horizontal line whose endpoints are marked by upward pointing arrows. This is the interval over which Halle et al. (1957) computed spectra for the stop burst. The Fourier spectra shown at the bottom of the figure are computed for the 0- to 11-kHz range. Each division along the frequency axis is a 1.0-kHz increment, each division along the intensity axis a 10–dB increment.

stop burst spectra, the important question is: How stable is the spectrum for a particular stop place of articulation when the following vowel (or any preceding or following segment) varies? If stop burst spectra vary in a significant way depending on the following vowel, the claim of unique spectral characteristics for the three different places of stop articulation may be difficult to defend. Vowel induced variation could result in highly variable stop burst spectra for a given place of articulation, with too little acoustic stability to serve as a reliable cue to place identification.

Figure 11–32 shows an example of a vowel effect on a burst spectrum. Two spectra are shown, both calculated for a 26-ms interval starting at the burst of the /t/ in /ɑti/ (light trace) and /ɑtu/ (dark trace). The analysis band is limited to 0 to 5 kHz and the spectra have been smoothed. The smoothing of the spectra,

which eliminates the detail of individual Fourier-spectrum components as if a continuous line were drawn to connect the many energy peaks while ignoring the dips and other details, was performed by calculating the LPC spectrum for the 26-ms interval (see Chapter 10). These two spectra have obvious differences, but are also very similar in an important way. The main difference between the spectra is the emphasis of lower frequencies for /tu/ as compared to /ti/. The /tu/ spectrum has rather large peaks at 2.8 and 3.7 kHz, whereas the /ti/ spectrum lacks dramatic peaks below 4.0 kHz but has steadily increasing energy up to roughly 5.0 kHz, where a peak is present. Stated more generally, the /t/ burst followed by /u/ has more low-frequency energy when compared to the /t/ burst followed by /i/, at least for this 0- to 5.0-kHz analysis band. From the perspective of coarticulation this makes

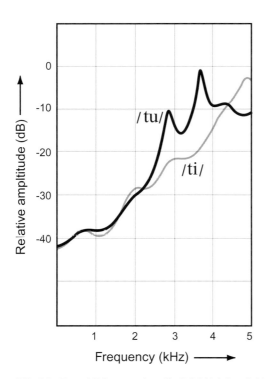

Figure 11–32. Two LPC spectra (0–5.0 kHz) for /t/ bursts produced before an /u/ (*dark line*) and an /i/ (*light line*). A comparison between these spectra shows the effects of vowel coarticulation on /t/ burst acoustics.

spectral variation in the burst spectrum due to speaker differences and coarticulation (that is, as a result of a particular stop being articulated with a variety of vowels) while preserving the more global spectral shape that was presumably the constant, or invariant acoustic characteristic of the stop burst. The templates were named *diffuse-falling* for bilabials, *diffuse-rising* for lingua-alveolars, and *compact* for dorsals. Examples of LPC spectra consistent with these templates are shown in Figure 11–33.

According to Blumstein and Stevens (1979), the diffuse-falling template fit most of the bilabial bursts, the diffuse-rising template the lingua-alveolar bursts, and the compact template the dorsal bursts. The diffuse-falling template had peaks between 0 and 5.0 kHz of roughly equivalent magnitude or with somewhat decreasing energy as frequency increased. In contrast, the diffuse-rising template showed peaks increasing in amplitude with increasing frequency. Both the diffuse-falling and diffuse-rising templates were likely to have multiple peaks of energy (energy diffusely spread across the spectrum), but with essentially opposite tilts: the falling template was tilted down and the rising template was tilted up. The compact template, however, had energy focused in a single, midfrequency peak somewhere between 1200 and 3500 Hz. Burst spectra shown in Figure 11–33 for the voiced stops /b/, /d/, and /g/, followed by the vowel /ɛ/, are more or less consistent with these descriptions. It is not too difficult to see the /b/ burst spectrum as flat or falling at higher frequencies, the /d/ burst as rising, and the /g/ burst as having a central peak of energy around 3.0 kHz. The stops from which these bursts were extracted were produced by one of the authors in V'CV frames, and the spectral analysis was derived from a 26-ms interval starting at the burst, just as in the Blumstein and Stevens study.

Blumstein and Stevens' (1979) description of place-specific spectral templates for stop consonant bursts is very much consistent with the more qualitative observations of Halle et al. (1957), reviewed above. Blumstein and Stevens, however, were the first scientists to quantify the *consistency* of these spectral templates in the classification of stop place of articulation. After the templates were finalized, six speakers produced 900 CV stops where C = /b,d,g,p,t,k/ and V = /i,e,a,o,u/, in all combinations and with each combination repeated five times (6 stops × 5 vowels × 5 repetitions × 6 speakers = 900 stops). Every stop, therefore, was produced with a wide variety of vowels to create a large amount of burst spectrum variation due to coarticulation. Stevens and Blumstein asked the following, two questions: Even with vowel-induced variation (see example in

sense because the formants of /u/ concentrate more energy in the low frequencies, whereas the formants of /i/ have more high-frequency concentration. These different concentrations of vowel energy influence the concentration of energy in the burst spectra.

The commonality in these two spectra is the steadily increasing energy from 0 to nearly 4.0 kHz, despite the difference in the location of prominent peaks. In this analysis band, both spectra are tilted to the higher frequencies. Perhaps the gross, upward tilt for /t/ bursts is the critical acoustic correlate to this place of articulation, and is always present even when the following vowel influences details of peak location and magnitude. The auditory system may be able to strip away "local" spectral detail and use the gross spectral shape to identify stop place of articulation.

In a classic acoustic phonetics study, Blumstein and Stevens (1979) attempted to demonstrate the uniqueness of such spectral shapes for the three different places of stop articulation. After examining for a small number of speakers LPC burst spectra for a 26-ms interval starting at the burst and for the 0- to 5.0-kHz analysis band, Blumstein and Stevens designed "spectral templates" for each of the three stop places of articulation. These templates were meant to allow

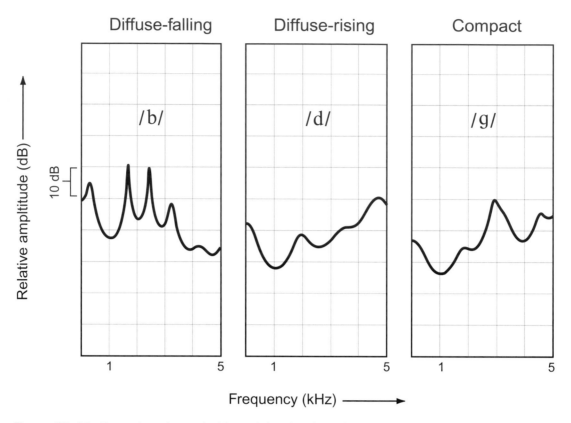

Figure 11–33. Examples of spectral templates for stop place of articulation, based on 26-ms burst spectra (LPC). The three templates—diffuse falling, diffuse rising, compact—were developed by Blumstein and Stevens (1979).

Figure 11–32) do the templates still capture a consistent spectral characteristic related to place? And are these consistencies found for different speakers? LPC spectra were prepared for each of the 900 stops and then *visually* classified by fitting each spectrum to each template and judging it as a match, or not a match. The results of this rather complicated procedure can be stated in simple terms, even if the interpretation is not so simple. Roughly 85% of the burst spectra were both correctly matched to the "correct" place template and correctly rejected by the "incorrect" templates. The last point needs some clarification. Each burst spectrum was compared to *each* template and a decision of "match" or "no match" was made. Blumstein and Stevens were looking for "match" when a burst spectrum from a particular place fit that place's template, and "no match" when the same burst was compared to the two other place templates. This implies that one burst spectrum might fit more than one of the three templates, and indeed this occurred in a small number of cases.

Is an 85% "correct match" and "correct rejection" performance good? Blumstein and Stevens (1979)

thought so, concluding that their visual spectrum-matching experiment demonstrated the existence of acoustic invariants for stop place of articulation, at least in CV syllables. Later experiments measuring different types of smoothed burst spectra also demonstrated successful classification of place of articulation (85–95% correct rates), either by visual matching or using automatic (statistical) classification procedures (Forrest et al., 1988; Kewley-Port, 1983; Kobatake & Ohtani, 1987; Nossair & Zahorian, 1991). The question, therefore, is not whether classification of stop place from burst spectra can be done with reasonable success, but *is the success good enough*? More generally, *why does the answer to this question matter*?

Acoustic Invariance and Theories of Speech Perception

The answer to the question of acoustic invariance for stop place of articulation is so important because of the profound role it has played in the development of theories of speech perception. Here, a brief summary of the issues is provided. More detail is provided in Chapter 12.

Early in the history of speech research, many speech scientists did not believe there were consistent acoustic characteristics for a given stop place of articulation. These scientists were convinced that the influence of different vowels on stop consonant acoustics was too great to allow something constant to remain in the acoustic signal that indicated reliably which place of articulation had been produced. Interestingly, this conclusion of "no acoustic invariance" (note the curious, double negative; despite the literary inelegance, this is a famous phrase in the speech science literature) was mostly derived from a series of well-known *perceptual* experiments conducted at the Haskins Laboratories (located originally in New York City, now for many years in New Haven, Connecticut). These experiments used a device called a *pattern-playback machine* to convert painted replicas of spectrographic patterns into sound. This device, described in more detail in Chapter 12, allowed an experimenter to create spectrographic patterns of any type to determine how these patterns, or variants of them, affected a listener's perception of sound identity.

When the Haskins scientists painted a pattern based on a real spectrogram, they typically did not reproduce every spectrographic detail. In a sense, the painted patterns were somewhat like stick figure or schematic representations of real spectrographic patterns. In the course of preparing these patterns, the scientists discovered something interesting. They could elicit perception of a stop-vowel syllable with a pattern having only F1-F2 transitions and following steady states. Stated otherwise, a painted representation of a burst was not necessary to create the auditory impression of a stop consonant (see Liberman, Cooper, Shankweiler, & Studdert-Kennedy, 1967, for a review of this work and relevant citations; and Story & Bunton, 2010, for a modern version and interpretation of this experiment).

Examples of two burstless, painted patterns are shown in Figure 11–34. The schematic F1 and F2 in both patterns contain transitions followed by a steady state, the latter defined as the interval during which the formant frequencies remain constant. When the pattern on the left was converted to sound and played to listeners, they heard /di/. The pattern on the right was heard as /du/. If the transition portions were eliminated and only the steady states played to listeners, they clearly heard the vowels /i/ (left) and /u/ (right).

Note in Figure 11–34 how different the F2 transition is for the perception of the /d/ in /di/ versus

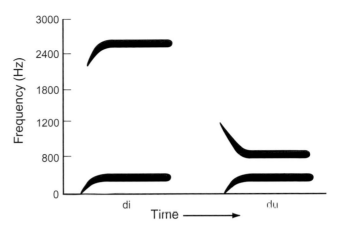

Figure 11–34. Burstless, painted patterns of formant transitions and steady states used in early Haskins Laboratories experiments to elicit perception of the consonant /d/ in two vowel environments. Adapted from Liberman et al. (1967).

/du/. The reader, after an examination of these two patterns, may have already asked the following question, relevant to the discussion of acoustic invariance: Why did two such different patterns of formant transitions result in the perception of the *same* stop consonant? The Haskins scientists determined, in fact, that for any place of articulation a wide variety of F2 transition patterns was associated with the perception of the same stop. The different F2 transitions depended on which vowel was paired with a particular stop consonant. If the vowel context had such a profound influence on the acoustic characteristics related to place of articulation of a stop, the Haskins scientists argued that there was no acoustic invariance for the place feature of stop consonants. This conclusion led to the development of a theory of speech perception, discussed more fully in Chapter 12, that downplays (if not eliminates) a primary role for auditory acoustic analysis in the perception of speech.

Blumstein and Stevens (1979), as well as other investigators who have had success in classifying stop place of articulation using the burst spectrum, argued against the position taken by the Haskins scientists. The demonstrated ability, in different studies, to assign 85 to 95% of burst spectra to the "correct" place of articulation seemed to point to a sufficient amount of acoustic invariance for the listener to use for important phonetic decisions, at least in the case of stop place of articulation. Researchers interested in the issue of acoustic invariance, or the lack of it, could reasonably argue that the Haskins studies were bound to find what appeared to be unmanageable variability in the acoustic properties of a given stop consonant. This is because the Haskins scientists focused almost all their attention on the transition patterns, not the spectrum of the burst interval, a classic case of looking for the right thing in the wrong place. In defense of the Haskins scientists, however, they did recognize the importance of the burst spectrum for *some* vowel contexts (Liberman et al., 1967), but never investigated the actual stability of those burst spectra in spoken utterances. The Haskins conclusions concerning the lack of acoustic invariance for stop acoustics were, in fact, based almost exclusively on perceptual, not production experiments.

A recent study has shown that a model of vocal tract acoustics has certain "hot spots" for stop consonant articulation and the resulting pattern of formant transitions into and out of the closure interval. Story and Bunton (2010) identified regions in and around the bilabial (/p, b/), lingua-alveolar (/t,d/), and dorsal (velar) (/k,g/) places of articulation that affect the pattern of F1, F2, and F3 transitions in unique and consistent ways, regardless of which vowel is adjacent to a particular stop. In this view, there is a nearly invariant, place-specific pattern in the *transitions* that is almost completely due to laws relating vocal tract configuration changes, from stops to vowels, to a pattern of formant frequency transitions. In effect, Story and Bunton's results suggest that not only did the Haskins' scientists ignore an acoustic event (the stop burst) that has some place-specific, invariant characteristics, but even the events deemed to be too variable across vowels (the transitions into and out of the closure interval) were not examined carefully enough, and in fact do have invariant characteristics.

Acoustic Invariance at the Interface of Speech Production and Perception

The issue of acoustic invariance has focused on stop consonants, but a more general question is the stability of the acoustic characteristics for *any* speech sound. A given sound may have very different acoustic characteristics, in both the temporal and spectral domains, depending on who produces the speech sample and the conditions under which it is produced. A speech sound has acoustic variability depending on the age, dialect, sex, size, and possibly race of the speaker. In addition, phonetic context, speaking rate, and speaking style can also have major effects on a speech sound's acoustic characteristics. If the acoustic characteristics of a speech sound are so variable, exactly what is meant by the term "acoustic invariance"?

The Haskins scientists apparently defined acoustic invariance in a very strict way. For them, almost any degree of acoustic variability for a particular aspect of a speech sound (such as the cues for place of articulation of stops) was an undesirable aspect of a communication signal. Scientists such as Blumstein and Stevens (1979), and several others who followed them, had a slightly looser approach to this problem. These scientists allowed that a sufficient degree of acoustic invariance was demonstrated when a relatively small percentage (5–15%) was misclassified according to their analysis criteria. This work has sometimes been criticized for two reasons, one having to do with the arbitrary nature of the analysis criteria, the second with the failure to explain the classification errors and how they are treated in the perception of speech.

The arbitrary analysis criteria can be illustrated with the following, simple questions: Does the 26-ms burst interval used by Blumstein and Stevens (1979) bear any relationship to the way the auditory system processes speech spectra? Is there good evidence for spectral shape analysis by the auditory system? Does the auditory system use a straightforward frequency analysis such as suggested by the work of Blumstein and Stevens, and others, or does it change the way frequency is represented as the signal travels the auditory pathways from the ear canal to the auditory cortex? These questions cannot be pursued in detail in this chapter, but it can be said that the answers to the questions are not simple. In short, speech acoustic analysis strategies may not always be well-matched to known aspects of auditory, and presumably speech perception, analysis. The linear frequency scales on the x-axis of the vowel or consonant spectra shown, for example, in Figures 11–1, 11–20, and 11–31, do not represent how the auditory system processes the range of low to high frequencies. In fact, the auditory system is much more capable of resolving frequency differences at the low end, as compared to the high end of these scales (stated in a different way, the 100-Hz difference between 200 and 300 Hz is analyzed by the auditory system much more finely than the 100-Hz difference between, say, 5500 and 5600 Hz). The second issue, of classification errors and how they are handled, has not been addressed in the series of articles on classification of stop burst spectra. Five to 15% does not seem like a lot of errors, but how often do listeners experience such perceptual errors when listening to speech? The answer is, not very often at all, unless speech is being produced and perceived in a very noisy environment or is heard by a listener with a hearing loss. So, how are classification errors explained within a perspective on "normal" speech perception?

An alternative view to this problem has been formulated by Lindblom (1990). For Lindblom, the issue is not the strict acoustic invariance of a particular speech sound, but rather how much its acoustic characteristics can vary and still remain distinctive relative to neighboring sounds. Lindblom (1990; see also Moon & Lindblom, 1994) pointed to the known variability in acoustic characteristics of speech sounds as an asset, not a liability, in a theory of speech production and perception. Speakers often vary the precision with which they produce sound segments. Under more formal circumstances, they produce speech very carefully, but in casual situations are likely to be rather imprecise. Formal speech styles, referred to in contemporary literature as "clear speech" (Ferguson & Kewley-Port, 2007), are characterized by acoustic characteristics of speech sounds that are maximally distinct from each other. However, casual speech styles decrease the distance between these acoustic characteristics, but leave them sufficiently distinct to retain their contrastive function. A good example of this effect would be the relative expansion and collapse of the F1-F2 vowel space under different speaking conditions (see Figure 11–7 and associated discussion). Variability in the acoustic characteristics of a class of speech sounds is allowable provided it does not compromise the speaker's

need to be understood and the listener's requirement for speech signals that meet the criterion of phonemic contrast. The speaker, according to Lindblom (1990), can actually calibrate just how much phonetic contrastivity a listener requires. Articulatory behavior is then adjusted to meet those requirements. This view seems much more consistent with natural communication situations than one in which a very narrow definition of acoustic invariance is required for the acoustic characteristics of speech sounds.

AFFRICATES

As noted in Chapter 9, affricates have aspects of both stop and fricative articulation. Affricates have not been studied extensively in English, and only a limited amount of work on vocal tract acoustics of affricates has been completed (see Stevens, 1993). What is known is that the frication interval of the English affricates /tʃ/ and /dʒ/ is longer than the frication interval of the stop component and shorter than the typical duration of the fricative component. Moreover, the stop closure duration of affricates typically is slightly shorter than the closure duration of singleton stops. A final point is that the place of articulation of the English affricates is slightly posterior to the place of articulation for lingua-alveolar stops and fricatives (Fletcher, 1989). This means that the frication spectrum and pattern of formant transitions into and out of an English affricate are likely to be different than the pattern for either lingua-alveolars or dorsals, as discussed above (see Stevens, 1998, for further information).

ACOUSTIC CHARACTERISTICS OF PROSODY

Prosody is a vast area of inquiry, encompassing intonation, rhythm, stress, pause, and even grammatical function. The relevant acoustic measures include phrase-level F0 and intensity contours, relative timing measures of multisyllabic utterances, and local (segmental) changes in F0, intensity, duration, and vowel quality that are used to signal syllable stress.

Phrase-Level F0 Contours

Figure 11–35 shows a spectrogram of close to 9 s of speech produced by an adult female reading a standard passage ("The Hunter Passage"; see Crystal &

Stops (Still) Win the Prize

On January 8, 2008, one of the authors searched the *Linguistics and Language Behavior Abstracts*, a database devoted to published papers in all aspects of linguistics, including phonetics. This search, conducted for the first edition of this textbook, was for papers published from 1950 to January 8, 2008, on different consonant classes, in any language. Keywords were entered into the "Abstract" dialog box, meaning the search engine was asked to return "hits" (published papers) for relevant publications. An updated search was conducted on October 4, 2012, for the current edition. The results, given by keyword and number of hits in parentheses with the first number representing the 2008 search and the second number the 2012 search, were stops (1658, 3965), fricatives (879, 1785), nasals (507, 2143), affricates (329, 566), and liquids (271, 648). As suggested in the previous and current editions of this textbook, stops are the glamour sounds in the phonetic beauty contest, but the dramatic increase in papers on nasals indicate they have nosed out fricatives for second place.

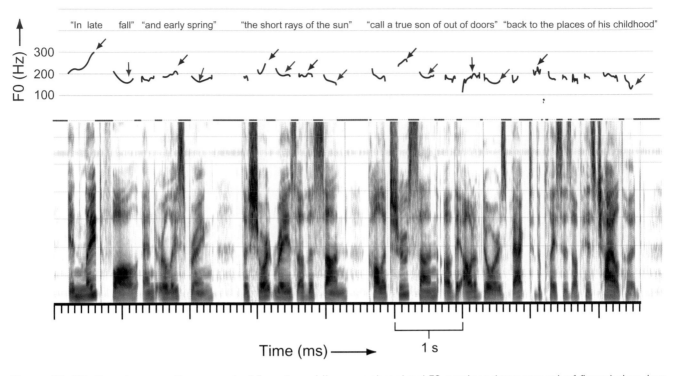

Figure 11–35. Spectrogram (*lower part of figure*) and time-synchronized F0 contour (*upper part of figure*) showing F0 variation across five phrases from a connected reading by an adult female. Within each phrase, the dark arrows point to the approximate location of the highest F0, the red arrow to the lowest F0. See text for additional information.

House, 1982). Immediately above the spectrogram is an F0 trace, generated automatically by TF32 and edited for obvious F0-estimation errors (see Chapter 10). The speaker read the following: "In late fall and early spring the short rays of the sun call a true son of the out of doors back to the places of his childhood." The phrases in this utterance, separated according to very coarse grammatical phrase rules, are shown in Figure 11–35 above the F0 trace. The orthographic transcription of each phrase extends roughly over the time span corresponding to the acoustic signal for the phrase. The organization of the F0 trace within each of these phrases is consistent with the description of phrase-level, F0 contours provided years ago by Lehiste (1970) in her famous book, *Suprasegmentals*. Lehiste noted that, for declarative phrases, an F0 peak typically occurs near the beginning of the phrase, followed by a gradually declining F0 to the lowest value at the end of the phrase. In Figure 11–35 the peak (highest) F0 values within a phrase are indicated by black arrows, the low F0 values by red arrows. Each "phrase" is a grammatical unit, and the peak F0 occurs near the beginning of the unit, often during the first content word. The lowest F0 within each phrase typically occurs during the

phrase-final word. The tendency of F0 to start high and then decline more or less steadily throughout an utterance is called *declination*. Each of the phrases in Figure 11–35 shows F0 declination; the details vary with each phrase, but the general pattern can be seen. Very similar observations of F0 patterns across grammatical phrases were made by Lea (1973) in his extensive study of read and spontaneous utterances.

In Figure 11–35, the highest F0 value (~300 Hz) throughout the *entire* utterance occurs at the beginning, during the first content word ("late"). The lowest F0 value (~120 Hz) of the utterance occurs on the final syllable of the final word ("childhood"). It seems the structure of this sequence of phrases may have been organized at a "supraphrase" level, as if a larger-scale declination was planned by the speaker across the sequence of several phrases. A half-decade following the publication of *Suprasegmentals*, Lehiste (1975) described this "supraphrase" declination of F0, as if a paragraph containing several phrases was organized as a prosodic unit with the individual phrases as subunits.

The speaker who produced the utterance in Figure 11–35 (not one of the authors) was not instructed to speak in a particular way. The F0 contour was produced by natural reading, and is a "real" reflection of how F0 was organized by this speaker within and across declarative phrases. The same pattern may not be seen, however, for every speaker and even for this particular speaker under different communication conditions. Phrase-level F0 contours can be highly variable, and may be affected by several linguistic and paralinguistic factors. The most obvious of these are the different F0 contours associated with declarative and interrogative utterances. An interrogative F0 contour typically has a *rising* F0 at the end of an utterance, not the falling F0 shown within and across the phrases in Figure 11–35. The utterance-final rise of F0 is a cue to the listener, along with other cues (lexical, syntactic, situational), that a question is being asked. F0 contours may also rise at the end of a declarative utterance when the speaker is intending to continue speaking. These F0 rises tend to be less dramatic than the rise for questions, but they are effective in signaling the listener that the talker is not finished (Lea, 1973). When a talker is finished and wants to signal the listener to respond, he or she is likely to produce a phrase-final F0 contour with a very steep and rapid fall.

F0 contours may also be modified by the level of stress produced on a specific syllable or syllables throughout a phrase or series of phrases. In English, multisyllabic words have lexical stress patterns (such as "frequency" /ˈfrikwənsi/ and "approach" /əˈproʊtʃ/) in which one or more syllables has greater stress than the other syllables. In words such as "frequency" and "approach," the stressed syllable typically has a greater F0 than the unstressed syllable or syllables. The magnitude of the F0 difference between stressed and unstressed syllables is highly variable across speakers (Howell, 1993; Sereno & Jongman, 1995). Syllables can also be stressed to focus attention on a specific word within an utterance. For example, in the utterance "Put these two back" (Wang, Kent, Duffy, & Thomas, 2005), speakers can add stress to any of the words (e.g., "Put THESE two back" versus "Put these TWO back") to signal their importance in conveying a message. This is called sentence stress (sometimes emphatic stress, or contrastive stress), and the syllable receiving extra emphasis typically has a higher F0 as compared to the syllable spoken without extra stress.

As in the case of lexical stress, the magnitude of the F0 difference between the emphatic and normally stressed syllable is quite variable across speakers (McRoberts, Studdert-Kennedy, & Shankweiler, 1995; Wang et al., 2005). More is said in the section titled "Stress" about the role of F0 in both lexical and sentence stress.

A phase-level F0 contour will also be affected, albeit at a subtle (but systematic) level, by the identity of the specific segments in a phrase. For example, all other things being equal, the F0 of high vowels is 7 to 15 Hz higher than the F0 of low vowels (Lea, 1973; and see Whalen & Levitt, 1995). Also, all other things being equal, the F0 following a voiceless consonant is up to 20 Hz higher than the F0 following a voiced consonant (Ohde, 1984; Silverman, 1987). These influences of segmental identity on F0 contours may appear to be small, but they change the form of the contour enough to allow listeners to detect them (Silverman, 1987).

Finally, F0 contours are subject to a variety of paralinguistic influences. The term *paralinguistics* is used to describe nonverbal aspects of speech, usually related to prosodic variation, that convey emotion and physiological status. Paralinguistic aspects of vocal communication can be thought of as a backdrop against which a message is transmitted. This vocal backdrop conveys a meaning in parallel to the meaning conveyed by the spoken words (for example, the same words can be spoken in a happy and sad way, that "way" transmitted by prosodic variations). Studies of variation in F0 contours with natural emotional variation are not easy because they require an experimenter to "be there" when there is an emotional change, and to identify reliably which emotional state is the correct description for a speaker. Scientists have tried to develop paralinguistic models of F0 contours by using actors to simulate different emotions and measuring the resulting variation in phrase-level F0. This work has revealed subtle changes between the F0 contours of simulated emotions such as anger, joy, and sadness (Bänziger & Scherer, 2005). "Sad" F0 contours tend to be flatter than angry or joyful F0 contours, but there is no clear evidence of sharp (categorical) distinctions between them (see review in Pell, 2001).

In summary, phrase-level F0 contours are subject to a number of influences, but the basic form of declarative and interrogative contours is clear, as are segmental influences on local F0 changes throughout an utterance. A general understanding of F0 contours and the influences on them is important because prosody plays a role in clinical issues. For example, F0 variation across words or phrases has been identified as a potentially important aspect of diagnosing developmental verbal apraxia (Shriberg et al., 2003) and characterizing neurogenic speech disorders in adults (Kent & Rosenbek, 1982). Treatment of persons with various speech disorders may have to account for paralinguistic influences on F0 contours, as in Parkinson disease where depression is known to be common.

Phrase-Level Intensity Contours

Phrase-level intensity contours have not been studied as extensively as F0 contours, but clinical considerations suggest the need for more data on this aspect of prosody. In a connected speech sample, an intensity contour varies over time primarily because consonants are less intense than vowels. A reasonable estimate of typical intensity differences between consonants and vowels is 7 to 14 dB. The degree to which consonants are less intense than vowels depends on many factors, including type of consonant and vowel, position of the consonant in a word, syllable stress level, overall vocal effort level, and sex of the speaker (Fairbanks & Miron, 1957). In more recent data from conversational speech, the standard deviation of intensity across utterances (pauses, and therefore "minimum" or theoretically zero intensity intervals, were excluded in this analysis) was found to be about 6.5 dB (Rosen, Kent, Delaney, & Duffy, 2006). This figure seems to be generally consistent with the 7- to 14-dB range reported by Fairbanks and Miron because the standard deviation reflects intensity variation across an utterance between relatively high-intensity vowels and lower intensity consonants (±1 standard deviation, a conventional way to estimate the "primary" variability of a measure, is 13 dB in this case). Figure 11–36 shows a relative intensity trace, scaled in decibels, for the same utterance shown in Figure 11–35. Selected relative intensities have been marked to show the typical differences between consonants (red arrows) and vowels (black arrows). For example, in the phrase "the short rays of the sun," the relative intensity of /ʃ/ is roughly 6 dB less than the following vowel, and the relative intensity of the /s/ is about 12 dB less than the following /ʌ/. Note also the very low, relative intensities of two stop closure intervals (upward-pointing, red arrows), consistent with a closed vocal tract that radiates little or no energy.

The clinical potential of phrase-level intensity contours is that a measure such as the standard deviation, described above, may serve as an index of the degree to which *segmental contrast* is maintained in a client's speech. In typical speech, acoustic boundaries between consonants and vowels are often "sharp," resulting in sudden changes in energy. The sharpness of these boundaries, or the sudden contrasts in energy between consonants and vowels, help listeners identify

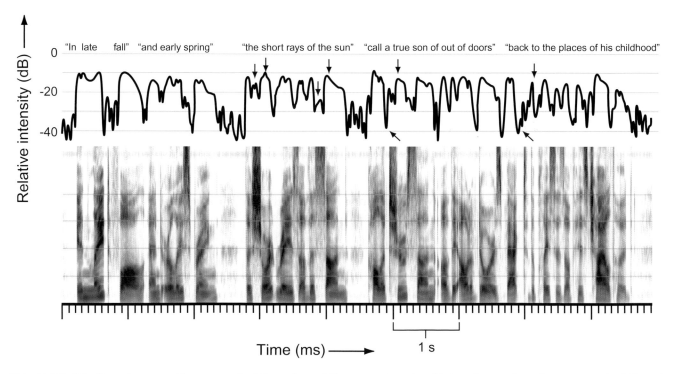

Figure 11-36. Spectrogram (*lower part of figure*) and time-synchronized intensity contour (*upper part of figure*) showing intensity variation across five phrases from a connected reading by an adult female. Selected vowel intensities are shown by downward-pointing, dark arrows; selected consonant intensities are shown by downward-pointing, red arrows. The two slanted, upward-pointing red arrows indicate intensities during stop closure intervals.

Paralinguistics Trivia, Literally

Paralinguistics is the branch of linguistics concerned with how utterances are spoken—their loudness, melody, rate, even voice quality. These utterance characteristics can convey mood, intent, and personality characteristics. Kimble and Seidel (1991) used a game of trivia to study the confidence with which people answered questions. They approached this as a paralinguistic question, hypothesizing that more confident answers (as rated by the responders) would have greater speech intensity (i.e., the answers would be louder) and be delivered faster than less confident answers. The data, as reported by Kimble and Seidel, supported the hypothesis. Casual observation suggests that politicians, bullies, and certain radio-show hosts already understand this effect.

segments. When these sharp boundaries are dulled, perhaps because a speaker does not make tight consonant constrictions or produces low-energy vowels, or because a person has a speech disorder, the listener's task becomes more difficult. In a sense, the listener loses the segmental landmarks that allow rapid and efficient sound identification and ultimately the ability to access the words that have been spoken (Stevens, 2002; Mattys & Liss, 2008).

Stress

English has multisyllabic words in which one syllable (sometimes two) is (are) stressed relative to the others. "Dictionary pronunciation," or more technically, "lexical stress," is basically a description of which syllables in a word are stressed, and which are not stressed. Lexically stressed syllables are often assumed to have higher F0, greater intensity, longer duration, and perhaps a less reduced vowel formant pattern as compared to unstressed syllables (Fry, 1955; Lea, 1973; Sereno & Jongman, 1995). This generalization applies not only to noun-verb pairs in which the segments are the same (such as noun "rebel" /ˈrɛbl̩/ versus verb "rebel" /rəˈbɛl/, or noun "survey" /ˈsɜrveɪ/ versus verb "survey" /sɚˈveɪ/), but also to the F0 pattern for a multisyllabic word such as "Escanaba" /ɛskəˈnɑbə/.

The same combination of acoustic variables may also be used for sentence stress, as defined above.

Kochanski, Grabe, Coleman, and Rosner (2005) reviewed the long history of research efforts to determine how the several acoustic variables associated with stress combine to produce a listener's perception of syllable prominence. The term *prominence* is sometimes used to refer to syllables that "stand out" in a perceived utterance. Prominence and stress are often used interchangeably, a practice followed in the current discussion.[19] As Kochanski et al. noted, many scientists have regarded the relative value of F0 or movement of the F0 contour (e.g., a rapid increase in F0) to be a primary correlate of stress. The evidence on which this claim is based, however, is slim and typically derived from unnatural speaking situations (single words, or highly formal sentence readings). Howell (1993) showed that different speakers use very different combinations of F0, intensity, duration, and vowel formant frequencies to produce stressed syllables in two-syllable words. Speakers did not follow a rule in choosing one phonetic "solution," such as raising F0, to make a syllable prominent. Similar variation across speakers in the use of F0, duration, and intensity for the production of lexical stress patterns can be found in data published by Sereno and Jongman (1995). Kochanski et al. (2005) examined various kinds of speech in British and Irish English, including spontaneous speech samples, in which prominent syllables were marked by two experienced phoneticians. They used statistical classifiers, as discussed above for classification of nasals, rhotics, stops, and fricatives, to determine which acoustic measures were most successful in identifying the prominent syllables. F0 measures had only a weak role in successful classification of prominent syllables. Syllable intensity and duration measures were far more successful in classifying the syllables marked as prominent.

The findings of Kochanski et al. (2005) are instructive for those clinical strategies or studies seeking to use stress to treat and understand speech disorders. Kochanski et al. argued that speakers are much more likely to use syllable intensity and duration, as compared to F0, to make a syllable prominent. Some studies have attempted to average acoustic measures related to stress to achieve a "composite" index of stress as a classifier of speech disorders. For example, Shriberg et al. (2003) averaged measures of F0, intensity, and duration to construct an acoustic index of lexical stress for bisyllabic word forms as a possible unique marker

---

[19]A technical difference between stress and prominence is that stress is phonological and prominence is phonetic. Presumably, there are several *phonetic* solutions to making a syllable prominent (F0, intensity, duration, vowel quality), and any one or a combination of these ways could satisfy the *phonological* requirement of stressing a particular syllable.

for children with apraxia of speech. The composite acoustic measure treated all acoustic measures related to stress as equal in the contribution to making a syllable prominent, an assumption not consistent with the information reviewed above. The inconsistency is not only in the potential greater contribution of intensity and duration, as compared to F0, to the perception of stress (Kochanski et al., 2005), but also in the very varied use of the measures across speakers to make a syllable prominent (Howell, 1993; Sereno & Jongman, 1995). Similarly, some studies (Penner, Miller, Hertrich, Ackermann, & Schumm, 2001) have evaluated the ability of speakers with Parkinson disease to use F0 as an indicator of sentence stress, but have not included other potentially acoustic correlates of prominence (intensity, duration, vowel quality) in their analyses. This may result in an incomplete representation of the prominence-producing capabilities of a group of speakers.

The point of this discussion is not to be overly critical of the cited studies. Rather, it is to highlight the complexity of stress/prominence, both as production and perception phenomena. A growing awareness of the importance of prosodic control to communication disorders requires a careful and complete understanding of the relevant phenomena (Blake, 2007; Caspar, Raphael, Harris, & Geibel, 2007; Lenden & Flipsen, 2007).

Rhythm

Rhythm is the patterning of segment or syllable durations across an utterance. If the unit of speech timing is taken to be a syllable, English is said to have a rhythm in which long- and short-duration syllables alternate with each other. The long syllables are the stressed ones, the unstressed syllables are the short ones. The alternation between long and short syllables is not usually a pattern of one long/one short/one long/one short (and so on), but rather a sequence of one long followed by several short syllables. Because of this repeating pattern of one stressed syllable followed by several unstressed syllables, English is referred to as a *stress-timed language*. A strict view of a stress-timed language requires the duration *between* stressed syllables in an utterance to be nearly constant. Stated otherwise, in a connected discourse, the time required to produce a stressed syllable and all the unstressed syllables that follow it is nearly identical to the time required to produce another stressed syllable and its following unstressed syllables. A simple example of this idea is shown in Figure 11–37, where a spectrogram of the utterance "Evaluate the preparation for the game" is shown together with a time-aligned phonetic transcription. The stressed syllables in this utterance (/væ/ in

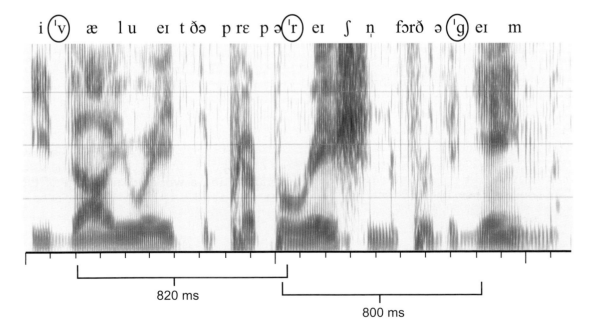

Figure 11-37. Spectrogram of the utterance, "Evaluate the preparation for the game" as an illustration of stress timing in English. The stress marks in the phonetic transcription show the stressed syllables of the succeeding phrases, and two stressed-syllable-plus-unstressed-syllable intervals are measured at the bottom of the spectrogram, one for the first "stress group," the next one for the second "stress group." See text for additional details.

"evaluate," /reɪ/ in "preparation," /geɪ/ in "game") are indicated in the phonetic transcription; the consonants preceding the stressed syllables are enclosed in ovals. At the bottom of the spectrogram two time intervals are shown, the first of 820 ms between the onset of the first glottal pulse of the stressed /æ/ and the first stressed /eɪ/, the second of 800 ms between the initial glottal pulses of the first and second stressed /eɪ/s. The nearly identical time intervals between the consecutive stressed intervals of this brief utterance seem consistent with the idea, stated above, of a stressed-time language. Note also the several short-duration, unstressed syllables following the first two stressed syllables. As Lehiste (1973) demonstrated, absolute *isochrony*—the phenomenon of equal time intervals between stressed syllables—does not exist, but speakers may approximate isochrony in production and listeners may hear these approximations as more isochronous than they really are (Lehiste, 1977).[20]

This brief summary of speech rhythm as an aspect of prosody is important because certain speech disorders exhibit rhythmic abnormalities. For example, speakers of English with diseases of the cerebellum may produce speech with a rhythm that distorts the tendency to isochrony by making *all* syllables roughly equal in duration. This eliminates the normal duration difference between stressed and unstressed syllables and results in perception of "metered" or "scanned" speech (Darley, Aronson, & Brown, 1975). In "scanned" speech, listeners report that each syllable sounds metered out in a fixed (relatively constant) time interval, as if a metronome were timing the speaker's output. Scientists interested in speech rhythm disorders have adopted an acoustic measure originally developed by Low, Grabe, and Nolan (2000) for use in second language acquisition (rhythmic differences between languages can cause substantial difficulty for the second language learner). This acoustic measure is called the *Pairwise Variability Index* (PVI). The formula for the PVI is available in Low et al.; here it is sufficient to describe the logic of the measure. If the vowels of consecutive syllables have very different durations, as would be expected in a stressed-timed language such as English, the measure reflects this with a "high-difference" value computed over many syllables. If, on the other hand, the vowels of consecutive syllables have very similar durations, as in ataxic dysarthria or syllable-timed languages (e.g., Spanish, for which the duration between consecutive syllables, rather than stressed syllables, is constant), the measure yields a "low-difference" value. The PVI is, therefore, an acoustic measure of the relative duration difference between consecutive syllables in connected speech. Measures such as the PVI show great potential as a diagnostic marker for different types of speech disorder (see Henrich, Lowit, Schalling, & Mennen, 2006; Liss, LeGendre, & Lotto, 2010; Liss, White, Mattys, Lansford, Lotto, Spitzer, & Caviness, 2009).

REVIEW

This chapter presented a review of acoustic phonetics data. Acoustic characteristics of segmental and suprasegmental (prosodic) components of speech production were summarized in a fair amount of detail. The interpretations of these measures were also discussed, and reference to clinical application of the measures was made when appropriate.

For the speech-language pathologist, there is much that can be learned and documented about an individual's speech production problem, using the techniques of acoustic phonetic analysis.

Acoustic phonetic analysis is noninvasive and a tremendous amount of scientific literature on typical speakers and speakers with disorders is available for comparison to a particular client's data.

Speech analysis can be implemented rather easily and relatively inexpensively on a desktop or laptop computer.

The audiologist who diagnoses and treats hearing loss with hearing aids or implantable devices should have a working knowledge of acoustic phonetics and its link to speech intelligibility.

Both speech-language pathologists and audiologists need to read the research literature to maintain a high-quality clinical practice.

Acoustic phonetics is an increasing presence in both the speech-language pathology and audiology literature, and a working knowledge of theory and data will serve the clinician well as she or he strives for excellence in service delivery.

REFERENCES

Assman, P., Nearey, T., & Hogan, J. (1982). Vowel identification: Orthographic, perceptual, and acoustical factors. *Journal of the Acoustical Society of America, 71*, 975–989.

Auzou, P., Özsancak, C., Morris, R., Jan, M., Eustache, F., & Hannequin, D. (2000). Voice onset time in aphasia, apraxia

---

[20]For advanced reading on the phenomenon of isochrony and rhythmic variation across language, see Port (2003) and White and Mattys (2007).

of speech and dysarthria: A review. *Clinical Linguistics and Phonetics, 14*, 131–150.

Bänziger, T., & Scherer, K. (2005). The role of intonation in emotional expression. *Speech Communication, 46*, 252–267.

Baum, S., & Blumstein, S. (1987). Preliminary observations on the use of duration as a cue to the syllable-initial fricative consonant voicing in English. *Journal of the Acoustical Society of America, 82*, 1073–1077.

Behrens, S., & Blumstein, S. (1988). Acoustic characteristics of English voiceless fricatives: A descriptive analysis. *Journal of Phonetics, 16*, 295–298.

Blake, M. (2007). Perspectives on treatment for communication deficits associated with right hemisphere brain damage. *American Journal of Speech-Language Pathology, 16*, 331–342.

Blumstein, S., & Stevens, K. (1979). Acoustic invariance in speech production: Evidence from measurements of the spectral characteristics of stop consonants. *Journal of the Acoustical Society of America, 66*, 1001–1017.

Bradlow, A. (1995). A comparative acoustic study of English and Spanish vowels. *Journal of the Acoustical Society of America, 97*, 1916–1924.

Bradlow, A., Torretta, G., & Pisoni, D. (1996). Intelligibility of normal speech I: Global and fine-grained acoustic-phonetic talker characteristics. *Speech Communication, 20*, 255–272.

Byrd, D. (1993). 54,000 American stops. *UCLA Working Papers in Phonetics, 83*, 97–116.

Calandruccio, L., Van Engen, K., Dhar, S., & Bradlow, A. R. (2010). The effectiveness of clear speech as a masker. *Journal of Speech, Language, and Hearing Research, 53*, 1458–1471.

Caspar, M., Raphael, L., Harris, K., & Geibel, J. (2007). Speech prosody in cerebellar ataxia. *International Journal of Language and Communication Disorders, 42*, 407–426.

Chaney, C. (1988). Acoustic analysis of correct and misarticulated semivowels. *Journal of Speech and Hearing Research, 31*, 275–287.

Chen, M. (1995). Acoustic parameters of nasalized vowels in hearing-impaired and normal-hearing speakers. *Journal of the Acoustical Society of America, 98*, 2443–2453.

Chen, M. (1997). Acoustic correlates of English and French nasalized vowels. *Journal of the Acoustical Society of America, 102*, 2360–2370.

Chen, Y., Robb, M., Gilbert, H., & Lerman, J. (2001). Vowel production by Mandarin speakers of English. *Clinical Linguistics and Phonetics, 15*, 427–440.

Cho, T., Jun, S.-A., & Ladefoged, P. (2002). Acoustic and aerodynamic correlates of Korean stops and fricatives. *Journal of Phonetics, 30*, 193–228.

Cho, T., & Ladefoged, P. (1999). Variation and universals in VOT: Evidence from 18 languages. *Journal of Phonetics, 27*, 207–229.

Chuang, H.-F., Yang, C.-C., Chi, L.-Y., Weismer, G., & Wang, Y.-T. (2012). Speech intelligibility, speaking rate, and vowel formant characteristics in Mandarin-speaking children with cochlear implant. *International Journal of Speech-Language Pathology, 14*, 119–129.

Clopper, C., Pisoni, D., & de Jong, K. (2005). Acoustic characteristics of the vowel systems of six regional varieties of American English. *Journal of the Acoustical Society of America, 118*, 1661–1676.

Craig, H., Thompson, C., Washington, J., & Potter, S. (2003). Phonological features of child African American English. *Journal of Speech, Language, and Hearing Research, 46*, 623–635.

Crystal, T., & House, A. (1982). Segmental durations in connected-speech signals: Preliminary results. *Journal of the Acoustical Society of America, 72*, 705–716.

Crystal, T., & House, A. (1988a). The duration of American-English vowels: An overview. *Journal of Phonetics, 16*, 263–284.

Crystal, T., & House, A. (1988b). The duration of American-English stop consonants: An overview. *Journal of Phonetics, 16*, 285–294.

Crystal, T., & House, A. (1988c). Segmental durations in connected-speech signals: Current results. *Journal of the Acoustical Society of America, 83*, 1553–1573.

Crystal, T., & House, A. (1988d). A note on the durations of fricatives in American English. *Journal of the Acoustical Society of America, 84*, 1932–1935.

Dalston, R. (1972). *A spectrographic analysis of the spectral and temporal acoustic characteristics of English semivowels spoken by three-year-old children and adults.* Doctoral dissertation, Northwestern University, Evanston, IL.

Dalston, R. (1975). Acoustic characteristics of English /w,r,l/ spoken correctly by young children and adults. *Journal of the Acoustical Society of America, 57*, 462–469.

Dang, J., & Honda, K. (1995). Acoustic characteristics of the paranasal sinuses derived from transmission characteristic measurement and morphological observation. *Journal of the Acoustical Society of America, 100*, 3374–3383.

Darley, F., Aronson, A., & Brown, J. (1975). *Motor speech disorders.* Philadelphia, PA: W. B. Saunders.

Davidsen-Nielsen, N. (1974). Syllabification in English words with medial sp, st, sk. *Journal of Phonetics, 2*, 15–45.

DeMerit, J.L. (1997). *Acoustic and perceptual effects of clear speech on duration-dependent vowel contrasts.* Unpublished doctoral dissertation, University of Wisconsin-Madison, Madison, WI.

Espy-Wilson, C. (1992). Acoustic measures for linguistic features distinguishing the semivowels /wjrl/ in American English. *Journal of the Acoustical Society of America, 92*, 736–757.

Espy-Wilson, C. (1994). A feature-based semivowel recognition system. *Journal of the Acoustical Society of America, 96*, 65–72.

Fairbanks, G., & Miron, M. (1957). Effects of vocal effort upon the consonant-vowel ratio within the syllable. *Journal of the Acoustical Society of America, 29*, 621–626.

Feng, G., & Castelli, E. (1996). Some acoustic features of nasal and nasalized vowels: A target for vowel nasalization. *Journal of the Acoustical Society of America, 99*, 3694–3706.

Ferguson, S., & Kewley-Port, D. (2007). Talker differences in clear and conversational speech: Acoustic characteristics of vowels. *Journal of Speech, Language, and Hearing Research, 50*, 1241–1255.

Fletcher, S. (1989). Palatometric specification of stop, affricate, and sibilant sounds. *Journal of Speech and Hearing Research, 32*, 736–748.

Forrest, K., Weismer, G., Hodge, M., Dinnsen, D., & Elbert, M. (1990). Statistical analysis of word-initial /k/ and /t/ produced by normal and phonologically disordered children. *Clinical Linguistics and Phonetics, 4*, 327–340.

Forrest, K., Weismer, G., Milenkovic, P., & Dougall, R. (1988). Statistical analysis of word-initial voiceless obstruents: Preliminary data. *Journal of the Acoustical Society of America, 84*, 115–124.

Fourakis, M. (1991). Tempo, stress, and vowel reduction in American English. *Journal of the Acoustical Society of America, 90*, 1816–1827.

Fox, R., & Nissan S. (2005). Sex-related acoustic changes in voiceless English fricatives. *Journal of Speech, Language, and Hearing Research, 48*, 753–765.

Fry, D. (1955). Duration and intensity as physical correlates of linguistic stress. *Journal of the Acoustical Society of America, 27*, 765–768.

Fujimura, O. (1962). Analysis of nasal consonants. *Journal of the Acoustical Society of America, 34*, 1865–1875.

Gay, T. (1968). Effect of speaking rate on diphthong formant movements. *Journal of the Acoustical Society of America, 44*, 1570–1573.

Gottfried, T., Miller, J., & Meyer, D. (1993). Three approaches to classification of American English diphthongs. *Journal of Phonetics, 21*, 205–229.

Granlund, S., Hazan, V., & Baker, B. (2012). An acoustic-phonetic comparison of the clear speaking styles of Finnish-English late bilinguals. *Journal of Phonetics, 40*, 509–520.

Halle, M., Hughes, G., & Radley, J.-P. (1957). Acoustic properties of stop consonants. *Journal of the Acoustical Society of America, 29*, 107–116.

Harrington, J. (1994). The contribution of the murmur and vowel to the place of articulation distinction in nasal consonants. *Journal of the Acoustical Society of America, 96*, 19–32.

Harris, K. (1958). Cues for the discrimination of American English fricatives in spoken syllables. *Language and Speech, 1*, 1–7.

Henrich, J., Lowit, A., Schalling, E., & Mennen, I. (2006). Rhythmic disturbance in ataxic dysarthria: A comparison of different measures and speech tasks. *Journal of Medical Speech-Language Pathology, 14*, 291–296.

Hillenbrand, J., Clark, M., & Nearey, T. (2001). Effects of consonant environment on vowel formant patterns. *Journal of the Acoustical Society of America, 109*, 748–763.

Hillenbrand, J., Getty, L., Clark, M., & Wheeler, K. (1995). Acoustic characteristics of American English vowels. *Journal of the Acoustical Society of America, 97*, 3099–3111.

Hillenbrand, J., & Nearey, T. (1999). Identification of resynthesized /hVd/ utterances: Effects of formant contour. *Journal of the Acoustical Society of America, 105*, 3509–3523.

Hirose, H. (1976). Posterior cricoarytenoid as a speech muscle. *Annals of Otology, Rhinology, and Laryngology, 85*, 334–343.

Hirose, H. (1977). Laryngeal adjustments in consonant production. *Phonetica, 34*, 289–294.

Hoffman, P., Stager, S., & Daniloff, R. (1983). Perception and production of misarticulated /r/. *Journal of Speech and Hearing Disorders, 48*, 210–215.

Holbrook, A., & Fairbanks, G. (1962). Diphthong formants and their movements. *Journal of Speech and Hearing Research, 5*, 38–58.

House, A. (1961). On vowel duration in English. *Journal of the Acoustical Society of America, 33*, 1174–1178.

Howell, P. (1993). Cue trading in the production and perception of vowel stress. *Journal of the Acoustical Society of America, 94*, 2063–2073.

Hughes, G., & Halle, M. (1956). Spectral properties of fricative consonants. *Journal of the Acoustical Society of America, 28*, 303–310.

Iskarous, K., Shadle, C. H., & Proctor, M.I. (2011). Articulatory-acoustic kinematics: The production of American English /s/. *Journal of the Acoustical Society of America, 129*, 944–954.

Jacewicz, W., & Fox, R. A. (2012). The effects of cross-generational and cross-dialectal variation on vowel identification and classification. *Journal of the Acoustical Society of America, 131*, 1413–1433.

Johnson, K. (2003). *Acoustic and auditory phonetics.* Oxford, UK: Blackwell.

Johnson, K., Ladefoged, P., & Lindau, M. (1993). Individual differences in vowel production. *Journal of the Acoustical Society of America, 94*, 701–714.

Jongman, A., Fourakis, M., & Sereno, J. (1989). The acoustic vowel space of Modern Greek and German. *Language and Speech, 32*, 221–248.

Jongman, A., Wayland, R., & Wong, S. (2000). Acoustic characteristics of English fricatives. *Journal of the Acoustical Society of America, 108*, 1252–1263.

Kent, R., & Rosenbek, J. (1982). Prosodic disturbance and neurologic lesion. *Brain and Language, 15*, 259–291.

Kessinger, R., & Blumstein, S. (1997). Effects of speaking rate on voice-onset time in Thai, French, and English. *Journal of Phonetics, 25*, 143–168.

Kewley-Port, D. (1983). Time-varying features as correlates of place of articulation in stop consonants. *Journal of the Acoustical Society of America, 73*, 322–335.

Kimble, C., & Seidel, S. (1991). Vocal signs of confidence. *Journal of Nonverbal Behavior, 15*, 99–105.

Kingston, J., & Diehl, R. (1994). Phonetic knowledge. *Language, 70*, 419–454.

Klatt, D. (1975). Vowel lengthening is syntactically determined in a connected discourse. *Journal of Phonetics, 3*, 129–140.

Klatt, D. (1976). Linguistic uses of segmental duration in English: Acoustic and perceptual evidence. *Journal of the Acoustical Society of America, 59*, 1208–1221.

Kobatake, H., & Ohtani, S. (1987). Spectral transition dynamics of voiceless stop consonants. *Journal of the Acoustical Society of America, 81*, 1146–1151.

Kochanski, G., Grabe, E., Coleman, J., & Rosner, B. (2005). Loudness predicts prominence: Fundamental frequency lends little. *Journal of the Acoustical Society of America, 118*, 1038–1054.

Krause, J., & Braida, L. (2004). Acoustic properties of naturally produced clear speech at normal speaking rates. *Journal of the Acoustical Society of America, 115*, 362–378.

Kuo, C. (2011). *Toward a systematic evaluation of vowel target events aross speech tasks.* Unpublished doctoral dissertation, University of Wisconsin-Madison, Madison, WI.

Kurowski, K., & Blumstein, S. (1984). Perceptual integration of the murmur and formant transitions for place of articulation in nasal consonants. *Journal of the Acoustical Society of America, 76*, 383–390.

Kurowski, K., & Blumstein, S. (1987). Acoustic properties for place of articulation in nasal consonants. *Journal of the Acoustical Society of America, 81*, 1917–1927.

Labov, W. (1991). The three dialects of English. In P. Eckert (Ed.), *New ways of analyzing sound change* (pp. 1–44). New York, NY: Academic Press.

Ladefoged, P. (2005). *Vowels and consonants* (2nd ed.). Oxford, UK: Blackwell.

Ladefoged, P., & Maddieson, I. (1996). *The sounds of the world's languages.* Oxford, UK: Blackwell.

Lam, J., Tjaden, K., & Wilding, G. (2012). Acoustics of clear speech: Effect of instruction. *Journal of Speech, Language, and Hearing Research.* Epub ahead of print.

Lea, W. (1973). Segmental and suprasegmental influences on fundamental frequency contours. In L. M. Hyman (Ed.), *Consonant types and tone* (pp. 15–70). Los Angeles, CA: University of Southern California.

Lehiste, I. (1964). Acoustical characteristics of selected English consonants. *International Journal of American Linguistics, 30*, 1–197.

Lehiste, I. (1970). *Suprasegmentals.* Cambridge, MA: MIT Press.

Lehiste, I. (1973). Rhythmic units and syntactic units in production and perception. *Journal of the Acoustical Society of America, 54*, 1228–1234.

Lehiste, I. (1975). The phonetic structure of paragraphs. In A. Cohen & S. Nooteboom (Eds.), *Structure and process in speech perception* (pp. 195–206). New York, NY: Springer-Verlag.

Lehiste, I. (1977). Isochrony reconsidered. *Journal of Phonetics, 5*, 153–163.

Lehiste, I., & Peterson, G. (1961). Transitions, glides, and diphthongs. *Journal of the Acoustical Society of America, 33*, 268–277.

Lenden, J., & Flipsen, P. Jr. (2007). Prosody and voice characteristics of children with cochlear implants. *Journal of Communication Disorders, 40*, 66–81.

Liberman, A., Cooper, F., Shankweiler, D., & Studdert- Kennedy, M. (1967). Perception of the speech code. *Psychological Review, 74*, 431–761.

Liberman, A., Delattre, P., Cooper, F., & Gerstman, L. (1954). The role of consonant-vowel transitions in the perception of stop and nasal consonants. *Psychological Monographs, 68*, 1–13.

Lindblom, B. (1963). Spectrographic study of vowel reduction. *Journal of the Acoustical Society of America, 35*, 1773–1781.

Lindblom, B. (1990). Explaining phonetic variation: A sketch of the H&H theory. In W. Hardcastle & A. Marchal (Eds.), *Speech production and speech modeling* (pp. 403–440). Dordrecht, Netherlands: Kluwer Academic.

Lisker, L. (1957). Closure duration and the intervocalic voiced-voiceless distinction in English. *Language, 33*, 42–49.

Lisker, L. (1986). "Voicing" in English: A catalogue of acoustic features signaling /b/ versus /p/ in trochees. *Language and Speech, 29*, 3–11.

Lisker, L., & Abramson, A. (1964). A cross-language study of voicing in initial stops. *Word, 20*, 384–442.

Liss, J. M., LeGendre, S., & Lotto, A. J. (2010). Disriminating dysarthria type from envelope modulation spectra. *Journal of Speech, Language, and Hearing Research, 53*, 1246–1255.

Liss, J. M., White, L., Mattys, S. L., Lansford, K., Lotto, A. J., Spitzer, S. M., & Caviness, J. N. (2009). Quantifying speech rhythm abnormalities in the dysarthrias. *Journal of Speech, Language, and Hearing Research, 52*, 1334–1352.

Liu, H-M., Tsao, F.-M., & Kuhl, P. (2005). The intelligibility of reduced vowel working space on speech intelligibility in Mandarin-speaking young adults with cerebral palsy. *Journal of the Acoustical Society of America, 117*, 3879–3889.

Löfqvist, A. (1980). Interarticulator programming in stop production. *Journal of Phonetics, 8*, 475–490.

Löfqvist, A., Baer, T., McGarr, N., & Story, R. (1989). The cricothyroid muscle in voicing control. *Journal of the Acoustical Society of America, 85*, 1314–1321.

Löfqvist, A., Baer, T., & Yoshioka, Y. (1981). Scaling of glottal opening. *Phonetica, 38*, 236–251.

Low, L., Grabe, E., & Nolan, F. (2000). Quantitative characterizations of speech rhythm: syllable-timing in Singapore English. *Language and Speech, 43*, 377–401.

Luce, P., & Charles-Luce, J. (1985). Contextual effects on vowel duration, closure duration, and the consonant/vowel ratio in speech production. *Journal of the Acoustical Society of America, 78*, 1949–1957.

Maddieson, I. (1997). Phonetic universals. In W. Hardcastle & J. Laver (Eds.), *The handbook of phonetic sciences* (pp. 619–639). Oxford, UK: Blackwell.

Marquardt, T., Reinhart, J., & Peterson, H. (1979). Markedness analysis of phonemic substitution errors in apraxia of speech. *Journal of Communication Disorders, 12*, 481–494.

Mattys, S. L., & Liss, J. M. (2008). On building models of spoken word recognition: When there is as much to learn from natural "oddities" as artificial normality. *Perception and Psychophysics, 70*, 1235–1242.

McRoberts, G., Studdert-Kennedy, M., & Shankweiler, D. (1995). The role of fundamental frequency in signaling linguistic stress and affect: Evidence for a dissociation. *Perception and Psychophysics, 52*, 159–174.

McWhorter, J. (2001). *The power of bable: A natural history of language.* New York, NY: Henry Holt.

Metz, D., Samar, V., Schiavetti, N., Sitler, R., & Whitehead, R. (1985). Acoustic dimensions of hearing-impaired speakers' intelligibility. *Journal of Speech and Hearing Research, 28*, 345–355.

Mielke, J. (2003). The interplay of speech perception and phonology: Experimental evidence from Turkish. *Phonetica, 60*, 208–229.

Milenkovic, P. (2001). *TF32.* Computer program. http://user pages.chorus.net/cspeech/

Moon, S-J., & Lindblom, B. (1994). Interaction between duration, context, and speaking style in English stressed vowels. *Journal of the Acoustical Society of America, 96,* 40–55.

Most, T., Amir, O., & Tobin, Y. (2000) The Hebrew vowels: Raw and normalized acoustic data. *Language and Speech, 43,* 295–308.

Narayanan, S. (1995). *Fricative consonants: An articulatory, acoustic, and systems study.* Doctoral dissertation. University of California, Los Angeles.

Narayanan, S., Alwan, A., & Haker, K. (1997). Toward articulatory-acoustic models for liquid approximants based on MRI and EPG data. Part I. The laterals. *Journal of the Acoustical Society of America, 101,* 1064–1077.

Nearey, T. M., & Assman, P. F. (1986). Modelling the role of inherent spectral change in vowel identification. *Journal of the Acoustical Society of America, 80,* 1297–1308.

Newman, R., Clouse, S., & Burnham, J. (2001). The perceptual consequences of within-talker variability in fricative production. *Journal of the Acoustical Society of America, 109,* 1181–1196.

Norman, L. (1973). Rule addition and intrinsic order. *Minnesota Working Papers in Linguistics and Philosophy of Language, 1,* 135–159.

Nossair, Z., & Zahorian, S. (1991). Dynamic spectral shape features as acoustic correlates for initial stop consonants. *Journal of the Acoustical Society of America, 89,* 2978–2991.

Ohala, J. (1980). *The acoustic origin of the smile.* Paper presented at the 100th meeting of the Acoustical Society of America, Los Angeles.

Ohde, R. (1984). Fundamental frequency as an acoustic correlate of stop consonant voicing. *Journal of the Acoustical Society of America, 75,* 224–230.

Pell, M. (2001). Influence of emotion and focus location on prosody in matched statements and questions. *Journal of the Acoustical Society of America, 109,* 1668–1680.

Penner, H., Miller, N., Hertrich, I., Ackermann, H., & Schumm, F. (2001). Dysprosody in Parkinson's disease: An investigation of intonation patterns. *Clinical Linguistics and Phonetics, 15,* 551–566.

Peterson, G., & Barney, H. (1952). Control methods used in a study of the vowels. *Journal of the Acoustical Society of America, 24,* 175–184.

Picheny, M., Durlach, N., & Braida, L. (1985). Speaking clearly for the hard of hearing I: Intelligibility differences between clear and conversational speech. *Journal of Speech and Hearing Research, 28,* 96–103.

Picheny, M., Durlach, N., & Braida, L. (1986). Speaking clearly for the hard of hearing II: Acoustic characteristics of clear and conversational speech. *Journal of Speech and Hearing Research, 29,* 434–446.

Platt, L., Andrews, G., & Howie, P. (1980). Dysarthria of adult cerebral palsy. II. Phonemic analysis of articulation errors. *Journal of Speech and Hearing Research, 23,* 41–55.

Port, R. (2003). Meter and speech. *Journal of Phonetics, 31,* 599–611.

Pruthi, T., & Espy-Wilson, C. (2004). Acoustic parameters for automatic extraction of nasal manner. *Speech Communication, 43,* 225–239.

Qi, Y., & Fox, R. (1992). Analysis of nasal consonants using perceptual linear prediction. *Journal of the Acoustical Society of America, 91,* 1718–1726.

Repp, B. (1986). Perception of the [m]-[n] distinction in CV syllables. *Journal of the Acoustical Society of America, 79,* 1987–1999.

Robb, M. P., & Chen, Y. (2009). Is /h/ phonetically neutral? *Clinical Linguistics and Phonetics, 23,* 842–855.

Rong, P., & Kuehn, D. P. (2010). The effect of oral articulation on the acoustic characteristics of nasalized vowels. *Journal of the Acoustical Society of America, 127,* 2543–2553.

Rosen, K., Kent, R., Delaney, A., & Duffy, J. (2006). Parametric quantitative acoustic analysis of conversation produced by speakers with dysarthria and healthy speakers. *Journal of Speech, Language, and Hearing Research, 49,* 395–411.

Seitz, P., McCormick, M., Watson, I., & Bladon, A. (1990). Relational spectral features for place of articulation in nasal consonants. *Journal of the Acoustical Society of America, 87,* 351–358.

Sereno, J., & Jongman, A. (1995). Acoustic correlates of grammatical class. *Language and Speech, 38,* 57–76.

Serrurier, A., & Badin, P. (2008). A three-dimensional articulatory model of the velum and nasopharyngeal wall based on MRI and CT data. *Journal of the Acoustical Society of America, 123,* 2335–2355.

Shriberg, L., Campbell, T., Karlsson, H., Brown, R., McSweeny, J., & Nadler, C. (2003). A diagnostic marker for childhood apraxia of speech: The lexical stress ratio. *Clinical Linguistics and Phonetics, 17,* 549–574.

Silverman, K. (1987). *The structure and processing of fundamental frequency contours.* Doctoral dissertation, Cambridge University.

Smiljanić, R., & Bradlow, A. (2005). Does clear speech enhance the voice onset time contrast in Croatian and English? *Journal of the Acoustical Society of America, 118,* 1900.

Smiljanić, R., & Bradlow, A. R. (2008). Stability of temporal contrasts in conversational and clear speech. *Journal of Phonetics, 36,* 91–113.

Smiljanić, R., & Bradlow, A. (2011). Bidirectional clear speech perception benefit for native and high-proficiency non-native talkers and listeners: Intelligibility and accentedness. *Journal of the Acoustical Society of America, 130,* 4020–4031.

Stathopoulos, E., & Weismer, G. (1983). Closure duration of stop consonants. *Journal of Phonetics, 11,* 395–400.

Stevens, K. (1993). Modelling affricate consonants. *Speech Communication, 13,* 33–43.

Stevens, K. (1998). *Acoustic phonetics.* Cambridge, MA: MIT Press.

Stevens, K. (2002). Toward a model for lexical access based on acoustic landmarks and distinctive features. *Journal of the Acoustical Society of America, 111,* 1872–1891.

Stevens, K., Fant, G., & Hawkins, S. (1987). Some acoustical and perceptual correlates of nasal vowels. In R. Channon

& L. Shockey (Eds.), *In honor of Ilse Lehiste* (pp. 241–254). Dordrecht, Netherlands: Foris.

Stevens, K., & House, A. (1963). Perturbation of vowel articulations by consonantal context: An acoustical study. *Journal of Speech and Hearing Research, 6*, 111–128.

Story, B. H., & Bunton, K. (2010). Relation of vocal tract shape, formant transitions, and stop consonant identification. *Journal of Speech, Language, and Hearing Research, 53*, 1514–1528.

Summerfield, Q. (1975). How a full account of segmental perception depends on prosody and vice versa. In A. Cohen & S. Nooteboom (Eds.), *Structure and process in speech perception* (pp. 51–66). New York, NY: Springer- Verlag.

Tabain, M. (1998). Non-sibilant fricatives in English: Spectral information above 10 kHz. *Phonetica, 55*, 107–130.

Tabain, M. (2001). Variability in fricative production and spectra: Implications for the hyper- and hypo- and quantal theories of speech production. *Language and Speech, 44*, 57–94.

Tjaden, K., & Turner, G. (1997). Spectral properties of fricatives in amyotrophic lateral sclerosis. *Journal of Speech, Language, and Hearing Research, 40*, 1358–1372.

Tjaden, K., & Wilding, G. (2004). Rate and loudness manipulations in dysarthria: Acoustic and perceptual findings. *Journal of Speech, Language, and Hearing Research, 47*, 766–783.

Tsao, Y.-C., & Weismer, G. (1997). Interspeaker variation of habitual speaking rate: Evidence for a neuromuscular component. *Journal of Speech, Language and Hearing Research, 40*, 858–866.

Turner, G., Tjaden, K., & Weismer, G. (1995). The influence of speaking rate on vowel space and speech intelligibility for individuals with amyotrophic lateral sclerosis. *Journal of Speech, Language, and Hearing Research, 38*, 1001–1013.

Umeda, N. (1975). Vowel duration in American English. *Journal of the Acoustical Society of America, 58*, 434–445.

Umeda, N. (1977). Consonant duration in American English. *Journal of the Acoustical Society of America, 61*, 846–858.

Van Santen J. (1992). Contextual effects on vowel duration. *Speech Communication, 11*, 513–546.

Wang, Y., Kent, R., Duffy, J., & Thomas, J. (2005). Dysarthria associated with traumatic brain injury: Speaking rate and emphatic stress. *Journal of Communication Disorders, 38*, 231–260.

Watson, C., & Harrington, J. (1999). Acoustic evidence for dynamic formant trajectories in Australian English vowels. *Journal of the Acoustical Society of America, 106*, 458–468.

Weismer, G. (1980). Control of the voicing distinction for intervocalic stops and fricatives: Some data and theoretical considerations. *Journal of Phonetics, 8*, 427–438.

Weismer, G. (1984). Acoustic analysis strategies for the refinement of phonological analyses. In M. Elbert, D. Dinnsen, & G. Weismer (Eds.), Phonological theory and the misarticulating child. *ASHA Monographs, 22*, 30–52.

Weismer, G. (2006). Speech disorders. In M. Traxler & M. Gernsbacher (Eds.), *Handbook of psycholinguistics* (pp. 93–124). Oxford, UK: Blackwell.

Weismer, G., Dinnsen, D., & Elbert, M. (1981). A study of the voicing distinction associated with omitted, word-final stops. *Journal of Speech and Hearing Research, 46*, 320–327.

Weismer, G., & Ingrisano, D. (1979). Phrase-level timing patterns in English: Effects of emphatic stress location and speaking rate. *Journal of Speech and Hearing Research, 22*, 516–533.

Weismer, G., Jeng, J-Y., Laures, J., Kent, R., & Kent, J. (2001). Acoustic and intelligibility characteristics of sentence production in neurogenic speech disorders. *Folia Phoniatrica et Logopaedica, 53*, 1–18.

Weismer, G., & Martin, R. (1992). Acoustic and perceptual approaches to the study of intelligibility. In R. Kent (Ed.), *Intelligibility in speech disorders* (pp. 67–118). Amsterdam, The Netherlands: John Benjamin.

Westbury, J. (1994). *X-ray microbeam speech production database user's handbook.* University of Wisconsin, Madison.

Whalen, D., & Levitt, A. (1995). The universality of intrinsic F0 of vowels. *Journal of Phonetics, 23*, 349–366.

White, L., & Mattys, S. (2007). Rhythmic typology and variation in first and second languages. In P. Prieto, J. Mascaró, & M.-J. Solé (Eds.), *Segmental and prosodic issues in romance phonology.* Current Issues in Linguistic Theory series (pp. 237–257). Amsterdam , The Netherlands: John Benjamin.

Whitehill, T., Ciocca, V., Chan, J., & Samman, N. (2006). Acoustic analysis of vowels following glossectomy. *Clinical Linguistics and Phonetics, 20*, 135–140.

Zue, V., & LaFerriere, M. (1979). Acoustic study of medial /t,d/ in American English. *Journal of the Acoustical Society of America, 66*, 1039–1050.

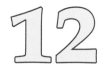

Speech Perception

INTRODUCTION

Speech perception is a multifaceted and complicated topic that depends in important ways on information presented in Chapters 8–11, but also has its own jargon and theoretical paraphernalia. The complications occur partly because there are several competing theories of speech perception, and partly because it is not always clear how experimental data bear on a choice between those theories. The same data, or at least the same general form of data, can in some cases be used to support two theories that provide opposing accounts of speech perception. This is somewhat different from speech acoustics, where a single theory seems to explain the major phenomena and the relation of data to theory is fairly straightforward.

The goal of this chapter is to present a review of speech perception that has potential relevance to clinical applications. Because history is very important to a proper understanding of the scientific study of speech perception, the early days of speech perception research are reviewed to show how these beginnings dictated the course of thinking in the area for the past half-century, indeed to the present day. The major theories of speech perception are reviewed, together with selected experiments whose results are consistent (or inconsistent) with these theories. The chapter concludes with comments about speech intelligibility as a special form of speech perception with direct relevance to clinical practice.

EARLY SPEECH PERCEPTION RESEARCH AND CATEGORICAL PERCEPTION

Scientists in the late 19th and early 20th century had thoughts about speech perception, as reviewed in an interesting article by Cole and Rudnicky (1983).

But systematic work in this area, and the creation of speech perception research as a flourishing scientific discipline, began in the late 1940s and early 1950s when scientists at Haskins Laboratories employed an early kind of speech synthesizer to perform experiments on the perception of speech. The scientists who developed the synthesizer—Franklin Cooper, Alvin Liberman, and John Borst—were already familiar with the spectrogram, which at that time was a relatively new way to display speech acoustic events. Cooper, Liberman, and Borst (1951) described a machine that allowed them to take natural spectrographic features of speech, such as vowel formant frequencies, formant transition characteristics, and stop burst spectra, and manipulate them in small steps for presentation to listeners. Such a device, they reasoned, would allow them to identify the important acoustic cues for the identification of specific speech sounds.

A diagram of this speech synthesizer, called a *pattern-playback* machine, is shown in Figure 12–1. The machine used the principle that fluctuations in light can be transformed into sound waves, under the proper conditions. Figure 12–1 shows how a light source was directed at a rotating wheel that was a circular film negative. On this film negative were a series of rings arranged in a way to produce frequencies from 120 Hz to 6000 Hz, in a consecutive-integer harmonic series. This is why the rotating circle was called a "tone wheel." A spectrographic pattern was painted on a transparent sheet (such as the overhead transparencies used in classroom presentations before the advent of computer-based presentations) and mounted on a movable surface that was exposed to light coming through the tone wheel. As light passed through the harmonic rings on the film negative and the painted spectrogram was transported by a moving belt, the dark parts of the spectrogram reflected certain of the "light frequencies" generated by the wheel, whereas the clear parts of the spectrogram generated no reflection. The movement

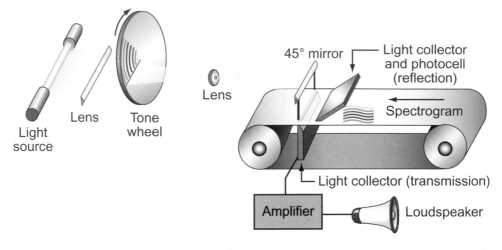

Figure 12–1. Schematic drawing of the pattern-playback machine, an early speech synthesizer used by scientists at Haskins Laboratories to do speech perception research. See text for details.

of the belt simulated the time aspect of speech. The reflected light frequencies, changing over time as the belt moved, were transmitted to a device that converted the reflections to sound (the light collector in Figure 12–1). These sound waves were amplified and output by a loudspeaker, producing spectrographic representations of speech sounds that had been painted on the transparent sheet.

The key to understanding how the device was used to create small changes in spectrographic patterns is this: The clear sheet on which the spectrographic representation was painted could reflect whatever pattern the investigator desired; any type of "speech signal" could be painted, and the question asked: How is this pattern heard? For example, Cooper and his colleagues (1951) performed an early set of experiments with the pattern-playback machine in which they discovered that a two-formant pattern with proper F1 and F2 transitions could elicit the perception of stop-vowel syllables, even though stop bursts were *not* included in the painted pattern. Such patterns—like stick figure representations of real speech signals—are shown in Figure 12–2 for the voiced (top) and voiceless (bottom) set of English stop consonants. The portion of the signals between the dotted, vertical lines shows the transitions, or changing formant frequencies as a function of time. The steady states of F1 and F2 were painted to elicit perception of the vowel /ɑ/. For the voiceless stops, the F1 transition was "cut back" in time relative to the F2 transition. More is said about this later.

When the top patterns in Figure 12–2 were transported by the moving belt and their reflected light

converted over time to sound, most listeners heard the left-most pattern as /bɑ/, the middle pattern as /dɑ/, and the right-most pattern as /gɑ/. Cooper and his colleagues selected these patterns to mimic the ones they had seen in spectrograms of natural speech; they already knew the F2 transition was different for the three places of stop consonant articulation in English, at least when the stops were followed by /ɑ/. The finding that a *burstless* pattern could elicit the perception of these stop consonants, with the correct place of articulation dependent on the pattern of transitions shown in Figure 12–2, was somewhat of a surprise.

The /bɑ/-/dɑ/-/gɑ/ Experiment

Cooper and his colleagues (1951) then asked the logical question: What happens to listeners' perception when the *starting frequency* of F2 is changed in small and systematic steps over a large range of frequencies? Using the pattern-playback machine, the scientists painted a series of two-formant patterns varying only in the starting frequency of F2. The result was a series, or *continuum* of stimuli, like those shown in Figure 12–3.

Each of these two-formant stimuli is labeled with a number, ranging from –6 to +6. The stimulus labeled 0 had no transition, and the two *endpoint* stimuli had the most extreme F2 transitions—that is, transitions covering the widest range of frequencies but moving in opposite directions. Stimulus –6 had the lowest starting frequency and, therefore, an extensive, rising F2 transition (where the transition starts at a lower frequency

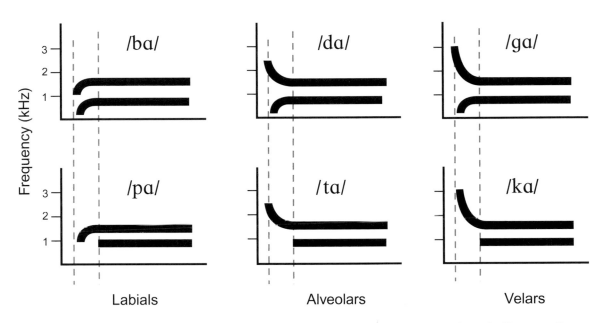

Figure 12-2. Two-formant, painted patterns used in pattern-playback experiments. These patterns, like stick figure representations of real spectrograms, were heard as stop-vowel syllables (*top*, /ba/, /da/, /ga/; *bottom*, /pa/, /ta/, and /ka/ from left to right), even though there was no stop burst painted as part of the pattern.

and moves to a higher one). Stimulus +6 had the highest starting frequency and, therefore, a very extensive, falling F2 transition. The other features of these stimuli were constant across the entire continuum, including the rising F1 transition and the voice bar preceding it (the voice bar ensured that all stops would be heard as voiced). The previous discussion of the three patterns in Figure 12–2 suggests that endpoint stimulus –6 was heard as /ba/ and endpoint stimulus –6 as /ga/. How did listeners respond to the other stimuli along the continuum?

When Cooper and his colleagues (1951) performed this experiment, they first obtained *identification data* from listeners. In the identification experiment, listeners were asked to label the presented stimuli. Listeners had three labels from which to choose: /b/, /d/, or /g/. Each stimulus was presented several times to each member of a crew of listeners, and the results were plotted as the percentage of /b/, /d/, or /g/ responses across the series of stimuli. A typical plot of the results is shown in Figure 12–4.

In this plot, stimulus number (see Figure 12–3) is on the *x*-axis, which is also labeled "F2 starting frequency" because the different stimulus numbers indicate different starting frequencies. The percentage of /b/ (pink boxes), /d/ (white boxes), and /g/ (blue boxes) judgments for each stimulus number is on the *y*-axis. A quick glance at these identification results

shows that stimuli from –6 to –3 were heard almost exclusively as /b/, stimuli from –1 to +2 as /d/, and stimuli from +4 to +6 as /g/. A few stimuli, such as –2 and +3, were ambiguous, but –2 was only ambiguous for /b/ and /d/ responses (no /g/ responses) and +3 was only ambiguous for /d/ and /g/ responses (no /g/ responses).

The take-home message from this experiment was that relatively continuous variation of the physical stimulus—the starting frequency of the F2 transition—did not result in a continuous change in the perceptual response. Rather, place of articulation seemed to be perceived *categorically*, with a series of adjacent stimuli yielding one response, as in the case of stimuli –6 through –3 producing a percept of /b/, until a sudden change in response pattern at the next step along the continuum (e.g., at stimulus –2).

Categorical Perception: Some General Considerations

The finding that stop place of articulation was perceived categorically, not continuously, has had a profound effect on speech perception research and theory. The meaning of categorical perception is discussed here more thoroughly before returning to the interpretation of the /ba/-/da/-/ga/ experiment described above.

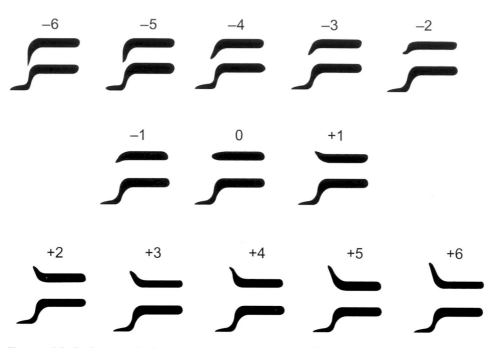

Figure 12–3. Series of stimuli painted for pattern-playback experiments on the effect of F2 transition starting frequency on perception of stop consonant place of articulation. Stimulus "–6" had the lowest F2 starting frequency, and stimulus "+6" had the highest F2 starting frequency. Each stimulus from "–6" to "+6" increased the F2 starting frequency by a small increment. The flat portion in each stimulus preceding the F1 transition ensured that the stop was heard as voiced. After Liberman, Harris, Hoffman, and Griffith (1957).

Categorical perception is demonstrated when continuous variation in a physical stimulus is perceived in a discontinuous (i.e., categorical) way. The study of psychological reactions to variations in physical stimuli is called *psychophysics*. Categorical perception is an example of a psychophysical phenomenon. A schematic illustration of categorical perception, and how it contrasts with the psychophysical phenomenon of *continuous perception*, is shown in Figure 12–5.

Both graphs in Figure 12–5 show hypothetical relationships between a continuously varying physical variable (*x*-axis) and a perceptual (psychological) response (*y*-axis). The perceptual response is a number assigned by the perceiver to the magnitude or quality of each stimulus along the physically varying continuum. This is why the *y*-axis is labeled "Psychological scale value." In the left-hand graph, each change of the physical variable from a lower to higher value elicits a corresponding change in the perceiver's mind and, therefore, on the number scale. This results in the straight-line, 45-degree function relating the changes

in the physical stimulus to changes on the psychological scale. The function in the left-hand graph is labeled "continuous perception" because a given increment along the physical scale always results in the same increment along the perceptual scale.

The right-hand graph shows a different relationship. Here the continuous variation of the physical stimulus is exactly the same as in the left-hand graph, but the perceptual response is much different. The initial change in the physical stimulus, beginning at the lowest values, produces *no change* in the psychological scale value; the variations in the physical stimulus result in a constant psychological scale value. The listener treats the different stimuli as belonging to a single psychological event. When the stimulus reaches the value indicated by the first vertical dotted line, the perceptual scale value "jumps" to a higher value, where it stays even as the physical stimulus continues to increase to higher values. The same thing happens at the second dotted line, where the perceptual scale value jumps to yet another higher value.

Identification

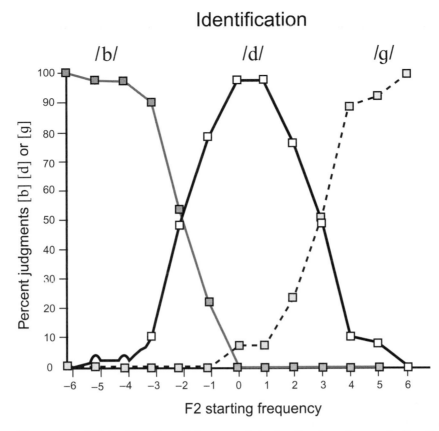

Figure 12-4. Identification (labeling) data for the two-formant stimuli shown in Figure 12–3 and described in text. The x-axis is labeled "F2 starting frequency" but the values along the axis are the stimulus numbers shown in Figure 12–3. The y-axis is the percent judgments of /b/, /d/, or /g/. /b/ labels as a function of F2 starting frequency (stimulus number) are shown by pink boxes, /d/ labels by white boxes, /g/ labels by blue boxes. See text for interpretation. Figure adapted from Liberman et al. (1957).

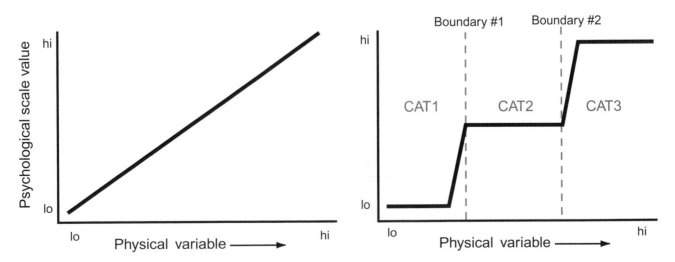

Figure 12-5. Two schematic graphs showing the difference between continuous (*left*) and categorical (*right*) psychophysical functions. Variation in the physical stimulus is shown on the x-axes, variation in the psychological reaction on the y-axes. See text for discussion.

The vertical dotted lines in the right-hand graph are labeled "Boundary 1" and "Boundary 2." The lines indicate locations along the physical stimulus continuum where a small change in the value of the stimulus results in a sudden and large change in the perceptual response. The function in the right-hand graph shows categorical perception, because the two boundaries separate the psychological reaction to a continuously varying stimulus into three categories, labeled CAT1, CAT2, and CAT3. In categorical perception, the *same* increment along the physical stimulus produces very different psychological responses, depending on whether the increment is within a category, or straddling a category boundary. Within a category, a small change along the physical continuum leads to little or no difference in the psychological response. Exactly the same change *across* a category boundary, however, causes a major change in the psychological response.

This simple description of the difference between continuous and categorical perception applies directly to the pattern-playback results shown in Figure 12–4. The F2 starting frequency was changed more or less continuously from low to high values, but listeners heard only categories, not smoothly changing speech events. The categorical labeling functions shown in Figure 12–4 are entirely consistent with the schematic illustration of categorical perception shown in Figure 12–5. Small changes in the F2 starting frequency, starting from the lowest value, all yielded /b/ responses. At a certain point along the physical continuum of F2 starting frequencies the *same* change resulted in a sudden shift to /d/ responses. The perception of place of articulation for stop consonants appeared to be categorical when the F2 starting frequency was the physical variable of interest.

Labeling Versus Discrimination

One more experiment was required to verify the categorical perception of stop consonant place of articulation. The categorical perception functions shown in Figure 12–4 were from an experiment in which listeners heard a stimulus and attached a label to it. Listeners were told to label the stimuli as /b/, /d/, or /g/. The resulting categorical perception functions may have reflected nothing more than the listeners being limited to just these three categories as responses. For example, listeners were not permitted to respond, "This stimulus sounds as if it is midway between a /b/ and /d/ (or between a /d/ and /g/)," even though it is possible some stimuli sounded this way. If such responses were available to the listeners, the functions may not have looked as categorical as those shown in Figure 12–4.

To address this potential problem, the labeling experiment was followed by a *discrimination experiment*. As indicated above in the discussion of Figure 12–5, in a true categorical perception function, an increment of fixed magnitude in the physical stimulus may result in either no psychological change, or a large psychological change, depending on where the increment is located along the entire physical continuum. A fixed physical increment between two stimuli, located within a category determined by a labeling experiment, should produce little or no psychological change. The same increment located *across* a category boundary should produce a large psychological change. In a discrimination experiment, a true categorical perception function is determined when listeners cannot discriminate two different stimuli chosen from within a category, but easily discriminate two stimuli chosen *across* a category boundary (one chosen from one category, the other from the adjacent category). *The physical difference between the two stimuli is the same in both cases, but the psychological reaction to the difference between the stimuli is radically different.*

Cooper and his colleagues (1951) performed these discrimination experiments after they demonstrated what appeared to be categorical labeling functions for place of articulation, as cued by F2 starting frequency. The discrimination experiments produced the expected results. When listeners were asked if two stimuli (presented one after the other) were the same or different, they said "same" when the stimuli were chosen from within a category determined in the labeling experiment, and "different" when the stimuli were chosen from adjacent categories. This result was obtained even when the actual physical difference between the two judged stimuli was the same. The categorical labeling functions (see Figure 12–4) were confirmed by the discrimination experiment.

Categorical Perception: So What?

What was important about the demonstration of categorical perception for place of articulation? Liberman, Cooper, Shankweiler, and Studdert-Kennedy (1967), in their famous paper "Perception of the Speech Code," pointed to categorical perception as a cornerstone of the *motor theory of speech perception*. Listeners do not hear the continuous changes in F2 starting frequency, at least until a category boundary is reached, because they cannot *produce* continuous changes in place of articulation. Consideration of the different places of articulation for English stops shows why Liberman and his colleagues reasoned in this way. How do you produce a stop between a bilabial /b/ and a lingua-alveolar /d/? Or between a /d/ and dorsal /g/? The places of articulation for stops are essentially categorical, allowing no "in between" articulatory placements.[1]

The motor theory of speech perception was built on the idea that speech perception was constrained by speech production. In this view, a categorical production event, such as place of articulation for stops, limits speech perception to the same categories. Detection of acoustic differences within categories is therefore not possible. Liberman et al.'s (1967) focus on the role of speech production in speech perception, however, extended beyond the demonstration of categorical perception. Recall from Chapter 11 the discussion of pattern-playback experiments in which very different F2 transition patterns cued the perception of a single stop consonant (/d/, in the case covered in Chapter 11; see Figure 11–34). Liberman et al. reviewed several experiments in which a great deal of acoustic variability, primarily due to varying phonetic context, was associated with perception of a single stop consonant. In Chapter 11, this was described as the "no acoustic invariance" problem. Liberman et al. regarded the lack of acoustic invariance for a given stop consonant as a problem for a theory of speech perception in which listeners based their phonetic decisions directly on information in the acoustic signal. Instead, the constant factor in speech perception, at least for stop consonants, seemed to be the *articulatory* characteristics of a stop consonant. Yes, a stop such as /d/ may have varying acoustic characteristics—especially as seen in the F2 transition, and possibly also in the burst—depending on the identity of a preceding or following vowel, but the lingua-alveolar place of articulation remains constant across all phonetic contexts. For Liberman et al., it made more sense for listeners to base their phonetic decisions concerning a particular stop place of articulation on these constant articulatory characteristics, rather than the highly variable speech acoustic signal.

It is one thing to claim that speech is perceived by reference to articulation; it is another to say exactly how this is done. Liberman et al. (1967) argued for a species-specific mechanism in the brain of humans—a specialized and dedicated module for the perception of speech. An important component of this claim was the link between speech production and perception, specifically the "match" between the capabilities of the speech production and speech perception mechanisms. Part of this match was a notion of speech production as

Mirror, Mirror, in the Brain

When the motor theory was first proposed, the brain mechanisms for the (hypothesized) special module were unknown. Experiments were done to show that the likely location of the module was in the left hemisphere (Studdert-Kennedy & Shankweiler, 1970), but these were perception experiments and the inference to actual brain mechanisms involved a very long leap. Fast forward to the 21st century and the use of imaging and stimulation techniques to uncover brain function for complex behavior (like speech), and we have the concept of "mirror neurons." These are neurons that appear to be active during both the production and perception of action. When someone produces a gesture (such as a speech gesture), the *perceiver* of that gesture has greater activity in the neurons that are involved in *producing* the gesture! The motor neurons are said to "mirror" the perception of the gesture. Perhaps this is the brain basis of the species-specific, speech module proposed in motor theory (see Watkins & Paus, 2004).

an *encoded* form of communication. If there is encoding, there must be decoding, and this was provided by the special perceptual mechanism in the brain of humans. For Liberman et al. (1967), the tight link between speech perception and production was part of the evolutionary history of *Homo sapiens*.

There is more to the motor theory. Specifics are provided by Liberman et al. (1967) on how speech production is encoded in the acoustic signal emerging from a speaker's mouth, and how this signal is decoded by the human brain to recover articulatory behaviors. For the purposes of this chapter, these details are not critical and many of them have faced strong scientific challenges. What is critical are two general claims of the theory: (a) speech perception is a species-specific; human endowment; and (b) the speech acoustic signal associated with a given sound is far too variable to be useful for speech perception, but the underlying articulatory behavior is not, hence the claim that speech is perceived by reference to articulation.

---

[1]Perhaps this is not completely true. It seems as if stops can be made between the English locations for /d/ and /g/, by retroflexing the tongue and making the point of articulation posterior to the typical lingua-alveolar location (or anterior to the typical dorsal location for /g/; in fact, some languages have stops that are made in this way). Other "in between" possibilities can also be imagined.

Speech Perception Is Species Specific

The ability to speak is exclusive to humans. It makes sense that a theory of speech perception as a skill "matched" to speech production is regarded by many scientists as an exclusively human capability. The notion of coevolved mechanisms for production and perception of vocalizations, and especially of dedicated perceptual mechanisms "tuned" to species-specific vocalizations, is not limited to humans, however. There is evidence in monkeys, bats, and birds (and other animals) of perceptual mechanisms matched to the particular vocalizations produced by the animals (Andoni, Li, & Pollak, 2007; Davies, Madden, & Butchart, 2004; Miller & Jucszyk, 1989). The possible existence of such a match in humans is, consistent, in principle, with evolutionary principles derived from the study of vocal communication in other animals.

"In principle" evaluations of a theory are fine, but they do not go far enough. A theory should be testable, either by natural observation or experimentation. Karl Popper (2002a, 2002b), a famous philosopher of science, argued strongly that a theory can only be considered "scientific" if it can be disproved by a proper experiment. In other words, a theory has scientific value only if makes specific predictions that potentially can be shown to be untrue (can be "falsified") by a properly designed experiment. According to Popper, these experiment-based "falsifications" of a theory are the basis of scientific progress. Popper first published these ideas in the 1935 German edition of *The Logic of Scientific Discovery*. The book was published in English translation in 1959. Popper's ideas have had a profound influence on modern science in general, and very specifically on the motor theory of speech perception.

How can the motor theory be falsified? The scope of the present chapter does not allow a detailed answer to this question, but one can ask if there have been attempts to falsify the claims of the motor theory.

Categorical Perception of Stop Place of Articulation Shows the "Match" to Speech Production

The motor theory was criticized for failing to explain why certain individuals who could not speak (as in some cases of cerebral palsy, or other neurological diseases) were able to perceive speech in a normal way. This complaint was misguided, however, because the motor theorists never argued for the ability to *produce* speech as a requirement for normal speech perception abilities. To the contrary, the species-specific module for speech perception was thought to be innate (Liberman

& Mattingly, 1985)—a property of the human brain at birth. The demonstration of categorical perception in infants as young as 1 month of age was taken as evidence for this innate mechanism. These functions were very much like those obtained from adult listeners, even though infants do not produce speech. The categorical perception functions were obtained in infants by taking advantage of something infants do quite well, which is to suck for long periods of time. When infants suck for long periods of time, the strength of their suck varies with the degree of novelty in their environment. If things remain the same for a while, sucking is less intense. The introduction of a novel stimulus (something seen, heard, smelled) results in a sudden increase in suck strength, frequency, or both. Early studies of infant speech perception used sucking behavior to assess babies' reactions to speech stimuli within and across categories. Categorical perception functions, resembling quite closely those obtained from adults, were demonstrated in infants with the sucking paradigm. An excellent review of early infant speech perception research and methods is found in Eimas, Miller, and Jusczyk (1990).

What About Talking Birds?

The motor theory is species-specific to humans. The link between articulatory and speech perception capabilities is special because humans are the only species who produce speech sounds for communication. But wait. What about talking birds—mynahs, crows, budgerigars (small parrots, often called parakeets), and African Greys, for example. Talking birds produce speech using a very different apparatus from humans—they have no lips, and do not produce a sound source at the larynx but rather have a sound-producing mechanism deep in their chests called a syrinx. Yet the major question is not, "Can these birds articulate?" (because they obviously produce intelligible speech, even if mimicked), but "When they articulate, can they make *voluntary* adjustments to produce different speech sounds?" If the answer is, "Yes, they make such adjustments," then the species-specific claim of motor theory runs into some difficulty. Patterson and Pepperberg (1998) made just this claim for an African Grey parrot. An opposing view, that the speech produced by talking birds is nothing more than noninventive mimicry, was expressed by Lieberman (1996).

An apparent falsification of the motor theory was, ironically, a logical outgrowth of the findings in infants. If nonspeaking infants had categorical perception of sound contrasts, perhaps the same would be true of animals. Perhaps the reason infants showed the effect had little to do with a species-specific, speech perception mechanism, but instead reflected some general property of mammalian auditory systems. In fact, work by Kuhl and her colleagues (Kuhl, 1986; Kuhl & Miller, 1975; Kuhl & Padden, 1983) and others demonstrated categorical perception for voice-onset time (VOT) and stop place of articulation in chinchillas and monkeys, respectively. If categorical perception is the result of a special linkage between human speech production and perception, as claimed by Liberman et al. (1967), the existence of categorical speech perception in animals serves as a falsification of the linkage specifically, and the motor theory in general. A kinder interpretation of the animal data is that they raise questions about the motor theory, but do not falsify the theory in an absolute way. Miller and Jusczyk (1989) summarized this position thusly: "*In principle, there are many ways to arrive at the same classification of a set of objects. Hence, the fact that the animals can achieve the same classification does not prove that they use the same means to do so as humans*" (pp. 124–125). In other words, the data could turn out the same way in adult humans, human infants, and animals, but not necessarily as a result of a single, shared mechanism. This is an example of the same findings (categorical perception of speech signals) supporting opposing theoretical views.

Duplex Perception

The possibility of a special speech-perception module in the brains of humans does not, of course, eliminate the need for general auditory function. A host of everyday auditory perceptions requires analysis by mechanisms external to the speech module. Presumably, a speech signal "automatically" engages the speech module (the option is not available to "turn it off" for short periods of time, even if this would occasionally be a nice idea). Other auditory signals engage "general" (nonmodule) auditory mechanisms for analysis and perception. The idea of a separation[2] between mechanisms for speech perception versus general auditory perception was exploited experimentally to prove the existence of the speech module.

The schematic spectrograms in Figure 12–6 (adapted from Whalen & Liberman, 1987) illustrate the concept of *duplex perception*, the phenomenon in which the speech module *and* general auditory mechanisms seem to be activated simultaneously by one signal (Mann & Liberman, 1983; Whalen & Liberman, 1987). The upper graph shows a schematic spectrogram, with fixed patterns for F1 and F2, and two different transitions for F3. The steady-state formant frequencies are appropriate for the vowel /ɑ/, and the F1 and F2 transitions convey the impression of a stop consonant preceding the vowel. If this pattern is synthesized with a rising F3 transition, listeners hear /gɑ/. A falling F3 transition cues the perception of /dɑ/. The different perceptual effects of the rising versus falling F3 transition are consistent with naturally produced /gɑ/ and /dɑ/ syllables.

If the F3 transition portion (either the rising or falling one) is edited out from the schematic signal in the upper part of the Figure and played to listeners, the brief signal (~50 ms in duration) sounds something like a bird chirp or whistle glide. In the case of the transition for /g/, the pitch of this "chirp" rises quickly, and for /d/ it falls quickly. The isolated transitions are shown in the lower right-hand graph in Figure 12–6. Regardless of exactly how people hear these isolated transitions—as "chirps," quick frequency glides (*glissandi*, in musical terms), or outer space noises—they are *not* heard as having phonetic characteristics.

This situation suggests something of a perceptual mystery. Listeners hear the three-formant pattern at the top of Figure 12–6 as either /g/ or /d/, depending on whether the F3 transition is rising (/g/) or falling (/d/). But when that brief, apparently critical F3 transition is isolated from the spectrographic pattern and played to listeners, they hear something with absolutely no phonetic quality.

What do people hear when presented with the pattern *minus* the F3 transition? In Figure 12–6, this pattern is referred to as the "base," which listeners hear as a not-very-clear /d/, something different from the unambiguous /d/ heard when the falling F3 transition is in place.

Now the phenomenon of duplex perception, and its relationship to the concept of a special speech perception module in the brains of humans, can be explained. Consider the base and isolated transitions shown in Figure 12–6 as two separate signals, and imagine one of these signals (the base) delivered to one

---

[2]"Separation" may be too weak to describe what the motor theorists meant by a speech perception module. The motor theorists, and other cognitive scientists who investigated the role of modules in various aspects of cognition, viewed these mechanisms as dedicated to a single process, and isolated from other processes. The speech module envisioned by motor theorists was not only separable from other auditory processes, but there was no traffic between the two. Stated otherwise, the speech module was impermeable to general auditory processes, and vice versa.

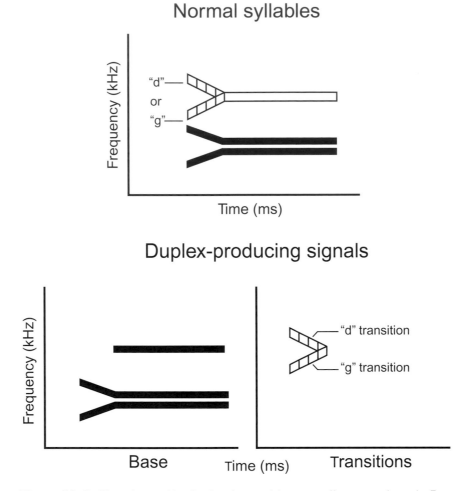

Figure 12-6. Signals used in duplex (speech) perception experiments. Top graph shows three-formant patterns, with fixed patterns for F1 and F2. The third formant has either a rising transition (producing a percept of /ga/) or falling transition (producing a percept of /da/). When these F3 transitions are presented alone, as shown in the lower right-hand panel of the figure, they sound like rising or falling bird "chirps" or whistles. When the three-formant pattern is presented without the F3 transition (the base, lower left-hand panel of the figure), listeners typically hear an indistinct /da/ (as compared to the very clear /da/ heard when the falling F3 transition is in place). Playing the base into one ear, and an F3 transition into the other ear, results in simultaneous perception of the "good" syllable (either /da/ or /ga/, depending on which F3 transition is played) plus the nonspeech "chirp." The same effect can be produced with both signals in one ear and the isolated F3 transition played at a fairly high level. The "duplex" in "duplex perception" is the simultaneous perception of a speech and nonspeech event, from the same signal.

ear, and the other (an isolated transition) delivered to the other ear. This experimental arrangement is shown in the cartoon of Figure 12–7, where the "base" is sent to a listener's right ear and one of the "isolated transitions"—either the one appropriate to /g/, or /d/—is sent to the left ear. The isolated F3 transition is delivered to the left ear with proper timing relative to the F1

and F2 transitions in the base, meaning the transition is sequenced properly in time relative to the base (as in the top graph of Figure 12–6, showing the "complete" patterns for either /d/ or /g/).

What did listeners hear when the experiment depicted in Figure 12–7 was performed? Mann and Liberman (1983), among others, showed that listeners

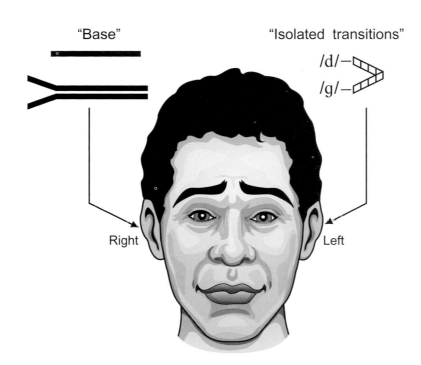

Figure 12-7. Cartoon showing how duplex perception experiment was performed. The base was delivered to one ear, the isolated F3 transition to the other ear. Alternatively, both signals were delivered to the same ear and the presentation level of the isolated transition was raised until listeners heard both the "good" syllable and the chirp.

heard a "good" /dɑ/ or /gɑ/ (depending on which F3 transition was played) *plus* a chirp! The simultaneous perception from the same signal of two events—speech and nonspeech—suggested the term "duplex perception." Duplex perception seemed to show the human listener operating simultaneously in the special speech mode and in the general auditory mode. The perception of the "good" /dɑ/ or /gɑ/ was the result of the "base" and the "isolated transition" combining somewhere in the nervous system, automatically engaging the speech mode of perception. At the same time, the isolated F3 transition was processed as a chirp by general auditory mechanisms. The F3 transition, therefore, did double duty, engaging two different kinds of hearing mechanism at the same time. One of those mechanisms, according to Mann and Liberman (1983) and Whalen and Liberman (1987), could only be the specialized speech perception module proposed as the centerpiece of the motor theory.

In many ways, this experimental finding seemed to be a strong endorsement of a species-specific module for perceiving speech. What other explanation could account for why the same signal (the F3 transition) evoked two simultaneous perceptions, one clearly phonetic and consistent with previous studies on the role

of the transition in cuing /g/ or /d/, the other clearly nonphonetic and consistent with the direction of the frequency glide (rising versus falling)? Even though duplex perception seemed like ironclad evidence for a special mode for perceiving speech, distinct from general auditory processes, the results of an experiment reported by Fowler and Rosenblum (1991) cast doubt on this interpretation.

Fowler and Rosenblum (1991) recorded the acoustic signal produced by the closing of a metal door. They computed a spectrum of this acoustic event, like the one shown in the upper graph of Figure 12–8. Then they separated the spectrum into two parts, a lower-frequency part (from 0 to 3.0 kHz) and a higher frequency part (from 3.0 to 11.0 kHz; see lower left and lower right graphs in Figure 12–8). This separation was accomplished by filtering the original signal to get the 0- to 3.0-kHz and 3.0- to 11.0-kHz parts. Fowler and Rosenblum presented these three signals (the original, "full" signal; the 0- to 3.0-kHz part; and the 3.0-to 11.0-kHz part) to listeners for separate identification. Listeners reported hearing a metal door closing or some "hard collision" for the full signal (upper graph of Figure 12–8), a duller, wooden door-closing sound for the 0- to 3.0-kHz signal (lower left graph, Figure 12–8),

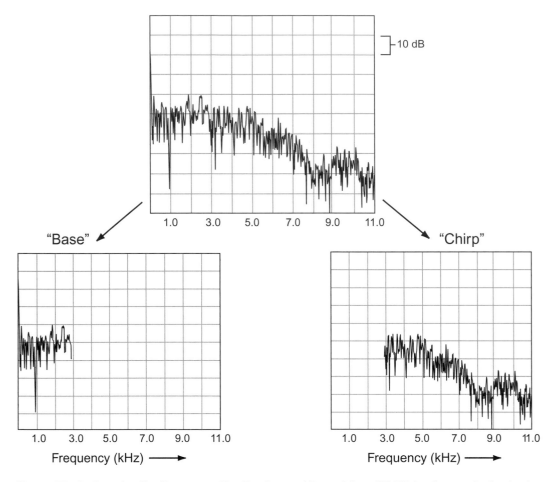

Figure 12–8. Spectra like those used by Fowler and Rosenblum (1991) to demonstrate duplex perception for nonspeech events. Top spectrum is of a slamming metal door. The bottom two spectra are the result of filtering the top spectrum in two ways: (a) to allow only the frequencies from 0 to 3.0 kHz to be heard (*bottom, left*), and (b) to allow only the frequencies from 3.0 to 11.0 kHz to be heard (*bottom, right*). The 0- to 3.0-kHz spectrum is analogous to the base, the 3.0- to 11.0-kHz spectrum is analogous to the chirp. When the two bottom signals are played at the same time and the 3.0- to 11.0-kHz signal has sufficient intensity, listeners hear a slamming metal door and a shaking can of rice (or jangling keys) at the same time, demonstrating duplex perception for nonspeech signals.

and a shaking can of rice, a tambourine, or jangling keys for the 3.0- to 11.0-kHz signal (lower right graph, Figure 12–8).

Fowler and Rosenblum (1991) took advantage of a finding reported by Whalen and Liberman (1987) for their next experimental move: Whalen and Liberman had obtained duplex perception for /dɑ/ and /gɑ/ syllables in which the "base" and "chirp" (isolated third formant transition, as in Figure 12–6) were played into the *same* ear, but the "chirp" was raised in intensity relative to the "base." When the "chirp" intensity was relatively low in comparison with the "base," listeners heard a good /dɑ/ or /gɑ/ depending on which F3

transition was used, but as the F3 "chirp" was increased in intensity a threshold was reached at which listeners heard both a good /dɑ/ or /gɑ/ *plus* a "chirp." In other words, they perceived the signal as duplex, just as in the earlier experiments described above in which the "base" and "chirp" were in opposite ears. Fowler and Rosenblum repeated this experiment except with the 0- to 3.0-kHz signal as the "base" and the 3.0- to 11.0-kHz signal as the "chirp." Relatively low "chirp" intensities produced a percept of a slamming metal door, consistent with the percept elicited by the original, intact signal (top spectrum in Figure 12–8). As the "chirp" intensity was raised, a threshold was reached at which listeners heard the slamming metal door *plus* the shaking can of rice/tambourine/ jangling keys. Fowler and Rosenblum (1991) thus evoked a duplex percept exactly parallel to the one described above for /dɑ/ and /gɑ/, except in this case for nonspeech sounds.

If the original duplex perception findings (Liberman & Mattingly, 1985; Mann & Liberman, 1983; Whalen & Liberman, 1987) seemed to provide compelling evidence for a special speech perception module in humans, the demonstration of duplex perception for a slamming metal door is devastating evidence *against* the idea of the speech module. As Fowler and Rosenblum (1991) pointed out, if the phonetic member of duplex perception was taken as the output of a special speech module, the slamming metal door percept in response to presentation of the two lower signals in Figure 12–8 had to be taken as evidence of a special human module for the perception of such doors being slammed shut. It is not ridiculous to imagine a human biological endowment for perceiving speech signals as an evolutionary adaptation, but it is impossible to imagine an adaptive advantage for modular (automatic) processing of the sound of a slamming metal door. Perhaps there is a special biological endowment for perceiving speech, but duplex perception is not the critical test for its existence.

Acoustic Invariance

The lack of acoustic invariance for speech sounds was an important catalyst for the development of the motor theory of speech perception. As discussed in Chapter 11, Blumstein and Stevens (1979) performed an acoustic analysis of stop burst acoustics that led them to reject this central claim of the motor theorists. Blumstein and Stevens used the stop burst spectrum to classify correctly 85% of word-initial stop consonants in a variety of vowel contexts. They regarded this finding as a falsification of the motor theorists' claim that there was too much context-conditioned acoustic variability to allow listeners to establish a consistent and reliable link between speech acoustic characteristics and phonetic categories. For the motor theorist, consistency associated with speech sound categories was found in the underlying articulatory gestures for specific sounds, even when the context of a sound was changed. For the motor theorist, the "underlying articulatory gesture" was the neural code for generating the gesture. This code was assumed to be "fixed" for a particular gesture, regardless of its phonetic context. Whatever changes occurred to the *actual* articulatory gesture—the collective movements of the lips, tongue, mandible, and so forth—were not relevant to the motor theory. In the motor theory, perception of speech depended on these more abstract neural commands, higher up in the process, so to speak, that were not coded for phonetic context. These invariant commands were assumed to be part of the special speech module.

The falsification of the lack of acoustic invariance for sound categories is a bit more involved than a simple demonstration of consistency between a selected acoustic measure (such as the shape of a burst spectrum) and a particular sound. Liberman and Mattingly (1985), in a very fine review of why they believed the acoustic signal was not consistent enough to establish and maintain speech sound categories in perception (where "categories" = "phonemes"), identified a whole set of complications with so-called "auditory theories" of speech perception. Auditory theories claim that information in the speech acoustic signal is sufficient, and sufficiently consistent, to support speech perception. These theories regard the auditory mechanisms for speech perception to be the same as mechanisms for the perception of environmental sounds, music, or any acoustic signal. One specific auditory perspective on speech perception (Diehl, Lotto, & Holt, 2004; Kingston & Diehl, 1994) claims that speakers control their speech acoustic output to produce speech signals well-matched to auditory processing capabilities.

Why were Liberman and Mattingly (1985) so adamant in rejecting auditory theories of speech perception? First, Liberman and Mattingly pointed to what they termed "extraphonetic" factors that cause variation in the acoustic characteristics of speech sounds. These factors include (among others) speaking rate and speaker sex and age. The speaker sex/age issue is particularly interesting because the same vowel has widely varying formant frequencies depending on the size of a speaker's vocal tract. An auditory theory of speech perception either requires listeners to learn all these different formant patterns, or employs some sort of cognitive process to place all formant patterns on a single, "master" scale. This issue, of how one hears the same vowel (or consonant) when so many different-sized vocal tracts produce it with different formant frequencies, is called the "speaker normalization" issue (interesting papers on speaker normalization are found in Johnson and Mullenix, 1997; see also Adank, Smits, & van Hout, 2004). The motor theory, however, finesses this problem by arguing that the perception of different formant transition patterns is mediated by a special mechanism that extracts intended articulatory gestures and "outputs" these gestures as the percepts. For example, the motor theory assumes that the intended gestures (the neural code for the gestures) for the vowel in the word "bad" are roughly equivalent for men, women, and children, even if the outputs of their different-sized vocal tracts are not. The special speech perception module registers the same intended gesture for all three speakers, and hence the same vowel perception. The motor theory makes the speaker normalization problem go away.

A second reason to reject auditory theories, according to Liberman and Mattingly (1985), is the interesting case of trading relations in the acoustic cues for a given sound category. For any given sound, there are at least several different acoustic cues whose values can contribute to the proper identification of the sound. As Liberman and Mattingly pointed out, none of these individual values are necessarily critical to the proper identification of a sound segment, but the *collection* of the several values may be. More interesting for the present discussion, among these several cues, the acoustic value of one can be "offset" by the acoustic value of another to yield the same phonetic percept. For example, Figure 12–9 shows spectrograms of a single speaker's production of the words "say" and "stay." These two words can be described as a minimal-pair opposition defined by the presence or absence of the stop consonant /t/. In "stay" (but not "say") there is the obvious silent closure interval of approximately 60 to 90 ms, but the "say"-"stay" opposition also involves a subtle difference in the starting frequency of the F1 transition for /eɪ/. Figure 12–9 shows the F1 starting frequency in "stay" to be somewhat lower than the starting frequency in "say" (compare frequen-

cies labeled "F1 onset"). The lower starting frequency in "stay" is consistent with theoretical and laboratory findings of F1 transitions pointing toward the spectrographic baseline — that is, 0 Hz — at the boundary of a stop consonant and vowel (Fant, 1960).

In an often cited experiment, Best, Morrongiello, and Robson (1981), took advantage of these two cues to the difference between "say" and "stay" — the closure interval, and the lower F1 starting frequency following the stop closure — to demonstrate the "trading relations" phenomenon. Figure 12–10 shows the kinds of stimuli used by Best et al. to make their point. The gray, stippled interval represents the voiceless fricative /s/, the narrow rectangles the closure intervals for /t/, and the two solid lines the F1-F2 trajectories for /eɪ/. Best et al. synthesized these sequences in two ways, one with an F1 starting frequency of 230 Hz (Figure 12–10, left side), the other with an F1 starting frequency of 430 Hz (Figure 12–10, right side). Best et al. changed the duration of the stop closure interval between 0 (no closure interval) and 136 ms, sometimes with the lower F1 starting frequency, and sometimes with the higher frequency, and discovered something interesting. When the pattern was synthesized with one of the longer closure intervals, close to 136 ms, listeners clearly heard the sequence as "stay." When the pattern was synthesized with a very short or nonexistent closure interval, "say" was heard. None of this is surprising and is consistent with the real spectrographic patterns shown in Figure 12–9.

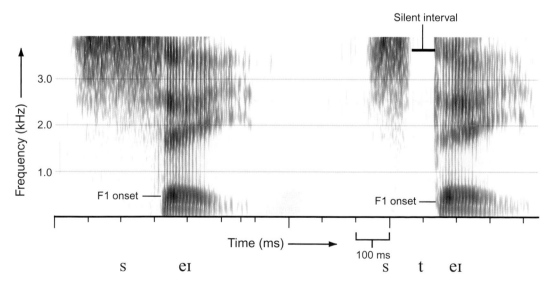

Figure 12-9. Spectrograms of the utterances "say" and "stay" showing two acoustic differences that distinguish the syllables with and without the /t/ One difference is the presence of the silent (closure interval) for /t/ (*right*), the other is the slightly lower F1 starting frequency in "stay," as compared to "say." See text for details.

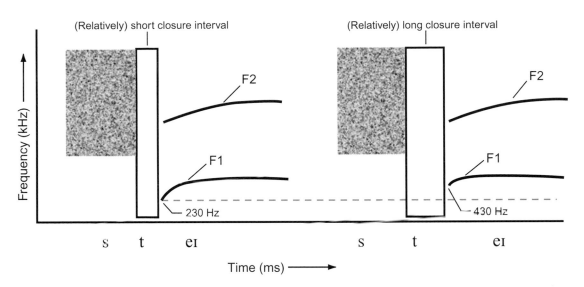

Figure 12–10. Two schematic spectrograms, showing how two different cues can "trade off" against each other to maintain a single phonetic percept. The phonetic percept is the presence of the stop consonant /t/ between an /s/ and /eɪ/. The two cues manipulated in these schematic spectrograms are: (a) the duration of the closure interval (the width of the narrow rectangles), and (b) the starting frequency of the F1 transition. Longer closure intervals and lower F1 starting frequencies tend to produce more /t/ responses. The tendency for more /t/ responses with longer closure intervals can be offset by a higher starting frequency for F1. In the left spectrogram, a shorter closure requires a lower F1 starting frequency for the /t/ percept. In the right spectrogram, which shows a longer closure interval, the F1 starting frequency can be higher.

The interesting findings occurred when the length of the closure interval between the /s/ and /eɪ/ was rather short (~30–50 ms) and resulted in roughly equal "say" and "stay" responses (that is, the presence or absence of a /t/ was ambiguous). Best et al. determined that when the F1 starting frequency was the higher one (430 Hz in Figure 12–10), a longer closure interval was required for listeners to hear "stay." When the F1 starting frequency was the lower one (230 Hz in Figure 12–10), a shorter closure interval allowed the listeners to hear "stay." In other words, the two cues to the presence of a /t/ between the /s/ and /eɪ/—closure interval duration and the F1 starting frequency—seemed to "trade off" against each other to produce the same

---

Speech Synthesis and Speech Perception

The pattern-playback machine allowed speech scientists to synthesize speech signals, but the quality of these signals was—let's be gracious—not particularly good. Developments in computer technology, knowledge of acoustic phonetics, and programming sophistication have greatly improved speech synthesis. Current synthetic speech signals are so good they sometimes cannot be distinguished from natural speech. These developments have allowed speech perception researchers to make very fine adjustments in signals to learn about speech perception while avoiding the problem of the fuzzy speech signals produced by the pattern-playback machine. In 1987, Dennis Klatt from the Massachusetts Institute of Technology published a wonderful history of speech synthesis, and provided audio examples of synthetic speech signals from 1939 to 1987 (Klatt, 1987). You can hear these examples at http://www.cs.indiana.edu/rhythmsp/ASA/Contents.html

percept—a /t/ between the fricative and the following vowel. Both patterns shown in Figure 12–10 produced the same percept of a "good" /t/. There was a "trading relation" between the two cues to the presence or absence of /t/ between the /s/ and /eɪ/.

For Liberman and Mattingly (1985), the trading relations phenomenon proved the point about the inability to connect a particular acoustic characteristic with a particular sound category. The potential, multiple acoustic cues to a given phonetic category were simply too numerous to be used by a listener to develop and maintain the category identification. In the particular case of "say"-"stay," the lower versus higher F1 starting frequency, or the precise value of the closure interval, was not by itself sufficient to serve as an acoustic constant of a phonetic category. The *collection* of these several cues, however, was a reflection of the underlying gesture for the sound category. Small variations in one cue could be compensated for by variations in a different cue, but in the end the sum of these various cues yielded a single percept which was the phonetic category (e.g., a /t/ associated with a constant and consistent articulatory gesture). In support of Liberman and Mattingly's theoretical cause, trading relations have been demonstrated for many different phonetic distinctions. It is not just a "say"-"stay" phenomenon (see Repp [1982] and Repp and Liberman [1987] for excellent reviews of trading relations in phonetic perception).

The Competition: General Auditory Explanations of Speech Perception

An obvious approach to understanding speech perception is to regard the speech acoustic signal as a sufficiently rich source of information for a listener's needs. In this view, the speech acoustic signal contains reliable, learnable information for a listener to identify the sounds, words, and phrases intended by a speaker. A *general auditory explanation* of speech perception seems simple, and perhaps the logical starting point —like a default perspective—for scientists who study speech perception. In fact, contrary to this apparent logic, general auditory explanations have fought an uphill scientific battle since the motor theory was formulated in the 1950s.

The information presented above described the reasons for the development of the original and revised motor theories of speech perception. Those reasons led to one overarching assumption concerning speech perception. A special perceptual processor is required because general auditory mechanisms were not up to

the task of perceiving speech (Remez, Rubin, Berns, Pardo, & Lang [1994] offer yet another perspective on the essential difference between perceiving speech and nonspeech sounds). In contrast, a central theme of general auditory explanations of speech perception is that special perceptual mechanisms are not required. Indeed, the speech acoustic signal is assumed to be processed in precisely the same way as other acoustic signals.

As in the published work on the motor theory, a set of reasons in support of a general auditory account of speech perception has been carefully articulated in the scientific literature. These are summarized below.

Sufficient Acoustic Invariance

As noted earlier, Blumstein and Stevens (1979) demonstrated a fair degree of acoustic consistency for stop consonant place of articulation, and many of the successful, automatic classification experiments described in Chapter 11 imply something consistent in the acoustic signal for vowels, diphthongs, nasals, fricatives, and semivowels. Recall from Chapter 11 that Lindblom (1990) argued for a more flexible view of speech acoustic variability. In this view, listeners do not need *absolute* acoustic invariance for a speech sound, but only enough to maintain discriminability from neighboring sound classes.

General auditory accounts of speech perception rely on this more flexible view of acoustic distinctiveness for the perception of speech sounds. Presumably, an initial front-end acoustic analysis of the speech signal by general auditory mechanisms is supplemented by higher level processing which can resolve any ambiguities in sound identity. The front-end analysis is like a hypothesis concerning the sequence of incoming sounds, and the higher-level processes include knowledge of the context in which each sound is produced, plus syntactic, semantic, and pragmatic constraints on the message. Clearly, listeners bring more to the speech perception process than just a capability for acoustic analysis. These additional sources of knowledge considerably loosen the demand for strict acoustic invariance for each sound segment.

Scientists often refer to the front-end part of this process as "bottom-up" processing, and the higher level knowledge part of this process as "top-down" processing. Stevens (2005) has proposed a speech perception model in which bottom-up, auditory mechanisms analyze the incoming speech signal for segment identity and top-down processes resolve ambiguities emerging from this front-end analysis. When an account of speech perception is framed within the general cognitive abilities of humans and includes top-down processes, a role for general auditory analysis in the perception of speech becomes much more plausible (Lotto & Holt, 2006). Clearly, the lack of strict acoustic invariance for a particular speech sound cannot be used as an argument against a role for general auditory mechanisms in speech perception.

Replication of Speech Perception Effects Using Nonspeech Signals

Many categorical perception effects have been demonstrated using synthetic speech stimuli. Several of these experiments were reviewed above. There have also been many demonstrations of similar effects using nonspeech signals. Categorical perception of speech signals has been a centerpiece of the original and revised motor theory. The demonstration of the same effects with nonspeech signals, however, seems to damage the proposed link between speech production and speech perception implied by findings of categorical perception for speech signals.

The approach employed by scientists interested in a general auditory theory of speech perception is to take a categorical perception experiment using speech signals and reproduce the effect using nonspeech signals. If the nonspeech experiment turns out the same way as the speech experiment, the categorical perception effect is attributed to auditory, not speech-special perceptual mechanisms. A famous example of such an experiment was published by Pisoni (1977) who showed that categorical perception functions for the voiced-voiceless contrast were probably due to auditory, not speech-special mechanisms.

Pisoni (1977) reviewed speech perception experiments in which labeling and discrimination data (as reviewed above) suggested categorical perception of voiced and voiceless stops. A typical set of data for this experiment is shown in Figure 12–11, where VOT is plotted on the x-axis and labeling (red points, left axis) and discrimination (blue points, right axis) are plotted as two y-axes. In this experiment, the stimulus is synthesized to sound like a stop-vowel syllable, and all features are held constant except for the VOT. Assume the transitions are synthesized to evoke perception of a bilabial stop, and that VOT is varied from lead values (negative VOT values) to long-lag values in 5-ms steps. For each VOT value, listeners are asked to label the stimulus as either /b/ or /p/. In the discrimination experiments, two stimuli from the VOT continuum are presented, always separated by 20 ms along the continuum (e.g., one stimulus with a VOT of 0 ms, the other

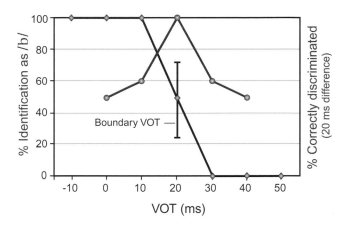

Figure 12–11. Labeling (identification) and discrimination functions for a VOT continuum, showing expected pattern for an interpretation of categorical perception of the voicing distinction for stops. The x-axis is VOT. Two y-axes are shown, one for identification (left y-axis, red points), one for discrimination (right y-axis, blue points). The categorical boundary, where the labeling function shifts rapidly between /b/ and /p/, is shown as 20 ms. Discrimination across this 20-ms boundary is 100%. Within the categories it is close to 50%. See Figure 12–12 and discussion in text.

with a VOT of 20 ms), and listeners are asked if they are the same or different. The results in Figure 12–11 show only /b/ labels for stimuli with VOT's from –10 ms to +15 ms, half /b/ and half /p/ for the stimulus with VOT of 20 ms, and all /p/ labels for stimuli with VOT = 30 ms or more. The change from /b/ to /p/ labels occurs quickly in the 20- to 30-ms range of VOTs, as required for an interpretation of categorical perception. The discrimination data (blue points) show perfect discrimination when the two VOT stimuli cross the labeling "boundary," but much poorer discrimination when the two stimuli are within a category, In short, these VOT data meet the requirements for categorical perception as reviewed above. The interpretation of categorical perception of VOT was consistent with the motor theory of speech perception. Speakers cannot produce continuous changes in VOT, so they cannot perceive them.

Pisoni (1977) knew that the synthesis of VOT differences for the same place of stop articulation involved variable asynchronies between two acoustic events. Re-examination of Figure 12–2 shows that the two-formant patterns for the three cognate pairs /ba-pa/, /da-ta/, and /ga-ka/ differ only in the onset time of the first formant relative to the second formant. Listeners were made to hear the voiceless member of each pair by delaying the onset of the first formant by approximately

50 ms relative to the onset of the second formant. A synthetic VOT continuum, such as the one just described, was generated in early studies by varying the starting time of the first format relative to the starting time of the second formant. Pisoni mimicked these asynchronies with nonspeech stimuli like those shown in Figure 12–12. Each stimulus consisted of a pair of sinusoids, one at a lower frequency (500 Hz), the other at a higher frequency (1500 Hz). Stimulus 1 shows the two tones with simultaneous onsets, which in a synthetic speech signal mimics simultaneous onset of the first two formant frequencies, or a VOT = 0 ms. Stimuli 2 through 6 have increasing asynchronies between the two tones, with the onset of the lower-frequency tone lagging that of the higher-frequency tone by increasing amounts. The stimulus progression from 2 through 6 mimics increasing, positive VOTs.[3]

Each two-tone stimulus was played to listeners who participated in both labeling and discrimination experiments. Pisoni (1977) found that unless the starting times of the two tones differed by more than 20 ms, listeners categorized (labeled) the two-tone pair as the same event. When the lower and upper tone began within 20 ms of each other, listeners treated them as the same event. A sudden change in the listeners' perception of the stimulus pairs occurred when the onset of the lower tone began at least 20 ms later than the onset of the higher tone. In Figure 12–12, stimuli 1 through 5 were heard as the "same" event, and stimulus 6 was heard as different. This 20-ms "boundary" for classifying the tone pairs as one event, versus another, was very close to the VOT boundary obtained when the first formant was delayed relative to the second formant. Based on these findings, Pisoni concluded that the VOT boundary for the experiments with *speech* signals did not reflect a special speech mechanism such as that proposed by motor theorists. Because the same boundary was demonstrated with nonspeech signals, it appeared to be a general property of auditory mechanisms (see Hirsh, 1959).

Many other experiments in which phonetic effects are mimicked with nonspeech signals have been reported in the literature (see Diehl et al., 2004, for a summary). In general, categorical perception effects or context effects demonstrated with speech signals can be demonstrated equally well when nonspeech signals (tones, noise intervals, etc.) mimic the speech condi-

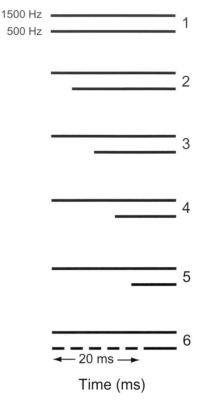

Figure 12–12. Illustration of stimuli used by Pisoni (1977) to demonstrate categorical perception of sinusoid tone pairs whose relative onsets simulated the VOT continuum shown in Figure 12–11. The onset of the lower-frequency sinusoid was either simultaneous with that of the higher-frequency sinusoid (stimulus 1), or was delayed in small steps (stimuli 2–6). Listeners labeled stimuli 1 through 5 as the same event, and could not discriminate between any of these tone pairs. Stimulus 6 was labeled as a different event from the other five, and was discriminated from them as well.

tions. Auditory theorists regard these findings as evidence for the ability of general auditory mechanisms to do the important, "front-end" work in speech perception. These theorists reject the idea of a special module for speech perception.

An interesting variation on this style of experiment has been reported by Laing, Liu, Lotto, and Holt (2012). These researchers showed that the categorization of a speech segment as /g/ or /d/ was affected by the frequency range of a sequence of tones (that is, *nonspeech*

---

[3]Readers will note that the manipulation of VOT in the synthetic speech signals of Figure 12–2, and the mimic signals illustrated in Figure 12–12, depend on modification of an acoustic variable that is somewhat different from the typical definition of VOT. VOT for natural speech signals is defined as the time difference between a stop burst and the onset of vocal fold vibration for the following vowel. The synthetic signals used to construct VOT continua, however, typically did not have a burst. Rather, the percept of the voiced-voiceless contrast could be elicited with the "F1 cutback" technique described in the text and illustrated in Figure 12–2.

signals) preceding the stop. The listeners' choice of /d/ vs. /g/ was affected *systematically* by whether the preceding tone sequence occupied a higher, versus lower, frequency range; this was not a random effect. A theory of speech perception that separates the mechanism for perceiving speech signals from the perceptual mechanism for other auditory signals is, plainly and simply, inconsistent with this finding. A motor theory of speech perception cannot explain why the frequency range of a sequence of tones has a systematic effect on the choice of a syllable as /d/ or /g/.

Animal and Infant Perception of Speech Signals

Auditory theorists point to the demonstration in animals of categorical perception for many speech sound contrasts, as well as the ability of animals to learn phonetic contrasts when properly trained, as evidence for the use of general auditory mechanisms in the perception of speech (Diehl, Lotto, & Holt, 2004; Kluender, 1994; Kluender & Kiefte, 2006). An argument for a special speech-perception mechanism in animals does not make sense because animals do not speak. The ability of animals to learn phonetic contrasts, when trained to do so, points to the ability of human infants to use their substantially more powerful cognitive resources to do the same thing. If infants can use phonetic input from their environment to develop sound categories, the logical appeal of a species-specific module for speech perception decreases dramatically. Saffran and Thiessen (2007) have summarized evidence for the human infant's use of phonetic data from the environment (e.g., speech produced by parents and others) in the development of phoneme categories. Saffran and Thiessen's viewpoint about such learning is consistent with the philosophy of auditory theorists, who believe general auditory mechanisms are used in speech perception. Saffran and Thiessen argue for general (not special) cognitive mechanisms in a child's learning of speech and language.

The Competition: Direct Realism

A theory of speech perception, called direct realism (Fowler, Galantucci, & Saltzman, 2003), is an alternative to both the motor theory and a general auditory approach. The direct realism perspective on speech perception is not easy to explain in the absence of substantial background information (which is not pursued here). Some scientists (Cleary & Pisoni, 2001) question the utility of direct realism as a theory because it is hard to understand how reasonable experimental tests can be made to support or refute it. In Popper's (2002a) terms, the specific predictions of direct realism, and the way in which those predictions might be falsified by experimental data, are not particularly clear. With these remarks in mind, a brief summary of direct realism is given here.

The direct realism perspective on speech perception takes its inspiration from the pioneering work of the psychologist J. J. Gibson (1904–1979). Gibson's theoretical and experimental focus was on visual perception, for which he rejected the idea of cognitively driven, "constructed" percepts (Gibson, 1968, 1979). Gibson did not like the idea of perception that had to be mediated by cognitive operations to produce a representation of the external world. Rather, he proposed the idea that animals, including humans, learn to perceive the visual layouts of environments directly, by linking the stimulation of their senses (by light waves, in the case of vision) with the sources of the stimulation. For example, perceivers learn the patterning of light reflected from a chair and sensed by their retina and

---

That Cute Cuddly Infant Is Actually a Statistical Model-Builder

Professor Jenny Saffran of the University of Wisconsin–Madison asks the question, "How do infants, when listening to connected speech, learn where one word ends and the next begins?" This clearly interesting question is even more compelling because speakers typically do not "mark" the ends and beginnings of words with special acoustic effects. The sounds all run together. So how do infants figure this out—how do they learn to identify where words end and begin? Saffran (2003) proposed that, over time, infants compile the phonetic input in their environment as a statistical model of which sound sequences are likely to begin words, to straddle words, and to end words. The model is basically a set of probabilities of which sound sequences are heard as word beginnings versus endings. Saffran pointed out that this kind of "statistical learning" is seen with all kinds of input—not just speech—and even among animals. This learning perspective on speech sound perception is very much at odds with the innate, species-specific mechanisms proposed by motor theorists.

other visual structures in the nervous system. These sensations are used to perceive the chair directly. In Gibson's view, there is no need for the perceiver to "process" and "encode" the light waves via cognitive operations whose output is a symbolic representation. Gibson coined the term "ecological psychology" for this view of perception and its scientific investigation. The term is consistent with a "realist" (i.e., ecologically valid) view of how organisms perceive things. For Gibson, much of the experimental psychologist's vocabulary, including terms found in information processing models such as "encoding" and "representation" (as examples), was not much more than a convenient set of descriptive terms. For Gibson, the terms did not have ecological validity—that is, they did not represent "real" things, "real" mechanisms that were the stuff of perception.

Motor theory requires operations of a special module to "convert" an unstable acoustic signal to a stable articulatory representation. A general auditory approach to speech perception requires some processing stages to match the incoming acoustics to stored templates or features (Klatt, 1989; Stevens, 2005). In both cases, cognitive operations of varying degrees of automaticity are required for perception of incoming sounds. Fowler (1986, 1996), the leading proponent of direct realism in speech perception, rejects cognitive "constructions" in the perception of speech sounds. That is, Fowler agrees with the Gibsonian idea that scientists should reject the idea of perception being driven by cognitive processes that produce an "output symbol." In the case of speech perception, the simplest example of such a symbol is a phoneme. She argues for direct perception of articulatory gestures. In this case, the speech acoustic signal is linked directly with the articulatory gesture that produced it. Listeners learn these links and do not need to construct the percepts of sounds. They literally hear articulatory gestures (or, on another interpretation, the sounds they hear *are* the articulatory gestures). The parallel with Gibson's (1969, 1970) view of visual perception is easy to see.

How is direct realism different from the motor theory? Both theories focus on perception of articulatory gestures, but motor theory requires a special, completely automatic mechanism (a module) to transform acoustic signals into articulatory mechanisms. Direct realism proposes no special mechanisms, and, in fact,

claims that the same principles apply to visual, auditory, and haptic (sense of touch) perception. In all cases, the source of the stimulation is what is perceived, without mediation by cognitive processing of the signals produced by that source.

How is direct realism different from an auditory approach to speech perception? This is a more interesting question, and one with a more complicated (and hotly debated) answer (see the exchange between Lotto and Holt [2006] and Fowler [2006]). The simplest answer is, in direct realism listeners hear the articulatory gestures, whereas in a general auditory approach listeners hear the acoustic signal.

Is there really a difference between these two? One difference, noted above, is that a general auditory approach presumably requires a listener to perform some kind of operation on the incoming speech acoustic signal such as matching it to a stored acoustic prototype, or transforming it to a more phonetically useful format (such as a binary or trinary feature, examples of which in English include the binary voicing opposition for stops or fricatives, and the trinary place opposition for stops), before it can be perceived as a particular sound. Direct realism, however, claims direct perception of the gestures that (in the language of direct realists) "structured" the acoustic signal. Perceptions are not "constructed" in direct realism—they are direct. In the comparison between these two approaches, is there an advantage of the direct realist perspective over the general auditory approach?[4]

As reviewed in Chapter 11, the speech acoustic signal for a given sound varies depending on its phonetic context (and other factors as well). For example, the /s/ spectra in the utterances [su] and [si] are quite different, because speakers typically produce some lip rounding during the /s/ in [su], but not [si]. The acoustic effect of lip rounding during the /s/ in [su] is to emphasize much lower frequencies in the aperiodic fricative spectrum, as compared to the /s/ spectrum in [si]. Direct realists argue that a general auditory approach to speech perception is cumbersome and overly complicated because a listener must learn and store all these different variants of spectra for a given sound. In direct realism, listeners are not burdened with this learning and storage problem because they "hear" the lingual fricative gesture combined, or coproduced, with the lip rounding gesture. Moreover, in direct realism the

---

[4]Many direct realists, including Fowler (Fowler et al., 2003), believe that their theory has the advantage of being preferable on *philosophical* grounds, in addition to any scientific advantages that may be demonstrated. This is to say that direct real ism unifies perceptual behavior across the senses, discards the (in their view) awkward theoretical constructs of much of cognitive psychology (such as the notion of mental representations, or specialized modules), and may be easier to integrate with general evolutionary theory than the "constructed perceptions" of so many psychological theories.

Growing Up in the 1950s and Speech Perception

Many of us who grew up in the 1950s went to the picture show every Saturday and sat through double features of perfectly awful science fiction movies. The music meant to convey the weirdness of on-screen aliens was equally awful, usually a kind of singing, multitonal whistling you might associate with attempts to tune in a distant radio station. Professor Robert Remez of Barnard University, and his colleagues, used such sounds to prove a point about speech perception. They looked at the first three formants of a natural utterance and mimicked their time-dependent frequency changes using sinusoids (you can hear these signals, plus the sentences they were based on, at http://www.haskins.yale.

edu/featured/sws/swssentences/sentences.html). When listeners heard these sounds, some described them as suggested above—weird outer space signals. But when people were told to listen to the signals as if they were speech, many heard the sentence as originally spoken, even though the signal was composed only of three time-varying sinusoids. Remez and his associates concluded that this finding disproved the idea of a speech-specific module that was *automatically* engaged by speech signals. It was as if listeners could hear the signals as speech, *if instructed to do so.* A dedicated speech perception module would not allow that kind of choice (see Pardo & Remez, 2006, pp. 207–208).

degree to which two articulatory gestures, such as lingual and labial gestures, are "coproduced" is perceived directly. In a general auditory approach, the large number of slight variations (for example, of how much of the /s/ in [su] is lip-rounded) presumably introduce acoustic variability for a given sound that may complicate the learning of speech sound categories and the mature form of speech perception. In short, direct realists see their theory of speech perception as much simpler than general auditory approaches.

A Tentative Summary

The research described above reveals a complicated, theory-driven view of possible mechanisms of speech perception. At least one of the theories—the motor theory of speech perception—requires a special human endowment in the brain to perceive speech. The other two theories reviewed, the so-called auditory theory, and the theory sometimes called direct realism, view speech perception as a process guided by brain mechanisms that are not specialized for speech, at least not in the strict sense of particular areas of brain tissue being "wired" exclusively, and innately, for the perceptual processing of speech sounds, words, and even different sentence forms.

What is the current state of this debate? The three theories, or positions stated above, have often been presented as mutually exclusive—if you believe one, you don't believe any of the others, even any parts of the others—but there have been recent attempts to merge some of the ideas behind at least two of these theories.

Scientists have taken advantage of developments in brain imaging techniques to study infants, who turn out to be good test cases for the unqualified idea of a completely innate mechanism for processing speech and language. If the mechanism for speech perception is a dedicated, human-specific module, lateralization to the left hemisphere of brain activity for speech perception (see Chapter 6) should be present at birth and remain more or less constant throughout the first year of life as the child passes from a prelingual to language-using creature. On the other hand, if speech perception skills have a fairly extensive basis in learning, with exposure to speech acoustic signals shaping the way the brain reacts to the processing of speech and language input, the degree of brain lateralization should shift across the first year of life. This shift might be from a more or less symmetrical pattern of brain activation around birth to an increasingly left-lateralized pattern as the child develops within a language environment over the first year of life. Minagawa-Kawai, Cristià, and Dupoux (2011) have recently reviewed the available evidence from brain imaging studies in infants listening to linguistic (and nonlinguistic) input, and concluded that there is a shift, over the first year of life, to the left-lateralized pattern observed in most adults. Based on this review, Minagawa-Kawai et al. (2011) argue for a hybrid theory of brain activity for speech perception. Babies, in this view, use the special computational skills of the left hemisphere to process speech signals and categorize them in a linguistically meaningful way. Notice the way the preceding sentence is written: the use of acoustic signals for speech perception is mentioned, as suggested by auditory theories, but so are "special computational skills" of the left hemisphere. The specialized computational skills mentioned by Minagawa-Kawai et al. may or may not be *speech*-specific, but they certainly are specific to constructing categories (such as those required for phonemic contrasts) and therefore have a particular specialty in the development of language skills. If this sounds like a game with words to avoid the "special speech module" idea, perhaps it is, but the point is the attempt to move from extreme and opposing theoretical positions to a middle view that recognizes the strengths of both extreme positions.

Speech Perception and Word Recognition

The three major theories (or approaches) discussed above are concerned with phonetic perception. They attempt to account for the way in which speech sounds are identified. Clearly, an important part of speech perception involves speech sound identification, but just as clearly the goal of speech perception is to recognize words, their combinations, and ultimately the message they convey.

Speech sound identification, however it is accomplished, is seen by many scientists as the "trigger" that initiates the process of word identification. A simple way to think about the link between sound and word identification is to imagine the lexicon as consisting of word "units" represented by strings of abstract phonological symbols (phonemes). In a very general sense, when the incoming sounds are identified and well-matched to one of these abstract, stored word units, spoken word recognition occurs.

This simple view glosses over some important details. First, it is known that spoken word recognition does not require a complete analysis of all sounds in a word. Listeners can make decisions concerning word identity before all the sounds are known, or even before any analysis of some remaining component sounds has been undertaken. This is especially the case for longer, multisyllabic words (Dahan & Magnuson, 2006; Nooteboom & van der Vlugt, 1988). In broad terms, spoken word recognition unfolds over time, by a *continuous* process as sound analysis and top-down information becomes increasingly available (Dahan & Gareth Gaskell, 2007; Grosjean, 1980). The ability of listeners to make correct word identifications in the absence of all the relevant "data" highlights the substantial role of top-down processing in spoken word recognition. Top-down processes may include, but are not limited to, a listener's knowledge of possible word candidates with a similar phonetic structure (see below) or similar frequencies of occurrence, the meaning of previously recognized words in an extended utterance, the topic under discussion, and even the identity of the person who is speaking.

Second, there is a fair amount of disagreement concerning the specific processes involved in transforming an initial sound analysis to the form of the abstract word representation. For example, when a man and woman speak the same word, the initial sound identification may have to be transformed to a common "acoustic space" before it can be mapped onto common abstract phonological symbols. Third, as described above and in Chapter 11, the acoustic signal for each sound is variable depending on such factors as dialect, speaking rate, speech style (formal vs. casual), and immediate phonetic context. How are these factors handled in moving from sound analysis to an abstract, phonological representation of words? Readers interested in pursuing these issues are encouraged to read Luce and McLennan (2005).

Theoretical challenges in understanding spoken word recognition may involve additional complications. The general concept of spoken word recognition described above, where an initial acoustic (or gestural) analysis of speech sounds is transformed to an abstract phonological code—a string of phonemes representing a word stored in the mental lexicon—implies a *loss* of information. The incoming acoustic signal contains information that is presumably irrelevant to the hypothesized, abstract phonological code. For example, allophonic variation (variant phonetic versions of the same phoneme, such as the aspirated and nonaspirated /p/s in [pʰɑt] and [tɑp]) is not typically thought to be part of the abstract representation, nor are such variables as speaker identity, speaking rate, or paralinguistics (e.g., the intonation contour signaling the emotional state of the speaker). Yet there is ample evidence from several sources (Goldinger, 1998; Sommers & Barcroft, 2006) that this kind of phonetic variation has a significant effect on spoken word recognition. For example, in an often-cited experiment, Mullenix, Pisoni, and Martin (1989) showed poorer recognition rates for a list of words read by a variety of talkers, as compared to a list read by a single talker. This result is very hard to square with a concept of spoken word recognition in which the goal is to match an input to an abstract, timeless (that is, discrete phoneme sequences), speaker-free phonological representation.

Phonological representations are typically thought to be faithful to the language—not to individual speakers of the language or to phonetic details of their sound productions. Perhaps the representations are faithful to both, and word recognition involves some significant level of phonetic information, even including different speaker voices and allophonic details.

Why Should Speech-Language Pathologists Care About Speech Perception?

Some of the information presented in this chapter may seem far removed from the daily concerns of speech-language pathologists. A good deal of research on speech perception, whether at the phonetic or word-recognition level, may appear both narrowly academic and exceedingly theoretical. In practice, however, the speech-language pathologist deals with these issues all the time. After all, clients engage the services of speech-language pathologists to be understood better—to be more intelligible. When a speech-language pathologist plans a program of remediation for a person with a speech disorder, the plan should include a goal of making the client's sounds and words more accessible to the listener. Commnication disorders are as much in the ear of the listener as they are in the mouth of the speaker. An understanding of speech perception processes in the typical listener can assist a speech-language pathologist in developing a remediation plan.

This claim seems obvious, but very often the speech-language pathologist directs therapeutic attention only to the client's speech production apparatus. For some clients this may be a reasonable approach, but for many others the needs of a typical listener can be factored into therapy efforts. Knowledge of these listening needs is the product of years of research on speech perception at the phonetic and word level.

An example may make this clear. Persons with damage to the cerebellum, a part of the brain that plays an important role in regulating sequential motor behavior (among other things), often have a speech disorder called ataxic dysarthria. *Dysarthria* is the term used for speech production disorders associated with damage to the central nervous system, and *ataxia* signifies a set of motor symptoms and signs associated with damage to the cerebellum. Among speakers of English, a frequent speech production sign in ataxic dysarthria is an inability to regulate the long-short-long-short patterning of syllable durations in a multisyllabic utterance (see Chapter 11). As it turns out, listeners use this patterning of syllable durations to make decisions concerning word onset locations (Cutler, Dahan, & van Donselaar, 1997). When listeners hear speech with an unusual pattern of syllable durations, their ability to identify word onsets, and, therefore, to access the words intended by the speaker, is compromised. In ataxic dysarthria, reduced word onset identification by normal listeners has been demonstrated and linked to the disruption in syllable timing patterns described above (Liss, Spitzer, Caviness, Adler, & Edwards, 2000). Unless a speech-language pathologist

understands something about the link between neural disease, speech timing problems, and lexical access as an important part of speech perceptual processing, therapy efforts may be directed primarily to a more traditional aspect of clinical management (such as speech sound therapy, or perhaps voice therapy; see Duffy, 1995). A focus on the speech timing issue may have a much greater benefit in improving the client's ability to make herself understood.

Another very concrete example of why a speech-language pathologist should be familiar with the basic principles of speech perception is to exploit knowledge concerning typical listening strategies, and thus maximize the effect of speech therapy. Most students know that standardized articulation tests evaluate the goodness of consonant production in the initial, medial, and final positions of a word. For example, articulation of the /b/ sound can be tested in word-initial position (e.g., "book"), word-medial position ("rabbit"), and word-final position ("tub"). In such a test, it is possible for the results to indicate a more substantial problem with word-final consonants as compared to word-initial consonants. These results could suggest a therapy plan initially aimed at practice on word-final consonants, but this plan is poorly matched to the needs of listeners. Speech perception research has shown that listeners typically use word onsets to recognize words in continuous speech (see review in Astheimer & Sanders, 2011). Extensive therapeutic effort devoted to the articulation of word-final consonants may result in

---

Speech Perception: A Lost Soul in Clinical Training Programs

It is an odd fact that material on speech perception is not a highlight of preclinical or masters-level training in speech-language pathology. At the least, training in speech perception should be emphasized as much as training in normal and disordered speech anatomy and physiology. Communication disorders are ultimately disorders in the listener's ear. A quick look at the clinical literature on voice disorders, craniofacial anomalies, motor speech disorders, developmental phonological disorders, and fluency disorders shows the degree to which perceptual judgments by clinicians and even family members of a client play a major role in understanding diagnosis and management of the disorder. Long live knowledge of speech perception theory in the speech-language pathologist's clinical toolbox!

well-produced consonants in that word position. If the results of speech perception research are to be believed, however, the effort may result in little improvement in the effective transmission of a message.

The idea of relating speech production problems in persons with various speech disorders to speech perception difficulties among everyday listeners is a huge and complex topic. Interested readers are referred to Weismer and Martin (1992), Liss (2007), and Weismer (2008) for reviews of some main issues in understanding how speech intelligibility is linked to specific speech production problems. The chapter now concludes with a brief section on speech intelligibility tests.

SPEECH INTELLIGIBILITY

The concept of speech intelligibility is well known to speech-language pathologists. Various speech intelligibility tests have been available to speech-language pathologists for many years, and are used routinely in clinical practice and research (Kent, 1992; Weismer, 2008; Yorkston, Beukelman, Strand, & Bell, 1999) A speech intelligibility score is clearly a measure of speech perception, but the design of specific speech intelligibility tests has rarely been guided by principles derived from speech perception theory.

Speech intelligibility tests were originally designed to measure the goodness of speech transmission over communication systems, such as telephone lines. Tests most often consisted of lists of single words, although sentence tests were also developed. These tests were intended to assess *only* the relationship between the acoustic characteristics of the speech signal and the percentage of words (or sentences) correctly heard by a group of listeners. Stated in a different way, the design of the tests was based on the assumption that under controlled conditions, the only variable contributing to the percentage intelligibility score was the integrity of the speech acoustic signal. Typically, the integrity of the speech signal was defined at the sound segment level. If the acoustic characteristics of individual speech sounds were in good shape, speech intelligibility scores were expected to be high. Disruption of speech sound acoustics, by a low presentation level, filtering (restriction of frequencies transmitted by the communication system), or competing noise, lowered the speech intelligibility score in proportion to the extent of the disruption (Weismer, 2008).

It is easy to see how this kind of information was extended past the evaluation of a communication system, to the case of a person with a *hearing* disorder. Speech intelligibility tests, in various forms, have been used for years in the determination of speech reception thresholds, speech discrimination scores, the fitting of hearing aids, and programming of implantable devices (Katz, 2002). Whereas early speech intelligibility tests were designed to evaluate communication systems, the application of such tests in clinical audiology demonstrated how the tests could be used in the case of the receiver (hearer) as well.

An extension of speech intelligibility tests to evaluate the *speaker* (sender) also makes sense. When speech is impaired and the communication system and receiver are in good shape, it seems logical that a speech intelligibility score serves as an index of the speaker's communication impairment. Speech intelligibility tests developed specifically for the evaluation of speech impairment were initially designed for persons with hearing impairment and dysarthria (Monsen, 1983; Weismer & Martin, 1992). Kent, Weismer, Kent, and Rosenbek (1989) reviewed these tests and concluded that most were merely indices of severity. Moreover, as demonstrated earlier by Monsen for speech intelligibility among persons with severe to profound hearing impairment, an intelligibility score depended on many factors extrinsic to the speaker. These factors included the identity of the listener (the degree of experience with the specific speech characteristics of persons with hearing impairment, or dysarthria) and the phonological and (in the case of sentence tests) syntactic complexity of the test utterances. Additional extrinsic factors also contribute variation to the speech intelligibility score for a particular individual with a speech impairment. In short, the statement, "Mr. Jones has a speech intelligibility score of 75%" is nearly impossible to interpret unless additional information is available about the test, the listening conditions (including the specific speech materials), and the listeners. This potential ambiguity in the meaning of a percentage value derived from a speech intelligibility test seemed to limit the utility of the measure even for simple estimates of speaker severity.[5]

"Explanatory" Speech Intelligibility Tests

Kent et al. (1989) had the idea to extend the interpretation of speech intelligibility testing by isolating the

---

[5]Such limitations could be eliminated by national or international standards for speech intelligibility testing of persons with speech disorders, but these do not exist.

particular phonetic problems that contributed to an intelligibility deficit. This idea emerged from a common clinical observation that two individuals with the same overall speech intelligibility score (e.g., 60%) may have very different reasons for their speech intelligibility deficits. For example, one individual's intelligibility deficit may be primarily a result of velopharyngeal incompetency, whereas another's may derive from problems with consonant place of articulation. The Kent et al. test was designed as a single-word, multiple choice instrument in which the response alternatives were related to the target by carefully manipulated phonetic contrasts. By analyzing not only the total number of incorrect words, but also the phonetic contrast errors underlying the incorrect choices, a profile of "vulnerable" contrasts—those frequently involved in word choice errors—was available. These "vulnerable" contrasts would be targeted in therapy because they presumably made a large contribution to the intelligibility deficit. In a sense, identification of "vulnerable" contrasts was like a prescription for primary attention in speech-language management. The concept of "vulnerable" contrasts also provided an explanation for why the same overall intelligibility score might be obtained for two individuals who sounded so differently. Even though the total number of words heard correctly by listeners was the same for these two persons, the speakers differed in their "vulnerable" contrasts, and, therefore, should have different therapy priorities.

Earlier in this section, the original speech intelligibility tests were described as a way to test the contribution of speech signal integrity to the goodness of a communication system. There is a direct link between this idea and the phonetic contrast approach to speech intelligibility testing, in which the *speaker* is the variable. In the original approach, speech intelligibility scores reflected the sum of the acoustic characteristics of speech sounds in the test words. Any degradation of the acoustic characteristics of a particular sound contributed to a decrease in an overall speech intelligibility score. The greater the number of sounds affected (degraded) by the communication system, the lower the intelligibility score. Similarly, the phonetic contrast approach of Kent et al. (1989) considered speech intelligibility as a sum of "good" phonetic contrasts produced by the speaker. The smaller the number of these "good" contrasts (the greater the number of "vulnerable" contrasts), the lower the speech intelligibility score. In addition, the ability to identify specific "vulnerable" contrasts was assumed to provide an explanation of the intelligibility deficit. This explanation was found in the speech production characteristics required to make a "good" contrast, which in the case of a speech intelligi-

bility deficit were sufficiently affected by some condition (anatomical, physiological, behavioral) to prevent the realization of the contrast.

Different individuals in fact, had different "vulnerable" contrasts revealed by the Kent et al. (1989) test (Weismer & Martin, 1992). Different "vulnerable" contrasts were seen in different dysarthria types and in some cases depended on the sex of the speaker (Kent et al., 1992). Although the concept of the Kent et al. (1989) test seems sound, there are problems in the interpretation of "vulnerable" contrasts. Specifically, the idea that the "good" phonetic contrasts sum up to produce the intelligibility score (much as the good acoustic characteristics sum up to show the integrity of a communication system) is overly simple. This is because the different phonetic contrasts, such as the high-low and front-back contrasts for vowels, the voiced-voiceless and palatal-alveolar contrasts for consonants, and the glottal-null (e.g., "hate" vs. "ate") contrast for syllable shape, are apparently *not* independent. A simple way to say this is, if one of these contrasts is revealed to be vulnerable by the Kent et al. (1989) test, the others will be as well (Weismer & Martin, 1992). Even though the contrasts may appear to have different "vulnerabilities" in different speakers or clinical populations, they are all highly correlated with each other and may not furnish the kind of prescription for management imagined when the test was developed.

The kinds of speech intelligibility tests described above are probably of greatest use when a single speaker's progress (or decline) is tracked across therapy or progression of a disease. In this case, all measures involve the same individual, who in a sense serves as his or her own control in evaluating the effects of management or disease progression. What is needed are measures of speech intelligibility motivated by more sophisticated knowledge of speech perception, and especially by factors that truly tap into language comprehension. For example, the ability of listeners to identify word onsets in connected speech produced by persons with speech disorders, and to access the lexicon to extract the meaning of a client's message, seems to be the next step in enhancing the clinical relevance of these measures of speech intelligibility.

Scaled Speech Intelligibility

Aspects of speech perception can be scaled. There is a long history of assigning numbers to reflect perceived magnitudes of speech perception characteristics (see review in Weismer, 2008); this is what is meant by perceptual scaling. Scaled speech perception characteristics may include (but are not limited to) speech intelligibility, speech normalcy, speech acceptability, naturalness, hypernasality, articulatory imprecision, and voice qualities such as breathiness, hoarseness, roughness, and strain. The present discussion is confined to the scaling of intelligibility, but the principles are applicable to scaling of any of these speech dimensions.

Speech intelligibility has been scaled often in the research literature, and routinely in clinical practice. Equal-appearing interval scales are those in which a certain range of numbers is spaced equally along a line, with the endpoints defined from normal to most severe. For example, seven-point, equal-appearing interval scales have been used to scale speech intelligibility in persons with dysarthria, with 1 = normal and 7 = most severely impaired (Darley, Aronson, & Brown, 1975). Listeners hear a speech sample (a word, a sentence, or even a paragraph reading) and assign a number along this range to correspond with their impression of the magnitude (the severity) of the speech impairment.

Equal-appearing interval scales are simple, can be administered quickly, and probably reflect the potential effects of all aspects of speech production (articulation, voice quality, prosody) on speech intelligibility. Single word tests such as the one described above, and even sentence intelligibility tests in which listeners write down the words they hear and intelligibility is expressed as a percentage of correctly heard words, are primarily dependent on the articulatory characteristics of segments making up the words and sentences. To the extent that factors such as voice quality and prosody (and perhaps other unknown factors) affect speech intelligibility, equal-appearing interval scales seem to have an advantage over percentage-correct measures by allowing nonsegmental factors to enter into a judge's estimate of speech intelligibility.

There are some problems with the use of equal-appearing interval scales in the scaling of speech intelligibility (or any speech percept). First, the equal steps between numbers along the scale may induce listeners to believe that a difference between, for example, a scale value of 4 and 5 is psychologically equivalent to the difference between 5 and 6. In other words, the "mapping" from the speech signal to the numbers on the scale is assumed to be more or less linear. The functions that related variation in a speech signal to a psychological impression of intelligibility are rarely linear, however. Some scientists therefore distrust equal-appearing interval scales because they seem to force this assumption on the listener. A second and related problem is the issue of floor and ceiling effects, and the manner in which the endpoints of the scale are anchored. Scientists and clinicians often use terms such

as "normal" and "most severe" to define the ends of the scale, or even provide recorded examples of an utterance they have decided represents "normal" intelligibility (1 on the scale) and "most unintelligible" (7 on the scale). These examples for the endpoints of a scale are called anchors. Unfortunately, there are no standards for anchors, and scientists and clinicians can and do argue about the best exemplars for the anchors. A typical problem with anchors is when a particular speech utterance is deemed by a listener to be more unintelligible than the "most unintelligible" anchor used to define the end of the scale, or "more intelligible" than the anchor defining the other end of the scale. The perception may be valid, but the listener has no way to represent the perception in numbers, because the ends of the scale have been "set in stone" and predefined. A floor effect occurs when the bottom (in this case, best intelligibility) of the number scale is not really the bottom of a particular listener's psychological response to a stimulus. A ceiling effect occurs when the predefined top (worst intelligibility) of the scale prevents a listener from representing the psychological magnitude of an utterance that he or she believes is more unintelligible than the anchor utterance used for that end of the scale. Floor and ceiling effects, and the use of equal-appearing intervals along the scale, may (and often do) distort the true underlying process of perceiving intelligibility variation.

Equal-appearing interval scales are not particularly reliable, either within judges or across judges. When the same judge scales the same utterances for speech intelligibility, at different times, an error of one scale value is often taken as an acceptable criterion for scaling reliability. This is because exact number matches using equal-appearing interval scales are not common, and some measurement error must be tolerated. However, because a difference of one number in the middle of the scale means three numbers can represent, in terms of reliability, the same percept—that is, a 3, 4, and 5 are taken as the same measurement of intelligibility, when the original scale value was 4—it is reasonable to question the intrinsic value of these scales. After all, on a 7-point scale an error across three numbers is a nearly 50% error relative to the entire scale.

A well-studied scaling technique that avoids the linearity and endpoint problems of equal-appearing interval scales is called direct magnitude estimation (DME). In DME listeners are told they will hear a sequence of speech stimuli varying in intelligibility, and their job is to assign numbers to each stimulus to reflect the magnitude of the speech intelligibility deficit. One version of DME uses an anchor stimulus, usually selected by the experimenter to represent a speech intelligibility deficit midway between perfectly intelligible and absolutely unintelligible. An alternate version of DME does not provide an anchor for the scaling exercise, but asks listeners to attach a number — any whole number — to the first stimulus, with all subsequent numbers using the previously assigned number as a reference. In either case of DME scaling, listeners are told to assign the numbers as *ratios* relative to a defined anchor, or to the immediately preceding stimulus. For example, in the case of anchored DME a speech sample midway between perfectly intelligible and perfectly unintelligible may be preassigned the number 10. The listener hears this anchor several times throughout the sequence of speech samples, to remind them of an intelligibility having a value of 10, and is told to assign a number to each of the undefined samples to reflect the intelligibility of that particular sample relative to the anchor. Because the listeners are asked to scale each sample as a ratio relative to the anchor, they are told to use the number 20 only if a particular sample sounds twice as intelligible as the anchor, and the number 5 only if the sample sounds half as intelligible as the anchor. Any subjective ratio is allowable, so any number can be assigned to a speech sample (not just half, or twice). When an anchor is not used, the ratio scaling is always done relative to the immediately preceding stimulus.

Readers may be surprised to learn that listeners can perform this task relatively easily and reliably, and that the anchored and unanchored versions of DME often produce very similar results for the same set of stimuli (see Schiavetti, 1992; and Weismer, 2008). DME is often viewed as a partial solution to the scaling problems associated with equal-appearing interval scales. In DME, there are no endpoints on the scale; a listener is free to use whatever range of numbers he or she chooses, eliminating the floor and ceiling effects imposed by an equal-appearing interval scale. Moreover, there is no linearity assumption, and in fact the ratio nature of DME is thought to be more consistent with the nonlinear relationships of many perceptual magnitudes to variations in a physical signal. Extensive studies of the reliability of DME are not available, but in at least one study original and repeat estimates of the same set of stimuli resulted in an average error of about 5% of the full scale of numbers (Turner & Weismer, 1993).

Like equal-appearing interval scales, DME provides a global estimate of speech intelligibility, meaning that the scale values are presumably affected by factors in addition to the articulatory component of segment identity. DME correlates well with estimates of intelligibility derived from single word tests, but as expected spreads out intelligibility estimates for speakers with very similar levels of single-word intelligibility (Weismer, Yunusova, & Bunton, 2012). The greater range of intelligibilities estimated by DME as compared to single word tests must be attributed to the DME values reflecting aspects of voice quality, prosody, and so forth. These speech production characteristics have minimal influence in single-word tests.

REVIEW

The modern era of speech perception research was initiated by experiments using the pattern-playback machine, a device that synthesized speech signals and was used to create small changes in the signals to evaluate the effect on listeners' phonetic decisions.

The motor theory of speech perception was based on the finding of categorical perception for stop consonant place of articulation.

Additional findings, including duplex perception and trading relations, were used to support the motor theory.

Motor theory was based on the idea that speech production and perception in humans were part of a special "code," and required a special mechanism in the brain for the perception of speech.

Categorical perception can be demonstrated in infants and animals, findings that may be interpreted as support for, or against, the motor theory.

The general auditory approach competes with motor theory as an explanation of speech perception and takes the perspective that the speech acoustic signal is sufficiently consistent to support speech sound perception, and that general auditory mechanisms (not special mechanisms) are used in the perception of speech signals.

Direct realism, a competing theory inspired by J. J. Gibson's ecological approach to perception, says that articulatory gestures are perceived directly (not by special mechanisms), and that listeners actually hear gestures, not acoustic representations of speech sounds that must be processed by cognitive mechanisms for proper recognition.

Recent results from the research literature suggest that both general auditory mechanisms and brain mechanisms with properties especially suited to the organization of linguistic input are used to perceive speech.

Speech perception involves not only the perception of speech sounds, but the use of those sounds to access words from the lexicon through a combination of bottom-up and top-down processes that probably account for the interplay between sound analysis and word choices in the understanding of a spoken message.

Speech intelligibility testing, a subtype of the general category of speech perception phenomena, has a clear role in speech-language pathology, even though specific tests have rarely been constructed according to principles derived from the speech perception literature.

The most common estimates of speech intelligibility use word or sentence tests, in which the scores are expressed as percentages of correctly heard words, or scaling techniques in which listeners attach numbers to the magnitudes of a speech intelligibility deficit.

REFERENCES

Adank, P., Smits, P., & van Hout, P. (2004). A comparison of vowel normalization procedures for language variation research. *Journal of the Acoustical Society of America, 116,* 3099–3107.

Andoni, S., Li, N., & Pollak, G. (2007). Spectrotemporal fields in the inferior colliculus revealing specificity for spectral motion in conspecific vocalizations. *Journal of Neuroscience, 27,* 4882–4893.

Astheimer, L.B., & Sanders, L.D. (2011). Pedictability affects early perceptual processing of word onsets in continuous speech. *Neuropsychologia, 49,* 3512–3516.

Best, C., Morrongiello, B., & Robson, R. (1981). Perceptual equivalence of acoustic cues in speech and nonspeech perception. *Perception and Psychophysics, 29,* 191–211.

Blumstein, S., & Stevens, K. (1979). Acoustic invariance in speech production: Evidence from measurements of the spectral characteristics of stop consonants. *Journal of the Acoustical Society of America, 66,* 1001–1017.

Cleary, M., & Pisoni, D. (2001). Speech perception and spoken word recognition: Research and theory. In E. Goldstein (Ed.), *Blackwell handbook of perception* (pp. 499–534). Oxford, UK: Blackwell.

Cole, R., & Rudnicky, A. (1983). What's new in speech perception? The research and idea of William Chandler Bagley, 1874–1946. *Psychological Review, 90,* 94–101.

Cooper, F., Liberman, A., & Borst, J. (1951). The interconversion of audible and visible patterns as a basis for research in the perception of speech. *Proceedings of the National Academy of Sciences, 37,* 318–325.

Cutler, A., Dahan, D., & van Donselaar, W. (1997). Prosody in the comprehension of spoken language: A literature review. *Language and Speech, 40,* 141–201.

Dahan, D., & Gareth Gaskell, M. (2007). The temporal dynamics of ambiguity resolution: Evidence from spoken word recognition. *Journal of Memory and Language, 57,* 483–501.

Dahan, D., & Magnuson, J. (2006). Spoken word recognition. In M. Traxler & M. Gernsbacher (Eds.), *Handbook of psycholinguistics* (2nd ed., pp. 249–283). New York, NY: Academic Press.

Darley, F., Aronson, A.E., & Brown, J. (1975). *Motor speech disorders*. Philadelphia, PA: Saunders.

Davies, N., Madden, J., & Butchart, S. (2004). Learning finetunes a specific response of nestlings to the parental alarm calls of their own species. *Proceedings of the Royal Society of London B, 271,* 2297–2304.

Diehl, R., Lotto, A., & Holt, L. (2004). Speech perception. *Annual Review of Psychology, 55,* 149–179.

Duffy, J. (1995). *Motor speech disorders: Substrates, differential diagnosis, and management*. St. Louis, MO: Mosby.

Eimas, P., Miller, J., & Jusczyk, P. (1990). On infant speech perception and the acquisition of language. In S. Harnad (Ed.), *Categorical perception: The groundwork of cognition* (pp. 161–195). Cambridge, UK: Cambridge University Press.

Fant, G. (1960). *Acoustic theory of speech production*. Hague, Netherlands: Mouton.

Fowler, C. (1986). An event approach to the study of speech perception from a direct-realist perspective. *Journal of Phonetics, 14,* 3–28.

Fowler, C. (1996). Listeners do hear sounds, not tongues. *Journal of the Acoustical Society of America, 99,* 1730–1741.

Fowler, C. (2006). Compensation for coarticulation reflects gesture perception, not spectral contrast. *Perception and Psychophysics, 68,* 161–177.

Fowler, C., Galantucci, B., & Saltzman, E. (2003). Motor theories of perception. In M. Arbib (Ed.), *The handbook of brain theory and neural networks* (pp. 705–707). Cambridge, MA: MIT Press.

Fowler, C., & Rosenblum, L. (1991). The perception of phonetic gestures. In I. Mattingly & M. Studdert-Kennedy (Eds.), *Modularity and the motor theory of speech perception* (pp. 33–59). Hillsdale, NJ: Lawrence Erlbaum.

Gibson, J. (1968). *The senses considered as perceptual systems*. Boston, MA: Houghton Mifflin.

Gibson, J. (1979). *The ecological approach to visual perception*. Boston, MA: Houghton Mifflin.

Goldinger, S. (1998). Echoes of echoes? An episodic theory of lexical access. *Psychological Review, 105,* 251–279.

Grosjean F. (1980). Spoken word recognition processes and the gating paradigm. *Perception and Psychophysics, 28,* 267–283.

Hirsh, I. (1959). Auditory perception of temporal order. *Journal of the Acoustical Society of America, 31,* 759–767.

Johnson, K., & Mullenix, J. (1997). *Talker variability in speech processing*. New York, NY: Academic Press.

Katz, J. (Ed.). (2002). *Handbook of clinical audiology* (5th ed.). Baltimore, MD: Lippincott Williams & Wilkins.

Kent J., Kent R., Rosenbek J., Weismer G., Martin R., Sufit R., & Brooks B. (1992). Quantitative description of the dysarthria in women with amyotrophic lateral sclerosis. *Journal of Speech and Hearing Research, 35,* 723–733.

Kent, R. (Ed.) (1992). *Intelligibility in speech disorders: Theory, measurement, and management*. Amsterdam, Netherlands: John Benjamin.

Kent, R., Weismer, G., Kent, J., & Rosenbek, J. (1989). Toward phonetic intelligibility testing in dysarthria. *Journal of Speech and Hearing Disorders, 54,* 482–499.

Kingston, J., & Diehl, R. (1994). Phonetic knowledge. *Language*, 70, 419–454.

Klatt, D. (1987). Review of text-to-speech conversion for English. *Journal of the Acoustical Society of America*, 82, 737–793.

Klatt, D. (1989). Review of selected models of speech perception. In W. Marslen-Wilson (Ed.), *Lexical representation and process* (pp. 169–226). Cambridge, MA: MIT Press.

Kluender, K. (1994). Speech perception as a tractable problem in cognitive science. In M. Gernsbacher (Ed.), *Handbook of psycholinguistics* (pp. 173–217). San Diego, CA: Academic Press.

Kluender, K., & Kiefte, M. (2006). Speech perception within a biologically realistic information-theoretic framework. In M. Traxler & M. Gernsbacher (Eds.), *Handbook of psycholinguistics* (2nd ed., pp. 153–199). London, UK: Elsevier.

Kuhl, P. (1986). Theoretical contribution of tests on animals to the special mechanisms debate in speech. *Experimental Biology*, 45, 233–265.

Kuhl, P., & Miller, J. (1975). Speech perception by the chinchilla: Voiced-voiceless distinction in alveolar plosive consonants. *Science*, 190, 69–72.

Kuhl, P., & Padden, D. (1983). Enhanced discriminability at the phoneme boundaries for place of articulation in macaques. *Journal of the Acoustical Society of America*, 73, 1003–1010.

Laing, E. J. C., Liu, R., Lotto, A. J., & Holt, L. L. (2012). Tuned with a tune: talker normalization via general auditory processes. *Frontiers in Psychology*, 3, 1–9.

Liberman, A., Cooper, F., Shankweiler, D., & Studdert-Kennedy, M. (1967). Perception of the speech code. *Psychological Review*, 74, 431–461.

Liberman, A., Harris, K., Hoffman, H., & Griffith, B. (1957). The discrimination of speech sounds within and across phoneme boundaries. *Journal of Experimental Psychology*, 54, 358–368.

Liberman, A., & Mattingly, I. (1985). The motor theory of speech perception revised. *Cognition*, 21, 1–36.

Lieberman, P. (1996). Some biological constraints on the analysis of prosody. In J. Morgan & K. Demuth (Eds.), *Signal to syntax: Bootstrapping from speech to grammar in early acquisition* (pp. 55–66). Hillsdale, NJ: Lawrence Erlbaum.

Lindblom, B. (1990). Explaining phonetic variation: A sketch of the H&H theory. In W. Hardcastle & A. Marchal (Eds.), *Speech production and speech modeling* (pp. 403–440). Dordrecht, Netherlands: Kluwer Academic.

Liss, J. (2007). The role of speech perception in motor speech disorders. In G. Weismer (Ed.), *Motor speech disorders* (pp. 187–219). San Diego, CA: Plural.

Liss, J., Spitzer, S., Caviness, J., Adler, C., & Edwards, B. (2000). Lexical boundary error analysis in hypokinetic and ataxic dysarthria. *Journal of the Acoustical Society of America*, 107, 3415–3424.

Lotto, A., & Holt, L. (2006). Putting phonetic context effects into context: A commentary on Fowler (2006). *Perception and Psychophysics*, 68, 178–183.

Luce, P., & McLennan, C. (2005). Spoken word recognition: The challenge of variation. In D. Pisoni & R. Remez (Eds.),

The handbook of speech perception (pp. 591–609). Malden, MA: Blackwell.

Mann, V., & Liberman, A. (1983). Some differences between phonetic and auditory modes of perception. *Cognition*, 14, 211–235.

Miller, J., & Jusczyk, P. (1989). Seeking the neurobiological basis of speech perception. *Cognition*, 33, 111–137.

Minagawa-Kawai, Y., Cristià, A., & Dupoux, E. (2011). Cerebral lateralization and early speech acquisition: A developmental scenario. *Developmental Cognitive Neuroscience*, 1, 217–232.

Monsen, R. (1983). The oral speech intelligibility of hearing-impaired talkers. *Journal of Speech and Hearing Disorders*, 48, 286–296.

Mullenix, J., Pisoni, D., & Martin, C. (1989). Some effects of talker variability on spoken word recognition. *Journal of the Acoustical Society of America*, 85, 365–378.

Nooteboom, S., & van der Vlugt, M. (1988). A search for a word-beginning superiority effect. *Journal of the Acoustical Society of America*, 84, 2018–2032.

Pardo, J., & Remez, R. (2006). The perception of speech. In M. Traxler and M. Gernsbacher (Eds.), *Handbook of psycholinguistics* (2nd ed., pp. 201–248). Amsterdam, Netherlands: Elsevier.

Patterson, D., & Pepperberg, I. (1998). Acoustic and articulatory correlates of stop consonants in a parrot and a human subject. *Journal of the Acoustical Society of America*, 103, 2197–2215.

Pisoni, D. (1977). Identification and discrimination of the relative onset time of two complex tones: Implications for voicing perception in stops. *Journal of the Acoustical Society of America*, 61, 1352–1361.

Popper, K. (2002a). *Conjectures and refutations: The growth of scientific knowledge*. London, UK: Routledge Classics.

Popper, K. (2002b). *The logic of scientific discovery*. London, UK: Routledge Classics.

Remez, R., Rubin, P., Berns, S., Pardo, J., & Lang, J. (1994). On the perceptual organization of speech. *Psychological Review*, 101, 129–156.

Repp, B. (1982). Phonetic trading relations and context effects: New experimental evidence for a speech mode of perception. *Psychological Bulletin*, 92, 81–110.

Repp, B., & Liberman, A. (1987). Phonetic category boundaries are flexible. In S. Harnad (Ed.), *Categorical perception: The groundwork of cognition* (pp. 89–112). Cambridge, UK: Cambridge University Press.

Saffran, J. (2003). Statistical language learning: Mechanisms and constraints. *Current Directions in Psychological Science*, 12, 110–114.

Saffran, J., & Thiessen, E. (2007). Domain-general learning capacities. In E. Hoff & M. Shatz (Eds.), *Handbook of language development* (pp. 68–86) Cambridge, UK: Blackwell.

Schiavetti, N. (1992). Scaling procedures for the measurement of speech intelligibility. In R.D. Kent (Ed.), *Intelligibility in speech disorders: Theory, measurement, management* (pp. 11–34). Amsterdam, Netherlands: John Benjamin.

Sommers, M., & Barcroft, J. (2006). Stimulus variability and the phonetic relevance hypothesis: Effects of variability in speaking style, fundamental frequency, and speaking rate on spoken word identification. *Journal of the Acoustical Society of America, 119,* 2406–2416.

Stevens, K. (2005). Features in speech perception and lexical access. In D. Pisoni & R. Remez (Eds.), *The handbook of speech perception* (pp. 125–155). Malden, MA: Blackwell.

Studdert-Kennedy, M., & Shankweiler, D. (1970). Hemispheric specialization for speech perception. *Journal of the Acoustical Society of America, 48,* 579–594.

Turner, G. S., & Weismer, G. (1993). Characteristics of speaking rate in the dysarthria associated with amyotrophic lateral sclerosis. *Journal of Speech and Hearing Research, 36,* 1134–1144.

Watkins, K., & Paus, T. (2004). Modulation of motor excitability during speech perception: The role of Broca's area. *Journal of Cognitive Neuroscience, 16,* 978–987.

Weismer, G. (2008). Speech intelligibility. In M. Ball, M. Perkins, N. Müller, & S. Howard (Eds.), *Handbook of clinical linguistics.* Oxford, UK: Blackwell.

Weismer, G., & Martin, R. (1992). Acoustic and perceptual approaches to the study of intelligibility. In R. Kent (Ed.), *Intelligibility in speech disorders: Theory, measurement, and management* (pp. 67–118). Amsterdam, Netherlands: John Benjamin.

Weismer, G., Yunusova, Y., & Bunton, K. (2012). Measures to evaluate the effects of DBS on speech production. *Journal of Neurolinguistics, 25,* 74–94.

Whalen, D., & Liberman, A. (1987). Speech perception takes precedence over nonspeech perception. *Science, 237,* 169–171.

Yorkston, K., Beukelman, D., Strand, E., & Bell, K. (1999). *Management of motor speech disorders in children and adults* (2nd ed.). Austin, TX: Pro-Ed.

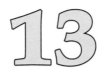

Swallowing

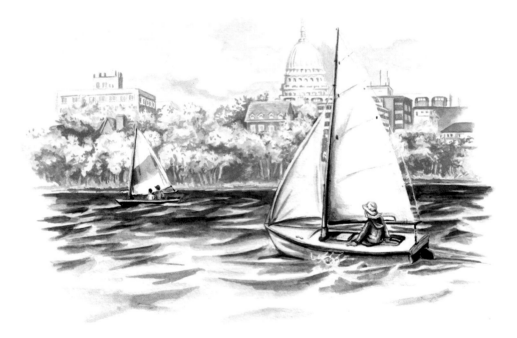

Scenario

She stepped on her skiff and things somehow felt a little different. There was no wind and the lake was as smooth as glass, yet she seemed to be gently rolling and pitching. The feeling was very brief and she thought nothing of it. By the time her skiff was rigged, the wind picked up, as if at her command. Lake Mendota and the signs of fall were especially calming to her. Her life was good. She had a new granddaughter to dote on, and her retirement from the university was coming into sight.

A week later she stumbled but caught herself as she walked into her living room. The incident was registered but then ignored. Within the next month she noticed occasional cramps in her legs and some twitching now and then in her right hand, just near the junction where her thumb and index finger came together. Probably nothing. But was it? She began to wonder only after she found herself struggling to get up out of an overstuffed chair in front of the television set. There was something wrong. It had crossed a threshold. She mentioned the events to her husband and they agreed that she should talk with her physician.

From this time on until her condition was diagnosed, other things about her movements began to concern her. She occasionally choked when eating, something she rarely did before. She seemed to tire more easily than usual. And she seemed to be losing some of the power in her voice. Within 3 months, a neurologist had fixed the diagnosis and the words were numbing. She had Lou Gehrig's disease or amyotrophic lateral sclerosis, and no matter which she chose to call it, her future was set. Only the time course and the manner of devastation were uncertainties.

Two years passed and her condition worsened. By then, she had moderate breathing discomfort, a wet and gurgly sounding voice, and her speech was difficult to understand in conversation. She had trouble swallowing and had lost much of her enjoyment of eating. She could no longer walk and was confined to a wheelchair during the day. All of her movements were slow and weak and she gave the impression of running on a dying battery. Her plight had rendered her almost completely dependent and only occasionally was her clear mind able to lift her above her quiet despair. Her best moments were when her new granddaughter was in sight.

She began to lose weight because of her swallowing problem, her speech was nearly unintelligible, and her breathing was becoming more of a struggle. Her neurologist referred her to a local medical center with the request that a speech-language pathologist evaluate her swallowing and speech and that a pulmonologist evaluate her breathing, both with an eye toward palliative management.

INTRODUCTION

Some of the most enjoyable activities of daily living involve eating and drinking. These include meals (where eating and drinking are the purpose of the activity), special events such as receptions (where eating and drinking enhance the celebration), and relaxation activities such as going to the movies (where eating popcorn and drinking soda are an integral part of the experience for some people). Figure 13–1 is a cartoon that depicts the anticipation of a good meal and the social context in which it is enjoyed.

The ease of eating and drinking is deceptive. They are complicated activities that require intricately coordinated actions of the lips, mandible, tongue, velum, pharynx, larynx, esophagus, and other structures. Because eating and drinking engage many of the same structures and much of the same airway as are used for speaking and breathing, it is not uncommon for there to be competition between these activities or for tradeoffs to occur when attempting to execute them simultaneously. For example, there are certain times when chewing must stop for speaking to occur and when speaking and breathing must stop for swallowing to occur.

The entire act of placing solid or liquid substance in the oral cavity, moving it backward to the pharynx, propelling it into the esophagus, and allowing it to make its way to the stomach is called deglutition. Although the word swallowing is sometimes used as a synonym for deglutition, swallowing actually includes only certain phases of deglutition. Nevertheless, to simplify the explanations that follow, the term swallowing is used in place of deglutition and is meant to include all phases of deglutition.

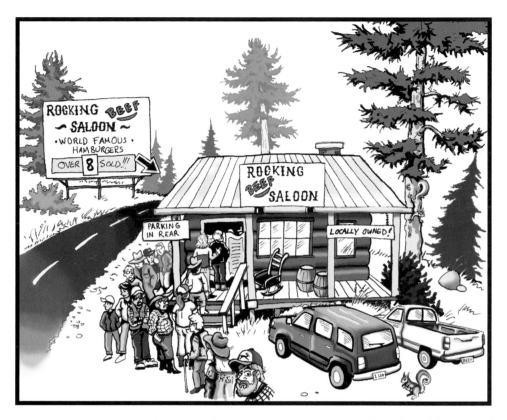

Figure 13–1. Cartoon depicting the anticipation of a good meal and the social context in which it is enjoyed.

ANATOMY

Figure 13–2 shows the structures that participate in swallowing. These structures extend from the lips to the stomach. Most of these same structures also participate in speech production; notable exceptions are the esophagus and stomach.

Breathing, Laryngeal, Velopharyngeal-Nasal, and Pharyngeal-Oral Structures

Structures within the breathing, laryngeal, velopharyngeal-nasal, and pharyngeal-oral subsystems participate in swallowing. These include the chest wall, vocal folds, ventricular folds, epiglottis, pharynx (laryngopharynx, oropharynx, nasopharynx), velum, tongue, mandible, and lips. Their anatomy is described in Chapters 2, 3, 4, and 5, and their functions during swallowing are described below. The anatomy of the esophagus and stomach is not covered in the other chapters and warrants attention here.

Esophagus

The esophagus is a flexible tube, about 20 cm long in adults, which runs from the lower part of the pharynx to the stomach. The esophagus begins below the base of the larynx and runs behind the trachea, pulmonary apparatus, and heart. It courses through the diaphragm (see Figure 2–6) and enters the abdominal cavity where it connects to the stomach. The esophagus is usually in a flattened state, but can stretch to accommodate substances passing through it. The cervical (upper) esophagus consists of striated (voluntary) muscle, whereas the thoracic (middle) esophagus comprises a mixture of striated and smooth (involuntary) muscle in its upper region and purely smooth muscle in its lower region. The abdominal (lower) esophagus is composed of only smooth muscle. The esophagus is lined with a thick layer of mucosa, beneath which lies connective tissue and glands that secrete mucus to aid in the movement of substances through it.

The esophagus is bounded at its upper end by the upper esophageal sphincter (sometimes called the

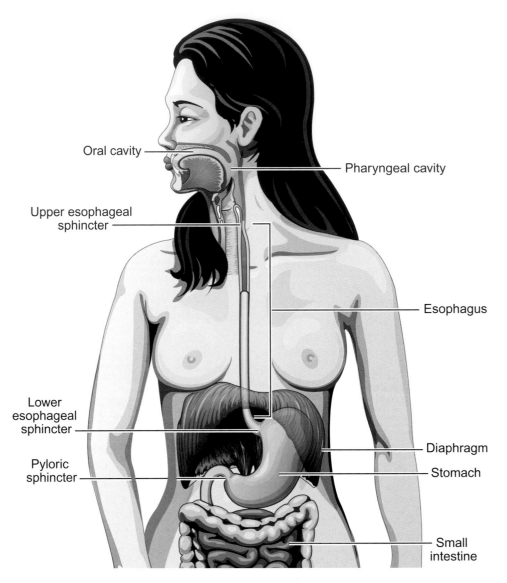

Oral cavity

Pharyngeal cavity

Upper esophageal
sphincter

Esophagus

Lower
esophageal
sphincter

Pyloric
sphincter

Diaphragm

Stomach

Small
intestine

Figure 13–2. Structures of the swallowing apparatus.

pharyngoesophageal segment, or PE segment) and at its lower end by the lower esophageal sphincter. These sphincters mark the entrance and exit of the esophagus, respectively, and are operationally defined as zones of high pressure, rather than as precise anatomical entities. It is uncertain which structures are responsible for creating these high-pressure zones. Nevertheless, indirect evidence suggests that the *cricopharyngeus* muscles of the pharynx (considered by some to be part of the *inferior constrictor* muscles) are the primary contributors to the contraction-relaxation pattern of the upper esophageal sphincter (Hila, Castell, & Castell, 2001).

Stomach

The stomach is a large, saclike structure that is made up of smooth muscle, mucosa, and other tissue. It is positioned on the left side of the abdominal cavity, against the undersurface of the diaphragm. The stomach connects to the esophagus via the lower esophageal sphincter and to the small intestine via the pyloric sphincter. After a typical meal, the stomach holds about a liter of solid and/or liquid substance, although it can stretch to hold much more if necessary. Gastric juices in the stomach break up ingested substances so that they can be absorbed into the body through the stomach lining.

America Regains the Mustard Yellow Belt

Holy stomach full! Japan's Takeru Kobayashi was the six-time hot-dog-eating world champion and ate 63 hot dogs and buns (six more than his personal best) on July 4, 2007 at Coney Island, New York. With more than 50,000 people in attendance and in the glare of national television cameras, Kobayashi lost his crown to Joey Chestnut of San Jose, California. Sanctioned by Major League Eating, the world governing body of all stomach-centric sport, Nathan's Famous International Fourth of July Hot Dog Eating Championship has been held each year on the 4th of July since 1916. In 2007, Chestnut put down an astounding 66 hot dogs and buns in just 12 minutes to set a new world's record. On July 4, 2012, Chestnut once again exceeded his personal best by ingesting 68 dogs and buns in 10 minutes and winning the men's competition for the sixth straight year. And, yes, there is a women's competition too. The women's 2012 winner was Sonya Thomas of Alexandria, Virginia, who took home her pink champion's belt and $10,000.

FORCES AND MOVEMENTS OF SWALLOWING

Although many of the structures that participate in swallowing are the same as those that are used for speaking, the forces and movements for the two activities are very different. In general, the forces are greater and many of the movements are slower during swallowing than during speech production.

To set the stage for understanding the forces and movements of swallowing, it is useful to begin by considering certain pressures associated with the resting state of the swallowing apparatus. These pressures are depicted in Figure 13–3 in the context of the swallowing apparatus at rest at the end of a tidal expiration. The pressure in the oral cavity is atmospheric. The pressure in the esophagus is below atmospheric (approximately -5 cmH$_2$O), because of the tendency of the pulmonary apparatus and chest wall to pull away from one another (the esophagus is in the chest wall). The pressure in the stomach is above atmospheric (approximately 5 cmH$_2$O) and results from the "muscle tone" of the wall of the stomach and the hydrostatic properties of the stomach contents. In contrast to these relatively low pressures, the pressures within the upper and lower esophageal sphincters are high (a typical range is 40 to 80 cmH$_2$O in the resting state). Their absolute magnitudes depend on the measurement approach used as well as a variety of physiological factors (Goyal & Cobb, 1981; Linden, Hogosta, & Norlander, 2007). The relatively high pressures in the upper and lower esophageal sphincters allow these regions to function like forcefully closed valves while at rest. It is important that the pressure in the lower esophageal sphincter remains substantially higher than the pressure in the stomach. Otherwise, substances from the stomach may reflux (flow back) into the esophagus.

Both passive and active forces contribute to swallowing. Passive force comes from many sources including: (a) the natural recoil of connective tissues (ligaments and membranes), cartilages, and bones, (b) the surface tension between structures in apposition, (c) the pull of gravity, and (d) aeromechanical factors. Active force results from the activation of breathing, laryngeal, velopharyngeal-nasal, and pharyngeal-oral muscles in various combinations. These contributions to active force are described in Chapters 2, 3, 4, and 5, and are discussed here as they relate to swallowing.

Forces and movements of swallowing can be considered in association with four phases of swallowing, as shown schematically in Figure 13–4. These are the oral preparatory phase, oral transport phase, pharyngeal transport phase, and esophageal transport phase and are used to describe the movement of a bolus through the oral, pharyngeal, and esophageal regions of the apparatus. Bolus is the word used to refer to the mass of solid substance (food) or the volume of liquid to be swallowed.

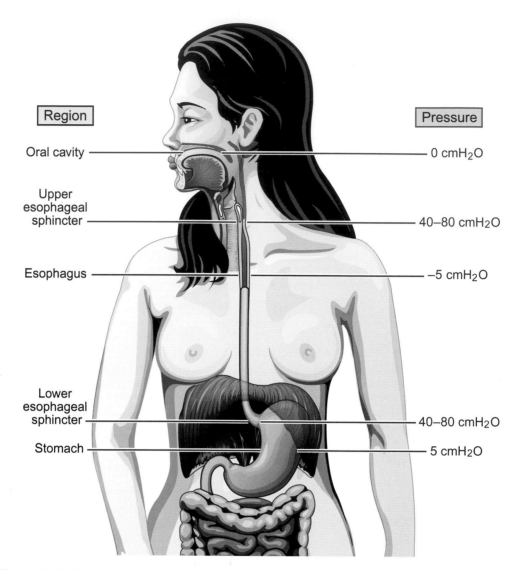

Figure 13–3. Relevant pressures associated with the resting state of the swallowing apparatus.

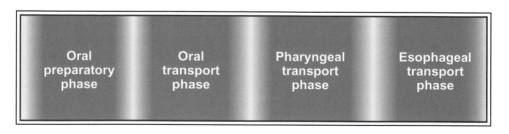

Figure 13–4. Schematic depiction of the four phases of swallowing.

Oral Preparatory Phase

The oral preparatory phase is depicted in Figure 13–5. This phase begins as solid or liquid substance makes contact with the structures of the anterior oral vestibule. The mandible lowers and the lips abduct to allow solid or liquid substance to enter. What happens next is largely dependent on the nature of the substance to be swallowed.

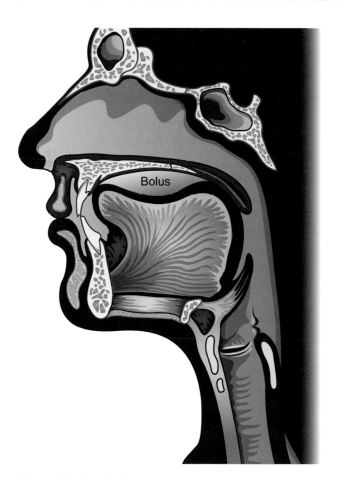

Figure 13–5. Oral preparatory phase of swallowing.

If the substance is liquid, the mandible elevates and the lips adduct, forming an anterior seal to contain the bolus. The bolus is contained in the anterior region of the oral cavity by actions of the tongue and other structures, and held there momentarily (usually on the order of 1 s). The anterior tongue depresses and the sides of the tongue elevate to form a "cup" for the bolus. The bolus may be cupped in one of two ways, depending on the person. Some people hold the bolus with the tongue tip elevated and contacting the back surface of the maxillary incisors, and other people hold the bolus on the floor of the oral cavity in front of the tongue. These two holding positions have been dubbed "dipper" and "tipper" type swallows (Dodds et al., 1989). The back of the tongue elevates to make contact with the velum to form a back wall that separates the oral from the pharyngeal cavities and helps to ensure that no substance can slip by and into the pulmonary airways. The velopharynx is open so that breathing can continue. Nevertheless, many people stop breathing momentarily (called the apneic interval) at this point

in the swallow, or even before the cup of liquid reaches the lips (Martin, Logemann, Shaker, & Dodds, 1994; Martin-Harris, Brodsky, Price, Michel, & Walters, 2003; Martin-Harris, Michel, & Castell, 2005b). This apneic interval serves to reduce the risk of aspiration (defined as invasion of substances below the vocal folds).

These initial events are quite different when the substance to be swallowed is solid, rather than liquid, because solid substances need to be masticated (chewed) into smaller pieces and mixed with saliva before being transported toward the esophagus. Saliva is an important ingredient to this process because it moistens the solid substance to help facilitate its transport as well as introduces enzymes that begin to break down the substance for digestion (see sidetrack Mmm Mmm Good!). Actions of the mandible (and teeth), lips, tongue, and cheeks grind and manipulate the solid substance into a cohesive bolus (lump) and position it on the surface of the anterior tongue. The lips may remain fully adducted (though this is not necessary) while the mandible moves to grind the bolus. During chewing, the mandible moves up and down, forward and backward, and side to side. This is in contrast to speech production, during which the mandible moves primarily up and down. The velum makes contact with the back part of the tongue to seal off the oral from the

---

Mmm Mmm Good!

"Mmm, mmm, good!" Does this make you think of steamy, chunky soup? Or, better yet, freshly baked cookies just out of the oven? Maybe your imagination is so good that your mouth actually starts to water. Which brings us to the point of this sidetrack: saliva. Saliva is produced by salivary glands and is critical to our ability to swallow and digest. Most saliva is swallowed alone (these are called "dry swallows"). During eating, saliva mixes with the food to moisten it for easier transport through oral, pharyngeal, and esophageal parts of the digestive tract and introduces enzymes that begin the digestive process. Do you have any idea how much saliva we produce? The answer is an amazing 1 to 2 liters of saliva every 24 hours! Although saliva production is continuous, its volume and content vary rhythmically; that is, saliva production has a circadian rhythm. Much less saliva is produced during sleep than during wakefulness. That's good. Better to save that saliva for the cookie-eating waking hours.

pharyngeal cavity to prevent the bolus from moving into the pharynx and larynx. The velopharynx is open during preparation of the bolus, and breathing may either continue or be interrupted by apnea (McFarland & Lund, 1995; Palmer & Hiiemae, 2003). The duration of the oral preparatory phase may last from as short as 3 s, when chewing a soft cookie, to as long as 20 s, when chewing a tough piece of steak.

At the end of the oral preparatory phase, the substance in the oral cavity is ready for consumption. Usually it is transported back toward the pharynx (oral transport phase) immediately. There are choices at this point, however, including that the substance can be: (a) savored for awhile by continued manipulation, (b) squirreled in the cheeks, or (c) expelled. In fact, the expulsion option is used when performing a "sham" feeding test to study the actions of the stomach in anticipation of receiving food.

Oral Transport Phase

Once the bolus is in the ready position (either the "dipper" or "tipper" position for liquids), it is usually transported back through the oral cavity, as illustrated in Figure 13–6. The tongue tip elevates and squeezes the bolus against the hard palate; then progressively more posterior regions of the tongue elevate and squeeze the bolus against the palate, moving the bolus back toward the pharynx. The tongue is an especially effective structure for moving and clearing the bolus because it behaves like a muscular hydrostat (in that it can move and change shape in an almost infinite number of ways—see Chapter 5). The force needed to propel the bolus varies with bolus viscosity. The lips usually press together firmly (although this is not necessary) and the cheeks are pulled inward slightly to keep the bolus positioned over the tongue. At the same time, the velum begins to elevate and the pharyngeal walls begin to constrict. The oral transport phase is short, generally lasting less than 0.5 second (Cook et al., 1994; Tracy et al., 1989).

Pharyngeal Transport Phase

The pharyngeal transport phase of the swallow is "triggered" once the bolus passes the anterior faucial pillars; the exact location of the trigger can vary, depending on the bolus type and the age of the individual. During this phase, depicted in Figure 13–7, several events occur rapidly and nearly simultaneously to move the

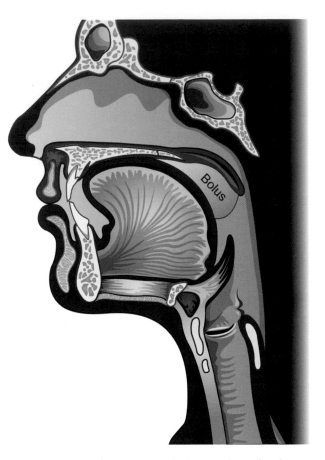

Figure 13-6. Oral transport phase of swallowing.

bolus quickly through the pharynx while protecting the airway. This phase is under "automatic" control, so that once triggered, it proceeds as a relatively fixed set of events that cannot be altered voluntarily (except in the magnitude and duration of the pressures generated). These events occur within about 0.5 s or less (Cook et al., 1994; Tracy et al., 1989) and include adjustments related to velopharyngeal closure, elevation of the hyoid bone and larynx, laryngeal closure, pharyngeal constriction, and opening of the upper esophageal sphincter, as described below.

The velopharynx closes like a flap-sphincter valve by elevation of the velum and constriction of the pharyngeal walls. This closure is forceful (more forceful than for speech production) so as to prohibit passage of substances into the nasopharynx.

The hyoid bone and larynx move upward and forward as a result of contraction of extrinsic tongue muscles (recall that several extrinsic muscles of the tongue attach to the hyoid bone). As the hyoid bone is pulled upward and forward, the larynx is pulled along with

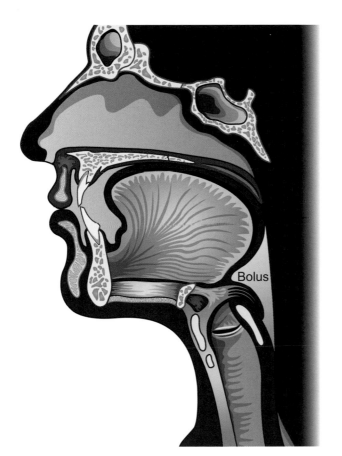

Figure 13–7. Pharyngeal transport phase of swallowing.

it via its muscular connections to the hyoid bone. In fact, because of these anatomical connections and the tendency to move as a unit, this group of structures is often called the hyolaryngeal complex. Elevation of the larynx also causes the pharynx to shorten.

Closure of the larynx for swallowing has been described as a folding of the laryngeal apparatus (Fink & Demarest, 1978) that forms a seal to the entrance of the trachea to protect the pulmonary airways. Closure occurs at multiple levels, which include the vocal folds, the ventricular folds, and the aryepiglottic folds and epiglottis. Both the vocal folds and ventricular folds adduct firmly, whereas the epiglottis is forced down over the laryngeal aditus like a trap door and serves as a first line of defense against substances entering the larynx and pulmonary airways. The epiglottis moves from a relatively upward pointing position, through a horizontal position, to a relatively downward pointing position. Both passive and active forces appear to be responsible for downward movement of the epiglottis during swallowing (Ekberg & Sigurjonsson, 1982; Fink

& Demarest, 1978; VanDaele, Perlman, & Cassell, 1995). The passive force derives from backward movement of the tongue and upward and forward movement of the hyoid bone and larynx, which mechanically deflect the epiglottis backward and downward. Upward and forward movement of the larynx simultaneously contributes to airway protection by tucking the larynx against the root of the tongue and deflecting the trachea away from the digestive pathway. The active force is somewhat less certain (Fink, Martin, & Rohrmann, 1979; Ramsey, Watson, Gramiak, & Weinberg, 1955; VanDaele et al., 1995), but is argued to derive from contraction of the *aryepiglottic* muscles (and possibly from vertically ascending lateral fibers of the *thyroarytenoid* muscles), which purportedly pull the epiglottis downward to complete the seal with the laryngeal aditus (Ekberg & Sigurjonsson, 1982). Whatever the relative contribution of passive and actives forces to downward displacement of the epiglottis, it can be stated with considerable certainty that the structure plays a key role in protection of the pulmonary airways during swallowing.

As the tongue propels the bolus into the pharynx, the pharynx undergoes segmental contraction (from top to bottom). The tongue root moves backward and the pharyngeal walls constrict to "squeeze" the bolus toward the esophagus. The bolus often divides at the epiglottis as it passes through the left and right epiglottic valleculae (lateral channels between the root of the tongue and the epiglottis) and into the left and right pyriform sinuses (recesses bounded by the pharynx and larynx), or it flows down one side or through the midline of the covered laryngeal aditus (Dua, Ren, Bardan, Xie, & Shaker, 1997; Logemann, Kahrilas, Kobara, & Vakil, 1989).

The final step of the pharyngeal transport phase of the swallow is the opening of the upper esophageal sphincter to allow the passage of the bolus into the esophagus. This is accomplished by relaxation of the *cricopharyngeus* muscles and simultaneous stretching of the esophageal opening by movement of the hyolaryngeal complex.

The bolus is propelled through the pharynx to the esophagus during the pharyngeal transport phase by a combination of mechanical (structural) forces and aeromechanical forces. The mechanical forces consist of the tongue pushing the bolus back into the pharynx and the pharynx contracting segmentally against the tongue root, as just described. The aeromechanical forces are in the form of regional air pressure changes that help to move the bolus along. Specifically, backward movement of the tongue and constriction of the pharyngeal walls serve to narrow the airway in that region and reduce the airway volume, thereby causing the air pressure to rise in that region. At the same time, dilation of the upper esophageal sphincter lowers the air pressure below the bolus. The pressure differential (higher pressure behind the bolus than in front of it) helps to drive the bolus toward its destination.

The pharyngeal transport phase of the swallow is invariably short and is characterized by a series of actions that move the bolus quickly through the pharynx and, at the same time, protect the pulmonary airways from invasion by substances. The final phase of swallowing is initiated as the bolus moves into the esophagus.

Esophageal Transport Phase

The esophageal transport phase, illustrated in Figure 13–8, begins when the bolus enters the upper esophageal sphincter and ends when it passes into the stomach through the lower esophageal sphincter. This phase may last anywhere from 8 to 20 s (Dodds, Hogan, Reid, Stewart, & Arndorfer, 1973). As described above, the bolus is pushed into the esophagus by muscles of the tongue and pharynx and by pressure differentials, and the upper esophageal sphincter opens so that the bolus can pass into the esophagus (the lower esophageal sphincter relaxes at the same time). The bolus is then propelled by peristaltic actions (alternating waves of contraction and relaxation) of the esophageal walls. Peristaltic contraction raises pressure behind the bolus and relaxation lowers pressure in front of the bolus creating the pressure differential needed to propel it toward the stomach. The nature of the peristaltic action varies somewhat depending on the nature of the bolus (solid or liquid), body position (relation of esophagus and bolus to gravity), and other factors. When a substance is left behind following the primary peristalsis, it is cleared by subsequent peristaltic action (called secondary peristalsis). Although the esophagus usually transports substances toward the stomach, it can also transport substances or gas away from the stomach (as in the case of vomiting or burping).

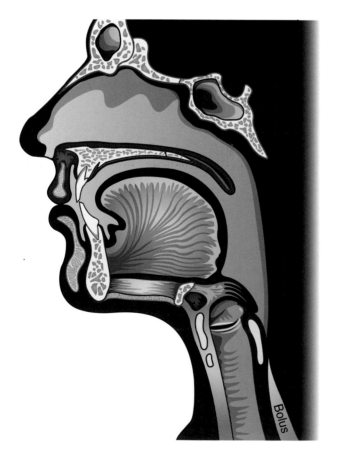

Figure 13–8. Esophageal transport phase of swallowing.

GERD and LPR

Your stomach is rich with chemicals that have about the same acidity as the battery acid in your car. That's right, that's the same battery acid that will burn a hole in your clothes if you splash some of it on you. GERD, an acronym for gastroesophageal reflux disease, is a chronic condition in which acid from the stomach backs up into the esophagus when the lower esophageal sphincter (the valve that separates the esophagus and stomach) fails to do its job properly. Although a certain amount of reflux (backflow) from the stomach into the esophagus is considered normal, too much can cause heartburn and the need to see a gastroenterologist (GI doctor). When stomach acid travels all the way through the esophagus and spills onto the larynx it is called laryngopharyngeal reflux, or LPR. LPR can irritate and erode laryngeal tissue. LPR can cause a hoarse voice, chronic cough, frequent throat clearing, and other problems that may lead to the need to seek help from an otolaryngologist (ENT doctor). Some helpful hints for avoiding GERD and LPR: Don't stuff yourself before you go to bed, lay off foods that make it worse, and sleep with your body inclined so that your head is higher than your feet.

Overlap of Phases

Although the phases of swallowing are described above as though they are discrete and occur one after the other, they can overlap. When eating a solid substance, for example, preparation of part of the bolus in the oral cavity may continue while another part of the bolus moves into the pharyngeal area, as illustrated in Figure 13–9. This partial bolus may remain in the epiglottic valleculae as long as 10 s before it merges with the remainder of the bolus and the pharyngeal transport phase of the swallow is triggered (Hiiemae & Palmer, 1999).

Overlap of phases is also apparent if swallowing is viewed in relation to the actions of individual structures, rather than in relation to the status of the bolus. Whereas the traditional description of swallowing (used in this chapter) focuses on the preparation and transport of the bolus to define the phases of swallowing, there are schema that attempt to segment physiological events along somewhat different conceptual lines and to categorize them across different levels of observation (Martin-Harris et al., 2005b). Such notions have emerged relatively recently and rely on the coordination of temporal events across structures that traditionally have been thought of in sequential terms. Schema that are based on cross-structure analyses speak to common and overlapping elements of swallowing behavior and hold promise for better understanding the function of the swallowing apparatus as a whole and interactions among its components.

BREATHING AND SWALLOWING

Protection of the pulmonary airways during swallowing is dependent, in large part, on the coordination of breathing and swallowing. Without such coordination, inspiration might occur just as a substance is being transported through the pharynx and that substance might be "sucked" through the larynx into the pulmonary airways (aspiration). This is avoided by closing the larynx, which arrests breathing for a brief period during the swallow. The risk of aspiration appears to be further reduced by timing the swallow in relation to the inspiratory-expiratory flow of the breathing cycle.

Swallowing usually occurs during the expiratory phase of the breathing cycle. During single swallows, the most common pattern is expiration-swallow-expiration; that is, expiration begins, the swallow occurs (accompanied by apnea), and then expiration continues (Martin et al., 1994; Martin-Harris, 2006; Nishino, Yonezawa, & Honda, 1985; Perlman, Ettema, & Barkmeier, 2000; Selley, Flack, Ellis, & Brooks, 1989; Smith, Wolkove, Colacone, & Kreisman, 1989). This pattern, shown in Figure 13–10, is the predominant one for swallowing over a broad range of bolus volumes and consistencies and under a variety of serving conditions, such as presenting a liquid bolus with a syringe, drinking from a cup or straw, or eating a solid substance (Preiksaitis & Mills, 1996; Wheeler-Hegland, Huber, Pitts, & Sapienza, 2009). This appears to be a protective mechanism for potentially "blowing" any foreign substance away from the pulmonary airways. Nevertheless, it is interesting to note that not every swallow is followed by expiration, and that some healthy individuals inspire occasionally immediately after a swallow. This is particularly prevalent in people over age 65 years (Martin-Harris et al., 2005a). Thus, it is not absolutely necessary to expire after swallowing.

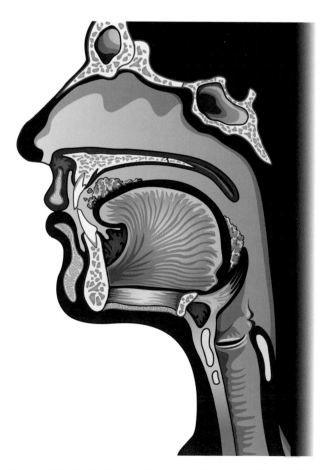

Figure 13–9. An illustration of eating, in which part of the bolus continues to be chewed while another part moves to the pharynx.

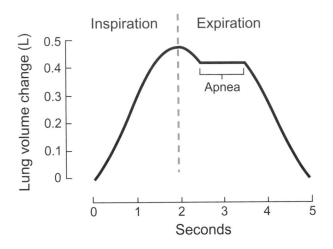

Figure 13-10. Swallow-related apnea (cessation of breathing) during expiration. This expiration-swallow-expiration pattern is typical of single swallows.

One Tug and Two Consequences

Breathing and swallowing cooperate in healthy individuals to prevent unwanted substances from entering the pulmonary airways. This cooperation can be more difficult with certain diseases. Chronic obstructive pulmonary disease (COPD) is one of these. A characteristic of this disease in advanced states is that the pulmonary apparatus expands and the diaphragm rides low and flat because air is trapped in the alveoli and airways. The abnormal positioning of the diaphragm has two potential consequences for swallowing. One is that a downward tug is placed on the larynx that tends to abduct the vocal folds and diminish their ability to protect the pulmonary airways. A second possible consequence is that the same downward tug lowers the laryngeal housing and tethers it from below. This means that the larynx may have difficulty moving up during a swallow because it has farther to go and because it must work against the downward pull of the diaphragm.

Although the apneic interval during swallowing typically lasts about 1 s, it can range from less than a second to several seconds (Klaun & Perlman, 1999; Martin et al., 1994; Martin-Harris et al., 2003, 2005a; Palmer & Hiiemae, 2003; Perlman et al., 2000; Preiksaitis & Mills, 1996). In some people, the duration of the apneic interval is influenced by variables such as bolus volume (Preiksaitis, Mayrand, Robins, & Diamant, 1992). Nevertheless, most of the variability in apnea duration can be attributed to variability in the onset of apnea relative to the eating or drinking event. For example, one person may stop breathing as the food or drink is approaching the mouth, whereas another person may continue to breathe until immediately before the larynx begins to elevate for the pharyngeal transport phase of the swallow (Martin et al., 1994). The apnea associated with swallowing can cause dyspnea (breathing discomfort) and a subsequent increase in ventilation, even in healthy people (Lederle, Hoit, & Barkmeier-Kraemer, 2012) and can be particularly uncomfortable and challenging in people with pulmonary disease (Hoit, Lansing, Dean, Yarkosky, & Lederle, 2011). When healthy people experience high respiratory drive (such as might occur during exercise or at high elevations), they tend to shorten the apneic interval during swallowing (Hårdemark Cedborg et al., 2010; in this study, high expiratory drive was created by breathing gas with a greater-than-usual amount of carbon dioxide). Shortening apnea in this way likely helps to minimize dyspnea. Another way that people apparently minimize dyspnea to breathe frequently during a series of swallows, such as when drinking a glass of water without stopping (Lederle et al., 2012).

Swallowing occurs at lung volumes that are almost always larger than the resting expiratory level (that is, the end-expiratory lung volume associated with resting tidal breathing), usually on the order of 10 to 20% larger (Lederle et al., 2012; Wheeler-Hegland et al., 2009; Wheeler-Hegland, Huber, Pitts, & Davenport, 2011). This lung volume range is one in which the passive (recoil) pressure of the breathing apparatus is positive, on the order of 5 to 10 cmH_2O (see Figure 2–17), and the tracheal pressures associated with swallowing generally fall in this recoil pressure range (Gross et al., in press). The fact that swallowing occurs at lung volumes that are larger than the resting size of the breathing apparatus, but still within the midrange of the vital capacity, appears to have several advantages. To begin, because swallows are produced at lung volumes where the tracheal pressure is positive, postswallow expirations are easily driven by the recoil pressure of the breathing apparatus. Furthermore, because swallows are produced at lung volumes that are only moderately large, there is no need to exert inspiratory muscular pressure to brake excessive positive recoil pressure that prevails at large lung volumes. In addition, by avoiding larger-than-necessary lung volumes, abductory force exerted on the vocal folds by the descent of the diaphragm is minimized (i.e., "tracheal tug," see Chapter 3).

A Sidetrack to a Sidetrack

The previous sidetrack focused on chronic obstructive pulmonary disease (COPD) and how certain mechanical consequences of advanced stages of the disease affect swallowing. These mechanical consequences are important contributors to swallowing problems, but there is another (perhaps less obvious) problem associated with COPD that may be equally important to swallowing. People with COPD are plagued by dyspnea (breathing discomfort), a condition that causes them to avoid activities that compete with their already strong drive to breathe. Most healthy people have no idea that they hold their breath when they swallow. But, for people with severe COPD, it's quite a different story. Eating may be an unpleasant chore because the swallowing associated with it may lead to "air hunger." Do everything you can to avoid COPD and your life will be happier. Have you quit smoking yet?

NEURAL CONTROL OF SWALLOWING

The neural control of swallowing is complex and not completely understood. Nevertheless, studies of humans and animals have offered important insights into how swallowing is controlled by the nervous system. Some of the salient features of that control are discussed below as they relate to peripheral nervous system and central nervous system participation.

Role of the Peripheral Nervous System in Swallowing

Nearly all the structures involved in swallowing are the same as those involved in speech production (the most notable exceptions being the esophagus and stomach). Those structures that participate in both swallowing and speech production are innervated by the spinal nerves and cranial nerves described in Chapters 2 through 6 and summarized in Table 13–1. As can

Table 13-1. Summary of Motor and Sensory Nerve Supply to the Breathing Apparatus, Laryngeal Apparatus, Velopharyngeal-Nasal Apparatus, and Pharyngeal-Oral Apparatus

APPARATUS	INNERVATION	
	MOTOR	SENSORY
Breathing	C1–C8, T1–T12, L1–L2	C1–C8, T1–T12, L1–L2
Laryngeal*	V, VII, X, XI, XII, C1–C3	X**
Velopharyngeal-Nasal	V, VII, Pharyngeal plexus***	V, VII, X
Pharyngeal-Oral	V, VII, XII, Pharyngeal plexus	V, VII, X

*Includes intrinsic, extrinsic, and supplementary laryngeal muscles.

**Sensory innervation of extrinsic and supplementary laryngeal muscles includes other cranial nerves, such as V and VII.

***The pharyngeal plexus is a network that includes cranial nerves IX, X, and possibly XI.

Note: Spinal nerves are designated by their segmental origins (C = cervical, T = thoracic, L = lumbar). Cranial nerves are V (trigeminal), VII (facial), IX (glossopharyngeal), X (vagus), XI (accessory), and XII (hypoglossal).

be seen in the table, half of the cranial nerves (6 of 12) and most of the spinal nerves (22 of 31) are potential participants in swallowing (and speech production). The cranial nerves are involved in swallowing through their innervation of the lips, mandible, tongue, velum, pharynx, and larynx, whereas the spinal nerves are primarily involved in breathing and its cessation as they relate to swallowing.

Peripheral innervation of the esophagus differs along its length. The upper (cervical) region is made up of striated muscle, the type of muscle found in other structures of the swallowing apparatus (lips, mandible, tongue, velum, pharynx, and larynx). The cervical region, which includes the upper esophageal sphincter, is innervated by the recurrent branch of the vagus nerve (cranial nerve X), the same branch that innervates most of the intrinsic muscles of the larynx. Thus, the same peripheral nerve is responsible for the simultaneous actions of closing the larynx and opening the upper esophageal sphincter. This means that there is a strong neural link between actions that serve to protect the airway and actions that allow substances to pass into the esophagus. This strong link has obvious advantages for the coordination of the normal swallow, but also has the disadvantage that damage to the recurrent branch of the vagus nerve can have serious consequences for both voice production and swallowing (Corbin-Lewis, Liss, & Sciortino, 2005).

In lower regions of the esophagus, where smooth muscle intermingles with striated muscle (thoracic esophagus) and where smooth muscle is the only type of muscle present (abdominal esophagus), a different form of neural control operates. This control comes from the autonomic nervous system, which is generally considered to be under automatic (as opposed to voluntary) control. The autonomic nervous system has two parts, the parasympathetic and sympathetic subdivisions. The parasympathetic subdivision is important for maintaining gastrointestinal motility so that a swallowed substance moves through the esophagus easily and quickly. In contrast, the sympathetic subdivision, best known for its importance in fight-or-flight responses to stressful situations, tends to inhibit gastrointestinal motility. This is one reason why gastrointestinal problems are associated with physical and emotional stress. Many of the nerve fibers of the autonomic nervous system travel with the vagus nerve.

Role of the Central Nervous System in Swallowing

Although swallowing and speech production are executed using many of the same peripheral nerves, the central nervous system control of these two activities is quite different. This means that a given structure, such as the tongue, is under one form of neural control during swallowing and under another form of neural control during speech production (see Chapter 6). Because of this, it is entirely possible to have central nervous system damage that impairs the function of a structure for speech production but not swallowing, and vice versa.

There are two major regions within the central nervous system that are responsible for the control of swallowing. One is in the brainstem and the other is in cortical and subcortical areas. The brainstem center is located primarily in the medulla, the structure that is contiguous with the uppermost part of the spinal cord. There are two main groups of brainstem neurons that participate in swallowing, one that appears to be primarily responsible for triggering the swallow and shaping its temporal pattern and another group that appears to allocate neural drive to the various motor nerves that participate in swallowing (Jean, 2001). The brainstem center has primary control over the more automatic phases of swallowing (pharyngeal and esophageal phases).

There are also cortical and subcortical regions that may contribute to the generation and shaping of swallowing behaviors. Cortical areas include the primary motor cortex, premotor cortex, and primary sensory cortex, among others, and subcortical areas include the insular cortex and the anterior ingulated cortex, with probable contributions from basal ganglia, thalamus, and cerebellum, among others (Humbert & Robbins, 2007). Activity from these areas has a strong influence over the control and modulation of the more voluntary phases of swallowing (oral preparatory phase, including mastication, and oral transport phase). However, studies of people with cortical damage from strokes indicate that the cortex may also exert influence over what have traditionally been thought of as the automatic phases (pharyngeal and esophageal phases) of swallowing (Martin & Sessle, 1993).

Afferent input is critical to the generation of a normal swallow. The sources of afferent input are numerous and include, but are not limited to, information related to: (a) muscle length and rate of length change, (b) muscle tension, (c) joint position and movement, (d) surface and deep pressures, (e) surface deformation, (f) temperature, (g) taste, and (h) noxious stimuli. Afferent activity is generated by receptors in the swallowing apparatus and sent to the brainstem, where such activity may trigger the motor output required to elicit the pharyngeal phase of the swallow or it may modulate the motor output to accommodate a larger-than-expected bolus. Afferent activity may also be sent on to subcortical regions (such as the thalamus) or cortical regions (such as the sensorimotor cortex) where it may be consciously perceived. Often the perception is a pleasant experience, such as savoring the flavor and texture of ice cream, or it may be unpleasant (see Figure 13–11 and sidetrack on Sphenopalatineganglioneuralgia).

Sphenopalatineganglioneuralgia

Boy, that sounds like something you wouldn't want to meet in the dark. But it comes from something really good. As a child (or even as an adult) you may have said the phrase, "I scream, you scream, we all scream for ice cream." Scream has a meaning of anticipation in this context, but it can also have a meaning of hurting. You know the feeling. You take a bite of ice cream and momentarily hold it against the roof of your mouth before you swallow it. Then suddenly you get an intense, stabbing pain in your forehead. What's up? The pain is caused as your hard palate warms up after you made it cold. Cold causes vasoconstriction (reduction in blood vessel diameter) in the region, which is followed by rapid vasodilation (increase in blood vessel diameter). It's the rapid vasodilation that hurts and gets your attention. The technical term for this pain is "sphenopalatineganglioneuralgia." The common term (and the one more easily pronounced) is "brain freeze." Fortunately, the pain lasts only a few seconds. Be thankful. There's all that ice cream still waiting to be eaten.

VARIABLES THAT INFLUENCE SWALLOWING

A number of variables influence swallowing. Some relate to the characteristics of the bolus, the swallowing mode, and the prevailing body position. There are also developmental and aging effects on swallowing, but essentially no influence of sex.

Bolus Characteristics and Swallowing

Although the act of swallowing occurs generally as described near the beginning of this chapter, the precise nature of the swallow is determined, in part, by what exactly is being swallowed. Bolus consistency, volume, and taste are three variables that have been found to influence the act of swallowing.

Consistency

One of the most important consistency contrasts that determines swallowing behavior is the difference between liquids and solids. Whereas a liquid bolus is usually held briefly in the front of the oral cavity before being propelled to the pharynx, a chewed solid bolus may be moved to the pharynx and left there for several seconds while the remainder of the bolus continues to be chewed (Hiiemae & Palmer, 1999; Palmer, Rudin, Lara, & Crompton, 1992; see Figure 13–9). Although this can also happen with liquids (Linden, Tippett, Johnston, Siebens, & French, 1989), it is much less common, except in cases where a combined liquid-and-solid bolus is chewed and swallowed (Saitoh et al.,

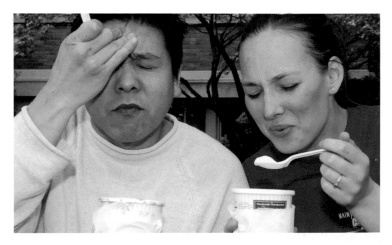

Figure 13–11. Sphenopalatineganglioneuralgia (or so-called "brain freeze") caused by placing something cold against the roof of the mouth. Image provided courtesy of the University of Cincinnati. Reproduced with permission.

2007), such as what might occur during mealtime eating (Dua et al., 1997).

Substances can be characterized on a viscosity continuum, ranging from substances as thin as water to substances as thick as pudding. Such differences in viscosity have been shown to influence swallowing; specifically, higher viscosity (thicker) substances (thick liquids or puree consistencies) tend to take longer to swallow than lower viscosity (thinner) substances (Chi-Fishman & Sonies, 2002; Im, Kim, Oommen, Kim, & Ko, 2012). This slowing is due to longer oral and pharyngeal phase events and longer upper esophageal sphincter opening durations (Dantas et al., 1990; Im et al., 2012). The swallowing of higher viscosity substances is also associated with larger tongue forces than the swallowing of lower viscosity substances (Chi-Fishman & Sonies, 2002; Miller & Watkin, 1996; Steele & van Lieshout, 2004). As might be predicted, it is more difficult to maintain a cohesive (single) bolus when swallowing thinner liquids as compared to thicker liquids. As a result, laryngeal penetration (where part of the bolus moves into the laryngeal vestibule, but remains above the vocal folds; Robbins, Hamilton, Lof, & Kempster, 1992) is more common when swallowing thin liquids than when swallowing thicker substances (Daggett, Logemann, Rademaker, & Pauloski, 2006).

It is also relevant to mention that swallowing occurs regularly throughout the day and night without the introduction of an external substance. These are called nonbolus swallows, dry swallows, or saliva swallows and they constitute the swallowing of saliva. These swallows are sometimes stimulated by pooling of saliva in the pharynx and can be initiated in the absence of oral preparatory and oral transport phases (Logemann, 1998).

Volume

It seems intuitive that the volume (size) of the bolus might affect the swallow and most studies indicate that, in fact, it does (Chi-Fishman & Sonies, 2002; Cook et al., 1989; Kahrilas & Logemann, 1993; Logemann et al., 2000; Logemann, Pauloski, Rademaker, & Kahrilas, 2002; Perlman, Palmer, McCullough, & VanDaele, 1999; Perlman, Schultz, & VanDaele, 1993; Tasko, Kent, & Westbury, 2002). When swallowing a larger bolus compared to swallowing a smaller bolus, tongue movements are generally larger and faster, hyoid bone movements begin earlier and are larger, pharyngeal wall movements and laryngeal movements are more extensive, and the upper esophageal sphincter opens earlier and stays open longer (Kahrilas & Logemann,

1993). This means that events related to tongue propulsion of the bolus, closing of the velopharynx, protection of the pulmonary airways, and opening of the upper esophageal sphincter are conditioned by bolus volume in ways that are more sustained and more vigorous for larger boluses than smaller boluses. Whether or not apnea is longer during the swallowing of larger (versus smaller) boluses has yet to be convincingly determined (Martin-Harris, 2006).

Despite the success of the adjustments made to accommodate a larger bolus, there tends to be a greater frequency of laryngeal penetration as bolus size increases, at least for liquid boluses. Specifically, part of the bolus penetrates the laryngeal vestibule more than twice as often when swallowing a 10-mL bolus than when swallowing a 1-mL bolus (Daggett et al., 2006). Nevertheless, when laryngeal penetration occurs in healthy individuals, the substance is almost always pushed away from the larynx and transported to the esophagus without being aspirated (going below the vocal folds).

Taste and Temperature

Taste and temperature contribute enormously to the enjoyment of the eating and drinking experience. Imagine, for a moment, eating a hot fudge sundae and how much of the pleasurable eating experience is derived from the special combination of vanilla and chocolate flavors and hot and cold temperatures.

Tastes include sweet, salty, sour, bitter, and other tastes (such as umami, meaning meaty or savory). Substances of different tastes (but of the same consistency and volume) may influence certain features of swallowing. For example, substances with taste (sweet, salty, sour), when compared to tasteless substances, are generally associated with higher peak tongue pressures (Pelletier & Dhanaraj, 2006) and faster and greater activation of selected swallow-related muscle regions (Ding, Logemann, Larson, & Rademaker, 2003). Sour tastes, in particular, appear to elicit more effortful swallows (greater amplitude muscle activity) than other tastes (Leow, Huckabee, Sharma, & Tooley, 2007; Palmer, McCulloch, Jaffe, & Neel, 2005). These behavioral effects of taste are associated with taste-related differences in brain function. For example, the ingestion of tasty liquids stimulates significantly more activity in certain cortical regions when compared to unflavored water (Babael et al., 2010). It should also be recognized that different tastes are accompanied by their associated smells, so that both the gustatory (taste) and olfactory (smell) senses are nearly always stimulated simultaneously.

Gutsy Stuff

Taste receptors in the tongue get all the press and all the credit for making things taste sweet—unsurprising, given that there are about 10,000 of them. Put a little sugar or artificial sweetener in your mouth and the taste receptors in your tongue will come to attention and tell your brain about it. But the taste of sweetness is not just limited to your mouth. Receptors that sense sugar and artificial sweetener have also been found in the gut (Margolskee et al., 2007). These gut receptors taste glucose in the same way that taste cells in your tongue signal sweetness to the brain. They've been found to influence the secretion of insulin and hormones that regulate blood sugar level and influence appetite. Those are two very important responsibilities. This is all very gutsy stuff and is touted by its discoverers as possibly leading to new treatment options for obesity and diabetes. Let's hope they're right.

The evidence that temperature affects normal swallowing is limited and contradictory. One study showed that a cold bolus delayed pharyngeal and laryngeal movements compared to a room-temperature bolus (Bisch, Logemann, Rademaker, Kahrilas, & Lazarus, 1994), and another study showed that a warm bolus reduced the level of suprahyoid muscle activation and the perception of "swallowing difficulty" compared to cooler boluses (Miyaoka et al., 2006). Other studies have shown no effects of temperature on swallowing.

Swallowing Mode

Much of the research on swallowing has focused on single swallows that were either cued ("Swallow now") or in which the bolus was introduced directly into the oral cavity with a syringe. Clearly, this is not how swallowing usually occurs in most situations. As the research base expands, there is growing evidence that sequential swallows differ from single swallows and that spontaneously initiated swallows differ from those that are elicited with an external cue, including the cue to swallow with greater-than-usual effort.

Single Versus Sequential Swallows

During eating and drinking, there are times when a swallow occurs in isolation. There are also times when swallows occur sequentially, one immediately after the other.

A swallow is characterized by the same major events whether produced singly or as part of a sequence—that is, the bolus is pushed back by the tongue, the velopharynx closes, the hyoid bone and larynx rise and close off the airway, the bolus is moved through the pharynx, and the upper esophageal sphincter opens to admit the bolus into the esophagus. Nevertheless, there are some subtle, yet important, differences between single swallows and sequential swallows that involve the relative timing of certain events and the nature of certain movements.

Although during both single and sequential swallows the tongue moves upward to the palate (front to back) to push the bolus backward, certain aspects of the movements differ under the two conditions (Chi-Fishman, Stone, & McCall, 1998). To begin, overall movement time is shorter during sequential swallows compared to single swallows, which may be accounted for by shorter contact times, faster movements, shorter movement distances, or some combination of these. Another special feature of sequential swallows is that certain movements that usually follow one another during a single swallow, such as tongue tip lowering and tongue body elevation, may occur simultaneously.

During a single swallow the hyolaryngeal complex rises and then falls back to its original (resting) position. In contrast, during sequential swallows, most studies have shown that the hyolaryngeal complex rises for the first swallow then falls, but only part way toward the resting position, before rising again for the next swallow (Chi-Fishman & Sonies, 2000; Daniels et al., 2004; Daniels & Foundas, 2001). The velum rises and falls in synchrony with the hyolaryngeal complex during sequential swallowing (Chi-Fishman & Sonies, 2000). The epiglottis either moves in synchrony with the hyolaryngeal complex or it remains down over the laryngeal airway throughout swallow cycles with the hyolaryngeal complex maintained in a partially elevated position (Daniels et al., 2004).

During sequential swallowing, successive boluses often merge in the epiglottic valleculae before the pharyngeal phase is triggered (Dua et al., 1997; Hiiemae & Palmer, 1999). When this happens, the airway tends to stay closed for liquid substances, but not for solid substances (Chi-Fishman & Sonies, 2000). Unsurprisingly, laryngeal penetration is more common during sequential swallows than for single swallows, but in healthy individuals, the penetrated substance is almost always cleared on the next swallow. As is the case with single swallows, the swallow apnea associated with sequential swallows is usually followed by expiration;

nevertheless, it is more common for inspiration to follow the apneic interval during sequential swallows than during single swallows (Lederle et al., 2012; Preiksaitis & Mills, 1996).

Esophageal behavior is also different for sequential versus single swallows. For example, during sequential drinking of water, the pressure associated with esophageal peristalsis is lower and the frequency of peristalsis is lower than during single swallows (Meyer, Gerhardt, & Castell, 1981).

Cued Versus Uncued Swallows

The majority of swallowing studies, including those performed for both research and clinical purposes, have been conducted using external cues to swallow (Daniels, Schroeder, DeGeorge, Corey, & Rosenbek, 2007). These are usually verbal cues ("Swallow now"), but they can also be visual or tactile cues. In contrast, the swallowing associated with eating and drinking in daily life is seldom accompanied by such cuing (unless you are a child whose caregiver is saying "Hurry up and drink your milk"). So, the question arises as to whether or not cuing alters the swallow. A study that addressed this question directly (Daniels et al., 2007) showed that under a cued condition, the substance (a single liquid bolus) is loaded into the anterior oral cavity and then moved somewhat back and held between the midline of the tongue and the hard palate in preparation for the cue. In contrast, in the noncued condition, the bolus is not held in position, but instead is moved immediately out of the anterior oral cavity as soon as loading is complete. This affects the values of timing measures associated with each of the phases of swallowing and has implications for how certain measures are obtained, but does not substantially alter the swallow otherwise.

Another form of cuing involves having a person voluntarily change the nature of the swallow. For example, an instruction such as, "Squeeze hard when you swallow" tends to elicit higher tongue and/or pharyngeal pressures (depending, in part, on the precise wording of the instruction) and greater muscle activation levels compared to swallows produced with usual effort (Steele & Huckabee, 2007; Wheeler-Hegland, Rosenbek, & Sapienza, 2008; Yeates, Steele, & Pelletier, 2010). Interestingly, effortful swallow maneuvers also appear to increase amplitudes of peristaltic pressure waves in regions of the esophagus containing smooth muscle, especially the region near the lower esophageal sphincter (Lever et al., 2007). Effortful swallow maneuvers, and other forms of conscious maneuvers, are often used as behavioral strategies to help clients with swallowing disorders (Leonard, Kendall, McKenzie, & Goodrich, 2008; Logemann, 1998).

Body Position and Swallowing

Certain details of swallowing change with body position. For example, whether in an upright body position or on "all fours" (on hands and knees, facing terra firma), swallowing usually occurs during the expiratory phase of the breathing cycle (McFarland, Lund, & Gagner, 1994). Nevertheless, there can be subtle changes in the onset time of the swallow within the expiratory phase. In an upright body position, the swallow usually occurs late in the expiratory phase, whereas when on "all fours," the swallow is more apt to occur earlier in the expiratory phase. It is unclear why this happens, but it may be related to the pull of gravity on the abdominal content, which, in turn, is transmitted to the larynx via its mechanical connections through the diaphragm and pulmonary apparatus (McFarland et al., 1994). As another example, a liquid bolus tends to arrive in the pharynx earlier during swallows produced in an upright body position than during swallows produced in a facedown position (Saitoh et al., 2007). This position-related timing difference does not appear to occur when swallowing a solid bolus (Palmer, 1998; Saitoh et al., 2007).

There are also differences between swallows produced in the supine body position versus those produced in upright body positions. For example, in a supine body position (compared to an upright body position): (a) the hyoid bone moves a greater distance anteriorly, the velum moves a smaller distance posteriorly, and the pharyngeal transport phase of the swallow is longer (Perry, Bae, & Kuehn, 2012), (b) pharyngeal pressure is more positive (Dejaeger, Pelemans, Ponette, & VanTrappen, 1994; Johnson, Shaw, Gabb, Dent, & Cook, 1995), (c) the upper esophageal sphincter pressure reaches its nadir (most subatmospheric pressure) slightly earlier (Castell, Dalton, & Castell, 1990), (d) the bolus flow through the upper esophageal sphincter is faster (Johnson et al., 1995), (e) peristaltic waves in the esophagus (particularly in its distal region) are slower and stronger, and (f) the pressure in the lower esophageal sphincter is higher (Sears, Castell, & Castell, 1990). It is not clear whether the timing of pharyngeal events is influenced by body position or not (Castell et al., 1990; Ingervall & Lantz, 1973; Johnson et al., 1995). The timing of sensory and motor events related to vocal fold activation before, during, and after the swallow appears to be unaffected by a change from upright to supine (Barkmeier, Bielamowicz, Takeda, & Ludlow, 2002).

Sword Throats

Sword swallowing is an ancient art that continues to be practiced. There is even a Sword Swallowers' Association International based in Antioch, Tennessee. The practice and ill effects of sword swallowing were discussed in an article in the prestigious *British Medical Journal* (Witcombe & Meyer, 2006). Major complications from sword swallowing are more likely when the swallower is distracted or swallows unusual swords. Sequelae can include perforation of the pharynx or esophagus, gastrointestinal bleeding, pneumothorax (collapsed lung), and chest pain (all of this is little wonder, we think). Novice sword swallowers must learn to desensitize the gag reflex, align the upper esophageal sphincter with the neck hyperextended, open the upper esophageal sphincter, and control retching as the blade is moved on toward the cardia. All in all it doesn't sound like fun to us. It also makes for a very long bolus.

Development and Swallowing

Infancy and childhood are times of significant anatomical and physiological development. Many of these developmental changes have been described in previous chapters (see sections on Development in Chapters 2, 3, 4, and 5). The focus here is on those that pertain to the development of swallowing.

There are many important anatomical changes that influence swallowing during the period from infancy through childhood. Some of these include the following (Arvedson & Brodsky, 2002): (a) the infant's tongue goes from nearly filling the oral cavity to filling only the floor of the oral cavity due to differential growth of oral structures; (b) the infant's oral cavity goes from being edentulous to having a full set of deciduous teeth; (c) the cheeks of the infant have fatty pads (sometimes called sucking pads) that eventually disappear to be replaced with muscle; (d) the infant goes from having essentially no oropharynx to having a distinct one as the larynx descends; and (e) the infant's larynx goes from being one-third adult size, with relatively large arytenoid cartilages and a high position within the neck, to the adult configuration and position. It is interesting to note that, although anatomical changes influence swallowing, the opposite is also true. That

is, because the forces exerted during swallowing and chewing are quite large, they have a profound influence on molding the oral and pharyngeal anatomy of the infant and young child.

Swallowing (of amniotic fluid) begins well before birth, as early as 12.5 weeks gestation (Humphrey, 1970). Interestingly, although many of the components of swallow are in place before birth, velopharyngeal closure during swallowing is not (Miller, Sonies, & Macedonia, 2003). Perhaps this is because the entire digestive tract is infused with amniotic fluid so that there is little consequence of having an open velopharynx (the amniotic fluid would infuse the nasal passages whether the velopharynx is open or closed). Immediately after birth, the velopharynx closes during swallowing and the infant exhibits a suckling pattern characterized by forward and backward (horizontal) movements of the tongue (Bosma, 1986; Bosma, Truby, & Lind, 1965). These tongue movements are accompanied by large vertical movements of the mandible and serve to draw liquid into the oral cavity. Around the age of 6 months, this suckling pattern converts to a sucking pattern, which is characterized by raising and lowering (vertical) movements of the tongue, firm approximation of the lips, and less pronounced vertical movements of the mandible. Sucking is stronger than suckling and allows the infant to pull in thicker substances, by creating a subatmospheric pressure within the oral cavity, and to begin the ingestion of soft food (Arvedson & Brodsky, 2002).

During the first few months of life, the infant relies on breast feeding (or nipple feeding from a bottle) for all nutritional intake. This form of feeding consists of suck-swallow or suck-swallow-breathe sequences, typically repeated several times (8 to 12 times) and followed by a rest period (several seconds). It was once thought that infants swallow and breathe at the same time, however, they do not. Although infants can continue breathing during the suck, they (like adults) stop breathing during the swallow (Wilson, Thach, Brouillette, & Abu-Osba, 1981), and their ventilation decreases as a result (Koenig, Davies, & Thach, 1990). During this period, several oral reflexes are active that aid in early feeding. These disappear around 6 months of age, with the exception of the gag reflex, which remains active throughout childhood and adulthood.

By about 6 months of age, infants are ready to begin eating solid foods with a spoon. Foods such as crackers and soft fruits and vegetables are introduced during the next few months. The basic patterns for chewing are in place by 9 months and continue to develop over the next few years of life (Green et al., 1997; Steeve, Moore, Green, Reilly, & Ruark McMurtrey,

2008). By 2 to 3 years of age, the child is able to eat regular table food.

Positive interactions between the infant and caregiver during periods of feeding are critical to development (Arvedson & Brodsky, 2002; Pitcher, Crandall, & Goodrich, 2008) and are associated with physical and emotional pleasure that can lead to healthy bonding and communication. As an infant grows, mealtimes should continue to be pleasurable experiences that provide needed nutrition and, when shared with others, also provide social stimulation.

Age and Swallowing

As with most physiological functions, swallowing changes with age across adulthood. The most robust age-related change is that swallowing becomes slower, particularly after age 60 years (Leonard & McKenzie, 2006; Logemann et al., 2002; Robbins et al., 1992; Sonies, Parent, Morrish, & Baum, 1988). Certain individual components of the swallow also tend to be delayed in older compared to younger adults. For example, the trigger for the pharyngeal transport phase is located closer to the esophagus in older adults (Robbins et al., 1992; Tracy et al., 1989) than in younger adults (Logemann, 1998). Also, it takes longer for the bolus to move through the pharynx and for the upper esophageal sphincter to open in older adults (Logemann et al., 2002; Mendell & Logemann, 2007; Robbins et al., 1992). The apneic interval during the swallow is generally longer in older adults than younger adults (Hirst, Ford, Gibson & Wilson, 2002), and the offset of the apneic interval occurs later (Martin-Harris et al., 2005a). Tongue movements are slower in older than younger adults (Steele & van Lieshout, 2009), though tongue pressures do not seem to change with age (Youmans, Youmans, & Stierwalt, 2009). Durational differences have also been associated with multiple movements of the tongue (rather than the single movement expected), more commonly seen in older adults than younger adults (Sonies et al., 1988).

An outcome of the age-related slowing of the swallow (combined with age-related reductions in sensory function; for example, see Malandraki, Perlman, Karampinos, & Sutton, 2011) is that the frequency of laryngeal penetration increases with age (Daniels et al., 2004; Robbins et al., 1992). Laryngeal penetration occurs in people over 50 years about twice as often as it occurs in adults under 50 years, and more frequently when swallowing liquids than when swallowing solids (Daggett et al., 2006). Although this appears to be a dangerous situation and a possible precursor to aspira-

tion, in healthy individuals the substance is moved out of the vestibule to be rejoined with the rest of the bolus (Daggett et al., 2006). Nevertheless, the risk of aspiration may be higher in senescent adults, compared to younger adults, because of their greater tendency to inspire immediately after swallowing (Martin-Harris et al., 2005a).

Sex and Swallowing

Several studies of swallowing have included participants of both sexes and some of these have revealed statistically significant differences in selected measures. Nevertheless, there do not appear to be consistent findings across studies that would lead to the conclusion that swallowing is different in men and women. Sex-related differences that have been reported are likely to be attributable to chance (such as that related to participant selection or statistical chance) or to variables other than sex (such as size and strength). Thus, given the current knowledge base, it seems safe to conclude that swallowing does not differ between the sexes in any consistent or important way and does not need to be taken into account in clinical endeavors.

MEASUREMENT OF SWALLOWING

Measurement of swallowing is not only critical to research endeavors, but has also become essential to clinical practice. Instrumental measurement of swallowing is especially important when considering that as many as half of the clients who aspirate do so "silently" (that is, without any signs of coughing or other signs of visible or audible struggle) (Logemann, 1998). In such cases, aspiration can only be detected through instrumental examination.

There are many instrumental approaches to measuring swallowing. Four of them are highlighted here —videofluoroscopy, endoscopy, ultrasonography, and manometry—because they have proven useful for both research and clinical applications and have direct relevance to the practice of speech-language pathology.

Videofluoroscopy

Videofluoroscopy, as applied to swallowing, involves the use of x-rays to image the swallowing apparatus while the person swallows substances mixed with barium sulfate. The barium is a contrast material that allows the bolus to be tracked visually as it travels through the oral, pharyngeal, and esophageal regions. The videofluoroscopic swallow study, often called a modified barium swallow (MBS) study, was first described by Logemann, Boshes, Blonsky, and Fisher (1977). The adjective "modified" is used to differentiate this study from a barium swallow study, which is conducted by a gastroenterologist to evaluate esophageal structure and function. This reflects one of the differences in scope of practice between the speech-language pathologist and gastroenterologist relative to evaluation and management of swallowing disorders (see section below on Clinical Professionals and Swallowing Disorders). Although the speech-language pathologist can screen for esophageal disorders, it is the gastroenterologist who diagnoses and treats those disorders.

A videofluoroscopic swallowing examination is usually conducted with the person seated in a specially designed chair. The examination is performed in a radiology laboratory, with a radiologist (or radiology technician) running the x-ray equipment and a speech-language pathologist directing the swallowing protocol. The examination protocol typically consists of the swallowing of a series of solid and liquid substances (mixed with barium or accompanied by ingestion of a barium capsule to provide contrast) that vary in volume and consistency. For example, the protocol might include the swallowing of thin liquid, nectar, and pudding in small and large servings and the chewing and swallowing of a cookie or cracker. The drinking of the thin liquid might be from a spoon, cup, straw, or a combination of these. The exact protocol depends on the nature of the research question or the nature of the client's swallowing complaint.

Figure 13–12 contains an example of a videofluoroscopic image of a healthy individual during the oral preparatory phase of swallowing. Although only one still frame is displayed there, the actual image is a moving image that can be viewed in real time, recorded, and played back at normal speed, slow speed, or even frame by frame. Images can be obtained using a lateral view (as in Figure 13–12) and a frontal view (not shown). Each view offers different advantages for capturing certain swallowing events.

A variety of temporal and spatial measurements can be made from the videofluoroscopic images. Temporal measurements are generally in the form of objective values. For example, measurements may be made of the time from the beginning of bolus movement from the oral cavity to its arrival at the upper esophageal sphincter or the time it takes the hyoid bone to reach its maximum upward excursion. Spatial measurements may be in the form of objective values, or they may

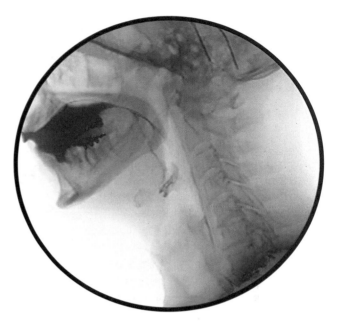

Figure 13–12. Videoflurosocopic image showing the oral preparatory phase of a swallow. From "Dynamic swallow studies: Measurement techniques," by R. Leonard and S. McKenzie in *Dysphagia assessment and treatment planning: A team approach* (2nd ed., p. 273). Edited by R. Leonard and K. Kendall, 2008, San Diego, CA: Plural Publishing, Inc. Copyright 2008 by Plural Publishing, Inc. Modified and reproduced with permission.

be in the form of judgments or ratings. For example, ratings may be made of the extent of velar elevation (on a scale of none to fully elevated) or extent of hyoid bone excursion (on a scale of none to normal). One of the most popular assessment tools, the Penetration-Aspiration Scale (Rosenbek, Robbins, Roecker, Coyle, & Wood, 1996), is an 8-point categorical rating scale that provides a description of events that indicate laryngeal penetration or aspiration (ranging from "Material does not enter the airway" to "Material enters the airway, passes below the vocal folds, and no effort is made to eject").

It is generally agreed that videofluoroscopy provides the most comprehensive evaluation of swallowing, and for many it is considered the "gold standard" of measurement. It has several advantages over other measurement approaches, including the following: (a) it provides relatively clear views of nearly all the important structures involved in swallowing and their movements, with the exception of the vocal folds; (b) it is possible to visualize barium-laced substances through the oral preparatory, oral transport, pharyngeal transport, and esophageal transport phases; (c) it is possible to view swallowing events from at least two

Chicken Dinner

Cancer had taken his tongue. He had no teeth. And signs of a stroke were on his face. His speech was remarkably good and arrangements were made to travel out of state with him to use special x-ray equipment that could reveal his compensations. The trip was by car and went well until a snowstorm forced an overnight stay. Dinner was instructive. To propel food toward his pharynx, he threw his head back in the way a chicken tosses its head when eating. Having no teeth helped him drink because he could touch his mandible to his maxilla and create a downward and backward sloping floor to his mouth. He poured liquids down this slope. When motion picture x-rays from his study were developed, they were enlightening. When he swallowed water, his epiglottis stood fully erect, as if at military attention, while liquid cascaded around it. He apparently hadn't read textbooks telling him how the epiglottis is always forced down over the larynx during swallowing.

different perspectives (lateral and frontal); and (d) it is possible to identify penetration and aspiration events. The major disadvantages of videofluoroscopy are that it requires exposure to radiation, it must be coordinated with radiology, and it cannot be conducted at bedside.

Endoscopy

Another way to visualize swallowing is with endoscopy. First described by Langmore, Schatz, and Olson (1988), this approach requires the use of a flexible fiberoptic endoscope, like the one used for visualizing the larynx and velopharynx (see Chapters 3 and 4). To view the swallowing apparatus, the endoscope is inserted through one of the nares (following the administration of topical anesthesia, if necessary), routed through the velopharyngeal port, and guided until its tip is positioned in the laryngopharynx. This approach has come to be known by the name of Flexible Endoscopic Evaluation of Swallowing (FEES). A FEES station is shown in Figure 13–13 (also see the lower part of Figure 3–50 in Chapter 3 which shows nasal insertion of a flexible endoscope).

The examination usually includes a preliminary viewing the velopharyngeal region, pharyngeal walls,

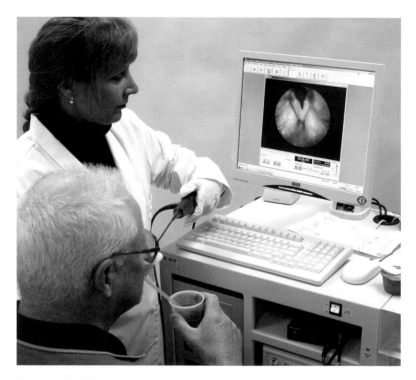

Figure 13–13. Fiberoptic endoscope used for evaluation of swallowing. Image provided courtesy of KayPENTAX, Montvale, NJ. Reproduced with permission.

back part of the tongue, epiglottis, aryepiglottic folds, epiglottic valleculae, pyriform sinuses, laryngeal vestibule, ventricular folds, vocal folds, and the inlet to the esophagus. Abnormalities in structure or color are noted and are used to help interpret abnormal swallow behaviors. Swallowing is evaluated in much the same way as for a videoflurosopic examination, by using solid and liquid substances of different consistencies and volumes (the major difference being that no barium is required). Descriptions provided by the speech-language pathologist might include the presence of substance remaining in the epiglottic valleculae or pyriform sinuses following the pharyngeal transport phase of swallowing, whether or not substance invaded the laryngeal vestibule (laryngeal penetration), and whether or not there is evidence that substance traveled below the vocal folds (aspiration).

Endoscopy offers certain advantages over other approaches to evaluating swallowing. To begin, the equipment is easily portable so that the examination can be done at bedside in a hospital, there is no exposure to x-rays and no need to use barium products, and it is possible to see structural and color abnormalities. In addition, the procedure can often be performed by a speech-language pathologist without the direct oversight of a physician or the aid of other health care professionals. Finally, the speech-language pathologist can observe the client eat an entire meal at the client's usual pace.

The major disadvantage of an endoscopic approach is that, during the pharyngeal transport phase of the swallow, there is a moment when the endoscopic view is blocked as the tongue and pharynx approximate. Also, there are some clients who cannot tolerate the procedure, including those with structural abnormalities such as a deviated nasal septum, hyperkinetic movement disorders, bleeding disorders, and certain cardiac conditions. Furthermore, it is sometimes difficult to detect penetration and aspiration with endoscopy. Nevertheless, one way to improve such detection is to infuse the swallowed substance with green dye. In this way, the endoscope can be directed into the laryngeal vestibule immediately following the swallow to look for any green substance that may have been deposited near or below the vocal folds.

When FEES is accompanied by sensory testing, it is called flexible Endoscopic Evaluation of Swallowing with Sensory Testing (FEESST) (Aviv et al., 1998). Sensory testing involves the delivery of brief air pressure pulses through the endoscope to the anterior wall of the pyriform sinus or the aryepiglottic folds, regions innervated by the superior laryngeal nerve (a sensory branch of cranial nerve X, vagus). In a healthy person,

this air pressure pulse elicits the laryngeal adductor reflex, a brainstem-mediated reflex that results in adduction of the vocal folds. This reflex is an important mechanism for protecting the lower airways from aspiration.

Ultrasonography

Another way to visualize swallowing events is with ultrasonography. The use of ultrasonography as it applies to the measurement of speech production is discussed in Chapter 5, and similar procedures can be applied to the measurement of swallowing. Briefly, ultrasonography requires the use of a transducer that generates and receives a high-frequency signal (sound waves). The transducer is pressed against the skin (usually on the undersurface of the mandible) and the signal is transmitted through the tissue toward the airway. When the signal encounters air, it reflects back. The receiver senses the returning sound waves and the resultant signal is processed to provide an image of the outline of the proximal border of the airway.

Ultrasonography is applied to the measurement of swallowing much less frequently than are videofluoroscopy and flexible endoscopy. Nevertheless, it can offer some valuable information especially in relation to the behavior of the tongue (Stone & Shawker, 1986), lateral pharyngeal walls (Miller & Watkin, 1997), and other structures by way of images obtained in sagittal, frontal, and transverse planes. It may also be a useful biofeedback tool in the management of oral preparatory phase behavior (Shawker & Sonies, 1985). Its major limitation is that aspiration cannot be detected.

Manometry

Manometry refers to the measurement of pressure. In the context of swallowing, two types of manometric measurement approaches are of interest. One allows for measurement of pressure in the pharyngeal and upper esophageal sphincter regions and one allows inferences to be made regarding the temporal relationship between swallowing events and breathing events.

Technological advances have made manometric measurements of pharyngeal and upper esophageal sphincter events more accurate and have, therefore, made valuable additions to understanding swallowing events related to normal and disordered swallow. A high-resolution manometric device comprises approximately three dozen miniature pressure sensors positioned in the pharynx and upper esophageal sphincter (or all of them positioned in the esophagus).

The output signals can provide information about the magnitude of the pressures generated during the pharyngeal propulsive wave, the squeezing pressures exerted within the upper esophageal sphincter, and the magnitude of relaxation (pressure drop) of the upper esophageal sphincter during the passage of the bolus. Concurrent videofluoroscopic imaging can be used with manometry for more accurate interpretation of the pressure signals (Hila et al., 2001; Logemann, 1998). Although manometric measurements can be used to assess pharyngeal function as well tongue function, they are most often used to evaluate esophageal function. This form of manometry is conducted under the direction of a gastroenterologist (see section below on Clinical Professionals and Swallowing Disorders) and is typically accompanied by simultaneous videofluoroscopic imaging of the esophagus (barium swallow study).

A different type of pressure measurement can be used to determine the relationship between swallowing and breathing. This is nasal air pressure that is sensed near the anterior nares using a small, double-barreled catheter connected to a pressure transducer. During nasal breathing, this pressure is below atmospheric for inspiration and above atmospheric for expiration. When nasal pressure is recorded simultaneously with videofluoroscopic imaging, it is possible to infer the temporal relationships among certain swallowing events and inspiration, expiration, and apnea (Martin-Harris et al., 2005a; Perlman, He, Barkmeier, & Van Leer, 2005). A brief negative pressure is routinely observed during swallowing; this has been interpreted to reflect a pressure drop associated with a widening of the pharynx near the end of the pharyngeal transport phase of the swallow (not a breathing-related event) (Brodsky, McFarland, Michel, Orr, & Martin-Harris, 2012).

SWALLOWING DISORDERS

Another word for swallowing disorder is dysphagia (pronounced dis-FAY-juh). Dysphagia comes in many forms and can have many different causes. Occasionally it can have a functional cause (no known physical cause), but more commonly it has an organic (physical) cause.

There are times when a person complains of swallowing difficulty, and yet no physical cause can be identified. This is usually diagnosed as psychogenic dysphagia and is often associated with the complaint of a "lump in the throat" and the sensation that swallowed food (solid substance) does not move quickly enough through the esophagus. People with psychogenic dysphagia have different psychological profiles than people with eating disorders, such as bulemia or anorexia (Barofsky & Fontaine, 1998), and a special subcategory called phagophobia, meaning fear of swallowing, has been identified (Shapiro, Franko, & Gagne, 1997). However, some have cautioned that psychogenic dysphagia may be overdiagnosed and that it is prudent to suspect undetected physical causes until they are completely ruled out (Ravich, Wilson, Jones, & Donner, 1989).

Organic dysphagia can have structural, neurogenic, and systemic or other causes. Structural causes include tumors (malignant or benign), diverticula (abnormal pouches in the wall of a structure), osteophytes (bone spurs on the spine that can press on the esophagus), deformation caused by surgical removal of tissue or trauma, congenital malformations, and tracheostomy (a surgically created opening at the front of the neck), among others. Dysphagia can also have neurogenic causes such as stroke, degenerative diseases (such as Parkinson disease and muscular dystrophy), and traumatic brain injury. Systemic or other causes of dysphagia might include scleroderma (causing weakening of the esophageal tissue), immune deficiency disease, pulmonary disease, drug-induced or radiation-induced xerostomia (dry mouth), or gastroesophageal reflux disease (see sidetrack on GERD and LPR).

Dysphagia can also be categorized as oropharyngeal dysphagia and esophageal dysphagia. Oropharyngeal dysphagia is due to impairment of the oral preparatory, oral transport, and/or pharyngeal transport phases of swallowing, and esophageal dysphagia is due to impairment of the esophageal phase of swallowing. Although these categories are not mutually exclusive (someone can have both oropharyngeal dysphagia and esophageal dysphagia), this is an important dichotomy because it has implications regarding which health care professionals are responsible for evaluation and management of the dysphagia (discussed in the next section). Two general types of conditions that constitute common causes of oropharyngeal dysphagia are oral or pharyngeal cancer (either due to the presence of a tumor or to surgical removal of malignant tissue, such as glossectomy), and strokes, traumatic injuries, and degenerative diseases that impair regions of the central and/or peripheral nervous system that control swallowing. Common causes of esophageal dysphagia are esophageal strictures (narrowings), impaired esophageal peristalsis, poor relaxation of the lower esophageal sphincter, and gastroesophageal reflux disease.

There are significant consequences of dysphagia that make accurate evaluation and appropriate management critical to quality of life, and sometimes to life itself. For example, dysphagia can be accompanied by pain (called odynophagia) that requires treatment to bring relief. Even more importantly, dysphagia and can result in malnutrition and dehydration from inadequate ingestion of food and liquid. It can also cause pneumonia when unwanted substance is aspirated into the pulmonary apparatus. When dysphagia is so severe as to pose such risks, it may be necessary to use a non-oral (tube-feeding) approach to sustain life.

CLINICAL PROFESSIONALS AND SWALLOWING DISORDERS

Evaluation and management of swallowing disorders requires a team of health care professionals. Team members may include a speech-language pathologist, radiologist, gastroenterologist, otolaryngologist, dietitian, occupational therapist, and others, depending on the nature of the swallowing disorder.

The speech-language pathologist is responsible for the evaluation and behavioral management of oropharyngeal dysphagia (swallowing disorders involving the oral preparatory, oral transport, and pharyngeal transport phases). Usually the speech-language pathologist is asked by a physician to evaluate a client with a potential swallowing disorder. The speech-language pathologist may begin by performing a bedside swallowing evaluation, which includes a case history interview, a physical examination of the swallowing structures, and visual, auditory, and tactile observation of the client during swallowing of water and possibly other substances. If a problem is suspected, the speech-language pathologist will perform a videofluoroscopic swallowing examination (modified barium swallow study) in collaboration with a radiologist. During the swallow study, the speech-language pathologist may screen for esophageal problems, and if any are noted, a gastroenterologist is notified. Alternatively or additionally, a fiberoptic endoscopic evaluation of swallowing may be conducted, a procedure that can usually be performed by the speech-language pathologist independently. Behavioral management is in the purview of the speech-language pathologist and might include the teaching of postural strategies to improve swallowing, diet (consistency) recommendations, therapeutic exercises (to improve strength and coordination of

swallow-related structures), and counseling regarding the swallowing disorder.

The radiologist has a limited, but critical, role in the evaluation of swallowing. Specifically, the radiologist is responsible for the instrumental aspects of modified barium swallow studies and barium swallow studies and, in some instances, may help in their interpretation.

Whereas the speech-language pathologist focuses on the oral preparatory, oral transport, and pharyngeal transport phases of swallowing, the gastroenterologist focuses on the esophageal transport phase of swallowing. Evaluation approaches used by the gastroenterologist include barium swallow studies, esophageal endoscopy, esophageal manometry, and other procedures that provide information about the structure and function of the esophagus and stomach. Management approaches used by gastroenterologists are usually pharmaceutical or surgical.

An otolaryngologist (also called an ear, nose, and throat physician) is responsible for evaluating oral, pharyngeal, nasal, and laryngeal structures for pathology. An otolaryngologist may diagnose pharyngeal cancer and surgically remove it or diagnose vocal fold paralysis and treat it by surgical medialization (inserting a substance in the vocal fold to move it toward the midline of the airway). Vocal fold paralysis is sometimes associated with aspiration.

A dietitian is often critical in developing menus that meet the caloric and nutritional needs of clients with swallowing disorders. Whereas the speech-language pathologist recommends the best consistencies and volumes of the solid and liquid substances for a client, the dietician helps determine whether or not the client is able to meet nutritional needs solely through oral ingestion or whether nonoral supplementation (tube feeding) should be requested. It falls to the client and the client's physician to decide whether or not nonoral feeding will be used.

Many clients, particularly infants and children, require the expertise of an occupational therapist. An occupational therapist can provide devices, compensatory strategies, and behavioral therapy to improve the ability to self-feed. For example, the occupational therapist might provide special utensils and cups to facilitate the client's ability to eat and drink independently.

There are many other health care professionals that may be involved in the evaluation and management of a client with a swallowing disorder. For example, if the cause of the dysphagia is neural, a neurologist will be a critical member of the team. Similarly, if dysphagia is associated with pulmonary disease, a pulmonologist and respiratory therapist will be involved in the client's management. A dentist or prosthodontist might participate in the care of clients with swallowing disorders if dental or other oral structural problems are contributing factors, such as in clients with oral cancer, cleft palate, or structural abnormalities associated with a congenital syndrome. A physical therapist might be needed to help the client achieve the best posture for eating and drinking. Nurses and nurses' aides often screen for swallowing problems, alerting the physician of any problem noted, and helping to carry out the management plan. Clearly, it is critical that health care professionals representing many disciplines collaborate to determine the nature of a swallowing problem and how best to manage it.

REVIEW

Eating and drinking involve intricately coordinated actions of the lips, mandible, tongue, velum, pharynx, larynx, esophagus, and other structures.

The act of placing solid or liquid substances in the oral cavity, moving it backward to the pharynx, propelling it into the esophagus, and allowing it to make its way to the stomach is called deglutition.

The term swallowing is ingrained as a synonym for deglutition, and is used as such in this chapter, although swallowing technically involves only part of the deglutition process.

Many of the important anatomical and physiological components of the speech production apparatus, discussed in Chapters 2 through 6 of this text, are also important anatomical and physiological components of the swallowing apparatus.

The esophagus is a muscular tube that extends from the lower border of the pharynx to the stomach and is bounded at its two ends by high-pressure valves (the upper esophageal sphincter and the lower esophageal sphincter) that govern the passage of solid and liquid substances into and out of the structure.

The stomach is a liter-sized sac whose upper end connects to the esophagus through the lower esophageal sphincter and whose lower end connects to the small intestine through the pyloric sphincter.

The forces of swallowing are greater and the movements of swallowing are generally slower than those associated with speech production.

Passive forces of swallowing come from the natural recoil of structures, surface tension between structures in apposition, gravity, and aeromechanical factors, whereas active forces result from the activation of breathing, laryngeal, velopharyngeal-nasal, and pharyngeal-oral muscles in various combinations.

Different pressure gradients are critical to the swallowing process and are influenced by pressures existing within the oral cavity, the upper esophageal sphincter, the esophagus, the lower esophageal sphincter, and the stomach.

The forces and movements associated with the act of swallowing can be categorized in four phases that include an oral preparatory phase, oral transport phase, pharyngeal transport phase, and esophageal transport phase.

The oral preparatory phase involves taking solid or liquid substances in through the oral vestibule and manipulating it within the oral cavity to prepare the bolus (lump of solid or liquid volume) for passage.

The oral transport phase involves movement of the bolus (or a part of it) through the oral cavity toward the pharynx by rearward propulsion.

The pharyngeal transport phase is usually "triggered" when the bolus passes the anterior faucial pillars, and results from a combination of compressive actions that force the bolus downward toward the esophagus.

The esophageal transport phase pushes the bolus through the esophagus toward the stomach by a series of peristaltic waves of muscular contraction and relaxation that progress down the muscular tube and which are followed by secondary waves that clear the esophagus.

Swallowing usually occurs during expiration at lung volumes that are somewhat larger than the resting expiratory level, and is associated with a brief apneic interval (cessation of breathing).

The neural control of swallowing is vested in the brainstem and in other higher brain centers that oversee automatic and voluntary aspects of the different phases of swallowing.

Characteristics of the bolus can influence the swallowing pattern, including bolus consistency, bolus volume, and the taste evoked by the bolus.

The mode of swallowing has an impact on the swallowing process, with differences observed for single swallows versus sequential swallows, cued swallows versus spontaneous swallows, and with dependencies on how the solid or liquid substance is presented and what instructions are given.

Details of the swallowing pattern may change with changes in body position, including when swallowing occurs during the breathing cycle, the timing of certain swallowing events, and the magnitudes of certain pressures.

The development of swallowing is rapid and complex and moves through different sucking and chewing patterns toward adult-like eating and drinking behaviors, and carries with it important developmental processes related to social and emotional development.

Age influences swallowing in that the overall duration of the swallow increases in older individuals and the spatial and temporal coordination among certain structures of the swallowing apparatus undergo modification.

Sex of the individual makes little difference to the nature of swallowing.

Several methods are used to measure swallowing events, including videofluoroscopy (which uses x-rays to image all phases of swallowing), endoscopy (which uses a flexible endoscope to image the pharyngeal, laryngeal, and esophageal regions), ultrasonography (which uses ultrasound to image the structures of swallowing), and manometry (which uses pressure transducers to sense pressure change in the pharynx and/or esophagus, or air pressure change at the nares).

A swallowing disorder (also called dysphagia) may be characterized as oropharyngeal dysphagia or esophageal dysphagia and may have no apparent physical cause or, more commonly, has structural, neurogenic, or systemic causes.

Some of the more important clinical professionals who work with individuals with swallowing disorders include speech-language pathologists, radiologists, gastroenterologists, otolaryngologists, dietitians, and occupational therapists.

Scenario

There was no cure. No way to slow it down. There was nothing but nature and the ticking of time. Her referral to a speech-language pathologist had given her helpful strategies for drinking and eating more safely. Crackers, steak, and her beloved honey-roasted cashews gave way to pudding, oatmeal, and thick soups. She concentrated on taking small bites and on tucking her chin when she swallowed. She maintained her weight for a period of time, but her swallowing problem worsened. She choked often and came to dislike eating altogether, a combination that led to weight loss at a dangerous rate. Re-evaluation by the speech-language pathologist revealed that she was aspirating frequently. The medical option of choice was a feeding tube. She resisted but with the urging of her family she agreed to have a tube inserted into her stomach through which nutrition and hydration could be delivered safely. She was allowed to drink water as long as it was pure and her mouth was clean.

As time went by, breathing became the focus of her existence. She felt starved for air and would tend to exhaust herself to satisfy her air hunger. Eventually she could no longer breathe on her own and was placed on a positive-pressure ventilator by her pulmonologist. The ventilator evoked mixed feelings. She had sadness at the thought of being "on life support," but relief at no longer struggling to breathe. By this time, all attempts to maintain her residual speech were abandoned and she had transitioned to a "talking computer" that enabled her to carry on conversations with her family and the few friends who were comfortable enough with her condition to visit her. Nothing else was as important as this connection to the people she loved.

She left one quiet morning with a nurse sleeping at her side. She had been saying goodbyes in various forms for months. The time she chose was sometime between 4:00 and 5:00 AM, that mystical span when so many choose to steal away. The air was still and the lake was as smooth as glass.

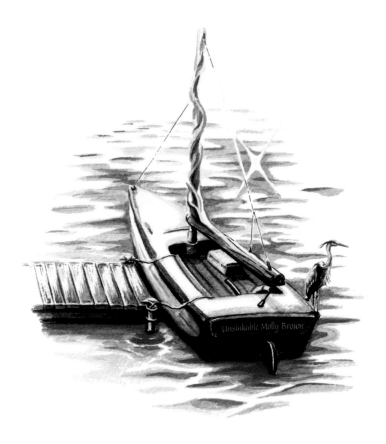

REFERENCES

Arvedson, J., & Brodsky, L. (2002). *Pediatric swallowing and feeding: Assessment and management* (2nd ed.). Clifton Park, NY: Thomson Learning (Singular Publishing Group).

Aviv, J., Kim, T., Thomson, J., Sunshine, S., Kaplan, S., & Close, L. (1998). Fiberoptic endoscopic evaluation of swallowing with sensory testing (FEESST) in healthy controls. *Dysphagia, 13,* 87–92.

Babael, A., Kern, M., Antonik, S., Mepant, R., Ward, B., Li, S-J., Hyde, J., & Shaker, R. (2010). Enhancing effects of flavored nutritive stimuli on cortical swallowing network activity. *American Journal of Physiology: Gastrointestinal and Liver Physiology, 299,* G422–G429.

Barkmeier, J., Bielamowicz, S., Takeda, N., & Ludlow, C. (2002). Laryngeal activity during upright vs. supine swallowing. *Journal of Applied Physiology, 93,* 740–745.

Barofsky, I., & Fontaine, K. (1998). Do psychogenic dysphagia patients have an eating disorder? *Dysphagia, 13,* 24–27.

Bisch, E., Logemann, J., Rademaker, A., Kahrilas, P., & Lazarus, C. (1994). Pharygeal effects of bolus volume, viscosity, and temperature in patients with dysphagia resulting from neurologic impairment and in normal subjects. *Journal of Speech and Hearing Research, 37,* 1041–1059.

Bosma, J. (1986). Development of feeding. *Clinical Nutrition, 5,* 210–218.

Bosma, J., Truby, H., & Lind, J. (1965). Cry motions of the newborn infant. *Acta Paediatrica Scandinavica, 163,* 63–91.

Brodsky, M., McFarland, D., Michel, Y., Orr, S., & Martin-Harris, B. (2012). Significance of nonrespiratory airflow during swallowing. *Dysphagia, 27,* 178–184.

Castell, J., Dalton, C., & Castell, D. (1990). Effects of body position and bolus consistency on the manometric parameters and coordination of the upper esophageal sphincter and pharynx. *Dysphagia, 5,* 179–186.

Chi-Fishman, G., & Sonies, B. (2000). Motor strategy in rapid sequential swallowing: New insights. *Journal of Speech, Language, and Hearing Research, 43,* 1481–1492.

Chi-Fishman, G., & Sonies, B. (2002). Effects of systematic bolus viscosity and volume changes on hyoid movement kinematics. *Dysphagia, 17,* 278–287.

Chi-Fishman, G., Stone, M., & McCall, G. (1998). Lingual action in normal sequential swallowing. *Journal of Speech, Language, and Hearing Research, 41,* 771–785.

Cook, I., Dodds, W., Dantas, R., Kern, M., Massey, B., Shaker, R., & Hogan, W.. (1989). Timing of videofluoroscopic, manometric events, and bolus transit during the oral and pharyngeal phases of swallowing. *Dysphagia, 4,* 8–15.

Cook, I., Weltman, M., Wallace, K., Shaw, D., McKay, E., Smart, R., & Butler, S.. (1994). Influence of aging on oral-pharyngeal bolus transit and clearance during swallowing: Scintigraphic study. *American Journal of Physiology, 266,* G972–G977.

Corbin-Lewis, K., Liss, J., & Sciortino, K. (2005). *Clinical anatomy and physiology of the swallow mechanism.* Clifton Park, NY: Thomson Delmar Learning.

Daggett, A., Logemann, J., Rademaker, A., & Pauloski, B. (2006). Laryngeal penetration during deglutition in normal subjects of various ages. *Dysphagia, 21,* 270–274.

Daniels, S., Corey, D., Hadskey, L., Legendre, C., Priestly, D., Rosenbek, J., & Foundas, A.. (2004). Mechanism of sequential swallowing during straw drinking in healthy young and older adults. *Journal of Speech, Language, and Hearing Research, 47,* 33–45.

Daniels, S., & Foundas, A. (2001). Swallowing physiology of sequential straw drinking. *Dysphagia, 16,* 176–182.

Daniels, S., Schroeder, M., DeGeorge, P., Corey, D., & Rosenbek, J. (2007). Effects of verbal cue on bolus flow during swallowing. *American Journal of Speech-Language Pathology, 16,* 140–147.

Dantas, R., Kern, M., Massey, B., Dodds, W., Kahrilas, P., Brasseur, J., Cook, I., & Lang, I. (1990). Effect of swallowed bolus variables on oral and pharyngeal phases of swallowing. *American Journal of Physiology, 258,* G675–G681.

Dejaeger, E., Pelemans, W., Ponette, E., & VanTrappen, G. (1994). Effect of body position on deglutition. *Digestive Diseases and Sciences, 39,* 762–765.

Ding, R., Logemann, J., Larson, C., & Rademaker, A. (2003). The effects of taste and consistency on swallow physiology in younger and older healthy individuals: A surface electromyographic study. *Journal of Speech, Language, and Hearing Research, 46,* 977–989.

Dodds, W., Hogan, W., Reid, D., Stewart, E., & Arndorfer, R. (1973). A comparison between primary esophageal peristalsis following wet and dry swallows. *Journal of Applied Physiology, 35,* 851–857.

Dodds, W., Taylor, A., Stewart, E., Kern, M., Logemann, J., & Cook, I. (1989). Tipper and dipper types of oral swallows. *American Journal of Roentgenology, 153,* 1197–1199.

Dua, K., Ren, J., Bardan, E., Xie, P., & Shaker, R. (1997). Coordination of deglutitive glottal function and pharyngeal bolus transit during normal eating. *Gastroenterology, 112,* 73–83.

Ekberg, O., & Sigurjonsson, S. (1982). Movement of epiglottis during deglutition: A cineradiographic study. *Gastrointestinal Radiology, 7,* 101–107.

Fink, B., & Demarest, R. (1978). *Laryngeal biomechanics.* Cambridge, MA: Harvard University Press.

Fink, B., Martin, R., & Rohrmann, C. (1979). Biomechanics of the human epiglottis. *Acta Otolaryngologica, 87,* 554–559.

Goyal, R., & Cobb, B. (1981). Motility of the pharynx, esophagus, and esophageal sphincters. In L. Johnson (Ed.), *Physiology of the gastrointestinal tract* (pp. 359–390). New York, NY: Raven Press.

Green, J., Moore, C., Ruark, J., Rodda, P., Morvee, W., & VanWitzenburg, M. (1997). Development of chewing in children from 12 to 48 months: Longitudinal study of EMG patterns. *Journal of Neurophysiology, 77,* 2704–2716.

Gross, R., Carrau, R., Slivka, W., Gisser, R., Smith, L., Zajac, D., & Sciurba, F. (in press). Deglutitive subglottic air pressure and respiratory system recoil. *Dysphagia.*

Hårdemark Cedborg, A., Bodén, K., Witt Hedström, H., Kuylenstierna, R., Ekberg, O., Eriksson, L., & Sundman, E. (2010). Breathing and swallowing in normal man—effects of changes in body position, bolus types, and respiratory drive. *Neurogastroenterology and Motility, 22,* 1201–e316.

Hiiemae, K., & Palmer, J. (1999). Food transport and bolus formation during complete feeding sequences on foods of different initial consistency. *Dysphagia, 14,* 31–42.

Hila, A., Castell, J., & Castell, D. (2001). Pharyngeal and upper esophageal sphincter manometry in the evaluation of dysphagia. *Journal of Clinical Gastroenterology, 33,* 355–361.

Hirst, L., Ford, G., Gibson, G., & Wilson, J. (2002). Swallow-induced alterations in breathing in normal older people. *Dysphagia, 17,* 152–161.

Hoit, J., Lansing, R., Dean, K., Yarkosky, M., & Lederle, A. (2011). Nature and evaluation of dyspnea in speaking and swallowing. *Seminars in Speech and Language, 32,* 5–20.

Humbert, I., & Robbins, J. (2007). Normal swallowing and functional magnetic resonance imaging: A systematic review. *Dysphagia, 22,* 266–275.

Humphrey, T. (1970). Reflex activity in the oral and facial area of the human fetus. In J. Bosma (Ed.), *Second symposium on oral sensation and perception* (pp. 195–233). Springfield, IL: Charles C. Thomas.

Im, I., Kim, Y., Oommen, E., Kim, H., & Ko, M. (2012). The effects of bolus consistency in pharyngeal transit duration during normal swallowing. *Annals of Rehabilitation Medicine, 36,* 220–225.

Ingervall, B., & Lantz, B. (1973). Significance of gravity on the passage of bolus through the human pharynx. *Archives of Oral Biology, 18,* 351–356.

Jean, A. (2001). Brain stem control of swallowing: Neuronal network and cellular mechanisms. *Physiological Reviews, 81,* 929–969.

Johnson, F., Shaw, D., Gabb, M., Dent, J., & Cook, I. (1995). Influence of gravity and body position on normal oropharyngeal swallowing. *American Journal of Physiology, 269,* G653–G658.

Kahrilas, P., & Logemann, J. (1993). Volume accommodation during swallowing. *Dysphagia, 8,* 259–265.

Klaun, M., & Perlman, A. (1999). Temporal and durational patterns associating respiration and swallowing. *Dysphagia, 14,* 131–138.

Koenig, J., Davies, A., & Thach, B. (1990). Coordination of breathing, sucking, and swallowing during bottle feedings in human infants. *Journal of Applied Physiology, 69,* 1623–1629.

Langmore, S., Schatz, K., & Olson, N. (1988). Fiberoptic endoscopic evaluation of swallowing safety: A new procedure. *Dysphagia, 2,* 216–219.

Lederle, A., Hoit, J., & Barkmeier-Kraemer, J. (2012). Effects of sequential swallowing on drive to breathe in young, healthy adults. *Dysphagia, 27,* 221–227.

Leonard, R., Kendall, K., McKenzie, S., & Goodrich, S. (2008). The treatment plan. In R. Leonard & K. Kendall (Eds.), *Dysphagia assessment and treatment planning: A team approach* (2nd ed., pp. 295–336). San Diego, CA: Plural.

Leonard, R., & McKenzie, S. (2006). Hyoid-bolus transit latencies in normal swallow. *Dysphagia, 21,* 183–190.

Leow, L., Huckabee, M., Sharma, S., & Tooley, T. (2007). The influence of taste on swallowing apnea, oral preparation time, and duration and amplitude of submental muscle contraction. *Chemical Senses, 32,* 119–128.

Lever, T., Cox, K., Holbert, D., Shahrier, M., Hough, M., & Kelley-Salamon, K. (2007). The effect of effortful swallow on the normal adult esophagus. *Dysphagia, 22,* 312–325.

Linden, M., Hogosta, S., & Norlander, T. (2007). Monitoring of pharyngeal and upper esophageal sphincter activity with an arterial dilation balloon catheter. *Dysphagia, 22,* 81–88.

Linden, P., Tippett, D., Johnston, J., Siebens, A., & French, J. (1989). Bolus position at swallow onset in normal adults: Preliminary observations. *Dysphagia, 4,* 146–150.

Logemann, J. (1998). *Evaluation and treatment of swallowing disorders* (2nd ed.). Austin, TX: Pro-Ed.

Logemann, J., Boshes, B., Blonsky, E., & Fisher, H. (1977). Speech and swallowing evaluation in the differential diagnosis of neurologic disease. *Neurologia, Neurocirugia, and Psiquiatria, 18*(2–3 Suppl.), 71–78.

Logemann, J., Kahrilas, P., Kobara, M., & Vakil, N. (1989). The benefit of head rotation on pharyngo-esophageal dysphagia. *Archives of Physical Medicine and Rehabilitation, 70,* 767–771.

Logemann, J., Pauloski, B., Rademaker, A., Colangelo, L., Kahrilas, P., & Smith, C. (2000). Temporal and biomechanical characteristics of oropharyngeal swallow in younger and older men. *Journal of Speech, Language, and Hearing Research, 43,* 1264–1274.

Logemann, J., Pauloski, B., Rademaker, A., & Kahrilas, P. (2002). Oropharyngeal swallow in younger and older women: Videofluoroscopic analysis. *Journal of Speech, Language, and Hearing Research, 45,* 434–445.

Malandraki, G., Perlman, A., Karampinos, D., & Sutton, B. (2011). Reduced somatosensory activations in swallowing with age. *Human Brain Mapping, 32,* 730–743.

Margolskee, R., Dyer, J., Kokrashvili, Z., Salmon, K., Ilegems, E., Daly, K., Ninomiya Y., Mosinger, B., & Shirazi-Beechey, S. (2007). T1R3 and gustducin in gut sense sugars to regulate expression of Na+-glucose cotransporter 1. *Proceedings of the National Academy of Sciences, 104,* 15075–15080.

Martin, B., Logemann, J., Shaker, R., & Dodds, W. (1994). Coordination between respiration and swallowing: Respiratory phase relationships and temporal integration. *Journal of Applied Physiology, 76,* 714–723.

Martin, R., & Sessle, B. (1993). The role of the cerebral cortex in swallowing. *Dysphagia, 8,* 195–202.

Martin-Harris, B. (May 16, 2006). Coordination of respiration and swallowing. *GI Motility Online.*

Martin-Harris, B., Brodsky, M., Michel, Y., Ford, C., Walters, B., & Heffner, J. (2005a). Breathing and swallowing dynamics across the adult lifespan. *Archives of Otolaryngology-Head and Neck Surgery, 131,* 762–770.

Martin-Harris, B., Brodsky, M., Price, C., Michel, Y., & Walters, B. (2003). Temporal coordination of pharyngeal and laryngeal dynamics with breathing during swallowing:

Single liquid swallows. *Journal of Applied Physiology, 94,* 1735–1743.

Martin-Harris, B., Michel, Y., & Castell, D. (2005b). Physiologic model of oropharyngeal swallowing revisited. *Otolaryngology-Head and Neck Surgery, 133,* 234–240.

McFarland, D., & Lund, J. (1995). Modification of mastication and respiration during swallowing in the adult human. *Journal of Neurophysiology, 74,* 1509–1517.

McFarland, D., Lund, J., & Gagner, M. (1994). Effects of posture on the coordination of respiration and swallowing. *Journal of Neurophysiology, 72,* 2431–2437.

Mendell, D., & Logemann, J. (2007). Temporal sequence of swallow events during the oropharyngeal swallow. *Journal of Speech, Language, and Hearing Research, 50,* 1256–1271.

Meyer, G., Gerhardt, D., & Castell, D. (1981). Human esophageal response to rapid swallowing: Muscle refractory period or neural inhibition? *American Journal of Physiology, 241,* G129–G136.

Miller, J., Sonies, B., & Macedonia, C. (2003). Emergence of oropharyngeal, laryngeal and swallowing activity in the developing fetal upper aerodigestive tract: An ultrasound evaluation. *Early Human Development, 71,* 61–87.

Miller, J., & Watkin, K. (1996). The influence of bolus volume and viscosity on anterior lingual force during the oral stage of swallowing. *Dysphagia, 11,* 117–124.

Miller, J., & Watkin, K. (1997). Lateral pharyngeal wall motion during swallowing using real time ultrasound. *Dysphagia, 12,* 125–132.

Miyaoka, Y., Haishima, K., Takagi, M., Haishima, H., Asari, J., & Yamada, Y. (2006). Influences of thermal and gustatory characteristics on sensory and motor aspects of swallowing. *Dysphagia, 21,* 38–48.

Nishino, T., Yonezawa, T., & Honda, Y. (1985). Effects of swallowing on the pattern of continuous respiration in human adults. *American Review of Respiratory Disease, 132,* 1219–1222.

Palmer, J. (1998). Bolus aggregation in the oropharynx does not depend on gravity. *Archives of Physical Medicine and Rehabilitation, 79,* 691–696.

Palmer, J., & Hiiemae, K. (2003). Eating and breathing: Interactions between respiration and feeding on solid food. *Dysphagia, 18,* 169–178.

Palmer, P., McCulloch, T., Jaffe, D., & Neel, A. (2005). Effects of a sour bolus on the intramuscular electromyographic (EMG) activity of muscles in the submental region. *Dysphagia, 20,* 210–217.

Palmer, J., Rudin, N., Lara, G., & Crompton, A. (1992). Coordination of mastication and swallowing. *Dysphagia, 7,* 187–200.

Pelletier, C., & Dhanaraj, G. (2006). The effect of taste and palatability on lingual swallowing pressure. *Dysphagia, 21,* 121–128.

Perlman, A., Ettema, S., & Barkmeier, J. (2000). Respiratory and acoustic signals associated with bolus passage during swallowing. *Dysphagia, 15,* 89–94.

Perlman, A., He, X., Barkmeier, J., & Van Leer, E. (2005). Bolus location associated with videofluoroscopic and respirodeglutometric events. *Journal of Speech, Language, and Hearing Research, 48*, 21–33.

Perlman, A., Palmer, P., McCullough, T., & VanDaele, D. (1999). Electromyographic activity from human laryngeal, pharyngeal, and submental muscles during swallowing. *Journal of Applied Physiology, 86*, 1663–1669.

Perlman, A., Schultz, J., & VanDaele, D. (1993). Effects of age, gender, bolus volume, and bolus viscosity on oropharyngeal pressure during swallowing. *Journal of Applied Physiology, 75*, 33–37.

Perry, J., Bae, Y., & Kuehn, D. (2012). Effect of posture on deglutitive biomechanics in healthy individuals. *Dysphagia, 27*, 70–80.

Pitcher, J., Crandall, M., & Goodrich, S. (2008). Pediatric clinical feeding assessment. In R. Leonard & K. Kendall (Eds.), *Dysphagia assessment and treatment planning: A team approach* (2nd ed., pp. 117–136). San Diego, CA: Plural.

Preiksaitis, H., Mayrand, S., Robins, K., & Diamant, N. (1992). Coordination of respiration and swallowing: Effect of bolus volume in normal adults. *American Journal of Physiology, 263*, R624–R630.

Preiksaitis, H., & Mills, C. (1996). Coordination of respiration and swallowing: Effects of bolus consistency and presentation in normal adults. *Journal of Applied Physiology, 81*, 1707–1714.

Ramsey, G., Watson, J., Gramiak, R., & Weinberg, S. (1955). Cinefluorographic analysis of the mechanism of swallowing. *Radiology, 64*, 498–518.

Ravich, W., Wilson, R., Jones, B., & Donner, M. (1989). Psychogenic dysphagia and globus: Reevaluation of 23 patients. *Dysphagia, 4*, 35–38.

Robbins, J., Hamilton, J., Lof, G., & Kempster, G. (1992). Oropharyngeal swallowing in normal adults of different ages. *Gastroenterology, 103*, 823–829.

Rosenbek, J., Robbins, J., Roecker, E., Coyle, J., & Wood, J. (1996) A penetration-aspiration scale. *Dysphagia, 11*, 93–98.

Saitoh, E., Shibata, S., Matsuo, K., Baba, M., Fujii, W., & Palmer, J. (2007). Chewing and food consistency: Effects on bolus transport and swallow initiation. *Dysphagia, 22*, 100–107.

Sears, V., Castell, J., & Castell, D. (1990). Comparison of effects of upright versus supine body position and liquid versus solid bolus on esophageal pressures in normal humans. *Digestive Diseases and Sciences, 35*, 857–864.

Selley, W., Flack, F., Ellis, R., & Brooks, W. (1989). Respiratory patterns associated with swallowing: Part I. The normal adult pattern and changes with age. *Age and Ageing, 18*, 168–172.

Shapiro, J., Franko, D., & Gagne, A. (1997). Phagophobia: A form of psychogenic dysphagia. A new entity. *Annals of Otolaryngology, Rhinology, and Laryngology, 106*, 286–290.

Shawker, T., & Sonies, B. (1985). Ultrasound biofeedback for speech training. *Investigative Radiology, 20*, 90–93.

Smith, J., Wolkove, N., Colacone, A., & Kreisman, H. (1989). Coordination of eating, drinking, and breathing in adults. *Chest, 96*, 578–582.

Sonies, B., Parent, L., Morrish, K., & Baum, B. (1988). Durational aspects of the oral-pharyngeal phase of swallow in normal adults. *Dysphagia, 3*, 1–10.

Steele, C., & Huckabee, M. (2007). The influence of orolingual pressure on the timing of pharyngeal pressure events. *Dysphagia, 22*, 30–36.

Steele, C., & van Lieshout, P. (2004). Influence of bolus consistency on lingual behaviors in sequential swallowing. *Dysphagia, 19*, 192–206.

Steele, C., & van Lieshout, P. (2009). Tongue movements during water swallowing in healthy young and older adults. *Journal of Speech, Language, and Hearing Research, 52*, 1255–1267.

Steeve, R., Moore, C., Green, J., Reilly, K., & Ruark McMurtrey, J. (2008). Babbling, chewing, and sucking: Oromandibular coordination at 9 months. *Journal of Speech, Language, and Hearing Research, 51*, 1390–1404.

Stone, M., & Shawker, T. (1986). An ultrasound examination of tongue movement during swallowing. *Dysphagia, 1*, 78–83.

Tasko, S., Kent, R., & Westbury, J. (2002). Variability in tongue movement kinematics during normal liquid swallow. *Dysphagia, 17*, 126–138.

Tracy, J., Logemann, J., Kahrilas, P., Jacob, P., Kobara, M., & Krugler, C. (1989). Preliminary observations on the effects of age on oropharyngeal deglutition. *Dysphagia, 4*, 90–94.

VanDaele, D., Perlman, A., & Cassell, M. (1995). Intrinsic fibre architecture attachments of the human epiglottis and their contributions to the mechanism of deglutition. *Journal of Anatomy, 186*, 1–15.

Wheeler-Hegland, K., Huber, J., Pitts, T., & Davenport, P. (2011). Lung volume measured during sequential swallowing in healthy young adults. *Journal of Speech, Language, and Hearing Research, 54*, 777–786.

Wheeler-Hegland, K., Huber, J., Pitts, T., & Sapienza, C. (2009). Lung volume during swallowing: Single bolus swallows in healthy young adults. *Journal of Speech, Language, and Hearing Research, 52*, 178–187.

Wheeler-Hegland, K., Rosenbek, J., & Sapienza, C. (2008). Submental sEMG and hyoid movement during Mendelsohn maneuver, effortful swallow, and expiratory muscle strength training. *Journal of Speech, Language, and Hearing Research, 51*, 1072–1087.

Wilson, S., Thach, B., Brouillette, R., & Abu-Osba, Y. (1981). Coordination of breathing and swallowing in human infants. *Journal of Applied Physiology, 50*, 851–858.

Witcombe, B., & Meyer, D. (2006). Sword swallowing and its side effects. *British Medical Journal, 333*, 1285–1287.

Yeates, E., Steele, C., & Pelletier, C. (2010). Tongue pressure and submental surface electromyography measures during noneffortful and effortful saliva swallows in healthy women. *American Journal of Speech-Language Pathology, 19*, 274–281.

Youmans, S., Youmans, G., & Stierwalt, J. (2009). Differences in tongue strength across age and gender: Is there a diminished strength reserve? *Dysphagia, 24*, 57–65.

Name Index

Subject Index